The Breast

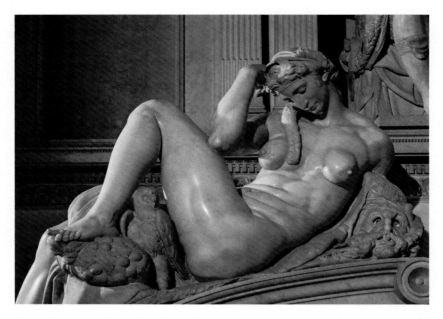

Carved in the 1520s by Michelangelo, the sculpture *Night* has been on display in the Medici Mortuary Chapel in the Church of San Lorenzo in Florence, Italy for hundreds of years. After nearly five hundred years and many comments on its appearance, the left breast of *Night* has undergone renewed scrutiny. Close observation reveals a mass in the medial aspect of the breast, slight skin puckering adjacent to the mass, and diffuse swelling of the nipple-areola complex—characteristics of locally advanced breast cancer. None of Michelangelo's numerous other depictions of the female breast share these characteristics. Stark and Nelson* concluded that Michelangelo knew that breast cancer was a fatal illness and that he therefore chose it to memorialize his patron Giuliano de' Medici, whose remains reside in the crypt covered by the sculpture. Giuliano died from a protracted wasting illness, possibly tuberculosis; *Night*, they concluded, was an allegory to that illness. Referring to *Night* and its three companion sarcophagi, Michelangelo imagines them conversing: "Day and Night speak, and say, 'We with our swift course have brought Duke Giuliano to death.'" In a sonnet written in 1545, Michelangelo has *Night* say, "I prize my sleep, and more my being stone/As long as Hurt and Shamefulness endure."

Michelangelo was known to have access to human autopsy specimens and, no doubt, had observed the gross morphology of breast cancer. His depiction of breast cancer in *Night* represents one of the first works of art to accurately depict this disease.

James J. Stark, MD, FACP
Professor of Clinical Internal Medicine
Eastern Virginia Medical School
Medical Director, Cancer Program, Maryview Medical Center
Suffolk, VA

Art credit:

Michelangelo Buonarroti (1475–1564)

The figure of Night, from the tomb of Giuliano de' Medici (1478–1516), Duke of Nemours and son of Lorenzo il Magnifico. Marble, 1521–1534.

S. Lorenzo, Florence, Italy

© Erich Lessing/Art Resource, NY

---

*Stark JJ, Nelson JK: The breasts of "Night": Michelangelo as oncologist. N Engl J Med 343:1577–1578, 2000.

KIRBY I. BLAND, MD

Fay Fletcher Kerner Professor and Chair
Department of Surgery
Deputy Director, UAB Comprehensive Cancer Center
University of Alabama School of Medicine
Birmingham, Alabama

EDWARD M. COPELAND III, MD

Distinguished Professor
Department of Surgery
University of Florida College of Medicine
Gainesville, Florida

VOLUME ONE

The Breast
Comprehensive Management of Benign and Malignant Diseases

Fourth Edition

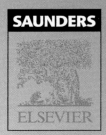

SAUNDERS

ELSEVIER

SAUNDERS
ELSEVIER

1600 John F. Kennedy Blvd.
Ste 1800
Philadelphia, PA 19103–2899

THE BREAST: COMPREHENSIVE MANAGEMENT
OF BENIGN AND MALIGNANT DISORDERS

ISBN: 978-1-4160-5221-0

Notice

Knowledge and best practice in this field are constantly changing. As new research and experience broaden our knowledge, changes in practice, treatment, and drug therapy may become necessary or appropriate. Readers are advised to check the most current information provided (i) on procedures featured or (ii) by the manufacturer of each product to be administered, to verify the recommended dose or formula, the method and duration of administration, and contraindications. It is the responsibility of the practitioner, relying on his or her own experience and knowledge of the patient, to make diagnoses, to determine dosages and the best treatment for each individual patient, and to take all appropriate safety precautions. To the fullest extent of the law, neither the Publisher nor the Editors assume any liability for any injury and/or damage to persons or property arising out or related to any use of the material contained in this book.

The Publisher

Library of Congress Cataloging-in-Publication Data

The breast : comprehensive management of benign and malignant diseases/[edited by] Kirby I. Bland, Edward M. Copeland III.—4th ed.
   p. ; cm
   Includes bibliographical references and index.
   ISBN 978-1-4160-5221-0
   1. Breast—Cancer—Treatment. 2. Breast—Diseases—Treatment. I. Bland K. I. II. Copeland, Edward M.
   [DNLM: 1. Breast Diseases—therapy. 2. Breast Neoplasms—therapy. WP 900 B828 2009]
   RC280.B8B7134 2009
   618.1′906—dc22

2009014220

Publishing Director: Judith Fletcher
Developmental Editor: Roxanne Halpine
Project Manager: David Saltzberg
Design Direction: Steve Stave

Working together to grow
libraries in developing countries

www.elsevier.com | www.bookaid.org | www.sabre.org

ELSEVIER   BOOK AID International   Sabre Foundation

Printed in Canada.

Last digit is the print number: 9 8 7 6 5 4 3 2 1

Sanford H. Barsky, MD
The Donald A. Senhauser Endowed Chair of Pathology
Department of Pathology
The Ohio State University
Columbus, Ohio

William J. Gradishar, MD
Professor of Medicine and Director of Breast Oncology
Robert H. Lurie Comprehensive Cancer Center
Northwestern University Feinberg School of Medicine
Chicago, Illinois

Abram Recht, MD
Professor
Department of Radiation Oncology
Harvard Medical School
Senior Radiation Oncologist and Deputy Chief
Department of Radiation Oncology
Beth Israel Deaconess Medical Center
Boston, Massachusetts

Marshall M. Urist, MD
Champ Lyons Professor and Vice Chair
Department of Surgery
University of Alabama at Birmingham
Birmingham, Alabama

Contributors

Doreen Agnese, MD
Assistant Professor of Surgery, The Ohio State University, Columbus, OH
12 *Extent and Multicentricity of in Situ and Invasive Carcinoma*

Kathleen Gardiner Allen, MD
Surgical Associates of West Florida, Clearwater, FL
52 *Biology and Management of Lobular Carcinoma in Situ of the Breast*

Raheela Ashfaq, MD, FCAP, FASCP
Professor of Pathology; Charles T. Ashworth Professor of Pathology and Gynecology; Director OncoDiagnostics Laboratory; University of Texas Southwestern Medical Center, Dallas, TX
4 *Discharges and Secretions of the Nipple*

Thomas R. Aversano, MD
Associate Professor of Medicine, Johns Hopkins Medical Institutions, Baltimore, MD
80 *Management of Pericardial Metastases in Breast Cancer*

Sanford H. Barsky, MD
The Donald A. Senhauser Endowed Chair of Pathology, The Ohio State University College of Medicine, Columbus, OH
10 *In Situ Carcinomas of the Breast: Ductal Carcinoma in Situ and Lobular Carcinoma in Situ*
11 *Infiltrating Carcinomas of the Breast: Not One Disease*
16 *Digital Automation of Breast Biomarker Immunocytochemistry*
29 *Stem Cells, the Breast, and Breast Cancer*
87 *Inflammatory Breast Cancer*

Lawrence W. Bassett, MD
Professor, University of California at Los Angeles, Los Angeles, CA
36 *Breast Imaging*
38 *Stereotactic Breast Biopsy*

Elisabeth K. Beahm, MD, FACS
Associate Professor, Department of Plastic and Reconstructive Surgery, University of Texas M.D. Anderson Cancer Center, Houston, TX
69 *Surgical Procedures for Advanced Local and Regional Malignancies of the Breast*

Samuel W. Beenken, MD
Consultant, Oncology Writings, Montevallo, AL
5 *Etiology and Management of Benign Breast Disease*
7 *Gynecomastia*
42 *Evolution of the Surgical Management of Breast Cancer*

Honnie R. Bermas, MD
Fox Valley Surgical Associates, Appleton, WI
74 *Local Therapy for the Intact Breast Primary in the Presence of Metastatic Disease*

Therese B. Bevers, MD
Associate Professor, Clinical Cancer Prevention; Medical Director, Cancer Prevention Center and Prevention Outreach Programs, University of Texas M.D. Anderson Cancer Center, Houston, TX
86 *Clinical Management of the Patient at Increased or High Risk*

Mehret Birru, BA
Medical Student, University of Pittsburgh School of Medicine, Pittsburgh, PA
20 *Primary Prevention of Breast Cancer*

Kirby I. Bland, MD, FACS
Fay Fletcher Kerner Professor and Chair, Department of Surgery; Deputy Director Comprehensive Cancer Center, University of Alabama at Birmingham, Birmingham, AL
1 *History of the Therapy of Breast Cancer*
2 *Anatomy of the Breast, Axilla, Chest Wall, and Related Metastatic Sites*
3 *Breast Physiology: Normal and Abnormal Development and Function*
5 *Etiology and Management of Benign Breast Disease*
7 *Gynecomastia*
9 *Congenital and Acquired Disturbances of Breast Development and Growth*
42 *Evolution of the Surgical Management of Breast Cancer*
43 *Indications and Techniques for Biopsy*
44 *General Principles of Mastectomy: Evaluation and Therapeutic Options*
45 *Halsted Radical Mastectomy*
46 *Modified Radical Mastectomy and Total (Simple) Mastectomy*
47 *Breast Conservation Therapy for Invasive Breast Cancer*
50 *Wound Care and Complications of Mastectomy*

Abenaa M. Brewster, MD, MHS
Assistant Professor, University of Texas M.D. Anderson Cancer Center, Houston, TX
72 *Locally Advanced Breast Cancer*

Louise A. Brinton, PhD
Chief, Hormonal and Reproductive Epidemiology
  Branch, National Cancer Institute, Rockville, MD
37 *Interval Breast Cancer: Clinical, Epidemiologic,
  and Biologic Features*

Malcolm V. Brock, MD
Assistant Professor of Surgery, Division of Thoracic
  Surgery, Johns Hopkins University School of
  Medicine, Baltimore, MD
78 *Diagnosis and Management of Pleural Metastases
  in Breast Cancer*

Mai N. Brooks, MD, FACS
Greater Los Angeles Veterans Affairs, Los Angeles, CA
32 *Angiogenesis in Breast Cancer*

Thomas A. Buchholz, MD, FACR
Professor and Chair, Department of Radiation
  Oncology, University of Texas M.D. Anderson
  Cancer Center, Houston, TX
61 *Radiation Therapy for Locally Advanced Disease*

Helena R. Chang, MD, PhD
Professor of Surgery; Director, Revlon/UCLA Breast
  Center, University of California at Los Angeles,
  Los Angeles, CA
46 *Modified Radical Mastectomy and Total (Simple)
  Mastectomy*

Bhishamjit S. Chera, MD
University of Florida, Gainesville, FL
79 *Management of Central Nervous System Metastases
  in Breast Cancer*

C. Denise Ching, MD
Fellow of Surgical Oncology, University of Texas M.D.
  Anderson Cancer Center, Houston, TX
59 *Percutaneous Ablation: Minimally Invasive Techniques
  in Breast Cancer Therapy*

Maureen A. Chung, MD, PhD
Associate Professor of Surgery, Rhode Island Hospital;
  Brown University, Providence, RI
54 *Therapeutic Value of Axillary Node Dissection and
  Selective Management of the Axilla in Small Breast
  Cancers*
58 *Surgical Management of Early Breast Cancer*

Hiram S. Cody III, MD
Professor of Clinical Surgery, The Weill Medical
  College of Cornell University; Attending Surgeon,
  Memorial Sloan-Kettering Cancer Center,
  New York, NY
56 *Detection and Significance of Axillary Lymph Node
  Micrometastases*
81 *Bilateral Breast Cancer*

Edward M. Copeland III, MD, FACS
Distinguished Professor, University of Florida College
  of Medicine; Distinguished Professor of Surgery,
  Shands Hospital at the University of Florida,
  Gainesville, FL
6B *Clinical Management of Mastitis and Breast Abscess and
  Idiopathic Granulomatous Mastitis*
8 *Benign, High-Risk, and Premalignant Lesions of the Breast*
44 *General Principles of Mastectomy: Evaluation and
  Therapeutic Options*
45 *Halsted Radical Mastectomy*
46 *Modified Radical Mastectomy and Total (Simple)
  Mastectomy*
57 *Intraoperative Evaluation of Surgical Margins in
  Breast-Conserving Therapy*
83 *Local Recurrence, the Augmented Breast, and the
  Contralateral Breast*

Charles E. Cox, MD, FACS
McCann Foundation Endowed Professor of Breast
  Surgery; CEO, Breast Health CRISP, University of
  South Florida College of Medicine; Medical Director
  ASC, Carol and Frank Morsani Center for Advanced
  Health Care, Tampa, FL
23 *Assessment and Designation of Breast Cancer Stage*
51 *Lymphedema in the Postmastectomy Patient:
  Pathophysiology, Prevention, and Management*

Massimo Cristofanilli, MD
Associate Professor, University of Texas M.D. Anderson
  Cancer Center, Houston, TX
73 *Detection and Clinical Implications of Occult Systemic
  Micrometastatic Breast Cancer*

David T. Curiel, MD, PhD
Director, Division of Human Gene Therapy, Gene
  Therapy Center, University of Alabama at
  Birmingham, Birmingham, AL
31 *Gene Therapy for Breast Cancer*

Laurie W. Cuttino, MD
Assistant Professor, Virginia Commonwealth University,
  Richmond, VA
62 *Radiotherapy and Ductal Carcinoma in Situ*
66 *Accelerated Partial Breast Irradiation*

Jorge I. de la Torre, MD
Professor of Surgery, Division of Plastic Surgery;
  Program Director, Plastic Surgery Residency Program,
  University of Alabama at Birmingham;
  Director, Center for Advanced Surgical Aesthetics;
  Section Chief, Plastic Surgery, Birmingham VA
  Medical Center, Birmingham, AL
48 *Breast Reconstruction following Mastectomy*
49 *Macromastia and Reduction Mammaplasty*

Jennifer F. De Los Santos, MD
Associate Professor, University of Alabama at
  Birmingham; Medical Director, The Kirklin Clinic
  at Acton Road Comprehensive Cancer Center,
  Birmingham, AL
47 *Breast Conservation Therapy for Invasive Breast Cancer*

Mohammad S. Diab, MD
Auxillary Faculty, The Ohio State University,
Columbus, OH; Associate, Group Health Associates,
Cincinnati, OH
15 *Primary and Secondary Dermatologic Disorders
of the Breast*

Mary L. Disis, MD
Professor, University of Washington, Seattle, WA
33 *Immune Recognition of Breast Cancer*

William C. Dooley, MD, FACS
Director of Surgical Oncology, Oklahoma
University Health Sciences Center, Oklahoma
City, OK
40 *Breast Ductoscopy*

William D. DuPont, PhD
Professor of Biostatistics and Preventive Medicine,
Vanderbilt University School of Medicine,
Nashville, TN
26 *Risk Factors for Breast Carcinoma in Women with
Proliferative Breast Disease*

Philip L. Dutt, MD
Novato, CA
12 *Extent and Multicentricity of in Situ and Invasive
Carcinoma*

Timothy J. Eberlein, MD
Bixby Professor and Chair, Department of Surgery;
Spencer T. and Ann W. Olin Distinguished
Professor, Alvin J. Siteman Cancer Center,
Washington University School of Medicine;
Surgeon-in-Chief; Barnes-Jewish Hospital,
St. Louis, MO
34 *Immunology and the Role of Immunotherapy in Breast
Cancer: Human Clinical Trials*

Mary Edgerton, MD, PhD
Assistant Professor, Departments of Pathology and
Biomedical Informatics, Vanderbilt University Medical
Center, Nashville, TN
12 *Extent and Multicentricity of in Situ and Invasive
Carcinoma*

Mahmoud El-Tamer, MD
Associate Professor of Clinical Surgery; Program Director
of Breast Fellowship, Columbia University; Attending,
New York-Presbyterian Hospital, New York, NY
22 *Patterns of Recurrence in Breast Cancer*

William B. Farrar, MD
Professor of Surgery and The Arthur G. James/Richard J.
Solove Chair of Surgical Oncology, The Arthur
G. James Cancer Hospital/Richard J. Solove
Research Institute at The Ohio State University,
Columbus, OH
12 *Extent and Multicentricity of in Situ and Invasive
Carcinoma*

Regina M. Fearmonti, MD
Resident, Department of Surgery, Division of Plastic,
Reconstructive, Maxillofacial, and Oral Surgery, Duke
University Medical Center, Durham, NC
69 *Surgical Procedures for Advanced Local and Regional
Malignancies of the Breast*

M. Judah Folkman, MD*
Department of Surgery, Children's Hospital and Harvard
Medical School, Boston, MA
32 *Angiogenesis in Breast Cancer*

Gary M. Freedman, MD
Member, Fox Chase Cancer Center, Philadelphia, PA
65 *Breast-Conserving Therapy for Invasive Breast Cancers*
67 *Radiation Complications and Their Management*

Eric R. Frykberg, MD
Professor of Surgery, University of Florida Shands
Medical Center, Jacksonville, FL
42 *Evolution of the Surgical Management of Breast Cancer*

Thomas A. Gaskin III, MD
Attending Surgeon, Princeton Baptist Health Center,
Birmingham, AL
90 *Rehabilitation*

Mary Gemignani, MD, MPH
Instructor of Obstetrics and Gynecology, Department of
Surgery, Weill Medical College of Cornell University;
Associate Attending Surgeon, Breast Surgery and
Gynecology Services, Memorial Sloan-Kettering
Cancer Center, New York, NY
84 *Carcinoma of the Breast in Pregnancy and Lactation*

William E. Gillanders, MD
Associate Professor of Surgery, Washington University
School of Medicine, St. Louis, MO
34 *Immunology and the Role of Immunotherapy in Breast
Cancer: Human Clinical Trials*

Armando E. Giuliano, MD
Director, John Wayne Cancer Institute Breast Center
at Saint John's Health Center; Chief of Science
and Medicine, John Wayne Cancer Institute, Santa
Monica, CA
55 *Lymphatic Mapping and Sentinel Lymphadenectomy
for Breast Cancer*

Peter S. Goedegebuure, PhD
Research Associate Professor, Washington University
School of Medicine, St. Louis, MO
34 *Immunology and the Role of Immunotherapy in Breast
Cancer: Human Clinical Trials*

Julie Gold, MD
Clinical Fellow in Medical Oncology and Hematology,
Dana-Farber Cancer Institute, Boston, MA
76 *Chemotherapy for Metastatic Breast Cancer*

*Deceased.

Mehra Golshan, MD
Assistant Professor of Surgery, Harvard Medical School;
    Director of Breast Surgical Services, Dana-Farber
    Cancer Institute/Brigham and Women's Hospital
    Boston, MA
35 *Examination Techniques: Roles of the Physician and
    Patient in Evaluating Breast Disease*

William J. Gradishar, MD
Professor of Medicine, Northwestern University Feinberg
    School of Medicine; Director of Breast Oncology,
    Robert H. Lurie Comprehensive Cancer Center,
    Chicago, IL
68 *Adjuvant Chemotherapy for Early-Stage Breast Cancer*

Stephen R. Grobmyer, MD
Assistant Professor of Surgical Oncology, University of
    Florida; Chief of Breast, Melanoma, Sarcoma, and
    Endocrine Services, Shands Hospital, Gainesville, FL
6B *Clinical Management of Mastitis and Breast Abscess
    and Idiopathic Granulomatous Mastitis*
 8 *Benign, High-Risk, and Premalignant Lesions of the Breast*
57 *Intraoperative Evaluation of Surgical Margins in
    Breast-Conserving Therapy*

Baiba J. Grube, MD
Associate Professor, Yale University School of Medicine;
    Yale–New Haven Hospital, New Haven, CT
55 *Lymphatic Mapping and Sentinel Lymphadenectomy
    for Breast Cancer*

Seema Harichand-Herdt, MD
Fellow of Hematology and Oncology, Emory University,
    Atlanta, GA
77 *Endocrine Therapy for Breast Cancer*

J. Garrett Harper, MD
Resident in General Surgery, Medical College of Georgia,
    Augusta, GA
83 *Local Recurrence, the Augmented Breast, and the
    Contralateral Breast*

Yasmin Hasan, MD
Instructor, Department of Radiation and Cellular
    Oncology, Universiy of Chicago Medical Center,
    Chicago, IL
66 *Accelerated Partial Breast Irradiation*

Mary H. Hohenhaus, MD
Clinical Instructor, Division of General Internal
    Medicine, Alpert Medical School of Brown University;
    Medical Director, Fain Primary Care Clinic,
    The Miriam Hospital, Providence, RI
89 *Management of Menopause in the Breast Cancer Patient*

Gabriel N. Hortobagyi, MD
Professor and Chair, Department of Breast Medical
    Oncology, University of Texas M.D. Anderson Cancer
    Center, Houston, TX
72 *Locally Advanced Breast Cancer*

J. Harrison Howard, MD
Surgical Resident, Department of Surgery, University of
    Alabama at Birmingham Hospital, Birmingham, AL
 9 *Congenital and Acquired Disturbances of Breast
    Development and Growth*

Christopher P. Hsu, MD
University of California at Los Angeles, Los Angeles, CA
36 *Breast Imaging*

Alana G. Hudson, PhD
University of Pittsburgh, Pittsburgh, PA
19 *Epidemiology of Breast Cancer*

Kelly K. Hunt, MD
Professor of Surgery; Chief of Surgical Breast Section,
    University of Texas M.D. Anderson Cancer Center,
    Houston, TX
59 *Percutaneous Ablation: Minimally Invasive Techniques
    in Breast Cancer Therapy*
69 *Surgical Procedures for Advanced Local and Regional
    Malignancies of the Breast*

Anamaria Ioan, MD
PhD candidate, University of Southern California,
    Los Angeles, CA
28 *Molecular Oncology of Breast Cancer*

Rafael E. Jimenez, MD
Senior Associate Consultant, Mayo Clinic,
    Rochester, MN
14 *Paget's Disease of the Breast*

Joyce E. Johnson, MD
Department of Pathology, Vanderbilt University School
    of Medicine, Nashville, TN
12 *Extent and Multicentricity of in Situ and Invasive
    Carcinoma*

Virginia G. Kaklamani, MD, DSc
Assistant Professor, Northwestern University, Chicago, IL
68 *Adjuvant Chemotherapy for Early-Stage Breast Cancer*

Amer Karam, MD
Breast Surgery Service, Memorial Sloan-Kettering Cancer
    Center, New York, NY
84 *Carcinoma of the Breast in Pregnancy and Lactation*

Nina J. Karlin, MD
Assistant Professor of Medicine; Senior Associate
    Consultant, Mayo Clinic Arizona, Scottsdale, AZ
17 *Breast Lymphoma*

Rena B. Kass, MD
Assistant Professor of Surgery; Surgical Director of the
    Breast Program, Penn State Hershey Medical Center,
    Hershey, PA
 3 *Breast Physiology: Normal and Abnormal Development
    and Function*
 5 *Etiology and Management of Benign Breast Disease*

Paramjeet Kaur, MD
Associate, Department of Surgery, Frankford
  Hospital, Jefferson Health System,
  Philadelphia, PA
51 *Lymphedema in the Postmastectomy Patient:*
  Pathophysiology, Prevention, and Management

Kenneth A. Kern, MD, MPH
Professor of Clinical Surgery, University of California
  at San Diego; Director, Oncology Clinical
  Development, Pfizer Global Research and
  Development, San Diego, CA
94 *Delayed Diagnosis of Symptomatic Breast Cancer*

Seema A. Khan, MD
Professor of Surgery, Northwestern University Feinberg
  School of Medicine; Director, Bluhm Family
  Program for Breast Cancer Early Detection &
  Prevention, Robert H. Lurie Comprehensive Cancer
  Center, Chicago, IL
74 *Local Therapy for the Intact Breast Primary in the*
  Presence of Metastatic Disease

John V. Kiluk, MD
Assistant Professor of Surgery, University of South
  Florida; Assistant Member, Breast Program, Moffitt
  Cancer Center, Tampa, FL
23 *Assessment and Designation of Breast Cancer Stage*

Paula Kim, MD
CEO and Founder, Translating Research Across
  Communities, Green Cove Springs, FL
92 *Patient and Family Resources*

Jessica Kirwan, MA
Editor, Department of Radiation Oncology, University of
  Florida, Gainesville, FL
79 *Management of Central Nervous System Metastases*
  in Breast Cancer

V. Suzanne Klimberg, MD
Muriel Balsam Kohn Chair in Breast Surgical
  Oncology, University of Arkansas for Medical
  Sciences; Director, Breast Cancer Program,
  Winthrop P. Rockefeller Cancer Institute,
  Little Rock, AR
3 *Breast Physiology: Normal and Abnormal Development*
  and Function
5 *Etiology and Management of Benign Breast Disease*

Merieme Klobocista, MD
Clinical Instructor, University of Southern California,
  Los Angeles, CA
28 *Molecular Oncology of Breast Cancer*

Kara C. Kort, MD
Assistant Professor of Surgery, SUNY Upstate Medical
  University, Syracuse, NY
6A *Subareolar Breast Abscess: The Penultimate Stage*
  of the Mammary Duct-associated Inflammatory Disease
  Sequence

Helen Krontiras, MD
Associate Professor of Surgery, University of Alabama at
  Birmingham, Birmingham, AL
47 *Breast Conservation Therapy for Invasive Breast Cancer*
50 *Wound Care and Complications of Mastectomy*

E. James Kruse, DO
Assistant Professor of Surgery, Medical College of
  Georgia, Augusta, GA
83 *Local Recurrence, the Augmented Breast, and the*
  Contralateral Breast

Henry Kuerer, MD, PhD, FACS
Professor and Director of Training Program, University
  of Texas M.D. Anderson Cancer Center, Houston, TX
70 *Solitary Metastases*

Jane W. Lee, MD
Resident Fellow, University of California at Los Angeles,
  Los Angeles, CA
36 *Breast Imaging*

A. Marilyn Leitch, MD
Professor of Surgery, University of Texas Southwestern
  Medical Center, Dallas, TX
4 *Discharges and Secretions of the Nipple*

Huong T. Le-Petross, MD, FRCPC
Assistant Professor of Radiology; Radiologist, Breast and
  Body Imaging, University of Texas M.D. Anderson
  Cancer Center, Houston, TX
85 *Unknown Primary Presenting with Axillary*
  Lymphadenopathy

Judith L. Lightsey, MD
Assistant Professor of Radiation Oncology, University
  of Florida; Shands Hospital, Gainesville, FL
75 *Management of Bone Metastases in Breast Cancer*

Jennifer A. Ligibel, MD
Instructor in Medicine, Harvard Medical School; Staff
  Physician, Dana-Farber Cancer Institute, Boston, MA
91 *Psychosocial Consequences and Lifestyle Interventions*

D. Scott Lind, MD
Professor and Chief of Surgical Oncology, Medical
  College of Georgia, Augusta, GA
83 *Local Recurrence, the Augmented Breast, and the*
  Contralateral Breast

Stanley Lipkowitz, MD, PhD
Senior Investigator, Laboratory of Cellular and
  Molecular Biology, Center for Cancer Research,
  National Cancer Institute, Bethesda, MD
37 *Interval Breast Cancer: Clinical, Epidemiologic,
  and Biologic Features*

James N. Long, MD
Assistant Professor, University of Alabama at
  Birmingham; Attending, Plastic, Hand, and
  Reconstructive Surgery, Children's Hospital
  of Birmingham and Cooper Green Hospital;
  Director, Plastic, Hand, and Reconstrcutive Surgery,
  Birmingham Veterans Administration Medical Center,
  Birmingham, AL
48 *Breast Reconstruction following Mastectomy*
49 *Macromastia and Reduction Mammaplasty*

Richard Love, MD
Professor of Internal Medicine and Public Health, The
  Ohio State University, Columbus, OH; Senior
  Investigator, International Research, Office of the
  Director, National Cancer Institute, Bethesda, MD;
  Scientific Director, The International Breast Cancer
  Research Foundation, Madison, WI
87 *Inflammatory Breast Cancer*

Hailing Lu, MD, PhD
Acting Assistant Professor, University of Washington,
  Seattle, WA
33 *Immune Recognition of Breast Cancer*

Henry T. Lynch, MD
Chair, Preventive Medicine and Public Health; Professor
  of Medicine; Director of Creighton's Hereditary
  Cancer Institute, Creighton University School of
  Medicine, Omaha, NE
21 *Breast Cancer Genetics: Syndromes, Genes, Pathology,
  Counseling, Testing, and Treatment*

Jane Lynch, BSN
Instructor, Department of Preventive Medicine,
  Creighton University School of Medicine, Omaha, NE
21 *Breast Cancer Genetics: Syndromes, Genes, Pathology,
  Counseling, Testing, and Treatment*

Mary Mahoney, MD
Professor of Radiology, University of Cincinnati;
  Director of Breast Imaging, Barrett Cancer Center,
  Cincinnati, OH
38 *Stereotactic Breast Biopsy*

Anne T. Mancino, MD
Associate Professor of Surgery, University of Arkansas of
  Medical Sciences; Chief of General Surgery, Central
  Arkansas Veterans Healthcare System, Little Rock, AR
3 *Breast Physiology: Normal and Abnormal Development
  and Function*

Joseph N. Marcus, MD
Staff Pathologist, Missouri Baptist Medical Center,
  St. Louis, MO
21 *Breast Cancer Genetics: Syndromes, Genes, Pathology,
  Counseling, Testing, and Treatment*

Lawrence B. Marks, MD
Professor and Chair, Department of Radiation
  Oncology, University of North Carolina at Chapel
  Hill, Chapel Hill, NC
60 *Radiotherapy Techniques*

Shahla Masood, MD
Professor and Chair, Department of Pathology and
  Laboratory Medicine, University of Florida College
  of Medicine; Medical Director; Chief of Pathology,
  Shands Jacksonville Breast Health Center,
  Jacksonville, FL
39 *Cytopathology of the Breast*

Nicole Massoll, MD
Associate Professor of Pathology, University of Florida
  College of Medicine, Gainesville, FL
6B *Clinical Management of Mastitis and Breast Abscess and
  Idiopathic Granulomatous Mastitis*

John B. McCraw, MD
Professor of Plastic Surgery, University of Mississippi
  Medical Center, Jackson, MS
44 *General Principles of Mastectomy: Evaluation and
  Therapeutic Options*
48 *Breast Reconstruction following Mastectomy*

James McLoughlin, MD
Assistant Professor, Division of Surgical Oncology,
  Medical College of Georgia, Augusta, GA
83 *Local Recurrence, the Augmented Breast, and the
  Contralateral Breast*

Michael M. Meguid, MD, PhD
Professor of Surgery and Neuroscience/Physiology,
  SUNY Upstate Medical University, Syracuse, NY
6A *Subareolar Breast Abscess: The Penultimate Stage
  of the Mammary Duct-associated Inflammatory
  Disease Sequence*

Nancy P. Mendenhall, MD
University of Florida Proton Therapy Institute,
  Jacksonville, FL
71 *Locoregional Recurrence after Mastectomy*
75 *Management of Bone Metastases in Breast Cancer*

William M. Mendenhall, MD
Professor, Department of Radiation Oncology,
  University of Florida; Medical Director, Shands Davis
  Cancer Center, Gainesville, FL
79 *Management of Central Nervous System Metastases
  in Breast Cancer*

Jane Mendez, MD, FACS
Assistant Professor of Surgery, Boston University School
of Medicine; Attending, Boston Medical Center,
Boston, MA
70 *Solitary Metastases*

Lavinia P. Middleton, MD
Associate Professor, University of Texas M.D. Anderson
Cancer Center, Houston, TX
85 *Unknown Primary Presenting with Axillary
Lymphadenopathy*

Michael J. Miller, MD
Professor and Chief, Division of Plastic Surgery, The
Ohio State University, Columbus, OH
18 *Breast Implants and Related Methods of Breast-Modifying
Surgery*

Giselle J. Moore-Higgs, ARNP, PhDc, AOCN
Assistant Directior, Clinical Trials Office, University
of Florida Shands Cancer Center, Gainesville, FL
91 *Psychosocial Consequences and Lifestyle Interventions*

Anne W. Moulton, MD
Associate Professor, Warren Alpert School of
Medicine at Brown University; Internist, Women's
Health Associates; Rhode Island Hospital,
Providence, RI
89 *Management of Menopause in the Breast Cancer
Patient*

Ewa Mrozek, MD
The Ohio State University, Columbus, OH
87 *Inflammatory Breast Cancer*

Lisle Nabell, MD
Associate Professor of Medicine, University of Alabama
at Birmingham, Birmingham, AL
25 *Investigational Molecular Prognostic Factors for Breast
Carcinoma*

Jiho Nam, MD
Research Associate, Department of Radiation Oncology,
University of North Carolina at Chapel Hill, Chapel
Hill, NC
60 *Radiotherapy Techniques*

John E. Niederhuber, MD
Director, National Cancer Institute; Principal
Investigator, Tumor and Stem Cell Biology Group NCI
CCR, Bethesda, MD
37 *Interval Breast Cancer: Clinical, Epidemiologic, and
Biologic Features*

Patricia J. Numann, MD
Professor of Surgery; Director, Comprehensive Breast
Care Program; Medical Director, University Hospital,
Syracuse, NY
6A *Subareolar Breast Abscess: The Penultimate Stage
of the Mammary Duct-associated Inflammatory Disease
Sequence*

Albert Oler, MD, PhD
Formerly Assistant Professor of Pathology, SUNY Health
Science Center, Syracuse, NY
6A *Subareolar Breast Abscess: The Penultimate Stage of
the Mammary Duct-associated Inflammatory Disease
Sequence*

Ruth O'Regan, MD
Associate Professor of Hematology and Medical
Oncology; Director of Hematology Oncology
Fellowship; Director of Translational Breast Cancer
Research Program, Emory University, Atlanta, GA
77 *Endocrine Therapy for Breast Cancer*

David L. Page, MD
Professor of Pathology and Epidemiology, Vanderbilt
University Medical Center, Nashville, TN
 7 *Gynecomastia*
 8 *Benign, High-Risk, and Premalignant Lesions of the Breast*
12 *Extent and Multicentricity of in Situ and Invasive
Carcinoma*
26 *Risk Factors for Breast Carcinoma in Women with
Proliferative Breast Disease*

Juan P. Palazzo, MD
Professor of Pathology, Anatomy, and Cell Biology,
Jefferson Medical College; Attending Pathologist,
Thomas Jefferson University Hospital,
Philadelphia, PA
52 *Biology and Management of Lobular Carcinoma in Situ
of the Breast*

Ann H. Partridge, MD, MPH
Assistant Professor of Medicine, Harvard Medical School;
Medical Oncologist, Dana-Farber Cancer Institute,
Boston, MA
88 *General Considerations for Follow-Up*

Sara B. Peters, MD, PhD
Director of Dermatopathology; Associate Professor,
The Ohio State University Medical Center,
Columbus, OH
15 *Primary and Secondary Dermatologic Disorders of the Breast*

John Dung Hoang Pham, MD
Clinical Instructor; Staff Physician, The Ohio State
University Medical Center, Columbus, OH
15 *Primary and Secondary Dermatologic Disorders
of the Breast*

Vy Phan, PhD
Senior Fellow, University of Washington,
Seattle, WA
33 *Immune Recognition of Breast Cancer*

Raphael E. Pollock, MD, PhD
Professor and Chair, Department of Surgical Oncology;
Division Head of Surgery, University of Texas M.D.
Anderson Cancer Center, Houston, TX
69 *Surgical Procedures for Advanced Local and Regional
Malignancies of the Breast*

Elisa R. Port, MD, FACS
Assistant Professor, Weill Medical College of Cornell
 University; Assistant Attending Surgeon, Memorial
 Sloan-Kettering Cancer Center, New York, NY
81 *Bilateral Breast Cancer*

David Potter, MD, PhD
Associate Professor of Medicine, Division of
 Hematology/Oncology/Transplant, University of
 Minnesota Masonic Cancer Center,
 Minneapolis, MN
27 *Steroid Receptors in Breast Cancer*

Stephen P. Povoski, MD
Associate Professor of Surgery, The Arthur G. James
 Cancer Hospital and Richard J. Solove Research
 Institute and Comprehensive Cancer Center of
 The Ohio State University, Columbus, OH
10 *In Situ Carcinomas of the Breast: Ductal Carcinoma
 in Situ and Lobular Carcinoma in Situ*

Raquel Prati, MD
Visiting Assistant Professor, Revlon/UCLA Breast
 Center; Department of Surgery, Division of Surgical
 Oncology, University of California at Los Angeles,
 Los Angeles, CA
46 *Modified Radical Mastectomy and Total (Simple)
 Mastectomy*

Michael F. Press, MD, PhD
Harold E. Lee Chair in Cancer Research, University of
 Southern California, Los Angeles, CA
28 *Molecular Oncology of Breast Cancer*

Janet E. Price, DPhil
Associate Professor, University of Texas M.D. Anderson
 Cancer Center, Houston, TX
30 *Concepts and Mechanisms of Breast Cancer Metastasis*

Christopher A. Puleo, BS, PA-C
Physician Assistant in Cutaneous Oncology, H. Lee
 Moffitt Cancer Center and Research Institute,
 Tampa, FL
51 *Lymphedema in the Postmastectomy Patient:
 Pathophysiology, Prevention, and Management*

Abram Recht, MD
Professor of Radiation Oncology, Harvard Medical
 School; Deputy Chief and Senior Radiation
 Oncologist, Beth Israel Deaconess Medical Center,
 Boston, MA
63 *Radiotherapy and Regional Nodes*
64 *Postmastectomy Radiotherapy*

Katherine W. Reeves, PhD, MPH
Assistant Professor, School of Public Health and Health
 Sciences, University of Massachusetts, Amherst, MA
19 *Epidemiology of Breast Cancer*

James M. Reuben, PhD
Associate Professor, University of Texas M.D. Anderson
 Cancer Center, Houston, TX
73 *Detection and Clinical Implications of Occult Systemic
 Micrometastatic Breast Cancer*

Lynn J. Romrell, PhD
Professor and Associate Dean, Florida State University
 College of Medicine, Tallahassee, FL
2 *Anatomy of the Breast, Axilla, Chest Wall, and Related
 Metastatic Sites*
9 *Congenital and Acquired Disturbances of Breast
 Development and Growth*

Arlan L. Rosenbloom, MD
Division of Pediatric Endocrinology, University of
 Florida, Gainesville, FL
3 *Breast Physiology: Normal and Abnormal Development
 and Function*

Wendy S. Rubinstein, MD, PhD
Associate Professor of Medicine, Northwestern
 University Feinberg School of Medicine; Member,
 Robert H. Lurie Comprehensive Cancer Center,
 Chicago, IL; Medical Director, Center for Medical
 Genetics, NorthShore University Health System;
 Evanston, IL
21 *Breast Cancer Genetics: Syndromes, Genes, Pathology,
 Counseling, Testing, and Treatment*

Kathryn J. Ruddy, MD, MPH
Instructor in Medicine, Harvard Medical School; Medical
 Oncologist, Dana-Farber Cancer Institute, Boston, MA
88 *General Considerations for Follow-Up*

Kristen Sanfilippo, MD
Department of Internal Medicine, University of
 Pittsburgh Medical Center, Pittsburgh, PA
20 *Primary Prevention of Breast Cancer*

Alfredo A. Santillan, MD, MPH
Surgical Oncology Fellow, H. Lee Moffitt Cancer Center
 and Research Institute, Tampa, FL
23 *Assessment and Designation of Breast Cancer Stage*

Gordon F. Schwartz, MD, MBA, FACS
Professor of Surgery, Jefferson Medical College;
 Attending Surgeon, Thomas Jefferson University
 Hospital; Consultant Surgeon, Pennsylvania Hospital,
 Philadelphia, PA
52 *Biology and Management of Lobular Carcinoma in Situ
 of the Breast*

Heather Shah, MD
Hematology-Oncology Fellow, University of Alabama at
 Birmingham, Birmingham, AL
25 *Investigational Molecular Prognostic Factors for Breast
 Carcinoma*

Charles Shapiro, MD
Professor of Internal Medicine, The Ohio State
University Medical Center, Columbus, OH
11 *Infiltrating Carcinomas of the Breast: Not One Disease*

Angela Shen, MD
Department of Dermatology, Baylor College of
Medicine, Houston, TX
15 *Primary and Secondary Dermatologic Disorders
of the Breast*

Sherin Shirazi, MD
Attending Surgeon, LAC-USC Medical Center, Los
Angeles, CA; Attending Surgeon, Huntington Hospital,
Pasadena, CA
28 *Molecular Oncology of Breast Cancer*

Yu Shyr, PhD
Professor and Chief, Division of Cancer Biostatistics,
Vanderbilt University School of Medicine; Director,
Cancer Biostatistics Center; Ingram Professor of
Cancer Research, Vanderbilt-Ingram Cancer Center,
Nashville, TN
41 *Design and Conduct of Clinical Trials for Breast Cancer*

Melvin J. Silverstein, MD
Professor of Surgery, University of Southern California,
Los Angeles, CA; Medical Director, Breast Program,
Hoag Memorial Hospital Presbyterian, Newport
Beach, CA
53 *Ductal Carcinoma in Situ: Treatment Controversies
and Oncoplastic Surgery*

Jean F. Simpson, MD
Department of Pathology, Vanderbilt School of
Medicine, Nashville, TN
8 *Benign, High-Risk, and Premalignant Lesions of the Breast*

S. Eva Singletary, MD
Professor of Surgical Oncology, University of Texas M.D.
Anderson Cancer Center, Houston, TX
85 *Unknown Primary Presenting with Axillary
Lymphadenopathy*

Benjamin D. Smith, MD
Adjunct Assistant Professor, Department of Radiation
Oncology, University of Texas M.D. Anderson Cancer
Center, Houston, TX; Chief, Department of Radiation
Oncology, Wilford Hall Medical Center, Lackland
AFB, TX
61 *Radiation Therapy for Locally Advanced Disease*

Felicia E. Snead, MD
Assistant Professor, University of Florida Proton Therapy
Institute, Jacksonville, FL
71 *Locoregional Recurrence after Mastectomy*

Carrie L. Snyder, MSN, RN, APNG
Department of Preventive Medicine, Creighton
University, Omaha, NE
21 *Breast Cancer Genetics: Syndromes, Genes, Pathology,
Counseling, Testing, and Treatment*

Theresa V. Strong, PhD
Associate Professor, Division of Hematology/Oncology,
Department of Medicine; Gene Therapy Center,
University of Alabama at Birmingham,
Birmingham, AL
31 *Gene Therapy for Breast Cancer*

Toncred M. Styblo, MD
Associate Professor, Emory University School of
Medicine, Atlanta, GA
24 *Clinically Established Prognostic Factors in Breast
Cancer*

Marshall M. Urist, MD
Champ Lyons Professor and Vice Chair, Department of
Surgery, University of Alabama at Birmingham,
Birmingham, AL
43 *Indications and Techniques for Biopsy*

Mohan Uttarwar, MSCS, MSEE
President and CEO, BioImagene, Inc, Cupertino, CA
16 *Digital Automation of Breast Biomarker
Immunocytochemistry*

Luis O. Vasconez, MD
Vice Chair, Department of Surgery; Professor and
Director, Division of Plastic Surgery, University of
Alabama at Birmingham, Birmingham, AL
44 *General Principles of Mastectomy: Evaluation and
Therapeutic Options*
48 *Breast Reconstruction following Mastectomy*
49 *Macromastia and Reduction Mammaplasty*

Frank A. Vicini, MD, FACR
Professor, Oakland University, Rochester, MI
62 *Radiotherapy and Ductal Carcinoma in Situ*
66 *Accelerated Partial Breast Irradiation*

Victor G. Vogel, MD, MHS
Professor of Medicine and Epidemiology, University
of Pittsburgh; Medical Oncologist, Magee-Women's
Hospital; Co-Director, Biochemoprevention
Program, University of Pittsburgh Cancer Institute,
Pittsburgh, PA
19 *Epidemiology of Breast Cancer*
20 *Primary Prevention of Breast Cancer*

Paul E. Wakely Jr, MD
Professor, Department of Pathology, The Ohio State
University College of Medicine, Columbus, OH
13 *Mesenchymal Neoplasms of the Breast*

Terry J. Wall, JD, MD
Radiation Oncologist, St. Luke's Hospital of Kansas City,
Kansas City, MO
93 *Medical-Legal Aspects of Breast Care*

Max Wicha, MD
Distinguished Professor of Oncology, University
of Michigan; Director, University of Michigan
Comprehensive Cancer Center, Ann Arbor, MI
29 *Stem Cells, the Breast, and Breast Cancer*

David J. Winchester, MD
Clinical Professor of Surgery, University of
  Chicago School of Medicine, Chicago, IL;
  Chief, Division of Surgical Oncology and General
  Surgery, NorthShore University Health System,
  Evanston, IL
22 *Patterns of Recurrence in Breast Cancer*
82 *Cancer of the Male Breast*

David P. Winchester, MD
Professor of Surgery, Northwestern University Feinberg
  School of Medicine, Chicago, IL; Senior Attending
  Surgeon, Evanston Northwestern Healthcare,
  Evanston, IL
22 *Patterns of Recurrence in Breast Cancer*
82 *Cancer of the Male Breast*

Eric P. Winer, MD
Professor of Medicine, Harvard Medical School;
  Chief, Division of Women's Cancers, Dana-Farber
  Cancer Institute, Boston, MA
76 *Chemotherapy for Metastatic Breast Cancer*

William C. Wood, MD
Professor of Surgery, Emory University School of
  Medicine; Chief of Surgery, Emory University
  Hospital, Atlanta, GA
24 *Clinically Established Prognostic Factors in Breast Cancer*

Douglas Yee, MD
Professor, University of Minnesota Cancer Center,
  Minneapolis, MN
27 *Steroid Receptors in Breast Cancer*

Rex C.W. Yung, MD
Assistant Professor of Medicine and Oncology;
  Director of Pulmonary Oncology and Bronchology,
  Johns Hopkins University, Baltimore, MD
78 *Diagnosis and Management of Pleural Metastases
  in Breast Cancer*

Amelia Zelnak, MD
Instructor of Hematology and Oncology, Emory
  Winship Cancer Institute, Atlanta, GA
77 *Endocrine Therapy for Breast Cancer*

From an international perspective, all industrialized societies readily acknowledge the impact of breast disease in human society as a major epidemiologic issue that continues to expand exponentially. The biometry branch of the National Cancer Institute in the United States recognizes breast cancer as the most frequent carcinoma occurring in women. Furthermore, one of every three American women will consult a physician for breast diseases, and approximately one of every four women will undergo a breast biopsy. Of distinct demographic importance, the lifetime risk for one of every eight American women to develop an invasive carcinoma of the breast is significant and continues to grow. Moreover, current estimates suggest that the rapidly evolving diagnosis of ductal carcinoma in situ may represent as great as one fourth of all breast cancers diagnosed within the next two decades. All these demographic features support the concern of the epidemiologic increase for diagnosis of this neoplasm, and thus, the implementation of state-of-the-art therapies that follow.

With publication of the first edition of *The Breast* in 1991, the authors placed the diagnosis and therapy of breast disease in a working perspective, integrating contemporary, multidisciplinary oncologic principles and therapeutic approaches. The latter included surgery, radiation oncology, pathology, medical oncology, radiology, pharmacokinetics, genetics, transplantation, and biostatistics. These disciplines are synergistic in that they support the mission of hospice, social services, and psychosocial support teams to holistically treat all aspects of breast disease. Moreover, practitioners of each medical discipline have pursued an evolutionary process as new therapeutic modalities were added, which has enhanced clinical outcomes and patient care.

With publication of the second edition in 1998, and the third edition in 2004, unprecedented progress in the therapy of breast diseases was evident. Surgery and medicine have, in general, evolved very rapidly as a consequence of notable scientific events that include the following:

- Greater identification of breakthrough molecular and genetic subdisease process understanding with expansion of the knowledge base for phenotypically normal and abnormal (proliferative) disease processes (e.g., cancer genetics, cellular regulatory events in carcinogenesis, carcinoma initiation and disease progression, invasion and metastasis, molecular diagnostic and prognostic markers).
- DNA sequencing of the human genome with identification of mutational variance that affects genetic progression and phenotypic expression.
- Innovative therapeutic advents such as immunotherapy, gene therapy, bone marrow transplantation, angiogenesis inhibitors, and other technical

approaches that employ (and exploit) novel biologic discoveries.
- An emerging perspective that properly guides clinical outcomes research.
- Advances in surgical techniques and technology. At present, no other human organ system has had the integration of multimodal diagnostic and therapeutic approaches that are as recognized, focused, and successful as those that have been developed for breast neoplasms.

The fourth edition of *The Breast* has evolved into a comprehensive text that is highly readable for all medical researchers and clinicians. This tome reviews the basic tenets essential for diagnosis and therapy of the various benign and malignant disorders of the breast. The Editors have sought to develop the proper address of many recognized abnormalities presenting in the diagnosis and therapy of metabolic, physiologic, and neoplastic derangements of the organ. When we compare this edition with the first, second, and third editions, we consider the present text to be even more thorough, inclusive, and relevant to scientific and clinical achievements.

It is our considered opinion that this new edition provides the requirements necessary for young clinicians and scientists to acquire fundamental knowledge of basic, clinical, and laboratory concepts and techniques that will complement their oncology training. Integration of these principles with advancements in technologic, molecular, cellular, and biologic sciences represents the 21st century definition of each specialty involved with the care of breast disease. However, the ultimate measure of professional skill and effectiveness expected of us as clinicians in the management of breast diseases will be the quality that this text brings to bear on patient outcomes, as well as emotional and physical morbidity.

The fourth edition is not intended to replace standard textbooks of surgery, medicine, or biology, nor is this edition considered an encyclopedic recitation of the myriad of pathologic permutations that exist with various disorders of this organ site. The fourth edition of *The Breast*, however, should coexist with other major medical and surgical reference books. Each chapter is selectively organized and supported with notations of carefully selected journal articles, monographs, or chapters within major reference texts that the contributors of these specific subjects consider a valuable resource. Thus, this work represents a distillation of the herald contributions of innumerable physicians, physiologists, anatomists, geneticists, clinical scientists, and noted health-related workers who have devoted their careers and research to the management of various disorders of the breast.

The fourth edition comprises 21 sections and 95 chapters, with at least 30% additional and/or revised information when compared with the third edition. The opening section documents the historical aspects of breast disease, incorporating the major scientific contributions of investigators and surgeons of the 19th and 20th centuries. The sections that follow include pertinent physiology, anatomy, pathology, genetics, molecular biology, pharmacokinetics, surgery, radiation biology, medical oncology, and biostatistics. Throughout the fourth edition, authors and coauthors have supplemented the text with supportive history of the evolution and chronology of therapeutic principles. In addition, special sections are dedicated to the management of unusual and advanced presentations of the disease.

Additional chapters provide new approaches to the management of breast pain and the risk for carcinoma of the breast following hormonal replacement therapy; a chapter is included that defines patterns of recurrence. The evolution of precise staging evident with lymphatic mapping and sentinel lymph node biopsy has been addressed in depth and provides a new level of precise documentation of technique and outcomes as a consequence of the international experience with the technique since the completion of the second edition. The authors have also incorporated new approaches for gene therapy and counseling for genetic mutations, angiogenesis, immunology, and the evolving role for the immunotherapy of breast cancer. Furthermore, applications of nutritional management and evolving psychologic principles are incorporated in the text. Two chapters, again, are dedicated to addressing legal implications that relate to the management of breast disease. An additional chapter documents the nationwide resources available to both patients and practitioners. Chapters are also dedicated in this edition to covering the psychologic considerations of breast disease and its implications, which affect the patient, spouse, and family members.

With the evolution of this comprehensive reference, overlap will continue to exist among several chapters as a consequence of the dynamic interplay and expectations of medical and surgical practitioners involved with the diagnostic and therapeutic management of the cancer patient. However, the Editors have made every effort to minimize repetitious remarks and dedicated comments except where controversial or "state-of-the art" issues for management exist.

A salient attribute of the text includes the integration of basic science with translational research to emphasize efforts at transfer of knowledge from the bench laboratory to the bedside and the clinic. Only with evolving applications of phase II and phase III trials can the clinician objectively assess the therapeutic value of evolving technical and therapeutic management strategies. These translational research objectives will continue to evaluate promising chemotherapeutics, immunologic agents, inhibitors of angiogenesis, and additional molecularly engineered products that show promise in inhibiting neoplastic progression in this organ.

As previously noted, the authors are hopeful that the fourth edition of *The Breast* has achieved its developmental and scientific goals for assimilating and collating contemporary basic and clinical scientific data to provide clinicians and researchers with multidisciplinary principles used in practice for the treatment of diseases of the breast. The Editors gratefully acknowledge the opportunity provided by the immense challenge that has been entrusted to us by the publisher and are, again, hopeful that our diligence to this task has been properly served.

Kirby I. Bland
Edward M. Copeland III

Acknowledgments

The Editors are deeply indebted to the authors who have contributed to the fourth edition of *The Breast: Comprehensive Management of Benign and Malignant Diseases*. It is the view of the Editors and Associate Editors that this edition is the most comprehensive international reference on diseases of the breast. Both the Editors and Associate Editors have embellished pertinent clinical trials with basic and translational surgical science that has appropriate outcomes when applied in the clinics. Therefore we are deeply indebted to the Associate Editors for their efforts toward the completion of this comprehensive work.

The untold hours essential to properly prepare this treatise represent time taken from busy clinical practices, research laboratories, and our families. Thus the diligent efforts of the contributors to provide insightful state-of-the-art presentations are gratefully acknowledged. Furthermore, the updating of proper scientific knowledge by these contributors through their choice of selective illustrations, tables, and references to bring this text to its readable state of completeness and comprehensiveness is also praiseworthy.

The genesis of this tome began with the encouragement of Edward Wickland at Saunders. Special appreciation should also be paid to Louis Reines, former President of W.B. Saunders, who provided strong encouragement and support for initiation of the first, second, and third editions of this tome. The Editors wish to pay tribute to the diligent work by the staff members of Elsevier, Inc., who have made publication of the fourth edition possible. Judith A. Fletcher, Publishing Director, provided strong support for completion of this edition, which has been supervised in an extraordinary and skillful manner by Roxanne Halpine, developmental editor for the book, who was instrumental in overseeing the editorial process, procuring manuscripts, and scheduling. For these noteworthy contributions, the Editors and Associate Editors are most appreciative.

We further thank our editorial staff: Carol Ann Moore and Leslie B. Riley, who examined materials to ensure they were as flawless as possible. I am also grateful to all editorial assistants in the Department of Surgery at the University of Alabama at Birmingham, as well as our (KIB, EMC) former secretary and editorial assistant, Ervene Katz, of the University of Florida, who has retired since the publication of the third edition. We also express gratitude to Louis Clark and Jonathan Bland, the principal artists who skillfully prepared the illustrations and line drawings used throughout various chapters of the text.

The Editors and Associate Editors are all deeply appreciative of our Residents and Research Fellows in Surgery, Medicine, Pathology, and Radiation Oncology for their intellectual stimulation and their continual encouragement to proceed with development of the fourth edition. To the faculty and residents who have reviewed manuscripts, rendered opinions, and offered suggestions, we gratefully acknowledge their critiques, enlightening commentary, and sustained interest.

Finally, to all who were involved with the development of this text, inclusive of our immediate families and friends who expressed interest and encouragement in the completion of this textbook, we greatly appreciate your indulgence for the time allowed for us to pursue the ambitious goal of preparing what we consider to be a readable, comprehensive text that properly embraces the tenets essential for the diagnosis and therapy of breast diseases. The Editors and Associate Editors further realize that the goals organized and accomplished by the editorial staff and the publisher for the fourth edition could have been achieved only with the immense dedication to task that is evident in the contributions of the authors of each chapter, the artists, and our dedicated editorial assistants.

Kirby I. Bland
Edward M. Copeland III

Foreword

There are clinical textbooks for each medical specialty, and there are clinical textbooks that transcend specialties. The former are useful, but the latter are invaluable. Since its inception in 1991, *The Breast: Comprehensive Management of Benign and Malignant Disorders* has become the undisputed reference for anatomic, pathologic, genetic, immunologic, medical, and surgical aspects of neoplastic and non-neoplastic breast disease. This comprehensive text seamlessly integrates multidisciplinary diagnosis and management in a logical sequence of clearly written and well-referenced chapters from experts in the field.

Drs. Bland and Copeland, both internationally respected experts in breast disease, created *The Breast* as a comprehensive, readable presentation of the basic principles necessary for the diagnosis and treatment of various benign and malignant breast diseases. Their admirable success in part reflects the overall organization of the two-volume text: 95 chapters divided into 21 sections. Sections I through XIII cover breast anatomy, benign and premalignant lesions, pathology of malignancy, epidemiology, prognostic factors, molecular biology, screening and diagnosis, and surgical management. The remaining sections offer detailed, objective management guidelines for each stage of breast cancer, including surgical, radiologic, and systemic approaches. In addition, Volume Two includes genetics-based risk assessment; approaches to special presentations of breast cancer, such as breast cancer in pregnancy and axillary involvement without a known primary lesion; and an interesting discussion of medical-legal issues in breast cancer. Chapters are supported by carefully chosen treatment diagrams, figures, and tables; cross-referencing between chapters further increases ease of use.

My specialty is surgical oncology with a focus on melanoma, but an earlier edition of *The Breast* sits on my shelf and I reach for it when I need an authoritative, reliable reference on breast disease. I have used it to review the lymphatic physiology of the breast, the multidisciplinary management of systemic disease, the implications of recurrence in the reconstructed breast, and tumor markers of breast cancer, among other subjects. This text is an essential resource for all clinicians.

Improved treatments have reduced the mortality of breast cancer in the United States; it is now only the second highest cause of cancer deaths in women. However, every few minutes there is another diagnosis of breast cancer, and breast cancer remains the most frequent cancer in women, striking one of every eight females. These statistics mean that most clinicians will see patients with risk factors, signs, or symptoms of breast problems, and they must be prepared to give advice regarding the many different paradigms for management of benign or malignant breast disease. No diagnosis causes more emotion and fear in a woman than breast cancer, and no topic stimulates more multidisciplinary controversy than its optimum management. For these reasons, nonspecialists as well as specialists must maintain a high index of suspicion for possible malignancy and a high level of knowledge about breast disease. The fourth edition of *The Breast* will allow them to do so.

Donald L. Morton, MD, FACS
John Wayne Cancer Institute at Saint John's Health Center

Contents

SECTION I

History of the Therapy of Breast Cancer

chapter 1

History of the Therapy of Breast Cancer

KIRBY I. BLAND

Breast cancer, with its uncertain etiologies, has captured the attention of physicians throughout the ages. Despite centuries of theoretical meanderings and scientific inquiry, breast cancer remains one of the most dreaded of human diseases. The story of the efforts to cope with breast cancer is complex, and there is no happy ending as there is in diseases for which cause and cure have been found. However, progress has been made in lessening the horrors that formerly devastated the body and psyche.

This chapter records some of the key milestones in the development of the current understanding of the biology and therapy of breast cancer, which is based on the achievements and contributions of many doctors and scientists over many hundreds of years. Although the milestones listed here are important ones, the list is by no means comprehensive. This chapter is meant to be a useful reference to all people who would like to know more about the historical background of breast cancer and about the development of modern breast cancer therapy.

Ancient Civilizations

CHINESE

Huang Di, the Yellow Emperor, was born in 2698 BCE and subsequently wrote the *Nei Jing*, the oldest treatise of medicine, which gives the first description of tumors and documents five forms of therapy: spiritual care, pharmacology, diet, acupuncture, and the treatment of specific diseases.

EGYPTIAN

Imhotep, an Egyptian physician, architect, and astrologer, was born in 2650 BCE. He designed the first pyramid at Saqqara and was deified as the god of healing. The early Egyptians documented many cases of breast tumors, which were treated with cautery. To preserve their findings, the Egyptians etched their cursive script on thin sheets of papyrus leaf and also engraved or painted hieroglyphics on stone. Among six principal papyri, the most informative one with respect to diseases of the breast is that acquired by Edwin Smith (b. 1822) in 1862 and presented to the New York Historical Society at the time of his death. Dating to about 1600 BCE, it is a papyrus roll 15 feet long, with writing on both sides.[1] The front contains 17 columns describing 48 cases devoted to clinical surgery. References are made to diseases of the breast such as abscesses, trauma, and infected wounds. Case 45 is perhaps the earliest record of breast cancer, with the title *Instructions Concerning Tumors on His Breast* (Fig. 1-1). The examiner is told that a breast with bulging tumors, very cool to the touch, is an ailment for which there is no treatment.

BABYLONIAN

The Code of Hammurabi (ca. 1750 BCE) was commissioned in Babylon. Its 282 clauses provided the first laws that regulated medical practitioners and dealt with physicians' responsibilities and fees. At that time, internal medicine consisted mainly of a recitation of litanies and incantations against the demons of the earth, air, and water. Surgery consisted of opening an abscess with a bronze lancet. If the patient died or lost an eye during treatment, the physician's hands were cut off.

CLASSIC GREEK PERIOD (460 TO 136 BCE)

Medicine in Europe had its origins in ancient Greece. The scientific method and clinical advancement of medicine are credited to Hippocrates (b. 460 BCE), who also defined its ethical ideals. His basic philosophy was the linkage of four cardinal body humors (blood, phlegm, yellow bile, and black bile) with four universal elements (earth, air, water, and fire). Perfect health depended on a proper balance in the dynamic qualities of the humors. It was generally believed that blood was in the arteries and veins, phlegm in the brain, yellow bile in the liver, and black bile in the spleen. Hippocrates divided diseases into three general categories: those curable by medicine (most favorable), those not curable by medicine but curable by the knife, and those not curable by the

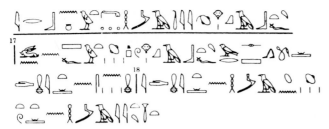

Figure 1-1   Recording of the earliest known case of breast cancer (1600 BCE). (From the Edwin Smith Papyrus. Published in facsimile and hieroglyphic transliteration with translation and commentary by James Henry Breasted. Birmingham, AL, The Classics of Medicine Library, 1984. Reprinted with permission.)

knife but curable by fire. The *Corpus Hippocraticum* deals with the treatment of fractures, tumors, surgical procedures, asthma, allergies, and diseases of the skin. A well-documented case history of Hippocrates describes a woman with breast cancer associated with bloody discharge from the nipple. Hippocrates associated breast cancer with cessation of menstruation, leading to breast engorgement and indurated nodules.

Alexandria on the Nile, founded by Alexander the Great in 332 BCE, became the focal point of Greek science during the third and second centuries BCE. More than 14,000 students studied various elements of Hellenistic knowledge there. This knowledge was contained in 700,000 scrolls in the largest library in antiquity, which was subsequently destroyed by Julius Caesar. Rudimentary anatomic studies were conducted and led to progress in the tools and techniques of surgery.

GRECO-ROMAN PERIOD (150 BCE TO 500 AD)

Following the destruction of Corinth in 146 BCE, Greek medicine migrated to Rome. During the preceding six centuries, the Romans had lived without physicians. They depended on medicinal herbs, assorted concoctions, votive objects, religious rites, and superstitions (Fig. 1-2).

Aurelius Celsus, a Roman born in 25 BCE, described the cardinal signs of inflammation (calor, rubor, dolor, and turgor). He wrote *De Medicina* around 30 AD, which contains an early clinical description of cancer. In it he mentions the breasts of women as one of the sites of cancer and describes a fixed irregular swelling with dilated tortuous veins and ulceration. He also delineates four clinical stages of cancer: early cancer, cancer without ulcer, ulcerated cancer, and ulcerated cancer with cauliflower-like excrescences that bleed easily. Celsus opposed treatment of the last three stages by any method, because aggressive measures irritated the condition and led to inevitable recurrence.

The Greek physician Leonides is credited with the first operative treatment for breast cancer in the first century AD. His method consisted of an initial incision into the uninvolved portion of the breast, followed by applications of cautery to stop the bleeding. Repeated incisions and applications of cautery were continued until the entire breast and tumor had been removed and the underlying tissues were covered with an eschar. With Roman influence and support, surgical instruments became highly specialized, as witnessed by the finding of more than 200 different instruments in the excavations of Pompei and Herculaneum (Figs. 1-3 and 1-4).

The greatest Greek physician to follow Hippocrates was Galen (b. 131 AD). He was born on the Mediterranean coast of Asia Minor, studied in Alexandria, and practiced medicine for the rest of his life in Rome. He is credited as the founder of experimental physiology, and his system of pathology followed that of Hippocrates.

Galen considered black bile, especially when it was extremely dark or thick, to be the most harmful of the four humors and the ultimate cause of cancer. He described breast cancer as a swelling with distended veins resembling the shape of a crab's legs. To prevent accumulation of black bile, Galen advocated that the patient be purged and bled. He claimed to have cured the disease in its early stage when the tumor was on the surface of the body and all the "roots" could be extirpated at surgery. The roots were not derived from the tumor but were dilated veins filled with morbid black bile. When removing the tumor, the surgeon had to be aware of the danger of profuse hemorrhage from large blood vessels. On the other hand, the surgeon was advised to allow the blood to flow freely for a while to allow the black blood to escape.

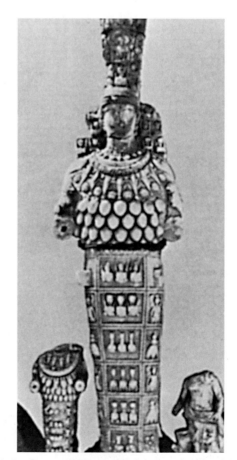

Figure 1-2   Statue of Diana of Ephesus, a fertility deity invoked by Roman women, displaying 20 accessory pectoral breasts. (From Haagensen CD: Diseases of the breast, 2nd ed. Philadelphia, WB Saunders, 1971.)

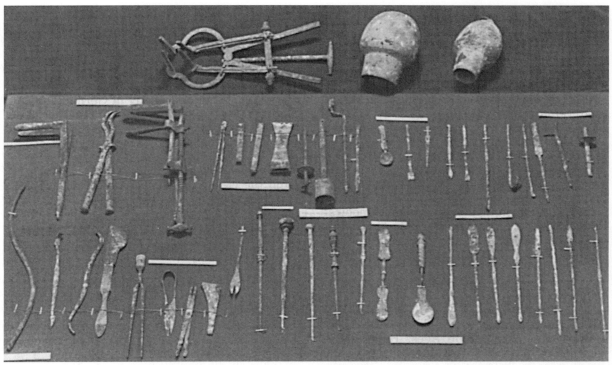

Figure 1-3 Surgical instruments (79 AD) from excavations of Pompei and Herculaneum. (Courtesy of the Archives of Thomas Jefferson University, Philadelphia, PA.)

Middle Ages

The Middle Ages may be considered the period between the downfall of Rome and the beginning of the Renaissance. The doctrine of the four humors, which formed the basis of Hippocratic medicine, was endowed with authority by Galen and governed all aspects of medical thinking throughout and beyond the Middle Ages. This influence can be traced in the Christian, Jewish, and Arabic traditions.

CHRISTIAN

From the Christian standpoint, the monks and clerics who constituted the educated class maintained medicine

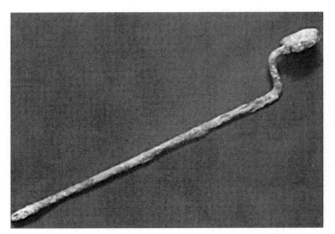

Figure 1-4 Roman cautery (79 AD) depicted from Figure 1-3.

in the Middle Ages. In 529, with the founding by Saint Benedict of the Monastery on Monte Cassino in central Italy, there arose a heightened interest in medicine in the scattered cloisters of the Roman Church. Monte Cassino fostered the teaching and practice of medicine, along with the copying and preserving of ancient manuscripts. Many satellite monasteries developed throughout Christendom in which the monks treated the sick and copied medical manuscripts. Subsequently, monastic schools spread under the Benedictines to England, Scotland, Ireland, France, Switzerland, and most of the European continent. The patron saint for breast disease was Saint Agatha. She had been a martyr in Sicily in the middle of the third century when her two breasts were torn off with iron shears because of resistance to the advances of the governor Quinctianus (Fig. 1-5). On Saint Agatha's day, two loaves of bread representing her breasts are carried in procession on a tray.

The Council of Rheims (1131) excluded monks and the clergy from the practice of medicine. From that time on, laymen increasingly carried on medical teaching and practice. Cathedral schools, although in clerical hands, profited from greater freedom than the monasteries had provided and enjoyed the intellectual contacts of the large cities. Further growth of cities in the eleventh and twelfth centuries led to the rise of universities, which led to the removal of medicine from monastic influence.

Paul of Aegina (b. 625) was an Alexandrian physician and surgeon famed for his *Epitomae Medicae Libri Septem*, which contained descriptions of trephining, tonsillotomy, paracentesis, and mastectomy. Lanfranc of Milan (b. 1250) was an Italian surgeon who worked in Paris and wrote *Chirurgia Magna*, which contained sections

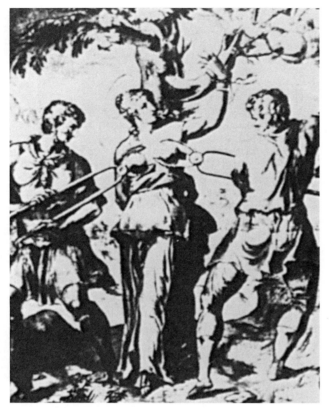

Figure 1-5 Martyrdom of Saint Agatha. (From Robinson JO: Treatment of breast cancer through the ages. Am J Surg 151: 317–333, 1986.)

on anatomy, embryology, ulcers, fistulas, and fractures, as well as sections on herbs and pharmacy and on cancer of the breast.

JEWISH

Jewish physicians were active at Salerno, Spain, as early as the ninth century. They achieved great distinction not only in the art of healing but also in their literary efforts. Popes, kings, and noblemen sought their services. In a time when poisoning of enemies and rivals was common, the Jews were considered the safest medical advisers. The Arabian rulers and Egyptian caliphs also preferred them to their Mohammedan physicians, who practiced magic and astrology in their treatment of disease.

Under the tolerant Moors of Spain and the early Christian rulers of Spain and Portugal, the Jews became leaders in the medical profession. The foremost among them was Moses Maimonides. Born in Cordova, Spain, in 1135, he studied medicine at Cairo and became the physician to Saladin, the Sultan of Egypt. In addition to his own medical treatise, he translated from Arabic into Hebrew the five volume *al-Quanum fil-Tib* of the Iranian physician Avicenna (b. 980), which was the authoritative encyclopedia of medicine during the Middle Ages. Maimonides also made a collection of the aphorisms of Hippocrates and Galen.

Jewish physicians remained prominent in Spain under the Western Caliphate until they were banished from the country in 1492. The Salerno School exploited them as teachers until it had enough indigenous talent to proceed without them. Even at Montpellier in southern France, the Jews were excluded in 1301. It would not be until the onset of the modern industrial age that they would again be admitted to citizenship throughout Europe and given university freedom, which once more liberated their brilliant medical talent.

ARABIC

Western society is indebted to Arabic scholars and physicians who valued and preserved the teachings and writings of their Greek predecessors. Without the intervention of the Arabs, the writings of the Greek physicians might have been lost. Baghdad, the capital of the Islamic Empire in Iraq, became the center for translation of the Greek authors. The library at Cordova had 600,000 manuscripts, and the one at Cairo had 18 rooms of books. The Tartars raided the library in Baghdad in 1260 and threw the books into the river.

Rhazes (b. 860), one of the great Arabic physicians, condoned excision of breast cancer only if it could be completely removed and the underlying tissues cauterized. He warned that incising a breast cancer would produce an ulceration. Haly ben Abbas, a Persian who died in 994, authored an encyclopedic work in medicine and surgery based on Rhazes and the Greek sources. He endorsed the removal of breast cancers with allowance for bleeding to evacuate melancholic humors, which were widely believed to predispose to cancer. He did not tie the arteries and made no mention of cautery. Avicenna was the successor to Haly ben Abbas and was known as the "Prince of Physicians." He was chief physician to the hospital at Baghdad and was the author of a vast scientific and philosophical encyclopedia, *Kitab-ash-shifa*, as well as the *al-Quanum fil-Tib*, both of which remained authoritative references for centuries.

Renaissance

The transition from the medieval to the modern era occurred in the latter part of the fifteenth century, with the introduction of gunpowder into warfare, the discovery of America, and the invention of the printing press. During this period, medical teaching flourished in universities in Montpellier, Bologna, Padua, Paris, Oxford, and Cambridge.

Andreas Vesalius (b. 1514) was a Flemish physician who revolutionized the study of medicine with his detailed descriptions of the anatomy of the human body, based on his own dissection of cadavers. While at the University of Padua, he wrote and illustrated the first comprehensive textbook of anatomy, *De Humani Corporis Fabrica Libri Septem* (1543). He recommended mastectomy for breast cancer and the use of sutures rather than cautery to control bleeding.

Ambrose Paré (b. 1510) studied medicine in Paris and through his war experience became the greatest surgeon of his time. His conservative surgical approach to cancer was detailed in *Oeuvres Complètes* (1575). He encouraged the use of vascular ligatures and avoidance of cautery and boiling oil. He condoned the excision of superficial breast cancers but attempted to treat other breast cancers through application of lead plates, which were intended to compress the blood supply and arrest tumor growth. He made the important observation that breast cancer often caused swelling of the axillary "glands." Michael Servetus (b. 1509), a Spaniard who studied in Paris, was burned at the stake for his heretical discovery that blood in the pulmonary circulation passes into the heart after having been mixed with air in the lungs. For cancer of the breast, Servetus suggested that the underlying pectoralis muscles be removed as well as the axillary glands described by Paré.

Wilhelm Fabry (b. 1560) is held in esteem as the "Father of German Surgery." His name was honored by the placement of a wreath at his statue in Hilden near Düsseldorf, Germany, by members of the International Society of the History of Medicine in 1986 (Fig. 1-6). He devised an instrument (Fig. 1-7) that compressed and fixed the base of the breast so that a knife could amputate it more swiftly and less painfully.[2] His text, *Opera*, included clear descriptions of breast cancer operations and illustrations of amputation forceps. He stipulated that the tumor should be mobile so that it could be removed completely, with no remnants being left behind. The other famous German surgeon of this period was Johann Schultes (b. 1595), known as Scultetus, who was an illustrator of surgery and inventor of surgical instruments. His book, *Armamentarium Chirurgicum*, which was published posthumously in 1653, contained illustrations of surgical procedures, one of which represented amputation of the breast. He used heavy ligatures on large needles, which transfixed the breast so that traction would facilitate its removal by the knife. Hemostasis was secured by cauterization of the base of the tumor (Fig. 1-8).

Because of the morbidity and mortality of breast cancer surgery and a paucity of competent surgeons, few breast amputations were actually performed. Nonsurgical remedies for breast cancer appeared in rudimentary scientific journals that were published toward the end of the century (Fig. 1-9).

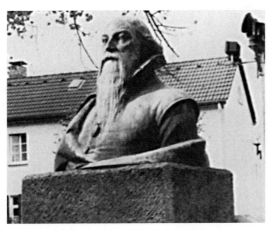

Figure 1-6 Statue of Wilhelm Fabry in Hilden, Germany. (Courtesy of Dr. Ellen Wiederhold, Burgermeister of Hilden.)

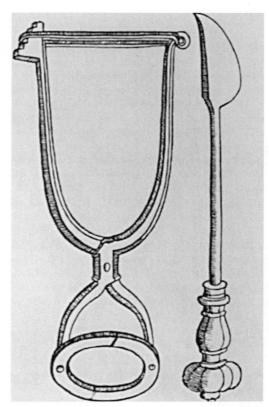

Figure 1-7 Mastectomy instruments of Fabry von Hilden in the late sixteenth century. (From Robinson JO: Treatment of breast cancer through the ages. Am J Surg 151:317–333, 1986.)

Eighteenth Century

The 1700s were slow to develop significant new concepts in pathology and physiology. The arbitrary separation of scirrhus and breast cancer in the doctrine of Galen was still thought to be correct. Many considered scirrhus to be a benign growth that under adverse circumstances could undergo malignant degeneration, whereas others regarded it as an existing stage of cancer. Most believed that scirrhus originated in stagnation and coagulation of body fluids within the breast (local cause). Others believed it to occur from a general internal derangement of the body juices (systemic cause). In accepting both causes, some authors wrote that the local cause could be a precipitating factor in a predisposed patient. Hermann Boerhaave (b. 1668) taught that Galen's yellow bile was blood serum rather than bile itself, that phlegm was serum that had been altered by standing, and that black bile was a part of a clot that had separated off and become a darker color. Thus, the four humors of Galen were only different components of the blood. Pieter Camper (b. 1722) described and illustrated the internal mammary lymph nodes, and Paolo Mascagni (b. 1752) did the same for the pectoral lymph nodes. Death caused by metastasis from breast cancer was not yet understood. If death was not caused by hemorrhage, it was ascribed to a general decomposition of the humors.

In Edinburgh, Scotland, which was strongly oriented to university teaching, the separation of surgeons from

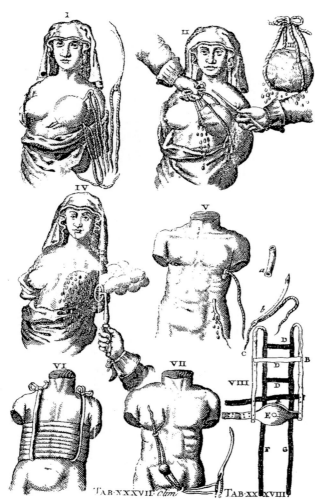

Figure 1-8 Mastectomy procedure of Scultetus in the seventeenth century. (From Robinson JO: Treatment of breast cancer through the ages. Am J Surg 151:317–333, 1986.)

barbers occurred by 1718. In London, where barber-surgeon guilds had existed, the separation occurred in 1745. A new era of British surgery began when William Cheselden (b. 1688), surgeon to St. Thomas' and St. George's Hospitals, first established private courses in anatomy and surgery. The Hunter brothers, John (b. 1728) and William (b. 1718), followed suit. These courses attracted students from all over the country, the continent, and America. John Hunter is credited as being the founder of experimental surgery and surgical pathology.

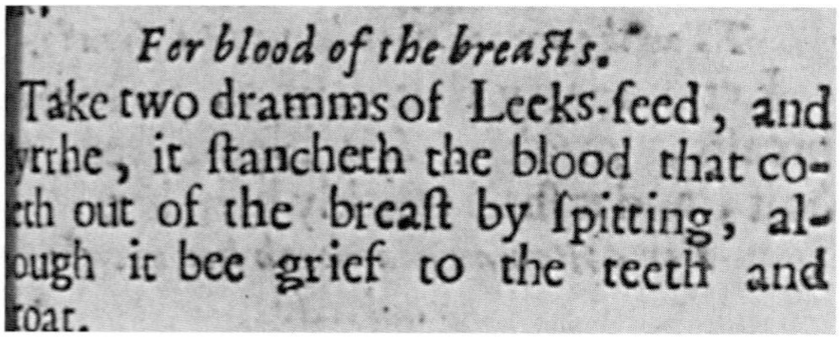

For blood of the breaſts.
Take two dramms of Leeks-feed, and
yrrhe, it ſtancheth the blood that co-
th out of the breaſt by ſpitting, al-
ough it bee grief to the teeth and
roat.

Figure 1-9 Home remedy "for blood of the breasts" (1664).

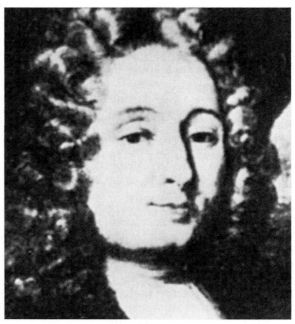

Figure 1-10 Henri François le Dran (1685–1770) noted that lymphatic spread worsened the prognosis of breast cancer. (From Robinson JO: Treatment of breast cancer through the ages. Am J Surg 151:317–333, 1986.)

Henri le Dran (b. 1685) of France (Fig. 1-10) concluded that cancer was a local disease in its early stages and that its spread to the lymphatic system signaled a worsened prognosis.[3] This was a courageous contradiction to the humoral theory of Galen, which had persisted for a thousand years and was to be upheld by many for two centuries to come. A colleague of le Dran, Jean Petit (b. 1674), first Director of the French Academy of Surgery, supported these principles. He advocated removal of the breast, the underlying pectoral muscle, and the axillary lymph nodes.[4] Another French surgeon, Bernard Pehrilhe, attempted to transmit cancer by injecting human breast cancer tissue into dogs.

The German surgeon Lorenz Heister (b. 1683) favored the use of a guillotine machine for breast tumors using the traction strings of Scultetus. This not only was rapid but also removed all the skin of the breast. Heister described the patient-surgeon relationship as follows: "Many females can stand the operation with the greatest courage and without hardly moaning at all. Others, however, make such a clamour that they may dishearten even the most undaunted surgeon and hinder the operation. To perform the operation, the surgeon should therefore be steadfast and not allow himself to become disconcerted by the cries of the patient."

Large numbers of mastectomies were performed during the early eighteenth century, but this number decreased during the second half of the century because of poor results and the indiscriminate mutilation that occurred with improper patient selection and with physician bias. In 1757 it was reported that in Amsterdam, a densely populated town with 200,000 inhabitants, "not six times a year a breast was amputated with reasonable chance of a cure."

Nineteenth Century

Breast surgery changed dramatically in the 1800s. William Morton introduced anesthesia in the United States in 1846, and Joseph Lister introduced the principle of antisepsis in England in 1867.

EUROPEAN SURGERY

At the beginning of the nineteenth century, the treatment for breast cancer remained in confusion. In 1811 Samuel Young in England revived the method of Paré, in which compression was used to cut off the blood supply of the tumor.[5] Nooth, another English surgeon, sprayed the breast with carbolic acid, which was a modified form of the ancient practice of cauterization.

James Syme (b. 1799) was a famous Scottish surgeon. His daughter married Sir Joseph Lister. Much of his breast surgery was performed before the use of anesthesia.[6] His third surgical apprentice, John Brown (b. 1810), wrote *Rab and His Friends* (1858), which contains a vivid description of breast surgery as performed by the then 28-year-old Syme in the Minto House Hospital of Edinburgh, Scotland.

> The operating theater is crowded; much talk and fun and all the cordiality and stir of youth. The surgeon with his staff of assistants is there. In comes Allie (the patient): one look at her quiets and abates the eager students. Allie stepped upon a seat, and laid herself on the table, as her friend the surgeon told her; arranged herself, gave a rapid look at James (her husband), shut her eyes, rested herself on me (Brown), and took my hand. The operation was at once begun; it was necessarily slow; and chloroform—one of God's best gifts to his suffering children—was then unknown. The surgeon did his work. The pale face showed its pain, but was still and silent. Rab's (a mastiff) soul was working within him; he saw that something strange was going on—blood flowing from his mistress, and she suffering; his ragged ear was up, and importunate; he growled and gave now and then a sharp impatient yelp; he would have liked to have done something to that man. But James had him firm, and gave him a glower from time to time, and an intimation of a possible kick—all the better for James, it kept his eye and his mind off Allie. It is over: she is dressed, steps gently and decently down from the table, looks for James; then turning to the surgeon and the students, she curtsies—and in a low, clear voice, begs their pardon if she has behaved ill. The students—all of us—wept like children; the surgeon helped her up carefully—and resting on James and me, Allie went to her room, Rab following. Four days after the operation what might have been expected happened. The patient had a chill, the wound was septic, and she died.[7]

Later in life Syme was able to operate with the patient under anesthesia. He felt it incumbent on the surgeon to search very carefully for axillary glands in the course of the operation but stated that the results were almost always unsatisfactory when the glands were involved, no matter how perfectly they seemed to have been removed. Sir James Paget (b. 1814) reported an operative mortality of 10% in 235 patients and among survivors, recurrence within 8 years. In 139 patients with scirrhus carcinoma, those who did not undergo surgery lived longer than those who did.[8] In 1874 Paget published *On Disease of the Mammary Areola Preceding Cancer of the Mammary Gland*, which described cancer of the nipple accompanied by eczematous changes and cancer of the lactiferous ducts (Paget's disease of the breast).[9]

Charles Moore (b. 1821) of the Middlesex Hospital in London championed the belief that the only possibility of cure for breast cancer was through wider and more extensive surgery, despite the frequent disastrous results (Fig. 1-11). His famous paper, *On the Influence of Inadequate Operation on the Theory of Cancer* (1867), was widely accepted.[10] He stressed that the tumor should not be cut and that recurrences originated as a result of dispersion from the primary growth and were not independent in origin. His operation called for removal of the entire breast, with special attention to removal of the skin in continuity with the main mass of the tumor. Moore did not advocate removal of the pectoralis major muscle.

The father of surgical antiseptic technique and one of England's most respected surgeons, Sir Joseph Lister (b. 1827), agreed with Moore's principles and advocated division of the origins of both pectoral muscles to gain better exposure of the axilla for the axillary gland dissection. His contribution of carbolic acid spray was not widely accepted for 15 to 20 years.[11] In 1877 Mitchell Banks of Liverpool, England, advocated removal of the axillary glands in all cases of surgery for breast cancer. He washed the wound with carbolic acid solution but avoided the spray because of its cooling effect on the patient.

Alfred-Armand-Louis-Marie Velpeau (b. 1795) of France, originally apprenticed to the blacksmith trade, later rose to become professor of clinical surgery at the Paris Faculty, which was established in 1834. In his *Treatise on Diseases of the Breast* (1854), he claimed to have seen more than 1000 benign or malignant breast tumors during a practice of 40 years.[12] In those times, once the cancer had been excised, the patient and surgeon parted company and follow-up was scanty. In 1844 Jean-Jacques-Joseph Leroy d'Etiolles (b. 1798) conducted a study of 1192 patients with breast cancer. He concluded

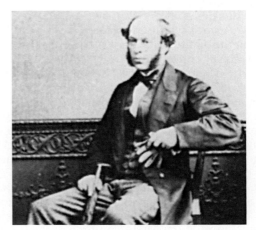

Figure 1-11 Charles Moore, British surgeon of the mid-nineteenth century, advocated wider and more extensive breast surgery. (From Robinson JO: Treatment of breast cancer through the ages. Am J Surg 151:317–333,1986.)

that mastectomy was more harmful than beneficial. The 1854 Congress of the Académie de Médecine discussed whether cancer should be treated at all.

New practices developed in Germany in 1875, when Richard von Volkmann (b. 1830) removed the entire breast, no matter how small the primary tumor, as well as the pectoral fascia, with an occasional thick layer of the underlying muscle, and the axillary nodes. Theodor Billroth (b. 1829) also removed the entire breast but wondered whether local excision of the tumor with a surrounding zone of normal tissue would not be adequate for small lesions. In fixed tumors, however, his resection included the pectoral fascia, along with a thick layer of the underlying muscle.[13] Ernst Kuster (b. 1839) of Berlin, Germany, recommended that the axillary fat be removed along with the axillary glands. Lothar Heidenhain (b. 1860), a pupil of Volkmann, recommended removal of the superficial portion of the pectoralis major muscle even if the tumor was freely mobile, but he also recommended that the entire muscle, with its underlying connective tissue, be removed if the tumor was fixed.[14] Concerning benign breast disease, Sir Astley Cooper (b. 1768), an eminent English surgeon, published *Illustrations of the Diseases of the Breast* in 1829, which clearly differentiated fibroadenomas from chronic cystic mastitis.

Other important milestones of the nineteenth century are as follows. In 1829 French gynecologist and obstetrician Joseph Récalmier introduced the term *metastasis* to describe the spread of cancer. In 1830 the English surgeon Everard Home (b. 1756) published a book on cancer, which contained the first illustrations of the appearance of cancer cells under the microscope. Heinrich von Waldeyer-Hartz (b. 1836) developed a histologic classification of cancers showing that carcinomas come from epithelial cells, whereas sarcomas come from mesodermal tissue. In 1865 Victor Cornil (b. 1837) described malignant transformation of the acinar epithelium of the breast. In 1893 the first description of loss of differentiation by cancer cells ("anaplasia") was made by David von Hensemann, a German pathologist.

AMERICAN SURGERY

In the nineteenth century, Philadelphia was the medical center of the United States. It harbored the country's oldest medical college, the University of Pennsylvania (founded in 1765), the Jefferson Medical College (founded in 1824), and more than 50 other medical schools. It had a permanent medical college for women, as well as one in homeopathy and one in osteopathy.

Joseph Pancoast (b. 1805) was a dexterous surgeon-anatomist, who in the flowery language of his era, was said "to have an eye as quick as a flashing sunbeam and a hand as light as floating perfume." His *Treatise on Operative Surgery*,[14] published in 1844 in the preanesthetic and preantiseptic era, illustrates a mastectomy (Fig. 1-12). The patient is awake, with eyes open, and is semireclining. An assistant compresses the subclavian artery above the clavicle with the thumb of one hand. Larger vessels in the wound are compressed with the

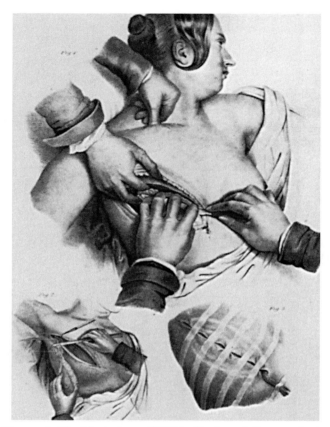

Figure 1-12 Mastectomy (1844) by Dr. Joseph Pancoast in the preanesthetic and preantiseptic era. En bloc removal with axillary lymphatic drainage.

thumb and index finger of the assistant's other hand. Ligatures are left long and brought through the lower pole of the wound, where they act as a drain and can be pulled out later as they slough off. In one of the smaller sketches, the axillary glands are shown in continuity with the breast, visualized through a single incision that extended into the axilla. This was the first illustration of en bloc removal of the breast with its axillary lymphatic drainage. Skin removal was scanty, with easy approximation of the wound using five wide adhesive strips.

Samuel D. Gross (b. 1805) was designated as "the greatest American surgeon of his time." His approach to cancer of the breast, however, was more conservative than that of Pancoast, his colleague. He described extirpation of the breast as "generally a very easy and simple affair." Using a small elliptical incision, he attempted to save enough skin for easy approximation of the edges of the wound. He aimed for healing by first intention, which was less likely if the wound were permitted to gape. In dealing with inordinately vascular tumors, he ligated each vessel but generally considered this as awkward and unnecessary. Glands in the axilla were removed only if grossly involved, in which case they were removed through the outer angle of the incision or through a separate one. The glands were enucleated with the finger or handle of the scalpel. It was his rule not to approximate the skin until 4 or 5 hours after the operation, "lest secondary hemorrhage should occur, and thus necessitate the removal of the dressings." In the sixth edition of his *System of Surgery* (1882), he devoted 30 pages to diseases of the breast.[15]

Samuel W. Gross (b. 1837) took a much more aggressive approach than that of his eminent father. He stated in 1887 that "no matter what the situation of the tumor may be, or whether glands can or cannot be detected in the armpit, the entire breast, with all the skin covering it, the paramammary fat, and the fascia of the pectoral muscle are cleanly dissected away, and the axillary contents are extirpated. It need scarcely be added that aseptic precautions are strictly observed."[16] Removal of all the skin of the breast led to its designation as the "dinner plate operation." Against the criticism that an open large wound resulted in granulations from which cancer would again develop, he said, "When fireplugs produce whales, and oak trees polar bears, then will granulations produce cancer, and not until then."

The younger Gross personally examined all the tumors he removed under the microscope. In 1879 he helped his father found the Philadelphia Academy of Surgery, the oldest surgical society in the United States. Following his premature death in 1889, his widow married William Osler. In her will of 1928, Lady Osler bequeathed an endowment for a lectureship at the Jefferson Medical College in honor of her first husband and his special interest in tumors.

D. Hayes Agnew (b. 1818) of the University of Pennsylvania wrote *Principles and Practice of Surgery* (1878), which endorsed Listerian antisepsis.[17] He shared the pessimistic view of many eminent surgeons of the time that few cancers were ever cured with surgery. The Agnew Clinic by Thomas Eakins (b. 1844) is a masterpiece of American art depicting a mastectomy performed in 1889 under conditions that would have been considered ideal for the time (Fig. 1-13).

Toward the later part of the nineteenth century, Philadelphia had to share its limelight with a number

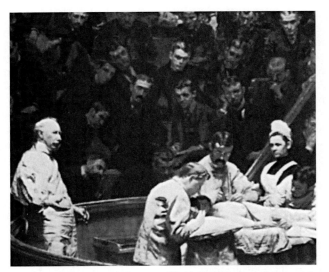

Figure 1-13 Eakins' Agnew Clinic (1889) depicting mastectomy under ideal conditions of the time. (Courtesy of University of Pennsylvania School of Medicine, Philadelphia, PA.)

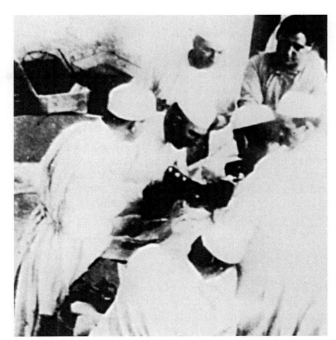

Figure 1-14 Dr. William S. Halsted performing a radical mastectomy. Note the absence of masks. (Courtesy of College of Physicians of Philadelphia, Philadelphia, PA.)

of other cities throughout the country, especially with Baltimore, where the recently organized Johns Hopkins Hospital Medical School produced a revolution in medical education and research. At that institution, William Halsted (b. 1852) recommended, "the suspected tissues [breast cancer] be removed in one piece lest the wound become infected by the division of tissue invaded by the disease, or by division of the lymphatic vessels containing cancer cells, and because shreds of cancerous tissue might be readily overlooked in a piecemeal extirpation." He advocated such wide removal of the skin that a graft would be required and recommended that the pectoralis major muscle be part of the en bloc specimen regardless of the size of the tumor.[18] Later, he went on to favor removal of the sheaths of the upper portion of the rectus abdominis, serratus anterior, subscapularis, latissimus dorsi, and teres major muscles.[19] Although there was nothing dramatically new in Halsted's operation, he placed it on a logical and scientific basis, spelled out the exact technique, and dispersed his principles widely throughout the profession (Fig. 1-14).

Another scholar of breast cancer and mastectomy techniques, Willie Meyer (b. 1854) of the New York Graduate School of Medicine, described a similar technique only 10 days after Halsted's published paper.[20] He advocated removal of the pectoralis minor muscle in addition to the major. His operation has been referred to as the *Willie Meyer modification of the Halsted procedure*. At the close of the nineteenth century, the Halsted radical mastectomy had been established as state-of-the-art for surgical treatment of breast cancer. This procedure was unchallenged for 70 years, until the advent of breast conservation methods.

In 1895, I. Cullen credited William Welch (b. 1850), a pathologist at Johns Hopkins, as being the first to use frozen section in the diagnosis of breast lesions.[21] Welch is stated to have used this procedure in 1891 on a patient who was found to have a benign breast tumor.

Twentieth Century

At the beginning of the twentieth century, it was evident that a higher cure rate for breast cancer would not be achieved through surgery alone. This lowering of surgical expectations stimulated scientific inquiry through epidemiologic studies, laboratory research, and statistical analysis of practical experiences with breast cancer surgery in its various pathologic stages.

SURGERY

The radical mastectomy described simultaneously by Halsted and Meyer, although extensive, did not include the supraclavicular and internal mammary nodes. In 1907, Halsted reported the removal of supraclavicular nodes in 119 patients.[22] In 44 patients with metastatic deposits, only two were alive and well after 5 years. In 1910, C. Westerman reported surgery involving a patient with local recurrence in which he disarticulated the arm and resected three ribs.[23] The thoracic wall defect was repaired with a pedicled flap. In two other cases, he carried out a partial excision of the thoracic wall and closed the defect with tissue from the contralateral healthy breast. These last two patients died within weeks, and the follow-up on the first was only for 1½ years. The surgeons discontinued these extensive operations within a few years because of the increased operative mortality and poor survival rates.

The internal mammary nodes were neglected until the third decade of the century. In 1927, William Handley (b. 1872) of the Middlesex Hospital directed attention to the frequency of internal mammary node involvement, especially when axillary lymph nodes were enlarged.[24] He reported the removal of internal mammary nodes as an extension of the radical mastectomy. After World War II, Jerome Urban and Owen Wangensteen, among others, advocated a "supraradical mastectomy," in which the dissection was carried into the mediastinum and the neck.[25,26]

The late Cushman Haagensen (Fig. 1-15) of Columbia-Presbyterian Medical Center in New York City dedicated his life to the surgical and pathologic study of breast diseases. He classified breast cancers in his patients according to size, clinical findings, and nodal status while establishing a breast unit where comprehensive data were maintained.[27] He was the first to propose self-examination of the breast and to suggest that lobular neoplasia (lobular carcinoma in situ) was not actual cancer. He distinguished this "marker of risk" from ductal carcinoma in situ.

In 1937, London surgeon Geoffrey Keynes demonstrated that less radical surgery was needed in breast cancer, with radiation giving equally good results. However,

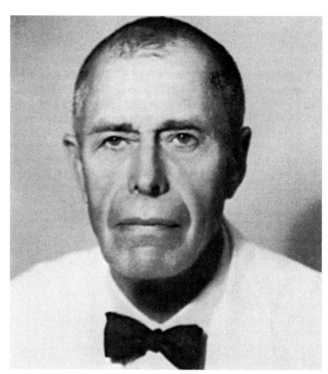

Figure 1-15 Dr. Cushman D. Haagensen, a strong advocate of radical mastectomy, who classified and analyzed breast cancer for half a century. (Courtesy of Dr. Gordon Schwartz.)

at the close of World War II, radical mastectomy remained the standard operation for breast cancer. In 1948, two reports appeared that were destined to change the management of breast cancer and become accepted as general principles in the management of localized disease. The first was the concept of modified radical mastectomy by D. Patey and W. Dyson from the Middlesex Hospital in London.[28] The second was treatment with simple mastectomy and radiotherapy, introduced by R. McWhirter of the University of Edinburgh.[29] Subsequent studies of patients treated with simple, radical, and modified radical mastectomies with or without radiotherapy revealed a striking similarity in survival rates. The contemporary trend (since 1970) has been breast conservation surgery followed by irradiation. Axillary dissection was confined to levels I and II lymph nodes.

In the later years of the twentieth century, Donald Morton (Fig. 1-16) and associates at the John Wayne Cancer Center in Santa Monica, California, developed the sentinel lymph node biopsy technique. It was originally proposed as an alternative to elective lymph node dissection for staging regional lymphatics in patients with cutaneous melanoma.[30] Subsequently, A. Giuliano investigated its use as an alternative to elective axillary lymph node dissection in patients with breast cancer.[31] Sentinel lymph node biopsy is now revolutionizing breast cancer staging and is redefining the indications for axillary dissection. In this application the technique uses lymphoscintigraphy and blue dye to localize the "sentinel" axillary lymph node, which is the node most likely to contain breast cancer metastases.

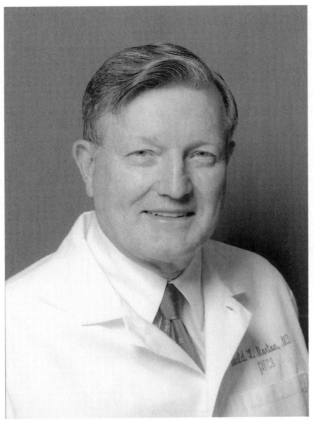

Figure 1-16 Dr. Donald L. Morton, John Wayne Cancer Center, Santa Monica, CA.

RADIOTHERAPY

Two months after the discovery of x-rays in 1895 by Wilhelm Roentgen (b. 1845), Emile Grubbe (b. 1875), a second-year medical student in Chicago, irradiated a patient with cancer of the breast. He protected the skin surrounding the lesion with tinfoil. He subsequently became the first professor of roentgenology at the Hahnemann Medical College of Philadelphia. In 1896 Hermann Gocht (b. 1869) of Hamburg, Germany, irradiated two patients with advanced cases of breast cancer while protecting the adjacent skin with flexible lead.[32] In 1898 Marie Curie and her husband Pierre discovered and isolated the radioactive elements polonium and radium. Their skin was burned as a result of working near these compounds, and in 1904 it was demonstrated that radium rays destroyed human cells.

In 1902, Guido Holzknecht (b. 1872) of Vienna, Italy, introduced a practical dosimeter. The therapeutic application of ionizing radiation soon followed. In 1902, Russian physician S. Goldberg successfully used radium in the treatment of cancer. In 1903, one of the first departments of radiotherapy for cancer was established at the Cancer Hospital in London, under the direction of J. Pollock. Georg Perthes (b. 1869), professor of surgery in Leipzig, Germany, in 1903 ascribed the "curative effect" of x-rays secondary to their inhibition of cell division.[33] Postoperative radiotherapy was initiated in many hospitals in America and Europe in the years before World War I. The equipment of the day permitted a maximum voltage of only 150 kV. Immediately after the war the voltages used increased, ranging from 170 to 200 kV.

In 1929, S. Harrington of the Mayo Clinic reported his follow-up of 1859 breast cancer cases irradiated between 1910 and 1923.[34] After analyzing his results, he expressed doubts about the value of ancillary radiotherapy. Even with improved equipment, controversy continued between enthusiasts and opponents of radiotherapy. George Pfahler (b. 1874) of Philadelphia recommended postoperative radiotherapy in all cases of breast cancer, starting 2 weeks after surgery. In his report of 1022 cases, he found no significant improvement in survival with stage I disease but did document an improved 5-year survival rate for patients with stage II disease.[35]

Radiotherapy as the sole therapeutic modality for breast cancer had been used for inoperable cases since the beginning of the twentieth century, but it was not until 1922 that a claim was made for its sole use in operable cases. William Stone (b. 1867) of New York City claimed the superiority of radiotherapy over radical surgery for the treatment of operable breast cancer. He based his conclusions on his experience with 10,000 cases. Geoffrey Keynes (b. 1887) of St. Bartholomew's Hospital in London reported in 1932 that radium can be used as a source of therapeutic irradiation.[36] After experience with this modality as an adjunct to surgery for breast cancer, he extended its use to being the sole treatment. He claimed a 5-year survival rate of 77% in the absence of enlarged axillary nodes and 36% with axillary involvement.

Supervoltage x-rays became available in the 1930s. At that time, François Baclesse (b. 1896) of Paris championed local excision of breast cancer, followed by radiotherapy. He reported cases studied between 1937 and 1953 at the Curie Foundation and concluded that for stage I and stage II cancers, his results were equal to those of radical mastectomy. In 1948, Robert McWhirter (b. 1904) proposed simple mastectomy followed by radiotherapy.[29] He argued that radical mastectomy for stage I disease was an overkill but was often inadequate for stage II disease, in which distant metastatic disease commonly developed. In the 1960s, even higher voltage x-rays were developed, along with the cobalt beam. In the late 1970s the development of the linear accelerator allowed the delivery of whole-breast radiotherapy of 4000 to 5000 cGy, with focal boost to the tumor bed to 6000 to 7000 cGy.

During the later part of the twentieth century, partial mastectomy ("lumpectomy"), axillary node dissection, and adjuvant breast irradiation played an increasingly important role in the therapy of early-stage breast cancer. The validity of breast conservation therapy was demonstrated through a series of carefully designed and controlled clinical trials coordinated through the National Surgical Adjuvant Breast and Bowel Project (NSABP). An American surgeon, Bernard Fischer (Fig. 1-17), served as chairman of the NSABP from 1967 to 1994 and since 1995 has been its scientific director. Fisher's systematic analyses brought breast cancer therapy into a new era and has set a standard for the investigation of therapies for other solid tumors.[37]

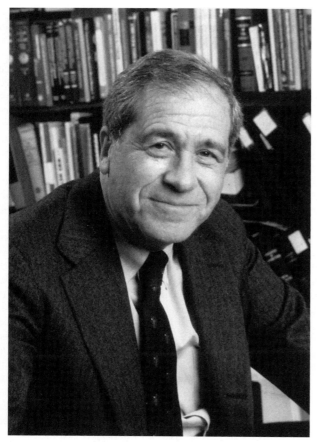

Figure 1-17 Dr. Bernard Fisher, National Surgical Adjuvant Breast and Bowel Project (NSABP), Pittsburgh, PA.

HORMONAL THERAPY

Hormonal treatment for breast cancer was considered even before the beginning of the twentieth century. In 1889, Albert Schinzinger (b. 1827) of Freiburg, Germany, proposed oophorectomy before mastectomy to produce "early aging" in menstruating women. This was based on his belief that the prognosis of breast cancer was worse in younger patients. In 1896 and again in 1901, George Beatson (b. 1848) of Glasgow, Scotland, reported three cases of advanced breast cancer that responded favorably to oophorectomy.[38] In 1900, S. Boyd performed the first combined oophorectomy and mastectomy for breast cancer. In 1905, the findings from a series of 99 patients with breast cancer treated by oophorectomy were presented at the Royal Medical and Chirurgical Society by a surgeon at the London Hospital, Hugh Lett.

In 1953, the late Nobel laureate and surgeon/urologist Charles Huggins (Fig. 1-18) of the University of Chicago advocated oophorectomy and adrenalectomy to remove the major sources of estrogens in the body.[39] Some patients with breast cancer responded with dramatic remissions, whereas others remained unaffected. In the early 1950s, hypophysectomy for advanced breast cancer was recommended, with results similar to those of adrenalectomy. Clinical administration of hormones started in 1939, when P. Ulrich reported the beneficial

effect of testosterone in two cases of breast cancer.[40] In 1944, Alexander Haddow (b. 1912) of Edinburgh, Scotland, and his collaborators observed a favorable effect of synthetic estrogen in advanced breast cancer.[41] Edward Dodds of London synthesized stilbestrol in 1938.[42] I. Nathanson reported its effect on advanced breast cancer in 1946.[43] In the 1950s and 1960s, estrogens and androgens remained in active use. In 1973, W. McGuire demonstrated estrogen receptors in human breast tumors.[44] In 1975, K. Horowitz identified progesterone receptors in hormone-dependent breast cancer.[45] Since the 1980s, tamoxifen and other selective estrogen receptor modulators (SERMs) have been used for the treatment and prevention of breast cancer.

CHEMOTHERAPY

Adjuvant

The use of chemical compounds, especially arsenic, in the treatment of breast cancer dates to ancient times. However, Paul Ehrlich (b. 1854) is credited as being the "father of chemotherapy." He coined the designation chemotherapy and by 1898 had isolated the first alkylating agent. In a series of historic experiments, he methodically studied a group of compounds that led to the discovery of salvarsan in 1910, which successfully treated syphilis in rabbits.[46] It was not until just after World War II that his work was applied to the treatment of cancers.

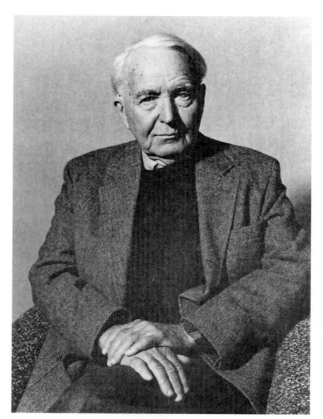

Figure 1-18 Dr. Charles B. Huggins, Nobel Laureate, University of Chicago, Chicago, IL.

During World War II, the U.S. Office of Scientific Research produced nitrogen mustard, an alkylating agent. A ship containing this substance blew up in the Naples, Italy, harbor, and the sailors who were exposed developed marrow and lymphoid hypoplasia. Experimental work with nitrogen mustard for the treatment of lymphosarcoma began at Memorial Hospital in New York City, but the results were withheld until the war secrecy ban was lifted in 1946. In that same year Frederick Phillips and Alfred Gilman demonstrated that nitrogen mustards could cause regression of certain lymphomas and leukemias.

Other antineoplastic drugs brought into clinical use were the purine and pyrimidine antagonists. In 1957, C. Heidelberger and collaborators reported the action of 5-fluorouracil, which has remained useful in the treatment of breast cancer.[47] In addition, the National Institutes of Health organized a cancer and chemotherapy national service. In 1958, patients were entered into a randomized, double-blind study using thiotriethylenephosphoramide, an alkylating agent. In 1963, E. Greenspan and his group in New York City were some of the first to engage in multidrug trials, using the antimetabolite methotrexate in combination with the alkylating agent thiotepa.[48]

Neoadjuvant

In the late 1970s and early 1980s, researchers first published the results of preliminary reports for induction chemotherapy (neoadjuvant chemotherapy) for locally advanced breast cancer. De Lena, Zucali, and Viganotti reported their findings of 110 patients with inoperable cancer treated with induction neoadjuvant regimens consisting of doxorubicin and vincristine.[49] Approximately 90% of patients had an objective response, of which 16% was complete, 55% was partial, and 19% was an "improvement." The 3-year overall survival rate of the treated patients was 53% in contrast to 41% for the historical control group not receiving chemotherapy.

Importantly, the trial by De Lena and associates[49] initiated interest in other neoadjuvant trials, principally for patients with inoperable disease.[50-53] In the 1983 report from the M.D. Anderson Cancer Center for a series of 52 patients with locally advanced breast cancer, three-cycle treatment with neoadjuvant chemotherapy that contained anthracyclines, the local therapy together with adjuvant therapy rendered 94% of patients free of disease for 2 years. Thereafter, Swain and colleagues[52] at the National Cancer Institute reported on the institute's experience with 76 patients with locally advanced disease treated with induction therapy until maximum clinical response was achieved. As previously, all these patients received adjuvant chemotherapy for at least 6 months with an objective response of 93%, with 43% complete, 44% partial, and 7% stable.

Similar induction chemotherapy response with neoadjuvant therapies has been compared with adjuvant chemotherapy trials in multiple randomized studies that included patients with locally advanced disease.[54-59] Importantly, the neoadjuvant chemotherapy arms had longer overall survival with a median follow-up of 34 months ($P = 0.04$). This trial[52] was one of the first to confirm that improved survival may reflect the benefit of chemotherapy in general rather than the specific application of the neoadjuvant chemotherapy protocol. Thus, outcomes of patients treated with neoadjuvant cytoreductive therapy were not worse than those who received adjuvant chemotherapy. Similar outcomes have been confirmed by Scholl and associates[55] from the Institut Curie, France, and Powles and colleagues[57] of the Royal Marsden Hospital, England, as well as the largest trial of neoadjuvant chemotherapy reported to date in the NSABP B-18, which randomized 1523 women with T_{1-3}, N_{0-1} operable breast cancer.[58,59] Overall, complete clinical responses were observed in 35% of patients, a clinical partial response in 44%, and stable disease in 17%. In comparison to the NSABP trial of adjuvant and neoadjuvant therapies, no differences in 5-year survival rates of disease-free survival, distant-disease-free survival, or overall survival were evident. Patients with T_3 disease had a survival rate equivalent to the rates of patients treated with adjuvant and neoadjuvant approaches. These similar outcomes have also been reported by the European Organization for Research and Treatment of Cancer (EORTC) Breast Cancer Cooperative Groups in an additional large randomized neoadjuvant chemotherapy trial of women with operable breast cancer.[60] These trials have demonstrated that neoadjuvant and adjuvant therapies produce equivalent outcomes. Although most studies have been conducted in patients with early-stage disease, some have included patients with locally advanced malignancies. The report by Hutcheon and colleagues[61] suggests that the addition of docetaxel to neoadjuvant regimens will improve survival for patients with locally advanced disease.[61]

Finally, the role of neoadjuvant hormonal therapy for locally advanced disease has been assessed in several studies, including those led by Veronesi,[62] Gazet,[63] Hoff,[64] and Ellis,[65] which have typically compared aromatase inhibitors and SERMS with ovarian ablation by medical and surgical measures. The majority of these studies have clearly demonstrated the benefit of neoadjuvant hormonal therapies in the subset of patients not treated with chemotherapy. For patients who can tolerate chemotherapy, however, it remains the standard of care. Although the role of ovarian suppression or ablation has been identified in the premenopausal patient, tamoxifen remains the standard endocrine therapy for the premenopausal individual with breast carcinoma with early-stage hormonal receptor–positive breast cancer. Bao and Davidson[66] acknowledge the uncertainty that exists regarding the optimal applications of endocrine therapy for premenopausal women who are estrogen receptor–positive. Clarke[67] has recently documented the journey along a hierarchy of evidence to show why research in ablation remains relevant in the management of these patients.

MAMMOGRAPHY

Before and after World War I, early diagnosis of breast cancer was difficult. Patients sought advice only when they felt a hard lump. Surgeons looked for skin retraction and inversion of the nipple and palpated the breast and axilla for masses. In 1913, a German surgeon, A. Salomon, used mammography to study 3000 amputated breasts and was able to differentiate scirrhus forms of breast cancer from nodular types.[68] He noted the microcalcifications in intraductal carcinomas but failed to appreciate their significance. In 1927, O. Kleinschmidt wrote a book in which he described mammography as an aid in diagnosis.[69]

Jacob Gershon-Cohen of Philadelphia studied x-ray mammary patterns from 1937 to 1948 and made notable progress in the accurate diagnosis of breast cancer. He tirelessly advocated the use of x-rays as an aid to clinical diagnosis and in 1948 was the first to demonstrate the feasibility of detecting occult carcinomas.[70] In 1962 at the M.D. Anderson Hospital and Tumor Institute, R. Egan described imaging of the breast with only two radiographic views. He reported a study of 2522 mammograms in which differentiation between benign and malignant tumors was made without the aid of clinical findings.[71] Since then, mammography has become the most important diagnostic tool for breast cancer.

BREAST RECONSTRUCTION

Iginio Tansini, Professor of Surgery of the University of Pavia in Italy, first described the latissimus dorsi flap in 1896.[72,73] In the early twentieth century, surgeons completed procedures performed without elevation of skin flaps, principally because the skin and subcutaneous tissue were sacrificed with en bloc resections. This left large circular defects centrally, which were repaired by skin grafts on occasion. The innovative approach of Tansini, which involved elevating the flap, allowed the early application of plastic surgical techniques following expiration measures of the Halsted radical procedure. Surgeons typically transposed anteriorly myocutaneous flaps with skin and latissimus dorsi for wound closures. In the early 1900s, it became evident that practitioners of rudimentary skin graft techniques more commonly favored using this technique rather than managing a large circular defect, which ultimately required prolonged wound packing to allow for granulation to occur.[74] Later in the twentieth century, the enhancement of diagnostic techniques (e.g., radiographic, nuclear imaging, ultrasound) and downstaging of the primary tumor with chemotherapy allowed the use of extirpative procedures with primary closures.

Brown and McDowell[75] introduced the motorized dermatome in 1958, allowing very large skin grafts that could be meshed to expand for coverage of large surface area. This seminal innovation permitted surgeons to realize the sacrifice of involved skin, and with introduction of adjuvant radiotherapy, allowed enhancement of local control.

The Tansini latissimus dorsi myocutaneous flap was the prevailing reconstruction methodology following mastectomy in Europe until about 1920. However, Halsted made a grand tour of medical centers in Europe and stated: "Beware of the man with the plastic operation" because he considered the latissimus flap both "unnecessary and hazardous."[76] For several reasons,

principally the lack of the advent of blood transfusions, anesthetics, antibiotics, and intravenous fluids, Tansini's method did not further breast reconstructive surgery until the 1970s, when the pioneering efforts of McCraw, Vasconez, Hartramph, and others reintroduced the myocutaneous flap. This seminal contribution in pathophysiology and anatomy by McCraw and colleagues represented the single most important contribution to plastic surgery for reconstruction of ablative procedures in the past 75 years (Table 1-1). In 1982, Hartramph and associates first described application of the abdominal myocutaneous flap, which was an abdominal transverse rectus abdominis myocutaneous (TRAM) pedicle flap.[77] Thus, for 54 years (1920–1974), the Tansini procedure was completely abandoned, and myocutaneous flaps were not used for immediate reconstruction of the breasts until 1982.

Today, substantive remodeling of tissues for aesthetic, contour, and functional purposes is the primary goal of the plastic surgeon. The advancement in myocutaneous breast reconstruction followed introduction of silicone breast implants by Cronin and Gerow in 1964 and was thereafter popularized by a number of surgeons for 20 years.[78-82] The pioneering work of these two investigators was conducted in collaboration with Dow Chemical Company using silicone polymers. It was evident early that subpectoral placement of these implants enhanced results over those of the fibrous encapsulation of the implant placed beneath the thin mastectomy skin flaps. Early implant reconstruction failures were principally related to distortion of the breast contour (shape) referred to as *half grapefruit*, which describes the elevated, rounded, and firm implant. Subsequently, silicone implants were abandoned for several years because of concerns about fibromyalgia and immunologically related disorders. Although no firm, statistically objective reviews have confirmed silicone's harmful effects, this concern prompted a resurgence of the use of saline implants in the late 1980s and early 1990s. Today, a re-entry of silicone implants into the market with superior soft tissue coverage of shaped implants has allowed an improvement in outcomes, both physiologically and aesthetically.

TABLE 1-1
Historical Evolution of Breast Reconstruction

Date	Reconstructive Procedure
1896	Latissimus dorsi autogenous flaps
1900	Split/full-thickness skin grafts
1958	Skin grafts harvested with motorized Brown dermatome
1960s	Tubed skin flaps/silicone implants
1964	Silicone breast implants
1970s	Reintroduction of myocutaneous flaps
1982	Transverse rectus abdominis myocutaneous (TRAM) flap

Buzzelli RC, Forman DL, Heinrich JJ: Postmastectomy breast reconstruction: Helping patients decide whether—and when. J Am Academy Physician Assistants 21:26–30, 2003. Copyright 2008, American Academy of Physician Assistants and Haymarket Media Inc. Reproduced with permission.

CANCER BIOLOGY

The twentieth century saw unprecedented growth in our understanding of cancer biology, especially breast cancer biology. In the first part of the century, numerous observations were made concerning the development and behavior of cancer. In 1900, Leo Loeb experimentally transmitted cancer through several generations of animals. In 1911, Jean Clunet of France demonstrated the experimental production of cancer using x-rays. In 1920, an American pathologist, Albert Borders, classified cancers with regard to malignant potential on the basis of the state of differentiation of cancer cells. In 1932, the French physician Antoine Lacassagne demonstrated that breast cancer could be produced in animals with estrone benzoate. In 1944, P. Denoix of the Institut Gustav-Roussy in France proposed the tumor, node, metastasis (TNM) classification for cancer. In 1959, M. Macklin performed a comprehensive analysis of the role of hereditary factors in the predisposition to breast cancer.

The latter part of the twentieth century saw the development of molecular biology and the explanation of breast cancer development and behavior in terms of human genetics. In 1926, American geneticist Hermann Müller exposed fruit flies to x-rays and produced mutations and hereditary changes. He demonstrated that the mutations were the result of breakages in chromosomes and changes in individual genes. Hugh Cairns (b. 1922), a molecular biologist and virologist from Oxford University, showed that cancer developed from a single abnormal cell as a result of DNA mutation. Peter Vogt (b. 1932), a German-born American microbiologist from the University of Southern California, discovered oncogenes, which play a role in the normal growth of mammalian cells but can cause cancer through mutation. In 1970, David Baltimore, a New York City oncologist, announced his discovery of the enzyme reverse transcriptase, which can transcribe RNA into DNA, contributing greatly to our understanding of how viruses participate in the development of cancer. In 1978, David Lane, a professor of oncology at Dundee, Scotland, discovered the tumor-suppressor gene p53. Bert Vogelstein (b. 1949), a Baltimore oncologist and a pioneer in the study of the molecular basis of cancer, analyzed DNA from colon cancer cells and described mutation of three tumor suppressor genes: APC, DCC, and p53. Judith Folkman (b. 1933), an American surgeon, elucidated the importance of angiogenesis and opened the way for new therapy. In 1994, the first breast cancer gene, *BRCA1*, was identified, and in 1996, *BRCA2* was discovered. Building on these and other discoveries, the twenty-first century will undoubtedly see the development of genetically based therapies for breast cancer that will complement or replace the empirical therapies of the past.

REFERENCES

1. Breasted JH: The Edwin Smith surgical papyrus. Classics of Medicine Library, vol III. Chicago, University of Chicago Press, 1930.
2. Fabry W: Observationum et curationum chirurgicarum centuriae: Cent II. IA Huguetan, 1641.
3. le Dran F: Mémoire avec une précis de plusieurs observations sur le cancer. Mem Acad Roy Chir Paris 3:1, 1757.
4. Petit JL: Oeuvres complétes, section VII. Limoges, R. Chapoulard, 1837.
5. Young S: Minutes of cases of cancer and cancerous tendency successfully treated, with a preparatory letter addressed to the Governors of the Middlesex Hospital by Samuel Whitbread. London, E Coxe & Son, 1815.
6. Syme J: Principles of surgery. London, H Balliere, 1842.
7. Brown J: Horae subsecivae, 2nd ed. London, Adam & Charles Black, 1910.
8. Paget J: On the average duration of life in patients with scirrhus cancer of the breast, Lancet 1:62, 1856.
9. Paget J: On disease of the mammary areola preceding cancer of the mammary gland. St Bart Hosp Rep 10:87, 1874.
10. Moore C: On the influence of inadequate operations on the theory of cancer. R Med Chir Soc Lond 1:244, 1867.
11. Lister J: On the antiseptic principle in the practice of surgery. Lancet 11:95, 353, 668, 1867.
12. Velpeau AALM: Traité des maladies du sein et de la region mammaire. Paris, V Masson, 1854.
13. Volkmann R: Beitrage zur chirurgie. Leipzig, Breitkopf & Hartel, 1875.
14. Heidenhain L: Ueber die ursachen der localen krebsrecidive nach amputation mammae. Arch Klin Chir 39:97, 1889.
15. Gross SD: System of surgery, vol II, 5th ed. Philadelphia, Henry C Lea's Son, 1872.
16. Gross SW: An analysis of two hundred and seven cases of carcinoma of the breast. Med News 51:613, 1887.
17. Agnew DH: The principles and practice of surgery, vol III. Philadelphia, JB Lippincott, 1883.
18. Halsted WS: The results of operations for the cure of cancer of the breast performed at the Johns Hopkins Hospital from June 1889 to January 1894. Johns Hopkins Hosp Rep 4:297, 1894–1895.
19. Halsted WS: A clinical and histological study of certain adenocarcinomata of the breast. Ann Surg 28:557, 1898.
20. Meyer W: An improved method of the radical operation for carcinoma of the breast. Med Rec 46:746, 1894.
21. Cullen IS: A rapid method of making permanent specimens from frozen sections by the use of formalin. Bull Johns Hopkins Hosp 6:67, 1895.
22. Halsted WS: The results of radical operations for cure of cancer of the breast. Ann Surg 46:1, 1907.
23. Westerman CWG: Thoraxexcisie bij recidief van carcinoma mammae. Geneesk Med Lydschr 54:1681, 1910.
24. Handley WS: Parasternal invasion of the thorax in breast cancer and its suppression by the use of radium tubes as an operative precaution. Surg Gynecol Obstet 45:721, 1927.
25. Urban JA, Baker HW: Radical mastectomy in continuity with en bloc resection of the internal mammary lymph chain. Cancer 5:992–1008, 1952.
26. Wangensteen OH: Discussion to Taylor and Wallace: Carcinoma of the breast, fifty years' experience at the Massachusetts General Hospital. Ann Surg 132:838–843, 1950.
27. Haagensen CD: Diseases of the breast, 3rd ed. Philadelphia, WB Saunders, 1986.
28. Patey DH, Dyson WH: The prognosis of carcinoma of the breast in relation to the type of operation performed. Br J Cancer 2:7–13, 1948.
29. McWhirter R: The value of simple mastectomy and radiotherapy in the treatment of cancer of the breast. Br J Radiol 21:599–610, 1948.
30. Morton DL, Wen DR, Wong JH, et al: Technical details for intraoperative lymphatic mapping for early stage melanoma. Arch Surg 127:392–399, 1992.
31. Giuliano AE, Kirgan DM, Guenther JM, Morton DL: Lymphatic mapping and sentinel lymphadenectomy for breast cancer. Ann Surg 220:391–398, 1994.
32. Gocht H: Therapeutische verwendung der rontgenstrahlen. Fortschr Geb Roentgenstr 1:14, 1897.
33. Perthes GC: Ueber den einfluss der roentgenstrahlen auf epitheliale gewebe, insbesondere auf das carcinom. Langenbecks Arch Klin Chir 7:955, 1903.
34. Harrington SW: Carcinoma of the breast: Surgical treatment and results. JAMA 92:280, 1929.
35. Pfahler GE: Results of radiation therapy in 1,022 private cases of carcinoma of the breast from 1902 to 1928. AJR Am J Roentgenol 27:497, 1932.

36. Keynes GL: The radium treatment of carcinoma of the breast. Br J Surg 19:415, 1932.
37. Fisher B, Redmons C, Fisher ER: The contribution of recent clinical trials of primary breast cancer therapy to an understanding of tumor biology. Cancer 46(suppl 4):1009–1025, 1980.
38. Beatson GT: The treatment of cancer of the breast by oophorectomy and thyroid extract. BMJ 2:1145, 1901.
39. Huggins C, Doa TLY: Adrenalectomy and oophorectomy in the treatment of advanced carcinoma of the breast. JAMA 151:1388, 1953.
40. Ulrich P: Testosterone et son role possible dans le traitement de certains cancers du sein. Int Union Against Cancer 4:377, 1939.
41. Haddow A, Watkinson JM, Patterson D: Influence of synthetic estrogen upon advanced malignant disease. BMJ 2:393, 1944.
42. Dodds EC: Significance of synthetic estrogens. Acta Med Scand 90(suppl):141, 1938.
43. Nathanson IT: The effect of stilboestrol in advanced cancer of the breast. Cancer Res 6:484, 1946.
44. McGuire WL, De La Garza M: Similarity of estrogen receptors in human and rat mammary carcinoma. J Clin Endocrinol Metab 36:548–552, 1973.
45. Horowitz KB: Progesterone receptors and hormone dependent breast cancer, doctoral dissertation. Dallas, University of Texas Southwestern Medical School, 1975.
46. Ehrlich P: Closing notes on experimental chemotherapy of spirillosco. Berlin, J Springer, 1910.
47. Heidelberger C, Chaudhuri NK, Danneberg P, et al: Fluorinated pyrimidines, a new class of tumor inhibitory compounds. Nature 179:663–666, 1957.
48. Greenspan EM et al: Response of advanced breast carcinoma to the combination of the antimetabolic methotrexate and the alkylating agent thio-TEPA. Mt Sinai J Med 33:1, 1963.
49. De Lena M, Zucali R, Viganotti G: Combined chemotherapy radiotherapy approach in locally advanced breast cancer. Cancer Chemother Pharmacol 1:53–59, 1978.
50. Schick P, Goodstein J, Moor J, et al: Preoperative chemotherapy followed by mastectomy for locally advanced breast cancer. J Surg Oncol 22:278–282, 1983.
51. Perloff M, Lesnick GJ: Chemotherapy before and after mastectomy in stage III breast cancer. Arch Surg 117:879–881, 1982.
52. Swain SM, Sorace RA, Bagley CS, et al: Neoadjuvant chemotherapy in the combined modality approach of locally advanced nonmetastatic breast cancer. Cancer Res 47:3889–3894, 1987.
53. Hortobagyi GN, Blumenschein GR, Spanos W, et al: Multimodal treatment of locoregionally advanced breast cancer. Cancer 51:763–768, 1983.
54. Mauriac L, Durand M, Avril A, Dilhuydy JM, et al: Effects of primary chemotherapy in conservative treatment of breast cancer patients with operable tumors larger than 3 cm: Results of a randomized trial in a single centre. Ann Oncol 2:347–354, 1991.
55. Scholl SM, Fourquet A, Asselain B, et al: Neoadjuvant versus adjuvant chemotherapy in premenopausal patients with tumours considered too large for breast conserving surgery: preliminary results of a randomised trial: S6. Eur J Cancer 30A:645–652, 1994.
56. Semiglazov VF, Topuzov EE, Bavli JL, et al: Primary (neoadjuvant) chemotherapy and radiotherapy compared with primary radiotherapy alone in stage IIb-IIIa breast cancer. Ann Oncol 5:591–595, 1994.
57. Powles TJ, Hickish TF, Makris A, et al: Randomized trial of chemoendocrine therapy started before or after surgery for treatment of primary breast cancer. J Clin Oncol 13:547–552, 1995.
58. Fisher B, Brown A, Mamounas E, et al: Effect of preoperative chemotherapy on local-regional disease in women with operable breast cancer: Findings from National Surgical Adjuvant Breast and Bowel Project B-18. J Clin Oncol 15:2483–2493, 1997.
59. Fisher B, Bryant J, Woolmark N, et al: Effect of preoperative chemotherapy on the outcome of women with operable breast cancer. J Clin Oncol 16:2672–2685, 1998.
60. van der Hage JA, van de Velde CJ, Julien JP, et al: Preoperative chemotherapy in primary operable breast cancer: Results from the European Organization for Research and Treatment of Cancer Trial 10902. J Clin Oncol 19:4224–4237, 2001.
61. Hutcheon AW, Heys SD, Miller ID, et al: Improvements in survival in patients receiving primary chemotherapy with docetaxel for breast cancer: A randomised controlled trial (abstract). Breast Cancer Res Treat 69:298, 2001.
62. Veronesi A, Fructaci S, Tirelli U, et al: Tamoxifen therapy in postmenopausal advanced breast cancer: Efficacy at the primary tumor site in 46 evaluable patients. Tumori 67:235–238, 1981.
63. Gazet JC, Ford HT, Coombes RC: Randomised trial of chemotherapy versus endocrine therapy in patients presenting with locally advanced breast cancer (a pilot study). Br J Cancer 63:279–282, 1991.
64. Hoff PM, Valero V, Buzdar AU, et al: Combined modality treatment of locally advanced breast carcinoma in elderly patients or patients with severe comorbid conditions using tamoxifen as the primary therapy. Cancer 88:2054–2060, 2000.
65. Ellis MJ, Coop A, Singh B, et al: Letrozole is more effective neoadjuvant endocrine therapy than tamoxifen for ErbB-1- and/or ErbB-2-positive, estrogen receptor-positive primary breast cancer: Evidence from a phase III randomized trial. J Clin Oncol 19:3808–3816, 2001.
66. Bao T, Davidson NE: Adjuvant endocrine therapy for premenopausal women with early breast cancer. Breast Cancer Res 9:115, 2007.
67. Clarke MJ: Ovarian ablation in breast cancer, 1896 to 1998: Milestones along hierarchy of evidence from case report to Cochrane review. Br Medical J 317:1246–1248, 1998.
68. Salomon A: Beitrage zur pathologic und klinik der mammarcarcinom. arch klin Chir 105:573, 1913.
69. Kleinschmidt O: Brustdrüse. In Zweife P, Payr E (eds): Die klinik der bösartigen geschwülste. Leipzig, S Hirzel, 1927, pp 5–90.
70. Gershon-Cohen J: Atlas of mammography. New York, Springer-Verlag. 1970.
71. Egan RL: Experience with mammography in a tumor institution. Radiology 25:894, 1960.
72. Tansini I: Nuovo processo per 1=amputazione della mammaella per cancre. Reforma Medica 12:3, 1896.
73. Tansini I: Sopra ilmio nuovo processo di amputazione della mammaella. Reforma Medica 12:757, 1906.
74. Buzzelli RC, Forman DL, Heinrich JJ: Postmastectomy breast reconstruction: Helping patients decide whether—and when. J Am Acad Physician Assistants 16:25–30, 2003.
75. Brown JB, McDowell F: Skin grafting, 3rd ed. Philadelphia, 1958, Lippincott.
76. Maxwell GP: Iginio Tansini and the origin of the latissimus dorsi musculocutaneous flap. Plast Reconstr Surg 65:686–692, 1980.
77. Hartrampf CR, Scheflan M, Black PW: Breast reconstruction with a transverse abdominal island flap. Plast Reconstr Surg 69:216–225, 1982.
78. Broadbent TR, Woolf RM: Augmentation mammoplasty. Plast Reconstr Surg 40:517–523, 1967.
79. Dempsey WC, Latham WD: Subpectoral implants in augmentation mammoplasty. Plast Reconstr Surg 42:515–521, 1968.
80. Hester TR Jr, Nahai F, Bostwick J, Cukic J: A five-year experience with polyurethene-covered mammary prostheses for treatment of capsular contracture, primary augmentation mammoplasty, and breast reconstruction. Clin Plast Surg 15:569–585, 1988.
81. Pickrell KL, Puckett CL, Given KS: Subpectoral augmentation mammoplasty. Plast Reconstr Surg 60:325–336, 1977.
82. Pollock H: Polyurethane-covered breast implant. Plast Reconstr Surg 74:728–729, 1984.

SUGGESTED READINGS

Bordley J III, Harvey AM: Two centuries of American medicine, 1776–1976. Philadelphia, WB Saunders, 1976.
de Moulin D: A short history of breast cancer. The Hague, Martinus Nijhoff, 1983.
Garrison FH: An introduction to the history of medicine. Philadelphia, WB Saunders, 1929.
Grubbe EH: X-ray treatment: Its origin, birth and early history. St Paul, Bruce Publishing, 1949.
King LS: The medical world of the eighteenth century. Huntington, NY, RE Krieger, 1971.
Lee HSJ: Dates in oncology. Landmarks in medicine series. New York, Parthenon, 2000.
Levens P: The pathway to health, London, 1664. In special collections of Thomas Jefferson University Library. Philadelphia.
Pancoast J: Treatise on operative surgery. Philadelphia, Carey & Hart, 1844.
Riesman D: Medicine in the Middle Ages. New York, Paul B Hoeber, 1935.

SECTION II

Anatomy and Physiology of the Normal and Lactating Breast

chapter 2

Anatomy of the Breast, Axilla, Chest Wall, and Related Metastatic Sites

LYNN J. ROMRELL | KIRBY I. BLAND

Mammary glands, or breasts, are a distinguishing feature of mammals. They have evolved as milk-producing organs to provide nourishment to the offspring, which are born in a relatively immature and dependent state. The act of nursing the young provides physiologic benefit to the mother by aiding in postpartum uterine involution and to the young in transferring passive immunity. The nursing of the young is also of significance in the bonding between the mother and her offspring.

During embryologic development, there is growth and differentiation of the breasts in both sexes (for a review, see Morehead[1]). Paired glands develop along paired lines, the milk lines, extending between the limb buds from the future axilla to the future inguinal region. Among the various mammalian species, the number of paired glands varies greatly and is related to the number of young in each litter. In humans and most other primates, normally only one gland develops on each side in the pectoral region. An extra breast (polymastia) or nipple (polythelia) may occur as a heritable condition in about 1% of the female population. These relatively rare conditions also may occur in the male. When present, the supernumerary breast or nipple usually forms along the milk lines; about one third of the affected individuals have multiple extra breasts or nipples.

In the female the breasts undergo extensive postnatal development, which is correlated with age and regulated by hormones that influence reproductive function. By about 20 years of age, the breast has reached its greatest development, and by the age of 40, it begins atrophic changes. During each menstrual cycle, structural changes occur in the breast under the influence of ovarian hormone levels. During pregnancy and lactation, striking changes occur not only in the functional activity of the breast but also in the amount of glandular tissue. The actual secretion and production of milk are induced by prolactin from the pituitary and somatomammotropin from the placenta. With the changes in the hormonal environment that occur at menopause, the glandular component of the breast regresses, or involutes, and is replaced by fat and connective tissue.[2]

Gross Anatomic Structure— Surface Anatomy

FORM AND SIZE

The breast is located within the superficial fascia of the anterior thoracic wall. It consists of 15 to 20 lobes of glandular tissue of the tubuloalveolar type. Fibrous connective tissue forms a framework that supports the lobes, and adipose tissue fills the space between the lobes.[3] Subcutaneous connective tissue surrounds the gland and extends as septa between the lobes and lobules, providing support for the glandular elements, but it does not form a distinctive capsule around the components of the breast. The deep layer of the superficial fascia, which lies on the posterior (deep) surface of the breast, rests on the pectoral (deep) fascia of the thoracic wall. A distinct space, the *retromammary bursa*, can be identified surgically on the posterior aspect of the breast between the deep layer of the superficial fascia and the deep investing fascia of the pectoralis major and contiguous muscles of the thoracic wall (Fig. 2-1). The retromammary bursa contributes to the mobility of the breast on the thoracic wall. Fibrous thickenings of the connective tissue interdigitate between the parenchymal tissue of the breast. This connective tissue extends from the deep layer of the superficial fascia (hypodermis) and attaches to the dermis of the skin. These suspensory structures, called *Cooper's ligaments*, insert perpendicular to the delicate superficial fascial layers of the dermis, or corium, permitting remarkable mobility of the breast while providing support.

At maturity, the glandular portion of the breast has a unique and distinctive protuberant conical form. The base of the cone is roughly circular, measuring 10 to 12 cm in diameter and 5 to 7 cm in thickness. Commonly,

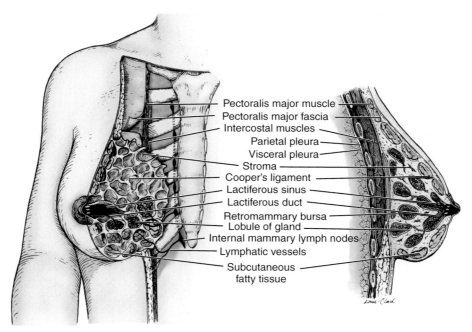

Pectoralis major muscle
Pectoralis major fascia
Intercostal muscles
Parietal pleura
Visceral pleura
Stroma
Cooper's ligament
Lactiferous sinus
Lactiferous duct
Retromammary bursa
Lobule of gland
Internal mammary lymph nodes
Lymphatic vessels
Subcutaneous
fatty tissue

Figure 2-1 A tangential view of the breast on the chest wall and a sectional (sagittal) view of the breast and associated chest wall. The breast lies in the superficial fascia just deep to the dermis. It is attached to the skin by the suspensory ligaments of Cooper and is separated from the investing fascia of the pectoralis major muscle by the retromammary bursa. Cooper's ligaments form fibrosepta in the stroma that provide support for the breast parenchyma. From 15 to 20 lactiferous ducts extend from lobules comprised of glandular epithelium to openings located on the nipple. A dilation of the duct, the lactiferous sinus, is present near the opening of the duct in the subareolar tissue. Subcutaneous fat and adipose tissue distributed around the lobules of the gland give the breast its smooth contour and, in the nonlactating breast, account for most of its mass. Lymphatic vessels pass through the stroma surrounding the lobules of the gland and convey lymph to collecting ducts. Lymphatic channels ending in the internal mammary (or parasternal) lymph nodes are shown. The pectoralis major muscle lies adjacent to the ribs and intercostal muscles. The parietal pleura, attached to the endothoracic fascia, and the visceral pleura, covering the surface of the lung, are shown.

breast tissue extends into the axilla as the axillary tail (of Spence). There is tremendous variation in the size of the breast. A typical nonlactating breast weighs between 150 and 225 g, whereas the lactating breast may exceed 500 g.[4,5] In a study of breast volume in 55 women, Smith and colleagues[6] reported that the mean volume of the right breast was 275.46 mL (SD = 172.65, median = 217.7, minimum = 94.6, maximum = 889.3) and the left breast was 291.69 mL (SD = 168.23, median = 224, minimum = 106.9, maximum = 893.9).

The breast of the nulliparous female has a typical hemispheric configuration with distinct flattening above the nipple.[7] The multiparous breast, which has experienced the hormonal stimulation associated with pregnancy and lactation, is usually larger and more pendulous. As noted, during pregnancy and lactation, the breast increases dramatically in size and becomes more pendulous. With increasing age, the breast usually decreases in volume, becomes somewhat flattened and pendulous, and is less firm.

EXTENT AND LOCATION

The mature female breast extends inferiorly from the level of the second or third rib to the inframammary fold, which is at about the level of the sixth or seventh rib, and laterally from the lateral border of the sternum to the anterior or midaxillary line. The deep or posterior surface of the breast rests on portions of the deep investing fasciae of the pectoralis major, serratus anterior, and

external abdominal oblique muscles and the upper extent of the rectus sheath. The axillary tail (of Spence) of the breast extends into the anterior axillary fold. The upper half of the breast, and particularly the upper outer quadrant, contains more glandular tissue than does the remainder of the breast.

Microscopic Anatomic Structure

NIPPLE AND AREOLA

The epidermis of the nipple and areola is highly pigmented and somewhat wrinkled. It is covered by keratinized, stratified squamous epithelium. The deep surface of the epidermis is invaded by unusually long dermal papillae that allow capillaries to bring blood close to the surface, giving the region a pinkish color in young, fair-skinned individuals. At puberty, the pigmentation of the nipple and areola increases and the nipple becomes more prominent. During pregnancy, the areola enlarges and the degree of pigmentation increases. Deep to the areola and nipple, bundles of smooth muscle fibers are arranged radially and circumferentially in the dense connective tissue and longitudinally along the lactiferous ducts that extend up into the nipple. These muscle fibers are responsible for the erection of nipple that occurs in response to various stimuli (for a review of the anatomy of the nipple and areola, see Giacometti and Montagna[8]).

The areola contains sebaceous glands, sweat glands, and accessory areolar glands (of Montgomery), which are intermediate in their structure between true mammary glands and sweat glands. The accessory areolar glands produce small elevations on the surface of the areola. The sebaceous glands (which usually lack associated hairs) and sweat glands are located along the margin of the areola. Whereas the tip of the nipple contains numerous free sensory nerve cell endings and Meissner's corpuscles in the dermal papillae, the areola contains fewer of these structures.[9] In a review of the innervation of the nipple and areola, Montagna and Macpherson[10] reported observing fewer nerve endings than described by other investigators. They reported that most of the endings were at the apex of the nipple. Neuronal plexuses are also present around hair follicles in the skin peripheral to the areola, and pacinian corpuscles may be present in the dermis and in the glandular tissue. The rich sensory innervation of the breast, particularly the nipple and areola,[11] is of great functional significance. The suckling infant initiates a chain of neural and neurohumoral events, resulting in the release of milk and maintenance of glandular differentiation that is essential for continued lactation.

INACTIVE MAMMARY GLAND

The adult mammary gland is composed of 15 to 20 irregular lobes of branched tubuloalveolar glands. The lobes, separated by fibrous bands of connective tissue, radiate from the *mammary papilla*, or *nipple*, and are further subdivided into numerous lobules. Those fibrous bands that connect with the dermis are the *suspensory ligaments of Cooper*. Abundant adipose tissue is present in the dense connective tissue of the interlobular spaces. The intralobular connective tissue is much less dense and contains little fat.

Each lobe of the mammary gland ends in a *lactiferous duct* (2 to 4 mm in diameter) that opens through a constricted orifice (0.4 to 0.7 mm in diameter) onto the nipple (see Fig. 2-1). Beneath the areola, each duct has a dilated portion, the *lactiferous sinus*. Near their openings, the lactiferous ducts are lined with stratified squamous epithelium. The epithelial lining of the duct shows a gradual transition to two layers of cuboidal cells in the lactiferous sinus and then becomes a single layer of columnar or cuboidal cells through the remainder of the duct system. Myoepithelial cells of ectodermal origin are located within the epithelium between the surface epithelial cells and the basal lamina.[12] These cells, arranged in a basketlike network, are present in the secretory portion of the gland but are more apparent in the larger ducts. They contain myofibrils and are strikingly similar to smooth muscle cells in their cytology.

In light microscopy, epithelial cells are characteristically seen to be attached to an underlying layer called the *basement membrane*. With electron microscopy, the substructure of the basement membrane can be identified. The inner layer of the basement membrane is called the *basal lamina*. In the breast, the parenchymal cells of the tubuloalveolar glands, as well as the epithelial and myoepithelial cells of the ducts, rest on a basement membrane or basal lamina. The integrity of this supporting

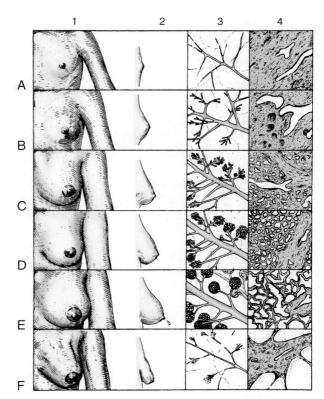

Figure 2-2 Schematic drawing illustrating mammary gland development. Anterior and lateral views of the breast are shown in columns 1 and 2. The microscopic appearances of the ducts and lobules are illustrated in columns 3 and 4, respectively. **A,** prepubertal (childhood); **B,** puberty; **C,** mature (reproductive); **D,** pregnancy; **E,** lactation; **F,** postmenopausal (senescent) state. (From Copeland EM III, Bland KI: The breast. In Sabiston DC Jr [ed]: Essentials of surgery. Philadelphia, WB Saunders, 1987.)

layer is of significance in evaluating biopsy specimens of breast tissue. Changes in the basement membrane have important implications in immune surveillance, transformation, differentiation, and metastasis.[13–16]

The morphology of the secretory portion of the mammary gland varies greatly with age and during pregnancy and lactation (Fig. 2-2). In the inactive gland, the glandular component is sparse and consists chiefly of duct elements (Fig. 2-3). Most investigators believe that the secretory units in the inactive breast are not organized as alveoli and consist only of ductules. During the menstrual cycle, the inactive breast undergoes slight cyclical changes. Early in the cycle, the ductules appear as cords with little or no lumen. Under estrogen stimulation, at about the time of ovulation, secretory cells increase in height, lumina appear as small amounts of secretions accumulate, and fluids and lipid accumulate in the connective tissue. Then, in the absence of continued hormonal stimulation, the gland regresses to a more inactive state through the remainder of the cycle.

ACTIVE MAMMARY GLANDS: PREGNANCY AND LACTATION

During pregnancy, in preparation for lactation, the mammary glands undergo dramatic proliferation and development. These changes in the glandular tissue are accompanied by relative decreases in the amount of

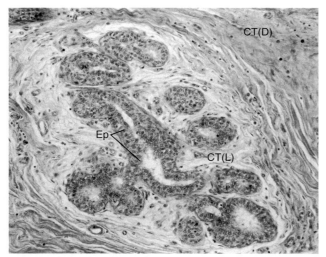

Figure 2-3 Inactive or resting human mammary gland. The epithelial (Ep) or glandular elements are embedded in loose connective tissue [CT(L)]. Within the lobule the epithelial cells are primarily duct elements. Dense connective tissue [CT(D)] surrounds the lobule. ×160. (Courtesy of Michael H. Ross, PhD, University of Florida College of Medicine, Gainesville, FL.)

connective and adipose tissue. Plasma cells, lymphocytes, and eosinophils infiltrate the fibrous component of the connective tissue as the breast develops in response to hormonal stimulation. The development of the glandular tissue is not uniform, and variation in the degree of development may occur within a single lobule. The cells vary in shape from low columnar to flattened. As the cells proliferate by mitotic division, the ductules branch and alveoli begin to develop. In the later stages of pregnancy, alveolar development becomes more prominent (Fig. 2-4). Near the end of pregnancy, the actual proliferation of cells declines and subsequent enlargement of the breast occurs through

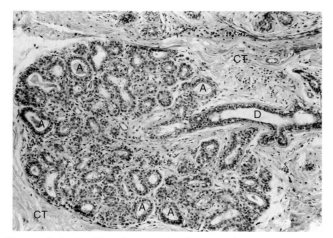

Figure 2-4 Proliferative or active (pregnant) human mammary gland. The alveolar elements of the gland become conspicuous during the early proliferative period (compare with Fig. 2-3). Within the lobule of the breast, distinct alveoli (A) are present. The alveoli are continuous with a duct (D). They are surrounded by highly cellular connective tissue (CT). The individual lobules are separated by dense connective tissue septa. ×160. (Courtesy of Michael H. Ross, PhD, University of Florida College of Medicine, Gainesville, FL.)

hypertrophy of the alveolar cells and accumulation of their secretory product in the lumina of the ductules.

The secretory cells contain abundant endoplasmic reticulum, a moderate number of large mitochondria, a supranuclear Golgi complex, and a number of dense lysosomes.[17,18] Depending on the secretory state of the cell, large lipid droplets and secretory granules may be present in the apical cytoplasm. Two distinct products produced by the cells are released by different mechanisms.[19] The protein component of the milk is synthesized in the granular endoplasmic reticulum, packaged in membrane-limited secretory granules for transport in the Golgi apparatus, and released from the cell by fusion of the granule's limiting membrane with the plasma membrane. This type of secretion is known as *merocrine secretion*. The lipid, or fatty, component of the milk arises as free lipid droplets in the cytoplasm. The lipid coalesces into large droplets that pass to the apical region of the cell and project into the lumen of the acinus prior to their release. As they are released from the cell, the droplets are invested with an envelope of plasma membrane. A thin layer of cytoplasm is trapped between the lipid droplet and plasma membrane as lipid is being released. It should be emphasized that only a very small amount of cytoplasm is lost during this secretory process, classically known as *apocrine secretion*.

The milk released during the first few days after childbirth is known as *colostrum*. It has low lipid content but is believed to contain considerable quantities of antibodies that provide the newborn with some degree of passive immunity. The lymphocytes and plasma cells that infiltrate the stroma of the breast during its proliferation and development are believed to be, in part, the source of the components of the colostrum. As the plasma cells and lymphocytes decrease in number, the production of colostrum stops and lipid-rich milk is produced.

HORMONAL REGULATION OF THE MAMMARY GLAND

Production of estrogens and progesterone by the ovary at puberty influences the initial growth of the mammary gland. Subsequent to this initial development, slight changes occur in the morphology of the glandular tissue with each ovarian, or menstrual, cycle. During pregnancy, the corpus luteum and placenta continuously produce estrogens and progesterone, which stimulate proliferation and development of the mammary gland. The growth of the glands is also dependent on the presence of prolactin, produced by the adenohypophysis; somatomammotropin (lactogenic hormone), produced by the placenta; and adrenal corticoids.

The level of circulating estrogens and progesterone drops abruptly at parturition with the degeneration of the corpus luteum and loss of the placenta. The secretion of milk is then brought about by increased production of prolactin and adrenal cortical steroids. A neurohormonal reflex regulates the high level of prolactin production and release. The act of suckling by the infant initiates impulses from receptors in the nipple; these impulses regulate cells in the hypothalamus. The impulses also cause the release of oxytocin in the neurohypophysis. The oxytocin stimulates the myoepithelial cells of the mammary glands, causing them to contract and eject milk.[20] In the absence of suckling, secretion of milk ceases and the glands regress and return to an inactive state.

After menopause, the gland atrophies, or involutes. As the release of ovarian hormones is diminished, the secretory cells of the alveoli degenerate and disappear, but some of the ducts remain. The connective tissue also demonstrates degenerative changes that are marked by a decrease in the number of stromal cells and collagen fibers.

Thoracic Wall

The thoracic wall is composed of both skeletal and muscular components. The skeletal components include the 12 thoracic vertebrae, the 12 ribs and their costal cartilages, and the sternum. The spaces between the ribs, the *intercostal spaces*, are filled with the *external, internal,* and *innermost intercostal muscles* and the associated *intercostal vessels* and *nerves* (Fig. 2-5). Some anatomists refer to the innermost layer as the *intima* of the *internal intercostal muscle*. The terminology chosen is of no particular consequence; the relationship that should be appreciated is that the intercostal veins, arteries, and nerves pass in the plane that separates the internal intercostal muscle from the innermost (or intimal) layer. The *endothoracic fascia*, a thin fibrous layer of connective tissue forming a fascial plane continuous with the most internal component of the investing fascia of the intercostal muscles and the adjacent layer of the periosteum, marks the internal limit of the thoracic wall. The parietal pleura rests on the endothoracic fascia.

It is important to recognize that the muscles and skeletal girdles of the upper extremities almost completely cover the thoracic wall anteriorly, laterally, and posteriorly. For the surgeon concerned with the breast, knowledge of the anatomy of the axilla and pectoral region is essential.

The 11 pairs of *external intercostal muscles* whose fibers run downward and forward form the most superficial

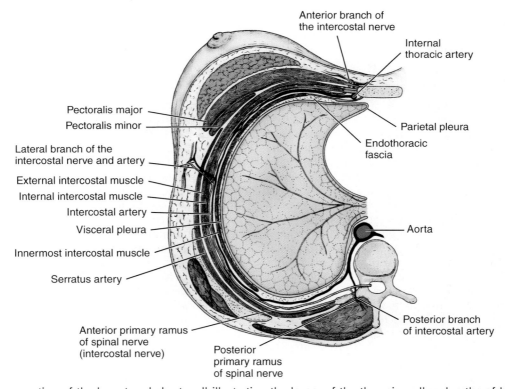

Figure 2-5 Cross section of the breast and chest wall illustrating the layers of the thoracic wall and paths of blood vessels and nerves. The intercostal muscles occur in three layers: external, internal, and innermost. The intercostal vessels and nerves pass between the internal and innermost layers. The posterior intercostal arteries arise from the aorta and pass anterior to anastomose with the anterior intercostal arteries that are branches of the internal thoracic artery. The veins are not shown but basically follow the course of the arteries. The intercostal nerves are direct continuations of the anterior primary rami of thoracic spinal nerves. They supply the intercostal muscles and give anterior and lateral branches that supply the overlying skin, including that of the breast. The breast lies superficial to the pectoralis major muscle and the underlying pectoralis minor muscle. The serratus anterior muscle originates from eight or nine fleshy digitations on the outer lateral surface of the ribs and inserts on the ventral surface of the medial (vertebral) border of the scapula. Parietal pleura attaches to the endothoracic fascia that lines the thoracic cavity. Visceral pleura covers the surface of the lungs. The thin channels in the substance of the lung represent lymphatic channels that convey lymph to pulmonary lymph nodes located in the hilum of the lung. Lymphatic channels draining the thoracic wall and overlying skin and superficial fascia are not illustrated but follow the path of the blood vessels that supply the region (see text).

layer (see later section on the innervation of the breast and Fig. 2-11). The muscle begins posteriorly at the tubercles of the ribs and extends anteriorly to the costochondral junction. Between the costal cartilages, the muscle is replaced by the *external intercostal membrane*. The fibers of the 11 pairs of *internal intercostal muscles* run downward and posteriorly. The muscle fibers of this layer reach the sternum anteriorly. Posteriorly, the muscle ends at the angle of the ribs and then the layer continues as the *internal intercostal membrane*. The *innermost intercostal muscles (intercostales intimi)* form the most internal layer and have fibers that are oriented more vertically but almost in parallel with the internal intercostal muscle fibers. The muscle fibers of this layer occupy approximately the middle half of the intercostal space. This is the least well developed of the three layers. It can best be distinguished by the fact that its fibers are separated from the internal intercostals by the intercostal vessels and nerves.

The *subcostalis* and *transversus thoracis muscles* are located on the internal surface of the thoracic wall. They occur in the same plane as the innermost intercostal muscles and are considered anterior and posterior extensions of this layer. The subcostal muscles are located posteriorly and have the same orientation as the innermost intercostal muscles. They are distinct because they pass to the second or third rib below (i.e., they pass over at least two intercostal spaces). Anteriorly, the *transversus thoracis muscles* form a layer that arises from the lower internal surface of the sternum and extends upward and laterally to insert on the costal cartilages of the second to sixth ribs (Fig. 2-6). These fibers pass deep to the internal thoracic artery and accompanying veins.

All of these muscles are innervated by the intercostal nerves associated with them. These nerves also give branches to the overlying skin. In a similar fashion, the intercostal vessels supply intercostal muscles and give branches to the overlying tissues. The intercostal nerves are direct continuations of the ventral primary rami of the upper 11 thoracic spinal nerves. As the nerves pass anteriorly, they give branches to supply the intercostal muscles. In addition, each nerve gives a relatively large lateral cutaneous branch, which exits the intercostal space along the midaxillary line near the attachment sites of the serratus anterior muscle on the ribs. The lateral cutaneous nerves then give branches that extend anteriorly and posteriorly. As the intercostal nerve continues anteriorly, it gives additional branches to the intercostal muscles. Just lateral to the border of the sternum the upper five intercostal nerves pierce the internal intercostal muscle and the external intercostal membrane to end superficially as the *anterior cutaneous nerves* of the chest. These nerves give rise to medial and lateral branches that supply the overlying skin. The lower six intercostal nerves continue past the costal margin into the anterior abdominal wall and are therefore identified as *thoracoabdominal nerves*.

The *intercostal arteries* originate in two groups: the anterior and posterior intercostal arteries. The *posterior intercostal arteries*, except for the first two spaces, arise from the thoracic aorta. The posterior intercostals for the first two spaces arise from the superior intercostal

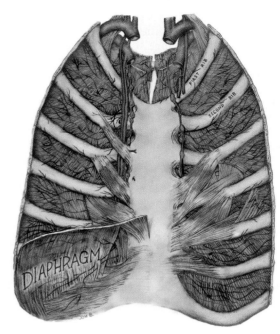

Figure 2-6 The anterior thoracic wall as viewed internally. The internal thoracic arteries and veins can be seen as they pass parallel to and about 1 cm from the sternal margin. Except in the upper two or three intercostal spaces, the transversus thoracic muscle lies deep to these vessels. The internal thoracic lymphatic trunks and associated parasternal lymph nodes accompany these vessels. Lymphatic channels located in the intercostal spaces convey lymph from the thoracic wall anteriorly to the parasternal nodes or posteriorly to the intercostal nodes.

arteries, which on the left and right sides branch from the costocervical trunk. The anterior intercostals are usually small paired arteries that extend laterally to the region of the costochondral junction. The anterior intercostal arteries of the upper five intercostal spaces arise from the internal thoracic (or mammary) artery; those of the lower six intercostal spaces arise from the musculophrenic artery. The anterior and posterior intercostal veins demonstrate a similar distribution. Anteriorly, they drain into the musculophrenic and internal thoracic veins. Posteriorly, the intercostal veins drain into the azygos and hemiazygos systems of veins.

The superficial muscles of the pectoral region include the *pectoralis major* and *minor muscles* and the *subclavius muscle*. The *pectoralis major muscle* is a fan-shaped muscle with two divisions. The clavicular division (or head) originates from the clavicle and is easily distinguished from the larger costosternal division that originates from the sternum and costal cartilages of the second through sixth ribs. The fibers of the two divisions converge laterally and insert into the crest of the greater tubercle of the humerus along the lateral lip of the bicipital groove. The *cephalic vein* serves as a convenient landmark defining the separation of the upper lateral border of the pectoralis major muscle from the deltoid muscle. The cephalic vein can be followed to the deltopectoral triangle, where it pierces the *clavipectoral fascia* and joins the axillary vein. The pectoralis major muscle acts primarily in flexion, adduction, and medial rotation of the arm at the shoulder joint. This action brings the arm across the chest. In climbing, the pectoralis major muscles, along with the latissimus dorsi muscles, function to elevate the trunk when the arms are fixed. The pectoralis major muscle is innervated by both the medial and the lateral pectoral nerves, which arise from the medial and lateral cords of the brachial plexus.

Located deep to the pectoralis major muscle, the *pectoralis minor muscle* arises from the external surface of the second to the fifth ribs and inserts on the coracoid process of the scapula. Although its main action is to lower the shoulder, it may serve as an accessory muscle of respiration. It is innervated by the medial pectoral nerve.

The *subclavius muscle* arises from the first rib near its costochondral junction and extends laterally to insert into the inferior surface of the clavicle. It functions to lower the clavicle and stabilize it during movements of the shoulder girdle. It is innervated by *the nerve to the subclavius muscle,* which arises from the upper trunk of the brachial plexus.

Axilla

Knowledge of the anatomy of the axilla and its contents is of paramount importance to the clinician. It is also essential that the surgeon be thoroughly familiar with the organization of the deep fascia and neurovascular relationships of the axilla.

BOUNDARIES OF THE AXILLA

The axilla is a pyramidal compartment between the upper extremity and the thoracic walls (Fig. 2-7). It is described as having four walls, an apex, and a base. The curved *base* is made of axillary fascia and skin. Externally, this region, the *armpit,* appears dome-shaped (and covered with hair after puberty). The *apex* is not a roof but an aperture that extends into the posterior triangle of the neck through the *cervicoaxillary canal.* The cervicoaxillary canal is bounded anteriorly by the clavicle, posteriorly by the scapula, and medially by the first rib. Most structures pass through the cervical axillary canal as they course between the neck and upper extremity. The *anterior wall* is made up of the pectoralis major and minor muscles and their associated fasciae. The *posterior wall* is composed primarily of the subscapularis muscle, located on the anterior surface of the scapula, and to a lesser extent by the teres major and latissimus dorsi muscles and their associated tendons. The *lateral wall* is a thin strip of the humerus, the bicipital groove, between the insertions of the muscles of the anterior and posterior walls. The *medial wall* is made up of serratus anterior muscle that covers the thoracic wall in this region (over the upper four or five ribs and their associated intercostal muscles).

CONTENTS OF THE AXILLA

The axilla contains the great vessels and nerves of the upper extremity. These, along with the other contents, are surrounded by loose connective tissue. Figure 2-7

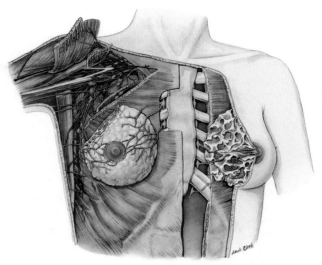

Figure 2-7 The anterior chest illustrating the structure of the chest wall, breast, and axilla. See text for details of the structure of the axilla and a description of its contents. On the right side, the pectoralis major muscle has been cut lateral to the breast and reflected laterally to its insertion into the crest of the greater tubercle of the humerus. This exposes the underlying pectoralis minor muscle and the other muscles forming the walls of the axilla. The contents of the axilla, including the axillary artery and vein, components of the brachial plexus, and axillary lymph node groups and lymphatic channels, are exposed. On the left side, the breast is cut to expose its structure in sagittal view. The lactiferous ducts and sinuses can be seen. Lymphatic channels passing to parasternal lymph nodes are also shown.

illustrates many of the key relationships of structures within the axilla. The vessels and nerves are closely associated with each other and are enclosed within a layer of fascia, the *axillary sheath.* This layer of dense connective tissue extends from the neck and gradually disappears as the nerves and vessels branch.

The axillary artery may be divided into three parts within the axilla.

1. The first part, located medial to the pectoralis minor muscle, gives one branch—the supreme thoracic artery that supplies the thoracic wall over the first and second intercostal spaces.
2. The second part, located posterior to the pectoralis minor muscle, gives two branches—the thoracoacromial artery and the lateral thoracic artery. The thoracoacromial artery divides into the acromial, clavicular, deltoid, and pectoral branches. The lateral thoracic artery passes along the lateral border of the pectoralis minor on the superficial surface of the serratus anterior muscle. Pectoral branches of the thoracoacromial and lateral thoracic arteries supply both the pectoralis major and minor muscles and must be identified during surgical dissection of the axilla. The lateral thoracic artery is of particular importance in surgery of the breast because it supplies the *lateral mammary branches.*
3. The third part, located lateral to the pectoralis minor, gives off three branches—the anterior and posterior circumflex humeral arteries, which supply the upper arm and contribute to the collateral

circulation around the humerus, and the subscapular artery. Although the latter artery does not supply the breast, it is of particular importance in the surgical dissection of the axilla. It is the largest branch within the axilla, giving rise after a short distance to its terminal branches, the subscapular circumflex and the thoracodorsal arteries, and it is closely associated with the central and subscapular lymph node groups. In the axilla, the thoracodorsal artery crosses the subscapularis and gives branches to it and to the serratus anterior and the latissimus dorsi muscles. A surgeon must use care in approaching this vessel and its branches to avoid undue bleeding that obscures the surgical field.

The *axillary vein* has tributaries that follow the course of the arteries just described. They are usually in the form of venae comitantes, paired veins that follow an artery. The *cephalic vein* passes in the groove between the deltoid and pectoralis major muscles and then joins the axillary vein after piercing the clavipectoral fascia.

Throughout its course in the axilla, the axillary artery is associated with various parts of the brachial plexus (Fig. 2-8). The cords of the *brachial plexus*—medial, lateral, and posterior—are named according to their relationship with the axillary artery. A majority of the branches of the brachial plexus arise in the axilla. The *lateral cord* gives four branches, namely, the *lateral pectoral nerve*, which supplies the pectoralis major; a branch that communicates with the medial pectoral nerve, which is called the *ansa pectoralis*[21]; and two terminal branches, the *musculocutaneous nerve* and the *lateral root of the median nerve*. Injury to the medial or lateral pectoral nerves, or the ansa pectoralis,[21] which joins them, may lead to loss of muscle mass and fatty necrosis of the pectoralis major or minor muscles,[22] depending of the level of nerve injury. The ansa pectoralis lies anterior to the axillary artery, making it vulnerable to injury during lymph node dissection in the axilla.

The *medial cord* usually gives five branches, the *medial pectoral nerve* (which supplies both the pectoralis major

and minor), the *median brachial cutaneous nerve*, the *medial antebrachial cutaneous nerve*, and two terminal branches—the *ulnar nerve* and the *lateral root of the median nerve*. The *posterior cord* usually has five branches. Three of these nerves arise from the posterior cord in the superior aspect of the axilla—the *upper subscapular*, the *thoracodorsal*, and the *lower subscapular*; the cord then divides into its two terminal branches—the *axillary* and *radial* nerves.

Two additional nerves are of particular interest to surgeons because they are vulnerable to injury during axillary dissection: the *long thoracic nerve*, which is a branch of the brachial plexus, and the *intercostobrachial nerve*. The *long thoracic nerve* is located on the medial wall of the axilla. It arises in the neck from the fifth, sixth, and seventh roots of the brachial and then enters the axilla through the cervicoaxillary canal. It lies on the surface of the serratus anterior muscle, which it supplies. The long thoracic nerve is covered by the serratus fascia and is sometimes accidentally removed with the fascia during surgery. This results in paralysis of part or all of the serratus anterior muscle. The functional deficit is an inability to raise the arm above the level of the shoulder (or extreme weakness when one attempts this movement). A second nerve, the *intercostobrachial*, is formed by the joining of a lateral cutaneous branch of the second intercostal nerve with the medial cutaneous nerve of the arm. This nerve supplies the skin of the floor of the axilla and the upper medial aspect of the arm. Sometimes, a second intercostobrachial nerve may form an anterior branch of the third lateral cutaneous nerve. This nerve is commonly injured in axillary dissection, resulting in numbness of the skin of the floor of the axilla and the medial aspect of the arm.

Lymph nodes are also present in the axilla. They are found in close association with the blood vessels. The lymph node groups and their location are described in the section on the lymphatic drainage of the breast.

AXILLARY FASCIAE

The anterior wall of the axilla is composed of the pectoralis major and minor muscles and the fascia that covers them. The fasciae occur in two layers: (1) a superficial layer investing the pectoralis major muscle, called the *pectoral fascia*, and (2) a deep layer that extends from the clavicle to the axillary fascia in the floor of the axilla, called the *clavipectoral* (or *costocoracoid*) *fascia*. The clavipectoral fascia encloses the subclavius muscle located below the clavicle and the pectoralis minor muscle (Fig. 2-9).

The upper portion of the clavipectoral fascia, the *costocoracoid membrane*, is pierced by the cephalic vein, the lateral pectoral nerve, and branches of the thoracoacromial artery. The medial pectoral nerve does not pierce the costocoracoid membrane but enters the deep surface of the pectoralis minor muscle, supplying it, and passes through the anterior investing layer of the pectoralis minor muscle to innervate the pectoralis major muscle. The lower portion of the clavipectoral fascia, located below the pectoralis minor muscle, is sometimes called the *suspensory ligament of the axilla*.

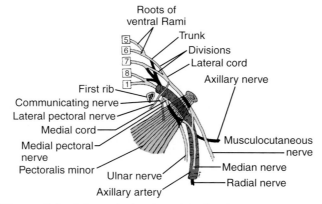

Roots of
ventral Rami
Trunk
5
6
7
Divisions
8
Lateral cord
1
Axillary nerve
First rib
Communicating nerve
Lateral pectoral nerve
Medial cord
Medial pectoral nerve
Musculocutaneous nerve
Pectoralis minor
Median nerve
Ulnar nerve
Radial nerve
Axillary artery

Figure 2-8 Schematic drawing of the brachial plexus illustrating its basic components. The cords are associated with the axillary artery and lie behind the pectoralis minor muscle. The names of the cords reflect their relationship to the artery. Compare with Figure 2-7 to identify the course of these structures in more detail.

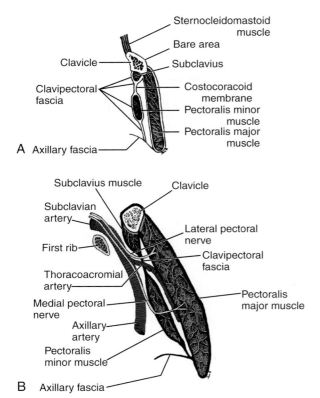

Figure 2-9 Sagittal sections of the chest wall in the axillary region. **A,** The anterior wall of the axilla. The clavicle and three muscles inferior to it are shown. **B,** Section through the chest wall illustrating the relationship of the axillary artery and medial and lateral pectoral nerves to the clavipectoral fascia. The clavipectoral fascia is a strong sheet of connective tissue that is attached superiorly to the clavicle and envelops the subclavius and pectoralis minor muscles. The fascia extends from the lower border of the pectoralis minor to become continuous with the axillary fascia in the floor of the axilla.

Halsted's ligament, a dense condensation of the clavipectoral fascia, extends from the medial end of the clavicle and attaches to the first rib (see Figs. 2-7 and 2-9A). The ligament covers the subclavian artery and vein as they cross the first rib.

Fascial Relationships of the Breast

The breast is located in the superficial fascia in the layer just deep to the dermis, the *hypodermis.* In approaching the breast, a surgeon may dissect in a bloodless plane just deep to the dermis. This dissection leaves a layer 2 to 3 mm in thickness in thin individuals in association with the skin flap. The layer may be several millimeters thick in obese individuals. The blood vessels and lymphatics passing in the deeper layer of the superficial fascia are left undisturbed.

Anterior fibrous processes, the *suspensory ligaments of Cooper,* pass from the septa that divide the lobules of the breast to insert into the skin. The posterior aspect of the breast is separated from the deep, or investing, fascia of the pectoralis major muscle by a space filled with loose areolar tissue, the *retromammary space* or *bursa*

(see Fig. 2-1). The existence of the suspensory ligaments of Cooper and the retromammary space allows the breast to move freely against the thoracic wall. The space between the well-defined fascial planes of the breast and pectoralis major muscle is easily identified by the surgeon removing a breast. Connective tissue thickenings, called *posterior suspensory ligaments,* extend from the deep surface of the breast to the deep pectoral fascia. Because breast parenchyma may follow these fibrous processes, it has been common practice to remove the adjacent portion of the pectoralis major muscle with the breast.

It is important to recognize, particularly with movements and variation in the size of the breast, that its deep surface contacts the investing fascia of other muscles in addition to the pectoralis major. Only about two thirds of the breast overlies the pectoralis major muscle. The lateral portion of the breast may contact the fourth through seventh slips of the serratus anterior muscle at its attachment to the thoracic wall. Just medial to this, the breast may contact the upper portion of the abdominal oblique muscle, where it interdigitates with the attachments of the serratus anterior muscle. As the breast extends to the axilla, it has contact with deep fascia present in this region.

BLOOD SUPPLY OF THE BREAST

The breast receives its blood supply from (1) perforating branches of the internal mammary artery; (2) lateral branches of the posterior intercostal arteries; and (3) several branches from the axillary artery, including highest thoracic, lateral thoracic, and pectoral branches of the thoracoacromial artery (Fig. 2-10). For reviews of the blood supply of the breast, see Cunningham,[23] Maliniac,[24] and Sakki.[25]

Branches from the second, third, and fourth anterior perforating arteries (Fig. 2-11, and see Fig. 2-10) pass to the breast as *medial mammary arteries.* These vessels enlarge considerably during lactation. The lateral thoracic artery gives branches to the serratus anterior muscle, both pectoralis muscles, and the subscapularis muscle. The lateral thoracic artery also gives rise to *lateral mammary branches* that wrap around the lateral border of the pectoralis major muscle to reach the breast. In the second, third, and fourth intercostal spaces, the posterior intercostal arteries give off *mammary branches;* these vessels increase in size during lactation.

The thoracodorsal branch of the subscapular artery is not involved in the supply of blood to the breast, but it is important to the surgeon who must deal with this artery during the dissection of the axilla. The central and scapular lymph node groups are intimately associated with this vessel. Bleeding that is difficult to control may result from cutting of branches of these vessels.

A fundamental knowledge of the pattern of venous drainage is important because carcinoma of the breast may metastasize through the veins and because lymphatic vessels often follow the course of the blood vessels. The veins of the breast basically follow the path of the arteries, with the chief venous drainage toward the axilla. The superficial veins demonstrate extensive anastomoses that may be apparent through the skin

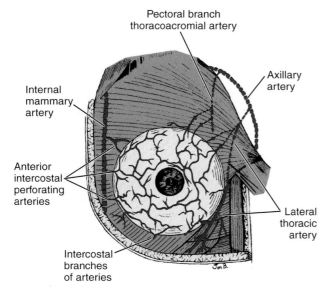

Figure 2-10 Arterial distribution of blood to the breast, axilla, and chest wall. The breast receives its blood supply via three major arterial routes: (1) medially from anterior perforating intercostal branches arising from the internal thoracic artery, (2) laterally from either pectoral branches of the thoracoacromial trunk or branches of the lateral thoracic artery (the thoracoacromial trunk and the lateral thoracic arteries are branches of the axillary artery), and (3) from lateral cutaneous branches of the intercostal arteries that are associated with the overlying breast. The arteries indicated with a *dashed line* lie deep to the muscles of the thoracic wall and axilla. Many of the arteries must pass through these muscles before reaching the breast.

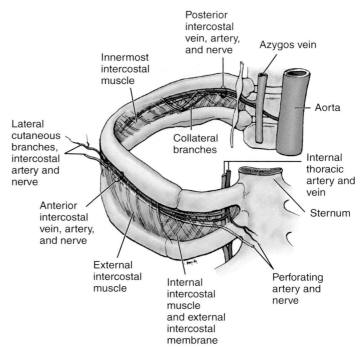

Figure 2-11 A segment of the body wall illustrating the relationship of structures to the ribs. Two ribs are shown as they extend from the vertebrae to attach to the sternum. The orientation of the muscle and connective tissue fibers is shown. The external intercostal muscle extends downward and forward. The muscle layer extends forward from the rib tubercle to the costochondral junction, where the muscle is replaced by the aponeurosis, called the external intercostal membrane. The internal intercostal muscle fibers with the opposite orientation can be seen through this layer. The innermost intercostal muscle fibers are present along the lateral half of the intercostal space. The intercostal nerve and vessels pass through the intercostal space in the plane between the internal and innermost (or intima of the internal) intercostal muscle layers. Anterior intercostal arteries arise from the internal thoracic artery; anterior intercostal veins join the internal thoracic vein. Posterior intercostal arteries arise from the aorta; posterior intercostal veins join the azygos venous system on the right and the hemiazygos system on the left. Lymphatics follow the path of the blood vessels. Anteriorly, lymphatics pass to parasternal (or internal mammary) nodes that are located along the internal mammary vessels; posteriorly, they pass to intercostal nodes located in the intercostal space near the vertebral bodies.

overlying the breast. The distribution of these veins has been studied by Massopust and Gardner[26] and Haagensen[27] using photographs taken in infrared light. Around the nipple, the veins form an anastomotic circle, the *circulus venosus*. Veins from this circle and from the substance of the gland transmit blood to the periphery of the breast and then into vessels joining the internal thoracic, axillary, and internal jugular veins.

Three principal groups of veins are involved in the venous drainage of the thoracic wall and the breast: (1) perforating branches of the internal thoracic vein, (2) tributaries of the axillary vein, and (3) perforating branches of posterior intercostal veins. Metastatic emboli traveling through any of these venous routes will pass through the venous return to the heart and then be stopped as they reach the capillary bed of the lungs, providing a direct venous route for metastasis of breast carcinoma to the lungs.

The *vertebral plexus of veins* (*Batson's plexus*) may provide a second route for metastasis of breast carcinoma via veins.[28–30] This venous plexus surrounds the vertebrae and extends from the base of the skull to the sacrum. Venous channels exist between this plexus and veins associated with thoracic, abdominal, and pelvic organs. In general, these veins do not have valves, making it possible for blood to flow through them in either direction. Furthermore, it is known that increases in intraabdominal pressure may force blood to enter these channels. These vessels provide a route for metastatic

emboli to reach the vertebral bodies, ribs, and central nervous system. These venous communications are of particular significance in the breast, where the posterior intercostal arteries are in direct continuity with the vertebral plexus.

Innervation of the Breast

Miller and Kasahara[31] have described the microscopic anatomic features of the innervation of the skin over the breast. They suggest that the specialization of the innervation of the breast, areola, and nipple is associated with the erection of the nipple[11] and flow of milk mediated through a neurohormonal reflex. As was explained previously, the act of suckling initiates impulses from receptors in the nipple that regulate cells in the hypothalamus. In response to the impulses, oxytocin is released in the neurohypophysis. The oxytocin stimulates the myoepithelial cells of the mammary glands, causing them to contract and eject milk from the glands. In the dermis of the nipple, Miller and Kasahara[31] found large numbers of multibranched free nerve endings; in the dermis of the areola and peripheral, Ruffini-like endings and Krause end-bulbs. The latter two receptor types are associated with tactile reception of stretch and pressure.

Sensory innervation of the breast is supplied primarily by the *lateral and anterior cutaneous branches of the second through sixth intercostal nerves* (see Fig. 2-11). Although the second and third intercostal nerves may give rise to cutaneous branches to the superior aspect of the breast, the nerves of the breast are derived primarily from the fourth, fifth, and sixth intercostal nerves. A limited region of the skin over the upper portion of the breast is supplied by nerves arising from the cervical plexus, specifically, the anterior, or medial, branches of the *supraclavicular nerve*. All of these nerves convey sympathetic fibers to the breast and overlying skin and therefore influence flow of blood through vessels accompanying the nerves and secretory function of the sweat glands of the skin. However, the secretory activity of the breast is chiefly under the control of ovarian and hypophyseal (pituitary) hormones.

The lateral branches of the intercostal nerves exit the intercostal space at the attachment sites of the slips of serratus anterior muscle. The nerves divide into anterior and posterior branches as they pass between the muscle fibers. As the anterior branches pass in the superficial fascia, they supply the anterolateral thoracic wall; the third through sixth branches, also known as *lateral mammary branches*, supply the breast. The lateral branch of the second intercostal nerve is of special significance because a large nerve, the *intercostal brachial*, arises from it. This nerve, which can be seen during surgical dissection of the axilla, passes through the fascia of the floor of the axilla and usually joins the medial cutaneous nerve of the arm. However, it is of limited functional significance. If this nerve is injured during surgery, the patient will have loss of cutaneous sensation from the upper medial aspect of the arm and floor of the axilla.

The anterior branches of the intercostal nerves exit the intercostal space near the lateral border of the sternum. These nerves send branches medially and laterally over the thoracic wall. The branches that pass laterally reach the medial aspect of the breast and are sometimes called *medial mammary nerves*.

Lymphatic Drainage of the Breast

LYMPH NODES OF THE AXILLA

The primary route of lymphatic drainage of the breast is through the axillary lymph node groups (Fig. 2-12, and see Fig. 2-7). Therefore, it is essential that the clinician understand the anatomy of the grouping of lymph nodes within the axilla. Unfortunately, the boundaries of groups of lymph nodes found in the axilla are not

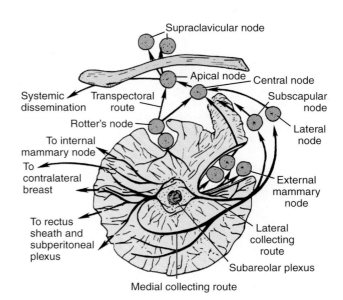

Figure 2-12 Schematic drawing of the breast identifying the position of lymph nodes relative to the breast and illustrating routes of lymphatic drainage. The clavicle is indicated as a reference point. See the text and Figure 2-14 to identify the group or level to which the lymph nodes belong. Level I lymph nodes include the external mammary (or anterior), axillary vein (or lateral), and scapular (or posterior) groups; level II, the central group; and level III, the subclavicular (or apical). The arrows indicate the routes of lymphatic drainage (see text).

well demarcated. Thus, there has been considerable variation in the names given to the lymph node groups. Anatomists usually define five groups of *axillary lymph nodes*[32,33]; surgeons usually identify six primary groups.[27] The most common terms used to identify the lymph nodes are indicated as follows:

1. The *axillary vein group*, usually identified by anatomists as the lateral group, consists of four to six lymph nodes that lie medial or posterior to the axillary vein. These lymph nodes receive most of the lymph draining from the upper extremity (Fig. 2-13). The exception is lymph that drains into the deltopectoral lymph nodes, a lymph node group sometimes called infraclavicular. The deltopectoral lymph nodes are not considered part of the axillary lymph node group but rather are outlying lymph nodes that drain into the subclavicular (or apical) lymph node group (see later discussion).

2. The *external mammary group*, usually identified by anatomists as the *anterior* or *pectoral group*, consists of four or five lymph nodes that lie along the lower border of the pectoralis minor muscle in association with the lateral thoracic vessels. These lymph nodes receive the major portion of the lymph draining from the breast. Lymph drains primarily from these lymph nodes into the central lymph nodes. However, lymph may pass directly from the external mammary nodes into the subclavicular lymph nodes.

3. The *scapular group*, usually identified by anatomists as the *posterior* or *subscapular group*, consists of six or seven lymph nodes that lie along the posterior

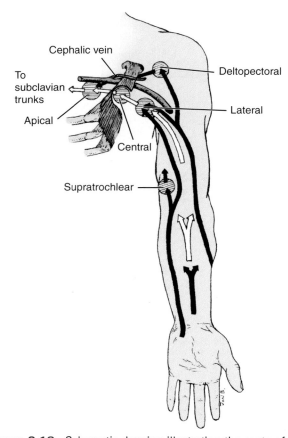

Figure 2-13 Schematic drawing illustrating the route of lymphatic drainage in the upper extremity. The relationship of this drainage to the major axillary lymph node groups is indicated by the arrows. All the lymph vessels of the upper extremity drain directly or indirectly through outlying lymph node groups into the axillary lymph nodes. The outlying lymph nodes are few in number and are organized into three groups: (1) supratrochlear lymph nodes (one or two, located above the medial epicondyle of the humerus adjacent to the basilic vein); (2) deltopectoral lymph nodes (one or two, located beside the cephalic vein where it lies between the pectoralis major and deltoid muscle just below the clavicle); and (3) variable small isolated lymph nodes (few and variable in number; may be located in the cubital fossa or along the medial side of the brachial vessels). Note that the deltopectoral lymph node group drains directly into the subclavicular, or apical, lymph nodes of the axillary group.

wall of the axilla at the lateral border of the scapula in association with the subscapular vessels. These lymph nodes receive lymph primarily from the inferior aspect of the posterior region of the neck, the posterior aspect of the trunk as far inferior as the iliac crest, and the posterior aspect of the shoulder region. Lymph from the scapular nodes passes to the central and subclavicular nodes.

4. The *central group* (both anatomists and surgeons use the same terminology for this group) consists of three or four large lymph nodes that are embedded in the fat of the axilla, usually posterior to the pectoralis minor muscle. They receive lymph from the three preceding groups and may receive afferent lymphatic vessels directly from the breast. Lymph from the central nodes passes directly to

the subclavicular (apical) nodes. This group is often superficially placed beneath the skin and fascia of the midaxilla and is centrally located between the posterior and anterior axillary folds. This nodal group is commonly palpable because of its superficial position and allows the clinical estimation of metastatic disease.[27,34]

5. The *subclavicular group*, usually identified by anatomists as the apical group, consists of 6 to 12 lymph nodes located partly posterior to the upper border of the pectoralis minor and partly superior to it. These lymph nodes extend into the apex of the axilla along the medial side of the axillary vein. They may receive lymph directly or indirectly from all the other groups of axillary lymph nodes. The efferent lymphatic vessels from the subclavicular lymph nodes unite to form the subclavian trunk. The course of the subclavian trunk is highly variable. It may directly join the internal jugular vein, the subclavian vein, or the junction of these two; likewise, on the right side of the trunk, it may join the right lymphatic duct, and on the left side, it may join the thoracic duct. Efferent vessels from the subclavicular lymph nodes may also pass to deep cervical lymph nodes.

6. The *interpectoral* or *Rotter's group*,[35] a group of nodes identified by surgeons[27] but usually not by anatomists, consists of one to four small lymph nodes that are located between the pectoralis major and minor muscles in association with the pectoral branches of the thoracoacromial vessels. Lymph from these nodes passes into central and subclavicular nodes.

Surgeons also define the axillary lymph nodes with respect to their relationship with the pectoralis minor muscle (Fig. 2-14).[34,36] These relationships are illustrated schematically in Figure 2-15. Lymph nodes that are located lateral to or below the lower border of the pectoralis minor muscle are called *level I* and include the external mammary, axillary vein, and scapular lymph node groups. Those lymph nodes located deep or posterior to the pectoralis minor muscle are called *level II* and include the central lymph node group and possibly some of the subclavicular lymph node group. Those lymph nodes located medial or superior to the upper border of the pectoralis minor muscle are called *level III* and include the subclavicular lymph node group.

Surgeons use the term *prepectoral* to identify a single lymph node that is only rarely found in the subcutaneous tissue associated with the breast or in the breast itself in its upper outer sector.[27] Haagensen reports finding only one or two prepectoral nodes each year among the several hundred mammary lesions studied.

SENTINEL LYMPH NODE BIOPSY

Several recent reviews[37–49] have discussed the potential benefits and risks of sentinel lymph node (SLN) identification and biopsy in breast cancer surgery and treatment. The basic principle of SLN biopsy is that the first lymph node that receives drainage from a tumor is the first site of lymphatic metastasis. The status of the SLN reflects

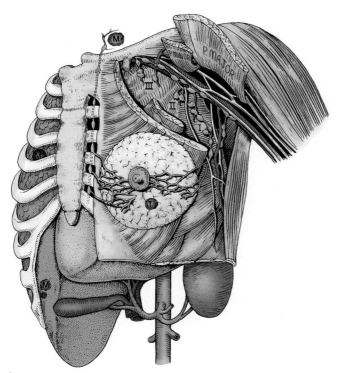

Figure 2-14 Lymphatic drainage of the breast. The pectoralis major and minor muscles, which contribute to the anterior wall of the axilla, have been cut and reflected. This exposes the medial and posterior walls of the axilla, as well as the basic contents of the axilla. The lymph node groups of the axilla and the internal mammary nodes are depicted. Also shown is the location of the long thoracic nerve on the surface of the serratus anterior muscle (on the medial wall of the axilla). The scapular lymph node group is closely associated with the thoracodorsal nerve and vessels. The Roman numerals indicate lymph node groups defined in Figure 2-15.

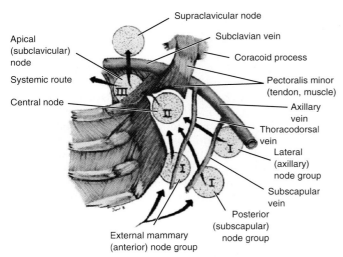

Figure 2-15 Schematic drawing illustrating the major lymph node groups associated with the lymphatic drainage of the breast. The Roman numerals indicate three levels or groups of lymph nodes that are defined by their location relative to the pectoralis minor. Level I includes lymph nodes located lateral to the pectoralis minor; level II, lymph nodes located deep to the muscle; and level III, lymph nodes located medial to the muscle. The arrows indicate the general direction of lymph flow. The axillary vein and its major tributaries associated with the pectoralis minor are included.

the status of the more distal lymph nodes along the lymphatic chain. The report by Lee and colleagues[39] on several studies showed that if only one lymph node has metastatic involvement, it is almost always the SLN; furthermore, in early stages of breast cancer it is often the only site of metastasis.

The three most important pathologic determinants of the prognosis of early breast cancer are the status of the axillary lymph nodes, histologic grade, and tumor size. For the past century, axillary lymph node dissection (ALND) has been an integral part of breast cancer management. The presence of axillary metastasis is associated with reduced disease-free and overall survival, and the number of involved axillary nodes has prognostic significance. SLN biopsy offers the possibility of optimal sampling of the axillary lymph nodes for the staging of breast cancer.

A number of techniques have been reported to optimize the identification of the SLN. The two main methods used are blue dye and/or radiolabeled material. In both methods the dye or radiolabeled material is injected around the tumor or deep in the overlying skin. With the blue dye, the location of the SLN is not known preoperatively, and the blue-stained lymphatics are followed intraoperatively to find the SLN. Use of radiolabeled material allows the tracer to be detected preoperatively with lymphoscintigraphy, or intraoperatively with a γ probe, or a combination of the two. Lee and colleagues[39] reported that in recent large studies, the SLN was identified 93% to 99% of the time. They also reported that in the larger series of studies, the false-negative SLN with metastasis elsewhere in the axilla was in the range of 1% to 11%.

Before SLN biopsy can be used to determine specific surgical approaches and the extent of adjuvant chemotherapy and regional radiation therapy, there must be consensus on the sensitivity of the method and the accepted false-negative rates. In his review, Von Smitten[41] reported rates of detection of sentinel nodes ranging from 66% to 100%, and false-negative rates of 17% to 0% have been reported. Von Smitten[41] suggested that a theoretical false-negative rate of 2% to 3% may be acceptable; Cody[37] suggested that a goal for surgeons and institutions using SLN biopsy may be at least 90% successful in finding the SLN with no more than 5% to 10% false-negative findings. In the case of SLN biopsy, as is true in most areas of medicine, the skill, expertise, and thoroughness of the pathologist who reads the specimen is of utmost importance.

Numerous recent reviews provide insight into the controversy with respect to SLN biopsy. A few recent articles are cited.[39,40,42–49] Many investigators have supported the positive aspect of more limited lymph node dissection by taking advantage of information gained via findings from carefully assessed SNL biopsy.

LYMPH FLOW

A conceptualization of lymphatic drainage of the breast is essential to the student of this organ's pathophysiology. Metastatic dissemination of breast cancer occurs predominantly by rich and extensive lymphatic routes that arborize in multiple directions through skin and mesenchymal (intraparenchymal) lymphatics. The delicate lymphatics of the corium are valveless; flow encompasses the lobular parenchyma and thereafter parallels major venous tributaries to enter the regional lymph nodes. This unidirectional lymphatic flow is pulsatile as a consequence of the wavelike contractions of the lymphatics to allow rapid transit and emptying of the lymphatic vascular spaces that interdigitate the extensive periductal and perilobular networks. As a consequence of obstruction to lymph flow by inflammatory or neoplastic diseases, a reversal in lymphatic flow is evident and can be appreciated microscopically as endolymphatic metastases of the dermis or breast parenchyma. This obstruction of lymphatic flow accounts for the neoplastic growth in local and regional sites remote from the primary neoplasm.

Lymphatic flow is typically unidirectional, except in the pathologic state, and has preferential flow from the periphery toward larger collecting ducts. Lymphatic capillaries begin as blind-ending ducts in tissues from which the lymph is collected; throughout their course these capillaries anastomose and fuse to form larger lymphatic channels that ultimately terminate in the thoracic duct on the left side of the body or the smaller right lymphatic duct on the right side. The thoracic duct empties into the region of the junction of the left subclavian and left internal jugular veins, whereas the right lymphatic duct drains into the right subclavian vein near its junction with the right internal jugular vein.

Anson and McVay[34] and Haagensen[27] acknowledged two accessory directions for lymphatic flow from breast parenchyma to nodes of the apex of the axilla: the *transpectoral* and *retropectoral routes* (see Fig. 2-12). Lymphatics of the transpectoral route (i.e., interpectoral nodes) lie between the pectoralis major and minor muscles and are referred to as *Rotter's nodes*. The transpectoral route begins in the loose areolar tissue of the retromammary plexus and interdigitates between the pectoral fascia and breast to perforate the pectoralis major muscle and follow the course of the thoracoacromial artery and terminate in the subclavicular (level III) group of nodes.

The second accessory lymphatic drainage group, the retropectoral pathway, drains the superior and internal aspects of the breast. Lymphatic vessels from this region of the breast join lymphatics from the posterior and lateral surfaces of the pectoralis major and minor muscles. These lymphatic channels terminate at the apex of the axilla in the subclavicular (level III) group. This route of lymphatic drainage is found in approximately one third of individuals and is a more direct mechanism of lymphatic flow to the subclavicular group. This accessory pathway is also the major lymphatic drainage by way of the external mammary and central axillary nodal groups (levels I and II, respectively).[27,34]

The recognition of metastatic spread of breast carcinoma into internal mammary nodes as a primary route of systemic dissemination is credited to the British surgeon R.S. Handley.[50] Extensive investigation confirmed that central and medial lymphatics of the breast pass medially and parallel the course of major blood vessels to perforate the pectoralis major muscle and thereafter terminate in the internal mammary nodal chain.

The internal mammary nodal group (see Figs. 2-6 and 2-14) is anatomically situated in the retrosternal interspaces between the costal cartilages approximately 2 to 3 cm within the sternal margin. These nodal groups also traverse and parallel the internal mammary vasculature and are invested by endothoracic fascia. The internal mammary lymphatic trunks eventually terminate in subclavicular nodal groups (see Figs. 2-6, 2-12, and 2-15). The right internal mammary nodal group enters the right lymphatic duct and the left enters the thoracic duct (Fig. 2-16). The presence of supraclavicular nodes (stage IV disease) results from lymphatic permeation and subsequent obstruction of the inferior, deep cervical group of nodes of the jugular-subclavian confluence. In effect, the supraclavicular nodal group represents the termination of efferent trunks from subclavian nodes of the internal mammary nodal group. These nodes are situated beneath the lateral margin of the inferior aspect of the sternocleidomastoid muscle beneath the clavicle and represent common sites of distant metastases from mammary carcinoma.

Cross-communication from the interstices of connecting lymphatic channels from each breast provides ready access of lymphatic flow to the opposite axilla. This observation of communicating dermal lymphatics to the contralateral breast explains occasional metastatic involvement of the opposite breast and axilla. Structures of the chest wall, including the internal and external intercostal musculature (see Fig. 2-11), have extensive lymphatic drainage that parallels the course of their major intercostal blood supply. As expected, invasive neoplasms of the lateral breast that involve deep musculature of the thoracic cavity have preferential flow toward the axilla. Invasion of medial musculature of the chest wall allows preferential drainage toward the internal mammary nodal groups, whereas bidirectional metastases may be evident with invasive central or subareolar cancers.

The lymphatic vessels that drain the breast occur in three interconnecting groups[51]: (1) a primary set of vessels originates as channels within the gland in the interlobular spaces and along the lactiferous ducts; (2) vessels draining the glandular tissue and overlying skin of the central part of the gland pass to an interconnecting network of vessels located beneath the areola, called the *subareolar plexus*[52]; and (3) a plexus on the deep surface of the breast communicates with minute vessels in the deep fascia underlying the breast. Along the medial border of the breast, lymphatic vessels within the substance of the gland anastomose with vessels passing to parasternal nodes.

Using autoradiographs of surgical specimens, Turner-Warwick[51] demonstrated that the main lymphatic drainage of the breast is through the system of lymphatic vessels occurring within the substance of the gland and not through the vessels on the superficial or deep surface. The main collecting trunks run laterally as they pass through the axillary fascia in the substance of the axillary tail. The subareolar plexus plays no essential part in the lymphatic drainage of the breast.[51] Using vital dyes,

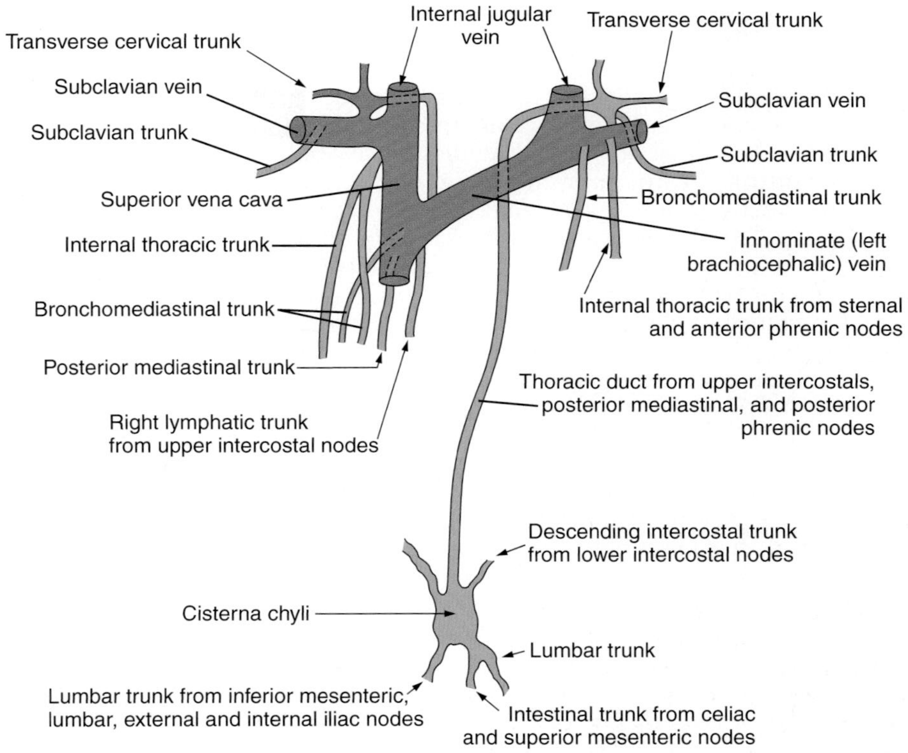

Figure 2-16 Schematic of the major lymphatic vessels of the thorax and the root of the neck. The thoracic duct begins at the cisterna chyli, a dilated sac that receives drainage from the lower extremities and the abdominal and pelvic cavities via the lumbar and intestinal trunks. Lymph enters the systemic circulation via channels that join the great veins of the neck and superior mediastinum. The lymphatic vessels demonstrate considerable variation as to their number and pattern of branching. A typical pattern is illustrated here. Most of the major trunks, including the thoracic and right lymphatic ducts, end at or near the confluence of the internal jugular with the subclavian veins.

Halsell and coworkers[53] demonstrated that this plexus receives lymph primarily from the nipple and the areola and conveys it toward the axilla. The lymphatics communicating with minute vessels in the deep fascia play no part in the normal lymphatic drainage of the breast and provide an alternative route only when the normal pathways are obstructed. More than 75% of the lymph from the breast passes to the axillary lymph nodes (see Fig. 2-12). Most of the remainder of the lymph passes to parasternal nodes. Some authorities have suggested that the parasternal nodes receive lymph primarily from the medial part of the breast. However, Turner-Warwick[51] reported that both the axillary and the parasternal lymph node groups receive lymph from all quadrants of the breast, with no striking tendency for any quadrant to drain in a particular direction.

Other routes for the flow of lymph from the breast have been identified. Occasionally, lymph from the breast reaches intercostal lymph nodes, located near the heads of the ribs (see later discussion). Lymphatic vessels reach this location by following lateral cutaneous branches of the posterior intercostal arteries. Lymph may pass to lymphatics within the rectus sheath or subperitoneal plexus by following branches of the intercostal and musculophrenic vessels. Lymph may pass directly to subclavicular, or apical, nodes from the upper portion of the breast. SLN biopsy has confirmed the direct metastasis from the breast to the supraclavicular nodes.

The skin over the breast has lymphatic drainage via the *superficial lymphatic vessels*, which ramify subcutaneously and converge on the axillary lymph nodes. The anterolateral chest and the upper abdominal wall above the umbilicus demonstrate striking directional flow of lymph toward the axilla. Lymphatic vessels near the lateral margin of the sternum pass through the intercostal space to the *parasternal lymph nodes*, which are associated with the internal thoracic vessels. Some of the lymphatic vessels located on adjacent sides of the sternum may anastomose in front of the sternum. In the upper pectoral region, a few of the lymphatic vessels may pass over the clavicle to *inferior deep cervical lymph nodes*.

The SLN biopsy identification is also providing better evidence of the paths of axillary lymphatic drainage of the breast. This technique is especially useful in identifying the lymphatic drainage into the parasternal or internal mammary lymph nodes.[38] The lymphatic vessels from the deeper structures of the thoracic wall drain primarily into parasternal, intercostal, or diaphragmatic lymph nodes (see later discussion).

LYMPH NODES OF THE THORACIC WALL

The lymphatic drainage of the skin and superficial tissues of thoracic and anterior abdominal walls is described in the section on the lymphatic drainage of the breast. Three sets of lymph nodes and associated vessels—*parasternal, intercostal,* and *diaphragmatic*—are involved in the lymphatic drainage of the deeper tissues of the thoracic wall:

1. The *parasternal,* or *internal thoracic, lymph nodes* consist of small lymph nodes located about 1 cm lateral to the sternal border in the intercostal spaces along the internal thoracic, or mammary,

vessels (see Figs. 2-1 and 2-6). The parasternal nodes lie in the areolar tissue underlying the endothoracic fascia that borders the space between the adjacent costal cartilages. The distribution of the nodes in the upper six intercostal spaces has been the subject of several studies since Stibbe's report in 1918 of an average total of 8.5 internal mammary nodes per subject, including both sides.[54] Stibbe reported that they usually occurred in the pattern of four on one side and five on the other. Each of the three upper spaces usually contained one lymph node, as did the sixth space. Often, there were no lymph nodes in the fourth or fifth space; an extra node usually was found in one of the upper three spaces on one of the sides. Soerensen[55] reported finding an average of seven nodes of minute size per subject in 39 autopsies, with an average of 3.5 on each side. Ju (as reported by Haagensen[27]) studied 100 autopsy subjects and found an average of 6.2 parasternal nodes per subject, with an average of 3.1 per side. A majority was found in the upper three spaces. However, in contradiction to Stibbe's findings, a lower but similar frequency of nodes was seen in all three of the lower intercostal spaces. Putti[56] studied 47 cadavers and found an average of 7.7 nodes per subject—again, with a majority of the nodes in the upper three spaces and many fewer in the lower spaces. Arão and Abrão[57] studied 100 autopsy specimens and found a much higher frequency of lymph nodes than had been previously reported. They found an average total of 16.2 per subject, with an average of 8.9 on the right side and 7.3 on the left. In 56.6% of the subjects, they found retromanubrial nodes between the right and left lymphatic trunks at the level of the first intercostal space. An average of 6.6 nodes were seen when the retromanubrial nodes were present.

2. The *intercostal lymph nodes* consist of small lymph nodes located in the posterior part of the thoracic cavity within the intercostal spaces near the head of the ribs (see Fig. 2-11). One or more may be found in each intercostal space in relationship with the intercostal vessels. These lymph nodes receive the deep lymphatics from the posterolateral thoracic wall, including lymphatic channels from the breast. Occasionally, small lymph nodes occur in the intercostal spaces along the lateral thoracic wall. Efferent lymphatics from the lower four or five intercostal spaces, on both the right and the left sides, join to form a trunk that descends to open into either the cisterna chyli or the initial portion of the thoracic duct. The upper efferent lymphatics from the intercostal nodes on the left side terminate in the thoracic duct; the efferent lymphatics from the corresponding nodes on the right side end in the right lymphatic duct.

3. The *diaphragmatic lymph nodes* consist of three sets of small lymph nodes (anterior, lateral, and posterior) located on the thoracic surface of the diaphragm.

The *anterior set of diaphragmatic lymph nodes* includes two or three small lymph nodes (also known as *prepericardial lymph nodes*) located behind the sternum at the base of the xiphoid process, which receive afferent lymphatics from the convex surface of the liver, and one or two nodes located on each side near the junction of the seventh rib with its costal cartilage, which receive afferents from the anterior aspect of the diaphragm. Afferent lymphatics also reach the prepericardial nodes by accompanying the branches of the superior epigastric blood vessels that pass from the rectus abdominis muscle and through the rectus sheath. Efferent lymphatics from the anterior diaphragmatic nodes pass to the *parasternal nodes*. This lymphatic channel is a potential route by which metastases from the breast may invade the parasternal region, with the potential for spread to the liver. As Haagensen[27] suggests, metastasis via this (rectus abdominis muscle) route most likely occurs only when the internal mammary lymphatic trunk is blocked higher in the upper intercostal spaces. When blockage occurs, the flow of lymph may be reversed and carcinoma emboli from the breast may reach the liver. It is significant to note that the autopsy subjects studied by Handley and Thackray,[50] who demonstrated this route of metastasis, had locally advanced breast carcinoma. Handley and Thackray[50] described the importance of the parasternal lymph nodes in carcinoma of the breast. Clearly, as Haagensen[27] and others have suggested, this route is not of importance in early cancer of the breast unless the primary tumor is located in the extreme lower inner portion of the breast where it overlies the sixth costal cartilage.

The *lateral set of diaphragmatic lymph nodes* consists of two or three small lymph nodes on each side of the diaphragm adjacent to the pericardial sac where the phrenic nerves enter the diaphragm. On the right side, they are located near the vena cava; on the left side, near the esophageal hiatus. Afferent lymphatic vessels reach these nodes from the middle region of the diaphragm; on the right side, afferent lymphatics from the convex surface of the liver also reach these nodes. Efferent lymphatics from the lateral diaphragmatic nodes may pass to the parasternal nodes via the anterior diaphragmatic nodes, to posterior mediastinal nodes, or to anterior nodes via vessels that follow the course of the phrenic nerve.

The *posterior set of diaphragmatic lymph nodes* consists of a few lymph nodes located adjacent to the crura of the diaphragm. They receive lymph from the posterior aspect of the diaphragm and convey it to posterior mediastinal and lateral aortic nodes.

LYMPH NODES OF THE THORACIC CAVITY

Three sets of nodes are involved in the lymphatic drainage of the thoracic viscera—*anterior mediastinal* (*brachiocephalic*), *posterior mediastinal*, and *tracheobronchial*. Although a knowledge of the lymphatic drainage of the thoracic viscera may not be particularly significant in treating carcinoma of the breast, it is important that one understand the system of collecting lymphatic trunks in this region (see Fig. 2-16), which all empty into the confluence of the internal jugular and subclavian veins.

For better comprehension of the pattern of lymphatic drainage in this region, a brief description of the regions and organs drained by the three thoracic lymph node groups is provided. The *anterior mediastinal group* consists of six to eight lymph nodes located in the upper anterior part of the mediastinum in front of the brachiocephalic veins and the large arterial trunks arising from the aorta. These correspond to the *retromanubrial nodes* as identified by Arão and Abrão.[57] The anterior mediastinal nodes receive afferent lymphatics from the thymus, thyroid, pericardium, and lateral diaphragmatic lymph nodes. Their efferent lymphatic vessels join with those from the tracheobronchial nodes to form the *bronchomediastinal trunks*.

The *posterior mediastinal group* consists of 8 to 10 nodes located posterior to the pericardium in association with the esophagus and descending thoracic aorta. They receive afferent lymphatics from the esophagus, the posterior portion of the pericardium, the diaphragm, and the convex surface of the liver. Most of their efferent lymphatic vessels join the thoracic duct, but some pass to *tracheobronchial nodes*.

The *tracheobronchial group* consists of a chain of five subgroups of lymph nodes—tracheal, superior tracheobronchial, inferior tracheobronchial, bronchopulmonary, and pulmonary—located adjacent to the trachea and bronchi, as is indicated by the descriptive names. The bronchopulmonary nodes are found in the hilus of each lung; the pulmonary nodes are found within the substance of the lung in association with the segmental bronchi. The tracheal nodes receive afferent lymphatics from the trachea and upper esophagus. The remaining nodes within this group form a continuous chain with boundaries of lymphatic drainage that are not well defined. The pulmonary and bronchopulmonary nodes receive afferent lymphatic vessels from the lungs and bronchial trees. The inferior and superior tracheobronchial nodes receive afferent lymphatic vessels from the lungs and bronchial trees. The inferior and superior tracheobronchial nodes receive

afferent lymphatic vessels from the bronchopulmonary nodes; the inferior tracheobronchial nodes also receive some afferent lymphatic vessels from the heart and posterior mediastinal organs. Efferent vessels from the subgroups of the tracheobronchial group pass sequentially to the level of the tracheal nodes. Efferents from the latter unite with efferents from parasternal and anterior mediastinal nodes to form the *right* and *left bronchomediastinal lymphatic trunks*. The left trunk may terminate by joining the thoracic duct, and the right trunk may join the right lymphatic duct. However, it is more common for the right and left trunks to open independently into the junction of the internal jugular and subclavian veins, each on their own side (see Fig. 2-16).

Venous Drainage of the Mammary Gland

Lymphatic drainage of the epithelial and mesenchymal components of the breast is the primary route for metastatic dissemination of adenocarcinoma of this organ. However, the vascular route for tumor embolization via venous drainage systems plays a major role in dissemination of neoplasms to the lung, bone, brain, liver, and so forth. The three groups of deep veins that drain the breast (Fig. 2-17) and serve as vascular routes include the following:

1. The *intercostal veins*, which traverse the posterior aspect of the breast from the second to the sixth intercostal spaces and arborize to enter the vertebral veins posteriorly and the azygos vein centrally to terminate in the superior vena cava.
2. The *axillary vein*, which may have variable tributaries that provide segmental drainage of the chest wall, pectoral muscles, and the breast.

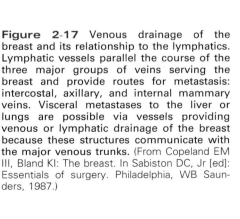

Figure 2-17 Venous drainage of the breast and its relationship to the lymphatics. Lymphatic vessels parallel the course of the three major groups of veins serving the breast and provide routes for metastasis: intercostal, axillary, and internal mammary veins. Visceral metastases to the liver or lungs are possible via vessels providing venous or lymphatic drainage of the breast because these structures communicate with the major venous trunks. (From Copeland EM III, Bland KI: The breast. In Sabiston DC, Jr [ed]: Essentials of surgery. Philadelphia, WB Saunders, 1987.)

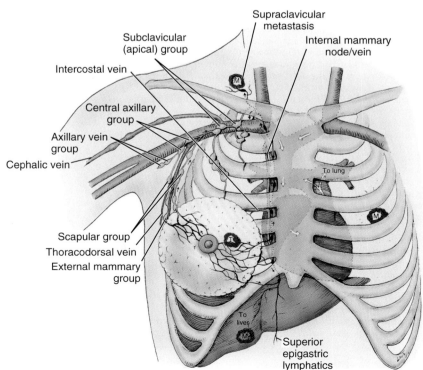

3. The *internal mammary vein perforators*, which represent the largest venous plexus to provide drainage of the mammary gland. This venous network traverses the rib interspaces to enter the brachiocephalic (innominate) veins. Thus, perforators that drain the parenchyma and epithelial components of the breast allow direct embolization to the pulmonary capillary spaces to establish metastatic disease.[27,34]

REFERENCES

1. Morehead JR: Anatomy and embryology of the breast. Clin Obstet Gynecol 25:353–357, 1982.
2. Helminen HJ, Ericsson JL: Studies on mammary gland involution. I. On the ultrastructure of the lactating mammary gland. J Ultrastruct Res 25:193–213, 1968.
3. Cowie AT: Overview of mammary gland. J Invest Dermatol 63:2–9, 1974.
4. Spratt JS: Anatomy of the breast. Major Probl Clin Surg 5:1–13, 1979.
5. Spratt JS Jr, Donegan WL: Anatomy of the breast. In Donegan WL, Spratt JS Jr (eds): Cancer of the breast, 3rd ed. Philadelphia, WB Saunders, 1979.
6. Smith DJ Jr et al: Breast volume and anthropomorphic measurements: Normal values. Plast Reconstr Surg 78:331–335, 1986.
7. Montagu A: Natural selection in the form of the breast in the female. JAMA 180:826–827, 1962.
8. Giacometti L, Montagna W: The nipple and areola of the human female breast. Anat Rec 144:191–197, 1962.
9. Sykes PA: The nerve supply of the human nipple. J Anat (Lond) 105:201, 1969.
10. Montagna W, Macpherson EA: Some neglected aspects of the anatomy of the human breasts. J Invest Dermatol 63:10–16, 1974.
11. Cathcart EP, Gairns FW, Garven HSD: The innervation of the human quiescent nipple, with notes on pigmentation, erection, and hyperneury. Trans R Soc Edinb 61:699–717, 1948.
12. Radnor CJ: Myoepithelium in the prelactating and lactating mammary glands of the rat. J Anat (Lond) 112:337–353, 1972.
13. Hoffman S, Dutton SL, Ernst H, et al: Functional characterization of antiadhesion molecules. Perspect Dev Neurobiol 2:101–110, 1994.
14. Stampfer MR, Yaswen P: Culture systems for study of human mammary epithelial cell proliferation, differentiation and transformation. Cancer Surv 18:7–34, 1993.
15. Thompson EW, Yu M, Bueno J, et al: Collagen induced MMP-2 activation in human breast cancer. Breast Cancer Res Treat 31:357–370, 1994.
16. Verhoeve D, Van-Marck E: Proliferation, basement membrane changes, metastasis and vascularization patterns in human breast cancer. Pathol Res Pract 189:851–861, 1993.
17. Tobon H, Salazar H: Ultrastructure of the human mammary gland. I. Development of the fetal gland throughout gestation. J Clin Endocrinol Metab 39:443–456, 1974.
18. Waugh D, Van Der Hoeven E: Fine structure of the human adult female breast. Lab Invest 11:220–228, 1962.
19. Wellings SR, Grunbaum BW, DeOme KB: Electron microscopy of milk secretion in the mammary gland of the C3H/Crgl mouse. J Natl Cancer Inst 25:423–437, 1960.
20. Linzell JL: The silver staining of myoepithelial cells particularly in the mammary gland, and their relation to ejection of milk. J Anat (Lond) 86:49–57, 1952.
21. Grife RM, Sullivan RM, Colborn GL: The ansa pectoralis: Anatomy and applications. Gainesville, FL, American Association of Clinical Anatomists, 2002.
22. Moosman DA: Anatomy of the pectoral nerves and their preservation in modified mastectomy. Am J Surg 139:883–886, 1980.
23. Cunningham L: The anatomy of the arteries and veins of the breast. J Surg Oncol 9:71–85, 1977.
24. Maliniac JW: Arterial blood supply of the breast. Arch Surg 47:329–343, 1943.
25. Sakki S: Angiography of the female breast. Ann Clin Res 6(suppl 12):1–47, 1974.
26. Massopust LC, Gardner WD: Infrared photographic studies of the superficial thoracic veins in the female. Surg Gynecol Obstet 91:717–727, 1950.
27. Haagensen CD: Anatomy of the mammary glands. In Haagensen CD (ed): Diseases of the breast, 3rd ed. Philadelphia, WB Saunders, 1986.
28. Batson OV: The function of the vertebral veins and their role in the spread of metastases. Ann Surg 112:138–149, 1940.
29. Batson OV: The role of the vertebral veins and metastatic processes. Ann Intern Med 16:38–45, 1942.
30. Henriques C: The veins of the vertebral column and their role in the spread of cancer. Ann R Coll Surg Engl 31:1–22, 1962.
31. Miller MR, Kasahara M: Cutaneous innervation of the human breast. Anat Rec 135:153–167, 1959.
32. Gray H: The lymphatic system. In Clemente CD (ed): Anatomy of the human body, 30th ed. Philadelphia, Lea & Febiger, 1985.
33. Mornard P: Sur deux cas de tumeurs malignes des mammelles axillaires aberrantes. Bull Mem Soc Chir Paris 21:487, 1929.
34. Anson BJ, McVay CB: Thoracic walls: Breast or mammary region. In Surgical anatomy, vol 1. Philadelphia, WB Saunders, 1971.
35. Grossman F: Ueber die Axillaren Lymphdrusen Inaug Dissert, Berlin, C. Vogt, 1986.
36. Copeland EM III, Bland KI: The breast. In Sabiston DC Jr (ed): Essentials of surgery. Philadelphia, WB Saunders, 1987.
37. Cody HS III: Clinical aspects of sentinel node biopsy. Breast Cancer Res 3:104–108, 2001.
38. Cserni G, Szekeres JP: Internal mammary lymph nodes and sentinel node biopsy in breast cancer. Surg Oncol 10:25–33, 2001.
39. Lee AH, Ellis IO, Pinder SE, et al: Pathological assessment of sentinel lymph-node biopsies in patients with breast cancer. Virchows Arch 436:97–101, 2000.
40. Nieweg OE, Rutgers EJ, Jansen L, et al: Is lymphatic mapping in breast cancer adequate and safe? World J Surg 25:780–788, 2001.
41. Von Smitten K: Sentinel node biopsy in breast cancer. Acta Oncol 13:33–36, 1999.
42. Motomura K, Egawa C, Komoike Y, et al: Sentinel node biopsy for breast cancer: Technical aspects and controversies. Breast Cancer,14:25–30, 2007.
43. Sato K, Shigenaga R, Ueda S, et al: Sentinel lymph node biopsy for breast cancer. J Surg Oncol 96:322–329, 2007.
44. Tangoku A, Seike J, Nakano et al: Current status of sentinel lymph node navigation surgery in breast and gastrointestinal tract. J Med Invest 54:1–18, 2007.
45. Veronesi P, Rodriguez-Fernandez J, Intra M: Controversies in the use of sentinel nodes: Microinvasion, post surgery and after preoperative systemic treatment. Breast 16(suppl 2):67–70, 2007.
46. Newman EA, Newman LA: Lymphatic mapping techniques and sentinel lymph node biopsy in breast cancer. Surg Clin North Am 87:353–364, 2007.
47. Nos C, Lesieur B, Clough KB, Lecuru F: Blue dye injection in the arm in order to conserve the lymphatic drainage of the arm in breast cancer patients requiring an axillary dissection. Ann Surg Oncol 14:2490–2496, 2007.
48. Rivers A, Hansen N: Axillary management after sentinel lymph node biopsy in breast cancer patients. Surg Clin North Am 87:365–377, 2007.
49. Rutgers EJ: Sentinel node biopsy: Interpretation and management of patients with immunohistochemistry-positive sentinel nodes and those with micrometastases. J Clin Oncol 26:698–702, 2008.
50. Handley RS, Thackray AC: The internal mammary lymph chain in carcinoma of the breast. Lancet 2:276–278, 1949.
51. Turner-Warwick RT: The lymphatics of the breast. Br J Surg 46:574–582, 1959.
52. Grant RN, Tabah EJ, Adair FF: The surgical significance of subareolar lymph plexus in cancer of the breast. Surgery 33:71–78, 1953.
53. Halsell JT et al: Lymphatic drainage of the breast demonstrated by vital dye staining and radiography. Ann Surg 162:221–226, 1965.
54. Stibbe EP: The internal mammary lymphatic glands. J Anat 52:527–564, 1918.
55. Soerensen B: Recherches sur la localisation des ganglions lymphatiques parasternaux par rapport aux espaces intercostaux. Int J Chir 11:501–509, 1951.
56. Putti F: Richerche anatomiche sui linfonodi mammari interni. Chir Ital 7:161–167, 1953.
57. Arão A, Abrão A: Estudo anatomico da cadeia ganglionar mamaria interna em 100 casos. Rev Paul Med 45:317–326, 1954.

Breast Physiology: Normal and Abnormal Development and Function

RENA B. KASS | ANNE T. MANCINO |
ARLAN L. ROSENBLOOM | V. SUZANNE KLIMBERG |
KIRBY I. BLAND

The mammary gland is composed of an epithelial system of ducts and lobuloalveolar secretory units embedded in a mesenchymally derived fat pad. The growth and morphogenesis of the epithelial structures of the breast occur in various stages and are associated with concurrent hormonal changes and affected by genetic mutations. Each stage reflects the effects of systemic hormones on the glandular epithelium as well as the paracrine effects of locally derived growth factors and other regulatory products produced in the stroma. Appreciating the relationship of epithelium to mesenchyme in normal growth is essential for understanding developmental abnormalities and factors that may lead to disease.

This chapter discusses the morphologic, hormonal, paracrine, and genetic changes of the breast. It also discusses the clinical correlates of the various stages of breast development, including that of the embryo, infancy and childhood, puberty, pregnancy, lactation, and menopause.

Embryology to Childhood

MORPHOLOGY

The breast of the human newborn is formed through 10 progressive fetal stages that begin in the sixth week of fetal development.[1] The mammary gland originates from the milk streaks, bilateral ectodermal thickenings that extend from the axilla to the groin. The ectoderm over the thorax invaginates into the surrounding mesenchyme, with subsequent epithelial budding and branching.[2,3] During the later part of pregnancy, this fetal epithelium further canalizes and ultimately differentiates to the end-vesicle stage seen in the newborn.[1] At term birth, the breast has six to eight widely patent ducts that empty at the nipple. Recent anatomical studies confirm a parallel bundle of an additional 25 smaller ducts with

distinct openings at the nipple surface.[4] All of these initial ducts contain one layer of epithelium and one layer of myoepithelial cells, terminating in a dilated blind sac. These so-called "ductules" are the precursors of future lobuloalveolar structures, the ultimate milk-producing units of the breast. Interestingly, despite the large number of actual ducts that drain onto the nipple, one fourth of the breast is drained by one duct and its branches and one half of the breast is drained by only three ducts.[4] Similar to the development of the ductal system, the subareolar lymphatic plexus also develops from the ectoderm.[5]

From birth until 2 years of age, there is wide individual variability in the morphologic and functional stages in the breast, with some neonates having more well-developed lobular structures and others with more secretory epithelial phenotypes.[6] The degree of morphologic differentiation does not correlate with functional ability. The ability of the entire ductal structure to respond to secretory stimuli may even occur in the rudimentary ductal systems.[6] Ultimately, in normal infant development, the differentiated glandular structures involute and only small ductal structures are left remaining within the stroma.[7]

During childhood, the ductal structures and stroma grow isometrically at a rate similar to that of the rest of the body until puberty.[6,8] The lymphatics grow simultaneously with the duct system, maintaining connection with the subareolar plexus.[5] As in the fetal stage, there are no morphologic differences between the sexes.[6]

HORMONES

The initial fetal stages of breast development are relatively independent of sex steroid influence. At birth the withdrawal of maternal steroids results in secretion of neonatal prolactin (PRL) that stimulates newborn breast secretion.

REGULATORY FACTORS AND POTENTIAL GENES

It is currently accepted that epithelial ductal proliferation into the mesenchyme is modulated by local factors, which regulate the epithelial-mesenchymal interaction. Many genes have been expressed in either the epithelium or mesenchyme during mammary embryogenesis, including fibroblast growth factor-7 (FGF-7),[9] FGF,[10] HOX,[11,12] tenascin-C,[13] syndecan-1, hedgehog network genes,[14,15] t-box family of transcription factors,[16] androgen receptor,[17] estrogen receptor,[15] transforming growth factor-α (TGF-α), TGF-β,[18] BCL-2,[6] and epidermal growth factor (EGF) receptor.[4] However, only Lef-1,[19] parathyroid hormone–related protein (PTHrP),[20] and the type 1 parathyroid hormone (PTH)/PTHrP receptor (PTHR-1) are required for mammary and nipple development. A deletion in any one of these can result in a failure of mammogenesis.

CLINICAL CORRELATES

During fetal development the extrathoracic milk streak typically regresses. Failure to completely regress can result in accessory nipple (*polythelia*) and mammary tissue (*polymastia*). The accessory mammary tissue, most often located in the axilla, may swell during pregnancy and if associated with a nipple may function during lactation.[21] Polythelia is most commonly seen on the thorax below healthy breasts. Rare instances of polymastia and polythelia occurring outside the mammary ridge in areas such as the posterior thigh, scapula, face, buttock, and vulva have been described and may be secondary to displaced embryonic crests.[22]

Although typically a purely cosmetic issue, studies have reported an association with genitourinary anomalies in 14.5% to 40% of polythelia cases,[23,24] and some suggest that a urologic workup, including renal ultrasound, be performed on diagnosis. Others have suggested an association with cardiovascular disorders including conduction delays.[23,25] Furthermore, aberrant breast tissue may harbor benign and malignant breast tumors and should be examined clinically.[23]

Mutations in the t-box family of transcription factors, normally activated during mammary embryogenesis, can result in *ulnar mammary syndrome* in humans. This may appear as *mammary hypoplasia, amastia* (lack of breasts), or an extra breast. These and other congenital abnormalities are further described in Chapter 9.

As previously described, PRL stimulates newborn breast secretion. This secretion, called *witch's milk*, contains water, fat, and debris; it occurs in 80% to 90% of infants, regardless of sex.[26,27] The secretion dissipates within 3 to 4 weeks as the influence of maternal sex hormones and PRL decreases. It should not be mechanically expressed, which could predispose to staphylococcal infection and result in breast bud destruction. The secretion may sequester at the nipple epithelium and resemble a pearl. This is called a lactocele and will resolve with time.[27]

Premature thelarche is breast development before 8 years of age without concomitant signs of puberty.

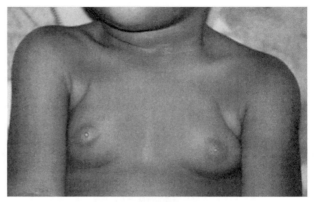

Figure 3-1 Premature thelarche. Fourteen-month-old child with breast development from birth. Height was at the 50th percentile without acceleration, and no other signs of sexual maturation were present. Breast development was considered Tanner stage 3 without nipple maturation. There had been some regression over the several months before this picture was taken.

Usually bilateral, it is most commonly seen within the first 2 years of life. It is believed to be the result of the persistence or increase in the breast tissue present at birth, and it resolves within 3 to 5 years with no adverse sequelae.[28] It has been suggested that although the initial stimulation of the infant breast may be secondary to maternal influences, the persistence of breast tissue may be related to infant hormones that may support breast growth. Persistent elevations of follicle-stimulating hormone (FSH), luteinizing hormone (LH), and estradiol in infants support this hypothesis (Figs. 3-1 and 3-2).[29]

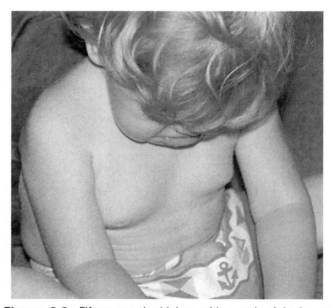

Figure 3-2 Fifteen-month-old boy with mostly right breast enlargement with galactorrhea. Prolactin levels varied from 58 to 100 ng/mL and were unrelated to the cessation of galactorrhea and reduction in breast size by 18 months. Magnetic resonance imaging of the brain was unremarkable at 15 and 21 months of age. Bromocriptine therapy suppressed prolactin levels and was associated with breast regression.

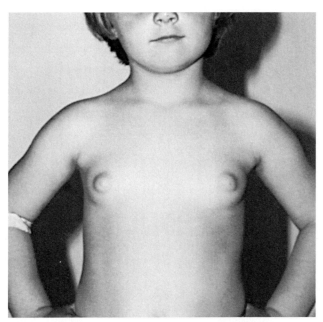

Figure 3-3 Three-and-a-half-year-old girl with central precocious puberty (adolescent levels of gonadotropins and estrogen). Breast development had been present for only a few months but included nipple maturation. Facial maturation was that of a 5- to 6-year-old child. Height age was 4½ years, and osseous maturation was 5 years, 9 months.

A second period of *premature thelarche* may occur after 6 years of age.[30] The reason for breast bud formation is unclear; because it can occur before the rise in estrogen levels, it is unlikely that estrogen is the key signal. Serum androgen levels,[31] free estrogen level,[32] altered

FSH secretion,[33] and altered serum insulin-like growth factor-I (IGF-I)–to–IGF-binding protein-3 ratios have been implicated as potential factors.[34] The breast tissue may persist or regress, but puberty occurs at the usual time and progresses normally. If assessment of bone age reveals no evidence of precocious puberty, no further evaluation is needed.[30]

Breast development before 8 years of age that is accompanied by other signs of puberty defines *precocious puberty*. Altered or premature gonadotropin-releasing hormone (GnRH) secretion may cause central precocious puberty (Fig. 3-3). Although more commonly idiopathic, central precocious puberty can be caused by cerebral infections and granulomatous conditions. Certain tumors, in particular hypothalamic hamartomas, can contain GnRH, and disrupt the inhibition of GnRH, or release TGF-α (a stimulant of GnRH), resulting in precocious puberty. Peripheral precocious puberty may result from the effects of estrogen from food,[35] from ovarian cysts, from constitutionally activated ovaries in McCune-Albright syndrome (a triad of café-au-lait spots, long-bone fibrous dysplasia, and precocious puberty), or in primary hypothyroidism (Fig. 3-4).[27] In addition to a history and physical examination, serum gonadotropin and sex steroid levels should be obtained in the workup of precocious puberty. High levels of both gonadotropins and sex steroids indicate central precocious puberty. Magnetic resonance imaging (MRI) or computed tomography (CT) scanning of the head can be performed to rule out a central lesion before treatment with GnRH analogs. Suppressed (low) levels of gonadotropins and high levels of sex steroids are consistent with peripheral precocious puberty.[36]

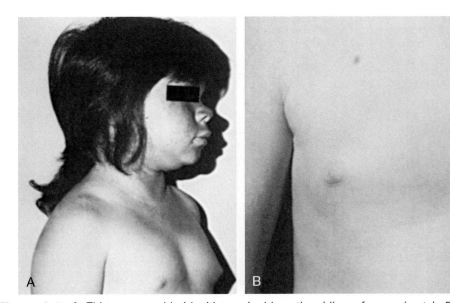

Figure 3-4 **A,** Thirteen-year-old girl with acquired hypothyroidism of approximately 5 years' duration, with Tanner stage 2 breast development despite osseous maturation of 8 years and comparable height age. **B,** Regression of breast development occurred within months of treatment with thyroid hormone. (Courtesy of Dr. A. Rosenbloom, Division of Pediatric Endocrinology, University of Florida, Gainesville, FL.)

Puberty

MORPHOLOGY

Thelarche, the beginning of adult breast development, marks the onset of puberty in the majority of white women and occurs at a mean age of 10 years; in African-American women it occurs at 8.9 years and is usually preceded by the appearance of pubic hair.[37] Changes in the breast contour and events in nipple development characterize the milestones in the staging system detailed by Tanner[38] (Fig. 3-5). However, these outward changes in the breast do not necessarily correlate with underlying structural events occurring with the new hormonal milieu of puberty.

The immature ductal system before puberty is believed to undergo a sequential progression to a mature lobuloalveolar system during adolescent development (Fig. 3-6). First, in the *ductal growth phase*, ducts elongate, ductal epithelium thickens, and periductal connective tissue increases. Stem cells in the ductal tree form club-shaped terminal end buds (TEBs), which are the site of the greatest rate of epithelial proliferation.[39,40] These TEBs are the lead point of advancement from the nipple into the peripheral mammary fat pad (mesenchyme). In the lobuloalveolar phase, these TEBs further divide and form alveolar buds. Within a few years after menarche, most likely with the onset of ovulation, clusters of 8 to 11 of these alveolar buds empty into terminal ductal lobular units. In early puberty, the terminal ductal lobular unit is termed a *virginal lobule or lobule type 1* (Lob 1).[41] Lob 1 is the predominant lobule found at this stage of development. Under the cyclic influence of ovarian hormones, some of the Lob 1 will undergo further division and differentiate into a lobule type 2 (Lob 2). In Lob 2 the alveolar buds become smaller but four times more numerous than those in Lob 1; these buds are termed *ductules* or *alveoli*. Lob 2 are present in moderate numbers during the late teens but then decline after the mid-20s.[42] Ultimately, the greatest number of lobules will be found in the upper outer quadrant.[43,44]

In the mature breast, the subareolar lymphatic plexus contains communications with both deep and superficial intramammary lymphatics and provides a high volume of lymphatic outflow to regional lymph nodes. In lymphatic studies, there appears to a consistent channel that originates from the subareolar plexus and extends to the regional lymph nodes, termed the *sentinel lymphatic channel*.[3]

During the human menstrual cycle the breast progresses through five histologic phases: *early follicular, follicular, luteal, secretory,* and ultimately *menstrual phase,* according to the characterizations of Vogel and colleagues[45] (Fig. 3-7). The *early follicular phase* occurs from day 3 to day 7 in a 28-day cycle. The alveoli are compact, with poorly defined lumina, and sit within a dense stroma. There appears to be only one epithelial cell type at this point. According to some, minimum volume is seen 5 to 7 days after menses.[21] However, a pilot study using MRI demonstrated the minimum volume to occur at day 11.[46] The *follicular phase* follows from day

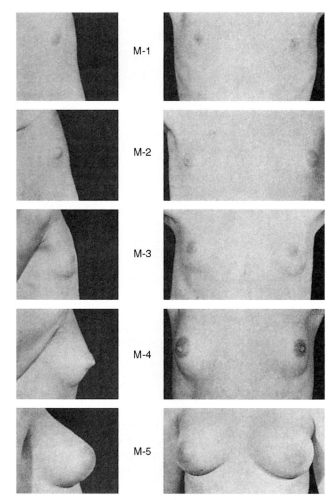

Figure 3-5 Stages of breast development. Stage 1 is preadolescent, with slight elevation of the papilla. In stage 2, there is elevation of the breast and papilla as a small mound, with an increase in size of the areola. Stage 3 is characterized by further enlargement of the breast. In stage 4 the areola and papilla form a secondary mound above the level of the breast. In stage 5, the areola recedes into the general contour of the breast. (From van Wieringen JD, et al: Growth diagrams 1965 Netherlands, Second National Survey on 0–24 year olds. Netherlands Institute for Preventive Medicine TNO. Groningen, Netherlands, Wolters-Noordoff, 1971.)

8 through day 14 and marks the progression of epithelial stratification into three cell types: the luminal, basal myoepithelial cell, and an intermediate cell. *Ovulation* initiates the *luteal phase*, which lasts from day 15 to day 29. In this phase, there is an overall increase in the size of the lobules resulting from alveoli luminal expansion with secretory products, an increase in the number of alveoli, ballooning of the myoepithelial cells with increased glycogen content, and stromal loosening. The maximum size of the lobules and number of alveoli within each lobule is reached in the *secretory phase,* from day 21 to day 27. This is consistent with MRI breast-volume data.[46] During this phase, there is active protein synthesis and apocrine secretion from the luminal epithelial cells. Peak mitotic activity occurs near day 22 to 24, after the progesterone peak and second estrogen peak.[47,48] The *menstrual phase* occurs on days 28 through

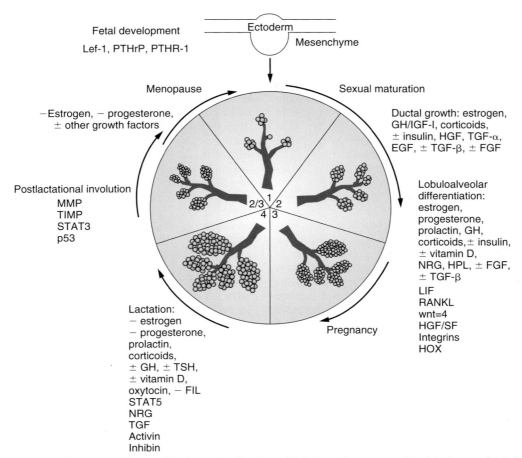

Figure 3-6 Regulatory influences on breast development. Numbers (1, 2, 3, etc.) correspond to lobule type (1, 2, 3, etc.). Ectoderm invaginates into mesenchyme during fetal development. Sexual maturation begins with the onset of puberty through periods of ductal and lobuloalveolar growth and is reflected in the formation of lobules type 1 and 2. Pregnancy initiates the formation of lobule type 3. Lactation, which follows, is associated with lobule type 4. Postlactational involution follows, with regression of lobules. Menopause is characterized by a majority of lobules type 1 and 2, similar to the virgin state. EGF, epidermal growth factor; FGF, fibroblast growth factor; FIL, feedback inhibitor of lactation; GH, growth hormone; HGF, hepatocyte growth factor; HPL, human placental lactogen; IGF-I, insulin-like growth factor-I; Lef-1, transcription factor Lef-1; MMP, metalloproteinase; NRG, neuregulin; PTH, parathyroid hormone; PTHR-1, PTH/PTHrP receptor type 1; PTHrP, parathyroid hormone–related peptide; TIMP, tissue inhibitor of metalloproteinase; TGF-α, transforming growth factor-α; TGF-β, transforming growth factor-β; TSH, thyroid-stimulating hormone. (Modified from Russo IH, Russo J: Role of hormones in mammary cancer initiation and progression. J Mammary Gland Biol Neoplasia 3:49, 1998; and Dickson R, Russo J: Biochemical control of breast development. In Harris J, et al [eds]: Diseases of the breast. Philadelphia, Lippincott Williams & Wilkins, 2000.)

Figure 3-7 Hormonal and histologic changes of the breast during the menstrual cycle. Maximal number of mitosis, breast volume, blood flow, and apoptosis follow the peak in progesterone. FSH, follicle-stimulating hormone; LH, luteinizing hormone. (Modified from Speroff L, Glass R, Kase N: Regulation of the menstrual cycle. In Speroff L, et al: Clinical gynecologic endocrinology and infertility. Baltimore, Lippincott Williams & Wilkins, 1999; and Simpson H, et al: Meta-analysis of sequential luteal-cycle-associated changes in human breast tissue. Breast Cancer Res Treat 63:171, 2000.)

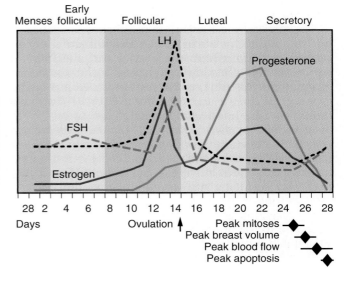

32 and is associated with the withdrawal of estrogen and progesterone. Apocrine secretion lessens and the lobules decrease in size, with fewer alveoli. Russo and Russo[42] suggest that each menstrual cycle fosters new budding that never fully returns to the baseline of the previous cycle. This positive proliferation continues until the mid-30s and plateaus until menopause, when regression is evident.

HORMONES

The pattern of release of GnRH from the hypothalamus initiates and regulates the secretion of FSH and LH seen with puberty. The initial immaturity of the hypothalamic-pituitary axis results in anovulatory cycles for the first 1 to 2 years after menses begin, subjecting the breast and the endometrium to the effects of unopposed estrogen. It is during this period of unopposed estrogen stimulation, considered an "estrogen window,"[49] that the *ductal growth phase* occurs (see Fig. 3-6).

The major hormonal influence on the breast at the onset of puberty is estrogen. A potent mammogen, estrogen primarily stimulates ductal growth but also increases fat deposition and contributes to later phases of development. Impaired ductal growth has been demonstrated in both mice lacking the functional gene for the estrogen receptor (ER) and mice treated with tamoxifen, an ER modulator.[50] The estrogen receptor ERα is thought to be the key mediator of estrogen effects, and in humans, has only been documented in luminal epithelium.[51] Despite its influential role, estrogen is unable to work independently. Lyon's classic experiments using oophorectomized, adrenalectomized, and hypophysectomized rodents demonstrated that a minimum combination of estrogen, growth hormone (GH), and corticoids are necessary to induce ductal growth.[52]

The effects of GH may be mediated by enhancing stromal secretion of IGF-I. IGF-I synergizes with estrogen to increase elongation and growth at the TEB[53] in a paracrine manner. In some reviews, glucocorticoids contribute to the maximal growth of ducts, but extensive ductal growth can occur in its absence.[54] Progesterone does not appear to be essential in early ductal growth.[55]

The precise mechanism that initiates ovulation is unclear, but it is postulated to be a combination of critical estrogen levels from the ovaries and alterations in FSH, LH, and gonadotropin levels.[56] The subsequent monthly progesterone secretion from the corpus luteum exposes the breast to the complete cyclic hormonal milieu of adulthood and facilitates the second phase of glandular growth, which is termed *lobuloalveolar growth*. Progesterone, working through the progesterone receptor (PR), is essential for lobuloalveolar development.[55,57,58] The ratio of the isoforms PR-A and PR-B may play a critical role in modulating the effect of progesterone.[57,58]

However, progesterone cannot independently bring the gland to maturity. Lyons, Li, and Johnson[52] demonstrated that prolactin, GH, estrogen, and glucocorticoids, in addition to progesterone, are necessary for full lobuloalveolar development.

PRL, a member of a multigene family including homologous GH and human placental lactogen (HPL), is also integral to lobuloalveolar development.[59] PRL-deficient knockout mice with adequate progesterone levels exhibited incomplete lobule formation.[60] PRL also works indirectly by facilitating progesterone's actions on the breast. PRL increases progesterone secretion from the corpus luteum by inhibiting progesterone's degradation enzyme, 20α-hydroxysteroid dehydrogenase.[61] In addition, PRL upregulates the PR in the mammary epithelium.[62] Estrogen contributes to lobuloalveolar development by upregulating PRs.[63] Insulin can bind to IGF-I receptors and may contribute to ductal or lobuloalveolar development, but it is not essential.[54,64,65]

Estrogen rises throughout the first half of the menstrual cycle and peaks at midcycle. After the LH surge, ovulation occurs with subsequent production of progesterone by the corpus luteum in the latter half of pregnancy. Progesterone peaks at the end of the third week, concurrently with a smaller second estrogen peak (see Fig. 3-7).

More recent meta-analysis of studies of mammary gland changes during the menstrual cycle reflects a trend of peak physiologic and histologic changes that chronologically follow the peak in progesterone. These changes include a peak in mitosis within 24 hours of the progesterone peak and estimated peaks of breast volume, epithelial volume, and surface temperature within 2 to 4 days after the progesterone peak.[66] These changes may in part explain the clinical signs and symptoms of fullness and tenderness that occur premenstrually. Apoptosis peaks just before menses, approximately 5 days after the progesterone peak[67] (see Fig. 3-7).

REGULATORY FACTORS AND POTENTIAL GENES

The effects of the aforementioned systemic hormones may be mediated through production of local growth factors (see Fig. 3-6). It has been suggested by Anderson and associates[51] that the effects of estrogen and progesterone are mediated by paracrine and juxtacrine factors such as leukemia inhibitory factor (LIF), RANKL, wnt-4, and EGF-like factors secreted by hormone receptor–containing cells as well as stromally derived factors such as IGF-I and IGF-II and FGF. This hypothesis is supported by the documentation that proliferating cells within the mammary epithelium contain neither ERα nor PR but instead are located commonly adjacent to the steroid receptor expressing cells.[68] The continued importance of the mesenchyme in epithelial proliferation and differentiation is evident in ductal and lobuloalveolar growth during puberty.

Hepatocyte growth factor (HGF)/scatter factor (SF) stimulates proliferation of luminal cells and induces branching morphogenesis in myoepithelial cells, resulting in enhanced ductal growth.[69,70] The mammary fibroblast in the breast mesenchyme is the likely source of HGF/SF, whereas its receptor, c-met, is localized to the ductal epithelium, illustrating its potential paracrine role.[71] Adhesion molecules, in particular α₂β₁ integrins, may facilitate HGF-induced branching.[70,72] Hydrocortisone, possibly through induction of the c-met receptor, enhances the tubulogenic effect of HGF and also enhances luminal formation.[69] This may partially explain the finding of Lyons, Li, and Johnson[52] that corticoids are necessary for ductal growth. Tubulogenic activity is not restricted to HGF. TGF-α and EGF induce an increase in duct length, but to a lesser degree.[73]

Neuregulins (NRGs), members of the EGF family of growth factors, are also secreted from the stroma. A specific NRG, heregulin, can activate the EGF receptor and contribute to lobuloalveolar growth and secretory activity.[74,75]

Diet may influence the composition of the mammary fat pad and may also affect glandular growth. Diets deficient in essential fatty acids result in impaired ductal growth and alveolar regression; in contrast, diets rich in unsaturated fat promote parenchymal growth and tumorigenesis and enhance the proliferative effects of EGF.[76–78] The vitamin D receptor, expressed in low levels in the mouse pubertal gland, is upregulated in pregnancy and lactation,[79] the time of lobuloalveolar development in mice, and is upregulated in response to cortisol, prolactin, and insulin.[80] One study has showed that vitamin D, acting through its receptor, appears to be essential in lobuloalveolar development because vitamin D receptor knockout mice had higher numbers of undifferentiated TEBs.[81]

The progression of the ductal epithelium through the mesenchymal stroma is also modulated by a constantly changing ratio of metalloproteinases (MMPs) that degrade the extracellular matrix and tissue inhibitors of metalloproteinase (TIMPs) that inhibit degradation of the extracellular matrix. MMPs may facilitate branching morphogenesis by releasing growth factors sequestered in the matrix. MMP can process TGF-α[82] and cleave IGF,[83] increasing their bioavailability. Continual basement membrane and stromal matrix remodeling are necessary to allow for ductal growth and lobuloalveolar expansion.

Finally, it has been suggested by some, that phosphatase and tensin homolog deleted from chromosome 10 (PTEN), a tumor suppressor gene, plays an essential role in controlling the proliferation and differentiation of mammary epithelial cells. Gang and colleagues[84] demonstrated that the mammary tissue of mice with a PTEN-deleted gene exhibited accelerated ductal extension, excessive side branching, and early lobuloalveolar development with subsequent early mammary tumors.

CLINICAL CORRELATES

Several *normal variants* may occur during pubertal development that may cause unnecessary concern. Development may be initially unilateral and can mimic an isolated breast mass. Biopsy should not be performed as it may result in permanent breast damage. It is also normal that final breast size may be asymmetric; this finding may be secondary to handedness.[30] Rapid growth of the breast may result in pink or white skin striae; these marks should not be confused with the purple striae of *Cushing's syndrome*, particularly if other classic signs of Cushing's syndrome are lacking. Periareolar

hair is common but should not be removed, because infection and irritation may ensue.[30]

Adolescent, juvenile, or *virginal hypertrophy* is a postpubertal continuation of epithelial and stromal growth that results in breasts that can weigh 3 to 8 kg. There can be ancillary breast tissue within the axilla.[85] The diagnosis should be limited to severe breast enlargement that results in skin ulceration or physical limitations. Although typically postpubertal, this type of hypertrophy can also be seen with pregnancy or severe obesity.[86] A familial pattern associated with congenital anonychia has also been described in prepubertal girls.[87] Hypertrophy usually involves both breasts but can be unilateral, suggesting the role of local factors in its cause. ER hypersensitivity,[88] use of the drug penicillamine,[89] and an inherited mutation in the PTEN gene[84] have been implicated in its etiology, with the latter being associated with a higher risk of malignant transformation (Cowden's disease).[84] Workup should include serum estradiol, PRL, FSH, LH, cortisol, somatomedin C, thyroid, and liver function tests, as well as urine 17-keto and hydroxysteroid levels. Typically, however, tests reveal no systemic hormonal imbalances. Discretely palpable masses should be worked up radiographically. Reduction mammaplasty is a treatment option, but hypertrophy may recur, and total mastectomy with reconstruction may ultimately be needed. In such cases, technical success has been achieved by some with nipple- and areolar-sparing techniques.[87] There has been limited experience with pharmaceuticals, including bromocriptine, tamoxifen, danazol, and medroxyprogesterone.[90,91]

Tuberous breast deformity, named because of the similarity of the affected breast appearance to a tuberous plant root, can also be seen during puberty. Most commonly, it presents as hypoplasia in the lower quadrants of a breast; however, it can affect all quadrants and can be associated with herniation of the areolar complex. It can be unilateral or bilateral. The lower pole of the deformed breast has a decreased number of ducts. Anomalies of the underlying fascia and inadvertent involution of the mammary ridge have been hypothesized as possible etiologies. Plastic surgical repair is suggested.[92]

In the adolescent male, *gynecomastia* occurs at age 13 to 14, when male pubertal changes and the sex hormones have established the male pattern.[93] It occurs in 70% of pubertal boys but rarely exceeds the Tanner B2 stage (elevation of the breast and papilla as a small mound)[29,36,94] (Fig. 3-8). Pubertal gynecomastia is usually resolved within several months to 2 years.[30] Generalized obesity can sometimes mimic gynecomastia. The primary complaint is concentric enlargement of breast tissue, but breast and nipple pain can occur in 25% of cases, with tenderness found in 40%. There is rarely a pathologic cause of adolescent gynecomastia, and histology typically reveals proliferation of the ductal and stromal tissue without evidence of lobuloalveolar formation.[6] An initial rise in estrogen levels, altered ratios of peripheral and central androgens to estrogens, increased diurnal periods of estrogen excess, peripheral aromatization of androgen,[29] and cyclo-oxygenase 2–induced aromatase overexpression[95] have been considered causal.

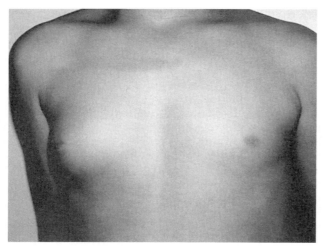

Figure 3-8 Nine-year-old boy with a 1-year history of right-sided gynecomastia. Health, growth, and hormone profile were all normal. Mastectomy was performed for psychologic reasons, and there was no recurrence of problems.

Higher circulating levels of leptin have been measured in pubertal boys with gynecomastia and may play a role in its pathogenesis either through stimulation of aromatase enzyme activity or producing a direct effect on mammary epithelial cells through the leptin or estrogen receptor.[96] Marijuana can cause gynecomastia, and its use should be ruled out.[97] Endocrinopathies, including *testosterone deficiency, LH receptor deficiency,* and *incomplete androgen insensitivity,* may result in breast formation (Fig. 3-9). Rarely, when treated with glucocorticoids, a genetic female completely virilized by congenital adrenal hyperplasia and raised as a male, will undergo adrenal androgen-directed release of suppression of gonadotropins and have breast development (Fig. 3-10).[27] Diagnosis begins with a good breast examination. Breast lipomas, neurofibromas, and carcinomas are more typically nonpainful and eccentrically located. Pubescent gynecomastia may also be the first sign of gonadal tumors[98,99]; therefore, an examination of the testes should also be performed. Serum levels of human chorionic gonadotropin, LH, testosterone, and estrogen can be obtained, with additional levels of prolactin and thyroid function tests if initial tests are abnormal. However, laboratory evaluation is typically reserved for prepubertal or postpubertal males. Cosmetic concerns

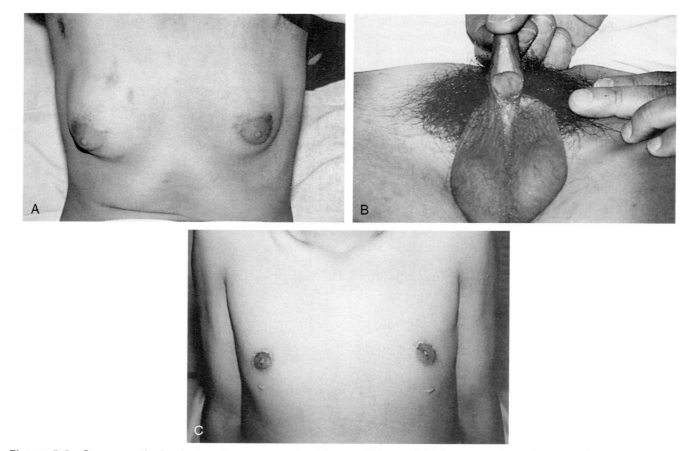

Figure 3-9 Gynecomastia developing at adolescence in a 16-year-old boy with high testosterone and estrogen levels as a result of partial androgen resistance. **A,** Tanner stage 5 breast development. **B,** Penoscrotal hypospadias with relatively small phallus and normal size testicles (this condition has been referred to in the past as Reifenstein's syndrome). **C,** One year after mastectomy. Complete mastectomy is necessary to avoid regeneration of breast tissue.

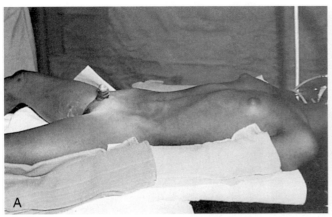
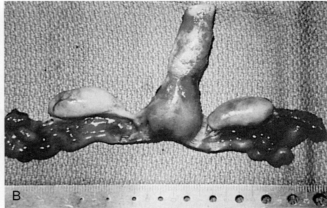

Figure 3-10   Ten-year-old boy with congenital adrenal hyperplasia (CAH) resulting from P-450$_{c21}$–hydroxylase deficiency. Diagnosed at age 3 as a male with CAH, he developed breasts at approximately 6 years of age, when his bone age was sufficiently advanced for normal sexual maturation. He was finally recognized to have no testicular tissue at 10 years of age; despite complete virilization of the urethra, it was realized that the patient was a genetic female. **A,** Appearance at age 10 years. **B,** Normal female internal genitalia removed at age 10 years. This was followed by dramatic loss of breast tissue. The patient was subsequently treated with testosterone replacement therapy and given testicular prostheses.

may lead to consideration of a subcutaneous mastectomy but should be performed only after any underlying organic cause has been ruled out. Although hormonal manipulation has been effective in some cases of postpubertal gynecomastia,[100] hormonal manipulation through the use of an aromatase inhibitor has not been found to be effective in pubertal boys.[101] The failure to respond to hormonal treatment may be secondary to histologic differences as well as to differences in Ki-67 activity seen between pubertal and postpubertal gynecomastia, which may confer sensitivity to treatment.[102]

Failure of estrogen production leads to insufficient development of the ductal system. Lack of estrogen can be related to primary ovarian failure or may result from *hypogonadotropism*. Primary ovarian failure may be the result of direct injury or torsion or may be associated with certain genetic syndromes (Table 3-1). The decreased estrogen level results in abnormal elevation of gonadotropin levels. The most common cause of primary ovarian failure is the Turner syndrome of gonadal dysgenesis. To prevent osteopenia and psychologic problems from sexual infantilism, cyclical estrogen therapy should not be unduly delayed (Figs. 3-11 and 3-12).[103] Intrinsic errors may also occur in aromatase activity and adrenal steroid biosynthesis resulting in failure of female development and virilization; this is most commonly caused by the P-450$_{c21}$–hydroxylase deficiency (Fig. 3-13).[103,104]

Hypogonadotropism may be caused by isolated gonadotropin insufficiency, brain tumors, and several genetic abnormalities. Chronic illness such as diabetes, hypothyroidism, Cushing's syndrome, or hyperprolactinemia can cause a functional hypogonadotropism. Malnutrition or low weight, such as that seen in high-performance athletes, can also cause a functional hypogonadotropism and delayed onset of puberty[105] (see Table 3-1).

Recent studies have demonstrated a positive correlation between tallness in pubertal girls (age 7 to 15)

and increased risk of future breast cancer. It has been suggested that this may be related to persistently high serum IGF levels in tall women.[106] Conversely, overweight children seem to have a decreased risk of breast cancer. It is possible that the fat-derived estrogens cause an earlier differentiation of the breast, decreasing malignant potential.[106]

TABLE 3-1
Failure of Estrogen Production

Primary Ovarian Failure
Direct Injury
Chemotherapy
Radiation
Autoimmune oophoritis
Galactosemia
Genetic Syndromes
Turner syndrome—loss of portion X chromosome
Gonadal dysgenesis with normal chromosomes

Hypogonadotropism
Direct Injury
Brain tumors
Radiation therapy to brain
Genetic Syndromes
Kallmann syndrome—midline facial, hyposmia
Histocytosis X
Bardet-Biedl—autosomal recessive syndrome
Prader-Willi—may get menarche with weight loss
Functional Hypogonadotropism
Chronic illness
Malnutrition
High-performance athlete

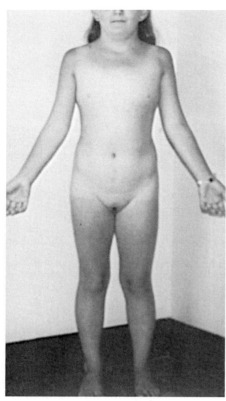

Figure 3-11 Fifteen-year-old girl with Turner syndrome (XO) demonstrating a shieldlike chest with widely separated hypoplastic nipples and lack of sexual maturation.

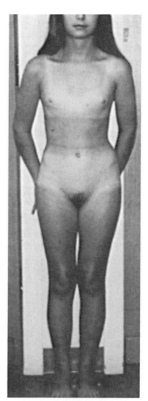

Figure 3-12 Nineteen-year-old girl with Turner syndrome caused by mosaicism (XO/XX) demonstrating hypoplastic widely spaced nipples and some breast development as a result of estrogen therapy.

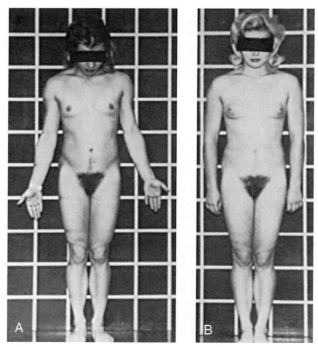

Figure 3-13 **A,** Sixteen-year-old girl with P450$_{c21}$-hydroxylase deficiency not previously recognized. This young woman had a large clitoris removed at age 3 years. She is muscular and has frontal temporal hairline recession, masculine facial features, and hair growth along the linea alba. She is hyperpigmented as a result of high adrenocorticotropic hormone levels. **B,** Following 10 months of hydrocortisone replacement therapy, with association of adrenal androgen production, which had been suppressing pituitary gonadotropin release. With gonadotropic stimulation of the ovaries, she underwent rapid breast development, with marked changes in subcutaneous fat and skin texture.

Pregnancy

MORPHOLOGY

Two phases occur during pregnancy to ultimately prepare the gland for lactation. The first phase, which occurs during early pregnancy, is the proliferation of the distal ducts to create more lobules and more alveoli within each lobule. There is considerable heterogeneity within the pregnant breast. Some lobular units may be resting while others expand with proliferative activity. This proliferation leads to the formation of more differentiated forms of lobules, lobule type 3 (Lob 3) and lobule type 4 (Lob 4). Lob 3 outnumbers the more primitive lobules by the end of the first trimester and can have up to 10 times the alveoli per lobules compared with Lob 1.[107] If the first term pregnancy occurs before the third decade of life, the number of Lob 3 significantly increases.[1] Lob 3 remains the dominant structure in all parous women until the fourth decade of life, after which it starts to decline and involute to Lob 1 and 2 after menopause (see Fig. 3-6).

By the midpoint of pregnancy, the lobuloalveolar framework is in place and differentiation of the lobular units into secretory units begins. Cell proliferation and formation of new alveoli are minimized, and the alveoli differentiate into acini. During the last trimester, the epithelial cells are filled with fat droplets, the acini distend with colostrum (an eosinophilic and proteinaceous secretion), and fat and connective tissue have largely been replaced by glandular proliferation. The increase in breast size during this period is secondary to distention of acini and increased vascularity.[108,109]

HORMONES

In the pregnant state, estrogen, progesterone, and PRL work in concert to prepare the breast for lactation (Fig. 3-14). As in puberty, PRL plays a continued role in lobuloalveolar differentiation. PRL increases beginning at 8 weeks and continues to rise throughout gestation and postpartum.[110,111] HPL, a member of the PRL family, is secreted during the second half of pregnancy. Although HPL has less bioactivity than PRL, by the end of gestation, the HPL concentration is approximately 30 times the concentration of PRL.[110] This suggests that HPL may contribute to the prolactin effects on lobuloalveolar development and final maturation of the gestational gland.[56]

The estrogen increase during gestation parallels that of PRL.[111,112] Estrogen is believed to be a direct and indirect modulator of prolactin secretion. First, estrogen induces the differentiation of anterior pituitary lactotrophs, which secrete PRL. Second, estrogen, through interaction with an estrogen-responsive element and an adjacent transcription factor–binding site, enhances PRL gene expression.[112–115] Finally, estrogen suppresses the secretion of the PRL inhibitory factor dopamine.[116]

With pregnancy, PRL primes the breast for lactation; however, initiation of lactogenesis is inhibited by the presence of progesterone. Although estrogen and progesterone are necessary for PRL receptor expression, paradoxically, progesterone reduces the binding and antagonizes the positive effects of PRL at its receptor.[117–119] Progesterone can directly suppress production of the milk protein casein by stimulating the production of a transcription inhibitor.[120]

REGULATORY FACTORS AND POTENTIAL GENES

As seen in puberty, NRG is expressed in the stroma of the mouse mammary gland during pregnancy.[74] In some in vivo models, NRG stimulated alveoli development and secretory activity, suggesting a potential role in mediating PRL. In other models (MMTV mice), however, NRG halted the progression of the lobuloalveolar system at the TEB stage, consistent with prolactin deficiency.[74,121] HRG α, a specific NRG, may play a critical role in lobuloalveolar development and subsequent lactogenesis.[75] Activins and inhibins, STAT5[122] (members of the TGF-β family) may also play a role in modulating glandular development. Mutations in these factors result in an inhibition of alveolar development during pregnancy.[122,123] Certain intracellular signaling molecules, including the transcription factors A-myb, c-erbB, hox9a, hox9b, hox9d, cell cycle protein cyclin D1,[124–127] RANK-L,[57] and slug transcription factor,[128] may play a role in the regulation of lobuloalveolar development. Deletions of the genes coding for several of these factors have caused impairment of lobuloalveolar development.[100–103]

With physiologic progression to puberty, proper balance between matrix-MMP,[129,130] and its inhibitor TIMP-1[106] initiates an important role in lobuloalveolar development during pregnancy and subsequent ability to lactate. For example, overexpression of TIMP caused a reduction in extracellular matrix remodeling and resulted in inhibition of lobuloalveolar development during pregnancy.[131]

CLINICAL CORRELATES

Gravid hypertrophy is the rapid and massive enlargement of the breast during pregnancy. Clinically and histologically it resembles that of *juvenile hypertrophy* discussed earlier. It may appear during a second pregnancy or after a normal first gestation. Its appearance is a risk factor for recurrence during future pregnancies.[91]

Epidemiologic studies suggest that early parity has a protective effect against breast cancer. In an attempt to explain the protective effect of parity, the proliferative activity, steroid receptors, angiogenic index, and protease inhibitors, serpin and MDGI were measured in the three types of lobules, Lob 1, Lob 2, Lob 3, in parous and nulliparous women.[132,133] Lob 1, the most undifferentiated lobule, had the highest rate of proliferation and highest percentage of cells that expressed both ERs and PRs. Of note, the cells that were highly proliferating were not the same population that expressed ER/PR receptors.[133] Lob 1 also had the highest angiogenic index, the number of blood vessels in relation to number of alveoli, and no expression of the protease inhibitors. In the progression from Lob 1 to Lob 3, proliferation, the percentage of lobules that are receptor positive, and

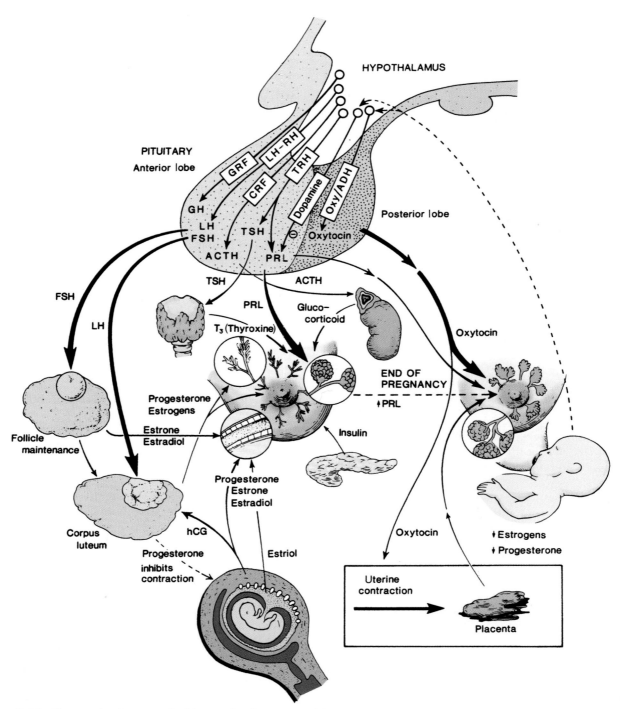

Figure 3-14 Neuroendocrine control of breast development and function. Luteinizing hormone–releasing hormone (LH-RH), also known as gonadotropin-releasing hormone (GnRH), from the hypothalamus stimulates the pituitary secretion of luteinizing hormone (LH) and follicle-stimulating hormone (FSH). Thyrotropin-releasing hormone (TRH) from the hypothalamus stimulates the release of prolactin (PRL), against the inhibitory control of dopamine from the hypothalamus. The pituitary gonadotropins stimulate ovarian synthesis and the release of progesterone and estrogen, which have mammotrophic effects. Pregnancy enhances the secretion of estrogen and progesterone from the corpus luteum during the first 12 weeks and subsequently from the placenta. After delivery, PRL secretion increases. Neural stimuli from suckling stimulates prolactin and oxytocin release. Milk let-down occurs. Other hormones are depicted that contribute to the growth and function of the mammary gland, including glucocorticoid, growth hormone (GH), insulin, and thyroxin. ACTH, Adrenocorticotropic hormone; ADH, antidiuretic hormone; CRF, corticotropin-releasing factor; GRF, growth hormone–releasing factor; hCG, human chorionic gonadotropin; TSH, thyroid-stimulating hormone.

the angiogenic index decreases, and there is expression of the protease inhibitors. Postmenopausal women who were parous ultimately had the same percentage of Lob 1 as the nulliparous women, but the proliferative index of Lob 1 in nulliparous women was higher than that of parous women. This difference persisted through menopause.[134-136] It has been suggested that cancer initiation involves the interaction of a carcinogen with undifferentiated, highly proliferating mammary epithelium,[1] and the Lob 1 of the nulliparous woman would seem to be a prime target.

Lactation

MORPHOLOGY AND PRODUCT

Whereas the first half of pregnancy is marked by significant ductal and lobuloalveolar proliferation and formation of Lob 3 structures and some Lob 4 structures, the second half of gestation involves the final maturation of the gland into the secretory organ of lactation. The ability to synthesize and secrete the milk product is termed *lactogenesis*. This is composed of two stages. Lactogenesis I is the synthesis of unique milk components. This portion of the phase is accompanied by morphologic changes in the alveolar epithelial cell with an increase in protein synthetic structures (i.e., rough endoplasmic reticulum, mitochondria, and Golgi apparatus). Complex protein, milk fat, and lactose synthetic pathways are activated, but minimal secretion into the alveoli lumina occurs.[26,109] Studies measuring urine lactose, an index of the breast's synthetic activity, have confirmed that this stage begins, in most mothers, between 15 and 20 weeks of gestation.[137] The alveoli distend with colostrum, an immature milk product, and along with increased vascularity contribute to the increase in breast volume seen in the latter part of gestation. Lob 4, formed during pregnancy, persists throughout lactation[63] (see Fig. 3-6).

Lactogenesis II is the initiation of significant milk secretion at or just after parturition[137] and is marked by a rise in citrate and α-lactalbumin.[54] The initial product is colostrum, which combines both nutritional elements and passive immunity for the infant. Transitional milk follows with less immunoglobulin and total protein. The ultimate product is mature milk that is composed of fat and protein suspended in a lactose solution. The fat, lactose, and protein are secreted in an apocrine fashion. Lactose and protein are also secreted in a merocrine fashion[26] (Fig. 3-15). Mature milk secretion begins 30 to 40 hours postpartum[137] and averages 1 to 2 ml/g of breast tissue per day. The rate of lactation remains constant for the first 6 months of lactation.[138-140] During lactation the *stromal lymphatics* increase in comparison to other periods. Interepithelial gaps widen, allowing for more direct uptake of particles and fluids and improved clearance from the breast.[141]

Following weaning, the breast involutes and returns to a state resembling that of prepregnancy. The lobules decrease in size, with a decrease in the number of alveoli per lobule. The ducts are not involved, in contrast with menopausal involution when both the lobules and ducts are reduced in number. There are two phases of postlactational involution. The first phase is reversible and is associated with the accumulation of milk. It is triggered by either physical distortion of the luminal epithelial cells or by accumulation of apoptosis-inducing factors in the milk.[142] The second phase is characterized by active tissue remodeling, including destruction of basement membranes and alveolar structure and irreversible loss of the differentiated function of the mammary gland.[143,144]

HORMONES

The physiologic importance of PRL and related peptides in mammary gland growth and differentiation is seen with lactation, the terminal state of differentiation of the mature mammary gland (see Figs. 3-14 and 3-15). PRL is the principal hormone for the synthesis of milk proteins and the maintenance of lactation.[8] Production of casein, the primary milk protein, does not occur in the absence of PRL.[56] This hormone is secreted in increasing amounts throughout pregnancy and peaks before delivery. However, the presence of the PRL inhibitory factor, luteal, and placental sex steroids, especially progesterone, prohibits PRL from achieving its full lactational effect.

Glucocorticoids work along with PRL to differentiate mammary epithelium and stimulate milk synthesis and secretion. Both glucocorticoids and their receptors are increased in late pregnancy and lactation. Progesterone binds the glucocorticoid receptor and acts as a glucocorticoid antagonist.[109]

After birth, in the background of dissipating progesterone, PRL, in concert with glucocorticoids, is able to initiate lactogenesis II. Neural stimuli from suckling enhance the release of PRL from the anterior pituitary gland. PRL then binds its membrane receptor. An intracellular portion of the receptor associates with Jak2, a tyrosine kinase, which ultimately phosphorylates STAT5a.[145] Isolated disruptions of STAT5a in mice have resulted in failure to lactate.[146] A dimeric complex of STAT5a couples with the glucocorticoid receptor, forming a ternary complex that then translocates to the nucleus and alters mRNA synthesis.[8] The mRNA of certain milk proteins can positively feedback on further gene expression (see Fig. 3-15).[147]

Several stimulatory secretagogues of prolactin have been enumerated, including estrogen,[148] hypothalamic peptides, thyrotropin-releasing hormone and vasoactive intestinal peptide,[149,150] and local factors EGF[151] and FGF.[152] Oral thyrotropin-releasing hormone may have benefits in improving lactation in women who occasionally breastfeed by increasing PRL levels. In these women, their baseline PRLs were lower than that of average fully breastfeeding women.[153] Extrapituitary synthesis of PRL occurs in the mammary gland and contributes to the high levels of the hormone secreted into the milk. Maturation of the newborn and fetal hypothalamic neuroendocrine system may be modulated by both PRL in the milk and PRL secreted into the amniotic fluid by the uterine decidua.[154]

Oxytocin is responsible for release of stored milk, commonly referred to as *milk let-down*. Oxytocin is secreted

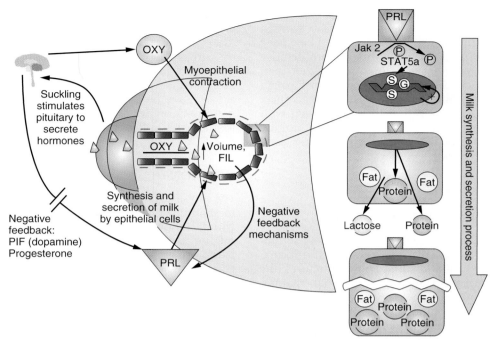

Figure 3-15 Control of lactation. Suckling stimulates the pituitary to secrete oxytocin (OXY), which causes myoepithelial contraction and milk release, and prolactin (PRL), which promotes synthesis and secretion of milk. Increased alveolar intraluminal volume, milk levels of feedback inhibitor of lactation (FIL), and systemic hormone (dopamine and progesterone) levels inhibit PRL action. Expanded view details PRL action on the epithelial cell. PRL binds its transmembrane receptor, activating the Jak-STAT pathway with resultant phosphorylation of STAT5a. A ternary complex of a STAT5a dimer (S-S) with a glucocorticoid receptor (G) forms and binds DNA in the nucleus, stimulating production of milk proteins. The mRNA of certain milk proteins can positively feedback on further gene expression. Complex protein, milk fat, and lactose synthetic pathways are activated. Lactose and some milk proteins can be secreted in a merocrine fashion. Other milk proteins and fats are stored in vesicles in the apex of the luminal epithelial cell. The proteins and fats are then secreted into the lumen along with the apical portion of the cell (apocrine secretion). PIF, PRL inhibitory factor.

from the posterior pituitary by a sensory stimulation from the nipple-areola complex, via T4, T5, and T6 sensory afferent nerve roots. Uniquely, it can be secreted in anticipation of nursing in the presence of a crying infant[56] and can be inhibited by pain and embarrassment.[27] Oxytocin stimulates contraction of the myoepithelial cells surrounding the acini and small ducts, resulting in an expulsion of milk into the lactiferous sinuses.

Lactogens of GH, PRL, and placental origin are structurally related hormones and may, to some extent, be interchangeable in function. Deficiency in one of them is not sufficient to cause lack of mammary gland development and function. For example, women with pituitary dwarfism who lack detectable GH, women who have had a pituitary adenoma removed with no subsequent rise in PRL during pregnancy or lactation,[155] and women with low levels of HPL[155] had normal pregnancies and were able to breastfeed.

Glucocorticoid and systemic lactogenic hormones act as survival factors both during lactation and through the phase of involution.[156] Decreasing levels of systemic hormones allow for increasing apoptosis and progression into the second phase of involution.

REGULATORY FACTORS AND POTENTIAL GENES

Cell-cell interactions play a regulatory role in lobuloalveolar development and milk synthesis. Alterations in the expression of E-cadherin in luminal epithelial cells and P-cadherin in myoepithelial cells[157] vary the onset of lobuloalveolar development and milk synthesis.[158,159] The role of hedgehog network genes in lactogenesis is still being elucidated.[14] Certain nuclear factor I proteins may also contribute to the control of lactation and involution.[160]

It has been noted that each breast has an independent rate of milk synthesis, suggesting a more important role for local factors in modulating function. Systemic factors, particularly PRL, do not appear to regulate the rate of milk synthesis. Luminal volume may contribute to synthesis rate by altering the interaction between the basement membrane and the lactocyte, leading to an inhibition of the PRL receptor.[161,162] Breast volume, however, is not the primary control of milk synthesis. Lactating goats, whose full breasts demonstrated a decrease in milk synthesis, had a resurgence of milk production when the milk was emptied and replaced isovolumetrically with a sucrose solution, suggesting that a compound within the milk was providing negative feedback. This intrinsic milk factor, the feedback inhibitor of lactation, is now thought to modulate local control of milk synthesis. This compound has been noted in many species, including women, and has been found to inhibit lactocyte differentiation, disrupt Golgi vesicle secretion, and inhibit protein synthesis in lactocytes.[163]

Involution requires active gene expression. *Milk stasis* is thought to initiate apoptosis of mammary epithelial cells through activation of p53- and Stat 3–mediated pathways (see Fig. 3-6).[164] During stage 1, there is upregulation of SGP-2, Stat 3, Fas antigen, WDNM1, and other TIMPs[165,166] and downregulation STAT5a and STAT5b.[166,167] During this first phase, local factors are sufficient to induce alveolar cell death, even in the presence of systemic lactogenic hormones. Insulin, dexamethasone, PRL, and their combinations did not affect expression of WDNM1 and SGP-2 genes. EGF, however, strongly inhibited the expression of WDNM1 and SGP2 in cell culture, and the addition of EGF with insulin completely protected the cells in culture from apoptosis.[168] Thus, EGF acts like a survival factor[168]; it is possible that loss of EGF induces gain of a death signal and leads to stage 1 of involution.

The second stage is characterized by the upregulation of MMPs gelatinase A and stromelysin-1 and serine protease urokinase-type plasminogen activator and downregulation of the inhibitor TIMP-1 and activation of proteinase-dependent pathways.[143] This change in ratio of MMP to TIMP, favoring MMP, is thought to correlate with the loss of expression of B-casein, a marker for milk production. The addition of TIMP-1 to change the ratio in the opposite direction favors cell survival and maintenance of secretory phenotype.[169] The role of other genes in lactational involution, TGF-α,[170] are currently being elucidated and may ultimately offer insight into the mechanisms of tumorigenesis.

CLINICAL CORRELATES

Chapman and Perez-Escamilla[171] have identified risk factors for *delayed onset of lactation*. These factors include lack of infant suckling, unscheduled cesarean delivery or vaginal delivery with prolonged stage 2 labor, and obesity. In these women, delay of lactogenesis II may be more than 72 hours postpartum. They should be encouraged to have frequent nursing sessions to potentially enhance the onset of lactation.[171] Progesterone, as described previously, inhibits the onset of lactogenesis II. Women who have portions of *retained placenta* may continue to have sufficient progesterone levels to inhibit their milk synthesis. The delay persists until the fragments are removed.[172,173] As described earlier, the exact role of insulin in lactogenesis is unclear; however, it has been observed that patients with *type 1 insulin-dependent diabetes mellitus* have a 24-hour delay in the onset of lactogenesis II. With assurance and prior knowledge of this information, these mothers can have success with breastfeeding.[172,173] Lactogenesis may also be affected by a high body mass index.[174]

Although it was once concluded that women with smaller breasts had *inadequate milk production* and less success with breastfeeding, this has now been disproved. New computerized topographical techniques (computer breast measurement) have allowed breast physiologists to study breast growth during pregnancy, short-term milk synthesis (between feeding intervals), and the degree of fullness without interrupting normal breastfeeding patterns.[137] Women with smaller-capacity breasts achieved lactational success by increasing the frequency of feedings and the degree of breast emptying with each feeding. Women with larger-capacity breasts have more flexibility in scheduling their feedings and can go longer at night without compromising their synthesis capabilities.[137]

Women who have minimal breast growth during pregnancy should not be dissuaded from breastfeeding. Women who had only small breast growth during pregnancy, with only a small increase in lactose in their urine, had compensatory growth during the first month postpartum. The growth during this month was equivalent to the growth of other women from conception to delivery.[137] Vigorous aerobic exercise should not be a deterrent to breastfeeding because it affects neither the volume nor the composition of breast milk.[175]

In the small subset of women who have lactational insufficiency secondary to low levels of prolactin, drugs such as metoclopramide have been shown to increase the secretion of PRL. Low levels of PRL should be documented and need to be measured 45 minutes after suckling. As mentioned, oral thyrotropin-releasing hormone may improve lactation in insufficient women noted to have low levels of PRL, although hyperthyroidism in the mother may be a side effect.[153] Lactational failure may be the first sign of *Sheehan's syndrome* (infarction of the pituitary gland with ensuing insufficiency of PRL and other hormones). Other rarer causes of lactational failure include lymphocytic hypophysitis, isolated hypoprolactinemia, or hypoprolactinemia as part of a generalized pituitary deficiency.[27]

Galactorrhea is the inappropriate secretion of milky fluid in the absence of pregnancy or breastfeeding for more than 6 months. The amount varies from minimal to excessive and may be produced spontaneously or require manual expression. White, clear, or yellowish fluid is produced from multiple ducts and may involve one or both breasts. Amenorrhea is often associated with galactorrhea,[176,177] but menses may be normal even in serious hormonal disorders. A variety of endocrine and nonendocrine disorders produce galactorrhea, involving either elevation of serum PRL levels or altered responsiveness to normal PRL levels.[178] In women, galactorrhea is usually seen when PRL levels reach 200 ng/ml, but in males it is rare to see galactorrhea even with much higher levels.[179]

Stress from exercise, surgery, sexual intercourse, or sleep can inhibit PRL inhibitory factor release, leading to an increase in PRL.[180] Drugs can stimulate PRL secretion either through direct stimulation of lactotrophs or by decreasing dopamine availability.[179,180] Drug-induced galactorrhea should resolve within 3 to 6 months after the drug is discontinued. Pituitary tumors and hypothalamic lesions may cause galactorrhea.[181] In hypothyroidism, excess thyrotropin-releasing hormone acts on the pituitary as a PRL-releasing factor and increases PRL secretion. Galactorrhea may also be associated with adrenal insufficiency,[182] Cushing's syndrome,[183] acromegaly,[184] renal failure,[185] or lung/renal tumors (ectopic PRL secretion).[186] The afferent neural pathways normally stimulated by suckling may also be stimulated with mastectomy, thoracotomy, spinal lesions, or herpes zoster.

The workup should include a detailed history and a fasting serum PRL level. If PRL levels are elevated and physiologic or pharmacologic causes are excluded, further workup is needed. A serum thyroid-stimulating hormone level should be measured and if elevated, it should be treated with thyroxin. High-resolution CT[187] or MRI should be obtained to exclude a pituitary tumor.

In patients with PRL levels less than 100 ng/ml and no evidence of a pituitary tumor, no treatment is needed. These patients should be followed with measurement of yearly PRL levels. If the patient wishes to become pregnant or desires cessation of galactorrhea, bromocriptine may be used. Of note, the presence of a prolactinoma does not contraindicate the use of oral contraceptives or pregnancy.[56]

Menopause

MORPHOLOGY

As the female approaches menopause, there is an increased number of Lob 1 and a decline in Lob 2 and Lob 3, with all women by the end of the fifth decade having mostly Lob 1. Independent of age, nulliparous women have 65% to 80% Lob 1, 10% to 35% Lob 2, and 0% to 5% Lob 3. Parous women, from postlactational involution to the fourth decade, have 70% to 90% of Lob 3. After the fourth decade their breasts start to involute, and after menopause the breakdown of lobular percentages are equivalent to those of nulliparous women (see Fig. 3-6).

Menopause otherwise progresses in much the same manner in both parous and nulliparous women. The climacteric phase from age 45 to 55 has a moderate decrease in glandular epithelium. This is followed by the postmenopausal phase, which typically occurs after age 50. During the postmenopausal phase, the glandular epithelium undergoes apoptosis, the interlobular stomal tissue regresses, and there is replacement by fat. The intralobular tissue is replaced by collagen. Menopausal involution results in reduction of the number of ducts and lobules. Fat intercalates the fibrous separations, so there are no well-defined quadrants or fascial planes. Lymphatic channels are also reduced in number.[5] Only residual islands of ductal tissue remain scattered throughout the fibrous tissue and fat.[26]

HORMONES

The ovarian hormones, estrogen and progesterone, have declined, and the ovarian androgens, androstenedione, testosterone, and dehydroepiandrosterone, become predominant.

REGULATORY FACTORS AND POTENTIAL GENES

Interestingly, little is known about factors responsible for this process.

CLINICAL CORRELATES

Age is considered a prominent risk factor for the development of breast cancer; most breast cancers (nearly two thirds) are seen in postmenopausal women. As discussed previously, postmenopausal women return to a high percentage of Lob 1, and in nulliparous women these Lob 1 cells have a higher proliferative index than that of parous women. Thus, postmenopausal women have ductile and lobular tissues that are more susceptible to interaction with carcinogens. Furthermore, the more highly proliferative cells in nulliparous women add to this risk. Diminished lymphatic capacity in postmenopausal women may impair localization of the sentinel lymph nodes and limit the utility of this technique in this higher risk group of women.[5]

REFERENCES

1. Russo J, Hu YF, Silva ID, Russo IH: Cancer risk related to mammary gland structure and development. Microsc Res Tech 52:204–223, 2001.
2. Cardiff RD, Wellings SR: The comparative pathology of human and mouse mammary glands. J Mammary Gland Biol Neoplasia 4:105–222, 1999.
3. Jolicoeur F: Intrauterine breast development and the mammary myoepithelial lineage. J Mammary Gland Biol Neoplasia 10:199–210, 2005.
4. Going JJ, Moffat DF: Escaping from Flatland: Clinical and biological aspects of human mammary duct anatomy in three dimensions. J Pathol 203:538–544, 2004.
5. Kern KA: Sentinel lymph node mapping in breast cancer using subareolar injection of blue dye. J Am Coll Surg 189:539–545, 1999.
6. Howard BA, Gusterson BA: Human breast development. J Mammary Gland Biol Neoplasia 5:119–137, 2000.
7. Anbazhagan R, Bartek J, Monaghan P, Gusterson BA: Growth and development of the human infant breast. Am J Anat 192:407–417, 1991.
8. Horseman ND: Prolactin and mammary gland development. J Mammary Gland Biol Neoplasia 4:79–88, 1999.
9. Cunha GR, Hom YK: Role of mesenchymal-epithelial interactions in mammary gland development. J Mammary Gland Biol Neoplasia 1:21–35, 1996.
10. Robinson GW: Identification of signaling pathways in early mammary gland development by mouse genetics. Breast Cancer Res 6:105–108, 2004.
11. Chen H, Sukumar S: Role of homeobox genes in normal mammary gland development and breast tumorigenesis. J Mammary Gland Biol Neoplasia 8:159–175, 2003.
12. Lewis MT: Homeobox genes in mammary gland development and neoplasia. Breast Cancer Res 2:158–169, 2000.
13. Chiquet-Ehrismann R, Mackie EJ, Pearson CA, Sakakura T: Tenascin: An extracellular matrix protein involved in tissue interactions during fetal development and oncogenesis. Cell 47:131–139, 1986.
14. Lewis MT, Veltmaat JM: Next stop, the twilight zone: Hedgehog network regulation of mammary gland development. J Mammary Gland Biol Neoplasia 9:165–181, 2004.
15. Robinson GW, Karpf AB, Kratochwil K: Regulation of mammary gland development by tissue interaction. J Mammary Gland Biol Neoplasia 4:9–19, 1999.
16. Bamshad M, Lin RC, Law DJ, et al: Mutations in human TBX3 alter limb, apocrine and genital development in ulnar-mammary syndrome. Nat Genet 16:311–315, 1997.

17. Sakakura T: Mammary embryogenesis. In Neville MC, Daniel CW (eds): The mammary gland: Development, regulation and function. New York, Plenum Press, 1987.

18. Osin PP, Anbazhagan R, Bartkova J, et al: Breast development gives insights into breast disease. Histopathology 33:275–283, 1998.

19. Ven Genderen C, Okamura R, Farinas I, et al: Development of several organs that require inductive epithelial-mesenchymal interactions is impaired in LEF-1 deficient mice. Genes Dev 8: 2691–2703, 1994.

20. Foley J, Dann P, Hong J, et al: Parathyroid hormone-related protein maintains mammary epithelial fate and triggers nipple skin differentiation during embryonic breast development. Development 128:513–525, 2001.

21. Osborne M: Breast development and anatomy. In Harris JR, Lippman ME, Morrow M, Osborne CK (eds): Diseases of the breast. Philadelphia, Lippincott Williams & Wilkins, 2000.

22. Leung W, Heaton JP, Morales A: An uncommon urologic presentation of a supernumerary breast. Urology 50:122–124, 1997.

23. Loukas M, Clarke P, Tubbs RS: Accessory breasts: A historical and current perspective. Am Surg 73:525–528, 2007.

24. Varsano IB, Jaber L, Garty BZ, et al: Urinary tract abnormalities in children with supernumerary nipples. Pediatrics 73:103–105, 1984.

25. Urbani CE: Supernumerary nipple and cardiocutaneous associations. J Am Acad Dermatol 50:e9 (author reply) e10, 2004.

26. McCarty KS Jr: Breast. In Sternberg SS (ed): Histology for pathologists. Philadelphia, Lippincott-Raven, 1997.

27. Rosenbloom A: Breast physiology: Normal and abnormal development and function. In Bland KI, Copeland EM III: The breast: Comprehensive management of benign and malignant diseases. Philadelphia, WB Saunders, 1998.

28. Mills JL, Stolley PD, Davies J, Moshang T Jr: Premature thelarche. Natural history and etiologic investigation. Am J Dis Child 135: 743–745, 1981.

29. Laurence DJ, Monaghan P, Gusterson BA: The development of the normal human breast. Oxf Rev Reprod Biol 13:149–174, 1991.

30. Sloand E: Pediatric and adolescent breast health. Lippincott's Prim Care Pract 2:170–175, 1998.

31. Murakami M, Kawai K, Higuchi K, et al: Correlation between breast development and hormone profiles in pubertal girls. Nippon Sanka Fujinka Gakkai Zasshi 40:561–567, 1988.

32. Radfar N, Ansusingha K, Kenny FM: Circulating bound and free estradiol and estrone during normal growth and development and in premature thelarche and isosexual precocity. J Pediatr 89:719–723, 1976.

33. Stanhope R: Studies of gonadotrophin pulsatility and pelvic ultrasound examinations distinguish between isolated premature thelarche and central precocious puberty. Eur J Pediatr 145: 190–194, 1986.

34. Sales DS, Moreira AC, Camacho-Hubner C, et al: Serum insulin-like growth factor (IGF)-I and IGF-binding protein-3 in girls with premature thelarche. J Pediatr Endocrinol Metab 16:827–833, 2003.

35. Bongiovanni AM: An epidemic of premature thelarche in Puerto Rico. J Pediatr 103:245–246, 1983.

36. Styne D: Puberty. In Greenspan, FS (ed): Basic and clinical endocrinology. New York, McGraw-Hill, 2001.

37. Herman-Giddens ME, Slora EJ, Wasserman RC, et al: Secondary sexual characteristics and menses in young girls seen in office practice: A study from the Pediatric Research in Office Settings network. Pediatrics 99:505–512, 1997.

38. Marshall WA, Tanner JM: Variations in pattern of pubertal changes in girls. Arch Dis Child 44:291–303, 1969.

39. Daniel C, Silberstein G: Postnatal development of the rodent mammary gland. In Neville MC, Daniel CW (eds): The mammary gland: Development, regulation, and function. New York, Plenum Press, 1987.

40. Russo IH, Medado J, Russo J: Endocrine influences on the mammary gland. In Jones T, Hunt E (eds): Integument and mammary glands. Berlin, Springer-Verlag, 1989.

41. Soderquist AM, Todderud G, Carpenter G: Elevated membrane association of phospholipase C-gamma 1 in MDA-468 mammary tumor cells. Cancer Res 52:4526–4529, 1992.

42. Russo J, Russo IH: Development of human mammary glands. In Neville MC, Daniel CW (eds): The mammary gland: Development, regulation, and function. New York, Plenum Press, 1987.

43. Shlykov IP, Chumachenko PA, Anokhina MA: Development of the female mammary gland at young ages (morphometric data). Arkh Anat Gistol Embriol 85:54–59, 1983.

44. Hutson SW, Cowen PN, Bird CC: Morphometric studies of age related changes in normal human breast and their significance for evolution of mammary cancer. J Clin Pathol 38:281–287, 1985.

45. Vogel PM, Georgiade NG, Fetter BF, et al: The correlation of histologic changes in the human breast with the menstrual cycle. Am J Pathol 104:23–34, 1981.

46. Hussain Z, Roberts N, Whitehouse GH, et al: Estimation of breast volume and its variation during the menstrual cycle using MRI and stereology. Br J Radiol 72:236–245, 1999.

47. Longacre TA, Bartow SA: A correlative morphologic study of human breast and endometrium in the menstrual cycle. Am J Surg Pathol 10:382–393, 1986.

48. Ferguson DJ, Anderson TJ: Morphological evaluation of cell turnover in relation to the menstrual cycle in the "resting" human breast. Br J Cancer 44:177–181, 1981.

49. Korenman SG: The endocrinology of breast cancer. Cancer 46(4 suppl):874–878, 1980.

50. Shyamala G: Progesterone signaling and mammary gland morphogenesis. J Mammary Gland Biol Neoplasia 4:89–104, 1999.

51. Anderson E, Clarke RB: Steroid receptors and cell cycle in normal mammary epithelium. J Mammary Gland Biol Neoplasia 9:3–13, 2004.

52. Lyons WR, Li CH, Johnson RE: The hormonal control of mammary growth and lactation. Recent Prog Horm Res 14:219–48, discussion 248–254, 1958.

53. Kleinberg DL: Early mammary development: growth hormone and IGF-1. J Mammary Gland Biol Neoplasia 2:49–57, 1997.

54. Topper YJ, Freeman CS: Multiple hormone interactions in the developmental biology of the mammary gland. Physiol Rev 60:1049–1106, 1980.

55. Lydon JP, DeMayo FJ, Funk CR, et al: Mice lacking progesterone receptor exhibit pleiotropic reproductive abnormalities. Genes Dev 9:2266–2278, 1995.

56. Speroff L, Glass RG, Kase NG: The breast: clinical gynecologic endocrinology and infertility. Philadelphia, Lippincott Williams & Wilkins, 1999.

57. Conneely OM, Jericevic BM, Lydon JP: Progesterone receptors in mammary gland development and tumorigenesis. J Mammary Gland Biol Neoplasia 8:205–214, 2003.

58. Lamote I, Meyer E, Massart-Leen AM, Burvenich C: Sex steroids and growth factors in the regulation of mammary gland proliferation, differentiation, and involution. Steroids 69:145–159, 2004.

59. Moore DD, Conkling MA, Goodman HM: Human growth hormone: A multigene family. Cell 29:285–286, 1982.

60. Ormandy CJ, Camus A, Barra J, et al: Null mutation of the prolactin receptor gene produces multiple reproductive defects in the mouse. Genes Dev 11:167–718, 1997.

61. Albarracin CT, Parmer TG, Duan WR, et al: Identification of a major prolactin-regulated protein as 20 α-hydroxysteroid dehydrogenase: coordinate regulation of its activity, protein content, and messenger ribonucleic acid expression. Endocrinology 134: 2453–2460, 1994.

62. Ormandy CJ, Graham J, Kelly PA, et al: The effect of progestins on prolactin receptor gene transcription in human breast cancer cells. DNA Cell Biol 11:721–726, 1992.

63. Russo IH, Russo J: Role of hormones in mammary cancer initiation and progression. J Mammary Gland Biol Neoplasia 3:49–61, 1998.

64. Friedberg SH, Oka T, Topper YJ: Development of insulin-sensitivity by mouse mammary gland in vitro. Proc Natl Acad Sci USA 67:1493–1500, 1970.

65. Forsberg JG, Jacobsohn D, Norgren A: Modifications of reproductive organs in male rats influenced prenatally or pre- and postnatally by an "antiandrogenic" steroid (Cyproterone). Z Anat Entwicklungsgesch 127:175–186, 1968.

66. Simpson HW, et al: Meta-analysis of sequential luteal-cycle-associated changes in human breast tissue. Breast Cancer Res Treat 63:171–173, 2000.

67. Dyrenfurth I: Temporal relationships of hormonal variables in the menstrual cycle. In Ferin M (ed): Institute for the study of human reproduction conference proceedings. New York, Wiley, 1974.

68. Clarke RB, Howell A, Potten CS, Anderson E: Dissociation between steroid receptor expression and cell proliferation in the human breast. Cancer Res 57:4987–4991, 1997.

69. Soriano JV, Pepper MS, Nakamura T, et al: Hepatocyte growth factor stimulates extensive development of branching duct-like structures by cloned mammary gland epithelial cells. J Cell Sci 108(Pt 2):413–430, 1995.

70. Berdichevsky F, Alford D, D'Souza B, Taylor-Papadimitriou J: Branching morphogenesis of human mammary epithelial cells in collagen gels. J Cell Sci 107(Pt 12):3557–3568, 1994.

71. Niranjan B, Buluwela L, Yant J, et al: HGF/SF: A potent cytokine for mammary growth, morphogenesis and development. Development 121:2897–2908, 1995.

72. Saelman EU, Keely PJ, Santoro SA: Loss of MDCK cell alpha 2 beta 1 integrin expression results in reduced cyst formation, failure of hepatocyte growth factor/scatter factor-induced branching morphogenesis, and increased apoptosis. J Cell Sci 108(Pt 11): 3531–3540, 1995.

73. Soriano JV, Pepper MS, Orci L, Montesano R: Roles of hepatocyte growth factor/scatter factor and transforming growth factor-β1 in mammary gland ductal morphogenesis. J Mammary Gland Biol Neoplasia 3:133–150, 1998.

74. Yang Y, Spitzer E, Meyer D, et al: Sequential requirement of hepatocyte growth factor and neuregulin in the morphogenesis and differentiation of the mammary gland. J Cell Biol 131:215–226, 1995.

75. Li L, Cleary S, Mandarano MA, et al: The breast proto-oncogene, HRGα regulates epithelial proliferation and lobuloalveolar development in the mouse mammary gland. Oncogene 21:4900–4907, 2002.

76. Abou-el-Ela SH, Prasse KW, Carroll R, et al: Eicosanoid synthesis in 7,12-dimethylbenz(a)anthracene-induced mammary carcinomas in Sprague-Dawley rats fed primrose oil, menhaden oil or corn oil diet. Lipids 23:948–954, 1988.

77. Welsch CW, O'Connor DH: Influence of the type of dietary fat on developmental growth of the mammary gland in immature and mature female BALB/c mice. Cancer Res 49:5999–6007, 1989.

78. Bandyopadhyay GK, Hwang S, Imagawa W, Nandi S: Role of polyunsaturated fatty acids as signal transducers: amplification of signals from growth factor receptors by fatty acids in mammary epithelial cells. Prostaglandins Leukot Essent Fatty Acids 48: 71–78, 1993.

79. Colston KW, Berger U, Wilson P, et al: Mammary gland 1,25-dihydroxyvitamin D3 receptor content during pregnancy and lactation. Mol Cell Endocrinol 60:15–22, 1988.

80. Mezzetti G, Barbiroli B, Oka T: 1,25-Dihydroxycholecalciferol receptor regulation in hormonally induced differentiation of mouse mammary gland in culture. Endocrinology 120:2488–2493, 1987.

81. Narvaez CJ, Zinser G, Welsh J: Functions of 1α,25-dihydroxyvitamin D(3) in mammary gland: from normal development to breast cancer. Steroids 66:301–308, 2001.

82. Gearing AJ, Beckett P, Christodoulou M, et al: Matrix metalloproteinases and processing of pro-TNF-α. J Leukoc Biol 57:774–777, 1995.

83. Fowlkes JL, Thrailkill KM, Serra DM, et al: Matrix metalloproteinases as insulin-like growth factor binding protein-degrading proteinases. Prog Growth Factor Res 6:255–263, 1995.

84. Li G, Robinson GW, Lesche R, et al: Conditional loss of PTEN leads to precocious development and neoplasia in the mammary gland. Development 129:4159–4170, 2002.

85. Frantz A: Endocrine disorders of the breast. In Wilson J (ed): Williams textbook of endocrinology. Philadelphia, WB Saunders, 1998.

86. Strombeck J: Types of macromastia. Acta Chir Scand Suppl 341:37–39, 1964.

87. Govrin-Yehudain J, Kogan L, Cohen HI, Falik-Zaccai TC: Familial juvenile hypertrophy of the breast. J Adolesc Health 35:151–155, 2004.

88. Morimoto T, Komaki K, Mori T, et al: Juvenile gigantomastia: report of a case. Surg Today 23:260–264, 1993.

89. Finer N, Emery P, Hicks BH: Mammary gigantism and D-penicillamine. Clin Endocrinol (Oxf) 21:219–222, 1984.

90. Lafreniere R, Temple W, Ketcham A: Gestational macromastia. Am J Surg 148:413–418, 1984.

91. Baker SB, Burkey BA, Thornton P, LaRossa D: Juvenile gigantomastia: presentation of four cases and review of the literature. Ann Plast Surg 46:517–525, discussion 525–526, 2001.

92. Latham K, Fernandez S, Iteld L, et al: Pediatric breast deformity. J Craniofac Surg 17:454–467, 2006.

93. Lee PA: The relationship of concentrations of serum hormones to pubertal gynecomastia. J Pediatr 86:212–215, 1975.

94. Braunstein G: Testes. In Greenspan FS (ed): Basic and clinical endocrinology, New York, McGraw-Hill, 2001.

95. Irahara N, Miyoshi Y, Taguchi T, et al: Possible involvement of aromatase overexpression induced by cyclo-oxygenase-2 in the pathogenesis of idiopathic gynecomastia. Endocr Res 31: 219–227, 2005.

96. Dundar B, Dundar N, Erci T, et al: Leptin levels in boys with pubertal gynecomastia. J Pediatr Endocrinol Metab 18:929–934, 2005.

97. Thompson DF, Carter JR: Drug-induced gynecomastia. Pharmacotherapy 13:37–45, 1993.

98. Kuhn JM, Mahoudeau JA, Billaud L, et al: Evaluation of diagnostic criteria for Leydig cell tumours in adult men revealed by gynaecomastia. Clin Endocrinol (Oxf) 26:407–416, 1987.

99. Kirschner MA, Cohen FB, Jespersen D: Estrogen production and its origin in men with gonadotropin-producing neoplasms. J Clin Endocrinol Metab 39:112–118, 1974.

100. Hanavadi S, Banerjee D, Monypenny IJ, Mansel RE: The role of tamoxifen in the management of gynaecomastia. Breast 15: 276–280, 2006.

101. Plourde PV, Reiter EO, Jou HC, et al: Safety and efficacy of anastrozole for the treatment of pubertal gynecomastia: a randomized, double-blind, placebo-controlled trial. J Clin Endocrinol Metab 89:4428–4433, 2004.

102. Kono S, Kurosumi M, Simooka H, et al: Immunohistochemical study of the relationship between Ki-67 labeling index of proliferating cells of gynecomastia, histological phase and duration of disease. Pathol Int 56:655–658, 2006.

103. Grumbach M: Disorders of sex differentiation. In Wilson J, Foster D (eds): Williams textbook of endocrinology. Philadelphia, WB Saunders, 1992.

104. Morishima A, Grumbach MM, Simpson ER, et al: Aromatase deficiency in male and female siblings caused by a novel mutation and the physiological role of estrogens. J Clin Endocrinol Metab 80:3689–3698, 1995.

105. Grumbach MM, Sytne D: Puberty: Ontogeny, neuroendocrinology, physiology, and disorders. In Wilson J, Foster D (eds): Williams textbook of endocrinology. Philadelphia,WB Saunders, 1992.

106. Hilakivi-Clarke L, Forsen T, Eriksson JG, et al: Tallness and overweight during childhood have opposing effects on breast cancer risk. Br J Cancer 85:1680–1684, 2001.

107. Russo J, Rivera R, Russo IH: Influence of age and parity on the development of the human breast. Breast Cancer Res Treat 23: 211–218, 1992.

108. McGreevy J, Bland K: The breast. In O'Leary JP (ed): Physiologic basis of surgery. Baltimore, Williams & Wilkins, 1996.

109. Kaplan CR: Endocrinology of the breast. In Mitchell GW (ed): The female breast and its disorders. Baltimore, Williams & Wilkins, 1990.

110. Tyson JE, Hwang P, Guyda H, Friesen HG: Studies of prolactin secretion in human pregnancy. Am J Obstet Gynecol 113:14–20, 1972.

111. Kletzky OA, Marrs RP, Howard WF, et al: Prolactin synthesis and release during pregnancy and puerperium. Am J Obstet Gynecol 136:545–550, 1980.

112. Tyson JE, Friesen HG: Factors influencing the secretion of human prolactin and growth hormone in menstrual and gestational women. Am J Obstet Gynecol 116:377–387, 1973.

113. Boockfor FR, Hoeffler JP, Frawley LS: Estradiol induces a shift in cultured cells that release prolactin or growth hormone. Am J Physiol 250(Pt 1):E103–E105, 1986.

114. Maurer RA: Estradiol regulates the transcription of the prolactin gene. J Biol Chem 257:2133–2136, 1982.

115. Barberia JM, Abu-Fadil S, Kletzky OA, et al: Serum prolactin patterns in early human gestation. Am J Obstet Gynecol 121: 1107–1110, 1975.
116. Cramer OM, Parker CR Jr, Porter JC: Estrogen inhibition of dopamine release into hypophysial portal blood. Endocrinology 104:419–422, 1979.
117. Kelly PA, Djiane J, Postel-Vinay MC, Edery M: The prolactin/growth hormone receptor family. Endocr Rev 12:235–251, 1991.
118. Murphy LJ, Murphy LC, Stead B, et al: Modulation of lactogenic receptors by progestins in cultured human breast cancer cells. J Clin Endocrinol Metab 62:280–287, 1986.
119. Simon WE, Pahnke VG, Holzel F: In vitro modulation of prolactin binding to human mammary carcinoma cells by steroid hormones and prolactin. J Clin Endocrinol Metab 60:1243–1249, 1985.
120. Lee CS, Oka T: Progesterone regulation of a pregnancy-specific transcription repressor to β-casein gene promoter in mouse mammary gland. Endocrinology 131:2257–2262, 1992.
121. Krane IM, Leder P: NDF/heregulin induces persistence of terminal end buds and adenocarcinomas in the mammary glands of transgenic mice. Oncogene 12:1781–1788, 1996.
122. Barash I: Stat5 in the mammary gland: controlling normal development and cancer. J Cell Physiol 209:305–313, 2006.
123. Robinson GW, Hennighausen L: Inhibins and activins regulate mammary epithelial cell differentiation through mesenchymal-epithelial interactions. Development 124:2701–2708, 1997.
124. Toscani A, Mettus RV, Coupland R, et al: Arrest of spermatogenesis and defective breast development in mice lacking A-myb. Nature 386:713–717, 1997.
125. Robinson GW, Johnson PF, Hennighausen L, Sterneck E: The C/EBPβ transcription factor regulates epithelial cell proliferation and differentiation in the mammary gland. Genes Dev 12: 1907–1916, 1998.
126. Chen F, Capecchi MR: Paralogous mouse Hox genes, Hoxa9, Hoxb9, and Hoxd9, function together to control development of the mammary gland in response to pregnancy. Proc Natl Acad Sci USA 96:541–546, 1999.
127. Sicinski P, Donaher JL, Parker SB, et al: Cyclin D1 provides a link between development and oncogenesis in the retina and breast. Cell 82:621–630, 1995.
128. Come C, Arnoux V, Bibeau F, Savagner P: Roles of the transcription factors snail and slug during mammary morphogenesis and breast carcinoma progression. J Mammary Gland Biol Neoplasia 9:183–193, 2004.
129. Sympson CJ, Talhouk RS, Alexander CM, et al: Targeted expression of stromelysin-1 in mammary gland provides evidence for a role of proteinases in branching morphogenesis and the requirement for an intact basement membrane for tissue-specific gene expression. J Cell Biol 125: 681–693, 1994.
130. Witty JP, Wright JH, Matrisian LM: Matrix metalloproteinases are expressed during ductal and alveolar mammary morphogenesis, and misregulation of stromelysin-1 in transgenic mice induces unscheduled alveolar development. Mol Biol Cell 6:1287–1303, 1995.
131. Alexander CM, Howard EW, Bissell MJ, Werb Z: Rescue of mammary epithelial cell apoptosis and entactin degradation by a tissue inhibitor of metalloproteinases-1 transgene. J Cell Biol 135 (Pt 1):1669–1677, 1996.
132. Russo J, Yang X, Hu YF, et al: Biological and molecular basis of human breast cancer. Front Biosci 3:D944–D960, 1998.
133. Russo J, Ao X, Grill C, Russo IH: Pattern of distribution of cells positive for estrogen receptor alpha and progesterone receptor in relation to proliferating cells in the mammary gland. Breast Cancer Res Treat 53: 217–227, 1999.
134. Russo J, Russo IH: Estrogens and cell proliferation in the human breast. J Cardiovasc Pharmacol 28 (Suppl) S19–S23, 1996.
135. Russo J, Russo IH: Role of differentiation in the pathogenesis and prevention of breast cancer. Endocr Rel Cancer 4:7–21, 1997.
136. Russo J, Russo IH: Role of hormone in human breast development: The menopausal breast. In Wreo B (ed): Progress in the management of menopause. London, Parthenon, 1997.
137. Cregan MD, Hartmann PE: Computerized breast measurement from conception to weaning: Clinical implications. J Hum Lact 15:89–96, 1999.
138. Kent JC, Mitoulas L, Cox DB, et al: Breast volume and milk production during extended lactation in women. Exp Physiol 84: 435–447, 1999.
139. Cox DB, Owens RA, Hartmann PE: Blood and milk prolactin and the rate of milk synthesis in women. Exp Physiol 81:1007–1020, 1996.
140. Hartmann P, Sherriff J, Kent J: Maternal nutrition and the regulation of milk synthesis. Proc Nutr Soc 54:379–389, 1995.
141. Ohtani O, Shao XJ, Saitoh M, Ohtani Y: Lymphatics of the rat mammary gland during virgin, pregnant, lactating and post-weaning periods. Ital J Anat Embryol 103(Suppl 1):335–342, 1998.
142. Marti A, Feng Z, Altermatt HJ, Jaggi R: Milk accumulation triggers apoptosis of mammary epithelial cells. Eur J Cell Biol 73: 158–165, 1997.
143. Lund LR, Romer J, Thomasset N, et al: Two distinct phases of apoptosis in mammary gland involution: proteinase-independent and -dependent pathways. Development 122:181–193, 1996.
144. Feng Z, Marti A, Jehn B, et al: Glucocorticoid and progesterone inhibit involution and programmed cell death in the mouse mammary gland. J Cell Biol 131:1095–1103, 1995.
145. Bole-Feysot C, Goffin V, Edery M, et al: Prolactin (PRL) and its receptor: Actions, signal transduction pathways and phenotypes observed in PRL receptor knockout mice. Endocr Rev 19: 225–268, 1998.
146. Liu X: Stat5a is mandatory for adult mammary gland development and lactogenesis. Genes Dev 11:179–186, 1997.
147. Altiok S, Groner B: β-Casein mRNA sequesters a single-stranded nucleic acid-binding protein which negatively regulates the β-casein gene promoter. Mol Cell Biol 14:6004–6012, 1994.
148. Seyfred MA, Gorski J: An interaction between the 5′ flanking distal and proximal regulatory domains of the rat prolactin gene is required for transcriptional activation by estrogens. Mol Endocrinol 4:1226–1234, 1990.
149. Yan GZ, Pan WT, Bancroft C: Thyrotropin-releasing hormone action on the prolactin promoter is mediated by the POU protein pit-1. Mol Endocrinol 5:535–541, 1991.
150. Bredow S, Kacsoh B, Obal F, Jr., et al: Increase of prolactin mRNA in the rat hypothalamus after intracerebroventricular injection of VIP or PACAP. Brain Res 660:301–308, 1994.
151. Pickett CA, Gutierrez-Hartmann A: Ras mediates Src but not epidermal growth factor-receptor tyrosine kinase signaling pathways in GH4 neuroendocrine cells. Proc Natl Acad Sci USA 91:8612–8616, 1994.
152. Porter TE, Wiles CD, Frawley LS: Stimulation of lactotrope differentiation in vitro by fibroblast growth factor. Endocrinology 134:164–168, 1994.
153. Tyson JE, Perez A, Zanartu J: Human lactational response to oral thyrotropin releasing hormone. J Clin Endocrinol Metab 43: 760–768, 1976.
154. Ben-Jonathan N, Mershon JL, Allen DL, Steinmetz RW: Extrapituitary prolactin: Distribution, regulation, functions, and clinical aspects. Endocr Rev 17:639–669, 1996.
155. Franks S, Kiwi R, Nabarro JD: Pregnancy and lactation after pituitary surgery. Br Med J 1:882, 1977.
156. Li M, Liu X, Robinson G, et al: Mammary-derived signals activate programmed cell death during the first stage of mammary gland involution. Proc Natl Acad Sci USA 94:3425–3430, 1997.
157. Daniel CW, Strickland P, Friedmann Y: Expression and functional role of E- and P-cadherins in mouse mammary ductal morphogenesis and growth. Dev Biol 169:511–519, 1995.
158. Delmas V, Pla P, Feracci H, et al: Expression of the cytoplasmic domain of E-cadherin induces precocious mammary epithelial alveolar formation and affects cell polarity and cell-matrix integrity. Dev Biol 216: 491–506, 1999.
159. Radice GL, Ferreira-Cornwell MC, Robinson SD, et al: Precocious mammary gland development in P-cadherin-deficient mice. J Cell Biol 139:1025–1032, 1997.
160. Murtagh J, Martin F, Gronostajski RM: The nuclear factor I (NFI) gene family in mammary gland development and function. J Mammary Gland Biol Neoplasia 8:241–254, 2003.
161. Streuli CH, Schmidhauser C, Bailey N, et al: Laminin mediates tissue-specific gene expression in mammary epithelia. J Cell Biol 129:591–603, 1995.

162. Streuli CH, Edwards GM: Control of normal mammary epithelial phenotype by integrins. J Mammary Gland Biol Neoplasia 3: 151–163, 1998.

163. Daly SE, Owens RA, Hartmann PE: The short-term synthesis and infant-regulated removal of milk in lactating women. Exp Physiol 78:209–220, 1993.

164. Jerry DJ, Dickinson ES, Roberts AL, Said TK: Regulation of apoptosis during mammary involution by the p53 tumor suppressor gene. J Dairy Sci 85: 1103–1110, 2002.

165. Chapman RS, Lourenco PC, Tonner E, et al: Suppression of epithelial apoptosis and delayed mammary gland involution in mice with a conditional knockout of Stat3. Genes Dev 13:2604–2616, 1999.

166. Baik MG, Lee MJ, Choi YJ: Gene expression during involution of mammary gland (review). Int J Mol Med 2:39–44, 1998.

167. Philp JA, Burdon TG, Watson CJ: Differential activation of STATs 3 and 5 during mammary gland development. FEBS Lett 396:77–80, 1996.

168. Merlo GR, Basolo F, Fiore L, et al: p53-dependent and p53-independent activation of apoptosis in mammary epithelial cells reveals a survival function of EGF and insulin. J Cell Biol 128:1185–1196, 1995.

169. Talhouk RS, Bissell MJ, Werb Z: Coordinated expression of extracellular matrix-degrading proteinases and their inhibitors regulates mammary epithelial function during involution. J Cell Biol 118:1271–1282, 1992.

170. Schroeder MD, Rose-Hellekant TA, Sandgren EP, Schuler LA: Dysregulation of mammary Stats 1, 3 and 5 and PRL receptors by overexpression of TGF α. Mol Cell Endocrinol 175:173–183, 2001.

171. Chapman DJ, Perez-Escamilla R: Identification of risk factors for delayed onset of lactation. J Am Diet Assoc 99:450–454, quiz 455–456, 1999.

172. Neubauer SH, Ferris AM, Chase CG, et al: Delayed lactogenesis in women with insulin-dependent diabetes mellitus. Am J Clin Nutr 58:54–60, 1993.

173. Arthur PG, Kent JC, Hartmann PE: Metabolites of lactose synthesis in milk from diabetic and nondiabetic women during lactogenesis II. J Pediatr Gastroenterol Nutr 19:100–108, 1994.

174. Geddes DT: Inside the lactating breast: the latest anatomy research. J Midwifery Womens Health 52:556–563, 2007.

175. Dewey KG, Lovelady CA, Nommsen-Rivers LA, et al: A randomized study of the effects of aerobic exercise by lactating women on breast-milk volume and composition. N Engl J Med 330:449–453, 1994.

176. Sharp E: Historical review of a syndrome embracing utero-ovarian atrophy with persistent lactation. Am J Obstet Gynecol 30:411–414, 1935.

177. Forbes A: A syndrome, distinct from acromegamenorrhea, and low follicle-stimulating hormone excretion. J Clin Endocrinol 11:749, 1951.

178. Archer DF: Current concepts of prolacting physiology in normal and abnormal conditions. Fertil Steril 28:125–134, 1977.

179. Frantz A: Prolactin secretion in physiologic and pathologic human conditions measured by bioassay and radioimmunoassay. In Josimovich J, Cobo E (eds): Lactogenic hormones, fetal nutrition, and lactation, New York, Wiley, 1974.

180. Frantz AG: Prolactin. N Engl J Med 298:201–207, 1978.

181. Blackwell RE: Diagnosis and management of prolactinomas. Fertil Steril 43:5–16, 1985.

182. Kelver ME, Nagamani M: Hyperprolactinemia in primary adrenocortical insufficiency. Fertil Steril 44:423–425, 1985.

183. Mahesh VB, Pria SD, Greenblatt RB: Abnormal lactation with Cushing's syndrome—a case report. J Clin Endocrinol Metab 29:978–981, 1969.

184. Nabarro JD: Acromegaly. Clin Endocrinol (Oxf) 26:481–512, 1987.

185. Sievertsen GD, Lim VS, Nakawatase C, Frohman LA: Metabolic clearance and secretion rates of human prolactin in normal subjects and in patients with chronic renal failure. J Clin Endocrinol Metab 50:846–852, 1980.

186. Turkington RW: Ectopic production of prolactin. N Engl J Med 285:1455–1458, 1971.

187. Syvertsen A, Haughton VM, Williams AL, Cusick JF: The computed tomographic appearance of the normal pituitary gland and pituitary microadenomas. Radiology 133:385–391, 1979.

chapter 4

Discharges and Secretions of the Nipple

A. MARILYN LEITCH | RAHEELA ASHFAQ

Introduction and Definitions

Nipple discharge prompts the majority of women to seek immediate attention from their physician. Women view nipple secretions that are typically of nonlactational origin as potential indicators of breast cancer. Thus, it is critical for a physician caring for a woman with breast disease to have a comprehensive understanding of the physiology of breast secretions and the clinical significance of secretions and discharges. In this chapter, we review the pathophysiology of nipple discharge as well as the significance of breast secretions with respect to the risk of breast cancer. A review of the clinical management and evaluation of nipple discharge follows. This treatise includes a description of methods for collection and preparation of nipple fluid needed for optimum quality and best diagnostic results. In addition, a brief discussion of the role of ductoscopy is included.

The terms *discharge* and *secretion* of the nipple are defined as follows: *Discharge* is fluid that extrudes spontaneously from the nipple. *Secretion* is fluid present (existent) in mammary ducts that must be collected by nipple aspiration or by other measures that include conventional breast pump or massage and expression from the ductules (nonspontaneous secretion). Ductal lavage fluid (DLF) implies the application of saline washing from individual breast ducts with fluid retrieval via a microcatheter device.

The breast is a secretory gland that shows evidence of secretory activity under influence of maternal hormones initiated in the fetal stage (in utero) and under sex hormones during puberty and adult reproductive life. With the estrogen-progestin hormonal cycle, breast epithelium undergoes cellular proliferation in the estrogenic phase, followed by secretory activity. Breast tissue studies confirm cyclical changes related to follicular and luteal phases. Similar observations on changes in histologic pattern, cellular morphology, mitoses, and DNA content are evident.[1-4] Longacre and Bartow[5] found excessive lymphocytes, duct epithelial degenerative changes, and sloughing into duct lumens in the late secretory and early menstrual phases. Ferguson and Anderson[1] also confirm cell depletion through a process of apoptosis in this time interval, which peaks on day 28.

Objective measures of breast epithelial cyclical changes are provided by DNA quantitative cytochemistry previously described in tissue sections and with image cytometry of fine-needle aspiration (FNA) samples. In FNA biopsies, image cytometry using five nuclear features—area, circumference, boundary fluctuation, chromatin granularity, and stain intensity—successfully discriminated samples from women in *follicular phase* and those in *luteal phase*.[6] This approach, applied to the individual woman, was universally accurate in identifying the phase of the cycle. Concerned by the proliferative changes that mimic atypia or malignancy in the *postovulatory phase*, Malberger and colleagues recommended that FNA be used *only* in the *preovulatory phase*. These potentially confusing histologic changes in the sampled cells should be taken into account when evaluating cytologic features of nipple discharges and nipple fluid aspirates.

The functional unit of the breast is the terminal duct lobular unit (TDLU; Fig. 4-1).[7,8] Mammary secretions originate in the lobules. Lobules are connected by the intralobular ductals to the extralobular ductal system, which empties into the lactiferous sinus and onto the vestibule of the nipple. Anatomically, the breast has 15 to 20 segments, each with its unique drainage (Fig. 4-2). Nipple secretion is usually not clinically appreciated in nonlactating women, because dense keratotic debris obstructs passage into lactiferous sinuses. Such secretion is observed, however, in longitudinal planes of the duct lumen displayed in histologic sections of breast tissue. By removing the keratotic debris and using a simple nipple aspirator device, the physician may easily obtain fluid from a large proportion of women.[9-12] Researchers have also obtained secretions with use of a breast pump or with manual expression.[13-17]

NIPPLE ASPIRATION FLUID: CHARACTERIZATION AND SIGNIFICANCE

Many investigators have an interest in intraductal physiology and cytology as an indicator of risk of breast

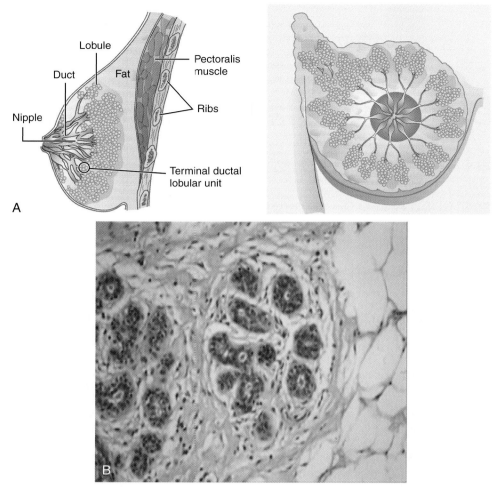

Figure 4-1   A, The breast duct lobular system. There are 15 to 20 ductal systems per breast. However, more recent studies have determined that the average breast nipple contains five to nine milk pores. Each pore corresponds to a central duct that projects back to the chest wall. Other orifices at the nipple are blind sebaceous glands. The ducts have lateral branches called lobules. At the far end of these branches are the terminal ductal lobular units, where milk is produced during lactation. Together, the duct and the lobules form the ductal lobular system. During lactation, the system distends with milk. But in the absence of lactation, the walls of the empty ducts are collapsed. **B,** Histology of the terminal ductal lobular unit. (**A,** Redrawn from art provided courtesy of Hologic, Inc. Original images by Jennifer Fairman, CMI.)

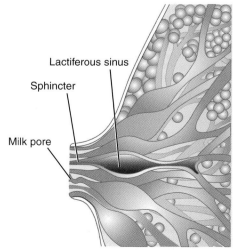

Figure 4-2   Anatomy of the breast duct. Within the duct, 1 to 2 centimeters beneath the surface of the nipple, is the lactiferous sinus. The duct also has a tiny sphincter. (Redrawn from art provided courtesy of Hologic, Inc. Original images by Jennifer Fairman, CMI.)

cancer. Many consider that breast cancer results from a cascade of sequential molecular and morphologic events that occur in the ductal epithelial cells. If that process can be detected *prior to* transition to a malignant phenotype, there is the opportunity for prevention strategies (Fig. 4-3). The methodologies for obtaining breast secretions and classifying cellular patterns, as well as the biochemical makeup of nipple aspiration fluid (NAF), are discussed in this section.

NAF is the simplest, least invasive, and least expensive method of sampling histologic alterations within the breast. Following cleaning of the nipple orifice to remove keratinous plugs, the breast is massaged from the base to the nipple. Using a modified breast pump (Fig. 4-4), suction is exerted to elicit the fluid. NAF appears as droplets on the nipple and is collected with small capillary tubes. Samples are usually pooled for examination to improve cellular yield.

Cytologic examination of the breast fluid has long been considered a potential aid in the detection of breast

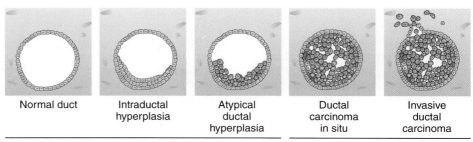

Figure 4-3 Multistep pathogenesis of breast cancer. Breast cancer is believed to be the result of the progressive molecular and morphologic changes that develop in ductal epithelial cells. These changes have been studied extensively. (Redrawn from art provided courtesy of Hologic, Inc. Original images by Jennifer Fairman, CMI.)

Normal duct | Intraductal hyperplasia | Atypical ductal hyperplasia | Ductal carcinoma in situ | Invasive ductal carcinoma

Predict and prevent   Detect and treat

disease and is not a new technique. In 1914, Nathan was the first to diagnose a mammary carcinoma on the basis of malignant cells in a nipple discharge. Saphir (1950),[18] Ringrose (1966),[17] and Masukawa (1966)[3] later reported the cytologic criteria for the diagnosis of chronic mastitis, intraductal papillomas, and carcinoma based on stained smears of spontaneous nipple discharge.

Following the successful application of the cervical smear (Pap smear) for the diagnosis of cervical cancer, George Papanicolaou more vigorously tested and developed the concept of a "Pap smear" for breast cancer. In 1950, Papanicolaou began a study to investigate normal, atypical, and malignant breast epithelia. This subsequently resulted in determination of the role of cytologic smears for the diagnosis of breast cancer, the diagnostic value of microscopic examination of the nipple secretions, the proportion of asymptomatic women from whom breast secretions could be obtained with a consideration of using breast secretion smears in screening for mammary carcinoma, and the value of studying aspirates of breast cysts.[16]

In this study, Papanicolaou examined breast aspirates in 917 asymptomatic patients. Using a hand breast pump, secretions were obtained unilaterally in 171 (18.5%) and bilaterally in 74 (8.1%). Premenopausal women yielded a higher percentage of fluid than postmenopausal women, with the highest percentage found in women 20 to 39 years of age. Four occult carcinomas and one ductal carcinoma in situ (DCIS) were discovered. Papanicolaou also sought to

define "normal" cytologic findings in nipple fluid. The two cell types most often encountered were foam cells and duct epithelial cells. Scant histiocytes and lymphocytes were also present.

Papanicolaou concluded that careful examination of the breast for secretions can be incorporated into the regular physical examination of the patient.[16] In the 1970s, using a modified breast pump, Sartorius and associates attempted nipple aspiration in 1503 women with suspected breast disease and 203 asymptomatic volunteers. They developed the histologic classification to define cytologic changes; it required a minimum of 50 to 100 cells for diagnosis.[10] Diagnostic categories included the following:

- Normal: all duct lining cells uniform in size and staining characteristics
- Hyperplasia: excessive number of ductal groups with multilayering and slight variations in size and shape, but without significant nuclear abnormality and a constant nucleocytoplasmic ratio
- Atypical hyperplasia: criteria similar to that used for hyperplasia but with greater variation in nuclear size and shape, abnormal distribution of chromatin and increased nuclear: cytoplasmic ratio and prominent nucleoli
- Suspected carcinoma: criteria similar to atypical hyperplasia but with marked nuclear abnormality, chromatin clearing, nuclear membrane irregularity, and nucleoli

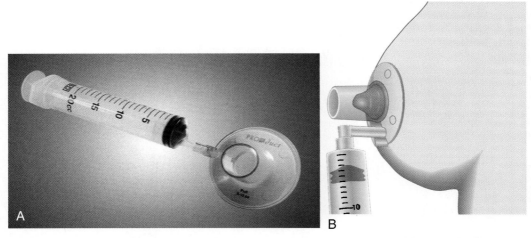

Figure 4-4 **A,** Breast pump used for obtaining nipple aspirate fluid. **B,** Nipple aspiration using a modified pump. Gentle suction is applied to draw the fluid. (**B,** Redrawn from art provided courtesy of Hologic, Inc. Original images by Jennifer Fairman, CMI.)

See Figure 4-5 for examples of nipple fluid cytology and corresponding histology.

Of the 203 asymptomatic volunteers, NAF was obtained in 163 (80%), with adequate cellular samples obtained in 48.7%. Of the 1503 women with breast disease, NAF with adequate cellularity was obtained in 825 (54.9%); 11.2% yielded fluid without adequate cells. Women 31 to 50 years of age (65%) gave cellular samples, and those older than 60 years of age yielded less fluid. Of the 825 women who yielded fluid, 237 were classified as high-risk based on factors such as family history and history of prior breast surgery. A significantly larger percentage of high-risk women had abnormal cytology compared with the normal risk group. This association was seen more frequently in women older than 40 years of age. The women categorized in abnormal cell categories were asymptomatic and without palpable masses. Thereafter, Sartorius used a technique of ductography in 469 women with 223 evaluable cases and confirmed that a cytologic diagnosis of hyperplasia correlated with papillomas. Those in the atypical hyperplasia category revealed duct wall abnormalities and frequently had a histologic diagnosis of sclerosing adenosis, florid adenosis, and atypical intraductal hyperplasia. There were two cases of DCIS and two of occult invasive carcinoma. Twenty-seven women with suspected carcinoma had the following histology: carcinoma (18), atypical papillomas (2), florid adenosis (1), sclerosing adenosis (4), and atypical hyperplasia (2). Sixty-seven women had carcinoma on entry; of these, 49 (73%) yielded no fluid. The investigators observed that as the lesion increased in size, there was *less* likelihood of detection with cytology. All seven lesions diagnosed by cytology were less than 1 cm. From their study, they concluded that presence of atypical cells in NAF strongly correlated with presence of breast disease and that NAF was able to detect occult carcinoma.[10]

Following the seminal work of Sartorius, Petrakis and King[19-22] further validated the association of atypical epithelial cells in NAF of asymptomatic women with histologically confirmed proliferative disease and atypical hyperplasia. This finding was particularly evident in high-risk women. These authors first proposed the finding of atypical cells in NAF as a possible marker to identify women at risk who would need close surveillance.

King and coworkers[22] conducted a cytologic-histologic correlation study of NAF using 82 women with cancer and 237 women subsequently diagnosed with benign breast disease. In this analysis of 134 samples (34 cancer; 100 noncancer), patients met the criteria for the presence of a minimum of 10 cells. Atypical hyperplasia in NAF was present in 80% of cancers and 39% of benign breast diseases. The diagnosis of cancer was made in only 21% of the cases. Subsequently, NAF was proposed as a novel, nascent approach to study breast cancer precursors but was not considered a diagnostic tool. Factors that affect NAF production in nonlactating women include age, existing proliferative breast disease, previous breast biopsy, and family history of breast cancer.

In a large prospective trial to determine breast cancer risk in relation to NAF, Wrensch and Petrakis[23] enrolled 2701 nonlactating women between 1973 and 1980 and reported their long-term follow-up (average, 12.7 years) in 1991. In this study, women who did not yield any fluid were described as the referent group because they represent the lowest risk of developing breast cancer. With follow-up at 87%, the study confirmed that women with atypical hyperplasia were 4.9 times more likely to

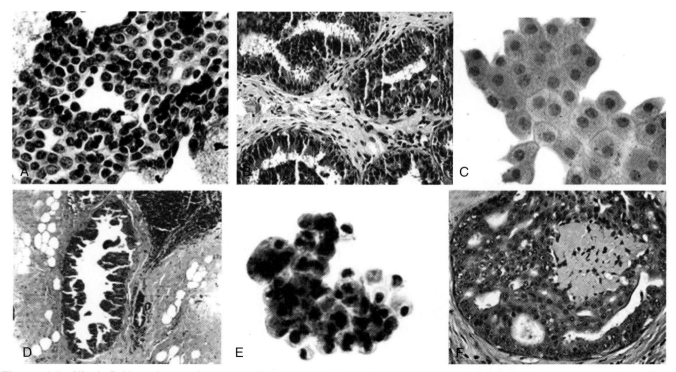

Figure 4-5 Nipple fluid cytology and corresponding histology. **A** and **B:** Epithelial hyperplasia. **C** and **D:** Apocrine metaplasia. **E** and **F:** High-grade ductal carcinoma in situ. (Courtesy of David Euhus, MD, UT Southwestern Medical Center.)

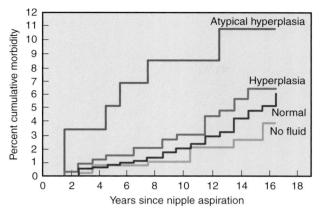

Figure 4-6 The occurrence of breast cancer in relation to the findings on cytology of nipple aspiration fluid. (From Wrensch MR, Petrakis NL, King EB, et al: Breast cancer incidence in women with abnormal cytology in nipple aspirates of breast fluid. Am J Epidemiol 135:130–141, 1992.)

develop breast cancer when compared with non–NAF-producing patients; this risk was 2.8 times more likely when compared with women with normal cytology (Fig. 4-6). The increase in the risk of breast cancer with abnormal cytology was more pronounced in younger (25–54 years) versus older (>55 years) women. Women with atypical NAF and family history of breast cancer were 18 times more likely to develop breast cancer compared to the referent groups, and they were 15 times more likely compared with those without atypia but positive family history. The study concluded that women with cytologic diagnosis of atypical hyperplasia experienced significant increase in risk of developing breast cancer.

In 2001, Wrensch and colleagues reported their findings on extended follow-up of 3627 volunteers. This study demonstrated that 3.5% of women developed breast cancer (median of 12 years follow-up), and 7.8% developed cancer in the median of 21 years follow-up. Again, women with NAF production were more likely to develop breast cancer than the non–NAF-producing group. This long-term follow-up data upheld their previous findings of increased risk for developing breast cancer related to abnormal cytology.[24]

More recently, Sauter and associates[25] used a modified breast pump to collect NAF in 177 patients with a success rate of 94%; evaluable cytology was obtained in 95%. NAF cytology correlated with increased risk of breast cancer. Birth control pills, hormone replacement therapy, or phase of menstrual cycle had no influence on NAF production. These authors were successful in obtaining NAF in postmenopausal women and advocated the use of NAF as a screening tool and as an intermediate marker for chemoprevention.[26]

Biochemical Composition of Nipple Aspiration Fluid

The noncellular component of the NAF has been studied for a number of biochemical substances and biomarkers. In a recent prospective study, NAF in women was prospectively evaluated (N = 192) for candidate proteins such as prostate-specific antigen (PSA), human glandular

kallikrein (hK2), basic fibroblast growth factor (bFGF), and cellular markers such as S-phase fraction, as well as for DNA index and cytology. The best breast cancer predictive model included cytology, bFGF, and age (88% sensitivity; 57% specificity). Incorporation of menopausal status to predict the optimal model of breast cancer indicates NAF hK2 or PSA and age to be 100% sensitive and 41% specific in premenopausal versus 93% sensitive and 12% specific in postmenopausal women.[27]

Recently, the focus for NAF has shifted from studying healthy volunteers or women with benign breast disease for comparison of NAF from carcinomatous breast to the healthy contralateral breast. Kuerer and coworkers prospectively determined the concentration of extracellular domain of Her2 in affected versus nonaffected breasts and found NAF Her2 levels to be highly correlative (r = 0.302; P = 0.038); tumors that overexpressed Her2 had higher Her2 levels in the affected versus the nonaffected breast.[28]

Moreover, NAF contains chemical substances of exogenous origin, such as caffeine, nicotine, pesticides, and orally ingested drugs. Approximately 10% of NAF samples have substances with mutagenic activity.[29] Additionally, endogenously derived proteins such as immunoglobulins, estrogen and progesterone, androgen, prolactin, PSA, and carcinoembryonic antigen have been detected.[29–31] Of these, a combination of Her2/neu (≤40 ng/mL) and carcinoembryonic antigen (≤400 ng/mL) was detected in all of the studied cancer patients, two of 2 with borderline lesions, two of 8 with papillomas, and two of 19 with fibrocystic disease.[27] The process of angiogenesis plays an important role in breast carcinogenesis and metastasis.[31–33] The substance bFGF is a potent angiogenic factor that can be detected in NAF. Control nipple fluid had significantly lower levels of bFGF (≤100 ng/mL) when compared with cancerous nipple fluids. This may serve as a potential diagnostic tool for breast cancer.[32–34]

MINIMALLY INVASIVE TECHNIQUES FOR DETERMINING RISK OF BREAST CANCER

Mammary Ductoscopy

Mammary ductoscopy has evolved over the past two decades. Earlier techniques were limited by suboptimal optics, resolution, large-caliber scopes and the inability to biopsy under direct visualization. Mammary ductoscopy represents a simple procedure performed under local anesthesia in an office setting or outpatient clinic setting. The endoscope is inserted through the ductal openings on the nipple surface following dilation of the duct orifice. The duct is infused with warm saline to widen and facilitate the passage of the endoscope. Mammary ductoscopy offers direct visualization of the lesion and the ability to combine the procedure with cytologic examination of ductal washings (lavage). Cytology obtained under direct visualization is more accurate than that obtained from simple discharges.

There is interest to enhance screening for breast cancer beyond standard mammography. Although mammography remains the gold standard for breast screening in women older than 40 years of age, the positive predictive value is low (25%).[35] Young women with dense breasts and those at high risk for developing breast cancer, such as those with BRCA1/BRCA2 mutations, usually undergo magnetic resonance imaging, which has been shown to be superior to mammography and ultrasound for screening of breast cancer.

Breast cancer arises in the TDLU. Therefore, it is conceivable that mammary ductoscopy could detect breast cancer earlier than mammography. Technical limitations of ductoscopy are related to breast anatomy. Going and Moffat[36] presented a three-dimensional model of breast anatomy that documents challenges of mammary ductoscopy. These investigations examined mastectomy specimens and found that the numbers of collecting ducts in the nipple (median, 27) are much greater than the number of nipple duct openings (typically 6 to 8 are identifiable).

Although the cytologic samples obtained through mammary ductoscopy have high specificity, ductoscopy lacks sensitivity. A reliable intraductal biopsy tool needs to be developed for histologic evaluation of these lesions. Another limitation is that 17% of invasive ductal carcinomas lack an intraductal component and may occlude the duct.[37] The future application of image analysis tools and molecular analyses together with this technique may serve to advance mammary ductoscopy from an investigational tool to a clinical procedure routinely used for risk assessment.

Ductal Lavage

Although quite promising, NAF cytology has major limitations in clinical screening because of the inconsistency of adequate cellular yield and the presumption that nipple aspiration fails to harvest cells from the distal portion of the duct-lobular system. To overcome these limitations, a new approach was developed in 1999 that allows collection of higher numbers of exfoliated cells from the TDLU. The ductal lavage (DL) procedure involves nipple aspiration using a modified suction cup to localize the NAF-yielding ducts. NAF-yielding ducts can subsequently be localized and cannulated using a microcatheter (Hologic, Inc.). Fluid-yielding ducts are infused with normal saline. Ductal effluent collected through the microcatheter is then analyzed cytologically (Fig. 4-7).

The DL technique was first attempted during a breast duct endoscopy study in which dilators were introduced into the ducts. Thereafter, a cannula (outer diameter, 0.4 mm) was inserted into the duct and saline was injected to wash the ductal lumen.[7] The washings were collected and studied cytologically. The technique was later refined with special development of a double-lumen catheter. Dooley and colleagues designed a prospective multicenter study to compare DL and nipple aspiration with regard to safety, tolerability, and outcomes for detection of abnormal cells.[38] The effluent was collected and cytologic preparations were performed using the millipore technique (also used in early NAF studies). The cytologic evaluation was performed by King and associates.[20,21] King functioned as the original pathologist for NAF studies. A total of 507 women were

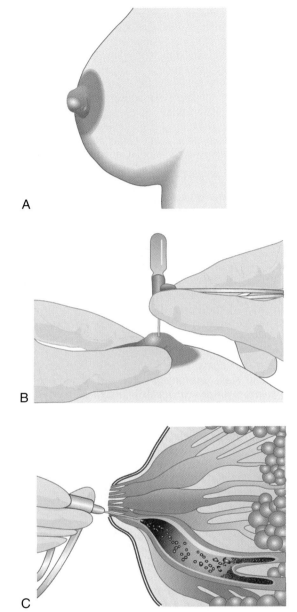

Figure 4-7 A–C, Ductal lavage technique. Once the ductal orifice has been located by the presence of a nipple aspirate fluid droplet, a flexible microcatheter is inserted about one-and-a-half centimeters into the duct through the duct's natural opening on the nipple surface. One to two cubic centimeters of lidocaine is then infused intraductally through the catheter to anesthetize the duct. Sometimes, to facilitate cannulation, the ductal orifice is first enlarged with multiple dilators. (Redrawn from art provided courtesy of Hologic, Inc. Original images by Jennifer Fairman, CMI.)

enrolled, 291 (57%) of whom had a history of breast cancer and 199 (39%) had a Gail risk of breast cancer of 1.7%. The minimum age was 52 years. Overall, the procedure was tolerated well. NAF was obtained in 417 women, and DL was performed in 383. On average, the NAF had 120 epithelial cells compared with 13,200 epithelial cells in the DL samples. Greater cellularity and high diagnostic yield was also noted in DL samples. Importantly, atypia was diagnosed in 24% of the DL versus 10% of NAF samples. Only ducts yielding NAF were targeted for DL (average 1.5 ducts/breast were lavaged). Currently, DL is limited to women who are at high risk for breast cancer.

Ductal Lavage Procedure. Preparation for the procedure is labor and time intensive; the technique requires breast massage for 30 minutes. A topical anesthetic (2.5% lidocaine and 2.5% prilocaine [EMLA]) is applied. Keratin plugs are removed from the nipple. The nipple suction device is used to obtain NAF and localize the ducts that can be cannulated. A grid can be used to record the location of the ducts for future reference. Usually 5 to 10 mL of saline are infused, collected, and submitted to a cytology laboratory in CytoLyt (Cytyc) solution. In the laboratory, a ThinPrep slide can be prepared and stained using the routine Papanicolaou stain. The diagnostic categories used for reporting ductal lavage cytology were developed by Wrensch and coworkers[23] and were further refined using the National Cancer Institute Consensus Conference Statement on breast FNAs.[39] The categories included the following:

- Insufficient cellular material for diagnosis. A minimum of 10 epithelial cells should be present per slide. The presence of macrophages alone does not render a specimen diagnostic.
- Benign. Samples categorized as benign contain 10 or more epithelial cells and variable number of other cellular components such as squamous cells, lymphocytes, and foamy macrophages. The benign duct epithelial cells are 10 to 15 μ in diameter and have a cyanophilic cytoplasm that may contain fine vacuoles. Ductal cells are more easily recognized in groups than in single cells, which are difficult to differentiate from lymphocytes. Cells may be arranged in monolayer sheets or strands.
- Mild atypia. In mild atypia, there is nuclear enlargement 1.5 to 3 times the normal ductal cell, and higher nuclear-cytoplasmic ratio. The nucleus may be hyperchromatic or hypochromatic and there may be nucleoli. Multilayering or complex and papillary architectural groups may be present and usually indicate hyperplastic changes.
- Marked atypia. The preceding abnormalities are more pronounced, nucleoli are more prominent, and nuclear membrane irregularities are easily appreciable.
- Malignant cells. Malignant cells on DL have obvious features of malignancy with high nuclear-cytoplasmic ratio, hyperchromasia, macronucleoli, and dyshesion (Figs. 4-8 and 4-9).

The diagnosis of malignancy on DL is uncommon, because the large majority of women who undergo the procedure have no palpable or mammographic

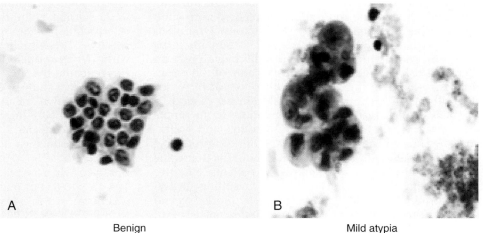

A   Benign

B   Mild atypia

Figure 4-8 A–D, Spectrum of cytology on nipple duct lavage.

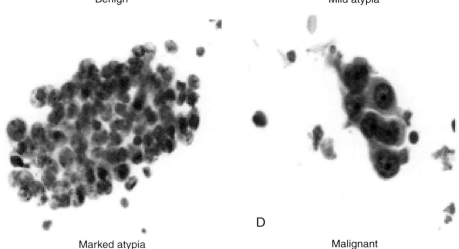

C   Marked atypia

D   Malignant

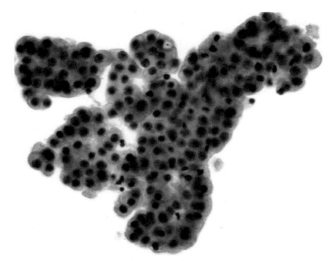

Figure 4-9 Cytologic features of intraductal papilloma on nipple duct lavage.

abnormality. Occasionally, however, a high-grade DCIS may be diagnosed in this manner. In Dooley's study, less than 1% of cases were diagnosed as malignant.[38]

Limitations of Ductal Lavage. The procedure is new and readily available in only a few clinical centers. The cost of disposables is high. Special expertise and training is required for the performance of DL. Cytologic interpretation may be variable and training is required for pathologists to become familiar with DL cytology. DL detects milder atypia than NAF (17% vs. 6%). It remains to be seen, however, as in NAF, whether mild atypia poses an increased risk. The negative predictive value of the procedure is not known (i.e., number of women at increased risk with negative DL who will develop breast cancer).

There are, however, important limitations to the nipple duct lavage (NDL) methodology. Maddux and colleagues[40] evaluated the atypia rate by NDL fluid-producing ducts compared with non–fluid-producing ducts and the atypia rate in high-risk versus low-risk patients. Fifty-five women with 226 ducts were lavaged, resulting in 136 ducts producing fluid versus 90 ducts producing no fluid. Of these, 44% had a Gail risk index greater than or equal to 1.7, and 56% had a Gail risk index less than 1.7%. Cytologic atypia was diagnosed in 34% of patients. The cytologic atypia rate was not statistically different in low-risk versus high-risk women based on a Gail index (33% vs. 35%; $P = 1$) or fluid-producing versus non–fluid-producing ducts (19% vs. 15%; $P = 0.61$), respectively. In this study, there was a higher atypia rate for fluid-producing ducts versus non–fluid-producing ducts (32% vs. 11%) in women at high-risk (Gail risk ≥ 1.7).

Another limitation of NDL is the lack of studies related to the performance characteristics of the procedure. It is possible that some atypical lavages may reflect underlying atypical hyperplasia, whereas others may reflect reversible physiologic changes. Johnson-Maddux and associates[41] proposed that persistent lavage atypia may be related to underlying pathology such as atypical duct hyperplasia while reversible atypia may be associated with physiologic changes. In a reproducibility study for NDL, Maddux and associates found marked atypia in 36% of breasts

with incident carcinoma and in 24% of benign breasts ($P = 0.19$). However, marked atypia was diagnosed more frequently in breasts with an incident carcinoma (22%) than in unaffected breasts (7%; $P = 0.01$). Interestingly, the insufficient sample rate was higher for ducts in breasts with an incident carcinoma (40%) than for ducts in breasts unaffected with carcinoma (27%; $P = 0.06$). Thirty-two patients with atypical lavage from the unaffected breast underwent repeat lavage at median 8.3 months, with atypia occurring in only 48%. Magnetic resonance imaging was abnormal in three of 24 breasts (13%); atypical lavage and DCIS was diagnosed in one patient.

NDL has been proposed as a secondary risk stratification procedure for women who are determined to be at increased risk for breast cancer. Atypia found in nipple aspirates, needle biopsies, or surgical biopsies may establish risk. Therefore, NDL is recommended only for risk stratification and not as a diagnostic procedure. However, in the study of Maddux and associates, marked atypia was more common in NDL samples from breasts with incident carcinoma (22%) than breasts with no carcinoma (6.8%). This is a higher atypia rate than reported previously. Marked atypia was also noted in 43% of unaffected breasts. However, reproducibility of atypia on repeat lavage ranges from 19% to 25% only.

The numbers of duct orifices (range, 11–48; mean, 27) present a challenge in reidentification with repeat lavage. Reproducibility is also affected by variables such as hormonal changes, number of cells and cytologic interpretation. The insufficient rate on repeat lavage was 29%.[41] The higher prevalence of lavage atypia, along with low reproducibility, limits the use of a single NDL in predicting the high risk of breast carcinoma.

In a recent study by Bushnaq and coworkers, 50 women without known breast carcinoma underwent NDL with lavage of all NAF-producing ducts and at least one non–NAF-producing duct.[42] The cytologic atypia was similar for NAF-producing ducts (19%) and non–NAF-producing ducts (15%; $P = 0.3$). No significant differences were observed when atypia was categorized as mild (13% vs. 10%; $P = 0.63$) or marked (6% vs. 4%; $P = 0.53$). Atypia was diagnosed in 34% of patients with a Gail risk of less than 1.7% versus 28% with Gail risk of greater than or equal to 1.7% ($P = 0.7$). This study concluded that limiting NDL to fluid-producing ducts in women with 5-year Gail risk of greater than or equal to 1.7% will reduce significantly the sensitivity for the population screened.

Ductal Lavage and Molecular Markers. In addition to routine cytology, DL may permit analysis of molecular markers associated with breast carcinoma.[34,43] Cytologic preparations of DL can be used for immunocytochemical analysis. Recent molecular cytogenetics analysis by King and colleagues[44] on 39 paired cases of ductal lavage and surgically excised breast lesions revealed interphase fluorescent in situ hybridization (FISH) cytogenetic changes on chromosomes 1, 8, 11, and/or 17 in 10 of 14 (71%) malignant tumors versus 2 of 18 (11%) from benign neoplasms (Fig. 4-10). This study confirms the potential utility of FISH as a future adjunctive technique. In another study by Yamamoto and associates,[45] DL was performed in women with nipple discharge and abnormal ductography. None of the

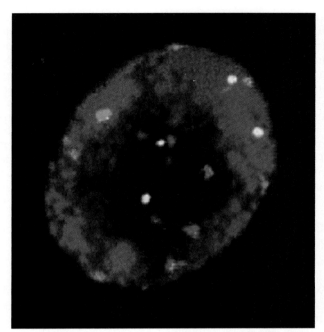

Figure 4-10 Interphase fluorescent in situ hybridization (FISH) for chromosomes 1 and 8. Chromosomes 11 and 17 can be used to determine aneusomy in breast cells. Normal cells are usually diploid, whereas malignant cells are aneuploid.

samples collected from 54 benign cases showed aneusomy for chromosomes 1, 11, and 17, giving a specificity of 100%, whereas aneusomy of at least three of these chromosomes was seen in all six malignant cases. In the future, the adjunctive use of FISH may be helpful in improving the discriminatory value of cytology.

Similarly, Evron and coworkers[46] performed methylation-specific polymerase chain reaction (PCR), or MSP, for cyclin D2, RAR B, and Twist genes on DL specimens. At least one of the genes was methylated in 96% of surgically excised primary tumors and 57% of DCIS, but not in normal breast tissue, resulting in high sensitivity and specificity. Thirty-seven women with biopsy-proven cancers underwent DL. On MSP, 17 of 20 women (85%) also had at least one gene methylated in the DL sample. All four women with negative DL were additionally observed to be negative by MSP. These data demonstrate the feasibility for the early detection of molecular markers in DL, which may possess a role in the early detection of breast cancer.

In the recent study by Euhus and colleagues,[43] investigators measured the prevalence of tumor suppressor gene methylation by quantitative multiplex methylation-specific PCR (QM-MSP) for cyclin D_2, APC, HIN1, RASSF1A, and RAR-β2. Methylation of at least two genes correlated with marked atypia in univariate analysis but not in multivariate analysis that was adjusted for sample cellularity and risk group stratification. This study concluded that both methylation and marked atypia are independently associated with highly cellular sampling, Gail index, and personal history of breast cancer. Based on cytology and methylation profiles, Euhus and colleagues concluded that NDL ipsilateral to a breast cancer rarely retrieves cancer cells (9%). It is apparent that NDL does not seem to be suitable for early detection of focal lesions such as carcinoma, and addition of molecular biomarkers does not resolve this issue. However, NDL may be useful for detection of more diffuse risk-associated field changes in the breast. Cytologic assessment of QM-MSP analysis of NDL samples may provide an approach for identifying high-risk women for monitoring the effects of chemopreventive strategies to reduce the risk of cancer.[43]

Ongoing investigations are exploring the proteome for unique signatures that can be exploited for diagnosis as well as risk determination. High throughput proteomic technologies such as surface enhanced laser desorption and ionization time of flight (SELDI-TOF) mass spectrometry have been used in a number of recent studies to generate unique signatures expressed in cancerous breasts and normal breasts. Using SELDI-TOF to examine NAF in 12 women with breast cancer and 15 healthy controls, Paweletz and associates identified unique proteomic patterns that were discriminatory between the two groups.[47] Using gel-based proteomics, Kuerer and coworkers detected 30 to 202 qualitative protein expression differences in NAF in the breast with cancer compared with the contralateral breast without cancer in the same patient.[48] Varnum and colleagues identified 64 proteins in NAF, including osteopontin and cathepsin D, which have been previously documented to vary with breast cancer status.[49]

Random Periareolar Fine-Needle Aspiration

Random periareolar FNA (RPFNA) is based on the premise that a widespread proliferative change in the breast might be detected by the technique.[50] Rather than detecting specific ducts that produce NAF, RPFNA detects field effect with the underlying presumption that women with atypia on RPFNA have a high density of proliferative changes and possess a higher *short-term risk* for breast cancer compared with women without atypia. RPFNA can be performed on four quadrants or even two quadrants as proposed by Fabian and associates[51] using local anesthesia, 21-gauge needle and a 12-mL syringe prewetted with RPM1. Four to five aspirations are performed. Samples are pooled and can be expressed directly into CytoLyt solution plus 1% of buffered formalin. The cell pellet is transferred to PreservCyt solution and monolayer slides prepared. In nonproliferative samples, cellularity ranges from 100 to 499 cells, and only one to two slides can be prepared, whereas in proliferative lesions cellularity exceeds 5000 cells. The procedure is low in cost and generally well tolerated with few minor complications (e.g., bleeding and hematoma formation), which can be minimized with appropriate precautions.

RPFNA has been shown to detect nonproliferative cytology in 30% of cases, hyperplasia in 49%, and hyperplasia with atypia in 21%. Premenopausal women and postmenopausal women on hormone replacement therapy have a higher ratio of atypia on RPFNA than postmenopausal women. At a median follow-up of 45 months, women with RPFNA hyperplasia and atypia were more likely to have developed DCIS and/or invasive carcinoma than women without atypia. This incidence, based on Gail risk scores, was 15% for high-risk versus 4% for low-risk groups.[50,51]

The technique is limited by high interobserver variance in the cytologic examination. However, Masood and coworkers developed a six category cytology scoring index depending on the degree of abnormality.[52] Nonproliferative samples scored 6 to 10, hyperplasia 11 to 14, and hyperplasia with atypia 15 to 18.

Genetic markers of imbalances such as loss of heterozygosity studies can be performed on FNA slides.[43] Also, biomarkers such as Ki 67, bcl2, and cyclin D-1 have also been attempted on samples obtained by RPFNA.[49]

Summary

The intraductal approach for diagnosis and risk assessment of breast cancer is an attractive alternative. The availability of cellular components for cytologic examination and evaluation with certain novel techniques provide an interesting paradigm in breast evaluation. Nipple aspiration and RPFNA are the least expensive. Nipple aspiration is limited by low cellularity, whereas RPFNA may have issues related to tolerability of the procedure as well as operator skill issues. DL, although more invasive, produces highly cellular material in the sample, but adoption has been slow because the procedure is expensive and the material is diluted, which may interfere with a biomarker approach. Duct endoscopy, although the most expensive and time-labor consuming, provides the best opportunity for integration into clinical practice because of its ability to identify specific lesions and ducts. Also, ductoscopy in conjunction with tissue sampling for cytologic and histologic examination and adjunctive use of FISH may improve yield for risk assessment and diagnosis. Perhaps the greatest promise for identifying unique biomarkers includes exploration of the proteome with novel molecular techniques that predict breast cancer risk and contribute to our understanding of the biology of breast cancer. The intraductal approach to breast cancer remains one of the most exciting novel developments of investigation and application.

Clinical Evaluation and Management of the Patient with Nipple Discharge

When a patient presents with nipple discharge, the physician must approach evaluation and treatment in a deliberate, systematic fashion. This depends on (1) the patient's history and presentation features, (2) the probability of an underlying malignancy versus a benign condition, and (3) additional data available on workup (Fig. 4-11).

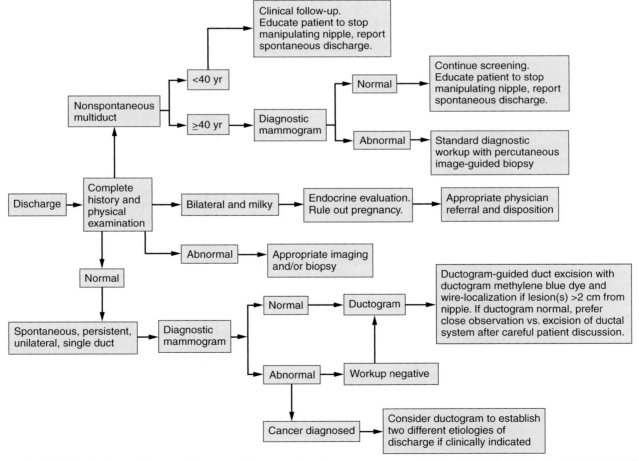

Figure 4-11   M.D. Anderson Cancer Center algorithm for evaluation and management of patients with nipple discharge. (From Cabioglu N, Hunt KK, Singletary SE: Surgical decision making and factors determining a diagnosis of breast carcinoma in women presenting with nipple discharge. J Am Coll Surg 196:354–364, 2003.)

FREQUENCY AND ETIOLOGY OF NIPPLE DISCHARGE

Spontaneous nipple discharge is the chief complaint in 3% to 6% of women presenting to breast specialty services.[53] In a series of 10,000 encounters, Seltzer reported that only 3% were the result of nipple discharge. Of those, one third occurred in women older than 50 years of age.[54] However, nipple discharge may not always be reported by the patient. Newman and colleagues[55] found spontaneous discharge in 10% of 2685 women seen for routine examination. The great majority of nipple discharges are caused by benign conditions (Table 4-1). Papillomas or papillomatosis are the most frequent causes of pathologic nipple discharge. The frequency of cancer as etiology of nipple discharge varies in reported series. This may be related to the nature of the medical/surgical or gynecologic practice and whether it is heavily weighted to cancer patients. Also, in some series, the patients ultimately undergoing surgery were highly selected and thus would be expected to have a higher proportion of cancers. In the series reported by Florio,[56] only those patients with abnormal cytology had surgical resection of the duct. Cabioglu[57] studied patients at the M.D. Anderson Cancer Center of which 20% with nipple discharge were diagnosed with cancer; this incidence of cancer is lower in other series.[53,58-60] Benign papillomas and duct ectasia are more common in younger women, and cancer is more common in older women.[61]

The clinical significance of nipple discharge and the appropriate decision making for its management is most important in the absence of a palpable mass. Kilgore and associates[62] found no palpable mass in 35% of carcinomas associated with nipple discharge, whereas Funderburk and Syphax[63] found no palpable mass in 82% cases of nipple discharge.

Cancers infrequently present as an isolated discharge. Chaudary and coworkers[64] reported that only 16 of 2476 (0.6%) cancers presented with isolated discharge. Devitt,[65] however, reported discharge associated with 2% of all breast cancers. Seltzer reported that 9% of patients older than 50 years of age presenting with nipple discharge had breast cancer compared with only 1% of those younger than 50 years of age.

Intraductal Papilloma

Papillomas are benign epithelial lesions, with supporting stroma, growing within ducts, that are independent of the ductal walls. Most common is the solitary intraductal papilloma located in the major ducts near the nipple. A single papilloma is rarely associated with cancer. Histologically, papillomas are arborizing lesions with papillary fronds lined by epithelial and myoepithelial cells (Fig. 4-12). Occasionally, papillomas may have areas of atypical hyperplasia, which has been shown to increase the risk of subsequent cancer.[66] Intraductal papillomas are typically regarded as clonal proliferations of a precursor cell with the ability to differentiate into epithelial and myoepithelial cells.

Less common are peripheral papillomas. Ohuchi and colleagues[66] reported that 6 of 25 patients with multiple peripheral papillomas had associated DCIS. In their

TABLE 4-1

Etiology of Pathologic Nipple Discharge

Study	No. of Patients	Cancer (%)	Papilloma/ Papillomatosis (%)	Duct Ectasia/Fibrocystic Conditions (%)	Atypia (%)	Other Benign Conditions (%)
Adair[a]	108	47.2	45.3	—	—	7.4
Madalin[b]	100	1	58	25	—	16
Urban[c]	435	8	45	36.5	—	10.5
Murad[d]	267	21	35	42	—	—
Leis[e]	586	14.3	48.1	4.8	18.2	14.6
Dawes[f]	39	12.8	64.1	23.1	—	—
Florio[g,*]	94	26.6	59.5	2.1	—	11.8
King[h]	50	8	42	50	·	—
Cabioglu[i]	94	20.2	66	—	—	13.8
Lau[j]	118	9.3	57.6	—	—	33.1
Adepoju[k]	168	12	48	14	11	16
Vargas[l]	68	5.8	57	32.4	—	4.4

*Only patients with suspicious cytology had operative intervention.
[a]Data from Adair FE: Sanguineous discharge from the nipple and its significance in relation to cancer. Ann Surg 91:197–209, 1930.
[b]Data from Madalin HE, Clagett OT, McDonald JR: Lesions of the breast associated with discharge from the nipple. Ann Surg 46:751–763, 1957.
[c]Data from Urban JA, Egeli RA: Non-lactational nipple discharge. CA Cancer J Clin 28:130–140, 1978.
[d]Data from Murad TM, Contesso G, Mouriesse H.[61]
[e]Data from Leis HP: Management of nipple discharge. World J Surg 13:736–742, 1989.
[f]Data from Dawes LG, et al.[87]
[g]Data from Florio MG, et al.[56]
[h]Data from King TA, et al.[60]
[i]Data from Cabioglu N, et al.[84]
[j]Data from Lau S, et al.[58]
[k]Data from Adepoju LJ, et al.[59]
[l]Data from Vargas HI, et al.[53]

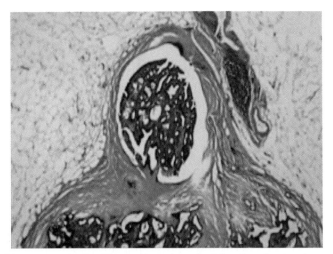

Figure 4-12 Papilloma. Note the arborizing fronds of an intraductal papilloma lined by epithelial cells.

series of 77 patients with papillary lesions, Cardenosa and Eklund[67] reported that 18% of patients have multiple peripheral papillomas. Only one of these patients had nipple discharge as a presenting symptom.

Nipple adenoma or florid papillomatosis of the terminal portion of lactiferous ducts is also associated with bloody nipple discharge. However, because of the proximity to the nipple, the lesion may have nests of squamous metaplasia. Occasionally, intraductal papillary carcinoma and invasive ductal carcinoma may arise in nipple adenomas. Treatment is by simple excision and may require localization assisted by ultrasound or mammography.

Papillary-type lesions are also seen at the confluence of major ducts late in pregnancy and in the early postpartum period; this presentation accounts for the bloody secretions sometimes seen during pregnancy.[68] These lesions have no association with cancer.

Duct Ectasia

Ectasia is a dilation of ducts with loss of elastin in duct walls and the presence of chronic inflammatory cells, especially plasma cells, around duct walls. Theories of causation range from transudation of secretions sequestered in ducts dilated from previous pregnancy to primary periductal inflammation. Up to 60% of nipple discharges associated with duct ectasia contain bacteria (*Enterococcus*, anaerobic *Streptococcus*, *Staphylococcus aureus*, and *Bacteroides*), but whether infection is the primary cause or a secondary supercontamination is unknown.[69] Duct ectasia does not indicate predisposition to cancer. Cytologically/histologically the duct contents are comprised of proteinaceous debris, lipid-containing histiocytes (Fig. 4-13), cholesterol crystals, and calcification (duct ectasia). Nipple discharge is present in 20% of the cases. Most cases are seen in premenopausal women.[70]

Lactational Bloody Nipple Discharge

Pregnancy is associated with significant proliferative alterations in the breast tissue. The "normal" cytology

of breast secretions during pregnancy is characterized by increased cellularity compared with the resting breast, particularly in the late months of pregnancy. Cell types are the same as those found in the absence of pregnancy but show some differences in the proportions of various cells. Epithelial cell clusters are numerous and sometimes possess a configuration suggesting a papillary structure. In the late third trimester and after childbirth, neutrophils are abundant.[1-6,20,71-76]

Holmquist and Papanicolaou[76] found an unexpectedly large number of ductal epithelial cells in patients during pregnancy and lactation. The groups of cells were papillary in structure and similar to papillary fronds from intraductal papilloma.

Kline and Lash[77] studied the cytology of breast secretions obtained during the third trimester from 50 pregnant women (16 to 39 years of age). This study was prompted by the erroneous interpretation of cytologic findings during pregnancy based on the papillary groupings and changes similar to those described by Holmquist and Papanicolaou.[76] In the Kline and Lash study,[77] 43 of the 50 women had papillary groupings, whereas the remaining seven had only foam cells and leukocytes. Tissue from four biopsies obtained in the third trimester of pregnancy revealed "tufts" of cells forming "spurs" or invaginations into duct and alveolar lumens with similar structures that were desquamated into lumina and were similar to clusters of cells found in the breast secretions. The observed "spurs" were closely associated with the formation of new alveoli. Delicate capillary networks within these tufts of cells could be easily traumatized, causing blood to appear in breast secretions.

Blood may be found in secretions from pregnant and lactating patients in the absence of clinically evident lesions.[68,77] These findings justify observation of nipple discharges in pregnant or lactating women but only after confirmation of the absence of suspicious clinical or radiologic findings.

Nonbreast Etiology

Drugs and hormonal disorders may be associated with nipple discharge. Disorders of hormone production,

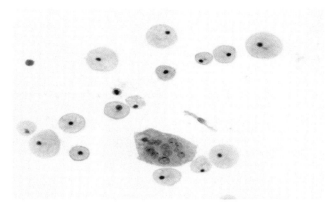

Figure 4-13 Cytologic examination of the nipple discharge may reveal foamy histiocytes only.

including anovulatory syndromes,[78] may induce pathophysiologic responses in the breast.

Prolactinemia from a pituitary adenoma may initiate nipple discharge. Although discharge has been reported in nearly one half of patients with this pituitary neoplasm, the 2.2% reported by Newman's group is probably more representative of the frequency of prolactin tumors in patients with discharge.[55] Normal serum prolactin levels are less than or equal to 20 µg/mL. If values are repeatedly elevated, thin-section computed tomography of the sella turcica of the calvarium is indicated. Patients with only moderate elevation often have normal radiologic results, but they should be followed closely. With advanced prolactin tumors, examination confirms loss of visual fields and/or a possible history of infertility.

Because the breast lacks a biologic feedback mechanism, prolonged secretory responses may follow short, often unrecognized, surges in circulating prolactin.[66] Furthermore, transient rises in prolactin may explain the nipple discharge in situations such as breast stimulation (especially as in nursing or nipple manipulation), chest trauma, or after thoracotomy.

Large doses of tranquilizers (e.g., phenothiazines, reserpine, methyldopa) can induce lactation. Hooper and coworkers[79] noted galactorrhea in 24 of 100 psychiatric inpatients; of those with galactorrhea, 23 of the 24 were taking major tranquilizers. Lactation ceases following discontinuation of drug usage and may not return with smaller doses.[78] Alterations in nipple secretions may also be related to industrial or agricultural exposure to estrogens.[80]

HISTORY

In assessing the clinical significance of a nipple discharge, it is important to take a careful history to characterize the nature (content) and origin of the discharge. The most important factor in the history is whether the discharge is spontaneous or elicited. The index of suspicion for a pathologic discharge is greater when the patient complains of a (spontaneous) discharge first noted as a stain on her clothing. Previously, patient education in breast self-examination has emphasized observation for a nipple discharge as same may be a sign of cancer. Women often manipulate the nipple quite vigorously in checking for a discharge. It is common that one or more drops of liquid can be expressed from about half of women during their reproductive years. Generally, a discharge that occurs only with manipulation does not require further evaluation. However, the presence of a significant amount of clear, bloody, or serous fluid on a routine physical examination with compression or during a mammogram requires further evaluation. If the discharge occurred when the patient manipulated the breast, it may be instructive to the examiner to have the patient demonstrate the discharge.

It is also important to ascertain whether the discharge is bilateral or unilateral or comes from a single duct or multiple ducts. The color and consistency of the observed discharge should be determined. The patient should be queried as to whether the discharge was associated with painful swelling of the breast, a mass, skin changes or nipple deformities.

In addition, it is necessary to query the patient with regard to trauma to the breast or chest wall and to take a detailed history of current medications. Breast discharge can be a response to a variety of stimuli other than underlying breast disease. The patient should be queried regarding previous history of endocrine problems.

EXAMINATION

Examination should identify the duct or ducts producing the discharge, its color and nature, and the location of the trigger point (quadrant of origin) that on compression causes the discharge. The patient should be carefully examined for other signs of breast pathology such as a mass, skin changes of the nipple–areola complex, nipple inversion, or retraction. The number of ducts producing discharge is almost as useful a guide as spontaneous discharge. Discharges from multiple ducts are rarely malignant, whereas single-duct discharge indicates a risk of malignancy. Ciatto and colleagues[81] report that single-duct discharge has a relative risk of 4.07 (confidence interval, 2.7 to 6) of malignancy compared with an asymptomatic population, whereas multiductal or bilateral discharges harbor risks similar to those of the general population. Murad and associates[61] report that none of their patients with cancer had bilateral discharges.

Leis and coworkers[82] describe four types of discharge—serous, serosanguineous, sanguineous, and watery—that in ascending frequency (6.3%, 11.9%, 24%, and 45.5%, respectively) are more likely to be associated with cancer. However, although only 24% of bloody discharges were related to a cancer, 45% of all of the cancers did have a bloody discharge. In a review of 386 nipple discharges without associated mass, 177 (46%) were bloody. Of patients with benign disease, 38% had bloody discharge, compared with 69% in women with carcinoma. Kilgore and colleagues[62] classify serous or bloody discharge as pathologic and discharge with evidence of secretory products as physiologic. Funderburk and Syphax[63] found serous or bloody fluid in 106 of 167 of samples (63%) and milky, colored, or clear fluid in 61 of 167 (37%). The serous or bloody fluids were associated with carcinoma, papilloma, or other papillary lesions in 74% of cases (78 of 106); fibrocystic changes in 22%; and duct ectasia, drugs, and other conditions in 4%. The majority (94%) of fluids with secretory components were associated with fibrocystic change and other nonproliferative breast lesions, whereas only 6% (4 of 61) were associated with papilloma.

Elicited fluid should be tested for occult blood even if it appears nonbloody. Chaudary's group[64] tested for heme with laboratory test sticks (as used for urine dip testing). Test sticks detect as few as 5 to 15 red blood cells/mL, which would not be visible as bloody fluid. All 16 patients with cancer had hemoglobin in nipple secretions; however, positive predictive value is low because 107 of 132 intraductal papillomas and 67 of 94 duct ectasias also had hemoglobin in the discharge. Blood may also be present in nipple secretions in as great as 20% of women during normal pregnancy.[77,83]

Single-duct discharges typically have a trigger point on the breast where pressure induces a discharge. This trigger point should be identified and documented in the patient's chart before planning surgery (see subsequent discussion). The patient is examined in a standard position, preferably supine with the ipsilateral hand behind the head. Direct digital pressure is then applied to sequential points around the areola by the examiner until the site where pressure elicits the maximum discharge identified. It is rarely necessary to squeeze the nipple to elicit a pathologic nipple discharge. Should the physician be unable to elicit the discharge, it is minimally distressful to ask the patient to squeeze the nipple in a final attempt to elicit the discharge.

Clinical breast examination is important as discharge associated with cancer often is accompanied by a mass. Devitt[65] found in his series of patients with discharge that 8 of 10 women with cancer had palpable masses; 1 patient had nipple distortion but no mass. Leis and associates[81] reported palpable masses in 88.1% of 67 patients with nipple discharge and cancer. However, discharge with mass is still more likely to be benign. Florio and coworkers[56] report cancer in only 10% of women with discharge and a mass. King and colleagues[60] identified cancer in only three of 11 women with discharge who had an abnormal mammogram. Cabioglu and associates reported that six of 19 women with malignant nipple discharge had a mass on physical examination.[84]

IMAGING EVALUATION

Mammography should be performed in all patients with nipple discharge to seek a focal occult lesion and/or to estimate the extent of the abnormality with identification of a palpable mass on examination. The mammogram may be normal in as many as 60% to 83% of patients with spontaneous nipple discharge.[67,85] Mammographic findings[5,16–18] include benign-appearing circumscribed masses of various sizes (typically retroareolar in location), a solitary dilated retroareolar duct, and calcifications (Fig. 4-14). There is controversy regarding the additional radiographic studies that are warranted to evaluate nipple discharge.[86,87] When radiographic studies are negative, one cannot assume that there is no intraductal pathology. Ultrasound of the central breast can be performed to identify dilated ducts with intraductal lesions. However, it is critical to have confidence that the lesion identified by ultrasound is in fact associated with the discharge. Cabioglu and associates identified sonographic abnormalities in 40% of patients with papilloma and in 60% of patients with cancers.[85] An abnormal ultrasound was associated with a 5.5-fold relative risk for breast cancer in patients with a nipple discharge. Rissanen and coworkers evaluated the value of ultrasound in localizing intraductal lesions in patients with nipple discharge.[88] Ultrasound demonstrated intraductal lesions in 36 of 52 patients (69%), ductal dilatation in 6 patients (12%), and no lesion in 10 patients (19%). Although only 20% of malignant lesions demonstrated an ultrasound abnormality, 80% of papillomatous lesions were associated with an ultrasound abnormality. When these abnormalities are identified, the surgical procedure can be used to target the suspected source. Examples of intraductal lesions seen on ultrasound are shown in Figure 4-15.

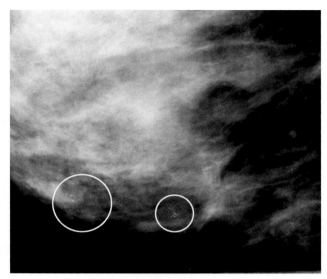

Figure 4-14 Mammogram in patient with spontaneous copious nipple discharge. Microcalcifications are suspicious and in area of tortuous ducts identified on ductogram. Final pathology is ductal carcinoma in situ. (Courtesy of Phil Evans, MD, UT Southwestern Medical Center.)

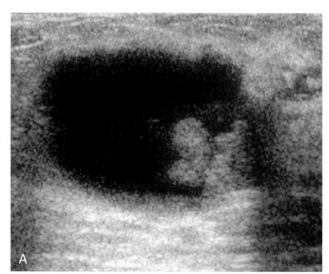
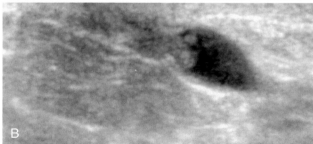

Figure 4-15 A, Ultrasound showing intracystic papilloma. **B,** Ultrasound showing intraductal papilloma filling a duct. (Courtesy of Ralph Wynn, MD, UT Southwestern Medical Center.)

The nipple ducts can be accessed with contrast injection, visualization by ductoscopy, or lavage. Technical issues common to the three techniques include adequate anesthesia and success of the duct cannulation. Topical anesthetic agents, such as 2.5% lidocaine and 2.5% prilocaine (EMLA), anesthetize the nipple in 45 to 60 minutes. Careful injection of local anesthesia near the base of the nipple is effective. Care is taken to avoid distortion or hemorrhage in the nipple-areolar complex as the creation of tortuosity of the duct at the base of the nipple from hemorrhage may inhibit duct cannulation. The nipple can be gently stretched and pushed to allow passage of instrumentation.

Ductography–Galactography

Ductography or galactography can be performed to define the intraductal abnormality. Ductography involves cannulation of the discharging duct with a small catheter or 30-gauge blunt tip needle (often with a 90-degree bend near the tip).[89] The cannula is introduced into the discharging orifice following activation of discharge with compression at the edge of the nipple–areola complex. It may be necessary to elevate the nipple between the thumb and forefinger to facilitate cannulation of the duct. The cannula is attached to extension tubing with a 1- to 3-mL syringe. Full-strength water-soluble contrast iothalamate meglumine is injected.[90] Typically, the volume required to fill the duct is 0.2 to 0.3 mL. The injection should be discontinued if the patient has acute pain and should be done with low pressure to avoid extravasation. The cannula is then taped to the skin. Mammograms are performed immediately while the contrast material is in the breast ducts. Magnification views in the craniocaudad and medial-lateral oblique projection are obtained. If an intraductal lesion is not identified, the cannula can be removed from the duct orifice, because it may be obscuring a lesion at the distal duct or nipple ampulla.

Allergic reactions to the injection of contrast into the ductal system are very rare compared with intravenous (IV) injections of similar agents. However, patients with a prior history of rash and itching with IV contrast should be premedicated with diphenhydramine and steroids. Patients with a history of anaphylactic reactions to IV contrast should not undergo ductography.

If ductography fails because of inability to cannulate the duct, several strategies can be undertaken. Schwab and colleagues described a technique of applying a local anesthetic (lidocaine) spray typically used for mucosal anesthesia.[91] The operator waits 5 minutes to attempt cannulation, which allows for relaxation of the nipple and areola. In the series of 47 patients, Schwab reported that cannulation of the duct initially failed in 8 patients. With application of the lidocaine spray, they were able to successfully cannulate the nipple duct all 8 patients. Berna-Serna and associates reported the use of lidocaine and prilocaine cream application 45 to 60 minutes prior to ductography.[92] Outcomes of patients receiving the topical anesthetic cream are encouraging. With use of anesthetic cream, all 27 patients had successful ductography. Four of 19 patients experienced unsuccessful duct cannulation when no anesthetic cream was used.

Magnification of the nipple–areola complex is another strategy for facilitating duct cannulation. The application of warm moist compresses may augment relaxation of the nipple–areola complex. Another

maneuver that can be undertaken involves placement of a 2-0 polypropylene suture into the discharging orifice as a guide over which the cannula is introduced.[93] Hou and coworkers report successful cannulation of discharging ducts in 105 consecutive patients using this technique.[94] Success with ductography varies significantly. Sharma and colleagues report failure of ductography in 33% of the 148 patients in whom it was attempted.[95]

Ductograms commonly reveal intraductal lesions within several centimeters of the nipple. Ductographic findings include (1) a cutoff sign or ductal obstruction, (2) ductal dilatation, (3) filling defects, (4) irregularity of the ductal wall, (5) ductal narrowing, and (6) distortion of the ductal arborization (Figs. 4-16 to 4-18).

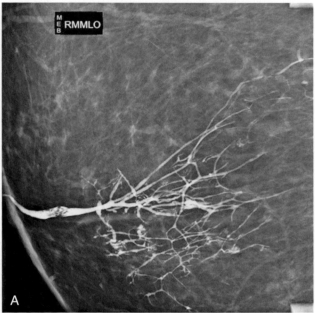

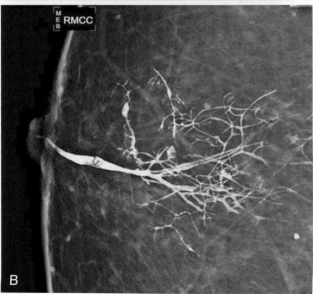

Figure 4-16 **A,** Ductogram with multiple filling defects magnified CC view. **B,** Ductogram with multiple filling defects magnified MLO view. (Courtesy of Phil Evans, MD, UT Southwestern Medical Center.)

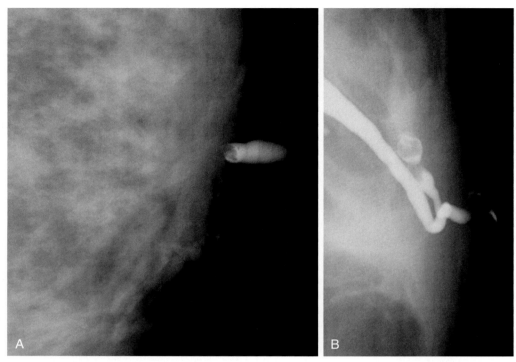

Figure 4-17   A, Ductogram with "cutoff" or duct obstruction. Diagnosis of papilloma. **B,** Ductogram with filling defect. Diagnosis of papilloma. (Courtesy of Ralph Wynn, MD, UT Southwestern Medical Center.)

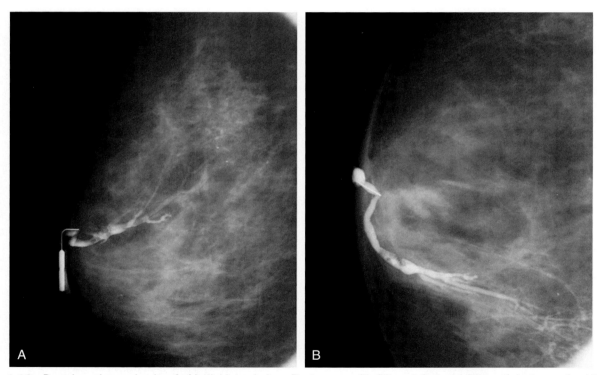

Figure 4-18   Ductal carcinoma in situ. **A,** Medial-lateral view. Ductogram with filling defect and filling of ducts proximal to lesion, with injecting needle in place. **B,** Craniocaudad view. (**A,** Courtesy of Ralph Wynn, MD, UT Southwestern Medical Center.)

Although the duct may have arborization into the deeper breast, the duct excision may be more limited if the lesion is solitary in the distal ductal region. Dawes and associates reported that 20% of ductograms demonstrated one or more lesions greater than 3 cm from the nipple.[87] Cardenosa and Eklund identified abnormalities in 32 of 35 (91%) galactograms obtained to investigate spontaneous nipple discharge, which ultimately were shown to be caused by solitary papillomas.[67] Ten patients (29%) showed expansion or distortion of the duct; 10 ducts (29%) were completely obstructed. Eight patients (23%) had filling defects, three had irregularity of the duct wall (including one with associated obstruction), and one showed ductal ectasia. Woods and coworkers observed filling defect(s) on 92% of diagnostic ductograms.[85] Tabar and colleagues reported that all of 18 women with cancer were identified by ductography but that only 50% had a mass lesion on routine mammograms.[90] Berni and de Guili, however, report only 79% accuracy of ductography, based on pathologic findings in patients who went on to surgical biopsy after ductography.[96]

Dinkel and associates[70] support the latter view that galactography should be used primarily to estimate the extent of a lesion rather than to presume to rule out cancer. They correlated preoperative galactography with pathology for 143 duct excisions, which included 11 women with cancer. Most commonly, cancer caused a filling defect or cutoff on galactography; however, only 6 of 90 patients with filling defects had cancer. Two cancers caused duct compression, and one was associated with duct ectasia. Importantly, in only 2 of 11 cancers was galactography normal.

Some authors advocate continued observation if the ductogram is negative.[97] However, others conclude that the false-negative rate is not acceptable.[87] Dawes and coworkers reported results of ductograms in 21 patients with pathologic discharge. Seven were normal. Four patients with a normal ductogram were shown to have a papilloma at the time of duct excision. Conversely, in four patients who had a filling defect on ductogram, no corresponding lesion was identified in the surgical specimen.

Other investigators have combined cytologic examination and galactography to select patients for biopsy.[56,98,99] They confirm that combined abnormal cytology and abnormal ductography findings indicate a high likelihood of either malignancy or a papilloma. However, this report provides minimal information on patients followed without biopsy.

Ductoscopy

Submillimeter fiberoptic scopes can be used to visualize the interior of the discharging duct.[100,101] The orifice of the duct that produces the discharge is dilated either with lacrimal probes or sequentially larger catheters. A fiberoptic scope is introduced into the dilated nipple orifice, manipulated through tortuous sections of the duct in the nipple, and then advanced into the ducts. As with other endoscopy techniques, fluid is gently introduced through the scope as it is advanced. Newer scopes can be introduced through a plastic sleeve, which serves both as a dilator and as an access to obtain washings. In a darkened room, the light of the scope can be seen through breast tissue. If a point of interest is identified, the skin can be marked over the spot of light to guide subsequent biopsy. Endoscopic findings may include an intraductal mass lesion, blood staining or injection in the wall of the duct, irregularity of the duct wall, duct obstruction, and scar.[102] Matsunaga

and colleagues classified intraductal lesions by type as hemispheric, papillary, and flat protrusion.[103,104] Intraductal papillomas were more likely to be hemispheric or papillary in shape; the flat protrusion configuration was more common in malignant lesions. Okazaki and associates described the surface of a normal duct as lustrous and smooth.[105] A cancer on the surface of the duct wall appeared white and slightly elevated.

Kothari and coworkers performed ex vivo mammary ductoscopy on 115 ducts in 35 mastectomy specimens.[106] Abnormalities were seen on 40% of ducts. The authors proposed a morphologic classification of endoluminal lesions. These include (1) obstructing endoluminal lesions; (2) epithelial surface abnormalities subdivided into premalignant and malignant epithelial proliferation versus inflammation; (3) papillomatous lesions—single or multiple; (4) intraductal scars, adhesions, and duct obliteration; and (5) intraductal calcifications. Sauter and colleagues reported a normal intraductal examination in one fourth of patients with spontaneous nipple discharge.[107] In a series of 88 patients undergoing endoscopy, Dooley and associates noted that 18% of patients had normal-appearing ducts on endoscopic examination.[108] The role of this technique in diagnosis of discharge and other lesions is under active investigation. The instrumentation has been refined dramatically since its introduction in the late 1980s to permit interventions via the scope, as well as enhanced visualization.

CYTOLOGIC EVALUATION

An adequate sample is the sine qua non for good results with for breast cytologic examination. The preparatory methods for this histopathologic technique include direct smears from spontaneous nipple discharge and the membrane filtration of NAF samples. Cytologic examination needs to be systematic and thorough, and a classification system should use terminology related to the anticipated histopathology.

Sample Collection

Spontaneous nipple discharge is expressed directly onto the glass slide, which is held at the opening of the duct, and then it is moved across the drop of fluid at the surface of the nipple to ensure a thin spread. This slide is then smeared with a second slide lengthwise. The slides are immersed immediately in the fixative of 95% ethanol. It is suggested that four to six smears be prepared from each discharge, because the material is often more cellular in the last drops of fluid. If blood-tinged fluid is observed to be emanating from one duct, its location should be noted and an attempt should be made to differentiate the sample from that duct separate from the remaining discharge. This can be accomplished by using a capillary pipette to collect the sample directly from the duct opening.[109]

Sample Preparation

Two important aspects of specimen preparation include the concentration of cells and recovery of cells. *Cell concentration* refers to increasing the number of cells per unit volume or area. *Cell recovery* is the efficiency of collecting cells per unit volume of sample or the percentage of total cells in a sample. In NAF samples, cell recovery is especially important because of the scant cellularity. If concentration techniques lead to a differential loss of cells, the preparation method may interfere with the diagnostic value of the sample.

Direct smears require no special laboratory preparation other than appropriate staining with Papanicolaou stain or other stains preferred by the laboratory.

NAF samples are concentrated and recovered on membrane filters. Millipore filters are preferred because of the anticipated high rate of cell recovery (approximately 80% of cells per sample) and the expected good-quality cytomorphology.[110]

Cytologic Examination

A complete and systematic examination of NAF, DLF, and breast discharge cytology by a cytotechnologist and pathologist with training and experience in this specialized area of cytopathology is required. Epithelial cells in NAF and breast discharge are often few and tend to be small, and significant cells or groups of cells can easily be missed. Qualitative assessment is made of the cellular composition, including types of cells and degree of cellularity. Cytologic evaluation is based on the changes in epithelial cells and accompanying cellular findings, and the final interpretation is considered following correlation with complete clinical data. It is essential that the clinician understand that a negative cytology does not exclude malignancy. Diagnostic terminology used for the cellular findings in NAF, DLF, and nipple discharge conforms to the expected lesion in subsequent biopsy. Morphologic terminology that is universally understood and consistent with standard nomenclature is preferred rather than systems that use nonspecific terms that are subject to a variety of interpretations.

The cytologic diagnosis of nipple discharge samples has been highly successful in the evaluation of breast cancer, Paget's disease of the nipple, and benign papilloma or papillary disease. Some examples of diagnostic results with nipple discharge appear in Table 4-2. Uei

and coworkers[111] analyzed the cytomorphology in NAF from both benign and malignant lesions. They noted some distinctive features in the structure of cell groups that improve the accuracy for diagnosis of breast cancer (41% to 66.3%) but also increased false-positive interpretations from 0.9% to 3.6%. Of interest is the finding of a disproportionate number of cases of ductal carcinoma in situ and the rare papillary carcinoma that exists in the presence of malignant nipple discharge.[16,22,63]

Papilloma was diagnosed cytologically by Papanicolaou and colleagues[16] in 34 of 43 (79%) of patients and was confirmed on tissue biopsy. Other investigators have reported similar success with the cytologic diagnosis of intraductal papilloma.[62]

Hou and associates[112] reported an improvement in results with cytology of single duct discharge in absence of a mass when they used an intraductal aspiration method. Adequate samples were obtained from 96.6% of patients, and intraductal aspiration is compared with 76% collected with the conventional method using pressure. Among 27 cancers in the series, 24 (88.9%) were correctly diagnosed with the aspiration sample; 33.3% were diagnosed using the conventional method.

DL is a technique that can improve cell retrieval and thereby improve on analysis of NAF.[38,112] Small amounts of fluid are washed into the duct using a catheter similar to that used for ductography. Fluid is collected as it drains, and cells are isolated and evaluated as for NAF. NAF cytologic examination is useful to demonstrate cancer or abnormal cytology. However, the high false-negative rate precludes using NAF cytology to exclude cancer.

Carty and coworkers[113] proposed use of a "triple test" for evaluation of nipple discharges. This is similar to the triple test used with FNA cytology of palpable masses. They do *not* perform surgical biopsy should clinical examination, mammography, and NAF cytologic examination prove to indicate a negative study. In a series of 56 women, 17 required biopsy using these criteria and 5 had malignancy. The authors followed 38 of the other 39 women for a minimum of 5 years, and the women had no further breast disease. However, 17 had additional nipple discharge on follow-up.

TABLE 4-2

Reported Results with Cytologic Examination of Nipple Discharge

Study	Year	No.	With Cancer	Positive Cytology		False-Positive Cytology	
				No.	Percent	No.	Percent
Papanicolaou[a]	1958	495	45	45	60	3	1
Kjellgren[b]	1964	216	25	21	89	15	8
Masukawa[c]	1966	94	16	6	43	1	1
Funderburk[d]	1969	182	7	6	86	—	—
Uei[e]	1980	190	80	53	66	4	4

[a]Data from Papanicolaou GN, et al.[16]
[b]Data from Kjellgren O: The cytologic diagnosis of cancer of the breast. Acta Cytol 8:216–223, 1964.
[c]Data from Masukawa T, Lewison EF, Frost JK.[3]
[d]Data from Funderburk WW, Syphax B.[63]
[e]Data from Uei Y, et al.[111]

Diagnosis and Surgical Intervention

Definitive diagnosis of the etiology of a nipple discharge is based on biopsy that should first be directed to any area identified by physical examination, mammography, or other studies. If no specific lesion is identified, duct excision should be undertaken for patients with a pathologic nipple discharge. The initial procedure described by Hadfield involved complete excision of the major ductal system with a conical tissue resection.[114] However, a more preferable procedure is microdochectomy, which involves a more directed excision of the discharging duct and its arborization into the breast. Surgical duct excision is both diagnostic and therapeutic for nipple discharge. Even benign discharges may be sufficiently bothersome to the patient that she would prefer duct excision to continued drainage of fluid from the nipple.

TECHNIQUE OF MICRODOCHECTOMY

Duct excision is an outpatient procedure performed with the patient under local anesthesia, usually with IV sedation (Fig. 4-19). A long-acting anesthetic agent is infiltrated at the site of the proposed incision, under the areola, and around the nipple. Injection into the nipple is unnecessary,

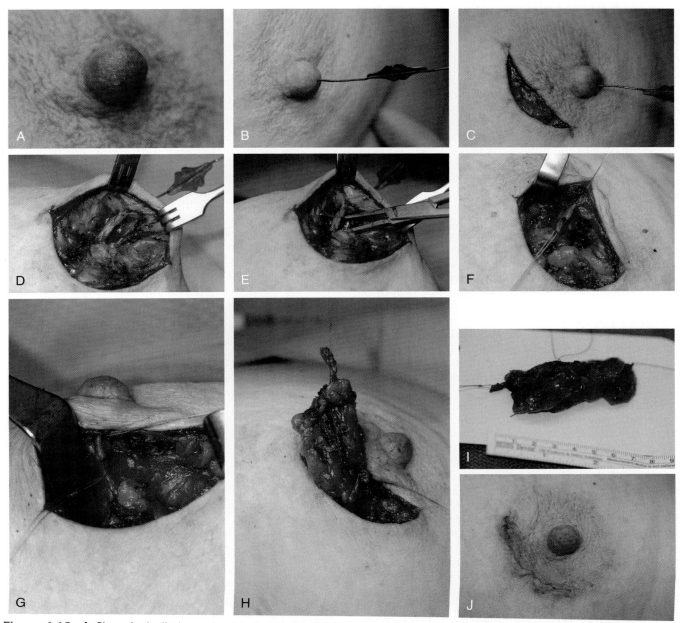

Figure 4-19   A, Clear nipple discharge, but it is Hemoccult positive. **B,** Lacrimal probe in discharging duct. **C,** Incision made at areolar edge corresponding to trigger point and palpable course of lacrimal probe. **D,** Cannulated duct dissected out. **E,** Cannulated duct dissected circumferentially. Duct ligated proximally (**F**) and distally (**G**). **G** shows the relationship to the visible nipple. **H,** Duct transected and gentle traction applied. **I,** Specimen. **J,** Circumareolar wound closure.

because the solution will diffuse from surrounding tissue. The discharge is elicited by pressing at the previously identified trigger point to identify the duct for cannulation with a lacrimal probe. The largest size probe that will accommodate the duct orifice should be used (see Fig. 4-19B). Alternatively, or together with placement of the lacrimal probe, the discharging duct can be injected with methylene blue via a 30-gauge catheter.

A circumareolar incision is made that should not encompass more than 50% of the circumference of the areola; this critical principle of surgical technique avoids devascularization of the nipple–areola complex. The incision centers on the trigger point or the pathology located by ductography or other studies (see Fig. 4-19C). The epicenter of the periareolar incision lies within the trigger point quadrant of the breast. The direction that the lacrimal probe takes on introduction may also guide the placement of the incision and direction of the dissection. Meticulous hemostasis is maintained. Using fine scissors or a 15-blade allows precise dissection. The edge of the areola is elevated with skin hooks, and dissection proceeds with the blade to raise a thick skin flap of the areolar skin toward the base of the nipple.

There are three methods to find the symptomatic duct: (1) palpation of the lacrimal duct probe through the tissue at the base of the nipple, (2) visually identifying the dilated duct by dissection posterior to the nipple, and (3) visually identifying the blue-stained duct when methylene blue is injected in the duct prior to making the skin incision. The identified duct is thereafter dissected superficially to the dermis of the nipple. Using a fine-tipped curved right-angle hemostat, the terminal duct is dissected circumferentially (see Fig. 4-19D). The lacrimal probe may be left in place to facilitate palpation of the extent of the duct (see Fig. 4-19E). However, if the lacrimal probe cannot be introduced more than one centimeter, it is preferable to ligate the duct at its termination on the nipple and transect the duct (see Fig. 4-19F and G). A suture can be placed through the proximal duct for gentle traction during the dissection into the deeper breast (see Fig. 4-19H). The dissection in the posterior breast planes involves dissecting out a pyramidal-shaped specimen of surrounding tissue (see Fig. 4-19I).[85]

The duct is usually within a segment of the breast that is denser than the contiguously adjacent tissue, often surrounded by either loose connective tissue or fatty tissue. The specimen increases in diameter as dissection extends into the deeper breast parenchyma. The extent of dissection into the posterior breast can be limited if the ductogram has revealed a lesion and the dissection can be tailored to fully encompass the lesion. If a dilated duct containing discharge is transected during dissection, it should be marked with a suture for later identification and excision.

If methylene blue has been injected into the duct, all blue-stained areas are generally removed. However, if an intraductal lesion has been identified by ductography or ultrasound in the immediate subareolar region, it is unnecessary to complete a segmental resection of the breast.

Van Zee and colleagues[115] confirmed that preoperative injection of dye facilitated excision. With methylene blue, they noted the pathology review explained the discharge in 100% of patients. However, without dye usage, they found pathology to account for only 67% of discharges.

In general, minimal local anesthesia is required for the dissection into the posterior breast. As wound closure is undertaken, attention should be directed to avoid the collapse of the nipple–areola complex into the soft tissue defect resulting from the resection (see Fig. 4-19J). It is often feasible to mobilize tissue on either side of the defect in the subareolar location and approximate it with absorbable interrupted sutures. The dermis and subcutaneous tissue are closed with interrupted absorbable sutures. The skin is then closed with a running subcuticular, absorbable suture.

The patient is advised to wear a bra for support for 72 hours. Vigorous activity should also be avoided during this period.

TECHNICAL MODIFICATIONS FOR DUCT EXCISION

In the circumstance of surgical biopsy for nipple discharge, there is concern as to whether the lesion is actually retrieved with the surgery. Baker and associates reported 30 cases of duct excision with ductogram abnormalities.[116] However, in six cases, the abnormalities identified on ductogram were not evident on the surgical pathology. This, perhaps, results from incorrect estimation of the depth of the dissection to encompass the ductal abnormality. Precise measurements to identify the distance of the lesion from the nipple are performed at the time the breast is compressed for mammography. Other proposed methods to ensure resection of the lesion include wire localization of abnormalities identified on ductogram, diagnostic mammogram, sonogram, and the novel application of intraoperative ductoscopy.

Chow and coworkers[117] described the performance of a ductogram on the day of surgery with placement of a localizing wire in the area of the identified ductal abnormality. A localization wire is placed while the contrast is still in the duct (Fig. 4-20). Because water-soluble contrast media

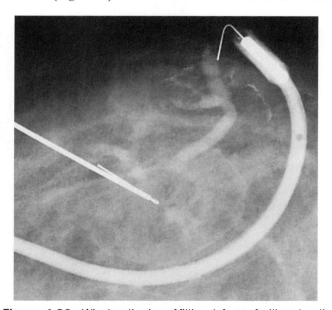

Figure 4-20 Wire localization of filling defect to facilitate localization of deeper lesion. Galactography combined with wire localization biopsy. The duct has an abrupt cutoff at the site of the lesion. The guidewire was placed while contrast media was within the duct. The contrast was not present at the time of the biopsy and could not be seen on the specimen radiograph. The lesion was a benign papilloma. (Courtesy of Edward A. Sickles, MD.)

does not usually persist in the duct, the specimen radiograph usually does not show any abnormality. Koskela and colleagues[118] described the use of wire localization when there is no mammographic or ultrasonographically identified lesion. The wire is placed with stereotactic guidance so that the tip is placed in the area of the abnormality identified on ductography. Rissanen and associates[88] reported using wire localization in 11 and 49 patients undergoing surgical resection for nipple discharge. Ultrasound-guided wire localization was used. They made the following clinical findings: (1) failure to cannulate the discharging duct, (2) preoperative ductogram identified a duct different from the one identified with the original diagnostic galactography, and (3) a positive ultrasound with a negative ductogram. There is no intraoperative means to verify removal of the pathologic tissue with these techniques, other than confirming that the localizing wire

tip is centrally located within the specimen with a margin of tissue circumferentially. A case study in the workup of nipple discharge (Fig. 4-21) demonstrates our approach to combining techniques to maximize assurance of resection of the pathologic lesions.

Dooley describes the technique for use of ductoscopy for intraoperative visualization of ductal abnormalities.[119] The discharging duct is cannulated with a 2-0 Prolene suture. The duct orifice is sequentially dilated using 26-, 24-, and 22-gauge catheters. Local anesthetic is instilled into the duct. The 0.9-mm fiberoptic endoscope is introduced. The ductal abnormalities are identified. The margin of resection of tissue is guided by transillumination from the scope. Twenty-seven patients with Hemoccult-positive spontaneous nipple discharge and negative mammography were taken to surgery for microductectomy. In 96% of cases, the intraductal

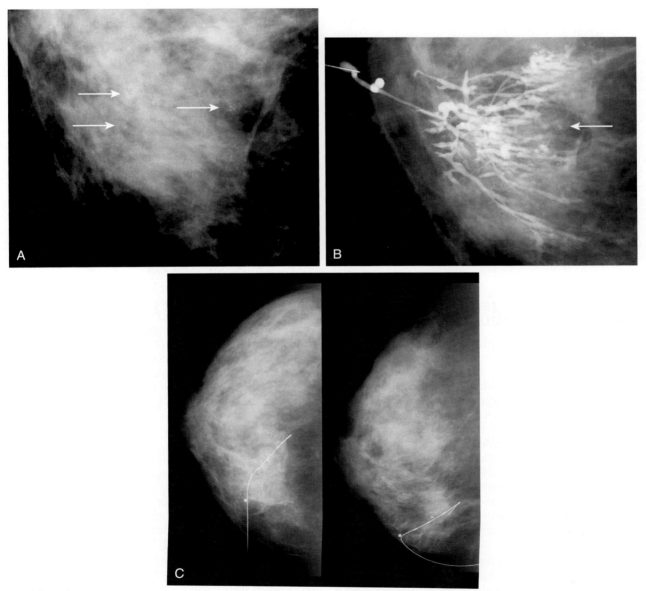

Figure 4-21 Case study. **A,** Nipple discharge workup included mammogram with microcalcifications deeper and more peripheral in medial breast shown at tips of *arrows.* **B,** Ductogram with multiple dilated ducts with extensive arborization in same area as microcalcifications. Stereotactic biopsy of microcalcifications revealed ductal carcinoma in situ. **C,** Our approach would be wire localization of the calcifications and placement of a lacrimal probe in the discharging duct at the time of surgery to confirm resection of the lesion causing discharge. (Courtesy of Phil Evans, MD, UT Southwestern Medical Center.)

lesion responsible for bleeding was identified. Multiple lesions were found in 70% of cases and often were deeper in the breast. Dooley noted coexistence of superficial papillomas with deeper DCIS lesions. Dietz and colleagues[120] described a series of 119 patients undergoing endoscopically guided duct excision. Cannulation of the discharging duct was successful in 88% of women, and endoscopy-directed resection was achieved in 87%. Cancer and hyperplasia were more likely to be correlated with failed duct cannulation. Similar to the report by Dooley, multiple lesions and those more than 4 cm from the nipple were noted in 22% of women. Dietz suggested that these lesions might have been left behind with standard microdochectomy. Ductoscopy was more accurate than preoperative ductography in identifying specific intraductal pathology (90% vs. 76%).

Moncrief and associates[102] compared ductoscopy-guided versus conventional surgical duct excision in 117 women with spontaneous nipple discharge. There was good correlation between the endoscopic findings and the pathologic diagnosis when an intraductal tumor was seen on ductoscopy, with 90% of 49 ducts demonstrating a papilloma or more severe pathology. The range of pathologic diagnoses was similar between the two procedures. The authors suggested that the gross appearance of the intraductal lesion cannot reliably distinguish between benign and malignant lesions. In the ductoscopy group, more peripheral lesions were identified, and multiple papillomas were more commonly found in the specimen. The potential advantage of ductoscopy-guided surgery is the identification of more peripheral lesions, which might impart a greater risk of breast cancer. Another potential advantage would be limitation of the extent of subareolar duct excision when resection is focused on the area of the lesion identified at ductoscopy rather than the entire duct. However, the authors did not provide data on the volume of tissue resected or preservation of subareolar ductal tissue.

MINIMALLY INVASIVE TECHNIQUES FOR BIOPSY OF INTRADUCTAL LESIONS

There is increasing interest in using nonsurgical techniques to biopsy intraductal lesions.[121] Govindarajulu and co-workers[122] reported on the use of ultrasound-guided mammotome biopsy for 77 patients with pathologic nipple discharge. The biopsy targeted a dilated duct only in 50% of cases and an intraductal lesion in 50%. A 3- to 5-cm segment of the duct was excised with the mammotome. Pathology results included papilloma (41%), epithelial hyperplasia (23%), chronic inflammation (29%), atypical ductal hyperplasia (1%), and malignancy (6%). Complications included recurrence of symptoms in 5% of patients, requiring duct excision or repeat mammotome resection. Six percent had a hematoma and a similar number had bleeding from the nipple. Long-term follow-up was not reported.

Beechey-Newman and colleagues[123] used ductoscopy with a microbrush technique to biopsy intraductal lesions in 50 patients presenting with nipple discharge. The microbrush has nylon bristles with a 0.55-mm diameter. The brush was inserted via a working channel in the scope,

and DL fluid was obtained after brushing. The patients underwent either microductectomy or total duct excision after ductoscopy. Thirty-three patients (66%) had an endoluminal lesion identified at ductoscopy. The microbrush was used to sample eight presumed papillary lesions. Of these, seven yielded papillary cells (87.5% sensitivity).

Hunerbein and colleagues[124,125] described a biopsy technique via a rigid ductoscope. The rigid scope has improved optics using fused gradient index lenses. The scope is introduced via a 0.9-mm needle with a lateral port for air insufflation. The introducer needle has a biopsy port to retrieve the specimen with suction. Biopsy via the ductoscope was successfully performed in 34 of 36 patients with nipple discharge and intraductal lesions. The specimen size was typically 1 mm. The results of the ductoscopic biopsies were more accurate than DL cytology. However, resection of lesions was not feasible.

Matsunaga and associates[126] reported on follow-up greater than 3 years for 70 patients undergoing 75 intraductal breast biopsy (IDBB) procedures with ductoscopy guidance. Thirty-six patients experienced resolution of nipple discharge after IDBB; another 13 had resolution after subsequent repeat IDBB. Thus, 70% of patients with nipple discharge had control of their symptoms. In 15 patients in whom bloody nipple discharge persisted, IDBB was repeated on several occasions. IDBB was less likely to be therapeutic in patients with multiple lesions. Two patients (3%) developed breast cancer 3 years after IDBB. Among 89 patients having a negative ductoscopic examination, 3 (4%) developed breast cancer, although the authors indicate that the cancer occurred in a different quadrant of the breast from that of the original lesion seen on ductography. Matsunaga points out that IDBB was less successful in diagnosing carcinoma, with only one third of patients with breast cancer having a positive IDBB.

For most series reporting minimally invasive techniques for diagnosis of nipple discharge, there is no long-term follow-up for the patients who did not have surgical duct excision after ductoscopic examination. In 10% to 12% of patients, ductoscopy is complicated by duct perforation.[102,123] It is important that patients undergoing minimally invasive techniques to evaluate spontaneous nipple discharge have long-term follow-up that provides a better understanding of the false-negative rate of these examinations.

OUTCOMES

The long-term outcome after the diagnosis of nipple discharge appears acceptable if cancer is not found in the initial evaluation. Early recurrence of the discharge may be related to evacuation of a seroma through the orifice of the transected duct. McPherson and Mackenzie[127] noted the recurrence of discharge in 5 of 72 patients at intervals of 2 weeks and 9 years after surgery. Cancer subsequently developed in three of the 72 patients, but two of the three lesions were in the contralateral breast and none of the three patients had recurrent discharge. Vargas and coworkers described a series of 157 patients presenting with nipple discharge, of which 82 were deemed to harbor a pathologic discharge.[53] There was no recurrence of nipple discharge at 18 months postoperatively in 63 patients who underwent duct excision. Lau and colleagues performed 118 duct excisions on 116 patients between 1995 and 2002, and none developed recurrent discharge.[58]

Summary

Spontaneous nipple discharges require a systematic evaluation to ascertain the etiology of the discharge. Although multiple additional studies, such as mammography, ultrasound, ductography and cytologic examination may be obtained, the definitive diagnosis is established with surgical excision of the involved duct. Ancillary tests, when positive, can provide invaluable information for planning the extent of surgical resection. When these tests are abnormal, the patient is commonly highly motivated to proceed with duct excision. The value of minimally invasive procedures to diagnose pathologic nipple discharge is not yet clearly defined; longer follow-up is required to evaluate outcomes. There continues to be interest in the evaluation of breast secretions obtained by NAF or DL to estimate breast cancer risk; however, these approaches remain investigational and, at present, are not incorporated into the routine management of nipple discharges.

REFERENCES

1. Ferguson DJ, Anderson TJ: Morphological evaluation of cell turnover in relation to the menstrual cycle in the "resting" human breast. Br J Cancer 44:177–181, 1981.
2. Masters JR, Drife JO, Scarisbrick JJ: Cyclic variation of DNA synthesis in human breast epithelium. J Natl Cancer Inst 58:1263–1265, 1977.
3. Masukawa T, Lewison EF, Frost JK: The cytologic examination of breast secretions. Acta Cytol 10:261, 1966.
4. Meyer J: Cell proliferation in normal human breast ducts, fibroadenomas, and other ductal hyperplasias measured by nuclear labeling with tritiated thymidine. Effects of menstrual phase, age, and oral contraceptive hormones. Hum Pathol 8:67–81, 1977.
5. Longacre TA, Bartow SA: A correlative morphologic study of human breast and endometrium in the menstrual cycle. Am J Surg Pathol 10:382–393, 1986.
6. Malberger E, Gutterman E, Bartfeld E, Zajicek G: Cellular changes in the mammary gland epithelium during the menstrual cycle. A computer image analysis study. Acta Cytol 31:305–308, 1987.
7. Love SM, Barsky SH: Breast-duct endoscopy to study stages of cancerous breast disease. Lancet 348:997–999, 1996.
8. Sartorius OW, Morris FL, Benedict DL, et al: Contrast ductography for recognition and localization of benign and malignant breast lesions: An improved technique. In Logan WW (ed): Breast carcinoma. New York, Wiley, 1977, pp 281–300.
9. Buehring GC: Screening for breast atypias using exfoliative cytology. Cancer 43:1788–1799, 1979.
10. Sartorius OW, Smith HS, Morris P, et al: Cytologic evaluation of breast fluid in the detection of breast disease. J Natl Cancer Inst 59:1073–1080, 1977.
11. Petrakis NL, Mason L, Lee R, et al: Association of race, age, menopausal status, and cerumen type with breast fluid secretion in nonlactating women, as determined by nipple aspiration. J Natl Cancer Inst 54:829–834, 1975.
12. Wynder EL, Lahti H, Laakso K, et al: Nipple aspirates of breast fluid and the epidemiology of breast disease. Cancer 56:1473–1478, 1985.
13. Jackson D: Cytological study of nipple secretions: an aid in the diagnosis of breast lesions. Tex State J Med 41:512, 1946.
14. Jackson D, Todd DA, Gorsuch PL: Study of breast secretion for detection of intramammary pathologic change and of silent papilloma. J Int Coll Surg 15:552–568, 1951.
15. Papanicolaou GN, Bader GM, Holmquist DG, Falk EA: Cytologic evaluation of breast secretions. Ann N Y Acad Sci 63:1409–1421, 1956.
16. Papanicolaou GN, Holmquist DG, Bader GM, Falk EA: Exfoliative cytology of the human mammary gland and its value in the diagnosis of cancer and other diseases of the breast. Cancer 11:377–409, 1958.
17. Ringrose CA: The role of cytology in the early detection of breast disease. Acta Cytol 10:373–375, 1966.
18. Saphir O: Cytologic examination of breast secretions. Am J Clin Pathol 20:1001–1010, 1950.
19. Petrakis NL: Physiologic, biochemical, and cytologic aspects of nipple aspirate fluid. Breast Cancer Res Treat 8:7–19, 1986.
20. King EB, Barrett D, King MC, Petrakis NL: Cellular composition of the nipple aspirate specimen of breast fluid. I. The benign cells. Am J Clin Pathol 64:728–738, 1975.
21. King EB, Barrett D, Petrakis NL: Cellular composition of the nipple aspirate specimen of breast fluid. II. Abnormal findings. Am J Clin Pathol 64:739–748, 1975.
22. King EB, Chew KL, Petrakis NL, Ernster VL: Nipple aspirate cytology for the study of breast cancer precursors. J Natl Cancer Inst 71:1115–1121, 1983.
23. Wrensch MR, Petrakis NL, King EB, et al: Breast cancer incidence in women with abnormal cytology in nipple aspirates of breast fluid. Am J Epidemiol 135:130–141, 1992.
24. Wrensch MR, Petrakis NL, Miike R, King EB: Breast cancer risk in women with abnormal cytology in nipple aspirates of breast fluid. J Natl Cancer Inst 93:1791–1798, 2001.
25. Sauter ER, Ross E, Daly M, et al: Nipple aspirate fluid: A promising non-invasive method to identify cellular markers of breast cancer risk. Br J Cancer 76:494–501, 1997.
26. Sauter ER, Ehya H, Mammen A, Klein G: Nipple aspirate cytology and pathologic parameters predict residual cancer and nodal involvement after excisional breast biopsy. Br J Cancer 85:1952–1957, 2001.
27. Sauter ER, Wagner-Mann C, Ehya H, Klein-Szanto A: Biologic markers of breast cancer in nipple aspirate fluid and nipple discharge are associated with clinical findings. Cancer Detect Prev 31:50–58, 2007.
28. Kuerer HM, Thompson PA, Krishnamurthy S, et al: High and differential expression of HER-2/neu extracellular domain in bilateral ductal fluids from women with unilateral invasive breast cancer. Clin Cancer Res 9:601–605, 2003.
29. Klein PM, Lawrence JA: Lavage and nipple aspiration of breast ductal fluids: a source of biomarkers for environmental mutagenesis. Environ Mol Mutagen 39:127–133, 2002.
30. Khan SA, Bhandare D, Chatterton RT Jr: The local hormonal environment and related biomarkers in the normal breast. Endocr Relat Cancer 12:497–510, 2005.
31. Sauter ER, Klein G, Wagner-Mann C, Diamandis EP: Prostate-specific antigen expression in nipple aspirate fluid is associated with advanced breast cancer. Cancer Detect Prev 28: 27–31, 2004.
32. Sauter ER, Nesbit M, Tichansky D, et al: Fibroblast growth factor-binding protein expression changes with disease progression in clinical and experimental human squamous epithelium. Int J Cancer 92:374–381, 2001.
33. Zhao Y, Verselis SJ, Klar N, et al: Nipple fluid carcinoembryonic antigen and prostate-specific antigen in cancer-bearing and tumor-free breasts. J Clin Oncol 19:1462–1467, 2001.
34. Dua RS, Isacke CM, Gui GP: The intraductal approach to breast cancer biomarker discovery. J Clin Oncol 24: 1209–1216, 2006.
35. Elmore JG, Barton MB, Moceri VM, et al: Ten-year risk of false positive screening mammograms and clinical breast examinations. N Engl J Med 338: 1089–1096, 1998.
36. Going JJ, Moffat DF: Escaping from Flatland: clinical and biological aspects of human mammary duct anatomy in three dimensions. J Pathol 203:538–544, 2004.
37. Badve S, Wiley E, Rodriguez N: Assessment of utility of ductal lavage and ductoscopy in breast cancer—a retrospective analysis of mastectomy specimens. Mod Pathol 16:206–209, 2003.
38. Dooley WC, Ljung BM, Veronesi U, et al: Ductal lavage for detection of cellular atypia in women at high risk for breast cancer. J Natl Cancer Inst 93: 1624–1632, 2001.

39. The uniform approach to breast fine-needle aspiration biopsy. NIH Consensus Development Conference. Am J Surg 174:371–385, 1997.

40. Maddux AJ, Ashfaq R, Naftalis E, et al: Patient and duct selection for nipple duct lavage. Am J Surg 188:390–394, 2004.

41. Johnson-Maddux A, Ashfaq R, Cler L, et al: Reproducibility of cytologic atypia in repeat nipple duct lavage. Cancer 103:1129–1136, 2005.

42. Bushnaq ZI, Ashfaq R, Leitch AM, Euhus D: Patient variables that predict atypical cytology by nipple duct lavage. Cancer 109:1247–1254, 2007.

43. Euhus DM, Bu D, Ashfaq R, et al: Atypia and DNA methylation in nipple duct lavage in relation to predicted breast cancer risk. Cancer Epidemiol Biomarkers Prev 16:1812–1821, 2007.

44. King BL, Tsai SC, Gryga M, et al: Detection of chromosomal instability in paired breast surgery and ductal lavage specimens by interphase fluorescence in situ hybridization. Clin Cancer Res 9:1509–1516, 2003.

45. Yamamoto D, Senzaki H, Nakagawa H, et al: Detection of chromosomal aneusomy by fluorescence in situ hybridization for patients with nipple discharge. Cancer 97:690–694, 2003.

46. Evron E, Dooley WC, Umbricht CB, et al: Detection of breast cancer cells in ductal lavage fluid by methylation-specific PCR. Lancet 357:1335–1336, 2001.

47. Paweletz CP, Trock B, Pennanen M, Tsangaris T: Proteomic patterns of nipple aspirate fluids obtained by SELDI-TOF: potential for new biomarkers to aid in the diagnosis of breast cancer. Dis Markers 17:301–307, 2001.

48. Kuerer KM, Goldknopf IL, Fritsche H, et al: Identification of distinct protein expression patterns in bilateral matched pair breast ductal fluid specimens from women with unilateral invasive breast carcinoma. Cancer 95:2276–2282, 2002.

49. Varnum SM, Covington CC, Woodbury RL, et al: Proteomic characterization of nipple aspirate fluid: Identification of potential biomarkers of breast cancer. Breast Cancer Res Treat 80:87–97, 2003.

50. Fabian CJ, Kimler BF, Mayo MS, Khan SA: Breast-tissue sampling for risk assessment and prevention. Endocr Relat Cancer 12:185–213, 2005.

51. Fabian CJ, Kimler BF, Zalles CM, et al: Short-term breast cancer prediction by random periareolar fine-needle aspiration cytology and the Gail risk model. J Natl Cancer Inst 92:1217–1227, 2000.

52. Masood S, Khalbuss WE: Nipple fluid cytology. Clin Lab Med 25:787–794, vii–viii, 2005.

53. Vargas HI, Vargas MP, Eldrageely K, et al: Outcomes of clinical and surgical assessment of women with pathological nipple discharge. Am Surg 72:124–128, 2006.

54. Seltzer MH: Breast complaints, biopsies, and cancer correlated with age in 10,000 consecutive new surgical referrals. Breast J 10:111–117, 2004.

55. Newman HF, Klein M, Northrup JD, et al: Nipple discharge. Frequency and pathogenesis in an ambulatory population. N Y State J Med 83:928–933, 1983.

56. Florio MG, Manganaro T, Pollicino A, et al: Surgical approach to nipple discharge: A ten-year experience. J Surg Oncol 71:235–238, 1999.

57. Cabioglu N, Krishnamurthy S, Kuerer HM, et al: Feasibility of breast-conserving surgery for patients with breast carcinoma associated with nipple discharge. Cancer 101:508–517, 2004.

58. Lau S, Kuchenmeister I, Stachs A, et al: Pathologic nipple discharge: Surgery is imperative in postmenopausal women. Ann Surg Oncol 12:546–551, 2005.

59. Adepoju LJ, Chun J, El-Tamer M, et al: The value of clinical characteristics and breast-imaging studies in predicting a histopathologic diagnosis of cancer or high-risk lesion in patients with spontaneous nipple discharge. Am J Surg 190:644–646, 2005.

60. King TA, Carter KM, Bolton JS, Fuhrman GM: A simple approach to nipple discharge. Am Surg 66:960–965, discussion 965–966, 2000.

61. Murad TM, Contesso G, Mouriesse H: Nipple discharge from the breast. Ann Surg 195:259–264, 1982.

62. Kilgore AR, Fleming R, Ramos MM: The incidence of cancer with nipple discharge and the risk of cancer in the presence of papillary disease of the breast. Surg Gynecol Obstet 96:649–660, 1953.

63. Funderburk WW, Syphax B: Evaluation of nipple discharge in benign and malignant diseases. Cancer 24:1290–1296, 1969.

64. Chaudary MA, Millis RR, Davies GC, Hayward JL: The diagnostic value of testing for occult blood. Ann Surg 196:651–655, 1982.

65. Devitt JE: Management of nipple discharge by clinical findings. Am J Surg 149:789–792, 1985.

66. Ohuchi N, Abe R, Kasai M: Possible cancerous change of intraductal papillomas of the breast. A 3-D reconstruction study of 25 cases. Cancer 54:605–611, 1984.

67. Cardenosa G, Eklund GW: Benign papillary neoplasms of the breast: Mammographic findings. Radiology 181:751–755, 1991.

68. Kline TS, Lash SR: The bleeding nipple of pregnancy and postpartum period: A cytologic and histologic study. Acta Cytol 8:336–340, 1964.

69. Bundred NJ, Dixon JM, Lumsden AB: Are the lesions of duct ectasia sterile? Br J Surg 72:844–845, 1985.

70. Dinkel HP, Trusen A, Gassel AM, et al: Predictive value of galactographic patterns for benign and malignant neoplasms of the breast in patients with nipple discharge. Br J Radiol 73:706–714, 2000.

71. Vogel PM, Georgiade NG, Fetter BF, et al: The correlation of histologic changes in the human breast with the menstrual cycle. Am J Pathol 104:23–34, 1981.

72. Dawson EK: A histological study of the normal mamma in relation to tumor growth, II: The mature gland in pregnancy and lactation. Edinb Med J 42, 1935.

73. Engel S: An investigation of the origin of the colostrum cells. J Anat 87:362–366, 1953.

74. Cole HA: The mammary gland of the mouse during the oestrous cycle, pregnancy and lactation. Proc R Soc Lond B Biol Sci 114:136–161, 1933.

75. Bloom W: A textbook of histology, 9th ed. Philadelphia, WB Saunders, 1968.

76. Holmquist DG, Papanicolaou GN: The exfoliative cytology of the mammary gland during pregnancy and lactation. Ann N Y Acad Sci 63:1422–1435, 1956.

77. Kline TS, Lash S: Nipple secretion in pregnancy. A cytologic and histologic study. Am J Clin Pathol 37:626–632, 1962.

78. Barnes AB: Diagnosis and treatment of abnormal breast secretions. N Engl J Med 275:1184–1187, 1966.

79. Hooper JH, Welch VC, Shackelford RT: Abnormal lactation associated with tranquilizing drug therapy. JAMA 178:506, 1961.

80. Mills JL, Jefferys JL, Stolley PD: Effects of occupational exposure to estrogen and progestogens and how to detect them. J Occup Med 26:269–272, 1984.

81. Ciatto S, Bravetti P, Cariaggi P: Significance of nipple discharge clinical patterns in the selection of cases for cytologic examination. Acta Cytol 30:17–20, 1986.

82. Leis HP Jr, Cammarata A, LaRaja RD, Higgins H: Breast biopsy and guidance for occult lesions. Int Surg 70:115–118, 1985.

83. Scott-Conner CE, Schorr SJ: The diagnosis and management of breast problems during pregnancy and lactation. Am J Surg 170:401–405, 1995.

84. Cabioglu N, Hunt KK, Singletary SE, et al: Surgical decision making and factors determining a diagnosis of breast carcinoma in women presenting with nipple discharge. J Am Coll Surg 196:354–364, 2003.

85. Woods E, Helvie MA, Ikeda DM, Mandell SH, et al: Solitary breast papilloma: Comparison of mammographic, galactographic, and pathologic findings. Am J Roentgenol 159:487–491, 1992.

86. Simmons R, Adamovich T, Brennan M, et al: Nonsurgical evaluation of pathologic nipple discharge. Ann Surg Oncol 10:113–116, 2003.

87. Dawes LG, Bowen C, Venta LA, Morrow M: Ductography for nipple discharge: No replacement for ductal excision. Surgery 124:685–691, 1998.

88. Rissanen T, Reinikainen H, Apaja-Sarkkinen M: Breast sonography in localizing the cause of nipple discharge: Comparison with galactography in 52 patients. J Ultrasound Med 26:1031–1039, 2007.

89. Slawson SH, Johnson BA: Ductography: How to and what if? Radiographics 21:133–150, 2001.

90. Tabar L, Dean PB, Pentek Z: Galactography: the diagnostic procedure of choice for nipple discharge. Radiology 149:31–38, 1983.

91. Schwab SA, Schulz-Wendtland R, Uder M, et al: Cutaneous application of local anaesthetic—a useful help in galactography. Eur Radiol 18:2085–2086, 2008.

92. Berna-Serna JD, Redondo MV, Duran I, Berna-Mestre JD: Galactography without discomfort using lidocaine/prilocaine anesthetic cream. Acta Radiol 49:22–24, 2008.

93. Hou MF, Huang TJ, Huang YS, Hsieh JS: A simple method of duct cannulation and localization for galactography before excision in patients with nipple discharge. Radiology 195:568–569, 1995.

94. Hou MF, Huang CJ, Huang YS, et al: Evaluation of galactography for nipple discharge. Clin Imaging 22:89–94, 1998.

95. Sharma R, Dietz J, Wright H, et al: Comparative analysis of minimally invasive microductectomy versus major duct excision in patients with pathologic nipple discharge. Surgery 138:591–596, discussion 596–597, 2005.

96. Berni D, De Giuli E: The value of ductogalactography in the diagnosis of intraductal papilloma. Tumori 69:539–544, 1983.

97. Funovics MA, Philipp MO, Lackner B, et al: Galactography: Method of choice in pathologic nipple discharge? Eur Radiol 13:94–99, 2003.

98. Dinkel HP, Gassel AM, Muller T, et al: Galactography and exfoliative cytology in women with abnormal nipple discharge. Obstet Gynecol 97:625–629, 2001.

99. Ohuchi N, Furuta A, Mori S: Management of ductal carcinoma in situ with nipple discharge. Intraductal spreading of carcinoma is an unfavorable pathologic factor for breast-conserving surgery. Cancer 74:1294–1302, 1994.

100. Dooley WC: Endoscopic visualization of breast tumors. JAMA 284:1518, 2000.

101. Shen KW, Wu J, Lu JS, et al: Fiberoptic ductoscopy for patients with nipple discharge. Cancer 89:1512–1519, 2000.

102. Moncrief RM, Nayar R, Diaz LK: A comparison of ductoscopy-guided and conventional surgical excision in women with spontaneous nipple discharge. Ann Surg 241:575–581, 2005.

103. Matsunaga T, Ohta D, Misaka T, et al: Mammary ductoscopy for diagnosis and treatment of intraductal lesions of the breast. Breast Cancer 8:213–221, 2001.

104. Escobar PF, Crowe JP, Matsunaga T, Mokbel K: The clinical applications of mammary ductoscopy. Am J Surg 191:211–2115, 2006.

105. Okazaki A, Hirata K, Okazaki M, et al: Nipple discharge disorders: Current diagnostic management and the role of fiber-ductoscopy. Eur Radiol 9:583–590, 1999.

106. Kothari A, Beechey-Newman N, Kulkarni D: Breast duct microendoscopy: A study of technique and a morphological classification of endo-luminal lesions. Breast 15:363–369, 2006.

107. Sauter ER, Ehya H, Klein-Szanto AJ: Fiberoptic ductoscopy findings in women with and without spontaneous nipple discharge. Cancer 103:914–921, 2005.

108. Dooley WC, Francescatti D, Clark L, Webber G: Office-based breast ductoscopy for diagnosis. Am J Surg 188:415–418, 2004.

109. Masukawa T: Improved cell collection technique in breast cytology. Cytotech Bull 7, 1970.

110. Barrett DL, King EB: Comparison of cellular recovery rates and morphologic detail obtained using membrane filter and cytocentrifuge techniques. Acta Cytol 20:174–180, 1976.

111. Uei Y, Watanabe Y, Hirota T, et al: Cytologic diagnosis of breast carcinoma with nipple discharge: Special significance of the spherical cell cluster. Acta Cytol 24:522–528, 1980.

112. Hou M, Tsai K, Lin H, et al: A simple intraductal aspiration method for cytodiagnosis in nipple discharge. Acta Cytol 44:1029–1034, 2000.

113. Carty NJ, Mudan SS, Ravichandran D, et al: Prospective study of outcome in women presenting with nipple discharge. Ann R Coll Surg Engl 76:387–389, 1994.

114. Hadfield J: Excision of major duct system for benign disease of the breast. Br J Surg 47:472–477, 1960.

115. Van Zee KJ, Ortega Perez G, Minnard E, Cohen MA: Preoperative galactography increases the diagnostic yield of major duct excision for nipple discharge. Cancer 82:1874–1880, 1998.

116. Baker KS, Davey DD, Stelling CB: Ductal abnormalities detected with galactography: Frequency of adequate excisional biopsy. AJR Am J Roentgenol 162:821–824, 1994.

117. Chow JS, Smith DN, Kaelin CM, Meyer JE: Galactography-guided wire localization of an intraductal papilloma: Case report. Clin Radiol 56:72–73, 2001.

118. Koskela A, Berg M, Pietilainen T, et al: Breast lesions causing nipple discharge: Preoperative galactography-aided stereotactic wire localization. AJR Am J Roentgenol 184:1795–1798, 2005.

119. Dooley WC: Routine operative breast endoscopy for bloody nipple discharge. Ann Surg Oncol 9:920–923, 2002.

120. Dietz JR, Crowe JP, Grundfest S, et al: Directed duct excision by using mammary ductoscopy in patients with pathologic nipple discharge. Surgery 132:582–587, discussion 587–588, 2002.

121. Pereira B, Mokbel K: Mammary ductoscopy: Past, present, and future. Int J Clin Oncol 10:112–116, 2005.

122. Govindarajulu S, Narreddy SR, Shere MH, et al: Sonographically guided mammotome excision of ducts in the diagnosis and management of single duct nipple discharge. Eur J Surg Oncol 32:725–728, 2006.

123. Beechey-Newman N, Kulkarni D, Kothari A, et al: Breast duct microendoscopy in nipple discharge: Microbrush improves cytology. Surg Endosc 19:1648–1651, 2005.

124. Hunerbein M, Raubach M, Gebauer B, et al: Ductoscopy and intraductal vacuum assisted biopsy in women with pathologic nipple discharge. Breast Cancer Res Treat 99:301–307, 2006.

125. Hunerbein M, Dubowy A, Raubach M, et al: Gradient index ductoscopy and intraductal biopsy of intraductal breast lesions. Am J Surg 194:511–514, 2007.

126. Matsunaga T, Kawakami Y, Namba K, Fujii M: Intraductal biopsy for diagnosis and treatment of intraductal lesions of the breast. Cancer 101:2164–2169, 2004.

127. McPherson VA, Mackenzie WC: Lesions of the breast associated with nipple discharge: Prognosis after local excision of benign lesions. Can J Surg 5:6, 1962.

SECTION III

Benign and Premalignant Lesions

chapter 5

Etiology and Management of Benign Breast Disease

V. SUZANNE KLIMBERG | RENA B. KASS |
SAMUEL W. BEENKEN | KIRBY I. BLAND

The aberrations of normal development and involution (ANDI) classification of benign breast disorder (BBD) provides an overall framework for benign conditions of the breast that encompasses both pathogenesis and the degree of abnormality.[1] It is a bidirectional framework based on the fact that most BBDs arise from normal physiologic processes (Table 5-1). The horizontal component defines BBD along a spectrum from normal to mild abnormality ("disorder") to severe abnormality ("disease"). The vertical component defines the pathogenesis of the condition. Together, these two components provide a comprehensive framework into which most BBDs can be fitted. This scheme was recommended by an international multidisciplinary working group in 1992.[2]

Breast Pain

Although mastalgia is one of the most commonly reported symptoms in women with breast complaints at dedicated breast clinics or general practice,[3] it is still underreported and poorly characterized. In a 1985 survey, nearly 66% of women reported having breast pain, of which 21% of cases were reported to be severe.[4] However, only 50% of women with breast pain had consulted a family physician,[4] and fewer still had visited a dedicated breast clinic. Because of the increasing awareness of breast cancer and the possibility that mastalgia may indicate disease, as well as the impact mastalgia has on the quality of life, more women than ever are seeking help for breast pain. Treatment usually balances management of relatively minor complaints with the side effects of treatment. More than 90% of patients with cyclic mastalgia and 64% of patients with noncyclic mastalgia can obtain relief by using a combination of nonprescription and prescription drugs.[5]

CLINICAL ASSESSMENT

The degree, severity, and relationship of breast pain to the menstrual cycle are best assessed with the use of a daily breast pain chart that uses a visual analog scale. This chart should be kept during at least two menstrual cycles. Mild breast pain (<3 on the scale) that lasts fewer than 5 days before a menstrual cycle is considered normal. The extent to which mastalgia disrupts the patient's normal lifestyle in terms of sleep, work, and sex provides a useful assessment of severity. A thorough history that includes diet, methylxanthine intake, and use of new medications (especially hormones, antidepressants such

TABLE 5-1

Aberrations of Normal Development and Involution Classification of Benign Breast Disease

	Normal	Disorder	Disease
Early reproductive years (age 15–25)	Lobular development Stromal development Nipple eversion	Fibroadenoma Adolescent hypertrophy Nipple inversion	Giant fibroadenoma Gigantomastia Subareolar abscess/mammary duct fistula
Mature reproductive years (age 25–40)	Cyclical changes of menstruation Epithelial hyperplasia of pregnancy	Cyclical mastalgia Nodularity Bloody nipple discharge	Incapacitating mastalgia
Involution (age 35–55)	Lobular involution	Macrocysts Sclerosing lesions	
	Duct involution/dilation sclerosis Epithelial turnover	Duct ectasia Nipple retraction Epithelial hyperplasia	Periductal mastitis/abscess Epithelial hyperplasia with atypia

as serotonin reuptake inhibitors, cardiac medications such as digoxin and cimetidine) should be taken,[6] and a history of recent stress should be recorded. Other conditions should be excluded, such as possible referred pain, such as shoulder bursitis; cervical radiculopathy; myocardial ischemia; lung disease; hiatal hernia; and cholelithiasis. Patients are reassured that they do not have breast cancer only after clinical examination and mammography are performed and reveal no malignancy.[4] Ultrasonography can be a useful adjunct to evaluate focal pain, especially in young dense breasts; 23% of patients have cysts or benign masses as the root cause.[7]

A study of 5319 patients by Leinster and colleagues showed that there was a higher incidence of "high-risk" mammographic patterns according to the Wolfe classification in premenopausal women with cyclic mastalgia. These patterns correlated with severity, duration, and need for treatment.[8] However, no study to date has reported an increased risk of breast cancer with cyclic mastalgia. Initial evaluation should exclude breast pain from localized benign lesions of the breast that may require needle aspiration or surgical therapy, such as painful cysts, fibroadenomas, subareolar duct ectasia, lipomas, and fibrocystic changes.

Classification

Classification of mastalgia provides a baseline measurement of pain and severity, dividing symptoms into the categories of cyclic mastalgia, noncyclic mastalgia, and chest wall pain. This distinction is important because presentation, occurrence of spontaneous remission, and likelihood of a response to treatment differs for these three conditions. A useful response is obtained in 92% of patients with cyclic mastalgia, 64% of those with noncyclic mastalgia,[4] and 97% of those with chest wall pain.[9]

Cyclic mastalgia accounts for approximately 67% of cases and usually is first seen during the third decade of life as dull, burning, or aching pain.[9] However, one breast is usually involved to a greater extent than the other, and the pain may be sharp and shooting, with radiation to the axilla or arm because of glandular entrapment of the intercostobrachial nerve. Cyclic mastalgia usually starts in the upper outer quadrant of the breast 5 days or more before the menstrual cycle, although severe pain can persist throughout the cycle. Exacerbation of symptoms just before menopause can occur. Resolution of symptoms at menopause occurs in 42% of women; however, spontaneous resolution prior to menopause occurs in only 14% of patients.[10]

Noncyclic mastalgia tends to occur much less frequently, in 26% of patients, and peaks during the fourth decade of life.[9] The duration of noncyclic mastalgia tends to be shorter, with spontaneous resolution occurring in nearly 50% of patients.[10] In contrast to cyclic mastalgia, noncyclic mastalgia is almost always unilateral. Exacerbations of pain occur for no apparent reason and are difficult to treat.

Mastalgia from other origins includes scapular bursitis,[9] costochondritis,[11] lateral extramammary pain syndrome,[12] cervical radiculopathy,[13] or other nonbreast causes. Chest wall pain from these etiologies is almost always felt either on the lateral chest wall or at the costochondral junction.[12]

Tietze syndrome, which commonly affects the second and third costochondral junctions, can manifest as focal medial breast pain.[14] Musculoskeletal inflammation, especially scapular bursitis, can present as referred pain to the breast and is often diagnosed by improvement with a scapular trigger point injection anesthetic and treatment with an injection of steroid.[9] Neurogenic pain is much more difficult to diagnose and treat. If pain of neurogenic origin is suspected, an empirical trial of amitriptyline or carbamazepine may be beneficial for diagnosis and treatment.

NOMENCLATURE

The term fibrocystic disease, of which mastalgia is the most common symptom, is unhelpful because it fails to delineate the full spectrum of disease. Postmortem studies of "normal" breast specimens indicate that fibrocystic changes occur in 50% to 100% of individuals.[15-17] The ANDI classification is used to classify BBDs, such as mastalgia, into those arising secondary to abnormalities of breast development, cyclic changes, or involution rather than as disease (see Table 5-1).[1]

Pathophysiology of Mastalgia

PATHOGENESIS AND ETIOLOGY

Epithelial and stromal activity, as well as regression, constantly occur within the breast. Fibrosis, adenosis, and lymphoid infiltration, commonly used to characterize mastalgia, cannot be correlated with clinical episodes.[1] Watt-Boolsen and colleagues found no histologic differences between women with cyclic and noncyclic mastalgia and asymptomatic patients.[18] Jorgensen and Watt-Boolsen reported fibrocystic changes in 100% of 41 women with breast pain who underwent breast biopsy.[19] Although a higher incidence of fibrocystic changes was seen in this cohort than in asymptomatic controls, the total incidence of breast abnormalities did not differ between groups. Attempts to demonstrate edema as the main cause of cyclic pain and nodularity have been unsuccessful. Cysts that commonly occur with ANDI and mastalgia are secondary to changes of involution, periductal inflammation, and fibrosis, which may narrow the ducts distally and cause proximal dilation.[1]

ENDOCRINE INFLUENCES

The natural history of mastalgia is clearly linked to the reproductive cycle, with onset at the age of menarche, monthly cycling, and cessation of symptoms at menopause. In a prospective study of reproductive factors associated with mastalgia, Gateley and colleagues reported that women with cyclic mastalgia were more likely to be premenopausal, to be nulliparous, or to have been at a young age when they had their first child.[5] However, theories of the exact hormonal events, including progesterone deficiency,[20] excess estrogen,[21] changes in the progestin-to-estrogen ratio,[22] differences in receptor sensitivity,[23] disparate follicle-stimulating hormone (FSH) and luteinizing hormone (LH) secretion,[24] low androgen levels,[25] and high prolactin (PRL) levels[26] have been difficult to prove or have not abated with hormone therapy.

Under normal circumstances, PRL exerts structural growth and secretory differentiation, mammary immune system development, and initiation and maintenance of milk secretion.[27] PRL secretion is episodic and shows circadian rhythm, with clustering of more intense episodes after midnight. In addition, PRL secretion has menstrual and seasonal variations.[28] These variations may, to some extent, account for the discrepancies in available reports.[25] Mastalgia may be related to an upward shift in the circadian PRL profile, a possible downward shift in menstrual profiles, and loss of seasonal variations.[28] Patients with mastalgia also show a heightened PRL secretion in response to thyrotropin-releasing hormone (TRH) antidopaminergic drugs[24] and may actively sequester iodine within their breast tissue as a result of an alteration in PRL control[29] (Fig. 5-1). In addition, stress can cause a rise in PRL response.[30]

Disturbances in the pituitary-ovarian steroid axis have long been associated with breast pain (see Fig. 5-1). However, numerous studies have not shown differences in estrogen and progesterone between asymptomatic controls and patients with mastalgia.[31-40] Available reports have measured estrogen over various time courses, from single midluteal phase samples to daily for an entire cycle. Clearly, circadian, menstrual, seasonal, or episodic changes could have been overlooked. More important, normal breast function is a balance between estrogen and progesterone, which is a part of the neuroendocrine control exerted by the hypothalamic-pituitary-gonadal axis (see Fig. 5-1). The theory of an inadequate luteal phase defect has never been confirmed. Three studies[31-33] demonstrate a significant decrease in luteal phase progesterone in women with mastalgia versus pain-free controls; however, four other comparable studies have not confirmed these results.[34-37] Nevertheless, an estrogen-progesterone imbalance could affect PRL secretion. An impairment of the normal ability to counteract estrogen-induced PRL release by increasing the central dopaminergic tone has been suggested as a cause of mastalgia.[41] Administration of naloxone has been shown to decrease PRL response to stress[42] (see Fig. 5-1).

NONENDOCRINE INFLUENCES

Serum studies in animals demonstrate that caffeine intake can increase PRL,[43] insulin,[44] and corticosterone[45] and can decrease thyroid-stimulating hormone, free triiodothyronine, and thyroxine.[43] Minton and associates[46,47] originally hypothesized that methylxanthines, either by inhibiting phosphodiesterase and breakdown of cyclic adenosine monophosphate (cAMP) or by increasing catecholamine release, increase cAMP, leading to cellular proliferation in the breast[48] (see Fig. 5-1). Tissue from patients with breast disease showed unchanged phosphodiesterase activity but appeared to have increased adenylate cyclase levels and increased responsiveness to the biochemical-stimulating effects of methylxanthines.[46,47]

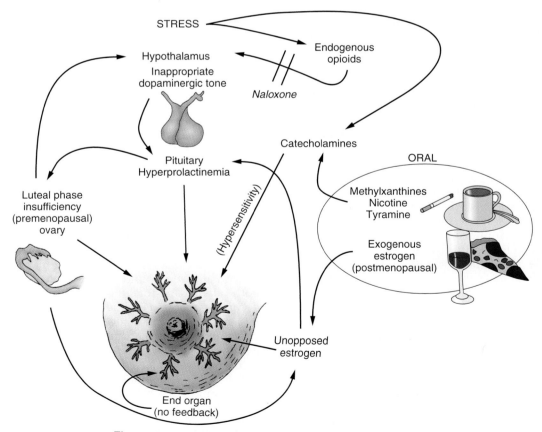

Figure 5-1 Suggested theories of causation of breast pain.

Caffeine itself has no direct effect on cAMP, but catecholamines can increase cAMP. Studies in Minton's laboratory have shown increased release of circulating catecholamines in response to caffeine consumption[49] (see Fig. 5-1). Indeed, studies by Minton and colleagues have shown "catecholamine supersensitivity" in patients with ANDI. There were significantly higher levels of β-adrenergic receptors in symptomatic patients (n = 21) than in asymptomatic controls (n = 13).[50] Basal receptors and stimulation of receptors, with isoprenaline or epinephrine, were higher in the symptomatic group. The increased activity and sensitivity of the β-adrenergic–adenylate cyclase system in symptomatic patients suggest a genetic predisposition for ANDI that is stimulated by the biochemical or hormonal effects of methylxanthines. Moreover, Butler and colleagues have been able to categorize patients genetically into fast and slow acetylators based on their caffeine metabolism.[51] Like the methylxanthines, a common biochemical effect of nicotine, tyramine, and physical and emotional stress is enhancement of catecholamine release and an increase of circulating catecholamines[50] (see Fig. 5-1). Arsiriy showed that women with mastalgia and ANDI had significantly higher levels of urinary catecholamines than did asymptomatic controls.[52] Studies have shown increased serum epinephrine and norepinephrine and decreased baseline dopamine levels in patients with cyclic as well as noncyclic mastalgia.[50] The increase or stimulation of adenylate cyclase activity in breast tissue appears to be an important step for triggering the intracellular cAMP-mediated events leading to symptomatic ANDI.[50] Randomized studies on smoking, tyramine, or stress reduction have not been performed.

The theory that fat increases endogenous hormone levels, and thus breast pain, has led to the performance of dietary fat-restriction studies.[53] In these studies, women with breast pain show lower levels of plasma essential fatty acid gamma-linolenic acid than do asymptomatic controls. It has been hypothesized that essential fatty acid deficiencies may affect the functioning of the cell membrane receptors of the breast by producing a supersensitive state.[54,55] High levels of saturated fats inhibit the rate-limiting delta-6 desaturation step between linoleic acid and gamma-linolenic acid. Catecholamines, diabetes, glucocorticoids, viral infections, and high cholesterol levels likewise limit this step.[54,55] Both with estrogen and progesterone receptors, a supersensitive state can be produced with a higher ratio of saturated to unsaturated fatty acids. Administration of essential fatty acids in the form of evening primrose oil (9% gamma-linolenic acid) bypasses the delta-6 desaturation step, leading to a gradual reduction in the proportions of the saturated fatty acids[54] and diminishing the abnormal sensitivity of the breast tissue. Likewise, Ghent and colleagues have theorized that the absence of dietary iodine may also render terminal intralobular duct epithelium more sensitive to estrogen stimulation.[56]

Management of Mastalgia

As might be anticipated, there is a long list of suggested modalities for the treatment of a ubiquitous entity whose cause is unknown and whose relationship to fibrocystic breast disease and cancer is poorly understood. Breast pain may resolve spontaneously, and 19% of patients have marked responses to placebo therapy. Therefore double-blind, placebo-controlled trials are required to prove the effectiveness of drugs in the treatment of mastalgia.[57] Gamma-linolenic acid, bromocriptine, danazol, luteinizing hormone–releasing hormone (LHRH) agonists, molecular iodine, and tamoxifen have all been shown by such trials to be of use in the treatment of breast pain. The safety and efficacy of these therapies, as well as less proven therapies, are discussed in the next section (Table 5-2).

NUTRITIONAL THERAPY

Nutritional factors have been less well documented than other modalities in the cause and treatment of breast pain. Although they are the least expensive and least prone to side effects, dietary changes are often the most difficult to institute in the noncompliant patient.

Methylxanthines

Chemicals classified as methylxanthines include caffeine, theophylline, and theobromine. These substances are found in coffee, tea, chocolate, and cola beverages, as well as in many respiratory medications and stimulants. Minton and colleagues reported complete disappearance of all palpable nodules, pain, tenderness, and nipple discharge 1 to 6 months after eliminating methylxanthines from the diet of 13 of 20 women (65%).[58] In a subsequent clinical trial involving 87 women, complete resolution was seen in 82.5%, with significant improvement in 15% of women abstaining from methylxanthines.[47] Resumption of methylxanthines was associated with recurrence of symptoms in this cohort. These data are supported by nonrandomized studies, including retrospective data from 90 pairs of twins[59] in which the twin with breast pain was found to be more likely to consume more coffee than the unaffected twin. Ernster and colleagues randomized 82 of 158 women to abstain from methylxanthine and 76 women to no dietary instruction.[60] Differences in clinically palpable breast findings were significantly less in the caffeine-abstaining group, but absolute changes were minor. Bullough and colleagues studied daily methylxanthine ingestion from drug and dietary sources by means of questionnaires from a sample of 102 women.[61] Fibrocystic breast disease assessed with mammography and breast pain were found to be positively correlated with both caffeine and total methylxanthine ingestion.

Minton reported evaluation of 315 patients with ANDI for a mean of 3 years (range, 1 to 11 years),[50] demonstrating improvement off caffeine and return of symptoms with resumption of caffeine intact. Other case-controlled studies, however, have not confirmed these clinical findings.[62–65] A study of an age- and race-matched cohort of approximately 3000 women who were a part of the Breast Cancer Detection Demonstration Project demonstrated no association between methylxanthine consumption and breast tenderness in women with fibrocystic disease

TABLE 5-2

Effectiveness of Interventions for Mastalgia

| Drug | Mastalgia | | | |
	Cyclical	Noncyclical	Combined	Side Effects
Methylxanthines[47]	—	—	83%	None
Dietary fat reduction[69]	90%	73%	83%	None
Molecular iodine[56]	—	—	65%	11%
Danazol[85]*	70%	31%	—	50%
Gestrinone[90]	—	—	55%	None
LHRH agonist[92]	—	—	81%	All
Thyroid replacement[95]	—	—	73%	None
Analgesics[103]	—	—	97%	3%
Tamoxifen[107]	90%	56%	—	65%[†]

LHRH, luteinizing hormone-releasing hormone.
*Low-dose regimen demonstrated a 55% complete response rate without side effects.
[†]Regimen is 20 mg of tamoxifen. On 10 mg, side effects and efficacy are lower.

or in controls.[66] Consumption of chocolate-containing foods and candies or caffeine-containing medication was not recorded. In a single-blind clinical trial of 56 women randomized to a control (no dietary restrictions), a placebo (cholesterol-free diet), and an experimental group (caffeine-free diet) for 4 months, Allen and Froberg showed that caffeine restriction did not lessen breast pain or tenderness.[67] Another factor is the significant difference in the length of withdrawal of caffeine seen between positive and negative studies. Minton's work has been criticized for lack of controls and blinding as well as the general instability of findings in patients with mastalgia.[68] An unflawed, large-scale, prospective, long-term study that would count methylxanthines from all sources and use reliable dependent variables to assess pain, either to prove or disprove the value of methylxanthine withdrawal, has yet to be performed. Until then, clinicians may want to suggest a methylxanthine-restricted diet, especially in light of its no cost, no side-effect status, and the other unwanted health consequences of caffeine.

Low Dietary Fat

As with breast cancer, mastalgia is less common in the East and in Eskimos, whose diets are notably lower in fat. Reduction of dietary fat intake (to <15% of total calories for 6 months) significantly improves cyclic breast tenderness and swelling.[53] In one study, Sharma and colleagues demonstrated significant elevations in high-density lipoprotein cholesterol and the ratio of high-density lipoprotein cholesterol to low-density lipoproteins, as well as a decrease in the ratio of total cholesterol to high-density lipoprotein cholesterol in 32 cyclic and 25 noncyclic mastalgia patients.[69] Response to a low-fat dietary regimen was significant only in the cyclic mastalgia group, suggesting that cyclic mastalgia may be from cyclic aberrations in lipid metabolism and that

dietary management may need to be pursued. A good or partial response was seen in 19 of 21 of the cyclic and 11 of 15 of the noncyclic patients. It is unclear what would lead to such a lipid profile abnormality—whether excessive intake, a genetic predisposition, or both. Nevertheless, dietary manipulation of this kind is difficult to achieve, is difficult to monitor, and requires a high degree of compliance.[70]

Evening Primrose Oil and Gamma-Linolenic Acid

Studies have shown that women with severe cyclic mastalgia have abnormal blood levels of some essential fatty acids,[71] which have been implicated in the control of PRL secretion and steroid hormone–receptor alterations.[23] Early clinical experience with evening primrose oil (EPO) produced a 58% response rate with cyclic mastalgia and a 38% response rate with noncyclic mastalgia.[5] Symptoms of pain and nodularity were significantly improved with EPO (3 g/day) in a placebo-controlled trial after 4 months, and treatment was associated with an elevation of essential fatty acids toward normal levels.[72] Two more recent randomized controlled trials have not supported or contradicted this earlier evidence of the efficacy of EPO in the treatment of mastalgia. In a large multicenter trial, Goyal and associates[73] evaluated mastalgia in 555 women and compared EPO plus antioxidants, EPO plus placebo antioxidants, antioxidants plus placebo EPO, and placebo antioxidants and placebo EPO. After 4 months, the investigators found no difference in recorded pain scores between women taking EPO plus vitamins versus placebo plus vitamins (15.2 vs. 14.9; $P = 0.3$). Similarly, Blommers and colleagues[74] found no significant difference between EPO and placebo in the frequency or severity of pain at 6 months. In this trial, 120 women were studied in four comparison groups: EPO plus placebo oil; fish oil plus placebo oil; fish oil plus EPO; and two placebo oils alone. Furthermore, a large recent meta-analysis performed by Srivastava and associates[75] reviewing the data from all randomized controlled trials using EPO revealed no significant beneficial effect of EPO over placebo. This new evidence in part, questions or refutes the utility of EPO as a first-line agent in the treatment of mastalgia, and the United Kingdom has withdrawn the prescription licence for EPO because of its lack of efficacy.[76]

Iodine

The exact influence of iodine on breast tissue is not understood. In contrast to iodides, which are thyrotrophic, Eskin and colleagues demonstrated that iodine is involved primarily in extrathyroidal activities, particularly in the breast.[77] Ghent and coworkers theorized that the absence of iodine may render the epithelium of the terminal intralobular ducts more sensitive to estrogen stimulation and proceeded to perform three studies.[56] In an uncontrolled study with sodium-bound iodide (313 volunteers for 2 years) and protein-bound iodide (588 volunteers for 5 years), subjects had 70% and 40% clinical improvement, respectively. The rate of side effects was high. In a prospective controlled crossover study, 145 patients in whom treatment with protein-bound iodide failed were given molecular iodine (0.08 mg/kg) and compared with 108 volunteers treated initially with molecular iodine. Objective improvement was noted in 74% of the patients in the crossover series and in 72% of those receiving molecular iodine as first-line therapy. The third part of the study was a controlled double-blind study in which 23 patients received molecular iodine (0.07 to 0.09 mg/kg) and 33 patients received placebo. In the treatment group, 65% had subjective and objective improvement. In the control group, 33% showed subjective placebo effect and 3% showed objective deterioration. Molecular iodine was found to be nonthyrotropic, without side effects, and beneficial for breast pain. In a randomized double-blind, placebo multicenter trial, Kessler[29] has since reported on the efficacy of Iogen for cyclical mastalgia. Iogen is a novel iodine formulation that generates molecular iodine (I_2), a substance thought to be less thyrotoxic on dissolution in gastric juices. In Kessler's study of 111 women with breast pain, 50% of patients reported a significant decrease in pain after 3 months in the 6-mg treatment group but not in the 1.5-mg and placebo groups.

ENDOCRINE THERAPY

Although it is difficult to prove, hormonal factors clearly play a role in the cause of cyclic mastalgia. This is evidenced by the fact that the condition manifests itself primarily during the ovulatory years, with symptoms that fluctuate during the course of the menstrual cycle, intensifying premenstrually and subsiding with menses.[78]

Androgens

Testosterone. One of the earliest effective hormonal treatments for mastalgia was testosterone injections. Its use has been limited by its adverse side effects. However, results from a placebo-controlled trial using 40 mg twice daily of the undecenoate oral form of testosterone demonstrated a reduction in mastalgia pain scores of 50%, with acceptable tolerance.[79]

Danazol. Danazol is an attenuated androgen and the 2,3-isoxazol derivative of 17α-ethinyl testosterone (ethisterone). Danazol competitively inhibits estrogen and progesterone receptors in the breast, hypothalamus, and pituitary[80]; inhibits multiple enzymes of ovarian steroidogenesis[81]; inhibits the midcycle surge of LH in premenopausal women; and reduces gonadotropin levels in postmenopausal women.[82] The precise mechanism of danazol in reducing breast pain is unknown. It is the only medication approved by the U.S. Food and Drug Administration (FDA) for the treatment of mastalgia.

In initial studies, a double-blind crossover trial comparing two dosages of danazol (200 vs. 400 mg/day) in 21 patients with mastalgia demonstrated significant decreases in pain and nodularity at both dosages.[83] Onset of response and side effects were higher with the higher dosage. Of the participants, 30% had amenorrhea and weight gain. There was significant reduction in mean pain scores and mammographic density using danazol in a randomized trial with daily treatments of 200 or 400 mg of danazol for 6 months.[84] Patients relapsed more quickly (9.2 vs. 12.2 months) and to a greater extent (67% vs. 52%) in women taking 200 versus 400 mg of danazol. Pye and colleagues treated 120 women in a nonrandomized fashion daily with 200 mg of danazol and found that 70% of patients with cyclic mastalgia and 31% of those with noncyclic mastalgia obtained a useful response.[85] Side effects were seen in 22% and were severe in 6%, with menstrual irregularity in up to 50% of patients. Because side effects of danazol are dose related, Harrison and colleagues[86] and Sutton and O'Malley[87] developed low-dose regimens. Patients responding to a dosage of 200 mg/day of danazol after 2 months were given a dosage of 100 mg/day for 2 months and then 100 mg every other day or 100 mg daily only during the second half of the menstrual cycle.[86] If previous reductions were well tolerated, the danazol was discontinued.[87] Symptoms were controlled without side effects at a total average monthly dose of 700 mg. Of 20 women, 13 (65%) of whom had experienced previous side effects, none reported side effects while taking this low dose. Some relief of pain was seen in all women, with a complete response maintained in 55%. Other reported side effects of danazol include muscle cramps, acne, oily hair, hot flashes, nervousness, hirsutism, voice change, fluid retention, increased libido, depression, headaches, and dyspareunia, which usually resolve after discontinuation of treatment. The drug is contraindicated in women with a history of thromboembolic disease. For women of childbearing age, adequate nonhormonal contraception is essential.

Gateley and colleagues reported a series of 126 patients with refractory mastalgia who had failed to respond to various first-line therapies.[88] The response rate of those with cyclic mastalgia treated with danazol as a second-line therapy was 57% and as a third-line therapy was 25%. Equivalent figures for noncyclic mastalgia were 24% and 21%, respectively. Danazol was confirmed to be the most effective therapy, regardless of the treatment sequence.

Recommendations for the administration of danazol are 100 mg twice daily for 2 months while the patient keeps a breast pain record. If no response or an incomplete response is obtained, the dose may be increased to 200 mg twice daily. If there is still no response, another drug should be tried. Therapy should not continue longer than 6 months (because side effects may develop), and the drug should be tapered, as described by Harrison and associates[86] and Sutton and O'Malley.[87]

Gestrinone. Gestrinone is an androgen derivative of 19-nortestosterone. As such, its mode of action and side effects are similar to those of danazol. However, side effects occur less frequently with the reduced dosage required for treatment (5 mg vs. 1400 to 4200 mg/week). With its androgenic, antiestrogenic, and antiprogestagenic properties, gestrinone may inhibit the midcycle gonadotropin surge and act directly on the pituitary gland, in the ovary, directly at the estrogen receptor of the mammary gland.[89]

In a multicenter trial evaluating the safety and efficacy of gestrinone,[90] 105 patients were randomized to receive gestrinone or placebo 2.5 mg twice weekly for 3 months. Of patients treated with gestrinone, 55% had a clinically favorable response, with a placebo effect of 25%. Complete resolution of symptoms with gestrinone occurred only in 22% of patients. Further trials with gestrinone have not been performed.

Others

Luteinizing Hormone–Releasing Hormone Agonist. The mechanisms of LHRH analogs are thought to be their antigonadotropic action and direct inhibition of ovarian steroidogenesis, which almost completely induce ovarian ablation, resulting in extremely low levels of the ovarian hormones estradiol, progesterone, androgens, and PRL. In a nonrandomized trial, Monosonego and colleagues[91] gave intramuscular LHRH agonist (3.75 mg as a monthly depot) to 66 patients during a 3- to 6-month period. A complete response was observed in 44% of the patients treated with an LHRH agonist alone, and a partial response was seen in 45%. Monthly injections of an LHRH analog resulted in an overall response rate of more than 81% in patients with both cyclic and noncyclic mastalgia. Side effects, which included hot flashes, myasthenia, depression, vaginal atrophy, decreased libido, visual disorders, and hypertension, were experienced by most participants but reportedly were not severe enough to require cessation of therapy.[92] Significantly, treatment with an LHRH agonist induced remarkable loss of trabecular bone.[93] For this reason, only short courses of LHRH analogs should be administered and only for acute and severe cases of mastalgia.

Thyroid Hormone. Data from in vitro studies have suggested that thyroid hormones may antagonize the effects of estrogen at the pituitary receptor levels of lactotrophs, such as TRH, although there is no conclusive support for this.[33] Relative estrogen dominance is suggested as a cause for the increase in PRL responsiveness to TRH in patients with mastalgia.

Kumar and colleagues[38] found a generalized abnormality of hypothalamic-pituitary axis in 17 patients with cyclic mastalgia compared with 11 controls by using a combined TRH and gonadotropin-releasing hormone test. The release of PRL, LH, and FSH was significantly greater in patients with cyclic mastalgia than in controls; estrogen and progesterone levels were normal. Carlson and coworkers showed a 50% response rate to thyroid hormone replacement in 16 of 18 patients with mastodynia who had elevated TRH-induced PRL responses; 13 of the patients had endemic goiter.[94] In 17 patients with mastalgia, Estes demonstrated that in patients given 0.1-mg doses of levothyroxine for 2 months, 47% obtained complete relief and 26% obtained partial relief without side effects.[95] A large, randomized, placebo-controlled trial of levothyroxine is needed before any recommendation is made for its use as a standard treatment.

NONENDOCRINE THERAPY

Bromocriptine

Results of recent studies point toward a PRL secretory hypersensitivity for estradiol in patients with cyclic mastalgia (see Fig. 5-1). Watt-Boolsen and colleagues[40] studied 20 women with cyclic mastalgia and compared them with 10 women who were asymptomatic. Basal serum PRL levels were significantly elevated, although within the normal range, in the mastalgia group versus controls. Cole and associates[26] have demonstrated that PRL is involved in the regulation of water and electrolyte balance in the nonlactating breast. An increase in serum PRL levels could possibly cause an influx of water and electrolytes in the breast, thus increasing tension and causing pain. Further support for this theory comes from Blichert-Toft and coworkers' observation that the breast becomes smaller, softer, and less tender during PRL-suppressive therapy.[96] However, PRL is probably not the only factor. In women with true hyperprolactinemia, levels of mammotrophic hormones are entirely different because ovarian steroid levels are suppressed. Bromocriptine is an ergot alkaloid that acts as a dopaminergic agonist on the hypothalamic-pituitary axis. One result of this action is suppression of PRL secretion.

Mansel and colleagues[97] reported a double-blind crossover study using bromocriptine in a group of patients with mastalgia. Lowered PRL levels associated with a significant clinical response were seen in patients with cyclic breast pain but not in those with noncyclic breast pain. In a double-blind controlled trial of danazol and bromocriptine, Hinton and associates[98] reported a clinical response with bromocriptine in two thirds of patients with cyclic pain but no response in patients with noncyclic pain. In contrast, Pye and coworkers[99] reported a minimal response rate of 20% with bromocriptine in patients with noncyclic mastalgia versus 47% in those with cyclic mastalgia. The European Multi-Center Trial of bromocriptine in cyclic mastalgia[100] confirmed the efficacy of bromocriptine. Side effects occurred in 45% of patients and were severe enough to warrant discontinuation of therapy in 11%. Side effects were reduced by an incremental buildup of doses over 2 weeks. However, reports of serious side effects of bromocriptine prescribed for lactation cessation, including seizures (63), strokes (31), and deaths (9), have resulted in its removal from the indication list of the FDA.[101] Bromocriptine has not been approved by the FDA for use in treating mastalgia. Despite its apparent effectiveness, because of the seriousness and frequency of the reported side effects, we do not recommend bromocriptine for use in mastalgia. A multicenter, double-blind, randomized study is underway in Europe to study a new, highly selective, potent, and long-lasting dopamine agonist, cabergoline. Initially used in lactation cessation, it appears to be better tolerated than bromocriptine and has the added advantage of only twice-weekly administration.[100]

Analgesics

In a retrospective questionnaire survey of 71 patients, a negligible response was seen to conium cream, phytolacca cream, metronidazole, aspirin, cyproterone acetate, and ibuprofen cream.[102] Recently, a prospective but nonrandomized trial administering nimesulide, an oral analgesic, was reported. All but 2 of 60 patients had a clinically useful response (97%) after 2 weeks of therapy. Of 60 patients, 28 (47%) had complete resolution of their symptoms. Two patients could not take the analgesic because of complaints of gastritis.[103] In a randomized control trial of 108 women, Diclofenac, a topical nonsteroidal drug, has been shown to be effective for the treatment of both cyclical and noncyclical mastalgia; but it is unavailable in the United States.[104]

Abstention from Medications

Onset of breast pain with the recent prescription of any medication should be suspect. This is particularly so with estrogen replacement therapy, and withdrawal of such can produce dramatic results. Tenderness caused by this therapy can be circumvented with initial low-dose therapy and dosage escalation or with short "drug holidays" when patients become symptomatic.

REFRACTORY MASTALGIA

Tamoxifen

Tamoxifen is an estrogen agonist-antagonist commonly used in the treatment of breast cancer. It is thought to competitively inhibit the action of estradiol on the mammary gland. In 1985, Cupceancu[105] first reported a noncontrolled prospective study of tamoxifen given for 10 to 20 days of the menstrual cycle at a dosage of 20 mg/day for up to six cycles; breast pain disappeared in 71% of patients and symptoms were ameliorated in 27%. Controlled trials at dosages of 10 and 20 mg/day produced greater than 50% reduction in mean pain scores in 90% of patients with cyclic mastalgia and in _%__ of those with noncyclic mastalgia.[106,107] The higher

dose was no more effective, but side effects were more prominent. In a double-blind, controlled, crossover trial of tamoxifen (20 mg/day) given during a 3-month period, pain relief was seen in 75% of patients receiving tamoxifen and in 22% of those receiving placebo. Major side effects included hot flashes (26%) and vaginal discharge (16%). In an effort to reduce side effects while maintaining efficacy, the tamoxifen dosage was lowered to 10 mg/day for 3 to 6 months. Side effects were seen in approximately 65% of patients taking 20 mg and in 20% of those taking 10 mg.[107] The efficacy of tamoxifen for the treatment of mastalgia is well supported by the recent meta-analysis of randomized controlled trials for mastalgia performed by Srisvastava and associates,[75] where tamoxifen achieved a relative risk of pain relief of 1.92. These results have led to their recommendation that tamoxifen should be used as a first-line agent for the treatment of breast pain. However, possible links between tamoxifen use and endometrial carcinoma have relegated its use only for patients in whom symptoms are severe and in whom all standard therapies have failed.

Gong and colleagues[108] have hypothesized that toremifene, a newer member of the family of selective estrogen receptor modulators, may be a better medication than tamoxifen for mastalgia. In comparison to tamoxifen as adjuvant endocrine therapy for breast cancer, toremifene has a comparable therapeutic effect, yet is associated with fewer adverse effects. In their double-blind, randomized control trial, patients treated for cyclical mastalgia with 30 mg daily of toremifene noted a 76.7% response rate as compared to a 34.8% response rate seen in placebo treatment ($P < 0.001$). The incidence of an intolerable adverse effect was not increased with toremifene therapy.

A recent study by Mansel and coworkers[109] evaluated the safety and efficacy of a topical gel containing the potent tamoxifen metabolite, afimoxifene (4-hydroxytamoxifen) for the treatment of cyclical mastalgia in premenopausal women. In their phase II trial, 130 women were randomized to placebo versus 2 or 4 mg of the transdermal agent for four menstrual cycles. After four cycles, patients in the 4-mg group were more likely to demonstrate improvements in pain ($P = 0.010$), tenderness ($P = 0.012$), and nodularity ($P = 0.017$) compared with placebo. Afimoxifene delivered percutaneously had 1000-fold lower serum levels than levels achieved after oral delivery of tamoxifen. There was no change in plasma hormone levels or any serious side effects in any of the treatment arms.

Trigger Point Injections for Scapular Bursitis Mimicking Severe Noncyclical Breast Pain

Because of the proximal location of the sclerotome supplying the shoulder and the extensive junction of afferent signals from this region to the dorsal horn of the spinal cord, location of symptoms may or may not correspond to the proximity of the pain source. As expected, pain may involve the shoulder, the scapular area, the arm, and more commonly unrecognized, the breast.[110] A thorough history and physical examination is essential for patients presenting with mastalgia, and it should be diagnostic when trigger points are found along the

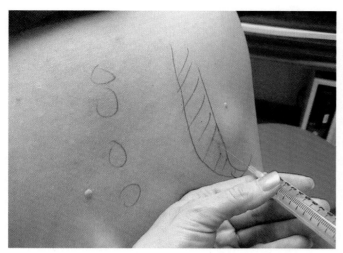

Figure 5-2 The most common site of a trigger point causing severe noncyclical breast pain, which is usually at the junction of the lower third and upper two thirds of the scapula.

medial scapular border. Injections containing a mix of lidocaine, bupivacaine, and steroids in the trigger point(s) result in relief within 15 minutes (Fig. 5-2).[9] In conjunction with daily heat to the bursa and nonsteroidal analgesics, this results in long-lasting relief in most patients.

Psychiatric Approaches

Lack of treatment for patients with mastalgia stems from the prevailing belief, as first proclaimed by Sir Astley Cooper, that all unexplained breast pain is a psychosomatic complaint seen in the neurotic female, not a real physiologic entity.[111] Indeed, in states of acute emotional stress, PRL is released and may form a physiologic basis for mastalgia (see Fig. 5-1). A study by Preece and colleagues found no difference between patients with cyclic and noncyclic mastalgia and those with varicose veins. However, a small subgroup of patients (5.4%) with treatment-resistant mastalgia had characteristics that were similar to those of a psychiatric patient group.[112] Jenkins and associates[113] hypothesized that patients with severe or resistant mastalgia are likely to exhibit psychiatric problems. To investigate this hypothesis, researchers had 25 patients with severe mastalgia complete a psychiatric evaluation using the Composite International Diagnostic Interview (CIDI) and a general health questionnaire. Based on the CIDI examination, 17 had current anxiety, 5 had panic disorders, 7 had somatization disorders, and 16 had current major depressive disorders. Jenkins suggested that in patients in whom "standard pharmacologic interventions" for mastalgia fail, evaluation by a psychiatrist and a trial of tricyclic antidepressants may be indicated.

Surgical Approaches

Surgery, such as a subcutaneous mastectomy[114] or excisional breast biopsy for mastodynia, is ill-advised and should be a tool of last resort. It should be offered only at the behest of the patient and then only after significant counseling. In general, surgical excision of localized

trigger spots is unsuccessful 20% of the time and runs the risk of replacing a painful area with a painful scar.[115]

Ineffective Treatments

Diuretics. Diuretics have never been tested in a double-blind, placebo-controlled trial. However, Preece and colleagues demonstrated that premenstrual fluid retention in patients with mastalgia is no different than in symptom-free controls, limiting the rationale for the use of diuretics.[116]

Progesterones. Studies by Maddox and associates (and others) using a randomized, controlled, double-blind, crossover design with 20 mg of medroxyprogesterone acetate during the luteal phase showed no benefit for the patient with mastalgia.[117]

Vitamins. Abrams[118] reported a favorable response to vitamin E in an uncontrolled trial nearly 30 years ago. In a small, prospective, double-blind, crossover study of the efficacy of vitamin E or placebo, 10 of 12 patients receiving 300 IU/day and 22 of 26 patients receiving 600 IU/day showed improvement after 4 weeks of taking vitamin E. Serum levels of dehydroepiandrosterone, but not estrogen or progesterone, were significantly higher in the responders to the drug before and normalized after administration of vitamin E. Meyer and associates[119] conducted a double-blind, placebo-controlled, crossover trial involving 105 women; randomly chosen ones received vitamin E (600 IU/day) for 3 months. Although 37% reported improvement while taking vitamin E, versus 19% reporting improvement with placebo, this was not statistically significant. Double-blind, placebo-controlled trials by London and coworkers[120] (128 patients receiving 150, 300, and 600 IU vitamin E for 2 months) and Ernster and colleagues[121] (73 patients receiving 600 IU for 2 months) reported no benefits from vitamin E.

Supplementation with vitamins B_1 and B_6[122,123] is thought to be of no benefit. A recent report by McFayden and associates[102] retrospectively reviewed treatment of 289 patients with pyridoxine (100 mg/day) for 3 months; 49% had a beneficial response, with only 2% reporting side effects. However, a double-blind controlled trial in 42 patients showed no benefit.

Vitamin A was first used for mastodynia by Brocq and colleagues in 1956 at a daily dose of 50,000 IU for 2 months, which led to significant reductions of pain.[124] In a small, nonrandomized trial in patients with symptomatic breast pain, 9 of 12 patients had marked pain reduction after 3 months of therapy with daily doses of 150,000 IU of vitamin A (all-trans retinal).[125] These results were associated with toxic effects often severe enough to stop or interrupt treatment. Santamaria and Bianchi-Santamaria developed a protocol of daily doses of 20 mg of beta-carotene interrupted with 300,000 IU of retinol acetate starting 7 days before each menstrual period and continuing for 7 days for each cycle.[126] Twenty-five patients with cyclic mastalgia were treated with this regimen for 6 months. Two patients had a complete response, and the remaining patients had a modest partial response. No side effects were reported. This regimen was not effective for noncyclic mastalgia.

Controlled trials have failed to demonstrate a role for vitamins in the treatment of breast pain.

SUMMARY

Figure 5-3 suggests a plausible algorithm for the treatment of breast pain.

Disorders of Development

Fibroadenoma. Fibroadenomas are predominantly seen in women 15 to 25 years of age. Parks showed that (1) hyperplastic lobules are histologically identical to fibroadenomas and can be found in virtually all breast tissues,[127] and (2) the epithelium and myoepithelium maintain a normal relationship.[128] Molecular biology studies show that fibroadenomas are polyclonal in keeping with hyperplasia, whereas phyllodes tumors are monoclonal in keeping with a neoplastic condition. Fibroadenomas are very responsive to hormonal stimulus enlarge during pregnancy or just prior to menses. Fifty percent stay the same or regress. Growth beyond 5 cm is considered a giant fibroadenoma. Fibroadenoma fits well into the ANDI classification: small fibroadenomas are normal, clinical fibroadenomas (1 to 3 cm) are a disorder of the normal process, and giant and multiple fibroadenomas fit in the disease end of the spectrum. Incidence of carcinoma arising in a fibroadenoma is about 2%.[129]

Fibroadenomatosis (fibroadenomatoid mastopathy). Fibroadenomatosis is a benign breast lesion with the composite histologic features of a fibroadenoma and fibrocystic changes that may represent a morphologic stage in the development of fibroadenomas. The lesion is characterized by microscopic fibroadenomatoid foci intermingled with dilated ducts, epitheliosis, and adenosis and was found in more than 10% of cases of BBD.[130]

Adolescent hypertrophy. Adolescent hypertrophy is associated with gross stromal hyperplasia at the time of breast development. The cause is unknown, but there is a hormonal basis to the condition. The spectrum from a small breast through massive hyperplasia fits the horizontal element of the ANDI concept: an excessively large breast is a disorder, whereas gigantomastia is at the disease end of the spectrum (Fig. 5-4). Cosmetic reduction is often warranted.[131]

DISORDERS OF INVOLUTION

Cyst Formation

Over a many-year period of cyclic changes, involution of stroma and epithelium is not always integrated, and disorders of the process are common. The exact mechanism of involution is not well understood, but it appears that involution of a lobular epithelium is dependent on the specialized stroma around it.[132] If the stroma involutes too quickly, the epithelial acini remain and can form microcysts, which are precursors of macrocyst formation (Fig. 5-5).[133]

Sclerosing Adenosis

Sclerosing adenosis can be considered a disorder of either the proliferative or the involutional phase of the

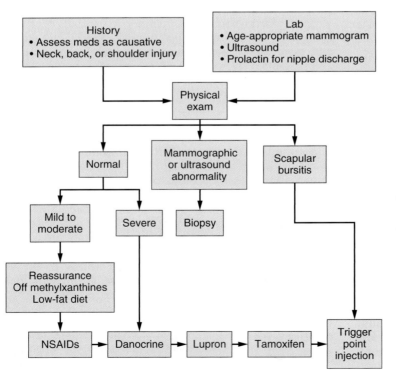

Figure 5-3 Algorithm of a plausible approach to mastalgia. NSAID, nonsteroidal anti-inflammatory drug.

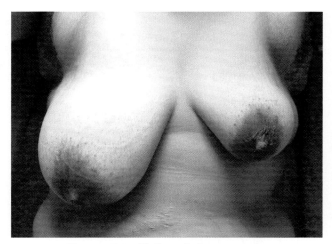

Figure 5-4   Unilateral gigantomastia.

breast cycle (or both) because of histologic changes that are both proliferative and involutional. Considering the complex interrelationship of the stromal fibrosis and epithelial regression that occur during involution, along with the concomitant cyclical change of ductal sprouting, it is not surprising that the characteristic distortion of epithelial acini by fibrous tissue seen in sclerosing adenosis is occasionally present.

Duct Ectasia and Periductal Mastitis

Duct ectasia is so common in the postmenopausal breast that it is considered part of the normal aging process and is present in nearly half of women older than 60 years of age.[134] The pathogenesis of duct ectasia is obscure but probably periductal mastitis, leading to weakening of the muscular layer of the ducts and secondary dilation, is the primary process.[135] The presenting symptoms of duct ectasia are nipple discharge, nipple retraction, inflammatory masses, and abscesses. Both duct dilation and duct sclerosis represent disorders of involution. Periductal fibrosis can occur in the absence of duct

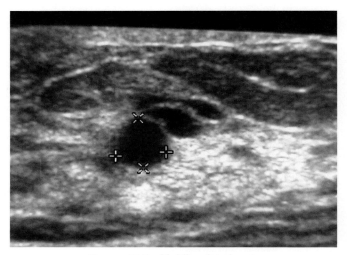

Figure 5-5   Multiloculated cyst.

ectasia or inflammation and probably represents part of the normal involutional process.[136]

Epithelial Hyperplasia

Parks showed that lobular and intraductal papillary hyperplasia is common in the premenopausal period and tends to regress spontaneously after menopause.[127] It is regarded as a disorder of normal involution. In an autopsy study, Kramer and Rush[137] found that 59% of women older than age 70 exhibited some degree of epithelial hyperplasia. Sloss, Bennett, and Clagett[138] concluded from another autopsy study, "the mere presence of blunt duct adenosis, apocrine epithelium and intraductal epithelial hyperplasia in the breast of women is insufficient to warrant such changes being called disease." However, studies by Page and colleagues[139] and Wellings, Jensen, and Marcum[140] have shown that the other end of the spectrum—atypical lobular hyperplasia and atypical ductal hyperplasia, particularly as seen in the terminal ductal lobular unit—is commonly associated with malignancy. Expression of estrogen receptor alpha in adjacent normal lobules doubles the breast cancer risk previously associated with epithelial hyperplasia lacking atypia.[141]

OTHER BENIGN BREAST DISORDERS

Nipple Inversion

Primary nipple inversion is a disorder of the development of the terminal ducts, preventing the normal protrusion of ducts and areola. Onset later in life can represent periductal fibrosis, but cancer must be excluded.[142]

Mammary Duct Fistula

Nipple inversion predisposes to terminal duct obstruction, leading to recurrent subareolar abscess and mammary duct fistula—the usual form of periductal mastitis seen in young women who smoke.[143]

Epithelial Hyperplasia of Pregnancy

Marked hyperplasia of the duct epithelium occurs in pregnancy. The papillary projections sometimes give rise to bilateral bloody nipple discharge. This will resolve, and only reassurance is necessary.

Benign Duct Papilloma

Benign duct papilloma is a common condition that occurs during the years of cyclical activity. It is the benign lesion with the highest risk of cancer that is most commonly ductal carcinoma in situ.[144]

Pathology of Benign Breast Disorders

The classification system developed by Page separates the various types of BBD into three clinically relevant groups: nonproliferative lesions, proliferative lesions without atypia, and proliferative lesions with atypia. This classification eliminates potentially confusing terminology and incorporates histologic criteria that are associated with an increased risk of the development of breast cancer and was adopted by the American College of Pathologists.[139,145] The histologic features of the breast biopsy specimen, together with the patient's personal and family history, establishes the relative risk of cancer. These data, combined with mammographic and physical examination findings, determine the management strategy and follow-up for the patient.[1]

NONPROLIFERATIVE LESIONS OF THE BREAST

Nonproliferative lesions of the breast account for approximately 70% of benign lesions and carry no increased risk of cancer.[139,140] Cysts and apocrine metaplasia, duct ectasia, mild ductal epithelial hyperplasia, calcifications, fibroadenomas, and related lesions are included in this category.

Cysts and Apocrine Metaplasia

Cysts are defined by the presence of fluid-filled epithelialized spaces.[146,147] Cysts in the breast vary greatly in size and number and can be microscopic or macroscopic. These lesions are almost always multifocal and bilateral, and they are almost never malignant. Cysts originate from the terminal duct lobular unit or from an obstructed ectatic duct. The typical macroscopic cyst is round, appears bluish (blue-domed cyst), and usually contains dark fluid ranging in color from green-gray to brown. The epithelium of the cyst is often flattened, and apocrine metaplasia of the epithelium lining the wall of the cyst is occasionally seen.

Duct Ectasia

Duct ectasia involves the large and intermediate ductules of the breast.[132] It is most often recognized by the presence of palpable dilated ducts filled with desquamated ductal epithelium and proteinaceous secretions. Periductal inflammation is a distinguishing histologic characteristic in this condition. The clinical significance of severe duct ectasia lies in its mimicry of invasive ductal carcinoma, but there is no demonstrated relationship to cancer risk.

Mild Ductal Epithelial Hyperplasia

The fundamental feature of epithelial hyperplasia is an increased number of nonstromal cells relative to what is normally observed two cell layers along the basement membrane.[139]

The diagnosis of epithelial hyperplasia of ductal tissue is often made by exclusion. It represents any epithelial hyperplasia that lacks lobular, apocrine, or atypical features. Mild and moderate epithelial hyperplasia are recognized primarily to distinguish them from the more marked changes of florid epithelial hyperplasia, which carries an increased risk of breast cancer[139,148] (Tables 5-3 and 5-4). A breast biopsy specimen showing mild hyperplasia does not imply any clinically significant risk of cancer, but studies have shown that 13% of these patients have a subsequent biopsy within 2 years and that 2% will have cancer.[149]

TABLE 5-3

Epithelial Hyperplasia of the Breast

Apocrine Type

Apocrine metaplasia (most commonly seen in the lining of cysts)

Ductal type

Sclerosing adenosis

Mild ductal hyperplasia

Moderate ductal hyperplasia

Florid ductal hyperplasia

ADH

Lobular Type

ALH

Ductal involvement of cells of ALH

ADH, atypical ductal hyperplasia; ALH, atypical lobular hyperplasia.
Modified from Consensus Statement: Is "fibrocystic disease" of the breast precancerous? Arch Pathol Lab Med 110:171–173, 1986; and Dupont WD, Page DL: Risk factors for breast cancer in women with proliferative breast disease. N Engl J Med 312:146–151, 1985.

Calcifications

Calcifications are common in the ductal, lobular, and stromal tissues of the breast. They can be macroscopic or microscopic and can be seen in blood vessels or lobules, free in the stroma, or associated with epithelium. Diffuse microcalcifications are commonly seen in sclerosing adenosis.[150,151]

Fibroadenoma and Related Lesions

Autopsy studies demonstrate that fibroadenomas are present in approximately 10% of women.[152] The peak incidence occurs between the second and third decades of life. However, these lesions are occasionally seen in the elderly. Fibroadenomas are benign well-marginated

TABLE 5-4

Risk for Development of Invasive Carcinoma

Lesion	Relative Risk
Nonproliferative lesions of the breast	No increased risk
Sclerosing adenosis	No increased risk
Intraductal papilloma	No increased risk
Florid hyperplasia	1.5- to 2-fold
Atypical lobular hyperplasia	4-fold
Atypical ductal hyperplasia	4-fold
Ductal involvement by cells of atypical ductal hyperplasia	7-fold
Lobular carcinoma in situ	10-fold
Ductal carcinoma in situ	10-fold

Data from Dupont WD, Page DL: Risk factors for breast cancer in women with proliferative breast disease. N Engl J Med 312:146–151, 1985; and Page DL, Vander Zwaag R, Rogers LW: Relation between component parts of fibrocystic disease complex and breast cancer. J Natl Cancer Inst 61:1055–1063, 1978.

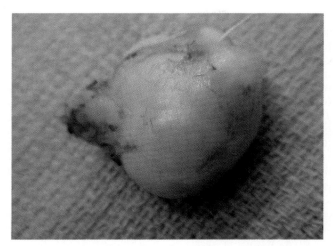

Figure 5-6 A well-marginated multilobulated fibroadenoma.

pseudoencapsulated tumors composed of abundant stroma and epithelial elements and display a wide spectrum of proliferative and nonproliferative histologic changes in as well as around adjacent tissue (Fig. 5-6).[153] Microscopically, fibroadenomas have both an epithelial and a stromal component. The histologic pattern depends on which of these components is predominant. Complex fibroadenomas are fibroadenomas harboring one or more complex features but can be managed similarly as the incidence or carcinoma is the same low 2%.[154]

Fibroadenomatosis is a benign breast lesion with the composite histologic features of a fibroadenoma and fibrocystic changes and is distinguished from the typical well-circumscribed fibroadenoma that may have fibrocystic changes. The lesion is present in about 10% of biopsy specimens and is characterized by microscopic fibroadenomatoid foci intermingled with dilated ducts, epitheliosis, and adenosis. The natural history of fibroadenomatosis is unknown but may represent a stage in the development of a fibroadenoma.[155]

Tubular adenomas present in young women as well-defined, freely mobile tumors that clinically resemble fibroadenomas being well-circumscribed tumors composed of benign epithelial elements with sparse stroma.[156] The sparse stroma is the histologic feature that differentiates adenomas from fibroadenomas, in which the stroma is abundant.[157] Lactating adenomas present during pregnancy or during the postpartum period. On microscopic examination, lactating adenomas have lobulated borders and are composed of glands lined by cuboidal cells that possess secretory activity identical to that normally observed in breast tissue during pregnancy and lactation.

Hamartoma is a rare benign tumor that can lead to unilateral breast enlargement without a palpable localized mass lesion. Histologically, a hamartoma consists of varying amounts of adipose, gland, fiber and smooth muscle tissue surrounding by a thin radiopaque pseudocapsule that can give a characteristic look on mammogram.[158] Multiple hamartomas are associated with Cowden's disease, which carries a higher risk of breast cancer.[159]

Adenolipomas/lipomas are very common and consist of sharply circumscribed nodules of fatty tissue that have normal lobules and ducts interspersed.[160] Microscopically, the fat is normal and the lobules and ducts are fairly evenly distributed throughout the tumor. They represent no increased risk of breast cancer.

PROLIFERATIVE BREAST DISORDERS WITHOUT ATYPIA

Proliferative breast disorders without atypia include sclerosing adenosis, intraductal papillomas, and florid ductal epithelial hyperplasia.

Sclerosing Adenosis

Sclerosing adenosis is a proliferation of glandular (stromal) elements that are increased in number relative to the basement membrane, resulting in an enlargement and distortion of lobular units.[150,161] The condition is characterized by an increased number of acinar structures and by fibrosis of the lobular stroma while the normal two-cell population along the enveloping basement membrane is maintained. The borders of the lesion are irregular but maintain its lobular architecture. Sclerosing adenosis commonly occurs in the context of multiple microscopic cysts and diffuse microcalcifications that makes screening mammography difficult.

Radial Scars and Complex Sclerosing Lesions

Radial scars and complex sclerosing lesions of the breast are characterized by central sclerosis and varying degrees of epithelial proliferation, apocrine metaplasia, and papilloma formation.[162] The term radial scar is reserved for smaller lesions (up to 1 cm in diameter), whereas complex sclerosing lesion is used for larger masses. Radial scars originate at the point of terminal duct branching. With the naked eye, the appearance is often unremarkable, but with magnification the characteristic histologic changes radiate from a central white area of fibrosis, which contains elastic elements. Radial scar imparts no increased risk of breast cancer above that of proliferative disease without radial scar.[162,163]

Florid Ductal Epithelial Hyperplasia

Florid hyperplasia is found in more than 20% of biopsy samples and thus is the most common proliferative lesion of the breast. It is associated with a minor increased risk of breast cancer.[139,161] This entity is characterized by an increase in cell number within the ducts, with a proliferation of cells that occupies at least 70% of the duct lumen. Architecturally, epithelial hyperplasia is either solid or papillary and is characterized by intracellular spaces that are irregular, slitlike, and variably shaped.

Intraductal Papillomas

Solitary intraductal papillomas are tumors of the major lactiferous ducts and are most commonly observed in premenopausal women. Commonly presenting features include a serous or bloody nipple discharge.[164,165] Grossly, these lesions are pinkish tan, friable, and usually attached to the wall of the involved duct by a stalk. Microscopically, they are composed of multiple branching papillae with a central fibrous vascular core that is lined by a layer of epithelial cells. It is often difficult to differentiate between benign papilloma and papillary cancer on frozen section. Multiple intraductal papillomas, which tend to occur in younger patients, are often peripheral and tend to be bilateral. Rizzo and colleagues recommend surgical excision of all intraductal papillomas identified on core needle biopsy because almost one fourth (24.5%) were upgraded to either atypical ductal hyperplasia or ductal carcinoma in situ (DCIS) and the majority of cases were asymptomatic.[166]

ATYPICAL PROLIFERATIVE LESIONS

Atypical proliferative lesions include both ductal and lobular lesions. These lesions have some, but not all, of the features of carcinoma in situ. At times, even the most experienced pathologists disagree as to whether a given lesion is atypical hyperplasia or carcinoma in situ.[167]

Lobular neoplasia of the breast represents a group ranging from risk lesions (atypical lobular hyperplasia and lobular carcinoma in situ [LCIS]) to invasive lobular carcinoma.[168]

Atypical Lobular Hyperplasia

As previously stated, atypical lobular hyperplasia fulfills some, but not all, of the criteria of lobular carcinoma in situ.[169] The cytology of atypical lobular hyperplasia is usually quite bland, with round, lightly stained eosinophilic cytoplasm. The uniformity and roundness of the cell population is pathognomonic of atypical lobular hyperplasia. The lobular unit is less than half filled with these cells, and no significant distortion of the lobular unit is present.[170] According to Page and colleagues, the risk of subsequent invasive cancer in women with atypical lobular hyperplasia is four times that of women who do not have this diagnosis[171–173] (see Table 5-4). The risk in the Vanderbilt cohort is approximately 10-fold in women with LCIS with a family history. Degnim and associates in the Mayo cohort did not find that family history further increased the risk of this breast lesion.[167] The incidence of atypical lobular hyperplasia present in benign biopsies is slightly greater than 1%, with the great majority of cases occurring in the perimenopausal period. As with atypical ductal hyperplasia, there appears to be an increased incidence in patients with a strong family history of breast cancer. Women with atypical lobular hyperplasia and a family history of breast cancer in a first-degree relative have a risk of invasive cancer twice that of the patient who presents with atypical lobular hyperplasia alone.

Atypical Ductal Hyperplasia

Atypical ductal hyperplasia is diagnosed when atypia is present and either the cytologic or architectural criteria for DCIS is absent. Page and coworkers[171] have emphasized that each of the following criteria must be met for a diagnosis of DCIS: (1) a uniform population of cells, (2) smooth geometric spaces between cells or micropapillary formation with uniform cellular placement, and (3) hyperchromatic nuclei. Atypical ductal hyperplasia has some, but not all, of these features. The natural history of atypical ductal hyperplasia suggests an intermediate risk (approximately fourfold) for the development of invasive cancer[171] (see Table 5-4). Women with atypical ductal hyperplasia who were followed for 15 years after breast biopsy alone developed invasive breast cancer about four times as often as women in the general population.[171,173] This relative risk translates into an absolute risk that 10% of women with atypical ductal hyperplasia will develop invasive carcinoma over a 10- to 15-year period following biopsy.

Clinical Features of Benign Breast Disorders

A useful classification system for BBD was described by Love, Gelman, and Silen[174] and is based on symptoms and physical findings. Six general categories were identified: physiologic swelling and tenderness, nodularity, mastalgia, dominant masses, nipple discharge, and breast infection.

PHYSIOLOGIC SWELLING AND TENDERNESS

Many women experience premenstrual tenderness, which is often associated with mild breast swelling. These changes are physiologic and generally limited to the reproductive years because they are hormonally regulated. They have been discussed previously.

NODULARITY

A cyclical pattern of diffuse lumpiness or nodularity is common and represents the responsiveness of breast parenchyma and stroma to circulating estrogenic and progestational hormones.[1,2,175] The nodularity can be finely granular or grossly lumpy, and it can involve the entire breast or a specific region. Patey coined the term *pseudolump* to describe a dominant area of lumpiness that coalesces into the surrounding breast tissue.[176]

DOMINANT MASSES

A dominant mass in the breast must be investigated to rule out cancer. Dominant masses that are benign include macroscopic cysts, galactoceles, and fibroadenomas.[132] As a general rule, discrete masses are aspirated with a needle to determine whether they are cystic or solid. If the lesion is cystic, the wall collapses with needle aspiration and the cyst is no longer palpable. If the lesion is solid, further evaluation to rule out cancer is mandatory.

NIPPLE DISCHARGE

Nipple discharge can be classified as galactorrhea or abnormal nipple discharge.[177] Galactorrhea is the spontaneous discharge of milklike fluid as a result of stimulation of the breast secondary to elevated PRL secretion from the pituitary. PRL levels can be elevated in patients who use oral contraceptives, in those with thyroid disease, and in those with a functional pituitary adenoma. Appropriate management includes thyroid tests and determination of the serum PRL level. Abnormal nipple discharge can be bloody or nonbloody. Takeda and colleagues noted that the presence of red blood cells or clusters of more than 30 ductal cells is suggestive of malignancy.[178] The most common causes of bloody discharge from the nipple are intraductal papilloma, duct ectasia, and less often cancer.

BREAST INFECTIONS

Excluding the postpartum period, infections of the female breast are rare. They are classified as intrinsic (secondary to abnormalities in breast architecture or function) or extrinsic (secondary to an infection in an adjacent organ or structure that involves the breast).[179] Intrinsic mastitis includes postpartum engorgement, lactational mastitis, and lactational breast abscess. Chronic recurrent subareolar abscesses occur primarily in women in the reproductive years and have a high incidence of squamous metaplasia of the involved ducts.[180] Antibiotics are generally not of therapeutic benefit in this setting, and resolution of the infection depends on excision of the chronically involved site. Acute mastitis associated with gross cysts is observed in the patient with macrocystic breasts who develops a localized area of redness, pain, edema, and fever (Fig. 5-7A). Because this entity mimics inflammatory cancer, the involved lesion is often aspirated or sampled by incisional biopsy for culture and histology (see Fig. 5-7B). Extrinsic infections develop secondary to an infectious process within the thoracic cavity or in the skin overlying the breast.

Most BBDs can be regarded as minor aberrations of normalcy, and hence they do not demand specific treatment. This being the case, any active management of these conditions is based on considerations such as an accurate diagnosis, the patient's concern, and interference with quality of life.

Treatment of Benign Breast Disease

CYSTS OF THE BREAST

Cysts represent dilated ducts. Simple cysts do not need to be aspirated by their very presence. If age-appropriate mammography and ultrasound demonstrates a benign cyst, then no further intervention is required. In fact, it is discouraged because it can cause future mammographic and ultrasound artifact.

Painful, complicated cysts and ones with multiple septae or ill-defined or fuzzy borders can be aspirated but require removal if that aspiration is either bloody or incomplete. An alternative approach is percutaneous removal. This approach obtains complete removal as well as tissue for examination. This is particularly useful for large macrocysts where aspiration is sure to be followed by reaccumulation. Percutaneous excision with a vacuum-assisted device can remove all the fluid as well as remove a piece of the cyst wall, preventing reaccumulation.

Multiple cysts and cyst aspirations are clinical markers of associated underlying histologic breast proliferation.[181] Women who have had multiple breast cysts aspirated have an increased risk of breast cancer, and they should be advised to practice regular self-examination, in addition to undergoing periodic clinical examination and age-appropriate mammography and ultrasound.[181,182]

FIBROADENOMA AND RELATED TUMORS

The consensus view is that women with fibroadenomas are not at significant increased risk for developing breast cancer.[183] Diagnosis is based on the combination of clinical examination, imaging, and nonsurgical tissue biopsy (the "triple" test). A clinical diagnosis of

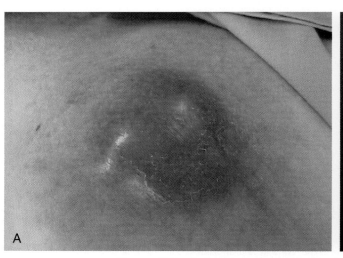
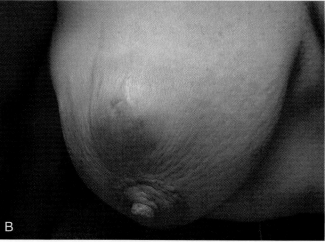

Figure 5-7   **A,** Breast abscess with skin changes, mimicking the breast cancer in **(B).**

fibroadenoma alone is unreliable and does not exclude malignancy, even in younger women. The choice of imaging is mammography; this should be combined with ultrasound in older women and ultrasound alone in younger women. Tissue biopsy, by either fine-needle aspiration or core biopsy, is the most accurate means of establishing the diagnosis. Traditionally, symptomatic fibroadenomas were treated by surgical excision, and this option should always be offered. There is increasing evidence that a conservative approach is safe and acceptable, provided the result of an adequate "triple" test is both negative for cancer and consistent with a fibroadenoma. Patients who choose conservative management need to be informed of the limitation of the tests, and they must be assessed promptly if there is symptomatic or clinical change.

Patients presenting with breast masses that are probably benign can be reliably diagnosed as having benign fibroadenomas using the "triple" negative test (normal clinical examination, benign imaging, and needle biopsy demonstrating fibroadenoma). There is increasing evidence that close follow-up for a period is acceptable.

The problem is noncompliance with close follow-up as well as patient anxiety. This has generated a plethora of ways to percutaneously remove fibroadenomas[184] or ablate them either by radiofrequency[185] or cryoablation.[186] Minimally invasive ablation or preferably removal under ultrasound guidance is an effective technique for the therapeutic management of these benign lesions; in the long run, this is probably more cost-effective, less labor-intense, and ultimately safer for these patients.

SCLEROSING ADENOSIS, RADIAL SCAR, AND COMPLEX SCLEROSING LESIONS

The diagnostic workup for radial scars, complex sclerosing lesions, and sclerosing adenosis is similar; workup involves stereoscopic or open biopsy depending on (1) the facilities and experience available and (2) the perceived risk of malignancy from the radiologic appearance. It is widely accepted that it is impossible to differentiate these lesions with certainty from cancer by mammographic features.[187]

THE DUCT ECTASIA AND PERIDUCTAL MASTITIS COMPLEX

There are many presentations and indications for surgery in patients with duct ectasia or periductal mastitis.

Nipple Discharge

Nonbloody, nonspontaneous, bilateral nipple discharge, typically from several ducts, is a benign condition with no increased cancer risk. It is not normally an indication for surgical treatment and often responds to decreased caffeine intake and cessation of smoking. Bloody nipple discharge is associated with a significant risk of cancer (20%), although bilateral bloody nipple discharge can be seen with pregnancy. In this setting, the operation of total duct excision has some advantages over more conservative procedures. In particular, it provides a good histologic specimen and relieves the patient's anxiety.

Correction of Nipple Inversion

Although the results are usually satisfactory, patients seeking correction for cosmetic reasons should be aware of the possibility of nipple necrosis, interference with sensation, inability to breastfeed, and the possibility that postoperative fibrosis will lead to late recurrent inversion. Because the benign condition results from shortening of the ducts, a complete division of the subareolar ducts is the only procedure that can correct it permanently.

Retroareolar Mass

The tender acute retroareolar mass of periductal mastitis often resolves spontaneously, so surgery is delayed if aspiration biopsy is suggestive of this diagnosis. When a mass persists for several weeks, the physician can treat it by performing a simple excisional biopsy. When an abscess is encountered during surgery, the surgeon can either undertake simple drainage with a view to further surgery should the problem recur or proceed immediately to total duct excision under appropriate antibiotic coverage.

Subareolar Abscess and Fistula

A subareolar abscess is confirmed with needle aspiration, which also provides a specimen for cytologic examination and bacterial culture.

Aspiration under antibiotic coverage is a reasonable alternative and has been advocated by Dixon.[188] In this setting, aspiration is facilitated by ultrasound guidance. Repeated aspirations are often necessary, and 40% of cases involving anaerobic bacteria recur after a short follow-up period. Others have advocated for a total nipple core biopsy or excision of the central nipple, including the obstructed ducts. This technique achieves a cure rate of 91% and an overall 95% satisfaction rate in the cosmetic outcome of the nipple,[180] and recent MRI studies have shown extensive tracking even to the opposite pole of the limbus.[189]

REFERENCES

1. Hughes LE, Mansel RE, Webster DJ: Aberrations of normal development and involution (ANDI): A new perspective on pathogenesis and nomenclature of benign breast disorders. Lancet 2:1316–1319, 1987.
2. Hughes LE, Smallwood J, Dixon JM: Nomenclature of benign breast disorders: Report of a working party on the rationalization of concepts and terminology of benign breast conditions. Breast 1:15, 1992.
3. Barton MB, Elmore JG, Fletcher SW: Breast symptoms among women enrolled in a health maintenance organization: Frequency, evaluation, and outcome. Ann Intern Med 130:651–657, 1999.
4. Maddox PR, Mansel RE: Management of breast pain and nodularity. World J Surg 13:699–705, 1989.
5. Gateley CA, Miers M, Mansel RE, Hughes LE: Drug treatments for mastalgia: 17 year experience in the Cardiff Mastalgia Clinic. J R Soc Med 85:12–15, 1992.
6. Smith RL, Pruthi S, Fitzpatrick LA: Evaluation and management of breast pain. Mayo Clin Proc 79:353–372, 2004.

7. Leung JW, Kornguth PJ, Gotway MB: Utility of targeted sonography in the evaluation of focal breast pain. J Ultrasound Med 21: 521–526, 2002.
8. Leinster SJ, Whitehouse GH, Walsh PV: Cyclical mastalgia: Clinical and mammographic observations in a screen population. Br J Surg 74:220–222, 1987.
9. Maddox PR, et al: Non-cyclical mastalgia: Improved classification and treatment. Br J Surg 76:901–904, 1989.
10. Davies EL, Gateley CA, Miers M, Mansel RE: The long-term course of mastalgia. J R Soc Med 91:462–464, 1998.
11. Gateley CA, Mansel RE: Management of painful nodular breast. BMJ 47:284–294, 1991.
12. Abramson DJ: Lateral extra mammary pain syndrome. Breast 6:2, 1980.
13. LaBan MM, Meerschaert JR, Taylor RS: Breast pain: Symptom of cervical radiculopathy. Arch Phys Med Rehabil 60:315–317, 1979.
14. Gregory PL: "Overuse"—an overused term? Sports Med 2:82–83, 2002.
15. Foote F, Stewart F: Comparative studies of cancerous versus noncancerous breasts. Ann Surg 121:6–53, 1945.
16. Davis H, Simons M, Davis J: Cystic disease of the breast: Relationship to cancer. Cancer 17:957–978, 1964.
17. Rush BF, Kramer WM: Proliferative histologic changes and occult carcinoma in the breast of the aging female. Surg Gynecol Obstet 117:425–432, 1962.
18. Watt-Boolsen S, Emus H, Junge J: Fibrocystic disease and mastalgia. Dan Med Bull 29:252–254, 1982.
19. Jorgensen J, Watt-Boolsen S: Cyclical mastalgia and breast pathology. Acta Chir Scand 151:319–321, 1985.
20. Mauvais-Jarvis P: Luteal insufficiency: A common pathophysiologic factor in the development of benign and malignant breast disease. In Bulbrook RD, Taylor DJ (eds): Commentaries on research in breast disease. New York, Alan R Liss, 1979.
21. Fechner RE: Benign breast disease in women on estrogen therapy. A pathologic study. Cancer 29:273–279, 1972.
22. Sitruk-Ware LR, Sterkers N, Mowszowicz I, Mauvais-Jarvis P: Inadequate corpus luteum function in women with benign breast diseases. J Clin Endocrin Metab 44:771–774, 1977.
23. Horrobin DF, Manku MS: Clinical biochemistry of essential fatty acids. In Horrobin DF (ed): Omega-6 essential fatty acids: Pathophysiology and roles in clinical medicine. New York, Wiley-Liss, 1990.
24. Kumar S, Mansel RE, Scanlon MF, et al: Altered responses of prolactin, luteinizing hormone and follicle stimulating hormone secretion to thyrotrophin releasing hormone/gonadotrophin releasing hormone stimulation in cyclical mastalgia. Br J Surg 71:870–873, 1984.
25. Brennan MJ, Wang DY, Hatward JL, et al: Urinary and plasma androgens in benign breast disease. Lancet 1:1076–1079, 1973.
26. Cole EM, Sellwood RA, England PC, Griffiths K: Serum prolactin concentrations in benign breast disease throughout the menstrual cycle. Eur J Cancer 13:597–603, 1977.
27. Robyn C: Endocrinological aspects of breast physiology. In Angeli A, Bradlow HL, Dogliotti L (eds): Endocrinology of cystic breast disease. New York, Raven, 1983.
28. Parker DC, Rossman LG, Vanderlaan ER: Sleep-related nychthemeral and briefly episodic variations in human plasma prolactin concentrations. J Clin Endocrinol Metab 36:1119–1124, 1973.
29. Kessler JH: The effect of supraphysiologic levels of iodine on patients with cyclic mastalgia. Breast J 10:328–336, 2004.
30. Dogliotti L, Faggiuolo R, Muccioli G, et al: Experimental and clinical evidences for a role of prolactin in human breast cancer and the possible usefulness of combining hypoprolactinemic drugs with standard hormonal treatments. In Baulier EE, Jacobell S, McGuire WL (eds): Endocrinology and malignancy. Carnforth, England, Parthenon, 1986.
31. Ayers J, Gidwani G: The "luteal breast" and hormonal and sonographic investigation of benign breast disease in patients with cyclic mastalgia. Fertil Steril 408:779–784, 1983.
32. Sitruk-Ware LR, Sterkers N, Mauvais-Jarvis P: Benign breast disease: Hormonal investigation. Obstet Gynecol 53:457–460, 1979.
33. Sitruk-Ware LR, Sterkers N, Mowszowicz I, et al: Inadequate corpus-luteal function in women with benign breast disease. Clin Endocrinol Metab 44:771–774, 1977.
34. Walsh P, McDicken IW, Bulbrook RD, et al: Serum oestradiol-17β and prolactin concentrations during the luteal phase in women with benign breast disease. Eur J Cancer Clin Oncol 20:1345–1351, 1984.
35. Walsh P, Bulbrook RD, Stell PM, et al: Serum progesterone concentration during the luteal phase in women with benign breast disease. Eur J Cancer Clin Oncol 20:1339–1343, 1984.
36. England P, Skinner LG, Cottrell KM, Sellwood RA: Sex hormones in breast disease. Br J Surg 62:806–809, 1975.
37. Golinger RC, Krebs J, Fisher ER, Danowski TS: Hormones and the pathophysiology of fibrocystic mastopathy: Elevated luteinizing hormone levels. Surgery 84:212–215, 1978.
38. Kumar S, Mansel RE, Hughes LE: Prolactin response to thyrotropin-stimulating hormone stimulation in dopaminergic inhibition in benign breast disease. Cancer 53:1311–1315, 1984.
39. Kumar S, Mansel RE, Wilson DW, et al: Daily salivary progesterone levels in cyclical mastalgia patients and their controls. Br J Surg 73:260–263, 1986.
40. Watt-Boolsen S, Andersen A, Blichert-Toft M: Serum prolactin and oestradiol levels in women with cyclical mastalgia. Horm Metab Res 13:700–702, 1981.
41. Angeli A, Fagiulo R, Berruti A: Abnormalities of prolactin secretion in patients with fibrocystic disease. In Dogliotti L, Mansel RE (eds): Fibrocystic breast disease. Aulendorf, France, Editio Cantor, 1986.
42. Pontiroli AE, Baio G, Stella L, et al: Effects of naloxone on prolactin, luteinizing hormone and cortisol responses to surgical stress in humans. J Clin Endocrinol Metab 55:378–380, 1982.
43. Spindel E, Arnold M, Cusack B, Wurtman RJ: Effects of caffeine on anterior pituitary and thyroid hormones in the rat. J Pharmacol Exp Ther 214:58–62, 1980.
44. Schlosber AJ, Fernstrom JD, Kopczynski MC, et al: Acute effects of caffeine injection on neutral amino acids and brain monoamine levels. Life Sci 29:173–183, 1981.
45. Krantz JC, Carr JC (eds): The pharmacologic principles of medical practice. Baltimore, Williams & Wilkins, 1969.
46. Minton JP, Foecking MC, Webster DJ, Matthews RH: Response of fibrocystic disease to caffeine withdrawal and correlation of cyclic nucleotides with breast disease. Am J Obstet Gynecol 135:157–158, 1979.
47. Minton JP, Abou-Issa H, Reiches N, Roseman JM: Clinical and biochemical studies on methyl xanthine-related fibrocystic disease. Surgery 90:299–304, 1981.
48. Bar H: Epinephrine and prostaglandin-sensitive adenyl cyclase in mammary gland. Biochem Biophys Acta 321:397–406, 1973.
49. Minton JP: Dietary factors in benign breast disease. Cancer Bull 40:44, 1988.
50. Minton JP, Abou-Issa H: Nonendocrine theories of etiology of benign breast disease. World J Surg 13:680–684, 1989.
51. Butler M, Lang NP, Young JF, et al: Determination of CYP1A2 and acetylator phenotypes in several human populations by analysis of caffeine urinary metabolites. Pharmacogenetics 2:116–127, 1992.
52. Arsiriy SA: Urine catecholamine content in patients with malignant and benign breast neoplasms. Vopr Onkol 15:50–53, 1969.
53. Boyd NF, McGuire V, Shannon P, et al: Effect of a low fat high-carbohydrate diet on symptoms of cyclical mastopathy. Lancet 2:128–132, 1988.
54. Horrobin DF, Manku MS: Clinical biochemistry of essential fatty acids. In Horrobin DF (ed): Omega-6 essential fatty acids: Pathophysiology and roles in clinical medicine. New York, Wiley-Liss, 1990.
55. Horrobin DF: The effects of gamma-linolenic acid on breast pain and diabetic neuropathy: Possible non-eicosanoid mechanisms. Prostaglandins Leukot Essent Fatty Acids 48:101–104, 1993.
56. Ghent WR, Eskin BA, Low DA, Hill LP: Iodine replacement in fibro-cystic disease of the breast. Can J Surg 36:453–460, 1993.
57. Hinton CP, Bishop HM, Holliday HW, et al: Double blind controlled trial of danazol and bromocriptine in the management of severe cyclical breast pain. Br J Surg 40:326–330, 1986.
58. Minton JP, Foecking MK, Webster DJ, Matthews RH: Caffeine, cyclic nucleotides and breast disease. Surgery 86:105–109, 1979.
59. Odenheimer DJ, Zunzunegui MV, King MC, et al: Risk factors for benign breast disease: A case controlled study of discordant twin. Am J Epidemiol 120:565–571, 1984.
60. Ernster VL, Mason L, Goodson WH 3rd, et al: Effects of caffeine-free diet on benign breast disease: A randomized trial. Surgery 91:263–267, 1982.

61. Bullough B, Hindei-Alexander M, Fetou HS: Methylxanthine and fibrocystic breast disease: A study of correlations. Nurse Pract 15:36–38, 1990.
62. Lubin F, Ron E, Wax Y, et al: A case-control study of caffeine and methyl xanthines in benign breast disease. JAMA 253:2388–2392, 1985.
63. Lawson D, Jick H, Rothman K: Coffee and tea consumption and breast disease. Surgery 90:801–803, 1981.
64. Marshall J, Graham S, Swanson M: Caffeine consumption and benign breast disease: A case control comparison. Am J Public Health 72:610–612, 1982.
65. Boyle CA, Berkowitz GS, LiVolsi VA, et al: Caffeine consumption of fibrocystic disease: A case control epidemiologic study. J Natl Cancer Inst 72:1015–1019, 1984.
66. Schaierer C, Brinton LA, Hoover RN: Methylxanthines in benign breast disease. Am J Epidemiol 124:603–611, 1986.
67. Allen SS, Froberg DG: The effect of decreased caffeine consumption on benign proliferative disease: A randomized clinical trial. Surgery 101:720–730, 1987.
68. Heyden S, Muhlbaier LH: Prospective study of fibrocystic breast disease and caffeine consumption. Surgery 96:479–484, 1984.
69. Sharma AK, Mishra SK, Salila M, et al: Cyclical mastalgia: is it a manifestation of aberration in lipid metabolism. Indian J Physiol Pharm 38:267–271, 1994.
70. Vobecky J, Simard A, Vobecky JS, et al: Nutritional profile of women with fibrocystic disease. Natl J Epidemiol 22:989–999, 1993.
71. Gateley CA, Maddox PR, Pritchard GA, et al: Plasma fatty acid profiles in benign breast disorders. Br J Surg 79:407–409, 1992.
72. Mansel RE, Pye JK, Hughes LE: Effects of essential fatty acids on cyclical mastalgia and non-cyclical breast disorder. In Horrobin DF (ed): Omega-6 essential fatty acids: Pathophysiology and roles in clinical medicine. New York, Wiley-Liss, 1990.
73. Goyal A, Mansel RE, and the Efamast Study Group: A randomized multicenter study of ganolenic acid (Efamast) with and without antioxidant vitamins and minerals in the management of mastalgia. Breast J 11:41–47, 2005.
74. Blommers J, de Lange-De Klerk ES, et al: Evening primrose oil and fish oil for severe chronic mastalgia: A randomized, double-blind, controlled trial. Am J Obstet Gynecol 187:1389–1394, 2002.
75. Srivastava A, Mansel RE, Arvind N, et al: Evidence-based management of mastalgia: A meta-analysis of randomised trials. Breast 16:503–512, 2007.
76. Srivastava N: Breast pain. Clin Evid 14:2190–2199, 2005.
77. Eskin BA: Etiology of mammary gland pathophysiology induced by iodine deficiency. In Medeiros-Neto G, Gaitan E (eds): Frontiers in thyroidology, vol II. Proceedings of the Ninth International Thyroid Congress, 1985, Sao Paolo, Brazil. New York, Plenum, 1986.
78. Andrews WC: Hormonal management of fibrocystic disease. J Reprod Med 35(suppl):87–90, 1990.
79. Laidlaw I. The Manchester Restandol trial. In Mansel RE (ed): Recent developments in the study of benign breast disease. Carnforth, England, Parthenon, 1992.
80. Chambers GC, Asch RH, Pauerstein CJ: Danazol binding and translocation of steroid receptors. Am J Obstet Gynecol 136: 426–429, 1980.
81. Barbier RS, Canick JA, Makris A, et al: Danazol inhibits steroidogenesis. Fertil Steril 28:809–813, 1977.
82. Greenblatt RB, Dmowski WP, Mahesh VB, Scholer HF: Clinical studies with the antigonadotrophin danazol. Fertil Steril 22: 102–112, 1971.
83. Hinton CP, Bishop HM, Holliday HW, et al: Double blind controlled trial of danazol and bromocriptine in the management of severe cyclical breast pain. Br J Surg 40:326–330, 1986.
84. Tobiasson T, Rasussen T, Döberl A, Rannevik G: Danazol treatment of severely symptomatic fibrocystic breast disease and long-term-follow-up: The Hjorring Project. Acta Obstet Gynecol Scand 123(suppl):159–176, 1984.
85. Pye JK, Mansel RE, Hughes LE: Clinical experience of drug treatments for mastalgia. Lancet 2:373–377, 1985.
86. Harrison BJ, Maddox PR, Mansel RE: Maintenance therapy of cyclical mastalgia using low-dose danazol. J R Coll Surg Edinb 34:79–81, 1989.
87. Sutton GLJ, O'Malley UP: Treatment of cyclical mastalgia with low dose short-term danazol. Br J Clin Pract 40:68–70, 1986.
88. Gateley CA, Maddox PR, Mansel RE: Mastalgia refractory to drug treatment. Br J Surg 77:1110–1112, 1990.
89. Snyder BW, Beecham GD, Winneker RC: Studies on the mechanism of action of danazol and gestrinone. Fertil Steril 51: 705–710, 1989.
90. Peters F: Multicentre study of gestrinone in cyclical breast pain. Lancet 339:205–208, 1991.
91. Monosonego J, et al: Fibrocystic disease of the breast in premenopausal women: Histohormonal correlation and response to luteinizing hormone releasing hormone analogue treatment. Am J Obstet Gynecol 164:1181–1199, 1991.
92. Hamed M, Caleffi M, Chaudary MA, Fentiman IS: LHRH analogue for treatment of recurrent and refractory mastalgia. Ann R Coll Surg Engl 72:221–224, 1990.
93. Dawood MY, Lewis V, Ramos J: Cortical and trabecular bone mineral content in women with endometriosis: effective gonadotrophin releasing hormone agonist and danazol. Fertil Steril 52: 21–26, 1989.
94. Carlson HE, Sawin CT, Krugman LG, et al: Effect of thyroid hormones on prolactin response to thyrotrophin releasing hormone in normal persons and euthyroid goiterous patients. J Clin Endocrinol Metab 47:275–279, 1978.
95. Estes NC: Mastodynia due to fibrocystic disease controlled with thyroid hormone. Am J Surg 142:764–766, 1981.
96. Blichert-Toft M, Henriksen OB, Mygind T: Treatment of mastalgia with bromocriptine: A double-blind crossover study. BMJ 1:237, 1979.
97. Mansel RE, Preece PE, Hughes LE: Double-blind trial of prolactin inhibitor bromocriptine in painful benign breast disease. Br J Surg 65:724–727, 1978.
98. Hinton CP, Bishop HM, Holliday HW, et al: A double-blind controlled trial of danazol and bromocriptine in the management of severe cyclical breast pain. Br J Surg 99:326–330, 1986.
99. Pye JK, Mansel RE, Hughes LE: Clinical experience of drug treatments for mastalgia. Lancet 2:373–377, 1985.
100. Mansel RE, Dogliotti L: A European multi-center trial of bromocriptine in cyclical mastalgia. Lancet 335:190–193, 1990.
101. Arrowsmith-Lowe T: Bromocriptine indications withdrawn. FDA Med Bull 24:2, 1994.
102. McFayden IJ, Forrest AP, Chetty U, Raab G: Cyclical breast pain: some observations and the difficulties in treatment. Br J Clin Pract 46:161–164, 1992.
103. Gabrielli G: Nimesulide in the treatment of mastalgia. Drugs 46 (suppl 1):137, 1993.
104. Colak T, Ipek T, Kanik A, et al: Efficacy of topical nonsteroidal antiinflammatory drugs in mastalgia treatment. J Am Coll Surg 196:525–530, 2003.
105. Cupceancu B: Short-term tamoxifen treatment in benign breast diseases. Endocrinologie 23:169–177, 1985.
106. Fentimen IS, Caleffi M, Brame K, et al: Double-blind controlled trial of tamoxifen therapy for mastalgia. Lancet 1:287–288, 1986.
107. Fentimen IS, Caelffi M, Hamed H, Chaudary MA: Studies of tamoxifen in women with mastalgia. Br J Clin Pract 43(suppl 68): 34–36, 49–53, 1989.
108. Gong C, Song E, Jia W, et al: A double-blind randomized controlled trial of toremifen therapy for mastalgia. Arch Surg 141: 43–47, 2006.
109. Mansel R, Goyal A, Nestour EL, et al: Afimoxifene (4-OHT) Breast Pain Research Group. A phase II trial of Afimoxifene (4-hydroxy-tamoxifen gel) for cyclical mastalgia in premenopausal women. Breast Cancer Res Treat 106:389–397, 2007.
110. Sizer PS, Phelps V, Gilbert K: Diagnosis and management of the painful shoulder. Part 2: Examination, interpretation, and management. Pain Pract 3:152–185, 2003.
111. Cooper A: Illustration of the diseases of the breast. London, Longman, Rees, Orme, Brown and Green, 1829.
112. Preece PE, Mansel RE, Hughes LE: Mastalgia: Psycho-neurosis or organic disease? BMJ 1:29–30, 1978.
113. Jenkins PI, Jamil N, Gateley C, Mansel RE: Psychiatric illness in patients with severe treatment-resistant mastalgia. Gen Hosp Psychiatry 15:55–57, 1993.
114. Salgado CJ, Mardini S, Chen HC: Mastodynia refractory to medical therapy: Is there a role for mastectomy and breast reconstruction? Plast Reconstr Surg 15;116:978–983, discussion 984–985, 2005.

115. Hinton CP: Breast pain. In Blamey RW (ed): Complications and management of breast disease. London, Bailliere & Tindall, 1986.
116. Preece PE, Mansel RE, Hughes LE: Mastalgia and total body water. BMJ 4:498–500, 1975.
117. Maddox PR, Harrison BJ, Horobin JM, et al: A randomized controlled trial of medroxyprogesterone acetate in mastalgia. Ann R Coll Surg Engl 72:71–76, 1990.
118. Abrams AA: Use of vitamin E in chronic cystic mastitis. N Engl J Med 272:1080–1081, 1965.
119. Meyer EC, Sommers DK, Reitz CJ, Mentis H: Vitamin E in benign breast disease. Surgery 107:549–551, 1990.
120. London RS, et al: Mammary dysplasia: A double-blind study. Obstet Gynecol 65:104–106, 1985.
121. Ernster VL, Goodson WH 3rd, Hunt TK, et al: Vitamin E in benign breast disease: A double-blind randomized clinical trial. Surgery 97:490–494, 1985.
122. Pye JK, Mansel RE, Hughes LE: Clinical experience of drug treatments for mastalgia. Lancet 2:373–377, 1985.
123. Smallwood J, Ah-Kye D, Taylor I: Vitamin B$_6$ in the treatment of premenstrual mastalgia. Br J Clin Pract 40:532–533, 1986.
124. Brocq P, Stora C, Bernheim L: De l'emploi de la vitamin A dans le traitement des mastoses. Ann Endocrinol (Paris) 17:193–200, 1956.
125. Band PR, Deschamps M, Falardeau M, et al: Treatment of benign breast disease with vitamin A. Prev Med 13:549–554, 1984.
126. Santamaria L, Bianchi-Santamaria A: Cancer chemo prevention by supplemental carotenoids and synergism with retinol in mastodynia treatment. Med Oncol 7:153–167, 1990.
127. Parks AG: The micro-anatomy of the breast. Ann R Coll Surgeons Engl 25:235–251, 1959.
128. Archer F, Omar N: The fine structure of fibroadenoma of the human breast. J Pathol 99:113–117, 1969.
129. Hassouna J, Damak T, Ben Slama A, et al: Breast carcinoma arising within fibroadenomas. Report of four observations. Tunis Med 85:891–895, 2007.
130. Hanson CA, Snover DC: Dehner fibroadenomatosis (fibroadenomatoid mastopathy): A benign breast lesion with composite pathologic features. Pathology 19:393–396, 1987.
131. Chang DS, McGrath MH: Management of benign tumors of the adolescent breast. Plast Reconstr Surg 120:13e–19e, 2007.
132. Azzopardi JG: Problems in breast pathology. Philadelphia, WB Saunders, 1979.
133. Miller WR, Dixon JM, Scott WN, Forrest AP: Classification of human breast cysts according to electrolyte and androgen conjugate composition. Clin Oncol 9:227–232, 1983.
134. Frants VK, Pickren JW, Melcher GW, Auchincloss H Jr: Incidence of chronic cystic disease in so-called "normal breasts," a study based on 225 postmortem examinations. Cancer 4:762–783, 1951.
135. Ammari FF, Yaghan RJ, Omari AK: Periductal mastitis. Clinical characteristics and outcome. Saudi Med J 23:819–822, 2002.
136. Elston CW, Ellis IO (eds): The breast, vol 13, 3rd. ed. of Symmer's Systematic Pathology. Edinburgh, Churchill Livingstone, 1998.
137. Kramer WM, Rush BF: Mammary duct proliferation in the elderly: A histological study. Cancer 31:130, 1973.
138. Sloss PT, Bennett WA, Clagett OT: Incidence in normal breasts of features associated with chronic cystic mastitis. Am J Pathol 33:1181, 1957.
139. Page DL, Vander Zwaag R, Rogers LW, et al: Relationship between component parts of fibrocystic disease complex and breast cancer. J Nat Cancer Inst 61:1055, 1978.
140. Wellings SR, Jensen HM, Marcum RG: An atlas of subgross pathology of the human breast with reference to possible precancerous lesions. J Nat Cancer Inst 55:231, 1975.
141. Gobbi H, Dupont WD, Parl FF, et al: Breast cancer risk associated with estrogen receptor expression in epithelial hyperplasia lacking atypia and adjacent lobular units. Int J Cancer 113:857–859, 2005.
142. Da Costa D, Taddese A, Cure ML, et al: Common and unusual diseases of the nipple-areolar complex. Radiographics 27:S65–S77, 2007.
143. Grant CS, Degnim A, Donohue J: Surgical management of recurrent subareolar breast abscesses: Mayo Clinic experience. Am J Surg 192:528–529, 2006.
144. Collins LC, Schnitt SJ: Papillary lesions of the breast: Selected diagnostic and management issues. Histopathology 52:20–29, 2008.
145. Consensus Meeting: Is "fibrocystic disease" of the breast precancerous? Arch Pathol Lab Med 110:171–173, 1986.
146. Hughes LE, Mansel RE, Webster DJT: Cysts of the breast. In Benign disorders and diseases of the breast: Concepts and clinical management. London, Bailliere Tindall, 1989.
147. Page DL, Anderson TJ: Cysts and apocrine change. In Page DL, Anderson TJ (eds): Diagnostic histopathology of the breast. New York, Churchill Livingstone, 1987.
148. Dupont WD, Page DL: Risk factors for breast cancer in women with proliferative breast disease. N Engl J Med 312:146–151, 1985.
149. Shin S, Schneider HB, Cole FJ Jr, Laronga C: Follow-up recommendations for benign breast biopsies. Breast J 12:413–417, 2006.
150. Page DL, Anderson TJ: Adenosis. In Page DL, Anderson TJ (eds): Diagnostic histopathology of the breast. New York, Churchill Livingstone, 1987.
151. Lehman CD, Rutter CM, Eby PR, et al: Lesion and patient characteristics associated with malignancy after a probably benign finding on community practice mammography. AJR Am J Roentgenol 190:511–515, 2008.
152. Hughes LE, Mansel RE, Webster DJT: Fibroadenoma and related tumors. In: Benign disorders and diseases of the breast: Concepts and clinical management. London, Bailliere Tindall, 1989.
153. Kuijper A, Mommers EC, van der Wall E, van Diest PJ: Histopathology of fibroadenoma of the breast. Am J Clin Pathol 115:736–742, 2001.
154. Sklair-Levy M, Sella T, Alweiss T, et al: Incidence and management of complex fibroadenomas. AJR Am J Roentgenol 190:214–218, 2008.
155. Chung A, Scharre K, Wilson M: Intraductal fibroadenomatosis: an unusual variant of fibroadenoma. Breast J 14:193–195, 2008
156. Moross T, Land AP, Mahoney L: Tubular adenoma of breast. Arch Pathol Lab Med 107:84–86, 1983.
157. Fechner RE: Fibroadenoma and related lesions. In Page DL, Anderson TJ (eds): Diagnostic histopathology of the breast. New York, Churchill Livingstone, 1987.
158. Wahner-Roedler DL, Sebo TJ, Gisvold JJ: Hamartomas of the breast: Clinical, radiologic, and pathologic manifestations. Breast J 7:101–105, 2001.
159. Uppal S, Mistry D, Coatesworth AP: Cowden disease: A review. Int J Clin Pract 61:645–652, 2007.
160. Spalding JE: Adenolipoma and lipoma of the breast. Guy's Hosp Rep 94:80, 1945.
161. Hartmann LC, Sellers TA, Frost MH, et al: Benign breast disease and the risk of breast cancer. N Engl J Med 353:229–237, 2005.
162. Sanders ME, Page DL, Simpson JF, et al: Interdependence of radial scar and proliferative disease with respect to invasive breast carcinoma risk in patients with benign breast biopsies. Cancer 106:1453–1461, 2006.
163. Berg JC, Visscher DW, Vierkant RA, et al: Breast cancer risk in women with radial scars in benign breast biopsies. Breast Cancer Res Treat 108:167–174, 2008.
164. Page DL, Anderson TJ: Papilloma and related lesions. In Page DL, Anderson TJ (eds): Diagnostic histopathology of the breast. New York, Churchill Livingstone, 1987.
165. Collins LC, Schnitt SJ: Papillary lesions of the breast: Selected diagnostic and management issues. Histopathology 52:20–29, 2008.
166. Rizzo M, Lund MJ, Oprea G, et al: Surgical follow-up and clinical presentation of 142 breast papillary lesions diagnosed by ultrasound-guided core-needle biopsy. Ann Surg Oncol 4:1040–1047, 2008.
167. Degnim AC, Visscher DW, Berman HK, et al: Stratification of breast cancer risk in women with atypia: A Mayo cohort study. J Clin Oncol 25:2671–2677, 2007.
168. Hanby AM, Hughes TA: In situ and invasive lobular neoplasia of the breast. Histopathology 52:58–66, 2008.
169. Simpson PT, Gale T, Fulford LG, et al: The diagnosis and management of pre-invasive breast disease: Pathology of atypical lobular hyperplasia and lobular carcinoma in situ. Breast Cancer Res 5:258–262, 2003.

170. Jensen RA, Dupont WD, Page DL: Diagnostic criteria and cancer risk of proliferative breast lesions. J Cell Biochem Suppl 17G: 59–64, 1993.
171. Page DL, Dupont WD, Rogers LW, Rados MS: Atypical hyperplastic lesions of the female breast: A long-term follow-up study. Cancer 55:2698–2708, 1985.
172. Dupont WD, Page DL: Risk factors for breast cancer in women with proliferative breast disease. N Engl J Med 312:146–151, 1985.
173. Page DL, Dupont WD, Rogers LW: Breast cancer risk of lobular-based hyperplasia after biopsy: "Ductal" pattern lesions. Cancer Detect Prevent 9:441–448, 1986.
174. Love SM, Gelman RS, Silen WS: Fibrocystic "disease" of the breast: A non-disease. N Engl J Med 307:1010–1014, 1982.
175. Bland KI, Copeland EM: Breast disease: physiologic considerations in normal benign and malignant states. In Miller T, Rowlands B (eds): The physiologic basis of modern surgical care. St Louis, Mosby, 1988.
176. Patey DH, Nurck AW: Natural history of cystic disease of breast treated conservatively. Br Med J 1:15–17, 1953.
177. Gray RJ, Pockaj BA, Karstaedt PJ: Navigating murky waters: A modern treatment algorithm for nipple discharge. Am J Surg 194:850–854, discussion 854–855, 2007.
178. Takeda T, et al: Cytologic studies of nipple discharges. Acta Cytol 26:35–36, 1982.
179. Moazzez A, Kelso RL, Towfigh S, et al: Breast abscess bacteriologic features in the era of community-acquired methicillin-resistant *Staphylococcus aureus* epidemics. Arch Surg 142:881–884, 2007.
180. Li S, Grant CS, Degnim A, Donohue J: Surgical management of recurrent subareolar breast abscesses: Mayo Clinic experience. Am J Surg 192:528–529, 2006.
181. Bundred NJ, West RR, Dowd JO, et al: Is there an increased risk of breast cancer in women who have had a breast cyst aspirated? Br J Cancer 64:953–955, 1991.
182. Dixon JM, McDonald C, Elton RA, Miller WR: Risk of breast cancer in women with palpable breast cysts: A prospective study. Edinburgh Breast Group. Lancet 353:1742–1745, 1999.
183. Houssami N, Cheung MN, Dixon JM: Fibroadenoma of the breast. Med J Aust 174:185–188, 2001.
184. Johnson AT, Henry-Tillman RS, Smith LF, et al: Percutaneous excisional breast biopsy. Am J Surg 184:550–554, discussion 554, 2002.
185. Fine RE, Staren ED: Percutaneous radiofrequency-assisted excision of fibroadenomas. Am J Surg 192:545–547, 2006.
186. Kaufman CS, Littrup PJ, Freeman-Gibb LA, et al: Office-based cryoablation of breast fibroadenomas with long-term follow-up. Breast J 11:344–350, 2005.
187. Berg JC, Visscher DW, Vierkant RA, et al: Breast cancer risk in women with radial scars in benign breast biopsies. Breast Cancer Res Treat 108:167–174, 2008.
188. Dixon JM: Outpatient treatment of non-lactational breast abscesses. Br J Surg 79:56, 1992.
189. Fu P, Kurihara Y, Kanemaki Y, et al: High-resolution MRI in detecting subareolar breast abscess. AJR Am J Roentgenol 188: 1568–1572, 2007.

Subareolar Breast Abscess: The Penultimate Stage of the Mammary Duct–associated Inflammatory Disease Sequence

MICHAEL M. MEGUID | KARA C. KORT |
PATRICIA J. NUMANN | ALBERT OLER

Historical Perspective and Terminology

The rational management of subareolar breast abscess, based on the understanding of its pathogenesis, has evolved over a long time. The vast array of terminology that has evolved over the years to describe both the clinical and histologic manifestations of this disease may have delayed an understanding of its pathogenesis. Terms such as *mastitis obliterans*,[1,2] *varicocele tumor of the breast*,[3] *periductal mastitis*,[4] *comedomastitis*,[5] *secretory cystic disease*,[6] *chronic pyogenic mastitis*,[7] and *plasma cell mastitis*[8] refer to the same disease process, each emphasizing a different perspective, and these, together with more recent terms, are summarized in Table 6A-1.

Birkett, in 1850, described a "morbid condition of the lactiferous ducts" (see Table 6A-1).[9] Bloodgood, in 1921, first documented the chronicity of this condition and its association with duct ectasia, blue-domed cyst, and periductal inflammation.[10] This disease was reported from different perspectives, based on clinical and microscopic observations (see Table 6A-1). In 1951, two milestone reports unified this clinical entity. In the first report, Zuska, Crile, and Ayres[11] emphasized the presence of a chronic, draining periareolar fistula associated with a breast abscess and proposed the pathogenesis to be (1) stasis of secretion in the duct, (2) dilation of lactiferous mammary duct, (3) ulceration of mammary duct epithelium with abscess formation, and (4) rupture of the abscess to form a draining sinus with a resulting fistula. They recommended excision of the tract with the involved "intranipple" portion of the duct. Their report established this to be a benign, noncancerous surgical condition that occurs frequently, is troublesome to both patient and surgeon, and is often mistaken for a recurrent primary inflammatory condition of the breast.[12,13]

In the second report, Haagensen correlated clinical and pathophysiologic findings.[14] He proposed an evolutionary disease process and coined the descriptive term *mammary duct ectasia* for the benign condition of the breast characterized by dilation of the subareolar terminal ducts, with lumen filled with desquamated cellular debris and associated periductal fibrosis and inflammation. He proposed stages in the pathogenesis of subareolar abscess, starting with dilation of major subareolar mammary ducts, followed by accumulation of cellular debris and material containing lipid. During this stage, the ductal epithelium was normal and there was no evidence of inflammation. As the disease progressed, the duct dilation extended into the peripheral breast tissue from the central subareolar region, and fibrosis and a periductal lymphocytic infiltrate were observed. The epithelium became atrophic and discontinuous; lipid material permeated the stroma; and an inflammatory reaction with necrosis, polymorphonuclear leukocytes, histiocytes, lymphocytes, and plasma cells supervened. Multiple ducts could be affected. Haagensen concluded

TABLE 6A-1

Nomenclature of Mammary Duct-associated Inflammatory Disease*

Term/Pathognomonic Factor	Investigators
Morbid condition of lactiferous duct	Birkett, 1850[a]
Mastitis obliterans	Ingier, 1909[b]
	Payne et al, 1943[c]
Chronic pyogenic mastitis	Deaver and McFarland, 1917[d]
Stale milk mastitis	Cromar, 1921[e]
Varicocele tumor of the breast	Bloodgood, 1923[f]
Plasma cell mastitis	Adair, 1933[g]
Involutional mammary duct ectasia with periductal mastitis	Foote, 1945[h]
Comedomastitis	Tice et al, 1948[i]
Periductal mastitis	Geschickter, 1948[j]
Chemical mastitis	Stewart, 1950[k]
Fistulas of lactiferous ducts	Zuska et al, 1951[l]
Mammary duct ectasia	Haagensen, 1951[m]
Squamous metaplasia	Patey and Thackray, 1958[n]
Secretory cystic disease of the breast	Ingleby, 1942[o]
	Ingleby and Gershon-Cohen, 1960[p]
Periductal mastitis/duct ectasia	Dixon, 1989[q]
Mammary duct-associated inflammatory disease sequence (MDAIDS)	Meguid et al, 1995[r]

*Terms used to describe the major conceptual milestones from early literature to current times. These terms reflect the different stages at which the pathology was described.
[a]Data from Birkett J.[9]
[b]Data from Ingier A: Uber obliterienende mastitis. Virchow's Arch Pathol Anat 198:338, 1909.
[c]Data from Payne RL, Strauss AF, Glasser RD.[2]
[d]Data from Deaver and McFarland.[7]
[e]Data from Cromar CDL: Correspondence. BMJ 1:363, 1921.
[f]Data from Bloodgood JC.[3]
[g]Data from Adair FE.[8]
[h]Data from Foote FW, Stewart FW: Comparative studies of cancerous versus noncancerous breasts. Ann Surg 121:197, 1945.
[i]Data from Tice GI, Dockerty MB, Harrington SW.[5]
[j]Data from Geschickter CF.[4]
[k]Data from Stewart FW: Tumors of the breast: AFIP fascicle 34. Washington, DC, Armed Forces Institute of Pathology, 1950.
[l]Data from Zuska JJ, Crile G Jr, Ayres WW.[11]
[m]Data from Haagenson CD.[14]
[n]Data from Patey DH, Thackray AC.[20]
[o]Data from Ingleby H.[6]
[p]Data from Ingleby H, Gershon-Cohen J: Comparative anatomy, pathology and roentgenology of the breast. Philadelphia, University of Pennsylvania Press, 1960.
[q]Data from Dixon JM.[19]
[r]Data from Meguid et al.[25]

that the preceding historical descriptions were all expressions of the same disease process at various stages.

In the 1960s, Bonser, Dossett, and Jull[15] and Dossett[16] challenged this pathogenesis and suggested that the periductal inflammation was responsible for the subsequent development of duct ectasia. Azzopardi,[17] in his monograph *Problems in Breast Pathology*, reiterated this view and favored the term *periductal mastitis*.

In the 1980s, Dixon and colleagues[18] introduced the term *periductal mastitis/duct ectasia*, and in agreement with Dossett and Azzopardi, they described the periductal inflammation as the primary event and the duct ectasia as a secondary phenomenon. They suggested that the hypothesis that infection follows stasis of secretions was incorrect.[18,19] They viewed mammary duct ectasia as an ill-conceived umbrella term for unrelated conditions that might lead to major surgery.

During the course of this intellectual struggle to come to terms with a condition often described as a nuisance by clinicians, the key observation of squamous metaplasia of a lactiferous duct was not given its due recognition. Patey and Thackray[20] noted that in six of their seven patients treated for mammary duct fistula, the portion of the associated duct from the fistulous tract to the nipple was partly or totally lined by squamous epithelium. The fistulous tract itself consisted of nonepithelialized granulation tissue. In the seventh patient the duct was lined by granulation tissue. Subsequently, Toker[21] reported the presence of a squamous lining in multiple ducts in a patient with a fistulous tract and concluded that the disease was the result of downward growth of squamous epithelium from the nipple into the subareolar mammary ducts. In 1970, Habif and associates[22] also observed squamous metaplasia in subareolar abscess.

Recent views put forward by Bundred and coworkers[23] and Dixon and colleagues[24] concerning the pathogenesis of this benign disease process propose that periductal inflammation is secondary to smoking and that duct ectasia is most likely an unrelated phenomenon. In contrast, our discussion of the pathogenesis of what we term the *mammary duct–associated inflammatory disease sequence* (MDAIDS) considers the interaction of various putative causal factors unifying the disease process while recognizing varied clinical expression. We see common elements in the spectrum of changes noted in MDAIDS. Furthermore, we believe in the original proposal by Haagensen that some form of mechanical obstruction, with associated retention of secretions, is at the core of the disease process, because (Table 6A-2) the frequency of asymptomatic dilatated ducts found incidentally in patients or at autopsy far exceeds the frequency of symptomatic duct dilation or ectasia.

Figure 6A-1 depicts our conceptualization of the disease process, from normal breast to a subareolar abscess and its sequelae, periareolar fistulas. MDAIDS is a more inclusive term that comprehensively describes the phases of this disease. This term encompasses the antecedent benign disease process (i.e., mammary duct ectasia), periductal inflammation/mastitis, the abscess, and its sequelae.

On the basis of our own histomorphologic observations[25] and those of others,[20–22] we postulate that squamous metaplasia of mammary duct epithelium, in association with duct ectasia, has a major role in this obstruction. Because the breast is a modified sweat gland, the presence of squamous metaplasia affects the accumulation of the continuously produced secretions and facilitates infection. This metaplasia initiates a cascade of changes whose molecular bases are beginning to be understood and that lead to the MDAIDS shown schematically in Figures 6A-1 and 6A-2. Also shown in

TABLE 6A-2

Frequency of Dilated Ducts as Incidental Findings at Operation or Autopsy and Frequency of Symptomatic Women and Men with MDAIDS

Investigators	Frequency (%)	All Patients with Breast Disease (n)	Average Age (Yrs)	Tissue Type
Asymptomatic (incidental and autopsy)				
Foote and Stewart, 1945[a]	38	200	42	Benign
	26	300	50	Carcinoma
Frantz et al, 1951[b]	25	225	62	"Normal breasts" postmortem
Sandison, 1956[c]	72*	800	75%, <80	Postmortem
Sandison, 1962[d]	6	500	No data	Postmortem
Tedeschi et al, 1963[e]	60	20	Postmenopausal	"Normal breasts" postmortem
Davies, 1971[f]	38	208	No data	Postmortem
Browning et al, 1986[g]	8.2	1256	46	Benign and malignant
Average = 29%		n = 3509		
Symptomatic MDAIDS				
Geschickter, 1948[h]	2.3	3107	40+	Benign
Sandison and Walker, 1962[i]	4.1	390	20–70	Benign
Bonser et al, 1961[j]	36	351	No data	Benign and malignant
Walker and Sandison, 1964[k]	12	283	48	Benign
Abramson, 1969[l]	2.1	857	No data	Benign and malignant
Frischbier and Lohbeck, 1977[m]	10.8	1256	No data	Benign and malignant
Thomas et al, 1982[n]	5.5	732	43	Benign
Dixon et al, 1983[o]	5.5	1963	All ages(<30–89)	Benign and malignant
Browning et al, 1986[g]	4.1	1256	47	Benign and malignant
Average = 5.9%		n = 10,195		

MDAIDS, mammary duct–associated inflammatory disease sequence.
*Includes duct ectasia and cysts. Includes 11% with duct ectasia observed on gross examination.
[a]Data from Foote FW, Stewart FW: Comparative studies of cancerous versus noncancerous breasts. Ann Surg 121:197, 1945.
[b]Data from Frantz VK, et al: Incidence of chronic cystic disease in so-called "normal breasts": A study based on 225 postmortem examinations. Cancer 4:762, 1951.
[c]Data from Sandison AT.[33]
[d]Data from Sandison AT: An autopsy study of the adult human breast, with special reference to proliferative epithelial changes of importance in the pathology of the breast, monograph 8. Bethesda, MD, National Cancer Institute, 1962.
[e]Data from Tedeschi LG, Ahari S, Byrne JJ: Involutional mammary duct ectasia and periductal mastitis. Am J Surg 106:517, 1963.
[f]Data from Davies JD: Periductal mastitis. Unpublished thesis, London, University of London, 1971.
[g]Data from Browning J, Bigrigg A, Taylor I.[79]
[h]Data from Geschickter CF.[4]
[i]Data from Sandison AT, Walker JC: Inflammatory mastitis, mammary duct ectasia, and mammillary fistula. Br J Surg 50:57, 1962/63.
[j]Data from Bonser GM, Dossett JA, Jull JW.[15]
[k]Data from Walker JC, Sandison AT.[114]
[l]Data from Abramson DJ.[82]
[m]Data from Frischbier HJ, Lohbeck HU: Fruhdiagnostik des Mammarkarzinomas. Lehrbuch und Atlas, Stuttgart, Georg Thieme, 1977.
[n]Data from Thomas WG et al.[76]
[o]Data from Dixon JM et al.[18]

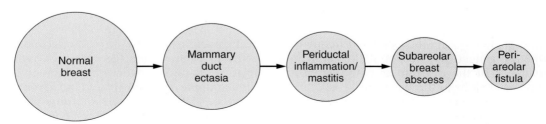

Figure 6A-1 The evolutionary stages of the mammary duct–associated inflammatory disease sequence (MDAIDS), from normal breast to its presentation of subareolar breast abscess and its sequela—periareolar fistula.

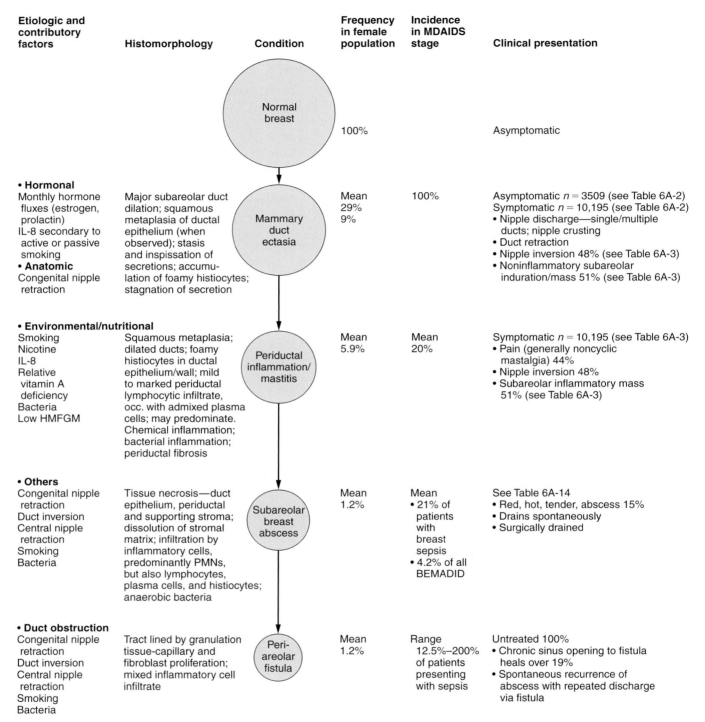

Figure 6A-2 Correlation between etiologic factors, histomorphologies, and clinical presentations of the mammary duct–associated inflammatory disease sequence (MDAIDS). Also shown is the estimated frequency of MDAIDS in the general female population and the calculated incidence of the different stages of MDAIDS as derived from the current literature.

Figure 6A-2 and Table 6A-3 are the estimated frequency of MDAIDS in the general female population and the calculated incidence of the different disease phases of MDAIDS, based on data from the literature.

Depending on a number of variables—the location and extent of the squamous metaplasia; the degree of impediment to secretion flow; the impact of hormonal (estrogen, prolactin), environmental (smoking), and local paracrine effects of cytokines secondary to smoking (active or passive); and the impact of nutritional factors (relative vitamin A deficiency), anatomic factors (congenital nipple retraction), and no doubt other factors yet to be defined—in one or more major subareolar and transnipple mammary ducts (or on occasion minor ducts in the peripheral breast tissue), varying degrees of duct ectasia, a primary chemically induced inflammatory

TABLE 6A-3

Frequency of Symptoms and Signs in Patients with MDAIDS as Summarized from the Literature

Specific Condition	Patients with MDAIDS (n)	Patients with Specific Condition (n)	Symptomatic (%)		References
			Occurrence	Range Of Occurrence	
Nipple Discharge					
Asymptomatic	103	8	8	—	79
Symptomatic	577	238	41	21–84	18,82,89,96,114,115,127*
Nipple Inversion/ Retraction					
Asymptomatic	103	7	7	—	79
Symptomatic	668	319	48	13–100	13,22,72,76,79,84,96,109,116,123,126,127[†]
Pain and Tenderness					
Asymptomatic	103	12	12	—	79
Symptomatic	183	84	44	11–106	79,89,96,114,116,128
Mass (Periareolar)					
Asymptomatic	103	33	32	—	79
Symptomatic	399	203	51	5–100	76,79,82,89,96,114[‡]
Abscess					
Asymptomatic	103	1	1	—	79
Symptomatic	803	124	15	8–28	79,90,96,115,125[§]
Fistula					
Asymptomatic	103	0	0	—	79
Symptomatic	176	34	19	12–67	79,82,90,96,102
Bilaterality					
Symptomatic	495	114	23	5–100	11,22,25,28,38,90,96,102,109,114,116,125,126,127[ǁ]

MDAIDS, mammary duct–associated inflammatory disease sequence.

*Additional data from Cromar CDL, Dockerty MB: Plasma cell mastitis. Proc Staff Meet Mayo Clin 16:775, 1941; Haagensen CD: Diseases of the breast, 2nd ed. Philadelphia, WB Saunders, 1971; Hartley MN, Stewart J, Benson EA: Subareolar dissection for duct ectasia and periareolar sepsis. Br J Surg 78:1187, 1991; and Urban JA: Excision of the major duct system of the breast. Cancer 16:516, 1963.

[†]Additional data from Cromar CDL, Dockerty MB: Plasma cell mastitis. Proc Staff Meet Mayo Clin 16:775, 1941; Haagensen CD: Diseases of the breast, 2nd ed. Philadelphia, WB Saunders, 1971; and Hartley MN, Stewart J, Benson EA: Subareolar dissection for duct ectasia and periareolar sepsis. Br J Surg 78:1187, 1991

[‡]Additional data from Cromar CDL, Dockerty MB: Plasma cell mastitis. Proc Staff Meet Mayo Clin 16:775, 1941; Haagensen CD: Diseases of the breast, 2nd ed. Philadelphia, WB Saunders, 1971; and Sandison AT, Walker JC: Inflammatory mastitis, mammary duct ectasia, and mammillary fistula. Br J Surg 50:57, 1962/63.

[§]Additional data from Hartley MN, Stewart J, Benson EA: Subareolar dissection for duct ectasia and periareolar sepsis. Br J Surg 78:1187, 1991; and Scholefield JH, Duncan JL, Rogers K: Review of a hospital experience with breast abscesses. Br J Surg 74:469, 1987.

[ǁ]Additional data from Ingleby H, Gershon-Cohen J: Comparative anatomy, pathology and roentgenology of the breast. Philadelphia, University of Pennsylvania Press, 1960.

reaction, and secondary bacterial growth, subsequently followed by infection and periductal inflammation occur. This concept is supported by the increased recognition and consensus that proper management of this disease entails use of a combination of antibiotics to cover aerobes and anaerobes and surgical excision of the involved duct and the periductal inflammation. On the basis of this evidence, we therefore believe the term MDAIDS is appropriate and correct.

Pathogenesis and Clinical Correlates

To fully appreciate the pathogenic process leading to *subareolar abscess* and its sequelae, familiarity with the normal structure and histologic appearance of the major subareolar lactiferous ducts, the ampulla, and the trans-nipple ducts is helpful. The breast is a modified sweat gland and thus produces a continuous, imperceptible discharge from the numerous orifices of the mammary ducts onto the nipple. This discharge is normally so small that it dries into a scarcely discernible crust on the nipple and is brushed away by the clothes.

As depicted in Figure 6A-3, the secretory acini of the lobular tissue in the periphery of the breast open into small (minor) intralobular ducts, which then drain into the major lobar ducts. Some 16 to 18 major mammary ducts draining acini are organized in lobular groupings surrounded by fibrofatty tissue, each separated by Cooper's ligaments. As each major mammary duct converges centrally onto and traverses the base of the nipple, it dilates to form a secretion-storing lactiferous ampulla, situated beneath the nipple areolar complex. From the

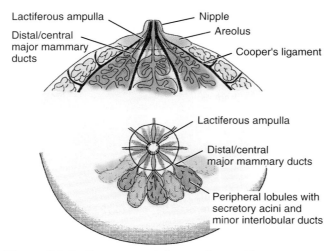

Figure 6A-3 Gross anatomic layout of normal breast structure.

ampulla, situated beneath the nipple–areola complex, each duct transverses the nipple and opens via a separate opening at the apex of the nipple. Thus, if there are 18 lobules with major ducts, there will be 18 separate openings for the major mammary ducts that open onto the apex of the nipple. Occasionally there are two major ducts draining the lobules, which converge into one ampulla.

As shown in the low-power view of a longitudinal section of the nipple (Fig. 6A-4), each duct is lined by a double layer of cells (inner cuboidal or low columnar epithelium) and an outer myoepithelial layer, whereas the ampulla and the final few millimeters of the intranipple duct terminating on the surface are lined by stratified squamous epithelium. The average frequency of dilated ducts found incidentally at surgery or autopsy is 29% (see Tables 6A-2 and 6A-3 and Fig. 6A-2). This far exceeds the average frequency of 5.9% in symptomatic females and males (see Table 6A-2) and suggests that a factor such as the relative imbalance of monthly hormone fluxes contributes to the development of early mammary duct ectasia.

In the literature on MDAIDS related to the pathologic process, several studies attribute ductal obstruction to squamous metaplasia or epidermalization of ductal columnar epithelium.[20–22,25] Based on these findings, our view of the evolution of MDAIDS, as postulated to correspond with the different histomorphologic changes, is shown schematically in Figure 6A-2.

Figure 6A-5A shows epidermalization of mammary duct epithelium. The squamous aplasia has progressed and has developed a granular layer (darkly stained subcorneal zone), which matures into keratin. This area of epidermalization is surrounded on either side by normal columnar epithelium consisting of a double layer of lining epithelial cells: the inner columnar and the outer flattened myoepithelial cells. At this stage, the symptoms may be discharge from one or more ducts, duct or nipple retraction, and/or subareolar induration (see Fig. 6A-2). As the disease progresses, the active granular layer (see Fig. 6A-5B) produces copious amounts of keratin, leading to obstruction of the major ducts by keratin plugs

(see Fig. 6A-5C). Following obstruction with keratin and cell debris, dilation of the duct and ampulla occurs because of the accumulation and stasis of secretory material from the acini. Clinically, the presenting symptom would be consistent with noncyclic mastalgia, nipple retraction, and/or subareolar induration (see Fig. 6A-2).

Finally, there is discontinuity or rupture of the thinned epithelial lining of the major duct, exposing the surrounding supporting stroma to the luminal contents and initiating chemically induced inflammation. In the process, the duct wall is permeated with lipid material, foamy histiocytes, and mild to marked periductal lymphocytic infiltrate, at times admixed with plasma cells (which may predominate). The keratin and the lipids of the secretions induce an inflammatory response—periductal inflammation, which presents clinically with symptoms of a subareolar inflammatory mass (see Fig. 6A-2). This milieu also serves as an excellent source for bacterial growth. The bacteria may be anaerobic or aerobic, from skin, endogenous breast flora, or oral contamination of the nipple.[26,27] Bacteria, both aerobic and anaerobic, can be cultured in more than 90% of breast tissue samples obtained at the time of augmentation or reduction mammoplasty.[26] Whether tissue

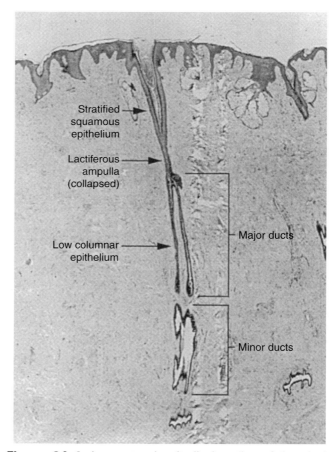

Figure 6A-4 Low-power longitudinal section of the nipple shows two major lactiferous ducts emptying into an ampulla (collapsed because of pathologic preparation) and then opening onto the surface of the nipple. (Modified from Meguid MM, Oler A, Numann PJ, Khan S: Pathogenesis-based treatment of recurring subareolar breast abscesses. Surgery 118:775–782, 1995.)

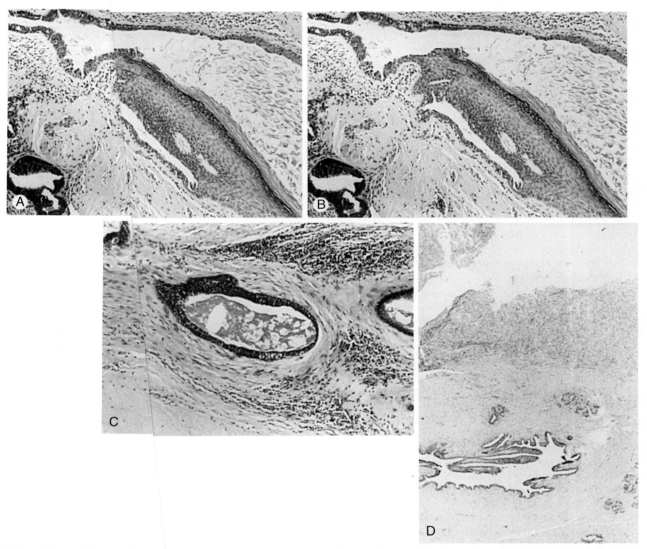

Figure 6A-5 Microscopic proc of squamous metaplasia of major lactiferous duct in series of patients. Epidermalization-metaplasia with granular layer and atin production (**A**), production of copious keratin (**B**), leading to keratin plugs (**C**) with ultimately acute and chronic inflammation (br abscess) (**D**). Abscess shown above a normal duct. (From Meguid MM, Oler A, Numann PJ, Khan S: Pathogenesis-based treatment of rec g subareolar breast abscesses. Surgery 118:775–782, 1995.)

samples are obtained from p in the mammary gland or superficially, the mai robic and anaerobic organisms cultured are coagle-negative staphylococci and propionibacteria, rectively.[26,27] Endogenous breast flora is similar to th resent on the skin[27] and is reflected in the incidence bacteria cultured in nonpuerperal subareolar breast cess specimens (see later in this chapter).[28] Coloniza of the tissue leads to an abscess beneath the areola (Fig. 6A-5D). Clinically, the patient may present wi an early subareolar abscess (see Fig. 6A-2) or, if process is more advanced and fluctuant, a sp neously draining abscess opening onto the vermilion rder of the areola. As the disease progresses, the absce ventually presents as a chronic sinus lined by granula tissue. On histologic examination, at varying distan from the opening of the fistula, the tract lined by gra ation tissue communicates with the main subaree duct lined by

squamous or epidermalized epithelium, usually packed behind the obstruction by desquamated keratin, debris that interferes with the normal drainage of secretion.[22]

The obstruction associated with epidermalization and the associated keratin debris is more severe and more rapid than that of squamous metaplasia or hormone imbalance (see following discussion). As a consequence, epidermalization of the mammary duct would induce changes that are more likely to be symptomatic earlier. In this rapidly changing mammary duct environment, as ectasia evolves with the presence of desquamated keratin flakes, epithelial injury and discontinuity are more likely. By its nature, keratin is very irritating and readily elicits an inflammatory response. The presence of keratin flakes in the retained secretions, in contact with the subepithelial stroma, greatly accentuates the periductal inflammation. Although this implies that these events occur in this sequence, as suggested by several studies,[20-22] the process probably occurs simultaneously but to different degrees in different large subareolar mammary ducts. Thus the presenting symptoms may not always follow the sequence depicted in Figure 6A-2.

Genesis of Mammary Duct–associated Inflammatory Disease Sequence

A schema of the interactions of the putative causal factors on the three basic disease phases of MDAIDS—namely, duct ectasia, squamous metaplasia, and abscess—is presented in Figure 6A-6. The molecular basis whereby ductal epithelium undergoes squamous metaplasia has been revealed via use of a knockout mice model (see reference 66). Initially, in 1958 Patey and Thackray[20] postulated that squamous metaplasia of the lactiferous ducts occurred secondary to a congenital anomaly of the duct system, because six of seven patients studied had congenital nipple inversion. However, today, it is well recognized that vitamin A is necessary for preserving the cellular differentiation of columnar epithelia. Vitamin A deficiency promotes squamous metaplasia/epidermalization, a development also associated with smoking. Increased interleukin 8 (IL-8) in alveolar capillary wall macrophages in lung tissue of smokers, as compared with controls, with its paracrine action stimulating polymorphonuclear cell migration, may contribute to the acute inflammatory response.[29] The course and evolution of the disease process leading to subareolar abscess, with its underlying histomorphologic alterations and clinical expression as MDAIDS (see Fig. 6A-2), depend on the impact of these two factors. Smoking shifts the metabolism of estrogen away from active metabolites[30] and induces lower serum prolactin levels.[31] Retinoic vitamin A promotes prolactin secretion,[32] implying that a deficiency of this vitamin could have an inhibitory effect on prolactin secretion.

HORMONAL INFLUENCES

The healthy infant often has transient breast enlargement of a few weeks' duration, and transient duct ectasia has been observed in some of these infants. The ectasia is attributed to transplacental passage of maternal hormones.[33] Symptomatic MDAIDS associated with bloody nipple discharge has been documented in infants and young children.[34-36] Of interest is the observation of a 100% increase in serum prolactin in a 3-year-old boy that was associated with MDAID.

Prolactin

Prolactin is essential for lactation participates in mammary growth through sensitization of the ductal epithelium to mitogenic synergism. Prolactin secretion is stimulated by estrogen and inhibited by drugs such as dopamine, the prolactin inhibitory factor.[38]

In several studies, MDAIDS has been reported to be associated with increased serum prolactin. The association of MDAIDS and prolactinemia has been seen in the setting of prolactin-secreting pituitary chromophobe adenoma,[39] breast cancer,[40] treatment with phenothiazine,[39] whose long-term can lead to hyperprolactinemia.[41] Phenothiazine can induce breast enlargement, lactation, amenorrhea, and gynecomastia.

Shousha and coworkers considered three possibilities for the association of MDS with increased serum prolactin: (1) a direct relationship, (2) unrelated events, and (3) a process secondary sudden decrease in serum prolactin. A decrease in serum prolactin has also been associated with smoking and may follow vitamin A deficiency.[31,32]

The impact of smoking on prolactin secretion has been investigated mainly with use of nicotine. This has biphasic effects depending on the dose and frequency of administration. One two doses of nicotine can stimulate prolactin secretion.[42] However, repeated doses inhibit prolactin secretion because of desensitization.

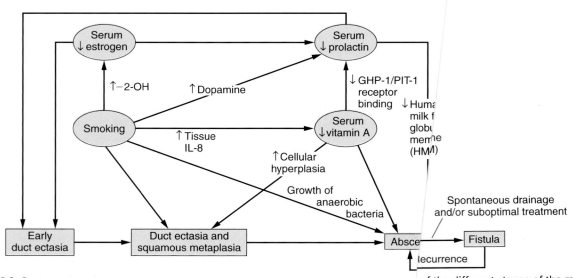

Figure 6A-6 Interplay of putative etiologic factors attributed as contributory to the evolution of the different stages of the mammary duct–associated inflammatory disease sequence (MDAIDS).

Berta and coworkers[31] evaluated the effect of smoking on the serum prolactin levels of fertile women who had not smoked for at least 12 hours and observed significantly lower serum prolactin levels in smokers than in nonsmokers. Male smokers also have a lower serum prolactin value than nonsmokers.[31]

Smoking acts via dopamine and serum prolactin levels on estrogen metabolism. Estrogen stimulates prolactin secretion.[30] Smoking induces a shift in estrogen metabolism that results in a decrease in peripherally active estrogen metabolites (see following discussion), possibly reducing prolactin secretion.[43]

A third pathway to lower serum prolactin levels may be a vitamin A deficiency or smoking (see later in this chapter). Recent studies in vitro suggest that retinoic acid activates the promoter responsible for the pituitary-specific GHP-1/Pit-1 transcription factor necessary for the expression of the prolactin gene.[32] Low serum levels of vitamin A would result in less receptor binding and thus less transcription of GHP-1/Pit-1.

Permanent decreases in serum prolactin or fluctuation to a subnormal physiologic concentration may be secondary to dopamine release, altered estrogen metabolism, or decreased serum binding of vitamin A receptor. This decrease in serum prolactin could promote MDAIDS, as proposed by Shousha and coworkers.[39] As to the mechanisms by which decreased serum prolactin would induce MDAIDS, we believe them to be alterations in secretions (composition and/or viscosity), resulting in stasis or affecting adhesion molecules.

Prolactin deficiency may also play a role in the initial stages of infection. As stated earlier, prolactin stimulates lactation. Breast milk contains lipid globules enclosed by fragments of the apical membrane of mammary secretory cells, referred to as human milk fat globule membrane (HMFGM).[44] These membrane fragments are not present in infant formulas; the addition of HMFGM inhibits adhesion of bacteria such as *Escherichia coli* to epithelial cells, and their absence facilitates sepsis.[45,46] It may be postulated that with decreased levels of prolactin, breast secretions of a nonlactating woman would also contain less HMFGM, thus facilitating adhesion of endogenous or exogenous bacteria to mammary epithelial cells and onset of infection.

Estrogen

Michnovicz and coworkers[30] showed that in persons who smoked at least 20 cigarettes per day, smoking stimulated the metabolic pathway of estradiol, leading to 2α-hydroxylation rather than to 16α-hydroxylation. 2α-Hydroxylated compounds are virtually devoid of peripheral estrogen activity. This increase in 2α-hydroxylation may result from the altered metabolism of steroid hormones following stimulation of hepatic P-450 microsomal enzymes by nicotine or other components of cigarette smoke.[47] Low levels of serum estrogen caused by nicotine and cotinine, its major metabolite, contribute to the conversion of testosterone to estradiol by aromatase.[48] From the results of these studies, we postulate that decreased estrogen activity impairs the hormonally controlled integrity of the breast duct epithelium.

NUTRITIONAL FACTORS

Vitamin A

Vitamin A deficiency induces keratinizing squamous metaplasia on multiple mucosal surfaces, including those of the head and neck region, bronchi, uterus, and cervix.[49] In the cervix, reserve cell proliferation, the precursor to squamous metaplasia, has been shown to be under the control of retinoids.[50]

There is increasing epidemiologic and experimental evidence that vitamin A or retinoids have a significant biologic effect on mammary duct epithelial cell proliferation and differentiation, of which insufficient levels result in the development of squamous metaplasia, possibly a pivotal event leading to MDAIDS (see Fig. 6A-6).

Vitamin A deficiency is implicated as a contributing factor in the development of infection. Vitamin A deficiency impairs blood clearance of bacteria and results in decreased phagocytic activity in vitro.[51] Increased bacterial binding to epithelial cells is observed with vitamin A deficiency.[52] For sepsis associated with MDAIDS, we postulate that the HMFGM is altered (see Fig. 6A-6). The apical surface of normal mammary duct epithelial cells consists of microvilli,[53] which are altered in various conditions.[54] In respiratory epithelium, this surface alteration induced by vitamin A deficiency can be observed by scanning electron microscopy before the appearance of squamous metaplasia, evident by optical microscopy.[55]

SMOKING

In 1988, Schafer, Furrer, and Mermillod[56] demonstrated the association between cigarette smoking and recurrent subareolar breast abscess. The relative risk of a recurrent subareolar breast abscess increased directly between light and heavy cigarette smokers, and 90% of all patients with recurrent breast abscess had been exposed to cigarette smoke for many years before the breast disorder was manifested.[56]

Various studies[23,24,57] have shown that severe periductal inflammation was more often associated with heavy smoking (>10 cigarettes per day) and younger age (Fig. 6A-7). These studies also noted an increased

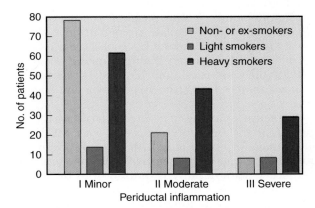

Figure 6A-7 Periductal inflammation and cigarette smoking in periductal mastitis ($P < 0.05$). (Modified from Bundred NJ, et al: In Mansel RE [ed]: Recent developments in the study of benign breast disease: Proceedings of the 5th International Symposium on Benign Breast Disease. London, 1993.)

incidence of mammary duct squamous metaplasia in smokers. Dixon and colleagues[24] performed a prospective analysis of 14,225 women, 4715 of whom were smokers. A prevalence of 2.28% (325 patients) of MDAIDS-related clinical symptoms was observed, and 54% of the patients were smokers.[24] When the severity of the disease process was correlated with smoking, only 28% of smokers had mammary duct ectasia. A significant increase in the percentage of smokers accounted for the subareolar abscess (87%) and periductal mastitis (88%) groups. The group with mammary duct fistula had the highest percentage of smokers (94%).[24] They also noted that an inflammatory response and its sequelae were associated with a younger age group.[24] On the basis of these analyses they postulated that clinical duct ectasia is likely to be totally unrelated to periductal mastitis.[24]

Conversely, the prospective data collected by Thomas, Williamson, and Webster[57] on 12,688 Welsh women did not uncover a significant difference in the percentage of smokers between patients with mammary duct ectasia (37%) and those with periductal mastitis (37.9%). In our smaller study of patients with recurrent subareolar breast abscesses, we found that 92% of them smoked, a percentage similar to that noted by Dixon's group.[24]

The molecular mechanisms by which smoking induces squamous metaplasia have yet to be identified, although their association is strong. Smoking-related squamous metaplasia of the bronchial mucosa is related to the intensity of tobacco use (packs per day) rather than to pack-years.[58] In the breast, within 30 minutes of smoking, nicotine and its metabolite cotinine are detected in the milk of lactating women.[59] In the nonlactating breast, glandular secretions are more concentrated, and in about 7% of women these secretions are mutagenic in the Ames tests and contain oxidized steroids and lipid peroxides.[60] These metabolites might be responsible for direct cellular injury leading to reactive squamous metaplasia.[60] Smoking reduces bioavailability of estrogen at target tissues by means of 2α-hydroxylation of estradiol, which may affect ductal cellular integrity.[30] In addition, nicotine and cotinine inhibit the aromatase-catalyzed conversion of testosterone to estrogen. A special class of estrogen derived from this reaction in humans is estradiol-17-sulfate and its metabolites, which originate from testosterone sulfate.[61] The metabolites 2-hydroxy- and 4-hydroxy estrogen-17-sulfate are potent lipid peroxidation antagonists.[61] The serum levels of these two metabolites may well be reduced during smoking. This would facilitate the cytotoxic injury induced by smoking and the development of reactive hyperplasia and squamous metaplasia.

Of interest, smoking may directly facilitate the development of the infection associated with MDAIDS. In vitro, smoke inhibits the growth of gram-positive cocci more than it does gram-negative rods. Smokers tend to have heavy gram-negative colonization of the mouth.[62] Those not infection-prone included more current smokers and persons with longer smoking experience.[63] Nevertheless, in a study of anaerobic respiratory infection,[64] heavy smoking and chronic lower airway infection were deemed to be pathogenic factors in the absence of aspiration; however, smoking does not appear to predispose

significantly to breast infection following mammary prosthesis.[65] Although the question has not been totally resolved, the possibility still exists that smoking may alter the composition of the endogenous flora in the mammary ducts and thus, in association with the previously discussed aberrations induced by prolactin and vitamin A deficiency, promote a bacterial infection.

Although the exact cause of MDAIDS is still unknown, certain contributing factors are becoming clearer. The repeated finding of squamous metaplasia has been well described in the literature.[22] Our own histomorphologic observations have also confirmed this finding.[25] Although it continues to make sense that squamous metaplasia and keratin plugging of lactiferous ducts may lead to obstruction and abscess formation, why the aforementioned process occurs remains unclear. Recent work by Li and colleagues[66] suggests that a genetic alteration may explain the predisposition of certain women to this difficult clinical problem. At least in animal models, alterations in many genes have been shown to alter mammary gland development and tumor formation.[67–69] More specifically, transforming growth factor-β (TGF-β) has been shown to play a role in mammary development and tumor formation.[70–72] The role of TGF-β in the development of mammalian mammary abscess has also been described by Li and colleagues. TGF-β signals are known to be regulated by a group of serine kinases known as Smad4 (a central mediator for TGF-β).[43] Specifically, with use of a Smad4 knockout mouse model, it has been shown that disruption of this gene repeatedly results in formation of mammary abscesses. This appears to be caused by transdifferentiation of normal mammary epithelium to squamous epithelium as a result of loss of TGF-β responsiveness. Histologic cross sectioning of these mice clearly showed increased proliferation of epithelial cells, keratinization, and squamous metaplasia associated with mammary abscess. This correlates almost precisely with the histologic picture seen in women with MDAIDS.

The preceding findings, although thus far shown only in a mouse model, promote a better understanding of the pathophysiology of human breast abscess as it relates to MDAIDS. It is hoped that further investigations will show a possible link between smoking or hormonal changes and these genetic alterations, which appear to be causally related to squamous metaplasia of the lactiferous duct.

Pathology of Mammary Duct–associated Inflammatory Disease Sequence

The least symptomatic stage consists of the earliest morphologic changes and includes mild mammary duct ectasia, foamy histiocytes with filling of duct lumens, and some degree of secretion stasis as granular flocculent intraluminal material distal to an area of squamous metaplasia. This can be quite focal and difficult to find histologically. In some of our more recent cases of early MDAIDS, this was present in only one or two serial histologic sections and was observed only by chance. In our more advanced cases of MDAIDS, the histologic evidence of squamous metaplasia and epidermalization was focal and not adjacent to the terminal end of the major mammary ducts.[25] The duct ectasia phase of MDAIDS is associated with changes in the periductal stroma, consisting of periductal fibrosis and fragmentation and disarray of (now) irregularly thick elastic fibers.[73] These stromal changes are found regardless of whether the duct ectasia occurs in the presence of periductal inflammation.[73] The presence of iron deposits suggests that intramural hemorrhage may have a role in the evolution of the disease process.

As the disease progresses, different degrees of histomorphologic changes are noted in association with the major and minor ducts. The major ducts exhibit increased ectasia and may contain dense inspissation of secretions and more pronounced periductal fibrosis. The minor ducts situated in the periphery of the breast tissue and the proximal parts of the lobules are dilated with foamy histiocytes or with homogeneous or granular secretions. Foamy histiocytes are seen permeating the ductal epithelium and surrounding stroma, which at first contains a mild lymphocytic inflammatory infiltrate. Less commonly, ducts are obliterated by fibrous tissue and even recanalized. Calcifications may occur. The presence of lipids in the stroma induces formation of lipid granulomas.

Subsequently, especially with infection, an abscess with a predominant acute inflammatory infiltrate may be observed. If the inflammation is more of the subacute or chronic type, the inflammatory exudate contains not only polymorphonuclear leukocytes but also lymphocytes, plasma cells, histiocytes, cell debris, and keratin. Although keratin was present in the intraluminal debris in most of our patients with abscesses, the inflamed segment of the duct was damaged so extensively that the foci of squamous metaplasia and epidermalization could no longer be found, even on examination of serial sections. This led us to conclude that if squamous metaplasia/epidermalization and ectasia affect only one inflamed duct, these changes may not be observed.

Clinical Overview of Mammary Duct–associated Inflammatory Disease Sequence

The incidence of MDAIDS is increasing. The entity is closely associated with the consumption of tobacco, which is on the increase among women,[74] a circumstance that may explain the increase in frequency. Currently, symptomatic MDAIDS represents approximately 20% of all benign conditions of the breast.[75]

Figure 6A-8 shows the age distribution of 186 patients with the clinical MDAIDS, combined from a couple of studies in the literature[19,76] in which this information was available and, for comparison, the age distribution of 1205 patients with operable breast cancer.[77] MDAIDS causes symptoms over a large age range, with the overall peak incidence between 40 and 49 years, although each symptom tends to peak at a different age (see following discussion).

The true incidence of the duct ectasia phase of MDAIDS can only be estimated because in most women it is subclinical or asymptomatic and is discovered only by chance at surgery (incidental) or autopsy. A degree of dilation of the major subareolar ducts is often seen during biopsy performed for both benign and malignant conditions of the breast. Thus asymptomatic duct ectasia of MDAIDS exists, but its clinical significance is uncertain. It is recognized, however, that many women have asymptomatic dilation of the major subareolar mammary ducts that becomes symptomatic only when infection supervenes and becomes part of the broad clinical syndrome of MDAIDS.

On the basis of the findings of several postmortem studies and incidental findings in histologic sections examined for other breast diseases (see Table 6A-2), the mean incidental frequency of MDAIDS appears to be approximately 30%. The mean incidence of symptomatic MDAIDS, based on a series of published studies, is approximately 6%. The pathologic process occasionally involves both breasts (usually with equal frequency).

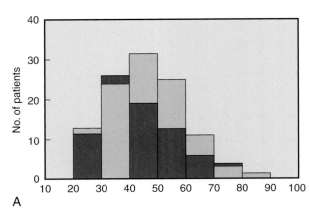

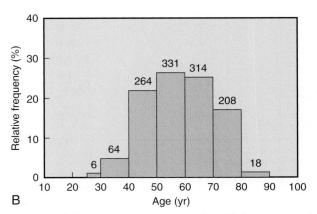

Figure 6A-8 **A**, Age distribution of 186 patients with clinical symptoms of the mammary duct–associated inflammatory disease sequence (MDAIDS). **B**, Age distribution of 1205 patients with operable breast cancer. (**A**, Yellow data from Thomas WG, Williamson RC, Davies JD, Webb AJ: The clinical syndrome of mammary duct ectasia. Br J Surg 69:423–425, 1982; and red data from Dixon JM: Periductal mastitis/duct ectasia. World J Surg 13:715–720, 1989. **B**, Data from the Yorkshire Breast Cancer Group: Br J Surg 1983.)

Table 6A-4 summarizes the major reported literature on the occurrence of MDAIDS in infants and males. Mammary duct ectasia also occurs in the breasts of elderly men who smoke (see Table 6A-4).[57] Consequently, mammary duct ectasia is not an involutionary disease as Haagensen asserted.[14] Clearly, this pathophysiologic condition is not limited to the female breast, a characteristic suggesting commonalities of etiologic and pathologic origin affecting mammary duct tissue.

The most common clinical presentation of the duct in MDAIDS is nipple discharge (Table 6A-5; see Fig. 6A-2). The reported prevalence averages 36% and ranges from 8% to 84%, depending on whether the patients are asymptomatic or symptomatic (see Table 6A-3), and

TABLE 6A-4

Males and Infants with MDAIDS Culled from World Literature

Investigators	Patient No.	Age (yr)	Clinical Features	Comments
Tedeschi and McCarthy, 1974[a]	1	57	Left breast tenderness, 3 cm indurated mass; discharge—0, adenopathy—0	No history of meds; excision biopsy; simple mastectomy; smoking history not noted
Mansel and Morgan, 1979[b]	2	62	Painful left subareolar breast mass; bloody nipple discharge; bilateral, painless nipple retraction during previous 2 yr; presented with draining left breast abscess	Total duct excision; smoking history not noted
	3	47	12-yr history recurrent right subareolar breast abscess with periareolar fistula; left breast and nipple normal	Simple mastectomy; smoking history not noted
	4	52	8-wk history tender left subareolar breast mass with intermittent discharge from periareolar fistula; right breast/nipple normal	No meds; antibiotics; subcutaneous mastectomy; smoking history not noted
Chan and Lau, 1984[c]	5	34	Right breast pain 1 wk; right nipple retracted with 2-cm, hard, tender subareolar mass; no nipple discharge; left breast normal	No meds; excision biopsy; smoking history not noted
McClure et al, 1985[d]	6	28	5-yr history swelling and occasional discomfort right breast; right breast enlarged; left breast normal	Phenotypically and karyotypically normal male; simple mastectomy; smoking history not noted
Ashworth et al, 1985[e]	7	50	2-mo history right subareolar breast mass; tender; no discharge; right subareolar abscess; left breast normal	No meds; major duct excision; smoking history not noted
Stringel et al, 1986[f]	8	3	Persistent bloody discharge right nipple; 1 yr later, bloody nipple discharge left breast	Normal endocrine workup, prolactin elevated; no meds; right subcutatenous mastectomy, then left subcutaneous mastectomy
	9	5 mo	Bloody nipple discharge left breast; intermittent for 3 mo; then stopped spontaneously	No meds
Thomas et al, 1993[g]	10	66	Breast abscess	20 cigarettes/day
	11	62	Bilateral periductal mastitis/breast abscess	15–20 cigarettes/day
	12	52	Periductal mastitis/mammary fistula	15 g tobacco/day
	13	51	Breast abscess	20 cigarettes/day
	14	44	Periductal mastitis/breast abscess	10 cigarettes/day
Lambert et al, 1986[h]	15		Fistula in male	Data not provided
Ekland and Ziegler, 1973[i]	16 and 17		Two males with subareolar breast abscess	Data not provided

MDAIDS, mammary duct–associated inflammatory disease sequence.
[a]Data from Tedeschi LG, McCarthy PE: Involutional mammary duct ectasia and periductal mastitis in a male. Hum Pathol 5:232, 1974.
[b]Data from Mansel RE, Morgan WP: Duct ectasia in the male. Br J Surg 66:660, 1979.
[c]Data from Chan KW, Lau WY: Duct ectasia in the male breast. Aust NZ J Surg 54:173, 1984.
[d]Data from McClure J, Banerjee SS, Sandilands DGD: Female type cystic hyperplasia in a male breast, Post Grad Med J 61:441, 1985.
[e]Data from Ashworth MT, Corcoran GD, Haqqani MT: Periductal mastitis and mammary duct ectasia in a male. Post Grad Med J 61:621, 1985.
[f]Data from Stringel G, Perelman A. Jiminez C.[36]
[g]Data from Thomas JA, Williamson MER, Webster DJT.[57]
[h]Data from Lambert ME, Betts CD, Sellwood RA: Mammillary fistula. Br J Surg 73:367, 1986.
[i]Data from Ekland DA, Zeigler MG.[116]

TABLE 6A-5

Predominant Symptoms of the Mammary Duct Ectasia Component of MDAIDS

	Symptomatic (n = 51)	Incidental (n = 103)
Nipple		
No discharge	13 (25%)	89 (86%)
Discharge	21 (41%)	7 (7%)
Inversion	5 (10%)	6 (6%)
Inversion + discharge	12 (24%)	1 (1%)
Pain		
None	17 (33%)	55 (53%)
Cyclical	21 (41%)	36 (35%)
Noncyclical	13 (25%)	12 (12%)
Lump		
None	21 (41%)	5 (5%)
Periareolar	23 (45%)	33 (32%)
Peripheral	7 (14%)	65 (65%)
Sepsis		
None	41 (81%)	102 (99%)
Abscess	4 (8%)	1 (1%)
Fistual	6 (12%)	0

MDAIDS, mammary duct–associated inflammatory disease sequence.
Modified from Browning J, Bigrigg A, Taylor I: Symptomatic and incidental mammary duct ectasia. J R Soc Med 79: 715–716, 1986.

the syndrome accounts for 11% of bloody and 13% of serous nipple discharges.[78] Bilateral symptoms occur in one third to one half of patients.[79] The discharge may come from one or more ducts. The color varies, often between ducts in the same breast. The discharge is sometimes grossly tinged or tests positive for occult blood. From studies of nipple discharge, the calculated frequency of bloody discharge is 64%.[18,78,80,81]

The other clinical symptoms are related primarily to the periductal inflammation and mastitis component of MDAIDS, which presents as noncyclic mastalgia and tenderness and occurs in approximately 44% of women with symptomatic MDAIDS (see Table 6A-3). Shown in Figures 6A-2, 6A-6, and 6A-16 are the factors thought to predispose to infection and to lead to the periductal mastitis component of MDAIDS. The presentation of the periductal inflammation and mastitis component spans a spectrum. At its minimum, the presentation is a subareolar tender mass, which occurs in 51% of women (see Table 6A-3). This mass may resolve spontaneously after 3 to 4 days but then recur at intervals of a few months or longer, a time sequence rarely seen with other breast conditions (see Fig. 6A-2). The inflammatory process is associated with foreshortening of the ducts, which results in partial or total nipple inversion. The reported incidence of nipple retraction/inversion varies widely, but the condition occurs in approximately 48% of symptomatic patients (see Table 6A-3). Often, patients present with multiple manifestations of MDAIDS. Thus, in one study with a 10% prevalence of nipple inversion, the condition was associated with a

discharge in 24%.[79] Pain of a noncyclic nature is associated with the inflammatory process and in various studies has occurred in approximately 44% of patients. At its worst presentation, the inflammation has progressed to a later stage of the MDAIDS, presenting as an obvious, large, florid red, hot, tender, fluctuant subareolar abscess that points at the vermilion border. Before the abscess either drains spontaneously or is drained surgically, it can be associated with pain, fever, and other signs of systemic sepsis. After spontaneous drainage, a persistent periareolar mammary duct fistula appears. Fistulas have been reported to occur in 12% to 67% of patients presenting with symptomatic MDAIDS (see Table 6A-3).[79,82] This is followed by the hallmark of this disease process—a recurrent subareolar abscess at a later date, either at the same site or in an adjacent segment of the breast. The frequency of treated recurrent breast abscess or fistula depends on the management of the disease but is estimated to occur in about one third of women. The study of Browning, Bigrigg, and Taylor[79] comparing symptomatic and incidental mammary duct ectasia tends to support these concepts. Many women have asymptomatic mammary duct ectasia. Symptomatic duct ectasia is secondary to infection that gives rise to sepsis, nipple changes, pain, and a subareolar mass (see Fig. 6A-2). These were the predominant features in patients in the study (see Table 6A-5), which included 51 who had symptoms of duct ectasia and 103 in whom the duct ectasia component of MDAIDS was found incidentally. This is the only study of its kind in the literature.

The term *MDAIDS* gives cohesion to a variety of conditions of the breast that until now appeared to be unrelated. The surgeon needs to be familiar with the pathophysiology of these conditions to avoid unnecessary surgery and to provide the patient with effective treatment.

Clinical Features Related to Management of Mammary Duct–associated Inflammatory Disease Sequence

NIPPLE DISCHARGE

Nipple discharge may be an early manifestation of MDAIDS. Table 6A-6 shows the causes of nipple discharge in 204 patients, based on the report by Tabar, Dean, and Pentek.[78] Physical examination revealed an ipsilateral palpable mass together with the discharge in only 29 of 204 patients. None of the patients with mammary duct ectasia had palpable masses or significant mammographic changes. Most of the women (88%) who had bloody discharge did not have cancer. Exfoliative cytologic examination was positive for only 11% (2 of 18) of patients with carcinoma. As in other series, the age distribution for patients with the mammary duct ectasia component of MDAIDS was 20 to 73 years; the median age was not given. Patients with cancer were older (see Fig. 6A-8 and Table 6A-6).

TABLE 6A-6

General Causes and Frequency of Nipple Discharge, Palpable Mass, and Age Distribution in 204 Patients

Histologic Disease	Types of Secretion (n)					Age (yr)		
	Cases	Milky	Greenish	Serous	Bloody	Total	Palpable Tumor (n)	Range	Mean
Fibrocystic disease	65	3	24	16	22	65 (32%)	14	20–58	43
Mammary duct ectasia	23		3	7	13	23 (11%)		20–73	53
Papilloma	68			20	48	68 (33%)	5	28–81	51
Papillomatosis	30			8	22	30 (15%)	3	36–77	53
Carcinoma	18			3	15	18 (9%)	7	40–78	59
Total	**204**	**3**	**27**	**54**	**120**	**204 (100%)**	**29**		

Modified from Tabár L, Dean PB, Péntek Z: Galactography: The diagnostic procedure of choice for nipple discharge. Radiology 149:31–38, 1983.

Clinical Features

The age distribution of 45 women presenting with intermittent nipple discharge, combined from three studies, is shown in Figure 6A-9; the peak age at which discharge occurred was the midforties.[80,81,83] In general, most women with nipple discharge have benign disease. Although nipple discharge may be an early manifestation of MDAIDS, other causes include mammary dysplasia, intraductal papilloma, intraductal carcinoma, and invasive carcinoma. Only 4% of women with nipple discharge have breast cancer,[74] although reports of incidence vary in the literature.[8,84-87]

An intermittent nipple discharge occurs in 8% to 84% of patients with MDAIDS; most patients are young, premenopausal women (see Table 6A-3). In Browning's study, nipple discharge occurred in only 8% of women with incidental duct ectasia but in 65% of symptomatic patients. The secretions vary from yellow, brown, or red to dark green, and the consistency varies from serosanguineous to toothpaste-like.[81,87,88] In the early stages, it may involve one ductal opening or one segment of the breast (Fig. 6A-10). At times, it may involve many ducts (Fig. 6A-11) and may be bilateral. Clinically, patients notice a stain on their clothes or bedsheets or expression of a discharge during routine breast self-examination. The occurrence of bilateral or multiple-duct, greenish or multicolored sticky discharge simultaneously with burning pain, itching, and swelling in the region of the nipple as the underlying disease process[87] strongly suggests the duct ectasia component of MDAIDS (see Fig. 6A-2). There is no relation to menstrual history, parity, or breast-feeding and no distinguishing factors as it relates to age at first pregnancy or menopause.

Investigation

A history should be obtained. The nature and quantity of the discharge, its spontaneity, and its relation to menstrual cycle, pregnancy, and occurrence of trauma should be determined. A number of medications, including agents for hormone replacement therapy, psychotropics, and antihypertensive drugs, as well as thyroid disorders and states of hyperprolactinemia, can cause nipple discharge. A persistent nipple discharge may be caused by hyperprolactinemia that is more often related to medications than to a pituitary adenoma (rare in clinical practice). Such physiologic discharges tend to be bilateral and multiductal in origin, and the secretion is clear to serous to milky and

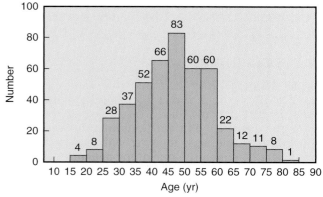

Figure 6A-9 Age distribution of 452 women with nipple discharge in nonmalignant breast disease culled from the literature. (Data from Fischermann K, Bech I, Foged P, et al: Nipple discharge. Diagnosis and treatment. Acta Chir Scand 135:403–406, 1969; Rimsten A, Skoog V, Stenkvist B: On the significance of nipple discharge in the diagnosis of breast disease. Acta Chir Scand 142:513–518, 1976; and Chaudary MA, Millis RR, Davies GC, Hayward JL: The diagnostic value of testing for occult blood. Ann Surg 196:651–655, 1982.)

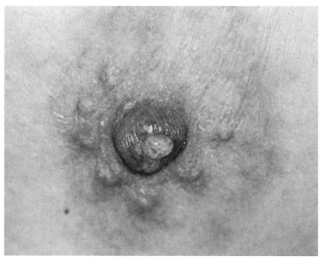

Figure 6A-10 Discharge from a single serosanguineous duct in a smoker. It was negative for occult blood.

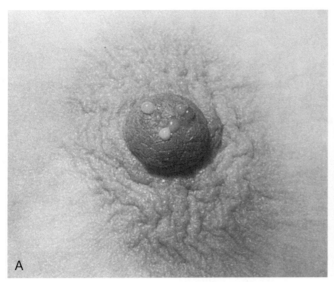
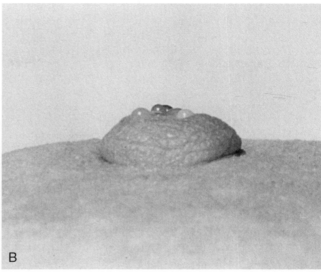

Figure 6A-11 **A** and **B**, Multiple-duct nipple discharge, varying from green to yellow. It was sticky and negative for occult blood. Patient was a heavy smoker and complained of persistent subareolar nipple burning.

negative for occult blood. In such cases, serum prolactin should be measured, and if the value is elevated an appropriate endocrine workup should be initiated. If it is normal, the patient should be observed with monthly follow-ups. The patient's smoking habits should be addressed because of the relationship of MDAIDS and heavy smoking (see Figs. 6A-6 and 6A-7).

The breast should be examined, and if a mass is identified, the duct or ducts from which the discharge comes should also be examined for masses. If a mass is identified, its management should be in accordance with that of a breast mass. In the absence of a mass, even if the nipple looks healthy, it should be inspected carefully while pressure is applied around the areola. Usually, pressure close to the areola and over the dilated subareolar mammary duct expresses the discharge. The site, the number of ducts, and the color of each discharge should be noted and recorded. The patient should express the nipple discharge to corroborate the physician's findings. Multiduct discharge indicates diffuse breast disease, often bilateral.

The clinical status of the subareolar ducts, as they course through the nipple, is assessed by gently palpating the ducts with the "finger-and-thumb" test, in which the intranipple and subnipple ducts are rolled between the tips of the finger and thumb (Fig. 6A-12A).

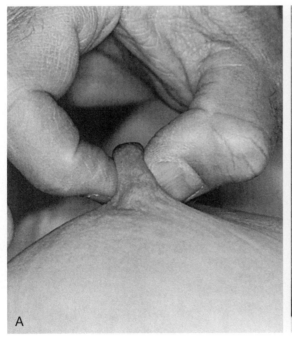
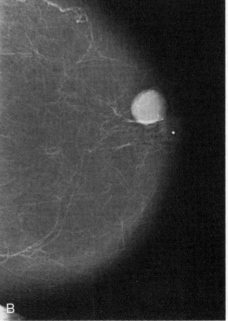

Figure 6A-12 **A**, The finger-and-thumb test to assess degree of inflammatory involvement and dilation of subareolar mammary ducts. **B**, Craniocaudal mammogram view of left breast. Small white dot is nipple marker. Large round lesion is a blue-domed cyst of a major subareolar mammary duct. The finger-and-thumb test was grossly positive.

The normal feel can be described as a "grooved sensation," in which each mammary duct is clearly palpable as a thin cord. In ectasia, the mammary ducts are thickened with various degrees of duct inflammation. If the nipple discharge is associated with significant periductal inflammation, axillary lymphadenopathy may be found.[89]

With progressive degrees of mammary duct inflammation and fibrosis, the finger-and-thumb test becomes progressively more positive, because the digits cannot be approximated below the nipple, indicating thickening of the mammary ducts or the presence of a blue-domed cyst. Eventually, as the disease progresses, the fingertips are separated by a firm, nontender mass that appears to be continuous with and inseparable from the nipple (see Fig. 6A-12B). Such a mass is either central to the subareolar area or deviated toward the side of the chronically diseased mammary ducts. For a woman older than 35 years with unilateral nipple discharge, a mammogram and ultrasound should be obtained to exclude cancer.

Several investigations should be done. First should be exfoliative cytologic evaluation of the discharge by Papanicolaou smear and Romanowsky's stain (methylene blue and eosin). Normal cytologic findings do not exclude an ongoing benign pathologic process or cancer. Typically, epithelial atypia is noted. A second study is bacteriologic culture of expressed discharge, a sample of which is obtained after cleaning of the nipple and surrounding areola with isopropyl alcohol. Two bacteriologic swab specimens should be taken: one for anaerobic culture and the other for aerobic culture.[90] In most cases (about 60%) involving nipple discharge associated with the duct ectasia component of MDAIDS, anaerobic bacteria are isolated from the nipple discharge and the ratio of anaerobes to aerobes is about 3:1.[28,90] Finally, the discharge should be tested for occult blood; in 64% of cases the test is positive.[18,26,78,80] An occult blood–positive discharge does not necessarily indicate cancer but suggests intraductal disease, whereas a clear discharge does not rule out cancer.[8,84–87,91]

If the cytologic analysis of a unilateral duct discharge is not contributory, or if the discharge tests positive for occult blood, ductography should be performed (Fig. 6A-13A). Ductography is a relatively simple technique whereby a small amount (0.1 to 1.5 mL) of sterile water-soluble contrast medium is injected into the discharging duct and the duct architecture is displayed mammographically. It is one way to rule out and determine the nature, extent, and location of intraductal lesions other than squamous metaplasia that are causing a discharge. It is particularly valuable when there are no other symptoms and neither physical examination nor mammography reveals the underlying cause. Successful visualization of duct lesions requires a skilled radiologist. Ductography repeated shortly before surgery with use of a mixture of 1% methylene blue dye and contrast medium demonstrates to the surgeon the status of the duct at operation, facilitating more precise and less radical surgery. Ultrasound is useful for visualizing the dilated ducts, their points of obstruction, and associated cysts (see Fig. 6A-13B). In more advanced cases, fine-needle aspiration (FNA) cytologic examination of the indurated mass should reveal foamy macrophages and inflammatory cells, and FNA of a mass for bacteriologic studies will reveal mixed flora with a major anaerobic component.[28,92–94]

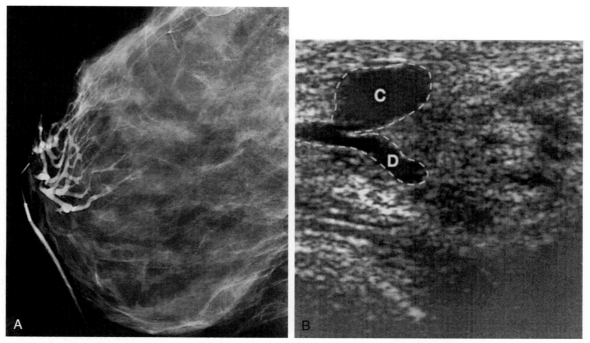

Figure 6A-13 **A,** Ductogram that was occult blood positive for a heavy smoker, showing multiple dilated and varicosed ducts. Pathology showed squamous metaplasia. **B,** Sonographic image showing a dilated duct (D) with obstruction and communicating cyst (C). (Courtesy of Beverly Spirt, MD, Department of Radiology, Breast Care Program, SUNY Health Science Center at Syracuse, NY.)

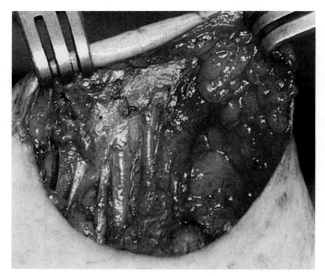

Figure 6A-14 Multiple dilated subareolar mammary ducts in a previous heavy smoker complaining of nipple discharge and pain. Pathologic analysis showed duct ectasia, periductal fibrosis, mild ductal epithelial hyperplasia, and chronic inflammatory infiltrate. Patient initially presented with multiple breast abscesses of the opposite breast 2 years previously while she was a smoker. Thereafter, she had stopped smoking.

Treatment Plan

In the absence of a subareolar induration or mass and in the presence of a normal mammogram, if a single duct is involved and if the discharge is purulent or green and sticky, the patient should be treated with antibiotics. These should cover both aerobes and anaerobes.[28,90,95] A suitable combination includes a cephalosporin and metronidazole, each at a dosage of 500 mg by mouth three times a day for 10 days. It is anticipated that the infection will improve, and thereafter the patient is observed. However, recurrent infection after antibiotic therapy alone is not infrequent; to avoid disappointment, this possibility should be communicated to the patient. Recurrence should be expected because the underlying disease process has not been eradicated and this process is not covered by the antibiotics. If the

discharge is not cleared by antibiotic therapy, a second 10-day course of antibiotics should be prescribed.

If the discharge is from multiple ducts and is persistent, is occult blood positive, and has not responded to antibiotic treatment, then on the basis of clinical judgment, surgery may be indicated. If during surgery the duct system as a whole is considered abnormal (Fig. 6A-14) or the presence of a blue-domed cyst (Fig. 6A-15) is noted, then the major subareolar mammary duct system should be excised.[96] A summary of the clinical evaluation and treatment is shown in Figure 6A-16.

MAMMARY DUCT–ASSOCIATED INFLAMMATORY DISEASE SEQUENCE-RELATED BREAST PAIN AND TENDERNESS

Continuous noncyclic breast pain and tenderness may also be an early manifestation of MDAIDS. It need not present after a mammary duct discharge in the sequence of MDAIDS-related symptoms (see Figs. 6A-2, 6A-6, and 6A-16). On occasion, it may be the presenting symptom. A comprehensive discussion of mastalgia and its management is included in Chapter 5.

Clinical Features

The age distribution of 272 women who presented with noncyclic mastalgia in two studies is shown in Figure 6A-17.[87,97] The peak symptoms occur in the mid-30s. Breast pain falls into three broad groups: costochondral pain, lateral chest wall pain, and cyclic or noncyclic breast pain (Fig. 6A-18). Two thirds of women with mastalgia have cyclic pain, and one third have noncyclic pain.[98] Noncyclic breast pain is a recognized symptom of the mammary duct ectasia phase of MDAIDS.[76] It appears to be related to periductal inflammation. In a study by Preece and colleagues,[99] 25% of 232 patients with mastalgia had pain related to the duct ectasia and the periductal inflammatory components of MDAIDS.

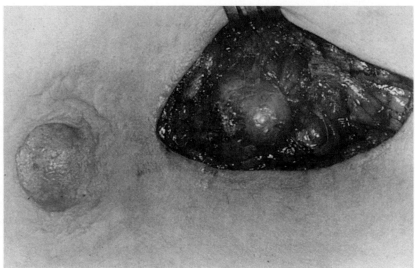

Figure 6A-15 Blue-domed cyst situated in lateral aspect subareolarly of the left breast. Pathologic analysis showed apocrine metaplasia, microcalcification, and papillomatosis.

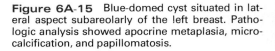

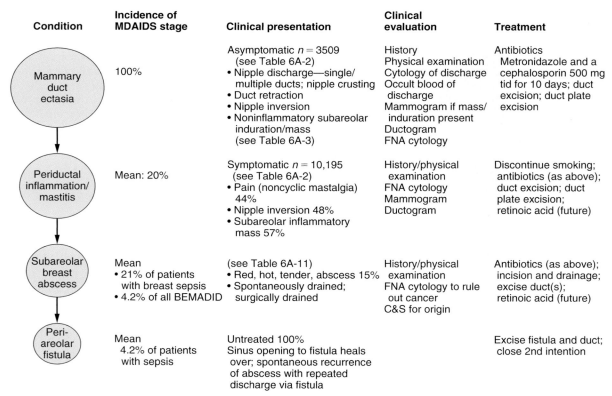

Condition	Incidence of MDAIDS stage	Clinical presentation	Clinical evaluation	Treatment
Mammary duct ectasia	100%	Asymptomatic *n* = 3509 (see Table 6A-2) • Nipple discharge—single/ multiple ducts; nipple crusting • Duct retraction • Nipple inversion • Noninflammatory subareolar induration/mass (see Table 6A-3)	History Physical examination Cytology of discharge Occult blood of discharge Mammogram if mass/ induration present Ductogram FNA cytology	Antibiotics Metronidazole and a cephalosporin 500 mg tid for 10 days; duct excision; duct plate excision
Periductal inflammation/ mastitis	Mean: 20%	Symptomatic *n* = 10,195 (see Table 6A-2) • Pain (noncyclic mastalgia) 44% • Nipple inversion 48% • Subareolar inflammatory mass 57%	History/physical examination FNA cytology Mammogram Ductogram	Discontinue smoking; antibiotics (as above); duct excision; duct plate excision; retinoic acid (future)
Subareolar breast abscess	Mean • 21% of patients with breast sepsis • 4.2% of all BEMADID	(see Table 6A-11) • Red, hot, tender, abscess 15% • Spontaneously drained; surgically drained	History/physical examination FNA cytology to rule out cancer C&S for origin	Antibiotics (as above); incision and drainage; excise duct(s); retinoic acid (future)
Peri-areolar fistula	Mean 4.2% of patients with sepsis	Untreated 100% Sinus opening to fistula heals over; spontaneous recurrence of abscess with repeated discharge via fistula		Excise fistula and duct; close 2nd intention

Figure 6A-16 Clinical evaluation and treatment of the mammary duct–associated inflammatory disease sequence (MDAIDS), showing incidences of the stages of MDAIDS.

The pain is quite exquisite. It is not a referred pain but arises from the breast itself. It is often continuous, characterized by burning, usually behind the nipple. It is also characterized by aching of both breasts and tenderness. It is unpredictable in occurrence and does not vary with the menstrual cycle.[100] In a study by Maddox of 33 patients, the mean duration of pain was about 36 months (range, 5 to 156 months).[101] Similarly, in the study by Preece and colleagues[99] of the 62 patients with noncyclic pain related to mammary

duct ectasia and periductal inflammation of MDAIDS, two thirds had had symptoms for 12 months or longer and only 5 of the 62 had had pain for less than 5 months on presentation. This pain comes on abruptly, is often worse in cold weather, is at the same site with serial visits, and disappears as suddenly as it appeared. Often, the history notes that the breast is "supersensitive." The patient's smoking habits should always be ascertained because of the evidence that noncyclic breast pain of MDAIDS is associated with heavy smoking (see Figs. 6A-6 and 6A-7).

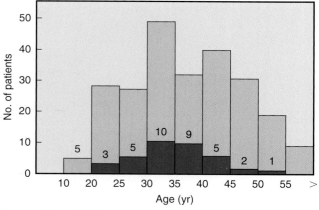

Figure 6A-17 Distribution by age of patients presenting with noncyclic breast pain. (Data from Maddox PR, Harrison BJ, Mansel RE, Hughes LE: Non-cyclical mastalgia: An improved classification and treatment. Br J Surg 76:901–904, 1989; and Preece PE: Mastalgia. Practitioner 226:1373–1382, 1982.)

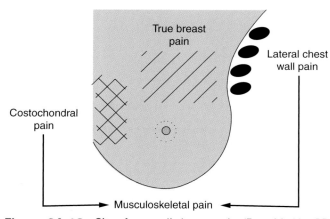

Figure 6A-18 Site of noncyclic breast pain. (From Maddox PR, Harrison BJ, Mansel RE, Hughes LE: Non-cyclical mastalgia: An improved classification and treatment. Br J Surg 76:901–904, 1989.)

MDAIDS-related noncyclic breast pain can be distinguished from cyclic breast pain by recording the type of pain for 3 months on charts. Cyclic breast pain is typically poorly localized and in most instances is bilateral. The pain is usually described as heavy, increasing in severity from midcycle onward and improving with menstruation yet varying in severity from cycle to cycle. The breast is tender to touch.

Noncyclic breast pain related to MDAIDS can be distinguished from chest wall pain by either tender costochondral junctions (Tietze's syndrome) or tenderness along the ribs (musculoskeletal pain). Musculoskeletal pain is unilateral in more than 90% of the cases and is localized along the chest wall and costochondral junction. In contrast with noncyclic breast pain of MDAIDS, the mean duration of symptoms with musculoskeletal pain is shorter: 14.7 months (range, 2 to 48 months).[101] This type of pain responds well to a combination of lidocaine and hydrocortisone injected into the musculoskeletal site.

Investigation

A detailed history of the pain should be obtained: its clinical features, character, relationship to menstruation, site, radiation, and duration and factors that exacerbate or relieve it. Through physical examination, costochondral pain and lateral chest wall pain should be ruled out. The breast should be palpated gently for intramammary lesions, nipple discharge, or a trigger point. Mammography should be performed. Radiographic features that can be associated with MDAIDS are coarse calcifications and the flame-shaped shadows of active periductal mastitis.[102–104]

In most patients, these findings are confined to the site of complaint. In addition, dilated ducts may be seen elsewhere in the breast or in the contralateral gland. For analysis of breast pain, ductography is seldom useful, and FNA cytology is neither rewarding nor cost effective.

Treatment Plan

With exclusion of obvious pathologic causes of pain, the patient is assured that there is no cancer; usually no active treatment is needed, but wearing a firm supporting bra 24 hours a day and taking a nonsteroidal anti-inflammatory drug or a mild analgesic for the duration of the pain often provides comfort (Table 6A-7).[98,100,105,106] Overall, 44% of patients with noncyclic mastalgia reported a lasting response (i.e., no return of symptoms within 6 months of finishing therapy).

If this fails, some women with noncyclic MDAIDS-related breast pain respond to drugs used for cyclic mastalgia (Table 6A-8). If their pain returns when treatment is stopped or the dose is reduced, these patients should undergo treatment again with the drug to which the original response was good. If the initial response was poor or if troublesome side effects occurred, the patient should be treated with a different drug. For a few patients with sufficiently severe noncyclic MDAIDS-related breast pain, excision of all the major subareolar mammary duct systems is warranted.

TABLE 6A-7
General Management of Mastalgia

1. Exclude cancer: Physical examination, mammography, and biopsy where indicated. For unremitting localized pain, follow frequently for at least 1 yr with repeat studies to exclude early cancer.

2. Adequate reassurance that the condition is benign will allow at least 85% of patients to accept and tolerate their pain. Those who require active treatment after reassurance are given a pain chart so that the pattern and severity of the pain can be monitored over the next 3 mo.

3. Noncyclic mastalgia can be treated with the expectation of an overall response rate of 44%. Individual drugs are no better than placebo, overall, but each drug appears to help a different group of patients. At present, there are no gudelines for predicting success for an individual drug. To reduce disappointment, patients should be warned before treatment of the low response rate. Most patients in this group, however, are willing to try any therapy with even a small chance of improvement, and they appreciate a frank assessment of the outcome.

4. Relapse is treated by recommencing the drug that was previously effective. With danazol, relapse may occur while the dose is being reduced or while the patient is taking maintenance doses. If the relapse is mild, a return to the previous dose may be sufficient to control the pain, but if symptoms are severe, return to the initial dose of 100 mg twice daily is usually necessary. Once the pain has been controlled, the dose can be reduced at monthly or 6-wk intervals to the maintenance dose for that patient. Symptoms are often exacerbated by emotional upheavals—bereavement and divorce in particular—althrough there is good evidence that the primary basis of the symptom is not psychologic in most cases.

5. Patients must be given adequate contraceptive advice, because drug treatment may interfere with the contraceptive pill and some patients' fertility may be enhanced by bromocriptine. Should pregnancy occur, the treatment must be discontinued immediately to avoide any untoward effects on the fetus.

Modified from Pye JK, Mansel RE, Hughes LE: Clinical experience of drug treatments for mastalgia. Lancet 2: 373–377, 1985.

NIPPLE RETRACTION AND SUBAREOLAR MASS AS RELATED TO MAMMARY DUCT–ASSOCIATED INFLAMMATORY DISEASE SEQUENCE

A change in nipple contour and retraction of an isolated opening of a nipple duct are among the early clinical features of MDAIDS. As the disease progresses, duct dilation and squamous metaplasia are accompanied by inflammatory changes and infiltration with lymphocytes. Periductal fibrosis with duct wall thickening occurs during chronic inflammation, and as ducts are destroyed and repaired, this leads to shortening of ducts and subsequent changes in nipple contour, flattening and retraction of the nipple, or deviation of the nipple (Fig. 6A-19). Although it is consistently publicized as an early sign of breast cancer, in most cases, nipple retraction is benign.

Mammary duct ectasia of MDAIDS is the most common pathologic cause of nipple inversion seen in well-breast clinics. In the series by Browning, Bigrigg, and

TABLE 6A-8

Drugs Used to Treat Cyclic Mastalgia

Agent	Action	Dose	Prevalence of Side Effects
Danazol	Antigonadotropin: acts on pituitary-ovarian axis	200 mg/day for 2–4 mo; discontinued or decreased to 100 mg/day for 2 mo; then 100 mg on alternate day for 2 mo	22%: abnormal menstrual cycle; headache; nausea; weight gain (6% severe)
Bromocriptine	Inhibits prolactin secretion	1.25 mg/day, increasing 1.25 mg every 7 day to a maximum of 2.5 mg/day for 2–4 mo, then stopped	33%: nausea; headaches; postural hypotension; constipation; depression (15% severe)
Evening primrose oil (rich in essential fatty acids)	Via prostaglandin pathways	6 capsules/day for 3–6 mo	2%: bloating; vague nausea

Data from Pye JK, Mansel RE, Hughes LE: Clinical experience of drug treatments for mastalgia. Lancet 2: 373–377, 1985.

Taylor,[79] the incidence varies from 10% to 24% in patients with symptomatic MDAIDS, depending on the presence of discharge. Nipple inversion was reported to be noted in 7% of women in whom the mammary duct ectasia component of MDAIDS was found incidentally.[79] Nipple retraction tends to be slowly progressive, with the retraction becoming more marked with time. The process continues until it is complete, and the entire nipple becomes inverted. The contralateral nipple may show similar changes, often lagging months or years in the development of retraction. In patients with mammary duct retractions, the incidence of bilaterality is approximately 15%.[106]

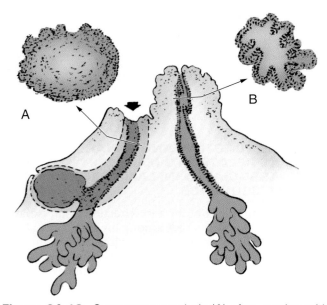

Figure 6A-19 Squamous metaplasia (**A**) often coexists with retraction of the nipple and plugging of the lactiferous duct with epithelial debris. Resulting suppuration breaks out at areolar margin. Dotted line designates margin of dissection recommended in core excision. In the normal situation (**B**), cuboidal epithelium and ductal continuity are maintained. Note pleating in lactiferous sinus. (From Powell BC, Maull KI, Sachatello CR: Recurrent subareolar abscess of the breast and squamous metaplasia of the lactiferous ducts: A clinical syndrome. South Med J 70: 935–937, 1977.)

When the continuity of the duct epithelium is broken, lipoid material escapes through the duct wall, leading to a marked yellowish gray induration of the surrounding tissue. The mass, with or without obvious inflammation, is firm and circumscribed. At this stage, nipple retraction and dimpling are often present, and consequently the lesion is frequently misdiagnosed as carcinoma. Pain and tenderness with repeated inflammatory changes, both occurring over a long period, tend to rule out such a diagnosis; however, this should be confirmed pathologically via biopsy.

In addition to the usual atrophic epithelial changes in the duct epithelium and inflammatory reaction in the duct wall, there may be a marked cellular inflammatory response. The inflammatory cells consist chiefly of lymphocytes and plasma cells or almost entirely of plasma cells (plasma cell mastitis). Phagocytic giant cells surround the lipoid material, and an infiltration of histiocytes occurs in the breast stroma.

Clinical Features

Nipple retraction is painless and of little consequence to the patient, except to rule out cancer. Presenting symptoms range from minor nipple abnormalities to complete nipple retraction. Minor degrees of nipple retraction occur early in disease[107] and in one study were present in up to 75% of patients presenting with periareolar inflammation.[108] When the degree of retraction is slight, it can be missed unless carefully sought. Marked retraction or nipple inversion occurs later and develops during the course of repeated periductal inflammation.[1] The earliest change detected is characterized by retraction of the central portion of the nipple, showing a slight elliptical pattern in a horizontal plane. Nipple retraction is commonly associated with slight spontaneous nipple discharge, which at this stage of the disease process is usually multiductal and multicolored, consistent with duct ectasia.

Investigation

A correct diagnosis of MDAIDS can be made on the basis of history and examination. Length of history and onset of symptoms is of great importance. The time course of the observed changes should be elicited and is critical for a correct diagnosis, as is obtaining a history of episodes of inflammation. Both point to an ongoing subclinical inflammatory process consistent with MDAIDS, because nipple retraction can develop after one or two inflammatory episodes. Long-standing nipple inversion arising at puberty or during pregnancy and lactation is always benign and is easily recognized. Usually it is bilateral, but not invariably, with a significant slitlike appearance and no deformity of the areolas or surrounding skin.

A surgical opinion is generally sought when nipple retraction is first noticed. Alternatively, patients are not aware of these long-standing nipple changes unless they are accompanied by discharge, pain, or a mass. Typically, the duration of retraction is long. Rees, Gravelle, and Hughes[107] reported on a series of 30 patients (25 to 75 years of age; mean, 52 years) with nipple retraction associated with the mammary duct ectasia phase of MDAIDS. The duration of retraction was 3 months to 16 months. The patient's smoking habits are important because of the evidence that nipple retraction of MDAIDS is associated with heavy smoking (see Figs. 6A-6 and 6A-7).

Next, the breast should be examined carefully and in different positions to characterize the pattern of nipple retraction and to assess features that favor the diagnosis of mammary duct ectasia/periductal inflammation or cancer.[107] On physical examination, a typical transverse central inversion of the nipple is seen (Fig. 6A-20). In MDAIDS, the nipple can usually be everted manually. The ability to evert the nipple, the presence of palpable ectatic mammary ducts felt as cords just beneath the nipple when performing the finger-and-thumb test (see Fig. 6A-12A), and the absence of a mass help exclude a diagnosis of cancer. The breast is examined for nipple discharge and to rule out other causes of nipple inversion. If a mass is present, its size and location should

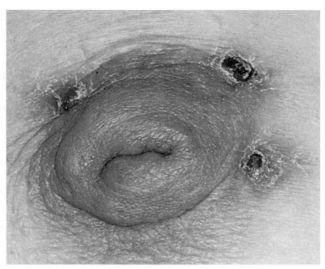

Figure 6A-21 Complete inversion of the central portion of the nipple, resulting in characteristic transverse nipple inversion with surrounding edema but without deformity of the remaining nipple. Patient also has signs of three periareolar fistulas.

be determined. In patients with long-standing and repeated episodes of subareolar inflammation, the central portion of the nipple becomes inverted and edematous (Fig. 6A-21).

Diagnostic difficulty arises in women who present usually in their 50s to 70s, with recent retraction of the nipple. Women older than age 40 years who present with sudden unilateral nipple retraction should be presumed to harbor a malignancy until proved otherwise. In MDAIDS, retraction of the nipples commonly precedes the development of the inflammatory reactions, especially in young women. With an acute breast abscess, the retraction is usually asymmetric. In contrast, with carcinoma the retraction is usually complete with distortion of the areolas, and there is seldom a serous or blood-stained discharge. Nipple retraction caused by carcinoma is a result of involvement of breast ducts by cancer, resulting in distortion because the cancer is commonly to one side, producing tilting or distortion of the nipple toward the tumor. The differences between nipple retraction of the mammary duct ectasia and periductal inflammation components of MDAIDS and that of carcinoma are detailed in Table 6A-9. Mammography and ultrasound are necessary to exclude carcinoma in the retroareolar area in all patients.

Treatment Plan

Treatment depends on the presence or absence of a mass.

Patient with No Mass. Younger patients with mammographically dense breasts are reassessed every 3 months. Older patients with fatty, atrophic breasts who have a negative mammogram are confidently assured that there is no serious disease and are seen every 6 months, with a repeat mammogram at 1 year.

Patient with Palpable Mass. FNA cytologic analysis of the mass should be performed to rule out carcinoma. In MDAIDS, FNA cytologic examination shows foamy

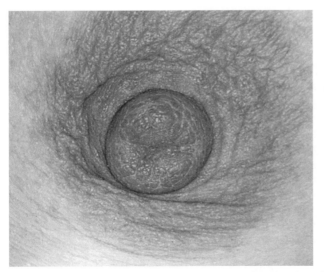

Figure 6A-20 Early central nipple inversion that developed during the previous 2 years in a smoker who was otherwise asymptomatic.

TABLE 6A-9

Differential Diagnosis of Nipple Retraction of the MDAIDS Phase with Mammary Duct Ectasia and Carcinoma (Conditions Could Coexist)

Clinical/ Investigative Feature	Mammary Duct Ectasia of MDAIDS	Carcinoma
History	>1 yr (present since puberty)	<1 yr
Pain (%)	33	<10
Discharge	Creamy, green	Serous, blood stained
Nipple (examine carefully)	Partial, central, symmetrical retraction, often bilateral	Complete unilateral retraction with deformity of areola
Mass	Tender, firm lesion with discrete outline	Nontender, hard lesion with ragged outline
Mammography	Excludes cancer; minor ductal dilatation; in multiparas, atrophic fatty, premenopausal or postmenopausal; seen as tubular densities, sometimes beaded, extending from base of nipple fanning out into breast disk; in younger patients, breast disk is dense, breast ducts are transradiant tubular shadows; smooth, coarse calcification, rounded or branched; within ducts; unilateral or bilateral nipple retraction	
Cytology	Foam cells	Malignant glandular cells
Ductography	Ectatic ducts	Intraluminal mass
Fine-needle aspiration	Cystic lesion, no residual mass, no blood on aspiration	Hard lesion; malignant glandular cells
Mass	Biopsy	Biopsy
Follow-up	No mass: re-examine every 4 mo and take annual mammogram	

MDAIDS, mammary duct–associated inflammatory disease sequence.

macrophages and inflammatory cells. If the mass is cystic, the fluid should be removed, tested for occult blood, and sent for cytologic examination. If the cytologic analysis is negative, the fluid contains no blood, and the mass disappears completely, management is similar to that for patients without a palpable mass. If there is a residual mass, excision biopsy is recommended. The subsequent management is based on the biopsy results. If the biopsy is negative for cancer, the patient should be followed up with repeat examinations and mammograms, initially at 4 months. The clinical evaluation and treatment are summarized in Figure 6A-16.

SUBAREOLAR BREAST ABSCESS AND RECURRENT SUBAREOLAR BREAST ABSCESS AS RELATED TO MAMMARY DUCT–ASSOCIATED INFLAMMATORY DISEASE SEQUENCE

In the sequence of the pathophysiology of MDAIDS outlined in Figures 6A-1, 6A-2, and 6A-16, the introduction of bacteria to the histopathologic stage of subareolar periductal inflammation leads to infection, manifesting ultimately as a subareolar breast abscess. Subareolar abscess is a challenging clinical entity. There are ample comments in the literature on the high incidence of persistence, recurrence, and bilaterality.[12,22,109,110]

Most reports on breast abscess identify mixed organisms with a major anaerobic component as the predominant bacterial flora in this disease. Table 6A-10 typifies

TABLE 6A-10

Spectrum of Bacteria Isolated from 29 Women with a Breast Abscess

Genus	Organisms (n)
Aerobes	
Staphylococcus*	24
Streptococcus	4
Bacillus	2
Corynebacterium	1
Escherichia	1
Proteus	1
Pseudomonas	2
Anaerobes	
Actinomyces	3
Clostridium	2
Fusobacterium	1
Mitsuokella	1
Bacteroides*	8
Lactobacillus	3
Eubacterium	3
Propionibacterium*	16
Peptostreptococcus*	34
Veillonella	2

*Predominant genus.
From Walker AP, Edmiston CE Jr, Krepel CJ, Condon RE: A prospective study of the microflora of nonpuerperal breast abscess. Arch Surg 123:908–911, 1988.

the spectrum of bacteria isolated from 29 women with breast abscesses.[28] Many of the anaerobic bacteria isolated are also commonly found in the vaginal vault, and prior vaginal manipulation leads to a hematogenous spread of these bacteria in a fashion comparable to the hematogenous, transient bacteremia that occurs with mastication. It has been reported that 10% of bacteremias that occur in the hospital are caused by anaerobes[94] and that even simple procedures such as sigmoidoscopy may lead to the presence of transient *Bacillus fragilis* in the blood.[111] The transient bacteremia following vaginal manipulation has been documented to be associated with anaerobic breast abscess.[112] In addition, facultative and obligate anaerobic microorganisms are also normal inhabitants of the oropharynx, and in smokers the flora of the oropharynx is predominantly anaerobic. This may be a source for subareolar mammary duct inoculation following oral stimulation of the breast,[28] and stagnant mammary duct secretions form an ideal medium for bacterial infection.

Finally, coagulase-negative staphylococci, normally present on the skin, adhere to the squamous epithelial cells derived from the galactophores or colonize the nipple skin and may be yet another source of the infection.[113] All of these sites may contribute to the endogenous bacterial flora of the normal breast.[26,27] Finally, as shown in Table 6A-4, these abscesses are not limited to females but also tend to occur in men who are heavy smokers, presumably also via hematogenous spread of oral bacteria secondary to mastication.

Anaerobic breast abscesses are usually seen in women of childbearing age with an inverted nipple and are due to underlying duct ectasia or chronic breast disease that provides a suitable nidus for the adhesion of these anaerobes.

Subareolar breast abscesses in the spectrum of MDAIDS are found in about 20% of patients with symptomatic MDAIDS undergoing surgery (Table 6A-11; see Fig. 6A-16). Both breasts are affected equally.[79] In approximately 10% of patients with subareolar abscess, the process is bilateral at presentation. Less frequent is the finding of multiple abscesses in one breast (see Fig. 6A-21) or an active small, acute, subareolar abscess with other areas of induration around the same nipple. Initially, a lesion can be a discrete tender lump with reddening of the skin that subsides spontaneously without

TABLE 6A-11

Frequency of Recurrence or Subareolar Breast Abscess after Operation for MDAIDS

Investigators	Patients with Local Breast Sepsis*/Total "Operated Patients"	Surgical Procedure	Recurrence/Outcome
Hadfield, 1960; 1968[a]	30/99	Excision major duct system	No recurrence (follow-up 1–7 yr)
Urban, 1963[b]	19/113	Excision major duct system	No recurrence (follow-up, 6 mo–14 yr)
Ekland and Zeigler, 1973[c]	38/–	Incision and drainage, 27; duct excision, 11	Total recurrence, 15 (40%); incision and drainage, 11/27 (41%); duct excision, 4/11 (36%)
Thomas et al, 1982[d]	9/78	Incision and drainage	Recurrence, 7/9 (78%); abscess and one fistula, 7 (78%) (2 [22%] eventually had simple mastectomy)
Browning et al, 1986[e]	11/51	Excisional biopsy, 51%	Needed further operation, 12 (24%)
		Formal duct excision, 41%	Reoperated for sepsis, 11 (45%)
		Nipple retraction, 6%	
		Mastectomy, 1%	
Scholefield et al, 1987[f]	28/–	Incision and drainage, 28	Further problems, 21 (75%), including 9 (32%) with fistulas
		Hadfield procedure (secondary operation), 6	No recurrence
Watt-Boolsen et al, 1987[g]	34/–	Incision and healing by granulation	Recurrence, 11/32 (34%) (10/11 fistulas; two patients lost to follow-up)
Hughes, 1989[h]	–/122	Subareolar dissection	Complication, 34 (28%)
Hartley et al, 1991[i]	13/46	Subareolar dissection	Recurrent sepsis, 8 (62%), including one fistula

MDAIDS, mammary duct–associated inflammatory disease sequence.
*Abscess and/or fistula.
[a]Data from Hadfield GJ[96] and Hadfield GJ.[115]
[b]Data from Urban JA: Excision of the major duct system of the breast. Cancer 16:516, 1963.
[c]Data from Ekland DA, Zeigler MG.[116]
[d]Data from Thomas WG, et al.[76]
[e]Data from Browning J, Bigrigg A, Taylor I.[79]
[f]Data from Scholefield JH, Duncan JL, Rogers K: Review of a hospital experience with breast abscesses. Br J Surg 74:469, 1987.
[g]Data from Watt-Boolsen S, Ramussen NR, Blichert-Toft M.[13]
[h]Data from Hughes L: Management of recurrent infection following surgery for periductal mastitis. Br J Clin Pract 43(suppl 68):81, 1989.
[i]Data from Hartley MN, Stewart J, Benson EA: Subareolar dissection for duct ectasia and periareolar sepsis. Br J Surg 78:1187, 1991.

TABLE 6A-12

Surgical Procedure and Frequency of Recurrence of Subareolar Breast Abscess or Fistula

Surgical Procedure	Investigator	Patients with Local Sepsis* (n)	Recurrence/Outcome
Excision of major duct system (Hadfield ductectomy)	Hadfield, 1960; 1968[a]	30	No recurrence
	Urban 1963[b]	19	No recurrence
	Thomas et al, 1982[c]	7[†]	2 (29%) recurrences
	Browning et al, 1986[d]	21[‡]	1 (4%) required further surgery
	Scholefield et al, 1987[e]	6[†]	"Took care of problem"
	Meguid et al, 1995[f]	11	No recurrence
Incision and drainage	Ekland and Zeigler, 1973[g]	27	15 (41%) recurrences
	Thomas et al, 1982[c]	9	7 (78%) recurrences
	Scholefield et al, 1987[e]	28	21 (75%) further problems, including 9 (32%) fistulas
	Watt-Boolsen et al, 1987[h]	32	11 (34%) recurrences, including 10 fistulas
Duct excision	Ekland and Zeigler 1973[g]	11	4 (36%) recurrences
	Browning et al, 1986[d]	26[‡]	11 (42%) repeat surgery
Subareolar dissection	Hartley et al, 1991[i]	13	8 (62%) recurrences, including 1 fistula

*Local sepsis (abscess and/or fistula).
[†]Secondary surgery after recurrence following incision and drainage.
[‡]Symptomatic (51 patietns, including 10 with local sepsis).
[a]Data from Hadfield GJ[96] and Hadfield GJ.[115]
[b]Data from Urban JA: Excision of the major duct system of the breast. Cancer 16:516, 1963.
[c]Data from Thomas WG, et al.[76]
[d]Data from Browning J, Bigrigg A, Taylor I.[79]
[e]Data from Scholefield JH, Duncan JL, Rogers K: Review of a hospital experience with breast abscesses. Br J Surg 74:469, 1987.
[f]Data from Meguid MM, et al.[25]
[g]Data from Ekland DA, Zeigler MG.[116]
[h]Data from Watt-Boolsen S, Ramussen NR, Blichert-Toft M.[13]
[i]Data from Hartley MN, Stewart J, Benson EA: Subareolar dissection for duct ectasia and periareolar sepsis. Br J Surg 78:1187, 1991.

drainage. In about half of the cases, however, there will be recurrence with eventual pointing, followed by either spontaneous or surgical drainage. Following only incision and drainage, the reported recurrence rate, as shown in Table 6A-12, varies from 34% to 78%.[13,76]

Recurrence reflects the inadequacy of the operative treatment provided for the initial presentation of a subareolar breast abscess (i.e., merely surgical incision and drainage), because it is not based on a conceptual understanding of the underlying disease process and abnormality, which persist after the local operative procedure.

Clinical Features

As shown in Figures 6A-1, 6A-2, and 6A-16, the penultimate stage in the pathophysiology of MDAIDS is a subareolar abscess, but there is considerable overlap in the sequence of the presenting symptoms. It is the ongoing active infection with an abscess that brings many patients with MDAIDS to the surgeon's attention; the antecedent disease process may have been sufficiently subclinical to have gone unnoticed or been forgotten by the patient except in hindsight. Subareolar breast abscess in relation to MDAIDS is a different lesion from a peripheral breast abscess or an abscess associated with lactation (Fig. 6A-22). Among 50 women with breast abscess, 38 had a subareolar abscesses and 12 had a peripheral abscess (Fig. 6A-23). The age ranges in several series of patients with only subareolar breast abscesses

for whom these data were available are combined in Table 6A-13. These agree with the age span shown in Figure 6A-23 and generally with those previously reported.[22,82,96,114,115] The general impression is that the peak incidence of subareolar abscess occurs in the fourth decade, predominantly in nonlactating premenopausal women.

Investigation

The characteristic features in the history are rapid onset of acute breast pain, tenderness, and swelling of the central subareolar tissue. There is no history of trauma, fibrocystic condition, or cancer. In our experience, a number of our patients who presented with an acute subareolar breast abscess had a history of antibiotic treatment for breast inflammation that occurred 3 to 4 days after a routine pelvic examination, as previously reported by Leach, Eykyn, and Phillips.[112] At the time they presented for surgery for the acute abscess, which occurred 3 to 4 months later, these patients were found to have gross evidence of duct ectasia, which must have been present but asymptomatic at the time of the pelvic examination.

In subacute cases, symptoms can exist for 1 week, whereas with chronic, poorly drained abscesses treated frequently with antibiotics, symptoms can last for more than 10 years. A medical history of similar problems that were treated either with antibiotics or, if the abscess was

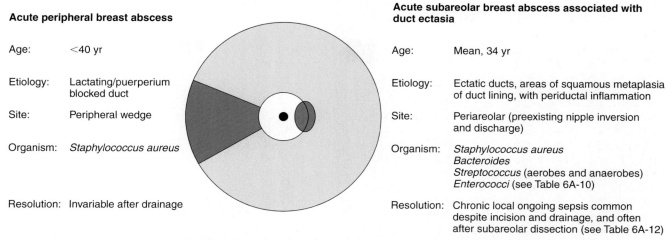

Acute peripheral breast abscess

Age: <40 yr

Etiology: Lactating/puerperium blocked duct

Site: Peripheral wedge

Organism: *Staphylococcus aureus*

Resolution: Invariable after drainage

Acute subareolar breast abscess associated with duct ectasia

Age: Mean, 34 yr

Etiology: Ectatic ducts, areas of squamous metaplasia of duct lining, with periductal inflammation

Site: Periareolar (preexisting nipple inversion and discharge)

Organism: *Staphylococcus aureus*
Bacteroides
Streptococcus (aerobes and anaerobes)
Enterococci (see Table 6A-10)

Resolution: Chronic local ongoing sepsis common despite incision and drainage, and often after subareolar dissection (see Table 6A-12)

Figure 6A-22 The main differences between an acute peripheral abscess and a subareolar abscess related to the mammary duct–associated inflammatory disease sequence (MDAIDS) are summarized. (Modified from Benson EA: Management of breast abscesses. World J Surg 13:753–756, 1989.)

well established, with surgical incision and drainage, is often reported. Alternatively, the subareolar abscess drained spontaneously. All acute and subacute symptoms usually resolved with treatment, and this is generally followed by an asymptomatic period, an interval of months to years of apparent resolution followed by recurrence.[22,116] Finally, the patient's smoking habits need to be determined because of the evidence that infectious complications of MDAIDS are associated with heavy smoking (see Figs. 6A-5 and 6A-6).

On physical examination the characteristic features are a florid acute abscess with local tenderness, swelling, erythema, sloughing of skin, and induration or a fluctuation (Fig. 6A-24). With chronic, recurrent abscesses a draining periareolar fistula is most often seen (Fig. 6A-25). On occasion, a purulent nipple discharge is observed.

The diagnosis is made on clinical grounds. In acute subareolar breast abscess, neither mammography, ultrasound, nor FNA cytologic analysis is warranted for diagnostic

purposes, although ultrasound can be useful when patients present with early symptoms (Fig. 6A-26). However, in women older than 40 years of age, these studies are warranted after resolution of the acute process, to rule out unsuspected underlying lesions.

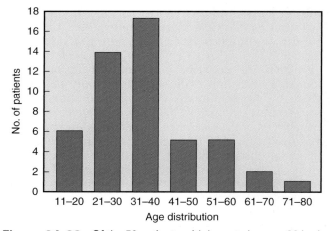

Figure 6A-23 Of the 50 patients with breast abscess, 38 had a subareolar breast abscess and 12 had a peripheral breast abscess. (Data from Ekland DA, Zeigler MG: Abscess in the nonlactating breast. Arch Surg 107:398–401, 1973.)

TABLE 6A-13				
Age of Patients with Breast Abscess Related to MDAIDS				
		Age (yr)		
Investigators	**Patients (n)**	**Range**	**Mean**	**Median**
Hadfield, 1960[a]	6	27–33	30	—
Abramson, 1969[b]	5	32–38	35	—
Caswell and Maier, 1969[c]	15	25–48	—	—
Habif et al, 1970[d]	146	20–59	36	—
Ekland and Zeigler, 1973[e]	38	14–72	34	—
Leach et al, 1979[f]	9	24–71	35	—
Golinger and O'Neal, 1982[g]	46	13–79	30	—
Watt-Boolsen et al, 1987[h]	34	15–92	—	—
Hartley et al, 1991[i]	13	18–78	—	—
Meguid et al, 1995[j]	24	26–61	—	33

MDAIDS, mammary duct-associated inflammatory disease sequence.
[a]Data from Hadfield GJ.[96]
[b]Data from Abramson DJ.[82]
[c]Data from Caswell HT, Maier WP.[109]
[d]Data from Habif DV, et al.[22]
[e]Data from Ekland DA, Zeigler MG.[116]
[f]Data from Leach RD, et al.[92]
[g]Data from Golinger RC, O'Neal BJ.[119]
[h]Data from Watt-Boolsen S, Ramussen NR, Blichert-Toft M.[13]
[i]Data from Hartley MN, Stewart J, Benson EA: Subareolar dissection for duct ectasia and periareolar sepsis. Br J Sug 78:1187, 1991.
[j]Data from Meguid MM, et al.[25]

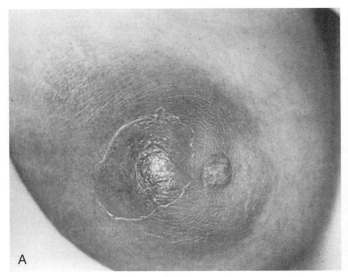

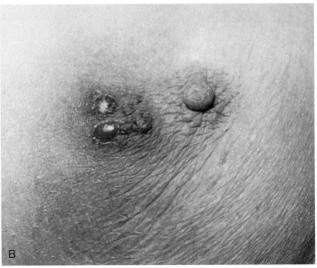

Figure 6A-24 **A,** A 38-year-old smoker presented with acute onset of right breast pain. There was no history of symptoms of the mammary duct–associated inflammatory disease sequence (MDAIDS). A red, hot, tender, fluctuant mass was observed. **B,** Another example of a subareolar breast abscess that is about to spontaneously discharge.

Treatment Plan

The approach to treatment of a primary (nonrecurrent) subareolar breast abscess should include consideration of its stage of development in the pathologic sequence outlined in Figures 6A-2 and 6A-16. If a patient presents with an established fistula with induration at the base of the sinus, the entire disease process should be excised, as described next.

Surgical Management. When a patient presents with a primary subareolar breast abscess, treatment should be determined by the degree of inflammation and the stage of abscess development.

Early Abscess. If the abscess is in its early stages (consisting of an indurated mass), a 2-week course of antibiotics consisting of a cephalosporin and metronidazole,

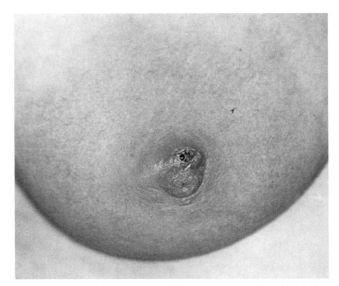

Figure 6A-25 A chronic draining mammary duct fistula in a 32-year-old woman with a history of abscesses. A tender subareolar mass was detected via the finger-and-thumb test. Note invagination of central portion of the nipple.

each at a dosage of 500 mg by mouth three times a day, is prescribed. Hot packs are recommended for comfort, and a well-fitted bra provides support and further comfort. The patient is scheduled for weekly appointments for follow-up until the process has resolved, and elective excision is planned for 2 to 4 weeks thereafter.

Mature Abscess. If the abscess is fluctuant or has already drained spontaneously, treatment with the patient under general anesthesia consists of making a wide incision to obtain effective drainage and to culture the pus. The patient is then given the two antibiotics for 10 days and monitored weekly to ensure satisfactory resolution with healing. Operative treatment of the abscess and the associated duct under general anesthesia is then planned for 4 to 6 weeks later.

If a patient presents with a recurrent subareolar abscess, the abscess should be incised and drained, as described in the following sections, with antibiotic coverage. After the acute phase has subsided, the major subareolar ducts should be totally excised with a technique similar to that proposed by Urban and Hadfield.[84,96] The distal intralobular ducts atrophy, thus dispelling any fear of complications arising during a subsequent pregnancy.

Whereas the conventional treatment for an acute subareolar breast abscess is surgical incision with drainage of the pus—optimally under general anesthesia in the operating room and with perioperative antibiotic coverage for both anaerobes and aerobes—it should be recognized that this is a temporizing measure in the subareolar abscess phase of MDAIDS. Another option, which can be used in the office setting instead of with general anesthesia, is to make the patient comfortable with oral sedation approximately 1 hour before the planned incision and drainage. Then, local analgesia of the incision site is obtained by freezing the skin over the abscess with topical ethyl chloride spray applied from far enough above the abscess to induce skin frosting and freezing. The incision is made through this

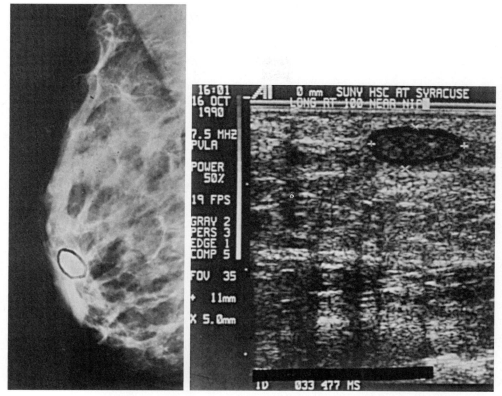

Figure 6A-26 Ultrasound imaging of early subareolar breast abscess.

frozen tissue. Use of conventional local anesthetic agents (e.g., lidocaine) is seldom effective in providing analgesia for the incision because of the low tissue pH in the inflamed skin tissue fluid. It should thus be avoided with an acute inflammatory process. A portion of the anterior abscess wall should be removed for pathologic examination because, although rare, a cancer could coexist.[116] The abscess may be extensive and multilocular and must be drained completely, but further exploration of the wound and excision of surrounding indurated tissue should be avoided so as not to destroy surrounding breast tissue or disfigure the breast. The pus should be cultured for both aerobic and anaerobic bacteria, and a Gram stain should be performed. Following irrigation of the abscess cavity, a small wick is placed to assist drainage and prevent premature skin closure. Tight packing should be avoided because it deforms the breast. Postoperatively, the two antibiotics should be continued. The healing process may take several weeks and should eventually be followed in 4 to 6 weeks by definitive surgery—major subareolar mammary duct excision (described later in this chapter).

Nonsurgical Management. Common usage of percutaneous FNA has introduced nonoperative treatment as a potential alternative, although the criteria for its use have not been defined. The argument given to support needle aspiration of the abscess cavity, coupled with treatment with systemic antibiotics, is that fistulization follows conventional treatment with incision and drainage. This is now a spurious argument, because it is recognized that incision and drainage are temporizing measures for an acute lesion that precede definitive duct surgery, thus avoiding fistulization.

Early reports noted that antibiotic therapy alone for subareolar breast abscesses resulted in complete resolution of only 3% of the infections in 181 breast abscesses because the antibiotics used were effective primarily against aerobes instead of both anaerobes and aerobes.[28,117] The overall success rate of nonsurgical management appears to be less than 50% in two reported series in which the long-term follow-up was inadequate.[95,118] Ignoring the possible role of duct abnormalities in the causation of breast infection leads to (1) inadequate treatment; (2) recurrent infections with periareolar fistulas; (3) mutilating deformities of the breast; and (4) radical breast surgery, including mastectomy.[119] Figure 6A-16 summarizes the clinical evaluation and treatment of subareolar breast abscess as it relates to MDAIDS.

PERIAREOLAR MAMMARY DUCT FISTULA AS RELATED TO MAMMARY DUCT–ASSOCIATED INFLAMMATORY DISEASE SEQUENCE

A periareolar fistula represents a sequela of treatment failure of the acute subareolar abscess and is the end-stage disease of MDAIDS (see Figs. 6A-1, 6A-2, and 6A-16). The periareolar mammary duct fistula is an established fistula, a chronically discharging lesion in the region of the areola, usually at the vermilion border (Fig. 6A-27; see Fig. 6A-21) but often at the base of the nipple (see Fig. 6A-25), which communicates with a

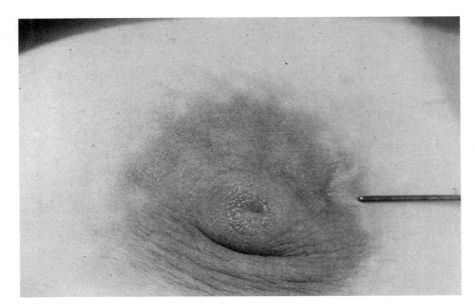

Figure 6A-27 Probe shows opening of chronic sinus at the vermilion border of the areola.

centrally situated major subareolar mammary duct (see Fig. 6A-19). The cause is related to varying degrees of obstruction of a major subareolar mammary duct, secondary to squamous metaplasia of the duct lining. This leads to an accumulation of secretions in acini that becomes infected, forming an acute subareolar abscess. Spontaneous discharge via the shortest and most direct route of least resistance is at the vermilion border. Occasionally, the discharge exits via the nipple. After the sinus has healed, in the vast majority of cases, a recurrent abscess appears and discharges once more along the same route, establishing a permanent fistulous tract. Until the underlying cause is removed, repeated episodes of infection are common and seldom self-limiting. This spectrum of MDAIDS and its sequelae is not limited to women but is also occasionally found in men (see Table 6A-4).

Clinical Features

The age range (mean and median) of patients who present specifically with periareolar mammary duct fistula, as reported in selected papers in the literature, is summarized in Table 6A-14. As expected, this corresponds to the age range of patients presenting with the other features of MDAIDS (i.e., nipple discharge, breast pain, varying degrees of nipple retraction, and acute subareolar abscess). As reported in the literature, the frequency of fistula related to a breast abscess varies from 4% to 20%, depending on whether one considers fistulas subsequent to treatment failure or patients with new fistulas.[79,82] In some reports, more patients presented with fistulas than with breast abscesses.[79,82] The overwhelming data show that most of the tracts studied are lined by granulation tissue.[20] In only a few was squamous

TABLE 6A-14					
Age of Patients Presenting with Periareolar Mammary Duct Fistula					
		Age (yr)			
Investigators	**Fistulas (n)**	**Range**	**Mean**	**Median**	**Comments**
Zuska et al, 1951[a]	5	29–40	34	—	1 patient had bilateral large ducts lined by squamous epithelium
Atkins, 1955[b]	35	21–63	34	—	7 bilateral lesions; 19 inverted nipples; 1 carcinoma; nonspecific granulation tissue
Abramson, 1969[c]	14	24–46	35	—	9 patients had previous surgery, 7 with duct ectasia, 2 with squamous metaplasia
Lambert et al, 1986[d]	52	19–63	31	30	1 male; 11 bilateral lesions; 3 patients had more than one fistula on same side
Bundred et al, 1987[e]	46	24–61	—	35	6 recurred after surgery without antibiotic coverage
Meguid et al, 1995[f]	116	26–61	—	33	All had previous incision and drainage

[a]Data from Zuska JJ, Crile G Jr, Ayres WW.[11]
[b]Data from Atkins HJB.[127]
[c]Data from Abramson DJ.[82]
[d]Data from Lambert ME, Betts CD, Sellwood RA: Mammillary fistula. Br J Surg 73:367, 1986.
[e]Data from Bundred NJ, et al.[126]
[f]Data from Meguid MM, et al.[25]

metaplasia found.[11] Often, communication with the underlying subareolar mammary duct can be demonstrated clearly via a lacrimal duct probe.

Investigation

The history should emphasize frequency and time intervals of antecedent acute subareolar abscesses or a subareolar inflammatory mass that had either discharged spontaneously or had been surgically incised and drained. This may also have occurred in the past in the contralateral breast. Other events preceding the fistula and their time course need to be ascertained, including nipple discharge, nipple retraction, a history of lactation, and breast biopsies. As stated earlier, inquiry into the patient's smoking habits is essential because of the evidence that periareolar mammary duct fistulas of MDAIDS are associated with heavy smoking (see Figs. 6A-6 and 6A-7).

On physical examination, the site and location of the fistula opening in the involved breast should be noted. Both breasts should be inspected to determine whether the nipples are retracted. Both breasts should be palpated gently and the finger-thumb test performed for subareolar masses (see Fig. 6A-12A), nipple discharge, or discharge from the fistula of the involved breast. Ipsilateral axillary adenopathy is often present. Mammography and ultrasonography are helpful in defining the nature of a small retroareolar mass (see Fig. 6A-12B) and detecting signs of prominent subareolar mammary ducts, periductal opacification, and coarse linear and irregular microcalcifications consistent with the radiologic features of MDAIDS.[103,120-123] Intuitively, one would think that a fistulogram would help define the anatomy, but strangely, the literature is lacking in reference to this procedure, although it is generally accepted for gastrointestinal fistulas.

Treatment Plan

Antibiotics—a cephalosporin and metronidazole, each at a dosage of 500 mg by mouth three times a day for 10 to 14 days—should be given to cover anaerobic and aerobic organisms if there are clinical signs of ongoing, low-grade, chronic infection. When the fistula is chronic and well established, the patient should undergo surgery, usually with general anesthesia and continued antibiotic coverage. The fistula tract into the subareolar-retronipple space should be excised, together with the duct (ductectomy) as it emerges through the nipple. The resulting wound is left open and loosely packed or closed primarily, with or without a drain, while further antibiotics are provided. A summary of the clinical evaluation and treatment is shown in Figure 6A-16. The surgical techniques are described in the following sections.

General Comments

The term *mammary fistula* was introduced by Atkins in 1955 to describe the fistulas of the subareolar mammary ducts reported by Zuska's group in 1951; they likened it to a fistula in ano.[48,59] It was Walker and Sandison[114] who stressed the association between subareolar abscess and the mammary duct ectasia component of MDAIDS. Other researchers[109,124,125] believe that the fistula originates and remains in the subepidermal glands, because they have failed to identify a communication with a mammary duct, either macroscopically or microscopically. This conservative view does not take into account the concept embodied in the MDAIDS. The fundamental lesion cannot always be determined from the histomorphologic slides because it is destroyed by the repeated acute—and persistent chronic—inflammation that commonly occurs.

Many patients suffer unnecessary pain and discomfort from recurrent sepsis because the diagnosis of a periareolar mammary duct fistula is not suspected. The patient whose breast is depicted in Figure 6A-21 was treated with a variety of systemic and topical antimicrobials by her primary care physician for more than 3 years for "recurrent skin furuncles," during which time her nipple progressively retracted. A high proportion of patients (as many as 60%) have retracted nipples, a known feature of the periductal inflammatory stage of MDAIDS.[126] Although on the basis of the work of Atkins it was initially thought that these are all of congenital origin, in our practice the time relation between retraction and periductal inflammation suggests that it is a consequence of repeated subareolar mammary duct inflammation and, as such, is closely associated with MDAIDS.[127]

Recurrences of mammary fistulas involve other ducts, particularly if only a single ductectomy is performed initially with the fistulectomy. Table 6A-15 shows the outcome of surgery for periareolar mammary duct fistula as reported by Bundred and coworkers.[126] For recurrent fistula, we recommend excision of all the major subareolar mammary ducts. In the past, recurrent fistulas and repeated infections have led to mastectomy.[76,96] The most common lesion is consistent with mammary duct ectasia and periductal mastitis,[21,120] although others have also reported granulomatous mastitis.[126]

TABLE 6A-15				
Treatment Outcome in 31 Surgeries for Periareolar Mammary Duct Fistula				
Procedure	Patients (n)	Successful Healing (n)	Prolonged Wound Discharge (n)	Recurrent Fistula (n)
Excision and packing	9	8	1	1
Primary closure alone	16	10	6	5
Primary closure with antibiotic coverage	6	6	0	0

From Bundred NJ, Dixon JM, Chetty U, Forrest AP: Mammillary fistula. Br J Surg 74:466–468, 1987.

Operative Techniques

DUCTECTOMY: WHEN ONE DUCT IS INVOLVED

With use of general anesthesia, a radial incision is usually made, starting from the middle of the nipple and encompassing the diseased duct. The incision is extended laterally through the areola and the vermilion border. The nipple is laid open and the duct is isolated and dissected out from its surroundings (Fig. 6A-28A). The dissection is carried down deep into the middle of the subareolar breast tissue (breast disk), encompassing the enlarged, firm, and inflamed ampulla and the distal duct tissue. The tissue is divided from the remaining breast by electrocoagulation, and the specimen is removed (see Fig. 6A-28B).

Reconstruction

After the diseased portion of the duct is removed, the nipple is carefully reconstructed with no. 4-0 absorbable suture material. The subcutaneous sutures are placed at three critical sites: (1) the circumferential edge of the apex of the nipple (Fig. 6A-29A), (2) the base of the nipple (see Fig. 6A-29A), and (3) the vermilion border of the areola (see Fig. 6A-29B). In patients who present with inverted nipples or a retracted nipple secondary to a previously drained chronic disease site, the nipple is everted and a fourth suture consisting of a purse-string or Z-suture with no. 4-0 Vicryl is placed inside the base of the nipple to prevent it from collapsing. This is done after placement of suture no. 2. Iodoform gauze of appropriate size is placed as a wick into the surgically created defect in the subareolar space and is exteriorized beyond the vermilion border through the lateral aspect of the incision (see Fig. 6A-29B). The patient is taught to change the wick daily. Antibiotics suitable for coverage against aerobes and anaerobes are selected

and prescribed for a course of 10 to 14 days. Figure 6A-29C shows the nipple–areola complex 3 weeks after operation.

RESECTION OF MAJOR MAMMARY DUCTS: WHEN MULTIPLE DUCTS ARE INVOLVED OR FOR RECURRENT SUBAREOLAR ABSCESS

A radial incision can be used similar to that described previously. Alternatively, a circumareolar incision is made below the areola (Fig. 6A-30A; see Fig. 6-14). Elevation of the nipple from the areola complex is performed with a knife (see Fig. 6A-30B). The major ducts are separated from the base of the nipple by passing a curved tonsil forceps or hemostat around the nipple base and dividing the ducts with a knife (see Fig. 6A-30C). The nipple base is then carefully cut down to remove all duct tissue (see Fig. 6A-30D). Care is taken to avoid devascularizing the nipple skin. A purse-string or Z-suture of no. 4-0 Vicryl is inserted through the nipple base to hold it everted without causing necrosis. The major subareolar duct system is then dissected out from the middle of the underlying breast tissue (breast disk; Fig. 6A-31; see Fig. 6A-30E). Hemostasis is achieved by electrocoagulation. The wound is irrigated. Primary closure of the subareolar space is performed to obliterate the dead space, and the skin is then closed with fine interrupted suture, absorbable suture with Vicryl, or nonabsorbable suture with fine nylon or Prolene, depending on the surgeon's preference (see Fig. 6A-30F). Any dilated ducts are electrocoagulated or ligated individually with no. 5-0 Vicryl. A drain is usually not required in the elective setting. The operation is performed with antibiotic coverage. The areolar skin is sutured in position with subcuticular, interrupted sutures (see Fig. 6A-30G). We prefer to leave the skin open for drainage or to approximate the skin edges with Steri-Strips to obtain the optimal cosmetic result. A firm dressing is placed over the breast. If a drain

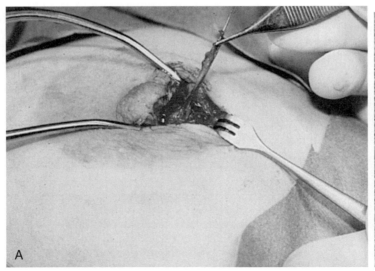

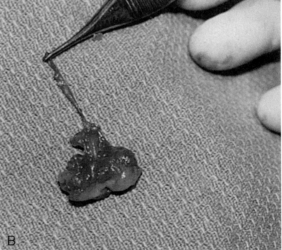

Figure 6A-28 **A,** A diseased major mammary duct has been dissected out from the nipple–areola complex. **B,** Enlarged, firm, inflamed lactiferous ampulla and distal ductal tissue. (From Meguid MM, Oler A, Numann PJ, Khan S: Pathogenesis-based treatment of recurring subareolar breast abscesses. Surgery 118:775–782, 1995.)

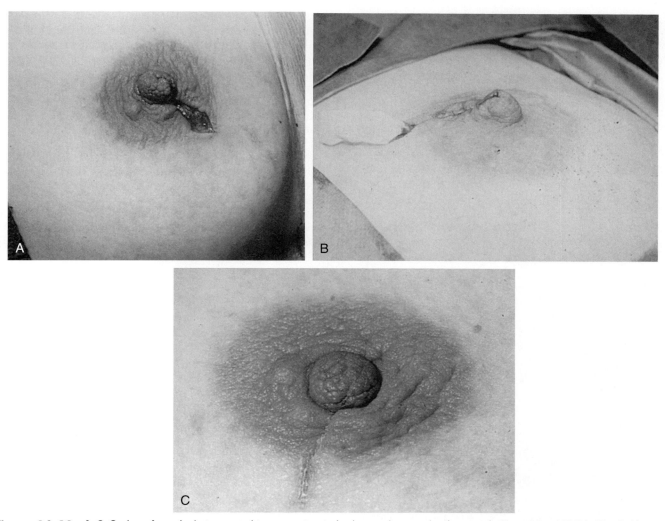

Figure 6A-29 **A–C,** Series of surgical steps used to reconstruct nipple–areola complex (see text). (From Meguid MM, Oler A, Numann PJ, Khan S: Pathogenesis-based treatment of recurring subareolar breast abscesses. Surgery 118:775–782, 1995.)

is used it is removed within 24 hours, and the patient is instructed to wear a well-fitted bra continuously. Patients undergoing surgery should be warned of the potential for recurrent problems and, possibly, loss of nipple sensation. Nipple necrosis is an uncommon complication of repeated surgery. Reasons for failure of surgery include inadequate removal of major duct tissue, either from the nipple base or from the breast disk itself, and failure to evert the nipple and remove the disease at its base.[1]

CHRONIC SUBAREOLAR BREAST ABSCESS WITH FISTULA

Either a radial or a subareolar incision can be used to encompass the sinus opening and the fistulous tract. The dissection is carried into the substance of the subareolar breast tissue and the tissue is removed en bloc (see Fig. 6A-30), together with the fistula tract. Injection of the fistula tract with 1% methylene blue before the start of the dissection is often helpful in identifying the corresponding major subareolar duct that

connects with the fistula. The wound is irrigated and closed as described earlier. Administration of antibiotics is continued postoperatively.

Peripheral Breast Abscess in Comparison to Mammary Duct–associated Inflammatory Disease Sequence

One fourth of all abscesses—at any age—are peripheral and present as a pink area in the periphery of the breast. The causes are various. Most common are abscesses related to lactation, folliculitis, and in postmenopausal women, diabetes. In the 3-year series by Petrek[128] of 18 postmenopausal women with breast abscess, half had adult-onset diabetes. These patients often presented without leukocytosis, pain, or accompanying cellulitis. Gallium-67 citrate in scintigraphy is used to detect latent breast abscesses.

Acute pyogenic abscess of the puerperium is becoming less common, whereas abscesses resulting from the duct

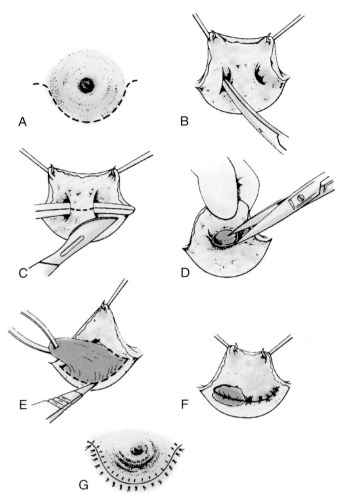

Figure 6A-30 **A–G,** Technique of subareolar dissection (see text). (From Hartley MN, Stewart J, Benson EA: Subareolar dissection for duct ectasia and periareolar sepsis. Br J Surg 78:1187–1188, 1991.)

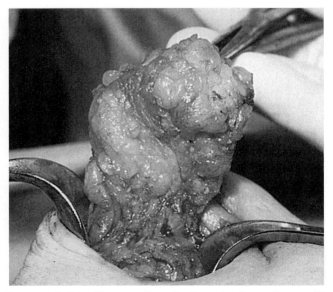

Figure 6A-31 Close-up view of subareolar tissue dissected in a patient following recurrent abscesses.

ectasia phase of MDAIDS have assumed increasing importance. Nevertheless, acute puerperal breast abscess still causes significant and occasionally serious morbidity. Figure 6A-22 shows the distinction between the two types of abscesses. They have different causes, bacteriology, presentations, and treatments. Puerperal abscess is an acute disease of the puerperium, and the pathogen is most often *Staphylococcus aureus*. It remains unclear whether the staphylococci are derived from the skin of the patient or from the mouth of her suckling infant. Perhaps both are sources of infection. The principal cause is blockage of a lactiferous duct or lactiferous ampulla with inspissated secretions and milk, resulting in retention of milk in the peripheral lobules of the breast drained by the blocked duct. This stagnant milk produces breast engorgement and is an excellent bacterial culture medium. The patient usually manifests systemic signs of sepsis, presenting with a fever, tachycardia, and leukocytosis; occasionally, septicemia occurs. Ipsilateral axillary lymphadenopathy is also found.

On physical examination, an exquisitely tender mass is usually present in the peripheral breast tissue. When early cellulitis is found, broad-spectrum antibiotic treatment produces resolution in most instances. If antibiotics are not given or if diagnosis is delayed, an abscess forms unless the blocked duct is rendered patent again by suckling.

Adequate incision and drainage with topical ethyl chloride spray or general anesthesia, with culture of the pus and antibiotic coverage, invariably produces rapid resolution.[129] The incision should be made over the site of maximum tenderness and kept within Langer's lines for optimal cosmesis. The abscess cavity should be explored and all the loculi broken down. In the appropriate age group, a biopsy specimen of the abscess wall is taken to rule out carcinoma. We have favored light packing of the abscess cavity. Although the matter has not been subjected to a randomized controlled clinical trial, others have preferred that the abscess be obliterated by deep mattress sutures and the patient treated with perioperative antibiotics without formal postoperative drainage. This technique has been shown to produce swifter healing with no more complications than formal drainage.[130] Total excision rather than drainage is recommended for smaller lesions. More recently, as discussed earlier, Ferrara and colleagues[118] recommended an attempt at needle aspiration as the primary procedure for selected cases of focal abscess—plus treatment with antibiotics. Antibiotics are continued for 10 days. In approximately 50% of women who develop acute puerperal breast abscess, lactation ceases spontaneously. For the others, there is no particular reason why breast-feeding should be stopped.

Occasionally unusual pathogens are the cause of abscess. One report described a silent *Mycobacterium chelonae* infection in a young woman who was immunocompromised by large doses of corticosteroids.[131] One of our patients with celiac disease and dermatitis herpetiformis over the legs, arms, and breast, immunosuppressed because of steroid therapy, developed a deep peripheral left breast abscess. This was initially incised and drained and then required treatment with simple mastectomy. Thereafter, she developed a right breast abscess, which was excised and allowed to heal by secondary intention. A case of severe recurrent breast abscess caused by *Corynebacterium minutissimum* resulted from a wound infection after breast biopsy performed through skin that was superficially infected with the same organism.[132] This required four drainage procedures before the infection was finally controlled with intravenous vancomycin and oral erythromycin.

Some cases of mastitis result from exogenous exposure to bacteria. Superficial folliculitis of the breast skin can occur, particularly in the Montgomery glands, and it is commonly caused by gram-positive organisms. This condition is optimally treated by cleansing with soap and water and repeated topical application of Bactroban (mupirocin) three times a day. The condition can also be self-limited and subside spontaneously within 3 or 4 days, although inadvertent use of steroids may cause rapid spread and predispose to invasive disease.[133] Outbreaks of *Pseudomonas aeruginosa* mastitis have been reported from inadequate chlorination of pools and hot tubs.[42] Buchanan and Kominos[134] reported a case of a deep peripheral breast abscess resulting from *P. aeruginosa* in a previously healthy premenopausal woman. The patient showed signs of systemic sepsis, with fever, leukocytosis, and erythema involving the lateral aspect of the breast. The abscess was incised and drained and the wound was left open; Iodophor packs were changed daily. Intravenous tobramycin and ticarcillin were also given, and the patient's condition responded in 2 weeks.

Ekland and Zeigler[116] reported a number of patients with peripheral breast abscess. All were females, ranging in age from 17 to 67 years (mean, 37.4 years). Duration of symptoms varied from 1 day to 4 weeks. Recent trauma was reported by three patients; two had active facial acne, one had a known epidermal cyst at the abscess site, and one had a history of paraffin injections in the affected breast. Insulin-dependent diabetes mellitus occurred in one patient and steroid-treated rheumatoid arthritis in another.

Treatment consisted of incision and drainage or excision. Specimens for bacterial cultures were obtained from 11 patients and were reported to yield no growth in six cultures, coagulase-positive staphylococci in three, coagulase-negative staphylococci in one, and *Proteus* organisms in one. Pathologic examination revealed predominantly acute and chronic inflammation. Other histologic abnormalities noted were epidermal cyst, intraductal papilloma, and cystic duct dilation with apocrine metaplasia in each of three specimens.

Idiopathic Granulomatous Mastitis

Idiopathic granulomatous mastitis (IGM) was first described histopathologically by Kessler and Wolloch in 1972.[135] This is a rare benign inflammatory disease of the breast of unknown etiology. It is similar to MDAIDS in that in advanced cases, the patient presents with fistulae or sinus formation in the breast, with abscesses and chronic suppuration, and the disease recurs in the form of chronic mastitis following

inadequate treatment.[136,137] It can be distinguished from MDAIDS in that of the approximately 160 cases reported in the literature, none presents with subareolar fistulas. Other differentiating features include presentation in women at a younger age (median age, 30s to 40s) and in parous women who generally have breast fed. It has been described in an 11-year-old girl, an 80-year-old woman, and in a male with gynecomastia.[138] In essence, IGM is a heterogeneous disease with variable clinical presentations, which poses a diagnostic dilemma. Thus, a high degree of clinical suspicion for IGM is needed to direct the workup and the management, which depends on the stage of clinical presentation.

In its early stages, IGM frequently presents as a painless, ill-defined, hard, nontender, unilateral mass that is difficult to differentiate from a cancer and usually without palpable axillary lymph adenopathy. Mammography is either nonspecific or may mimic breast cancer, whereas ultrasonography helps localize a related abscess in more advanced stages of IGM. In some cases, magnetic resonance imaging has been useful to rule out a cancer, showing normal breast parenchyma and ruling out a mass (Fig. 6A-32).[139-141] In patients with IGM, serum tumor markers (CA 15-3) are within normal limits. When a mass is present, core needle biopsy or repeated FNA shows a nonspecific inflammatory condition with atypical cells, which helps differentiate the lesion from a cancer. In the majority of cases reported in the literature, a FNA was the most dependable method of diagnosis. However, the definitive diagnosis depends on the availability and sophistication of diagnostic tools and trained staff to interpret the results. An excisional biopsy is recommended to obtain tissue for histologic diagnosis. In IGM, the tissue reveals granulomatous lesions (Fig. 6A-33) with no evidence of tubercle

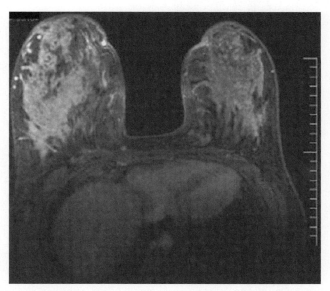

Figure 6A-32 An example of magnetic resonance image in a patient presenting with right idiopathic granulomatous mastitis. This T1-weighted subtraction image demonstrates no enhancing mass in either breast. There is breast asymmetry with the right breast larger than the left. (From Wilson JP, Massoll N, Marshall J, et al: Idiopathic granulomatous mastitis: In search of a therapeutic paradigm. Am Surg 73:798–802, 2007.)

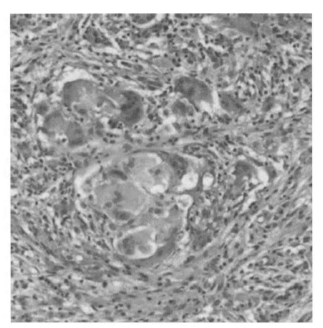

Figure 6A-33 Hematoxylin and eosin stain showing high magnification of multinucleated giant cells, fibrosis, and lymphocytes that have destroyed the lobule. (From Wilson JP, Massoll N, Marshall J, et al: Idiopathic granulomatous mastitis: In search of a therapeutic paradigm. Am Surg 73:798–802, 2007.)

formation and caseous necrosis. Cultures are sterile and show no growth. Thus, a wide local excision with free margin is the definitive treatment in early stages of IGM.

In an unusual report of a patient who presented with a mass in whom the workup was nondiagnostic but the initial FNA cytology was considered highly suspicious for cancer, a modified radical mastectomy was performed. This was colored by the fact that her identical twin had breast cancer. The final histologic diagnosis was granulomatous lobular mastitis with no evidence of malignancy.[142] However, other reports of mastectomies in patients with IGM also occur in the literature.

Patients with late stages of IGM usually present with a florid, inflammatory condition, including an ill-defined mass associated with signs of inflammation, pain, and redness (95%), and peau d'orange (40%).[141] The presence of one or more fistulae or sinus formation associated with abscesses or chronic suppuration may be among the presenting clinical features. The algorithm for the management of IGM is indicated in Figure 6A-34. A diagnostic biopsy is indicated and shows chronic lobulitis with granulomatous inflammation. The inflammatory lesion consists of polymorphonuclear leukocytes, epithelioid cells, plasma cells and multinucleated giant cells. Histopathology showing lobular distribution of granulomatous inflammation was observed in all cases. Recurrence, in the form of chronic mastitis, as late as a mean of 31 months or longer, has been described and therefore patients should be followed for a long period.

In patients with IGM, no past medical history of tuberculosis, sarcoidosis, or other infectious or granulomatous disease occurs. Similarly, no evidence of systemic immune abnormalities such as formation of autoantibodies or antigen-antibody complexes has been found.

Although the etiology remains undetermined, various postulates have been suggested. These include systemic autoimmune pathogenesis, as well as a localized immune response to extravasated secretions from the

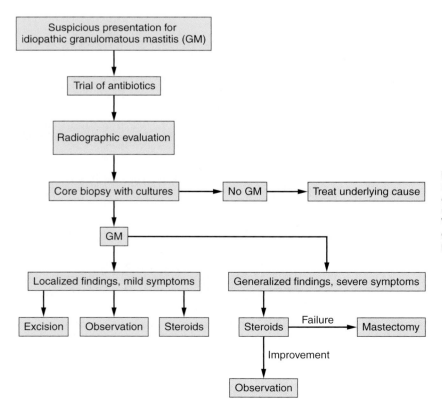

Figure 6A-34 Proposed algorithm for management of idiopathic granulomatous mastitis. Radiographic evaluation may entail mammography, ultrasound, or magnetic resonance imaging. (From Wilson JP, Massoll N, Marshall J, et al: Idiopathic granulomatous mastitis: In search of a therapeutic paradigm. Am Surg 73:798–802, 2007.)

lobules. IGM should be differentiated from other chronic inflammatory breast diseases, including mammary duct ectasia, Wegener's granuloma, sarcoidosis, tuberculosis, and histoplasmosis.

Summary

Our concept of the disease process leading to subareolar abscess is based on histomorphologic findings and disease management.[25] On the basis of our work and observations, we postulate an evolutionary process that begins with duct ectasia secondary to hormone imbalance. This mild duct ectasia is aggravated by the development of squamous metaplasia, which leads to duct obstruction and associated stasis of secretion, followed by inflammation. In part, the clinical and morphologic presentation of this disease process reflects the distribution of the aberrations along the duct system—thus the designation mammary duct–associated inflammatory disease sequence.

This approach is counter to that recently proposed by Dixon and Bundred and their colleagues, who believe duct ectasia and the inflammatory process are "likely to be totally unrelated."[18,19,23,24,75,90,103,121,126] Their position is based on the observation that, in their patient population, mastitis (1) is associated with an increased number of patients who smoke (whereas duct ectasia is not) and (2) occurs in a younger age group. However, in a prospective study of an equally large patient population, Thomas, Williamson, and Webster[57] did not observe a difference in the percentages of smokers who had mastitis and who had simple ectasia. Although most studies show that mastitis is more common in younger persons, it should be noted that symptomatic duct ectasia does occur in the same age group. The true incidence of simple duct ectasia is unknown because it is likely to be asymptomatic and is observed in women with other mammary diseases. Also lacking in the position taken by Dixon and Bundred and their coworkers is an explanation for a primary infectious etiology as the underlying cause of the mastitis; it appears that the stromal alterations are the same in patients who present with inflammation as in those with simple ectasia.[73]

Our hypothesis takes into consideration (1) the most likely causal factors, (2) the morphologic findings, and (3) the ample clinical experience and documentation that support the necessity for resecting the ducts to manage recurrent subareolar abscess after failed antibiotic therapy and incision and drainage. The molecular alterations in the duct epithelial cells that result from smoking, vitamin A deficiency, decreased serum prolactin, and inactive estrogen metabolites are still unknown and need to be investigated to enable us to gain a better understanding of the pathogenesis of MDAIDS. Morphologically, as in other organs, cellular alterations must occur before squamous metaplasia is recognizable by light microscopy. For example, there must be changes in the structure and organization of the duct cell microvilli,[54,55] which in some way must affect the function of the epithelium. The necessity to resect the ducts implies that the major distal ducts contribute to persistence of disease; thus, by extension, it can be postulated that the distal duct also has a role during the early stages of evolution of the disease.

Given our current state of knowledge, we view MDAIDS as a disease process related to altered duct epithelial function and structure, the latter evolving into squamous metaplasia. The squamous metaplasia acts as an obstruction, resulting in stasis of secretions, duct ectasia, and accumulation of inflammatory substances such as lipid and keratin. Depending on where along the duct system the obstruction lies and on the kind and degree of altered physiologic events that occur, MDAIDS can be either an asymptomatic entity (symptomatic simple duct ectasia) or an inflammatory process presenting as a subareolar abscess that may evolve into a mammary duct fistula (see Figs. 6A-1, 6A-2, and 6A-16).

Acknowledgments

We thank Ms. Deborah Rexine, Mr. George Reynolds, and Mr. Kenneth Peek for photographic service; Patricia Brady, RN, NP, Jane D'Antoni, RN, NP, for assisting with patient care; and Ms. Darlene Thompson for diligent editorial assistance.

REFERENCES

1. Hughes LE: Non-lactational inflammation and duct ectasia. Br Med Bull 47:272–283, 1991.
2. Payne RL, Strauss AF, Glasser RD: Mastitis obliterans. Surgery 14:719–724, 1943.
3. Bloodgood JC: Clinical picture of dilated ducts beneath the nipple frequently to be palpated as a doughy worm-like mass: The varicocele tumour of the breast. Surg Gynecol Obstet 36:486, 1923.
4. Geschickter CF: Diseases of the breast, 2nd ed. Philadelphia, JB Lippincott, 1948.
5. Tice GI, Dockerty MB, Harrington SW: Comedomastitis: A clinical and pathologic study of sata in 172 cases. Surg Gynecol Obstet 87:525–540, 1948.
6. Ingleby H: Normal and pathologic proliferation in the breast with special reference to cystic disease. Arch Pathol 33:573–588, 1942.
7. Deaver JB, McFarland J: The breast: Its anomalies, its diseases and their treatment. Philadelphia, Blakiston, 1917.
8. Adair FE: Plasma cell mastitis, a lesion simulating mammary carcinoma: A clinical and pathologic study with a report of ten cases. Arch Surg 29:735, 1933.
9. Birkett J: Diseases of the breast and their treatment. London, Kangman, 1850.
10. Bloodgood JC: The pathology of chronic mastitis of the female breast, with special consideration of the blue-domed cyst. Arch Surg 3:445–542, 1921.
11. Zuska JJ, Crile G Jr, Ayres WW: Fistulas of lactiferous ducts. Am J Surg 81:312–317, 1951.
12. Kilgore AR, Fleming R: Abscesses of the breast: Recurring lesions in the areolar area. Calif Med 77:191–192, 1952.
13. Watt-Boolsen S, Ramussen NR, Blichert-Toft M: Primary periareolar abscess in the nonlactating breast: Risk of recurrence. Am J Surg 153:571–573, 1987.
14. Haagensen CD: Mammary duct ectasia: A disease that may stimulate carcinoma. Cancer 4:749–761, 1951.
15. Bonser GM, Dossett JA, Jull JW: Human and experimental breast cancer. London, Pitman Medical, 1961.
16. Dossett JA: The normal breast, cystic disease and duct ectasia: A functional and histological study. MD thesis, London, University of London, 1959.
17. Azzopardi JG: Problems in breast pathology. London, WB Saunders, 1979.

18. Dixon JM, Anderson TJ, Lumsden AB, et al: Mammary duct ectasia. Br J Surg 70:601–603, 1983.
19. Dixon JM: Periductal mastitis/duct ectasia. World J Surg 13:715–720, 1989.
20. Patey DH, Thackray AC: Pathology and treatment of mammary-duct fistula. Lancet 2:871–873, 1958.
21. Toker C: Lactiferous duct fistula. J Pathol Bacteriol 84:143–146, 1962.
22. Habif DV, Perzin KH, Lipton R, et al: Subareolar abscess associated with squamous metaplasia of lactiferous ducts. Am J Surg 119:523–526, 1970.
23. Bundred NJ, Furlong A, El-Nakib L, et al: The aetiology of periductal mastitis. In Mansel RE (ed): Recent developments in the study of benign breast disease: Proceedings of the 5th International Royal College of Obstetricians Symposium on Benign Breast Disease. London, Parthenon, 1993, pp 207–214.
24. Dixon JM, Anderson TJ, Lumsden AB, et al: Smoking in patients with periductal mastitis and duct ectasia. In Mansel RE (ed): Recent developments in the study of benign breast disease: Proceedings of the 5th International Royal College of Obstetricians Symposium on Benign Breast Disease. London, Parthenon, 1993, pp 215–220.
25. Meguid MM, Oler A, Numann PJ, Khan S: Pathogenesis-based treatment of recurring subareolar breast abscesses. Surgery 118:775–782, 1995.
26. Ransjo U, Asplund OA, Gylbert L, Jurell G: Bacteria in the female breast. Scand J Plast Reconstr Surg 19:87–89, 1985.
27. Thornton JW, Argenta LC, McClathey KD, Marks MW: Studies on the endogenous flora of the human breast. Ann Plast Surg 20:39–42, 1988.
28. Walker AP, Edmiston CE Jr, Krepel CJ, Condon RE: A prospective study of the microflora of nonpuerperal breast abscess. Arch Surg 123:908–911, 1988.
29. Abul HT, Abul AT, Dashti HM, Behbehani AE: Comparison of local and systemic production of interleukin-8 in smoking and non-smoking patients with infectious lung disease. Med Principles Pract 5:19–24, 1996.
30. Michnovicz JJ, Hershcopf RJ, Naganuma H, Bradlow L: Increased 2-hydroxylation of oestradiol as a possible mechanism for the antiestrogenic effects of cigarette smoking. N Engl J Med 325:1305–1309, 1986.
31. Berta L, Frairia R, Fortunati N, et al: Smoking effects on the hormonal balance of fertile women. Hormone Res 37:45–48, 1992.
32. Sanchez-Pacheco A, Palomino T, Aranda A: Retinoic acid induces expression of the transcription factor GHF-1/Pit. 1 in pituitary prolactin– and growth hormone–producing cell lines. Endocrinology 136:5391–5398, 1995.
33. Sandison AT: Breast changes in fibrocystic disease of the pancreas. Lancet 1:691, 1956.
34. Berkowitz CD, Inkelish SH: Bloody nipple discharge in infancy. J Pediatrics 103:755–756, 1983.
35. Fenster DL: Bloody nipple discharge. J Pediatrics 104:640, 1984.
36. Stringel G, Perelman A, Jimenez C: Infantile mammary duct ectasia: A cause of bloody nipple discharge. J Pediatr Surg 21:671–674, 1986.
37. Kleinberg DL, Niemann W, Flamm E, et al: Primate mammary development: Effect of hypophysectomy, prolactin inhibition, and growth hormone administration. J Clin Invest 75:1943–1950, 1985.
38. MacLeod RM, Lehmyer JR: Studies on the mechanism of the dopamine-mediated inhibition of prolactin secretion. Endocrinology 94:1077–1085, 1974.
39. Shousha S, Backhouse CM, Dawson PM, et al: Mammary duct ectasia and pituitary adenomas. Am J Surg Pathol 12:130–133, 1988.
40. Franks S, Ralphs DNL, Seagroatt V, Jacobs HS: Prolactin concentrations in patients with breast cancer. Br Med J 4:320–321, 1974.
41. Kleinberg DL, Noel GL, Frantz AG: Galactorrhea: A study of 235 cases, including 48 with pituitary tumors. N Engl J Med 296:589–600, 1977.
42. Sharp BM, Beyer HS: Rapid desensitization of the acute stimulatory effects of nicotine on rat plasma adrenocorticotropin and prolactin. J Pharmacol Exp Ther 238:486–491, 1986.
43. Massagué J: TGF: beta signal transduction. Annu Rev Biochem 67:753–791, 1998.
44. Patton S, Keenan TW: The milk fat globule membrane. Biochim Biophys Acta 415:273–309, 1975.
45. Gothefors L, Olling S, Winberg J: Breast feeding and biological properties of faecal E. coli strains. Acta Paediatr Scand 64:807–812, 1975.
46. Schroten H, Hanisch FG, Plogmann R, et al: Inhibition of adhesion of S-frimbriated Escherichia coli to buccal epithelial cells by human milk fat globule membrane components: A novel aspect of the protective function of mucins in the nonimmunoglobulin fraction. Infect Immun 60:2893–2899, 1992.
47. Conney AH: Pharmacological implications of microsomal enzyme induction. Pharmacol Rev 19:317–366, 1967.
48. Barbieri RL, Gochberg J, Ryan KJ: Nicotine, cotinine, and anabasine inhibit aromatase in human trophoblast in vitro. J Clin Invest 77:1727–1733, 1986.
49. Mori S: Primary changes in eyes of rats which result from deficiency of fat-soluble A in diet. JAMA 79:197–200, 1922.
50. Darwiche N, Celli G, Sly L, et al: Retinoid status controls the appearance of reserve cells and keratin expression in mouse cervical epithelium. Cancer Res 53:2287–2299, 1993.
51. Ongsakul M, Sirisinha S, Lamb AJ: Impaired blood clearance of bacteria and phagocytic activity in vitamin A–deficient rats. Proc Soc Exp Biol Med 178:204–208, 1985.
52. Chandra RK, Wadhwa M: Nutritional modulation of intestinal mucosal immunity. Immunol Invest 18:119–126, 1989.
53. Spring-Mills E, Elias JJ: Cell surface differences in ducts from cancerous and noncancerous human breasts. Science 188:947–949, 1975.
54. Halter SA, Bradbury E, Mitchell WM: Diseases of the human breast: Selective isolation and exposure of epithelia and their correlative surface features and histopathology. Scan Electron Micros 3:139–145, 1978.
55. Biesalki HK: Vitamin A and ciliated cells: I. Respiratory epithelia. Z Ernahungswiss 25:114–122, 1986.
56. Schafer P, Furrer C, Mermillod B: An association of cigarette smoking with recurrent subareolar breast abscess. Int J Epidemiol 17:810–813, 1988.
57. Thomas JA, Williamson MER, Webster DJT: The relationship of cigarette smoking to breast disease: The Cardiff experience. In Mansel RE (ed): Recent developments in the study of benign breast disease: Proceedings of the 5th International Symposium on Benign Breast Disease. London, Parthenon, 1993.
58. Peters EJ, Morice R, Benner SE, Lippman S: Squamous metaplasia of the bronchial mucosa and its relationship to smoking. Chest 103:1429–1432, 1993.
59. Wynder EL, Hill P: Nicotine and cotinine in breast fluid. Cancer Lett 6:251–254, 1979.
60. Petrakis NL, Maack CA, Lee RE, Lyon M: Mutagenic activity in nipple aspirates of human breast fluid. Cancer Res 40:188–189, 1980.
61. Honjo H, Tanaka K, Yasuda J, et al: Serum estradiol 17-sulfate and lipid peroxides in late pregnancy. Acta Endocrinol 126:303–307, 1992.
62. Ertel A, Eng R, Smith SM: The differential effect of cigarette smoke on the growth of bacteria found in humans. Chest 100:628–630, 1991.
63. Taylor DC, Clancy RL, Cripps AW, et al: An alteration in the host-parasite relationship in subjects with chronic bronchitis prone to recurrent episodes of acute bronchitis. Immunol Cell Biol 72:143–151, 1994.
64. Ohnishi Y, Sawaki M, Mikasa K, Konishi M: Clinical study of anaerobic respiratory infection [in Japanese]. Kansenshogaku Zasshi J Jpn Assoc Infect Dis 67:336–341, 1993.
65. Brand KG: Infection of mammary prostheses: A survey and the question of prevention. Ann Plastic Surg 30:289–295, 1993.
66. Li W, Qiao W, Chen L, Xu X: Squamous cell carcinoma and mammary abscess formation through squamous metaplasia in Smad4/Dpc4 conditional knockout mice. Development 130:6143–6153, 2003.
67. Cardiff RD, Anver MR, Gusterson BA, Hennighausen L: The mammary pathology of genetically engineered mice: The consensus reports and recommendations from the Annapolis meeting. Oncogene 19:968–988, 2000.

68. Deng CX, Brodie SG: Knockout mouse models and mammary tumorigenesis. Semin Cancer Biol 11:387–394, 2001.
69. Henninghausen L, Robinson GW: Signaling pathways in mammary gland development. Dev Cell 1:467–475, 2001.
70. Derynck R, Akhurst RJ, Balmain A: TGF beta signaling in tumor suppression and cancer progression. Nat Genet 29:117–129, 2001.
71. Gorska AE, Joseph H, Derynck R, Moses HL: Dominant-negative interference of the transforming growth factor beta type II receptor in mammary gland epithelium results in alveolar hyperplasia and differentiation in virgin mice. Cell Growth Diff 9:229–238, 1998.
72. Jhappan C, Geiser AG, Kordon EC, Bagheri D: Targeting expression of a transforming growth factor beta 1 transgene to the pregnant mammary gland inhibits alveolar development and lactation. Ebo J 12:1835–1845, 1993.
73. Tedeschi LG, Byrne JJ: A histochemical evaluation of the structure of mammary duct walls. Surg Gynecol Obstet 114:559–562, 1982.
74. Holliday H, Hinton C: Nipple discharge and duct ectasia. In Blamey RW (ed): Management of breast disease. London, Tindall, 1986.
75. Bundred NJ, Dover MS, Coley S, Morrison JM: Breast abscesses and cigarette smoking. Br J Surg 79:58–59, 1992.
76. Thomas WC, Williamson RC, Davies JD, Webb AJ: The clinical syndrome of mammary duct ectasia. Br J Surg 69:423–425, 1982.
77. The Yorkshire Breast Cancer Group: Symptoms and signs of operable breast cancer, 1976–1981. Br J Surg 70:350–351, 1983.
78. Tabar L, Dean PB, Pentek Z: Galactography: The diagnostic procedure of choice for nipple discharge. Radiology 149:31–38, 1983.
79. Browning J, Bigrigg A, Taylor I: Symptomatic and incidental mammary duct ectasia. J R Soc Med 79:715–716, 1986.
80. Chaudary MA, Millis RR, Davies GC: Nipple discharge: The diagnostic value of testing for occult blood. Ann Surg 196:651–655, 1982.
81. Rimsten A, Skoog V, Stenkvist B: On the significance of nipple discharge in the diagnosis of breast disease. Acta Chir Scand 142:513–518, 1976.
82. Abramson DJ: Mammary duct ectasia, mammillary fistula and subareolar sinuses. Ann Surg 169:217–226, 1969.
83. Fischermann K, Bech I, Foged P, et al: Nipple discharge: Diagnosis and treatment. Acta Chir Scand 135:403–406, 1969.
84. Urban JA: Non-lactational nipple discharge. Ca Cancer J Clin 28:130–140, 1978.
85. Donnelly BA: Nipple discharge: Its clinical and pathologic significance. Ann Surg 131:342–355, 1950.
86. Kilgore AR, Fleming R, Ramos MM: The incidence of cancer with nipple discharge and the risk of cancer in the presence of papillary disease of the breast. Surg Gynecol Obstet 96:649–660, 1953.
87. Leis HP Jr, Pilnik S, Dursi J, et al: Nipple discharge. Int Surg 58:162–165, 1973.
88. Funderburk WW, Syphax B: Evaluation of nipple discharge in benign and malignant diseases. Cancer 24:1290–1296, 1969.
89. O'Brien PH, Kreutner A: Another cause of nipple discharge: Mammary duct ectasia with periductal mastitis. Am Surg 48:577–588, 1982.
90. Bundred NJ, Dixon JM, Lumsden AB, et al: Are the lesions of duct ectasia sterile? Br J Surg 72:844–845, 1985.
91. Seltzer MH, Perloff LJ, Kelley RI, et al: The significance of age in patients with nipple discharge. Surg Gynecol Obstet 131:519–522, 1970.
92. Leach RD, Eykyn SJ, Phillips I, et al: Anaerobic subareolar breast abscesses. Lancet 1:35–37, 1979.
93. Ingham HR, Freeman R, Wilson RG: Anaerobic breast abscesses. Lancet 1:164–165, 1979.
94. Wilson WR, Martin WJ, Wilkowske CJ, et al: Anaerobic bacteremia. Mayo Clin Proc 47:639–646, 1972.
95. Rosenthal LJ, Greenfield DS, Lesnick GJ: Breast abscess: Management in subareolar and peripheral disease. NY State J Med 81:182–183, 1981.
96. Hadfield GJ: Excision of the major duct system for benign disease of the breast. Br J Surg 47:472–477, 1960.
97. Preece PE: Mastalgia. Practitioner 226:1373–1382, 1982.
98. Maddox PR, Mansel RE: Management of breast pain and nodularity. World J Surg 13:699–705, 1989.
99. Preece PE, Mansel RE, Bolton PM, et al: Clinical syndromes of mastalgia. BMJ 2:670–673, 1976.
100. Griffith CDM, Dowle CS, Hinton CP, et al: The breast pain clinic: A rational approach to classification and treatment of breast pain. Postgrad Med J 63:547–549, 1987.
101. Maddox PR, Harrison BJ, Mansel RE: Non-cyclical mastalgia: An improved classification and treatment. Br J Surg 76:901–904, 1989.
102. Guyer PB: The use of ultrasound in benign breast disorders. World J Surg 13:692–698, 1989.
103. Evans KT, Gravelle IH: Mammography, thermography and ultrasonography in breast disease. London, Butterworths, 1973.
104. Gravelle IH, Lyons K: Radiological evaluation of benign breast disorders. World J Surg 13:685–691, 1989.
105. Hadfield GJ: The pathological lesions underlying discharges from the nipple in women. Ann R Coll Surg Engl 44:323–333, 1969.
106. Pye JK, Mansel RE, Hughes LE: Clinical experience of drug treatments for mastalgia. Lancet 2:373–377, 1985.
107. Rees BI, Gravelle IH, Hughes LE: Nipple retraction in duct ectasia. Br J Surg 64:577–580, 1977.
108. Dixon JM, Lee ECG, Greenall MJ: Treatment of periareolar inflammation associated with periductal mastitis using metronidazole and flucloxacillin: A preliminary report. Br J Clin Pract 42:78, 1988.
109. Caswell HT, Maier WP: Chronic recurrent periareolar abscess secondary to inversion of the nipple. Surg Gynecol Obstet 128:597–599, 1969.
110. Kleinfeld G: Chronic subareolar breast abscess. J Fla Med Assoc 53:21–24, 1966.
111. Lefrock JL, Ellis CA, Turchik JB, et al: Transient bacteremia associated with sigmoidoscopy. N Engl J Med 289:467–469, 1973.
112. Leach RD, Eykyn SJ, Phillips I: Vaginal manipulation and anaerobic breast abscesses. BMJ 282:610–611, 1981.
113. Brooker BE, Fuller R: The adhesion of coagulase-negative staphylococci to human skin and its relevance to the bacterial flora of milk. J Appl Bacteriol 57:325–332, 1984.
114. Walker JC, Sandison AT: Mammary duct ectasia: A clinical study. Br J Surg 51:350–355, 1964.
115. Hadfield GJ: Further experience of the operation for the excision of the major duct system of the breast. Br J Surg 55:530–535, 1968.
116. Ekland DA, Zeigler MG: Abscess in the nonlactating breast. Arch Surg 107:398–401, 1973.
117. Goodman MA, Benson EA: An evaluation of current trends in the management of breast abscesses. Med J Aust 1:1034–1039, 1970.
118. Ferrara JJ, Leveque J, Dyess DL: Nonsurgical management of breast infections in nonlactating women: A word of caution. Ann Surg 56:668–671, 1990.
119. Golinger RC, O'Neal BJ: Mastitis and mammary duct disease. Arch Surg 117:1027–1029, 1982.
120. Asch T, Frey C: Radiographic appearance of mammary-duct ectasia with calcification. N Engl J Med 266:86–87, 1962.
121. Dixon JM, Chetty U: The clinical syndrome of mammary duct ectasia. Br J Surg 70:57–58, 1983.
122. Ellerhorst-Ryan JM, Turba EP, Stahl DL: Evaluating benign breast disease. Nurse Practitioner 13:13, 16, 18, 1988.
123. Wood CB, Tsikos C, Keane P, et al: Ultrasound assessment response to therapy of clinically undetected breast cysts. Br J Clin Pract (suppl 68):102, 1989.
124. Caswell HT, Burnett WE: Chronic recurrent breast abscess secondary to inversion of the nipple. Surg Gynecol Obstet 102:439–442, 1956.
125. Maier WP, Berger A, Derrick BM: Periareolar abscess in the nonlactating breast. Am J Surg 144:359–361, 1982.
126. Bundred NJ, Dixon JM, Chetty U: Mammillary fistula. Br J Surg 74:466–468, 1987.
127. Atkins HJ: Mammary fistula. BMJ 2:1473–1474, 1955.
128. Petrek J: Postmenopausal breast abscess. South Med J 75:1198–1200, 1982.
129. Benson EA: Management of breast abscesses. World J Surg 13:753–756, 1989.
130. Benson EA, Goodman MA: Incision with primary suture in the treatment of acute peripheral breast abscess. Br J Surg 51:55–58, 1970.

131. Cua EJ, Oates E: Breast uptake of gallium-67 citrate in disseminated *Mycobacterium chelonae*. Clin Nucl Med 15:705–706, 1990.

132. Berger SA, Gorea A, Stadler, et al: Recurrent breast abscesses caused by *Corynebacterium minutissimum*. J Clin Microbiol 20: 1219–1220, 1984.

133. Bodey GP, Bolivar R, Fainstein V, et al: Infections caused by *Pseudomonas aeruginosa*. Rev Infect Dis 5:279–313, 1983.

134. Buchanan EB, Kominos SD: *Pseudomonas aeruginosa* mastitis: A case report. CMNEEJ 12:63, 1990.

135. Kessler E, Wolloch Y: Granulomatous mastitis: A lesion clinically simulating carcinoma. Am J Clin Pathol 58:642–646, 1972.

136. Going JJ, Anderson TJ, Wilkinson S, Chetty U: Granulomatous lobular mastitis. J Clin Pathol 40:535–540, 1987.

137. Salam IM, Alhomsi MF, Daniel MF, Sim AJ: Diagnosis and treatment of granulomatous mastitis. Br J Surg 82:214, 1995.

138. Bani-Hani KE, Yaghan RJ, Matalka II, Shatnawi NJ: Idiopathic granulomatous mastitis: Time to avoid unnecessary mastectomies. Breast J 10:318–322, 2004.

139. Yaghan RJ: The magnetic resonance image findings of idiopathic granulomatous mastitis. Saudi Med J 25:1715–1719, 2004.

140. Wilson JP, Massoll N, Marshall J, et al: Idiopathic granulomatous mastitis: In search of a therapeutic paradigm. Am Surg 73:798–802, 2007.

141. Baslaim MM, Khayat HA, Al-Amoudi SA: Idiopathic granulomatous mastitis: A heterogeneous disease with variable clinical presentation. World J Surg 31:1677–1681, 2007.

142. Imoto S, Kitaya T, Kodama T, et al: Idiopathic granulomatous mastitis: Case report and review of the literature. Jpn J Clin Oncol 27:274–277, 1997.

Clinical Management of Mastitis and Breast Abscess and Idiopathic Granulomatous Mastitis

STEPHEN R. GROBMYER | NICOLE MASSOLL | EDWARD M. COPELAND III

Mastitis and Breast Abscess

Patients with acute mastitis and abscess often represent a diagnostic and therapeutic challenge. There is currently no consensus on optimal management strategies. The principles that guide successful diagnosis, evaluation, and management are discussed presently.

PRESENTATION

Patients with acute breast infection typically present with one or more of the following symptoms: skin erythema, palpable mass, tenderness, fever, and/or pain.[1-3] Breast abscesses may occur in both the lactational and nonlactational setting.[4-8] Breast abscesses have been most commonly reported to occur in women between 20 and 50 years of age.[4,5,7,9] However, breast infections have also been reported in men,[9] postmenopausal women,[10] and children.[11] Postmenopausal patients with breast abscess often have a more indolent presentation and may lack many of the classical findings for breast abscess.[10] Abscesses may occur either centrally (subareolar or periareolar) or peripherally in the breast. Many authors have reported that a subareolar abscess is more common in nonlactating women,[1,4,7] and lactational abscesses are more common in the upper outer quadrant.[5,12] Conversely, two groups have reported that abscesses in nonlactating women occur in the periphery of the breast.[5,13]

BREAST INFECTION ASSOCIATED WITH OR FOLLOWING BREAST CANCER TREATMENT

Acute breast infection presenting as erythema, warmth, and/or purulent drainage from the wound may follow lumpectomy for breast cancer treatment.[14] The incidence of acute infection following lumpectomy may be reduced by reapproximation of the deep breast tissue when possible.[14] Delayed breast cellulitis[15] and abscesses have been reported to occur following operation, external beam radiation therapy,[16] and brachytherapy[17] for breast cancer. In this setting, breast infection may result from treatment-related impaired lymphatic drainage of the breast.[15]

There may be changes in the breast following breast biopsy, lymph node biopsy, or partial mastectomy that mimic breast infection or malignancy.[18] These changes, including mild erythema and edema of the breast, are thought to occur secondary to treatment-related disruption of breast lymphatics (breast lymphedema).[18] Recognition of this postoperative entity can be difficult but is important to limit overtreatment. Postoperative breast lymphedema is typically self-limited (1 month to 1 year).[18]

EVALUATION

Careful clinical examination is the cornerstone of diagnosis for acute breast infection. Findings on examination include a mass, erythema, skin warmth, skin thickening, and tenderness.[1-3] Ultrasound is a useful modality as an adjunct to physical examination to evaluate suspected acute breast infectious processes for the presence or absence of an associated abscess.[19-22] Ultrasound has a high sensitivity for the detection of an underlying breast abscess.[2] Many patients with breast abscess also have abnormal mammograms with nonspecific findings, including irregular mass, focal asymmetry, diffuse asymmetric density, circumscribed mass, and architectural distortion.[2] These findings in the acute setting may be difficult to differentiate from those findings associated with malignancy.[23] In addition, in the acute setting of suspected breast infection, mammography is often not possible secondary to breast pain and tenderness. Following successful medical, percutaneous, or surgical management of acute breast infection or abscess, mammography to exclude an underlying or associated malignancy may be performed and has been recommended by some authors[9] to exclude malignancy. However, the optimal timing of follow-up imaging and the yield of this practice has not been clearly elucidated.[9]

MICROBIOLOGY

Staphylococcus aureus is the most common organism associated with breast abscess. Other commonly reported causative organisms include *Pseudomonas aeruginosa*, *Staphylococcus epidermidis*, *Proteus*, *Serratia*, and *Bacterioides*.[1,4,5,24] Recently, an increase in methicillin-resistant *S. aureus* has been detected in community-acquired breast infections.[24] Twenty to 40% of breast abscesses are found to be sterile on culture.[1,4,5] Cigarette smoking has been associated with increased rates of anaerobic breast infections and increased rates of recurrent breast abscess.[25,26]

Breast abscess and mastitis have been reported in association with body art (nipple piercing and tattoos).[27,28] The incidence of breast infection associated with nipple piercing is most likely underreported.[28,29] Jacobs and colleagues have estimated the incidence to be as high as 10% to 20% in the months following the procedure.[28] Pathologic organisms that have been documented following piercing in this setting include aerobic, anaerobic, and mycobacterial infections.[29-32] In the management of breast abscess in patients with pierced nipples, particular attention should be given to obtaining cultures for these specific pathogens to help guide treatment decisions.

UNUSUAL BREAST INFECTIONS

A variety of unusual pathologic organisms have been documented in association with breast abscess, including *Actinomyces* species,[33] *Brucella*,[34] *Mycobacterium tuberculosis*,[35] *Fusarium solani*,[36] *Echinococcus*,[37] *Cryptococcus*,[38] and *Paragonimus*.[39] Many of these unusual infections are endemic to specific areas and specific patient populations, and they require special consideration in the appropriate clinical setting.

Necrotizing soft tissue infection and gangrene of the breast have rarely been reported.[40,41] Necrotizing soft tissue infections of the breast have been reported in association with anticoagulant treatment, trauma, and in the postpartum period.[42] Principles of management of necrotizing soft tissue infection are similar to necrotizing soft tissue infections of other areas and include early diagnosis, early and aggressive surgical management, and systemic antibiotics.[41-44] Because necrotizing soft tissue infections are most commonly polymicrobial in etiology, broad-spectrum antibiotics represent the best initial choice of antimicrobial coverage.[45]

BREAST MALIGNANCY PRESENTING AS MASTITIS AND ABSCESS

Breast cancer or other malignancies including squamous cell carcinoma or lymphoma may rarely present in association with breast abscess or with symptoms that mimic breast abscess.[46-52] This association has been primarily described in isolated case reports. Several retrospective studies have examined the incidence of cancer in larger series of patients undergoing management of breast abscess. Scott and associates[9] found an incidence of cancer of only 4% (n = 9) in a series of 229 patients who underwent routine biopsy of the abscess cavity; in all patients, there was a discrete mass in association with the abscess.[9] Christensen and coworkers[13] reported no cancer in association with the follow-up of 151 patients managed for breast abscess and followed for 2 years. The low rate of associated malignancy with breast abscess has led to the acceptance of percutaneous management for selected cases of breast abscess (see later discussion). However, failure of traditional management strategies to resolve symptoms of a "presumed" abscess should prompt tissue biopsies to exclude malignancy.

MANAGEMENT OF BREAST INFECTION

Antibiotics

In patients who present with signs and symptoms of mastitis or breast abscess and who are clinically suspected of having a breast infection, ultrasound is a very useful imaging modality for the detection of an intramammary fluid collection. For patients with no or a small fluid collection seen on ultrasound, a trial of oral antibiotics is warranted.[4,53] Initial choice of antibiotics is best directed by local antibiograms.[24] Failure to improve should prompt further evaluation with repeat ultrasound to evaluate for the development of an intramammary fluid collection requiring an alteration in the management strategy. A tissue biopsy may be necessary to exclude malignancy in some cases.

Surgical Incision and Drainage

The traditional approach to breast abscess involves surgical incision, disruption of septae, and open packing of wounds with or without administration of systemic antibiotics.[1,5] Suggested limitations to this approach may include need for general anesthesia, high cost, and cosmetic deformity.[4] In addition, surgical incision and drainage has been associated with recurrence rates between 10% and 38% requiring additional procedures.[54] A biopsy of the abscess cavity wall may be performed in conjunction with the incision and drainage and has been recommended by some authors[9]; however, the yield of this routine practice is not well defined. Again, following abscess resolution, some authors have recommended mammography and breast ultrasound to exclude malignancy.[9,13] However, the optimal timing and yield of this clinical practice has not been clearly delineated.

Aspiration

Numerous authors have suggested primary aspiration of breast lactational and nonlactational abscesses as an alternative to primary surgical management.[1,5,9,3,55–58] Potential benefits of aspiration as a primary management strategy include improved cosmesis, lack of requirement for general anesthesia, no requirement for wound packing, and decreased cost.[5,9] Reported success rates with single and multiple aspirations of breast abscess are 57% to 79% and 90% to 96%.[1,9,59] Patients who fail to improve with multiple aspirations or whose clinical condition deteriorates require operative drainage and/or tissue biopsy.

The reported technique of several authors involves use a 16-gauge needle (or larger if necessary) with aspiration and irrigation of the cavity through an area where the skin is not thinned from inflammation.[1,5] Use of ultrasound to guide aspiration may be helpful and associated with higher rates of success but is not required.[5,59] Most authors advocate treatment with oral antibiotics as a component of initial therapy for breast abscess managed with aspiration.[5,59,60] Cultures of aspirated fluid may be useful to guide antibiotic choice. Although some have suggested sending abscess fluid for cytology to exclude malignancy, the value of this practice is not well defined and it is not widely recommended.[60,61] Some authors have advocated instillation of antibiotics into the abscess cavity;[1,4] however, this practice is not widely accepted, and its benefit has not been clearly demonstrated. Some have advocated placement of an indwelling drain at the time of aspiration, but this practice is not widely used.[5,9] Following initial management, patients should undergo clinical reassessment to determine resolution of requirement for additional treatment (repeat aspiration or surgical drainage).[5] Median time to resolution of breast abscess with aspiration is 2 weeks (range, 1–7 weeks).[4]

Factors that have been associated with failure of aspiration include large size (>3 cm) and loculations.[1,5,59] Progression or failure of symptoms to improve with serial aspirations mandates surgical management as outlined previously.

Special Considerations for Lactational Mastitis and Abscesses

The highest incidence of lactational breast infection occurs in the first 12 weeks of the postpartum period.[5,62] The general principles for evaluation and management of breast infection outlined previously are applicable to lactational abscesses.[12,63] During treatment for lactational breast abscess, patients are encouraged to continue to drain the breast by either pumping the breast to prevent breast stasis and engorgement or breast feeding.[1,3,5] Breastfeeding from the infected side is thought to be safe for a healthy infant, although infants should be monitored for the development of infection.[64] In some cases, administration of antibiotics to the infant may be indicated.[64] Some authors have specifically cautioned against breastfeeding from the infected breast because of risk of infection transmission to the infant.[63,65] Galactoceles, which most commonly present at the cessation of lactation, may also become infected.[66] Management should be similar to other lactational abscesses and consists of drainage (percutaneous or open) and systemic antibiotics.

Chronic Subareolar Abscess

Chronic subareolar abscess results from chronic intermittent obstruction of the terminal ducts of the nonlactating breast.[7,67] This condition is characterized by recurrent abscesses and sinus formation.[68] Several authors have reported an association between cigarette smoking and chronic subareolar abscess.[25,26]

Simple incision and drainage of a chronic subareolar abscess may lead to temporary resolution of an acute infective process; however, this approach is associated with a high rate of recurrence.[7,67,69] Abscess drainage along with resection of the involved central ducts has been suggested to be a more definite treatment for chronic subareolar abscess associated with cure rates in excess of 90% and acceptable cosmesis.[7,8,67]

Authors' Recommendation for Breast Abscess Management

In the management of breast abscess, we in general prefer open drainage through a small incision to allow exploration of the wound and open packing. In our experience, breast abscess aspiration has not been extremely effective and many patients ultimately require open drainage. We have found that the cosmetic defect for surgically drained abscesses has been satisfactory. For acute subareolar abscesses that are often loculated, we surgically drain abscesses through two small incisions (on opposite sides of the areola) through which a temporary Penrose drain can be placed that exits both incisions. The tract that forms can be irrigated with saline, which aids healing by keeping the cavity clean and allowing healthy granulated tissue to develop.

For chronic subareolar abscesses, we often prescribe an extended course of oral antibiotics, often a month or longer, in attempt to sterilize chronically colonized ducts. If this does not alleviate symptoms, then an attempt to locate the offending duct can be explored. However, in our experience, this identification has been difficult and the ducts in the involved quadrant ultimately require excision. In patients who present with an acute infection and a history of chronic subareolar abscess, we prefer management of the acute infectious process with drainage prior to ductal excision.

Management of patients with a breast abscess is an "art," and each abscess has unique features that require familiarity by the treating physician. Even for a patient referred with chronic, recurring abscesses, we repeat the tissue conservative treatment that may have failed in the past, the purpose of which is to "get to know" the abscess and the patient. Breast abscesses are frustrating for the patient and for the treating physician. Knowing the personality of the patient is important because, on rare occasions, a simple mastectomy may be the last alternative to the patient's ability to live without recurrent breast abscesses.

Idiopathic Granulomatous Mastitis

Idiopathic granulomatous mastitis (IGM) is a uncommon chronic inflammatory condition of the breast that can clinically mimic bacterial abscess or breast cancer.[70] Patients with IGM may present with skin induration, tenderness, erythema, sinus tract formation, breast edema, and/or a masslike lesion[71,72] (Fig. 6B-1). The clinical presentation may clinically mimic mastitis, breast abscess, or malignancy. Depending on the clinical presentation, patients may appropriately be initially managed with antibiotics, attempted incision and drainage, biopsy, or excision. Failure of initial management strategies should prompt tissue biopsy (and breast imaging) to exclude malignancy and provide more information about the underlying pathologic process.

The diagnosis of IGM is one of exclusion. It is characterized by noncaseating granulomas (Fig. 6B-2), small abscesses, and inflammation of the lobules in the absence of specific infection (e.g., mycobacterial, mycotic, or parasitic), sarcoidosis, or foreign material.[70] Cultures of any associated fluid should be obtained to exclude an infectious etiology in those in whom the diagnosis of IGM is a consideration.[72]

The natural history of IGM is variable but often characterized by a chronic relapsing course. Management of patients with IGM can be very challenging, and numerous approaches have been described,[72] including observation, local excision, systemic steroids, and mastectomy. For patients with mild, localized symptoms of IGM, a trial of

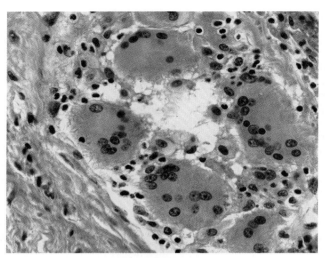

Figure 6B-2 Granulomatous lobular mastitis with central multinucleated histiocytes and peripheral lymphocytes.

observation, local excision, or steroids may be indicated.[72] Close clinical follow-up is indicated for patients being managed for IGM. For patients with progressive symptoms or those presenting with severe, generalized involvement of the breast a trial of steroids is warranted and may alleviate symptoms. Mastectomy may be indicated for patients with IGM who have intractable symptoms.[72]

REFERENCES

1. Leborgne F, Leborgne F: Treatment of breast abscesses with sonographically guided aspiration, irrigation, and instillation of antibiotics. AJR Am J Roentgenol 181:1089–1091, 2003.
2. Crowe DJ, Helvie MA, Wilson TE: Breast infection. Mammographic and sonographic findings with clinical correlation. Invest Radiol 30:582–587, 1995.
3. Dener C, Inan A: Breast abscesses in lactating women. World J Surg 27:130–133, 2003.
4. Imperiale A, Zandrino F, Calabrese M, et al: Abscesses of the breast. US-guided serial percutaneous aspiration and local antibiotic therapy after unsuccessful systemic antibiotic therapy. Acta Radiol 42:161–165, 2001.
5. Elagili F, Abdullah N, Fong L, et al: Aspiration of breast abscess under ultrasound guidance: Outcome obtained and factors affecting success. Asian J Surg 30:40–44, 2007.
6. Scholefield JH, Duncan JL, Rogers K: Review of a hospital experience of breast abscesses. Br J Surg 74:469–470, 1987.
7. Versluijs-Ossewaarde FN, Roumen RM, Goris RJ: Subareolar breast abscesses: Characteristics and results of surgical treatment. Breast J 11:179–182, 2005.
8. Maier WP, Au FC, Tang CK: Nonlactational breast infection. Am Surg 60:247–250, 1994.
9. Scott BG, Silberfein EJ, Pham HQ, et al: Rate of malignancies in breast abscesses and argument for ultrasound drainage. Am J Surg 192:869–872, 2006.
10. Petrek J: Postmenopausal breast abscess. South Med J 75:1198–1200, 1982.
11. Faden H: Mastitis in children from birth to 17 years. Pediatr Infect Dis J 24:1113, 2005.
12. Eryilmaz R, Sahin M, Hakan Tekelioglu M, et al: Management of lactational breast abscesses. Breast 14:375–379, 2005.
13. Christensen AF, Al-Suliman N, Nielsen KR, et al: Ultrasound-guided drainage of breast abscesses: Results in 151 patients. Br J Radiol 78:186–188, 2005.
14. Indelicato D, Grobmyer SR, Newlin H, et al: Association between operative closure type and acute infection, local recurrence, and disease surveillance in patients undergoing breast conserving therapy for early-stage breast cancer. Surgery 141:645–653, 2007.

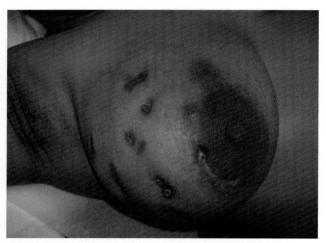

Figure 6B-1 Clinical appearance of right breast in a patient with granulomatous mastitis with classic chronic inflammatory changes and sinus formation. (Used with permission from Wilson JP: Idiopathic granulomatous mastitis: In search of a therapeutic paradigm. Am Surg 73:798–802, 2007.)

15. Indelicato DJ, Grobmyer SR, Newlin H, et al: Delayed breast cellulitis: An evolving complication of breast conservation. Int J Radiat Oncol Biol Phys 66:1339–1346, 2006.
16. Keidan RD, Hoffman JP, Weese JL, et al: Delayed breast abscesses after lumpectomy and radiation therapy. Am Surg 56:440–444, 1990.
17. Lopchinsky RA, Giles KA: Recurrent abscess after MammoSite brachytherapy. Breast J 10:536–538, 2004.
18. Loprinzi CL, Okuno S, Pisansky TM, et al: Postsurgical changes of the breast that mimic inflammatory breast carcinoma. Mayo Clin Proc 71:552–555, 1996.
19. Heywang SH, Lipsit ER, Glassman LM, et al: Specificity of ultrasonography in the diagnosis of benign breast masses. J Ultrasound Med 3:453–461, 1984.
20. Jackson VP: The role of US in breast imaging. Radiology 177:305–311, 1990.
21. Hayes R, Michell M, Nunnerley HB: Acute inflammation of the breast—the role of breast ultrasound in diagnosis and management. Clin Radiol 44:253–256, 1991.
22. Muttarak M: Abscess in the non-lactating breast: Radiodiagnostic aspects. Australas Radiol 40:223–225, 1996.
23. Reddin A, McCrea ES, Keramati B: Inflammatory breast disease: Mammographic spectrum. South Med J 81:981–984, 988, 1988.
24. Moazzez A, Kelso RL, Towfigh S, et al: Breast abscess bacteriologic features in the era of community-acquired methicillin-resistant *Staphylococcus aureus* epidemics. Arch Surg 142:881–884, 2007.
25. Schafer P, Furrer C, Mermillod B: An association of cigarette smoking with recurrent subareolar breast abscess. Int J Epidemiol 17:810–813, 1988.
26. Bundred NJ, Dover MS, Coley S, et al: Breast abscesses and cigarette smoking. Br J Surg 79:58–59, 1992.
27. Mayers LB, Judelson DA, Moriarty BW, et al: Prevalence of body art (body piercing and tattooing) in university undergraduates and incidence of medical complications. Mayo Clin Proc 77:29–34, 2002.
28. Jacobs VR, Golombeck K, Jonat W, et al: Mastitis nonpuerperalis after nipple piercing: Time to act. Int J Fertil Womens Med 48:226–231, 2003.
29. Bengualid V, Singh V, Singh H, et al: *Mycobacterium fortuitum* and anaerobic breast abscess following nipple piercing: Case presentation and review of the literature. J Adolesc Health 42:530–532, 2008.
30. Trupiano JK, Sebek BA, Goldfarb J, et al: Mastitis due to *Mycobacterium abscessus* after body piercing. Clin Infect Dis 33:131–134, 2001.
31. Pearlman MD: *Mycobacterium chelonei* breast abscess associated with nipple piercing. Infect Dis Obstet Gynecol 3:116–118, 1995.
32. Lewis CG, Wells MK, Jennings WC: *Mycobacterium fortuitum* breast infection following nipple-piercing, mimicking carcinoma. Breast J 10:363–365, 2004.
33. Attar KH, Waghorn D, Lyons M, et al: Rare species of actinomyces as causative pathogens in breast abscess. Breast J 13:501–505, 2007.
34. Erdem G, Karakas HM, Yetkin F, et al: Brucellar breast abscess. Breast 15:554–557, 2006.
35. Maroulis I, Spyropoulos C, Zolota V, et al: Mammary tuberculosis mimicking breast cancer: A case report. J Med Case Reports 2:34, 2008.
36. Anandi V, Vishwanathan P, Sasikala S, et al: *Fusarium solani* breast abscess. Indian J Med Microbiol 23:198–199, 2005.
37. Thurairatnam TP: Echinococcus breast abscess. Trop Doct 22:192, 1992.
38. Schouten WE, Damen M, Davids PH, et al: Cryptococcal breast abscess. Scand J Infect Dis 34:309–310, 2002.
39. Jun SY, Jang J, Ahn SH, et al: Paragonimiasis of the breast. Report of a case diagnosed by fine needle aspiration. Acta Cytol 47:685–687, 2003.
40. Alados JC, Perez M, Fontes J: Bacteriology of non-puerperal breast abscesses. Int J Gynaecol Obstet 48:105–106, 1995.
41. Delotte J, Karimdjee BS, Cua E, et al: Gas gangrene of the breast: Management of a potential life-threatening infection. Arch Gynecol Obstet 279:79–81, 2009.
42. Rege SA, Nunes Q, Rajput A, et al: Breast gangrene as a complication of puerperal sepsis. Arch Surg 137:1441–1442, 2002.
43. Elliott DC, Kufera JA, Myers RA: Necrotizing soft tissue infections. Risk factors for mortality and strategies for management. Ann Surg 224:672–683, 1996.
44. Rajakannu M, Kate V, Ananthakrishnan N: Necrotizing infection of the breast mimicking carcinoma. Breast J 12:266–267, 2006.
45. Elliott D, Kufera JA, Myers RA: The microbiology of necrotizing soft tissue infections. Am J Surg 179:361–366, 2000.
46. Wong C, Wright C, Colclough A, et al: Case report: Metaplastic carcinoma presenting as a breast abscess. Int Semin Surg Oncol 3:23, 2006.
47. Melamed JB, Schein M, Decker GA: Squamous carcinoma of the breast presenting as an abscess. A case report. S Afr Med J 69:771–772, 1986.
48. Wrightson WR, Edwards MJ, McMasters KM: Primary squamous cell carcinoma of the breast presenting as a breast abscess. Am Surg 65:1153–1155, 1999.
49. Gupta C, Malani AK: Abscess as initial presentation of pure primary squamous cell carcinoma of the breast. Clin Breast Cancer 7:180, 2006.
50. Kenwright DN, Gaskell D, Wakefield L, et al: Apocrine ductal carcinoma in situ of the breast presenting as a chronic abscess. Aust N Z J Surg 69:72–75, 1999.
51. Stanton MP, Cutress R, Royle GT: Primary non-Hodgkin's lymphoma of the female breast masquerading as a breast abscess. Eur J Surg Oncol 26:429, 2000.
52. Dawn B, Perry MC: Bilateral non-Hodgkin's lymphoma of the breast mimicking mastitis. South Med J 90:328–329, 1997.
53. Benson EA: Management of breast abscesses. World J Surg 13:753–756, 1989.
54. Watt-Boolsen S, Rasmussen NR, Blichert-Toft M: Primary periareolar abscess in the nonlactating breast: Risk of recurrence. Am J Surg 153:571–573, 1987.
55. Karstrup S, Nolsoe C, Brabrand K, et al: Ultrasonically guided percutaneous drainage of breast abscesses. Acta Radiol 31:157–159, 1990.
56. Hook GW, Ikeda DM: Treatment of breast abscesses with US-guided percutaneous needle drainage without indwelling catheter placement. Radiology 213:579–582, 1999.
57. O'Hara RJ, Dexter SP, Fox JN: Conservative management of infective mastitis and breast abscesses after ultrasonographic assessment. Br J Surg 83:1413–1414, 1996.
58. Dixon JM: Outpatient treatment of non-lactational breast abscesses. Br J Surg 79:56–57, 1992.
59. Schwarz RJ, Shrestha R: Needle aspiration of breast abscesses. Am J Surg 182:117–119, 2001.
60. Tan YM, Yeo A, Chia KH, et al: Breast abscess as the initial presentation of squamous cell carcinoma of the breast. Eur J Surg Oncol 28:91–93, 2002.
61. Ferrara JJ, Leveque J, Dyess DL, et al: Nonsurgical management of breast infections in nonlactating women. A word of caution. Am Surg 56:668–671, 1990.
62. Marchant DJ: Inflammation of the breast. Obstet Gynecol Clin North Am 29:89–102, 2002.
63. Scott-Conner CE, Schorr SJ: The diagnosis and management of breast problems during pregnancy and lactation. Am J Surg 170:401–405, 1995.
64. Betzold CM: An update on the recognition and management of lactational breast inflammation. J Midwifery Womens Health 52:595–605, 2007.
65. Eschenbach DA: Acute postpartum infections. Emerg Med Clin North Am 3:87–115, 1985.
66. Ghosh K, Morton MJ, Whaley DH, et al: Infected galactocele: A perplexing problem. Breast J 10:159, 2004.
67. Li S, Grant CS, Degnim A, et al: Surgical management of recurrent subareolar breast abscesses: Mayo Clinic experience. Am J Surg 192:528–529, 2006.
68. Lannin DR: Twenty-two year experience with recurring subareolar abscess and lactiferous duct fistula treated by a single breast surgeon. Am J Surg 188:407–410, 2004.
69. Meguid MM, Oler A, Numann PJ, et al: Pathogenesis-based treatment of recurring subareolar breast abscesses. Surgery 118:775–782, 1995.
70. Kessler E, Wolloch Y: Granulomatous mastitis: A lesion clinically simulating carcinoma. Am J Clin Pathol 58:642–646, 1972.
71. Baslaim MM, Khayat HA, Al-Amoudi SA: Idiopathic granulomatous mastitis: A heterogeneous disease with variable clinical presentation. World J Surg 31:1677–1681, 2007.
72. Wilson JP, Massoll N, Marshall J, et al: Idiopathic granulomatous mastitis: In search of a therapeutic paradigm. Am Surg 73:798–802, 2007.

chapter 7

Gynecomastia

SAMUEL W. BEENKEN | DAVID L. PAGE |
KIRBY I. BLAND

Gynecomastia is benign enlargement of the male breast due to proliferation of the glandular component. This common clinical condition, which may be unilateral or bilateral, presents as an incidental finding on routine physical examination, a painless unilateral or bilateral breast enlargement, or a painful and tender mass beneath the areolar region. This chapter focuses on the prevalence, clinical presentation, physiology, histopathology, pathophysiology, diagnosis, and treatment of gynecomastia. Finally, the specific clinical situations of gynecomastia in the pubertal male and in the aging male are reviewed to provide easily understood summaries of the complexities of this topic.

Prevalence

There are three distinct peaks in the age distribution of gynecomastia. The first peak is during the neonatal period when palpable breast tissue transiently develops in 60% to 90% of newborns because of the transplacental passage of estrogens.[1,2] The second peak is during puberty, with prevalence increasing at approximately 10 years of age and peaking between 13 and 14 years of age, followed by a decline during the later teenage years. See Table 7-1 for details. Pubertal gynecomastia is estimated to occur within 15 months after an increase in testicular size, the first sign of puberty.[3] The third peak is found in the adult population, with prevalence increasing at approximately 50 years of age and continuing into the eighth decade of life. See Table 7-2 for details.

Most patients seeking consultation for gynecomastia have idiopathic gynecomastia (approximately 25%) or acute/persistent gynecomastia due to puberty (25%), drugs (10% to 20%), cirrhosis/malnutrition (8%), or primary hypogonadism (8%). A lesser number have testicular tumors (3%), secondary hypogonadism (2%), hyperthyroidism (1.5%), or renal disease (1%).[1]

Clinical Presentation

The patient presents with a swelling of the breast, often unilateral, which is commonly tender. The patient may be concerned about the tenderness, the cosmetic appearance or the possibility of malignancy. Examination reveals a firm "donut" of retroareolar tissue, which is mobile. There is usually a clear demarcation of the firm breast tissue from the softer adjacent fat. The hallmark of gynecomastia is concentricity. If an eccentric mass is found, an alternate diagnosis should be considered, and mammography and biopsy should be performed.

Physiology

NORMAL DEVELOPMENT OF THE MALE BREAST

Male breast development in the fetus occurs in an analogous fashion to female breast development. By the ninth week of gestation, a recognizable nipple bud has formed from basal cells in the pectoral region. By the end of the third month, squamous epithelium invades the nipple bud and ducts develop, which connect to the nipple at the skin's surface. These become canalized and form lactiferous ducts. The blind ends of these ducts bud to form alveolar structures. At birth, with a decline in fetal prolactin, placental estrogen and placental progesterone, the infantile breast regresses until puberty.[4]

The breast tissues of both sexes appear histologically identical at birth and remain relatively quiescent during childhood, undergoing further differentiation at the time of puberty.[1,2] In the majority of males, transient proliferation of the ducts and surrounding mesenchymal tissue takes place during the period of rapid sexual maturation, followed by involution and ultimately atrophy of the ducts. In contrast, in females, the breast ductal and periductal tissues continue to enlarge and develop terminal acini, processes that require both estrogen and progesterone.[5] Supplementary information regarding key components of hormonal regulation of female breast development is presented in Table 7-3.

Because estrogens stimulate breast tissue and androgens antagonize these effects, gynecomastia has long been considered the result of an imbalance between these hormones.[6,7] The transition from the prepubertal to the postpubertal state is accompanied by a 30-fold increase in the concentration of testosterone, with only a threefold increase in estrogen levels.[8] Therefore, a relative imbalance between serum estrogen and androgen levels can exist during a portion of the pubertal process

TABLE 7-1

Prevalence of Gynecomastia in Pubertal Males

Study	Study Group	Criteria Used*	Age of Study Subjects (years)	No. of Study Subjects	No. (%) with Gynecomastia
Nydick[a]	Boy Scouts	≥5 mm	10–16	1865	722 (39)
Neyzi[b]	Turkish schoolboys	Firm subareolar tissue	9–17	993	70 (7)
Lee[c]	U.S. schoolboys	Firm subareolar disk	Pubertal boys	29	20 (69)
Fara[d]	Italian schoolboys	≥5 mm	11–14	681	228 (33)
Harlan[e]	U.S. youths	≥10 mm	12–17	3522	147 (4)
Moore[f]	Swiss youths	≥5 mm	8.5–17.5	135	30 (22)
Biro[g]	U.S. schoolboys	Palpable glandular tissue	10–15	377	183 (49)

*Measurements indicate the size of the subareolar mass on examination.
[a]Data from Nydick M, Bustos J, Dale JH Jr, Rawson RW: Gynecomastia in adolescent boys. JAMA 178:449–454, 1961.
[b]Data from Neyzi O, Alp H, Yalcindag A, Yakacikli S, et al: Sexual maturation in Turkish boys. Ann Hum Biol 2:251–259, 1975.
[c]Data from Lee.[13]
[d]Data from Fara GM, Del Corvo G, Bernuzzi S, et al: Epidemic of breast enlargement in an Italian school. Lancet 2:295–297, 1979.
[e]Data from Harlan WR, Grillo GP, Cornoni-Huntley J, Leaverton PE: Secondary sex characteristics of boys 12 to 17 years of age: the U.S. Health Examination Survey. J Pediatr 95:293–297, 1979.
[f]Data from Moore DC, Schlaepfer LV, Paunier L, Sizonenko PC: Hormonal changes during puberty. V. Transient pubertal gynecomastia: abnormal androgen-estrogen ratios. J Clin Endocrinol Metab 58:492–499, 1984.
[g]Data from Biro FM, Lucky AW, Huster GA, Morrison JA: Hormonal studies and physical maturation in adolescent gynecomastia. J Pediatr 116:450–455, 1990.
From Braunstein G: Gynecomastia. N Engl J Med 328:490–495, 1993. Copyright © 1993 Massachusetts Medical Society. All rights reserved.

and may result in gynecomastia. In an analysis of tissues from 30 males with gynecomastia, estrogen, progesterone, and androgen receptors were observed in 100%.[9]

NORMAL CIRCULATING MALE ESTROGEN CONCENTRATIONS

The adult testes secrete approximately 15% of the estradiol and less than 5% of the estrone in the circulation, whereas extragonadal tissues produce 85% of the estradiol and more than 95% of the estrone through the aromatization of precursors. The principal precursor of estradiol is testosterone, 95% of which is derived from the testes (Fig. 7-1). Androstenedione, an androgen secreted primarily by the adrenal gland, serves as a precursor of estrone formation. The important extraglandular sites of aromatization are adipose tissue, liver, and muscle. In addition, a substantial degree of interconversion between estrone and estradiol takes place through the action of the widely distributed enzyme 17-ketosteroid reductase, which also catalyzes the conversion of androstenedione to testosterone.[6,10,11]

TABLE 7-2

Prevalence of Gynecomastia in Adult Males

Study	Study Group	Criteria Used*	Age of Study Subjects (years)	No. of Study Subjects	No. (%) with Gynecomastia
Williams[a]	Autopsy	Histology	Adults	447	178 (40)
Nuttall[b]	U.S. military personnel	≥2 cm	17–58	306	109 (36)
Ley[c]	Contraceptive trial subjects	≥2 cm	19–39	63	22 (35)
Carlson[d]	Veterans	Not stated	Adults	100	32 (32)
Anderson and Gram[e]	Autopsy	Histology	Adults	100	55 (55)
Niewoehner and Nuttall[f]	Veterans	≥2 cm	27–92	214	140 (65)

*Measurements indicate the size of the subareolar mass on physical examination.
[a]Data from Williams MJ: Gynecomastia: its incidence, recognition and host characterization in 447 autopsy cases. Am J Med 34:103–112, 1963.
[b]Data from Nuttall FQ: Gynecomastia as a physical finding in normal men. J Clin Endocrinol Metab 48:338–340, 1979.
[c]Data from Ley SB, Mozaffarian GA, Leonard JM, Highley M, et al: Palpable breast tissue versus gynecomastia as a normal physical finding. Clin Res 28:24A, 1980.
[d]Data from Carlson HE: Gynecomastia. N Engl J Med 303:795–799, 1980.
[e]Data from Andersen JA, Gram JB.[154]
[f]Data from Niewoehner CB, Nuttall FQ.[14]
From Braunstein G: Gynecomastia. N Engl J Med 328:490–495, 1993. Copyright © 1993 Massachusetts Medical Society. All rights reserved.

TABLE 7-3

Hormonal Regulation of Female Breast Development

Hormone	Action
Estrogen	• Estrogen, acting through its receptor (ER), promotes duct growth.[a] • ER knockout mice display grossly impaired ductal development.[b] • Estrogen promotes GH secretion and increases GH levels, stimulating the production of IGF-1, which synergizes with estrogen to induce ductal development.
Progesterone	• Progesterone, acting through its receptor (PR), promotes alveolar development.[a] • PR knockout mice possess significant ductal development but lack alveolar development.[b] • Maximal alveolar proliferation occurs during the luteal phase of the female menstrual cycle when progesterone serum concentrations reach 10–20 ng/mL and estrogen concentrations are two to three times lower than in the follicular phase.[c] • Prolonged treatment of dogs with progesterones increases GH and IGF-1 serum concentrations.[d]
GH and IGF-1	• Neither estrogen alone nor estrogen plus progesterone can sustain breast development without other mediators such as GH and IGF-1. • GH effects on ductal growth are mediated through stimulation of IGF-1 as demonstrated by administration of estrogen and GH to IGF-1 knockout rats, which show significantly decreased mammary development when compared to age-matched IGF-1 intact controls.[e] • Combined estrogen and IGF-1 treatment in IGF-1 knockout rats restores mammary growth.[f] • GH-stimulated production of IGF-1 mRNA suggests that IGF-1 production in the stromal compartment of the mammary gland acts locally to promote breast development.[g]
Prolactin	• Prolactin stimulates epithelial cell proliferation only in the presence of estrogen and enhances lobuloalveolar differentiation only in the presence of progesterone. • Prolactin may be produced in normal mammary epithelial cells and breast tumors.[h]

GH, growth hormone; IGF-1, insulin growth factor-1.
[a]Data from Braunstein G: Gynecomastia. N Engl J Med 328:490–495; 1993.
[b]Data from Lubahn DB, Moyer JS, Golding TS: Alteration of reproductive function but not prenatal sexual development after insertional disruption of the mouse estrogen receptor gene. Proc Soc Natl Acad Sci U S A 90:11162–11166, 1993; Bocchinfuso WP, Korach MS: Mammary gland development and tumorigenesis in estrogen receptor knockout mice. J Mammary Gland Biol Neoplasia 90:323–334, 1997.
[c]Data from Santen R: Endocrinology, 4th ed. 3:2335–2341, 2001.
[d]Data from Mol JA, Van Garderen E, Rutteman GR, Rijnberk A: New insights into the molecular mechanism of progestin-induced proliferation of mammary epithelium: induction of the local biosynthesis of growth hormone in the mammary glands of dogs, cats, and humans. J Steroid Biochem Mol Biol 57:67–71, 1996.
[e]Data from Edmondson, Glass, and Soll,[8] and Bidlingmaier and Knorr.[9]
[f]Data from Kleinberg DL, Feldman, M, Ruan W: IGF-1: An essential factor in terminal end bud formation and ductal morphogenesis. J Mammary Gland Biol Neoplasia 5:7–17, 2000; Ruan W, Kleinberg DL: Insulin-like growth factor I is essential for terminal end bud formation and ductal morphogenesis during mammary development. Endocrinology 140:5075–5081, 1999.
[g]Data from Walden PD, Ruan W, Feldman M, Kleinberg DL: Evidence that the mammary fat pad mediated the action of growth hormone in mammary gland development. Endocrinology 139:659–662, 1998.
[h]Data from LeProvost F, Leroux C, Martin P, et al: Prolactin gene expression in ovine and caprine mammary gland. Neuroendocrinology 60:305–313, 1994; Steinmetz R, Grant A, Malven P: Transcription of prolactin gene in milk secretory cells of the rat mammary gland. J Endocrinology 36:305–313, 1993.

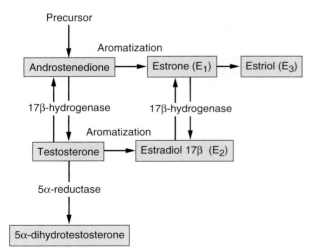

Figure 7-1 Potential pathways for androgen-estrogen interconversion in healthy men. (Modified from Gordon GG, Olivo J, Rafil F, Southren AL: Conversion of androgens to estrogens in cirrhosis of the liver. J Clin Endocrinol Metab 40:1018–1026, 1975.)

NEONATAL GYNECOMASTIA

Palpable enlargement of the male breast in the neonate is normal and occurs as a result of the action of prolactin, placental estrogens, and progesterones on the neonatal breast parenchyma. Although this breast enlargement usually regresses within a few weeks, it has been observed to persist for longer periods.[12]

PUBERTAL GYNECOMASTIA

Table 7-1 presents the prevalence of gynecomastia in pubertal males. Transient proliferation of the ducts and surrounding mesenchymal tissue takes place during this period of rapid sexual maturation, followed by involution and ultimately atrophy of the ducts. Gynecomastia is evident in as many as 69% of schoolboys in the United States.[13] For many of these boys, the enlarged breast(s) is asymmetric, tender, and psychologically disturbing (Fig. 7-2). However, by age 20, only a small percentage of these boys have a remaining palpable abnormality.

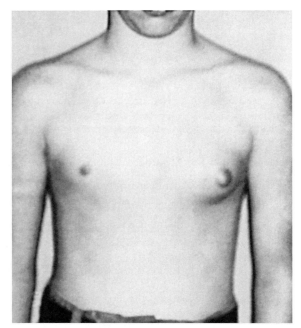

Figure 7-2 An 11-year-old boy with unilateral (left) gynecomastia at puberty.

SENILE GYNECOMASTIA

Table 7-2 presents the prevalence of gynecomastia in adult males. Senile gynecomastia occurs in 32% to 65% of adult males (Fig. 7-3), its prevalence correlates with the body fat content, and it does not require clinical evaluation unless symptomatic or of recent, rapid onset.[14] Plasma testosterone concentration values begin to fall at approximately 70 years of age.[15] In addition, there is concurrent elevation in the plasma sex hormone–binding globulin (SHBG), which causes a further fall in the free or unbound testosterone concentrations. A simultaneous increase in plasma luteinizing hormone (LH) may cause a concurrent increase in the rate of conversion of androgen to estrogen in peripheral tissues.[16] Hence, relative hyperestrinism is evident with a decrease in the plasma androgen-to-estrogen ratio (Fig. 7-4).

Histopathology

The histologic pattern of gynecomastia progresses from an early active phase (florid) to an inactive phase (fibrous), no matter what the cause. Grossly, there is a relatively sharp margin between breast tissue and surrounding subcutaneous fat. The few ductal structures of the male breast enlarge, elongate, and branch along with the encasing connective tissue.[17,18] This combined increase in glandular and stromal elements provides for a regular distribution of each element throughout the enlarged breast. Often, there is an increase in cell number relative to the basement membrane. The loose connective tissue that regularly outlines the ducts as a central feature of gynecomastia is prominent only in the earliest stage of the disease (Figs. 7-5 to 7-7). The fibroblasts within

this loose tissue are relatively large but lack atypical features and are not clustered, even though they appear more frequently immediately adjacent to the basement membrane of the ducts.

The epithelial cells are often increased to three or four in height. The cells are primarily cuboidal, without a prominence of basilar or myoepithelial cells. With greater cell numbers, there is a tendency toward a pattern mimicking "tufting," but these small areas, four to five cells in width, are the only foci of cell increase. This very slight hyperplasia, suggesting a papillary pattern, is often

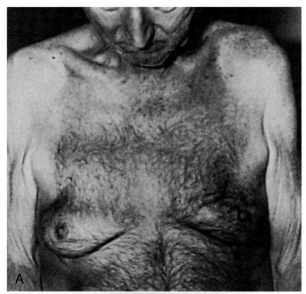

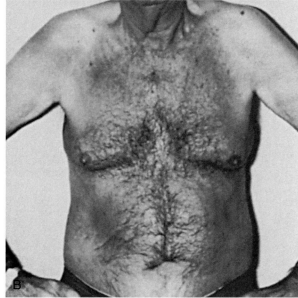

Figure 7-3 **A,** Senescent bilateral gynecomastia in an 85-year-old man. The patient had observed a gradual increase in the size of both breasts over the past 4 years. There are no breast masses, and the patient takes no medication. **B,** Senescent bilateral gynecomastia in a 72-year-old man with progressive enlargement of breasts over a 6-year period. The patient has no systemic diseases and takes no medications.

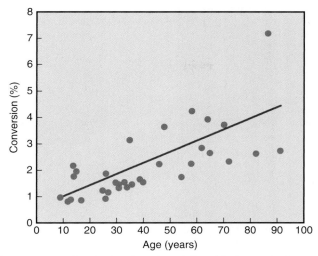

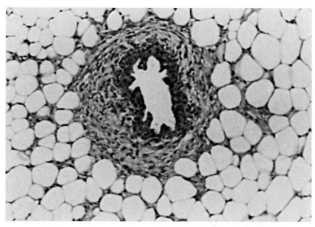

Figure 7-4 Graph showing the relationship between the conversion of circulating androstenedione to estrone in men as a function of age. (From Siiteri PK, MacDonald PC: Role of extraglandular estrogen in human endocrinology. In Greep RO, Astwood EB [eds]: Handbook of physiology. Washington, DC, American Physiological Society, 1975.)

Figure 7-7 From the florid phase of gynecomastia, this duct has elongated into surrounding fat. Note the cellular, young fibrous tissue ensheathing the duct and insinuating between fat cells.

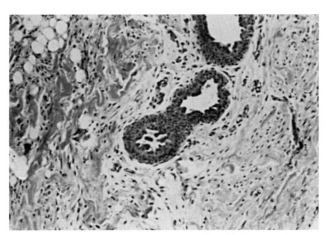

Figure 7-5 From the florid phase of gynecomastia, a tortuous duct passes through the center of the photograph. A richly vascular, loose connective tissue is present around the duct.

enhanced to produce long, narrow papillary proliferations of epithelial cells. These occasionally mimic atypical hyperplastic patterns except that the cells tend to have a regular placement, which differs from the pattern seen in well-developed atypical hyperplasia (Fig. 7-8; see Fig. 7-6).

The micropapillary pattern is the most common hyperplastic pattern seen with gynecomastia. With a frequent and even distribution throughout the specimen, these micropapillae are benign in appearance. When present only focally, the pattern resembles that of atypical hyperplasia or even carcinoma in situ. However, the presence of atypical ductal hyperplasia in the male breast is not well studied, and its clinical implications are unknown. In fact, these cytologic and histologic forms are only reminiscent of atypical ductal hyperplasia, not diagnostic of that condition. Focal squamous metaplasia also may be found, with islands of squamous metaplastic cells interspersed within the hyperplastic epithelial cells.[19] Foci of apocrine change may be seen but are even less common. The finding of lobular units in the male

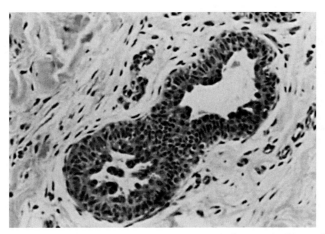

Figure 7-6 Seen at higher power, the duct (shown in Fig. 7-5) demonstrates hyperplastic epithelium. Note the increase in epithelial cell number over the basement membrane.

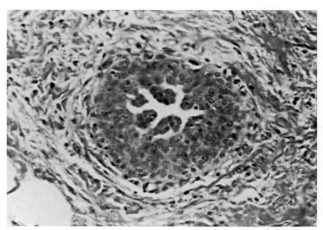

Figure 7-8 Hyperplasia of epithelial cells is evident in the many layers of cells. The micropapillary fronds that are present centrally are characteristic of the hyperplasia seen in gynecomastia.

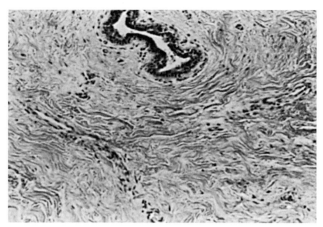

Figure 7-9 In the late or fibrous stage of gynecomastia, ductal elements are less prominent and a dense collagenous stroma is predominant.

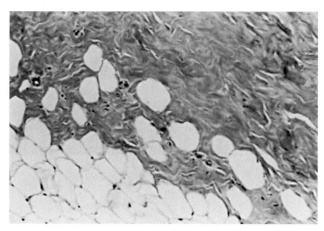

Figure 7-11 At the interface of mammary connective tissue with subcutaneous fats, there is an intermingling of elements. Note the density of the connective tissue in this case, which is of 6 years' duration.

breast is rare, being reported in 1 in 1000 cases.[20] The formation of lobular units has no known clinical correlate except that it seems to be somewhat more prevalent in florid gynecomastia.

Fibrous gynecomastia describes the later stage of gynecomastia and histologically has a dense collagenous stroma that contains relatively few fibroblasts (Figs. 7-9 to 7-11). This dense collagenous tissue is applied closely to delicate basement membrane regions surrounding sparse epithelial elements in which hyperplasia is usually absent. The loose pattern of periductal stroma that characterizes the florid stage of gynecomastia is lacking. Researchers used immunohistochemical techniques to show that the majority (89%) of gynecomastia specimens are estrogen receptor positive.[21] The investigators were unable to demonstrate an association between histopathologic staging of gynecomastia or hormonal parameters and estrogen receptor status.

Virtually any benign alteration found in the female breast (in particular, fibroadenoma and sclerosing adenosis) may be found in the male breast, although such changes are rare. Differentiating carcinoma of the male

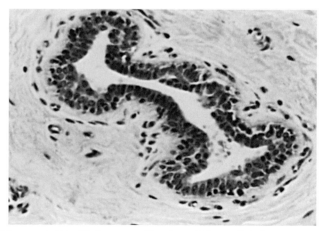

Figure 7-10 Higher magnification of Figure 7-9 demonstrates compact fibrous tissue applied almost directly on ductal basement membrane. There are fewer capillaries encircling the duct than in the more active earlier stages of gynecomastia.

breast from gynecomastia may be difficult clinically, but the problem is easily resolved with histologic or cytologic examination. There is significant discrepancy in the literature regarding the association of breast cancer and gynecomastia. Researchers identified an occult focus of cribriform intraductal carcinoma amid gynecomastia in a 20-year-old man.[22] Gynecomastia was present in 22% of cases of male breast cancer in West Africa.[23] Reports of an increased incidence of male breast cancer come from Egypt and Zambia, where gynecomastia is a common finding as a result of hyperestrogenism caused by liver fibrosis and malnutrition. Whether the unusual cases of atypical hyperplasia and carcinoma in the male breast are preceded by gynecomastia is unknown. The carcinomas in situ that are reported to occur in the male breast are most often the solid and comedo types, although complex cribriform patterns are also demonstrated.[24,25]

DNA was analyzed in patients with breast carcinoma, fibroadenoma, and gynecomastia.[26] Specifically, telomeric deletions and *HER2/neu* gene amplification were analyzed. *HER2/neu* amplification was observed in 26.8% of breast carcinoma specimens but not in patients with fibroadenoma or gynecomastia. Significant reductions in telomeric length and concentration were noted in all breast tissue compared with placental control DNA; in addition, no significant differences were noted between carcinoma, fibroadenoma, and gynecomastia.

Pathophysiology

As previously stated, most patients who present with possible gynecomastia have idiopathic gynecomastia or acute/persistent gynecomastia due to puberty, drugs, cirrhosis/malnutrition, or primary hypogonadism. A few have testicular tumors, secondary hypogonadism, hyperthyroidism, or renal disease.[1] Table 7-4 presents a comprehensive summary of the conditions commonly associated with gynecomastia.

TABLE	7-4
Conditions associated with Gynecomastia	

Estrogen Excess

Testicular neoplasms
Adrenal cortex neoplasms
Ectopic HCG production
Hermaphroditism
Hyperthyroidism
Liver cirrhosis
Recovery from starvation

Androgen Deficiency

Primary testicular failure
Secondary testicular failure
Androgen resistance syndromes
Increased aromatase activity
Chronic renal failure

Drug Related

HCG, human chorionic gonadotropin.

ESTROGEN EXCESS

Mechanisms of increased estrogen formation are presented in Figure 7-12.

Testicular Tumors

Testicular tumors can lead to increased blood estrogen levels by (1) estrogen overproduction, (2) androgen overproduction with aromatization in the periphery to estrogens, and (3) ectopic secretion of gonadotropins that stimulate otherwise normal Leydig cells.

Leydig's Cell Neoplasms. Leydig's cell neoplasms are relatively uncommon, constituting approximately 2% to 3% of all testicular neoplasms.[27] Such neoplasms are found in children as young as 2 years of age and in adults as old as 82 years of age.[28] The average age at diagnosis is between 20 and 60 years. Leydig's cell tumors account for up to 39% of non–germ cell tumors of the testes and 12% of the testicular neoplasms of children.[29-32]

Leydig's cell tumors of the testes are most often unilateral.[29,33] Sexual precocity is usually observed in children with these tumors and is accompanied by an increase in muscle mass and stature with advanced bone age in most patients. In children, Leydig's cell tumors are almost uniformly benign.

In adults, physical changes are less frequent, with endocrine signs noted in approximately 30% of adults with these tumors;[34] painful gynecomastia and decreased libido are the most common manifestations. Symptoms may precede the onset of a palpable testicular mass, particularly with Leydig's cell hyperplasia. Approximately 25% of the Leydig's cell tumors in adult men secrete predominantly estrogen.[31,32,35,36] For some patients, gynecomastia may be observed despite normal serum estrogen and testosterone levels. In these patients, gynecomastia may occur after in situ conversion of androstenedione to estrone in breast parenchyma, leading to increased tissue estrogen values without increasing serum levels.[37-40]

Malignant transformation of Leydig's cell tumors occurs in approximately 10% of patients, predominantly in adults and older men.[41,42] Gynecomastia associated with Leydig's cell tumors is more often seen when these tumors are benign, especially when 17-ketosteroid values are normal. Malignant Leydig's cell tumors usually demonstrate abnormal estrogen or androgen levels and are associated more frequently with elevated estrogens and 17-ketosteroid levels without gynecomastia.[41-43]

For patients with gynecomastia and increased circulating estrogen levels, pituitary suppression of LH release may initiate atrophy of the contralateral testis.[44] A prolonged plasma estradiol response to human chorionic gonadotropin (HCG) is a useful, although nonspecific, adjunct in the diagnosis of Leydig's cell tumors.[45]

Sertoli's Cell Tumors. Sertoli cell tumors comprise less than 1% of all testicular tumors and occur at all ages,

Normal

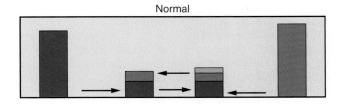

Increased estrogen secretion

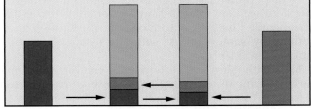

Increased substrate availability

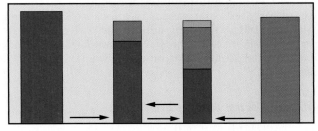

Increased peripheral aromatase

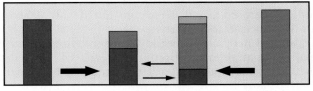

| Androstenedione | Estrone | Estradiol | Testosterone |

Figure 7-12 Gynecomastia as the result of increased estrogen formation can arise because of increased estrogen secretion into plasma by the adrenal or the testis, increased availability of substrate for peripheral conversion to estrogen, or an increased rate of aromatization within tissues. (From Wilson JD, Aiman J, MacDonald PC: The pathogenesis of gynecomastia. In Stollerman GH [ed]: Advances in internal medicine, vol 25. St Louis, Mosby, 1980.)

but one third occur in children younger than 13 years of age, usually in boys younger than 6 months of age. The tumors usually do not produce endocrine effects in children.

Gynecomastia is seen in 26% to 33% of individuals with benign Sertoli's cell tumors, and it rapidly regresses after orchiectomy.[46,47] In most cases, there was no elevation of estrogen or testosterone serum concentrations. Of five reported patients with malignant Sertoli's cell tumors and gynecomastia, two had elevated gonadotropin levels.[48]

Multifocal Sertoli's cell tumors in boys have been associated with the autosomal dominant syndrome of Peutz-Jeghers syndrome.[49-51] The increased risk of gonadal tumors for females with Peutz-Jeghers syndrome was recognized at an earlier date.[52]

The majority of Sertoli's cell tumors are benign, but as many as 10% can be malignant. Males with distant metastatic disease have been reported.[53,54]

Germ Cell Tumors. Germ cell tumors are the most common cancers in males between 15 and 35 years of age. They are divided into seminomatous and nonseminomatous subtypes. The theory of a common origin of germ cell tumors of the testes from embryonal carcinoma cells is supported by ultrastructural studies[55] and experimental production of teratoma from embryonal carcinoma explants.[56,57] Estrogen effects in men with germ cell neoplasms occur secondary to increased aromatization of testosterone and androstenedione into estrogens in peripheral sites.[58] Androstenedione, which has low androgenicity and is readily aromatized to estrone peripherally, may be produced in increased concentrations by some tumors, with the result of enhanced estrogen production.[16]

Men with germ cell tumors who exhibit gynecomastia have a higher mortality than those without gynecomastia.[59,60] After orchiectomy and chemotherapy, a 75% reduction in the number of men with gynecomastia is observed.[60]

Use of testicular ultrasound for detection and localization of early testicular masses in males with gynecomastia is essential. Any young adult male with unexplained gynecomastia, loss of libido, or impotence should have diagnostic testicular ultrasound for evaluation of occult tumors.[61,62]

Adrenal Cortex Neoplasms

The first childhood adrenal tumor was reported in 1865.[63] In a 48-year review of surgical experience at Roswell Park Memorial Institute, 153 adrenal cortical tumors were evaluated. They constituted only 0.04% of all the cancer cases evaluated.

Adrenal neoplasms should be suspected in any child with premature or inappropriate signs of virilization or feminization, especially if accompanied by evidence of hyperadrenocorticism or gynecomastia. Evidence of premature development of secondary sexual characteristics, such as enlarged penis, axillary hair, and pubic hair, may be seen in children with gynecomastia associated with tumors of the adrenal gland.[64]

An estrogen-producing adrenal tumor in an adult male was first reported in 1919.[65] In men, adrenal carcinomas that result only in feminization are very uncommon.[66]

However, neoplasms producing mixed syndromes, such as feminization and Cushing's disease, are almost always malignant.[67-69]

Ectopic Human Chorionic Gonadotropin Production

Carcinoma of the Lung. This disease may initiate an increase in serum chorionic gonadotropin values with simultaneous escalation in estrogen secretion.[70] Gonadotropins were identified in the urine of four male patients who died of bronchogenic carcinoma.[71] In three patients, gonadotropins were also present in tissue samples from the primary lung tumor. The appearance of gynecomastia in an adult male smoker should arouse suspicion of an underlying carcinoma of the lung. It has been proposed that the detection of HCG may be an aid in the diagnosis of bronchogenic carcinoma.[72]

Hepatocellular Carcinoma. This can also initiate gynecomastia via elevated serum HCG.[73] Normal hepatic parenchyma and primary hepatic neoplasms carry estrogen receptors. Hepatocellular carcinoma carries androgen receptors, whereas normal liver parenchyma cells do not.[74]

Hermaphroditism

True Hermaphroditism. True hermaphroditism occurs when an ovary and a testis or a gonad with mixed histologic features (ovotestis) is present. Four categories are recognized: (1) bilateral, with testicular and ovarian tissue (ovotestis) anatomically present on each side; (2) unilateral, with an ovotestis on one side and a normal ovary or testis on the contralateral side; (3) lateral, with a testis is evident on one side and an ovary on the opposite side; and (4) indeterminate, in which the clinical syndrome is expressed but the location and type of gonadal tissue is uncertain.[75]

Significant gynecomastia is evident at puberty in approximately 75% of individuals with true hermaphroditism. Approximately 50% of these individuals menstruate. For the phenotypic male with true hermaphroditism, menstruation presents as cyclic hematuria. Excess estradiol secretion relative to androgen production by the ovotestis is common.[76] Gonadal secretion of estradiol is observed in phenotypic men with feminization (gynecomastia and menstruation).[76,77]

Pseudohermaphroditism. 17-Ketosteroid reductase deficiency results in male pseudohermaphroditism with a marked overproduction of androstenedione and estrone as well as a decreased production of testosterone and estradiol. A late-onset form of testicular 17-ketosteroid reductase deficiency can cause gynecomastia and hypogonadism in men.[78]

Hyperthyroidism

In 1959, a review of the English literature found 26 cases of gynecomastia that had developed during clinical hyperthyroidism and then receded after re-establishment of the euthyroid state.[79] In most such cases, gynecomastia was bilateral.[80] The diffuse toxic goiter of Graves' disease is most commonly associated with gynecomastia.[80]

Both elevated estrogen and progesterone serum concentrations can be identified in men with hyperthyroidism.[81,82] These elevations decrease with re-establishment of the euthyroid state. Gynecomastia, which occurs in 20% to 40% of men with hyperthyroidism, may be due to elevated estrogens that results from a stimulatory effect of thyroxin on peripheral aromatase.[83]

Liver Cirrhosis

The evaluation of estrogen, testosterone, androstenedione, and cortisol concentrations and the percentage of binding of these steroids to plasma proteins demonstrated that alterations were most marked in patients with cirrhosis.[84] They were also evident to a lesser degree in patients with fatty metamorphosis of the liver and in normal aging patients.[84] Patients with cirrhosis showed an increase in estrone, a smaller increase in estradiol, a decrease in testosterone, and a rise in LH concentration. Cortisol concentration remained unchanged, whereas ratios of estradiol to testosterone and estrone to testosterone were augmented in patients with cirrhosis and were higher than those in healthy young subjects. The combination of elevated estrone and estradiol and reduced testosterone, which is strongly bound by increased SHBG, appeared to be responsible for gynecomastia and hypogonadism in chronic liver diseases. Other investigators have observed that plasma progesterone concentration is increased in 72% of men with nonalcoholic cirrhosis and gynecomastia when compared with healthy male controls.[85] However, this increase was not observed in men with alcoholic fatty change and alcoholic cirrhosis.

Gynecomastia is observed in approximately 40% of men with cirrhosis.[86–91] As stated, total plasma testosterone concentrations are lower than normal.[84,92–96] However, there is a far greater decline in the non–protein bound (biologically active) plasma testosterone.[81,87,94,97] This decrease appears to result from an increased concentration of SHBG.[98–101] The decreased concentration of plasma testosterone of men with cirrhosis is initiated by a reduction in testosterone synthesis by the testes; kinetic studies have confirmed that the production of testosterone is reduced by 75%.[102–104] In fact, 15% of the testosterone produced in males with cirrhosis is derived from peripheral conversion of circulating androstenedione (see Fig. 7-11).[103] There is disagreement about the relative roles of unbound (biologically active) plasma estradiol in men with cirrhosis and gynecomastia and the changes affecting testosterone concentrations, but the decline in non–protein bound (biologically active) plasma testosterone appears to be the most important factor.[105,106]

Recovery from Starvation

Gynecomastia produced by nutritional deprivation is well documented. Case-control studies of American prisoners of war during World War II demonstrated that 15% of males in Japanese prisoner-of-war camps developed gynecomastia.[107–109] Approximately one third of these cases occurred after release from prison, and other cases were associated with increases in the nutrition supplied during imprisonment. In most cases, gynecomastia was bilateral and disappeared within 5 to 7 months after release. Because many of the prisoners had fatty infiltration of the liver and spider angiomas, the pathogenesis is thought to be similar to that of gynecomastia in hepatic disease.[107]

ANDROGEN DEFICIENCY

Primary Testicular Failure

Klinefelter's Syndrome. Klinefelter's syndrome (XXY) was described more than four decades ago in adult phenotypic males with gynecomastia, hypergonadotropic hypogonadism, and azoospermia.[110] The chromosomal pattern XXY occurs in approximately 1 in 600 live births.[111] Klinefelter's syndrome represents the most common variant of male hypogonadism. However, the full spectrum of clinical findings, gynecomastia, eunuchoidism, and macro-orchidism does not emerge until the mid-teens and may never be fully expressed. By mid-puberty, affected individuals are uniformly hypergonadotropic and testicular growth ceases. After 15 years of age, serum testosterone concentrations remain in the low-normal range but serum estradiol values are increased, irrespective of the presence or absence of gynecomastia.[112] Although testicular biopsy during childhood reveals a reduced number of spermatogonia, tubular fibrosis and hyalinization of seminiferous tubules are not observed until mid-puberty.[113] Biochemical findings in the adult male include reduced levels of serum testosterone with high-normal or enhanced values of serum estradiol.[114]

It is estimated that carcinoma of the breast is 20 to 66.5 times more frequent in men with Klinefelter's than in the normal male population (Fig. 7-13).[115,116] Bilateral carcinoma of the breast has also been reported.[117]

Hereditary Defects of Androgen Biosynthesis. Multiple hereditary defects have been identified that result in defective androgen biosynthesis with incomplete

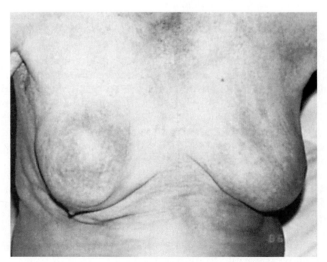

Figure 7-13 Advanced bilateral gynecomastia in a 70-year-old man. The patient also has a palpable, discrete mass in the right breast confirmed mammographically and on biopsy to be a carcinoma.

virilization of the male embryo.[118-122] The enzymes responsible for these failures in biosynthesis include 20,22-desmolase, 17,20-desmolase, 3β-hydroxysteroid dehydrogenase, 17α-hydroxylase, 17β-hydroxysteroid dehydrogenase, and 17-oxosteroid reductase. Each enzyme represents a critical pathway for the conversion of cholesterol to testosterone. As a consequence of the variability in the blockade of these enzymatic biochemical reactions, affected individuals have a profound escalation in gonadotropin secretion after negative feedback. For individuals with complete or partial deficiencies of 17β-hydroxysteroid dehydrogenase, feminization with gynecomastia develops in the early teens. Gynecomastia is also a common occurrence in male patients with 11-β-hydroxylase deficiency.[123] Deficiency of 17-oxosteroid reductase (see Fig. 7-1), causes elevation in estrone and androstenedione, which is then further aromatized to estradiol.[124]

Secondary Testicular Failure

Gynecomastia is common after testicular injury resulting from trauma, viral orchitis (mumps), or bacterial infections (e.g., tuberculosis, leprosy). The common pathogenic mechanism is functional revascularization of one or both testes. Mumps represents the most common cause of viral orchitis, although echovirus, lymphocytic choriomeningitis virus, and group B arboviruses, among others, have all been implicated in secondary testicular failure.[125,126] Testicular failure occurs in approximately 25% of men infected with the mumps virus; two thirds have unilateral orchitis. In a survey of 2000 adult men, atrophy of one or both testes was found in 2%; half of these men had had mumps.[125]

The use of chemotherapy and local radiation therapy as cancer treatment in children and adolescents can cause testicular failure. The testes of boys in early puberty are particularly susceptible to injury. Furthermore, radiation therapy to the hypothalamic-pituitary axis in children with brain tumors can result in gonadotropin deficiency or hyperprolactinemia, which, in turn, can result in gonadal insufficiency.

Androgen Resistance Syndromes

The androgen resistance syndromes are characterized by gynecomastia and varying degrees of pseudohermaphroditism. Androgens are not recognized by the peripheral tissues, including the breast and pituitary. Androgen resistance at the pituitary results in elevated serum LH levels and increased circulating testosterone. The increased serum testosterone is then aromatized peripherally, promoting gynecomastia.[127]

Reifenstein's Syndrome. First described in 1947, Reifenstein's syndrome (XY) is characterized by hypospadias, incomplete virilization, and maturational arrest during spermatogenesis, resulting in azoospermia.[128-130] Affected males have profound gynecomastia. Laboratory studies show elevated plasma LH and estradiol concentrations along with normal to high testosterone concentrations.

Kennedy Syndrome. Individuals with Kennedy syndrome, a neurodegenerative disease, have a defective androgen receptor.[131] In affected males, gynecomastia

is the combined result of decreased androgen responsiveness at the breast level and increased estrogen levels as a result of elevated androgen precursors of estradiol and estrone.

Increased Aromatase Activity

Estrogen effects on the breast may be the result of either circulating estradiol levels or locally produced estrogens. Aromatase P450 catalyzes the conversion of the C19 steroids, androstenedione, testosterone, and 16-α-hydroxyandrostenedione to estrone, estradiol, and estriol. Hence, an overabundance of substrate or increased enzymatic activity can increase estrogen concentrations and promote the development of gynecomastia.

The biologic effects of overexpression of the aromatase enzyme in male mouse transgenics caused increased mammary growth, histologic changes similar to gynecomastia, an increase in estrogen and progesterone receptors and an increase in downstream growth factors such as TGF-β and βFGF.[18,132] Use of an aromatase inhibitor leads to loss of the mammary gland phenotype.[133]

A familial form of gynecomastia has been discovered in which affected family members had elevated extragonadal aromatase activity.[134] Gain-of-function mutations in chromosome 15 have been reported to cause gynecomastia through the formation of cryptic promoters that lead to overexpression of aromatase.[135] Obesity may cause estrogen excess through increased aromatase activity in adipose tissue.

Chronic Renal Failure

Gynecomastia is common in uremic males, and 50% of males undergoing chronic hemodialysis develop gynecomastia.[136-141] Plasma LH and FSH concentrations are increased fourfold in men whose creatinine clearance rates are 4 mL per minute or less, whereas testosterone concentrations are only 30% of normal.[138] There is histologic damage to the testes, hypospermia, and a subnormal response to HCG administration, suggesting that secondary gonadal failure is the primary cause of gynecomastia.

DRUGS ASSOCIATED WITH GYNECOMASTIA

In a significant number of cases, gynecomastia is associated with drugs or chemicals that cause an increased estrogen effect on breast tissues. With some drugs or chemicals, the mechanism of action is known (Table 7-5), whereas with others it is unknown (Table 7-6). Known mechanisms include estrogen-like properties or binding of the estrogen receptor, stimulation of estrogen synthesis, supply of estrogen precursors for aromatases, damage to testicles, blockage of testosterone synthesis, blockage of androgen action, and displacement of estrogen from SHBG.

Known Mechanisms

Contact with estrogen vaginal creams can elevate circulating estrogen levels. Some of the creams contain synthetic

TABLE 7-5

Drugs associated with Gynecomastia: Known Mechanisms

Estrogen-like, or Binds the Estrogen Receptor	Stimulates Estrogen Synthesis	Supplies Precursors for Aromatase	Direct Testicular Damage	Blocks Testosterone Synthesis	Blocks Androgen Action	Displaces Estrogen from SHBG
Estrogen vaginal cream	Gonadotropins	Exogenous androgens	Busulfan	Ketoconazole	Flutamide	Spironolactone
Estrogen-containing embalming cream	Growth hormone	Androgen precursors (androstenedione, DHEA)	Nitrosourea	Spironolactone	Bicalutamide	Ethanol
Delousing powder Digitalis Clomiphene Marijuana			Vincristine Ethanol	Metronidazole Etomidate	Finasteride Cyproterone Zanoterone Cimetidine Ranitidine Spironolactone	

DHEA, dihydroepiandrosterone; SHBG, sex hormone–binding globulin.

estrogens; therefore, they may not be detected by standard estrogenic qualitative assays. An estrogen-containing embalming crème has been reported to cause gynecomastia in morticians.[142,143] Abuse of marijuana, a phytoestrogen, has also been associated with gynecomastia. It has been suggested that digitalis causes gynecomastia through its ability to bind to estrogen receptors.[144,145] The appearance of gynecomastia has been described in body builders and athletes after the administration of aromatizable androgens; gynecomastia results from the conversion of androgens to estrogens by peripheral aromatase enzymes.[146]

Drugs or chemicals cause decreased testosterone levels through direct testicular damage or by blocking testosterone synthesis or androgen action. Phenothrin, a component of delousing agents, possessing antiandrogenic activity, has been identified as the cause of an epidemic of gynecomastia among Haitian refugees in the early 1980s.[147] Chemotherapeutic agents, such as alkylating agents, cause Leydig cell and germ cell damage, resulting in primary hypogonadism. Flutamide, an antiestrogen used as treatment for prostate cancer, blocks androgen action in the peripheral tissues, whereas cimetidine blocks androgen receptors. Ketoconazole inhibits steroidogenic enzymes required for testosterone synthesis.

Spironolactone causes gynecomastia by several mechanisms. Like ketoconazole, it can block androgen production by inhibiting enzymes in the testosterone synthetic pathway (17-α-hydroxylase and 17-20-desmolase), but it can also block receptor binding of testosterone and dihydrotestosterone.[148] In addition to decreasing testosterone levels and biologic effects, spironolactone also displaces estradiol from SHBG, increasing free estrogen levels. Ethanol increases the estrogen-to-androgen ratio and also induces gynecomastia by multiple mechanisms: (1) increasing circulating levels of SHBG, which decreases free testosterone levels; (2) increasing hepatic clearance of testosterone; and (3) causing testicular damage.[149]

Unknown Mechanisms

Many drugs or chemicals are associated with gynecomastia through unknown mechanisms. They generally are listed by their category of known action: (1) cardiac agents and antihypertensives; (2) psychoactive drugs, including illegal street drugs such as amphetamines; (3) agents for infectious disease, including antivirals for human immunodeficiency virus (HIV); and (4) miscellaneous agents (see Table 7-6).

TABLE 7-6

Drugs associated with Gynecomastia: Unknown Mechanisms

Cardiac Drugs/Antihypertensives	Psychoactive Drugs	Infectious Disease Drugs	Other Drugs
Calcium channel blockers	Neuroleptics	Indinavir	Theophylline
ACE inhibitors	Diazepam	Isoniazid	Omeprazole
Amiodarone	Phenytoin	Ethionamide	Auranofin
Methyldopa	Tricyclic antidepressants	Griseofulvin	Diethylpropion
Reserpine	Haloperidol	HIV antivirals	Domperidone
Nitrates	Amphetamines		Penicillamine
			Sulindac
			Heparin

ACE, angiotensin-converting enzyme; HIV, human immunodeficiency virus.

Management of Gynecomastia

A primary concern in the evaluation of male breast enlargement is the possibility of male breast cancer. Although male breast cancer is rare, constituting only 0.2% of all male cancers, it must be included in the differential diagnosis of male breast enlargement, which also includes such disorders as neurofibroma, lymphangioma, hematoma, lipoma, and dermoid cyst. The risk of breast cancer in men with gynecomastia secondary to Klinefelter's syndrome is more than 20 times higher than in other men. Gynecomastia is otherwise not associated with an increased risk of breast cancer.[150]

On examination of the enlarged male breast, abnormalities such as asymmetry, firmness, or fixation of the breast tissue, dimpling of the overlying skin, retraction or crusting of the nipple, nipple discharge, or axillary lymphadenopathy require mammography and fine-needle biopsy for diagnosis.[151,152]

EVALUATION OF MALE BREAST ENLARGEMENT

The differentiation of gynecomastia from fatty enlargement of the breasts without glandular proliferation (pseudogynecomastia) is made by clinical examination. With the patient in a supine position, the examiner grasps the breast between the thumb and forefinger and gently moves the two digits toward the nipple. If gynecomastia is present, a firm or rubbery, mobile, disklike mound of tissue arising concentrically from beneath the nipple and areolar region will be felt. However, if the breast enlargement is caused by adipose tissue, no such disk of tissue is apparent.

Tender gynecomastia appearing during mid-to-late puberty requires only a history and physical examination, including careful palpation of the testicles. In the majority of boys, pubertal gynecomastia resolves spontaneously within 1 year. A 6-month return appointment can be scheduled. At times, the cosmetic and emotional consequences of pubertal gynecomastia warrant medical or surgical intervention.

Because gynecomastia is common in adult males, the presence of long-standing, stable breast enlargement requires minimal laboratory evaluation. A careful history, including the patient's use of medications, alcohol, and drugs such as marijuana and amphetamines, along with specific inquiry concerning the symptoms and signs of hepatic dysfunction, testicular insufficiency (decreased libido or impotence), and hyperthyroidism, most often uncovers the underlying cause of the gynecomastia. If no abnormalities are uncovered by a careful history and subsequent physical examination, laboratory assessment of hepatic, renal, and thyroid function is sufficient. As previously stated, medical or surgical intervention may be necessary based on the preferences of the patient.

Rapid onset and/or progressive gynecomastia in the adult male may require more extensive laboratory investigation. If no underlying cause of such gynecomastia is apparent from the history, physical examination, or the laboratory screening tests previously discussed, measurements of HCG, testosterone, and LH can determine the underlying cause (Fig. 7-14).

TREATMENT OF MALE BREAST ENLARGEMENT

If, during the evaluation process, an underlying cause for gynecomastia is identified, treatment is focused on the underlying cause; treatment can be as simple as stopping a medication. For gynecomastia with no known cause or for persistent gynecomastia following treatment of the underlying cause, medical and surgical therapies may be required.

Medical Therapy

Two concepts are integral to appropriate medical therapy of male breast enlargement: one, gynecomastia, especially pubertal gynecomastia, has a high rate of spontaneous regression;[151] and two, medical therapy is most effective during the active, proliferative phase of gynecomastia. After an interval of 12 months, there is increased stromal hyalinization, dilation of the ducts, and a marked reduction in epithelial proliferation.[153,154] The resulting fibrotic tissue responds poorly to medical therapy.

Danazol has been studied in several uncontrolled trials and at least one prospective placebo-controlled study. In the latter, gynecomastia cleared in 23% of the patients receiving danazol and 12% of the patients receiving placebo ($P < 0.05$).[155] The side effects of danazol include weight gain, edema, acne, muscle cramps, and nausea; these limit its usefulness.

Both clomiphene citrate and tamoxifen have been used for their antiestrogenic effects. An early study described reduction in breast size for 95% of males treated with clomiphene (50 mg/day).[156] However, a later study described a reduction in breast size for 36% of boys with pubertal gynecomastia treated with clomiphene (50 mg/day).[157] Subsequently, investigators described reduction in breast size for 64% of males treated with clomiphene (100 mg/day).[158] There were no side effects from the use of clomiphene in any of these clinical studies, although nausea, rashes, and visual problems have been noted when this drug is used in other settings. Tamoxifen (10 mg two times daily) has been studied in two randomized, double-blind studies and led to significant reduction in breast size and tenderness, without side effects.[159,160] A 3-month course of tamoxifen is a reasonable treatment strategy. Testolactone, an aromatase inhibitor, has been used in the treatment of pubertal gynecomastia and has resulted in decreases in breast size after 2 months of treatment.[161]

Surgical Therapy

The original surgical approach to gynecomastia was a simple mastectomy. However, the cosmetic results of this procedure were often unacceptable. Surgical treatment now depends on the extent of gynecomastia and the amount of associated adipose tissue. Mild or moderate

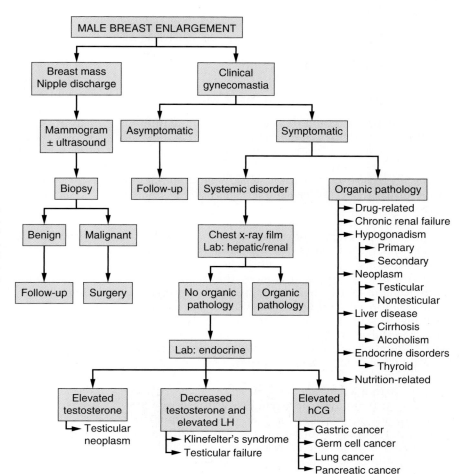

Figure 7-14 An algorithm for diagnostic approaches to the male patient with unilateral/bilateral breast mass(es) suspicious for gynecomastia. hCG, human chorionic gonadotropin; LH, luteinizing hormone. (Modified from Lucas LM, Kumar KL, Smith DL: Gynaecomastia: A worrisome problem for the patient. Postgrad Med 82:73, 1987.)

breast enlargement without skin redundancy can be dealt with by subcutaneous mastectomy through a periareolar incision.[162] Moderate or marked breast enlargement with skin redundancy can be dealt with by excising an ellipse of the areolar margin or by simple mastectomy with free nipple graft. A horizontal elliptical incision similar to that used for breast reduction procedures has been recommended for marked breast enlargement with skin redundancy and ptosis.[163]

Summary

Gynecomastia is a complex clinical entity. In review of some of the key, clinically relevant information presented in this chapter, pubertal gynecomastia and gynecomastia in the aging male are summarized in the following sections. For a more detailed discussion of these topics, see Braunstein GD.[164]

GYNECOMASTIA IN THE PUBERTAL MALE

An adolescent presenting with gynecomastia has physiologic pubertal gynecomastia in the great majority of cases. It generally appears at 13 or 14 years of age, lasts for 6 months or less, and then regresses. Fewer than 5% of affected boys have persistent gynecomastia, but this persistence is the reason that young men in their late teens or early 20s present for evaluation.

Other conditions to consider in adolescents and young adults with persistent gynecomastia are Klinefelter's syndrome, familial or sporadic excessive aromatase activity, incomplete androgen insensitivity, feminizing testicular or adrenal tumors, and hyperthyroidism.[135,165,166] Drug abuse, especially with anabolic steroids, but also with alcohol, marijuana, amphetamines, or opioids, also should be considered.[167]

Laboratory tests to determine the cause of pubertal gynecomastia without a history suggestive of an underlying pathologic cause and with an otherwise normal physical examination are unlikely to be revealing. On physical examination, careful attention must be paid to the testicles; any abnormality must be investigated using ultrasound techniques. If the gynecomastia should progress, evaluation of serum testosterone, LH, and HCG levels are appropriate.

If a specific cause of gynecomastia can be identified and treated, there may be regression of the breast enlargement. This regression most often occurs with discontinuation of an offending drug. If the gynecomastia is drug-induced, decreased tenderness and softening of the glandular tissue will usually be apparent within 1 month after discontinuation of the drug.

Because pubertal gynecomastia is self-limiting, no therapy is required in the great majority of cases. Persistent or progressive pubertal gynecomastia may cause emotional distress. In this circumstance, when there is no known cause after appropriate evaluation, simple surgical excision through a periareolar incision is sufficient.

The patient and his family must be made aware that flattening of the involved nipple may occur because of inadvertent removal of subcutaneous fat in addition to the offending breast tissue.

GYNECOMASTIA IN THE AGING MALE

Asymptomatic gynecomastia is found on examination in one third to two thirds of elderly men and at autopsy in 40% to 55% of men.[168] The condition has usually been present for months or years when it is first discovered during a physical examination. Histologic examination of the breast tissue in this setting usually shows dilated ducts with periductal fibrosis, stromal hyalinization, and increased subareolar fat.

The high prevalence of asymptomatic gynecomastia among older men raises the question of whether it should be considered to be pathologic or a part of the normal process of aging. It is likely that many cases of asymptomatic gynecomastia are due to the enhanced aromatization of androgens in subareolar fat tissue, resulting in high local concentrations of estrogens, as well as to the age-related decline in testosterone production.[169] Another possible cause is unrecognized exposure over time to unidentified environmental estrogens or antiandrogens.[170]

The pathophysiologic process of gynecomastia involves an imbalance between free estrogen and free androgen actions in the breast tissue; this imbalance can occur through multiple mechanisms. With aging, testosterone production declines. One study indicated that 50% of men in their 70s have a low free testosterone concentration.[171]

The first step in the clinical evaluation of the elderly male is to determine whether the enlarged breast tissue or mass is gynecomastia. Pseudogynecomastia is characterized by increased subareolar fat without enlargement of the breast glandular component. The differentiation between gynecomastia and pseudogynecomastia is made on physical examination. In the elderly population, breast cancer is also a concern. Nipple discharge is present in approximately 10% of men with breast cancer, but it is not expected with gynecomastia.[172] If the differentiation between gynecomastia and breast carcinoma cannot be made on the basis of clinical findings alone, the patient should undergo diagnostic mammography, which has 90% sensitivity and specificity for distinguishing malignant from benign breast diseases.[173]

There is no uniformity of opinion regarding what biochemical evaluation, if any, should be performed in an aging male with asymptomatic gynecomastia. In a retrospective study of 87 men with symptomatic gynecomastia, 16% had apparent liver or renal disease, 21% had drug-induced gynecomastia, and 2% had hyperthyroidism, whereas 61% were considered to have idiopathic gynecomastia. Forty-five of the 53 patients in the group with idiopathic gynecomastia underwent endocrine testing, of whom only 1 patient (2%) was found to have an endocrine abnormality—an occult Leydig-cell testicular tumor.[174]

Once the diagnosis of gynecomastia is established, it is important to review all medications, including over-the-counter drugs such as herbal products, which may contain phytoestrogens. Ingestion of sex steroid hormones or their precursors may cause gynecomastia through bioconversion to estrogens. Antiandrogens used for the treatment of prostate cancer, spironolactone, cimetidine, and one or more components of highly active antiviral therapy used for HIV infection (especially protease inhibitors) have been clearly shown to be associated with gynecomastia.[170,175-180] Several drugs used for cancer chemotherapy, particularly alkylating agents, can damage the testes and result in primary hypogonadism.

If an adult presents with unilateral or bilateral gynecomastia that has a rapid onset and is progressive, and if the patient's history and physical examination do not reveal the cause, HCG, LH, and testosterone should be measured. Many of the available measurements of testosterone have poor accuracy and precision, especially in men with testosterone levels at the low end of the normal range.[181] Measurement of these levels in the morning is recommended, because testosterone and LH secretion have a circadian rhythm, with the highest levels in the morning, as well as secretory bursts throughout the day. If the total testosterone level is borderline or low, free or bioavailable testosterone should be measured or calculated to confirm hypogonadism. Although such laboratory evaluation is prudent, no abnormalities are detected in the majority of patients.

If a specific cause of gynecomastia can be identified and treated during the painful proliferative phase, there may be regression of the breast enlargement. This regression most often occurs with discontinuation of an offending drug or after initiation of testosterone treatment for primary hypogonadism. If the gynecomastia is drug-induced, decreased tenderness and softening of the glandular tissue will usually be apparent within 1 month after discontinuation of the drug. However, if the gynecomastia has been present for more than 1 year, it is unlikely to regress substantially, either spontaneously or with medical therapy, because of the presence of fibrosis. In such circumstances, surgical removal, with or without liposuction, is the best option for cosmetic improvement.[182]

Tamoxifen

Although tamoxifen is not approved for the treatment of gynecomastia, this selective estrogen receptor modulator, administered orally at a dose of 20 mg daily for up to 3 months, has been shown to be effective in randomized and nonrandomized trials.[183-186] The result is partial regression of gynecomastia in approximately 80% of patients and complete regression in about 60%. Patients in whom tamoxifen is effective usually experience a decrease in pain and tenderness within 1 month. In a retrospective analysis of a series of patients with idiopathic gynecomastia, 78% of patients treated with tamoxifen had complete resolution of gynecomastia, compared with only 40% of patients receiving danazol.[183] In case series describing the use of tamoxifen for this condition in more than 225 patients, adverse events were uncommon.

Although tamoxifen has been used in men treated for prostate cancer, it is not approved by the U.S. Food and Drug Administration for this indication. However, it has been suggested that therapy with tamoxifen may prevent the development of gynecomastia in men receiving monotherapy with high doses of bicalutamide (Casodex) for prostate cancer. In a randomized, double-blind, controlled trial involving men receiving high-dose bicalutamide (150 mg per day),[187] gynecomastia occurred in 10% of patients who received tamoxifen at a dose of 20 mg daily, but it occurred in 51% of those who received anastrozole at a dose of 1 mg daily and in 73% of those who received placebo, over a period of 48 weeks. Mastalgia occurred in 6%, 27%, and 39% of these patients, respectively. In another trial involving 3 months of therapy, gynecomastia, mastalgia, or both occurred in 69.4% of patients receiving placebo, 11.8% receiving tamoxifen ($P < 0.001$ for comparison with placebo), and 63.9% receiving anastrozole (not significantly different from the rate in the placebo group).[188]

Among patients treated with bicalutamide alone, gynecomastia occurred in 68.6% and mastalgia occurred in 56.8%. These rates were significantly lower among patients receiving one 12-Gy fraction of radiation therapy to the breast on the first day of treatment with bicalutamide (34% and 30%, respectively), and they were further reduced among patients receiving bicalutamide and tamoxifen (8% and 6%, respectively).[189]

REFERENCES

1. Schmidt-Voigt J: Brustdruenschwellungen bei mannlichen Jugendlichen des Pubertatsalters (Pubertatsmakromastie). Z Kinderheilkd 62:590–606, 1941.
2. Hall PF: Gynaecomastia. Glebe, New South Wales, Australia, Australasian Medical, 1959.
3. Schydlower M: Breast masses in adolescents. Am Fam Physician 25:141–145, 1982.
4. Franz A, Wilson J: Williams textbook of endocrinology, 9th ed. St. Louis, WB Saunders, 1998, pp 877–885.
5. Wilson JD, Aiman J, MacDonald PC: The pathogenesis of gynecomastia. Adv Intern Med 25:1–32, 1980.
6. Rochefort H, Garcia M: The estrogenic and antiestrogenic activities of androgens in female target tissues. Pharmacol Ther 23:193–216, 1983.
7. Edmondson HA, Glass SJ, Soll SN: Gynecomastia associated with cirrhosis of the liver. Proc Soc Exp Biol Med 42:97–99, 1939.
8. Bidlingmaier F, Knorr D: Plasma testosterone and estrogens in pubertal gynecomastia. Z Kinderheilkd 115:89–94, 1973.
9. Sasano H, Kimura M, Shizawa S, et al: Aromatase and steroid receptors in gynecomastia and male breast cancer: an immunohistochemical study. J Clin Endocrinol Metab 81:3063–3067, 1996.
10. Smals AGH: Gynaecomastia. Neth J Med 31:47–51, 1987.
11. Weinstein RL, Kelch RP, Jenner MR, et al: Secretion of unconjugated androgens and estrogens by the normal and abnormal human testis before and after human chorionic gonadotropin. J Clin Invest 53:1–6, 1974.
12. Bronstein IP, Cassorla E: Breast enlargement in pediatric practice. Med Clin North Am 30:121, 1946.
13. Lee PA: The relationship of concentrations of serum hormones to pubertal gynecomastia. J Pediatr 86:212–215, 1975.
14. Niewoehner CB, Nuttall FQ: Gynecomastia in a hospitalized male population. Am J Med 77:633–638, 1984.
15. Snyder PF: Effect of age on the serum LH and FSH responses to gonadotropin-releasing hormone. In Geep RO, Aswood (eds): Handbook of physiology, vol 2, part 1. Baltimore, Waverly Press, 1973.
16. Siiteri PK, MacDonald PC: Role of extraglandular estrogen in human endocrinology. In Geep RO, Aswood (eds): Handbook of physiology, vol 2, part 1. Baltimore, Waverly Press, 1973.
17. Karsner HT: Gynecomastia. Am J Pathol 22:235, 1946.
18. Nicolis GL, Modlinger RS, Gabrilove JL: A study of the histopathology of human gynecomastia. J Clin Endocrinol Metab 32:173–178, 1971.
19. Gottfried MR: Extensive squamous metaplasia in gynecomastia. Arch Pathol Lab Med 110:971–973, 1986.
20. Bannayan GA, Hajdu SI: Gynecomastia: clinicopathologic study of 351 cases. Am J Clin Pathol 57:431–437, 1972.
21. Andersen J, Orntoft TF, Andersen JA, Poulson HS: Gynecomastia: Immunohistochemical demonstration of estrogen receptors. Acta Pathol Microbiol Immunol Scand 95:263–267, 1987.
22. Fodor PB: Breast cancer in a patient with gynecomastia. Plast Reconstr Surg 84:976–979, 1989.
23. Ajayi DO, Osegbe DN, Ademiluyi SA: Carcinoma of the male breast in West Africans and a review of world literature. Cancer 50:1664–1667, 1982.
24. Johnson RL: The male breast and gynaecomastia. In Page DL, Anderson TJ (eds): Diagnostic histopathology of the breast. New York, Churchill Livingstone, 1988.
25. Visfeldt J, Scheike O: Male breast cancer: Histologic typing and grading of 187 Danish cases. Cancer 32:985–990, 1973.
26. Odagiri E, Kanada N, Jibiki K, et al: Reduction of telomeric length and c-erbB-2 gene amplification in human breast cancer, fibroadenoma, and gynecomastia. Cancer 73:2978–2984, 1994.
27. Castle WN, Richardson JR Jr: Leydig cell tumor and metachronous Leydig cell hyperplasia: A case associated with gynecomastia and elevated urinary estrogens. J Urol 136:1307–1308, 1986.
28. Hemsell DL, Edman CD, Marks JF, et al: Massive extraglandular aromatization of plasma androstenedione resulting in the feminization of a prepubertal boy. J Clin Invest 60:455–464, 1977.
29. Brosman SA: Testicular tumors in prepubertal children. Urology 13:581–588, 1979.
30. Camin AJ, Dorfman RI, McDonald JH, Rosenthal IM: Interstitial cell tumor of the testis in a seven-year-old child. Am J Dis Child 100:389–399, 1960.
31. Mostofi FK, Price EB: Tumors of the testis in children. In Tumors of the male genital system, atlas of tumor pathology, series 2, fasc 16. Washington, DC, Armed Forces Institute of Pathology, 1973.
32. Symington T, Cameron KM: Endocrine and genetic lesions. In Pugh RCB (ed): Pathology of testes. Oxford, Blackwell, 1976.
33. Turner WR, Derrick FC, Wohltmann H: Leydig cell tumor in identical twins. Urology 7:194–197, 1976.
34. Caldamone AA, Altebarmakian V, Frank IN, Linke CA: Leydig cell tumor of the testis. Urology 14:39–43, 1979.
35. Mostofi FK, Price EB: Tumors of the testis. In Tumors of the male genital system, atlas of tumor pathology, series 2, part 8. Washington, DC, Armed Forces Institute of Pathology, 1973.
36. Mostofi FK, Price EB: Tumors of specialized gonadal stroma. In Tumors of the male genital system, atlas of tumor pathology, fasc. 8. Washington, DC, Armed Forces Institute of Pathology, 1973.
37. Brogard JM, Maurer C, Philippe E: Gyneácomastia et tumeur aá cellules de Leydig. Press Med 75:1253–1255, 1967.
38. Fligiel Z, Kaneko M, Leiter E: Bilateral Sertoli cell tumor of the testes with feminizing and masculinizing activity occurring in a child. Cancer 38:1853–1858, 1976.
39. Lucas LM, Kumar KL, Smith DL: Gynecomastia: A worrisome problem for the patient. Postgrad Med 82:73–76, 79–81, 1987.
40. Pierrepoint CG: The metabolism in vitro of dehydro epiandrosterone and hydroepiandrosterone sulphate by Sertoli cell tumours of the testis of two dogs with clinical signs of hyperoestrogenism. J Endocrinol 42:99, 1968.
41. Gabrilove JL: Some recent advances in virilizing and feminizing syndrome and hirsutism. Mt Sinai J Med 41:636–654, 1974.
42. Gabrilove JL, Freiberg EK, Leiter E, Nicolis GL: Feminizing and nonfeminizing Sertoli cell tumors. J Urol 124:757–767, 1980.
43. Davis S, DiMartino NA, Schneider G: Malignant interstitial cell carcinoma of the testis: Report of two cases with steroid profiles, response to therapy, and review of the literature. Cancer 47:425–431, 1981.
44. Selvaggi FP, Young RT, Brown DR, Dick AL: Interstitial cell tumor of the testis in an adult: Two case reports. J Urol 109:436–439, 1973.

45. Kuhn JM, Reznik Y, Mahoudeau JA, et al: hCG test in gynaecomastia: Further study. Clin Endocrinol 31:581–590, 1989.
46. Hopkins GB, Parry HD: Metastasizing Sertoli cell tumor. Cancer 23:463–467, 1969.
47. Richie JP: Neoplasms of the testis. In Campbell MF, Walsh PC (eds): Campbell's urology, vol 2, 6th ed. Philadelphia, WB Saunders, 1992.
48. Fligiel Z, Kaneko M, Leiter E: Bilateral Sertoli cell tumor of the testes with feminizing and masculinizing activity occurring in a child. Cancer 38:1853–1858, 1976.
49. Proppe KH, Scully RE: Large-cell calcifying Sertoli cell tumor of the testis. Am J Clin Pathol 74:607–619, 1980.
50. Wilson DM, Pitts WC, Hintz RL, Rosenfeld RG: Testicular tumors with Peutz-Jeghers syndrome. Cancer 57:2238–2240, 1986.
51. Young S, Gooneratne S, Straus FH 2nd, et al: Feminizing Sertoli cell tumors in boys with Peutz-Jeghers syndrome. Am J Surg Pathol 19:50–58, 1995.
52. Scully RE: Sex cord tumor with annular tubules: A distinctive ovarian tumor of the Peutz-Jeghers syndrome. Cancer 25:1107–1121, 1970.
53. Rosvoll RV, Woodard JR: Malignant Sertoli cell tumor of the testis. Cancer 22:8–13, 1968.
54. Kaplan GW, Cromie WJ, Kelalis PP, et al: Gonadal stromal tumors: A report of the prepubertal testicular tumor registry. J Urol 136:300–302, 1986.
55. Pierce GB Jr, Stevens LC, Nakane PK: Ultrastructural analysis of the early development of teratocarcinomas. J Natl Cancer Inst 39:755–773, 1967.
56. Stevens LC: Experimental production of testicular teratomas in mice. Proc Natl Acad Sci USA 52:654–661, 1964.
57. Stevens LC, Hummel KP: A description of spontaneous congenital teratomas in strain 129 mice. J Natl Cancer Inst 18:719–747, 1957.
58. Bardin CW: Pituitary-testicular axis. In Yen SSC, Jaffe RB (eds): Reproductive endocrinology. Philadelphia, WB Saunders, 1978.
59. Stephanas AV, Samaan NA, Schultz PN, Holoye PY: Endocrine studies in testicular tumor patients with and without gynecomastia. Cancer 41:369–376, 1978.
60. Tseng A, Horning SJ, Freiha FS, et al: Gynecomastia in testicular cancer patients: Prognostic and therapeutic implications. Cancer 56:2534–2538, 1985.
61. Hendry WS, Garvie WH, Ah-See WK, Bayliss AP: Ultrasonic detection of occult testicular neoplasms in patients with gynaecomastia. Br J Radiol 57:571–572, 1984.
62. Emory TH, Charboneau JW, Randall RV, et al: Occult testicular interstitial-cell tumor in a patient with gynecomastia: Ultrasonic detection. Radiology 151:474, 1984.
63. Ogle JW: Unusually large mass of carcinomatous deposit in one of the suprarenal capsules of a child. Trans Pathol Soc Lond 16:250, 1865.
64. Hayles AB, Hahn HB Jr, Sprague RG, et al: Hormone-secreting tumors of the adrenal cortex in children. Pediatrics 37:19–25, 1966.
65. Bittorf A: Nebennieren tumor and geschlechtsdrusenausfall beim mann. Berl Klin Wochenschr 56:776, 1919.
66. Wittenberg J: Computed tomography of the body. N Engl J Med 309:1224–1229, 1983.
67. Page DL, DeLellis RA, Hough AF Jr: Tumors of the adrenal. In Atlas of tumor pathology, second series, fasc 23. Washington, DC, Armed Forces Institute of Pathology, 1985.
68. Malchoff CD, Rosa J, DeBold CR, et al: Adrenocorticotropin-independent bilateral macronodular adrenal hyperplasia: An unusual cause of Cushing's syndrome. J Clin Endocrinol Metab 68:855–860, 1989.
69. Thompson NW, Cheung PSY: Diagnosis and treatment of functioning and nonfunctioning adrenocortical neoplasms including incidentalomas. Surg Clin North Am 67:423–436, 1987.
70. Smith LG, Lyubsky SL, Carlson HE: Postmenopausal uterine bleeding due to estrogen production by gonadotropin-secreting lung tumors. Am J Med 92:327–330, 1992.
71. Fusco FD, Rosen SW: Gonadotropin-producing anaplastic large-cell carcinomas of the lung. N Engl J Med 275:507–515, 1966.
72. Dailey JE, Marcuse PM: Gonadotropin secreting giant cell carcinoma of the lung. Cancer 24:388–396, 1969.
73. Stedman KE, Moore GE, Morgan RT: Estrogen receptor proteins in diverse human tumours. Arch Surg 115:244–248, 1980.
74. Iqbal MJ, Wilkinson ML, Johnson PJ, Williams R: Sex steroid receptor proteins in foetal, adult and malignant human liver tissue. Br J Cancer 48:791–796, 1983.
75. Van Niekerk WA: True hermaphroditism: An analytic view with a report of three new cases. Am J Obstet Gynecol 126:890–907, 1976.
76. Aiman J, Hemsell DL, MacDonald PC: Production and origin of estrogen in two true hermaphrodites. Am J Obstet Gynecol 132:401–409, 1978.
77. Gallegos AJ: Familial true hermaphroditism in three siblings: Plasma hormonal profile and in vitro steroid biosynthesis in gonadal structures. J Clin Endocrinol Metab 42:653–660, 1976.
78. Castro-Magana M, Angulo M, Uy J: Male hypogonadism with gynecomastia caused by late-onset deficiency of testicular 17-ketosteroid reductase. N Engl J Med 328:1297–1301, 1993.
79. Hall PH: Gynaecomastia. Monographs of the Federal Council of the British Medical Association in Australia, No. 2, 1959.
80. Larsson O, Sundbom CM, Astedt B: Gynaecomastia and diseases of the thyroid. Acta Endocrinol 44:133–138, 1963.
81. Chopra IJ, Tulchinsky D: Status of estrogen-androgen balance in hyperthyroid men with Graves' disease. J Clin Endocrinol Metab 38:269–277, 1974.
82. Nomura K, Suzuki H, Saji M, et al: High serum progesterone in hyperthyroid men with Graves' disease. J Clin Endocrinol Metab 66:230–232, 1988.
83. Chopra IJ: Gonadal steroids and gonadotropins in hyperthyroidism. Med Clin North Am 59:1109–1121, 1975.
84. Kley HK, Nieschlag E, Wiegelmann W, et al: Steroid hormones and their binding in plasma of male patients with fatty liver, chronic hepatitis and liver cirrhosis. Acta Endocrinol 79:275–285, 1975.
85. Baker HW, et al: Endocrine aspects of hepatic cirrhosis. Washington, DC, Fourth International Endocrine Congress (abstract), June 1972.
86. Baker HW, Burger HG, de Krester DM, et al: A study of the endocrine manifestations of hepatic cirrhosis. Q J Med 45:145–178, 1976.
87. Galväo-Teles A, Burke CW, Anderson DC, et al: Biologically active androgens and oestradiol in men with chronic liver disease. Lancet 1:173–177, 1973.
88. Lloyd CW, Williams RH: Endocrine changes associated with Laennec's cirrhosis of the liver. Am J Med 4:315–330, 1948.
89. Powell LW, Mortimer R, Harris OD: Cirrhosis of the liver: A comparative study of the four major aetiological groups. Med J Aust 1:941–950, 1971.
90. Southren AL, Gordon GG, Olivo J, et al: Androgen metabolism in cirrhosis of the liver. Metabolism 22:695–701, 1973.
91. Summerskill WH, Davidson CS, Dible JH, et al: Cirrhosis of the liver: A study of alcoholic and nonalcoholic patients in Boston and London. N Engl J Med 262:1–9, 1960.
92. Kley HK, Niederau C, Stremmel W, et al: Conversion of androgens to estrogens in idiopathic hemochromatosis: Comparison with alcoholic liver cirrhosis. J Clin Endocrinol Metab 61:1–6, 1985.
93. Van Thiel DH, Lester R, Sherins RJ: Hypogonadism in alcoholic liver disease: Evidence for a double defect. Gastroenterology 67:1188–1199, 1974.
94. Chopra IJ, Tulchinsky D, Greenway FL: Estrogen-androgen imbalance in hepatic cirrhosis: Studies in 13 male patients. Ann Intern Med 79:198–203, 1973.
95. Kent JR, Scaramuzzi RJ, Lauwers W, et al: Plasma testosterone, estradiol and gonadotrophins in hepatic insufficiency. Gastroenterology 64:111–115, 1973.
96. Pincus IJ, Rakoff AE, Cohn EM, Tumen EH: Hormonal studies in patients with chronic liver disease. Gastroenterology 19:735–754, 1951.
97. Mowat NAG, Edwards CR, Fisher R, et al: Hypothalamic-pituitary-gonadal function in men with cirrhosis of the liver. Gut 17:345–350, 1976.
98. Rosenbaum W, Christy NP, Kelly WG: Electrophoretic evidence for the presence of an estrogen-binding globulin in human plasma. J Clin Endocrinol Metab 26:1399–1403, 1966.
99. Rosner W: A simplified method for the quantitative determination of testosterone-estradiol-binding globulin activity in human plasma. J Clin Endocrinol Metab 34:983–988, 1972.

100. Vermeulen A, et al: Capacity of the testosterone-binding globulin in human plasma and influence of specific binding of testosterone on its metabolic clearance rate. J Clin Endocrinol Metab 29:1470, 1969.
101. Anderson DC: Sex-hormonal-binding globulin. Clin Endocrinol 3:69–96, 1974.
102. Gordon GG, Altman K, Southren AL, et al: Effect of alcohol (ethanol) administration on sex-hormone metabolism in normal men. N Engl J Med 295:793–797, 1976.
103. Gordon GG, Olivo J, Rafil F, Southren AL: Conversion of androgens to estrogens in cirrhosis of the liver. J Clin Endocrinol Metab 40:1018–1026, 1975.
104. Horton R, Tait JF: Androstenedione production and interconversion rates measured in peripheral blood and studies on the possible site of its conversion to testosterone. J Clin Invest 45:301–313, 1966.
105. Green JRB, Mowat MA, Fisher RA, Anderson DC: Plasma oestrogens in men with chronic liver disease. Gut 17:426–430, 1976.
106. Green JRB: Mechanism of hypogonadism in cirrhotic males. Gut 18:843–853, 1977.
107. Jacobs EC: Effects of starvation on sex hormones in the male. J Clin Endocrinol 8:227–232, 1948.
108. Klatskin G, Saltin WT, Humm FD: Gynecomastia due to malnutrition. Am J Med Sci 213:19, 1947.
109. Zubiran S, Gomez-Mont F: Endocrine disturbances in chronic human malnutrition. Vitam Horm 11:97–132, 1953.
110. Klinefelter HF, Reifenstein EC, Albright F: Syndrome characterized by gynecomastia, aspermatogenesis without aleydigism, and increased excretion of follicle-stimulating hormone. J Clin Endocrinol 2:615, 1942.
111. Gerald PS: Sex chromosome disorders. N Engl J Med 294:707–708, 1976.
112. Salbenblatt JA, Bender BG, Puck MH, et al: Pituitary-gonadal function in Klinefelter syndrome before and during puberty. Pediatr Res 19:82–86, 1985.
113. Ferguson-Smith MA: The prepubertal testicular lesion in chromatin-positive Klinefelter's syndrome (primary micro-orchidism) as seen in mentally handicapped children. Lancet 1:219–222, 1959.
114. Forti G, Giusti G, Borghi A, et al: Klinefelter's syndrome: A study of its hormonal plasma pattern. J Endocrinol Invest 2:149–154, 1978.
115. Cole EW: Klinefelter's syndrome and breast cancer. Johns Hopkins Med J 138:105, 1976.
116. Jackson AW, Muldal S, Ockey CH, O'Connor CH: Carcinoma of the male breast in association with the Klinefelter syndrome. BMJ 1:223–225, 1965.
117. Robson MC, Santiago Q, Huang TW: Bilateral carcinoma of the breast in a patient with Klinefelter's syndrome. J Clin Endocrinol Metabol 28:897–902, 1968.
118. Wilson JD, Aiman J, MacDonald PC: The pathogenesis of gynecomastia. Adv Intern Med 25:1–32, 1980.
119. Wilson JD, Harrod MJ, Goldstein JL, et al: Familial incomplete male pseudohermaphroditism, type 1: Evidence for androgen resistance and variable clinical manifestations in a family with the Reifenstein syndrome. N Engl J Med 290:1097–1103, 1982.
120. Bongiovanni AM: Congenital adrenal hyperplasia and related conditions. In Stanbury JB, Wyngaarden JB, Fredrickson DS (eds): The metabolic basis of inherited disease. New York, McGraw-Hill, 1978.
121. Griffin JE, Wilson JD: Hereditary male pseudohermaphroditism. Clin Obstet Gynecol 5:457–479, 1978.
122. Wilson JD, Goldstein JL: Classification of hereditary disorders of sexual development. Birth Defects Orig Art Ser 11:1–16, 1975.
123. Hochberg Z, Even L, Zadik Z: Mineralocorticoids in the mechanism of gynecomastia in adrenal hyperplasia caused by 11β-hydroxylase deficiency. J Pediatr 118:258–260, 1991.
124. Braunstein G: Aromatase and gynecomastia. Endocr Relat Cancer 6:315–324, 1999.
125. Riggs S, Sanford JP: Viral orchitis. N Engl J Med 266:990–993, 1962.
126. Kirkland RT, Bongiovanni AM, Cornfield D, et al: Gonadotropin responses to luteinizing releasing factor in boys treated with cyclophosphamide for nephrotic syndrome. J Pediatr 89:941–944, 1976.
127. Mathur R, Braunstein G: Gynecomastia: Pathomechanisms and treatment strategies. Hormone Research 48:95–102, 1997.
128. Amrhein JA, Klingensmith GJ, Walsh PC, et al: Partial androgen insensitivity: The Reifenstein syndrome revisited. N Engl J Med 297:350–356, 1977.
129. Reifenstein EC Jr: Hereditary familial hypogonadism. Proc Am Fed Clin Res 3:86, 1947.
130. Wilson JD, Harrod MJ, Goldstein JL, et al: Familial incomplete male pseudohermaphroditism, type 1: Evidence for androgen resistance and variable clinical manifestations in a family with the Reifenstein syndrome. N Engl J Med 290:1097–1103, 1982.
131. Hertl RJ, Wiebel J, Schafer H, et al: Feminizing Sertoli cell tumors associated with Peutz-Jeghers syndrome: An increasingly recognized cause of prepubertal gynecomastia. Plast Reconstr Surg 102:1151–1157, 1998.
132. Gill K, Kirma N, Ekmal RR: Overexpression of aromatase in transgenic male mice results in the induction of gynecomastia, and other biologic changes in mammary gland. J Steroid Biochem Mol Biol 77:13–18, 2001.
133. Li X, Warri A, Makela S, et al: Mammary gland development in transgenic male mice expressing human P450 aromatase. Endocrinology 143:4074–4083, 2002.
134. Berkovitz GD, Guerami, Brown TR, et al: Familial gynecomastia with increased extraglandular aromatization of plasma carbon 19-steroids, J Clin Invest 75:1763–1769, 1985.
135. Shozu M, Sebastian S, Takayama K, et al: Estrogen excess associated with novel gain-of-function mutations affecting the aromatase gene. N Engl J Med 8;348:1855–1865, 2003.
136. Freeman RM, Lawton RL, Fearing MO: Gynecomastia: An endocrinologic complication of hemodialysis. Ann Intern Med 69:67–72, 1968.
137. Gupta D, Bundschu HD: Testosterone and its binding in the plasma of male subjects with chronic renal failure. Clin Chim Acta 36:479–484, 1972.
138. Holdsworth MB, Atkins RC, de Kretser DM: The pituitary testicular axis in men with chronic renal failure. N Engl J Med 296:1245–1249, 1977.
139. Nagel TC, Freinkel N, Bell RH, et al: Gynecomastia, prolactin, and other peptide hormones in patients undergoing chronic hemodialysis. J Clin Endocrinol Metab 36:428–432, 1973.
140. Sawin CT, Longscope C, Schmitt GW, Ryan RJ: Blood levels of gonadotropins and gonadal hormones in gynecomastia associated with chronic hemodialysis. J Clin Endocrinol Metab 36:988–990, 1973.
141. Schmitt GW, Shehadeh I, Sawin CT: Transient gyneco mastia in chronic renal failure during chronic intermittent hemodialysis, Ann Intern Med 69:73–79, 1968.
142. Bhat N, Rosato E, Gupta P: Gynecomastia in a mortician: A case report. Acta Cytol 34:31–34, 1990.
143. Finkelstein J, McCully W, MacLaughlin D, et al: The mortician's mystery: Gynecomastia and reversible hypogonadotrophic hypogonadism in an embalmer. N Eng J Med 318:961–965, 1988.
144. Glass AR: Gynaecomastia. Endocrinol Metab Clin North Am 23:825–837, 1994.
145. Rifka SM, Pita JC, Vigersky RA, et al: Interaction of digitalis and spironolactone with human sex steroid receptors. J Clin Endocrinol Metab 46:338–344, 1978.
146. Caldaza L, Torres-Calleja JM, Martinez N: Measurement of androgen and estrogen receptors in breast tissue from subjects with anabolic steroid-dependent gynecomastia. Life Sci 69:1465–1479.
147. Brody SA, Loriaux DL: Epidemic of gynecomastia among Haitian refugees: Exposure to an environmental antiandrogen. Endocr Pract 9:370–375, 2003.
148. Thompson DF, Carter J: Drug-induced gynecomastia. Pharmacotherapy 13:37–45, 1993.
149. Mathur R, Braunstein GD: Gynecomastia: Differential diagnosis and management. Pediatr Clin North Am 37:1389–1404, 1990.
150. Waterfall NB, Glaser MG: A study of the effects of radiation on prevention of gynaecomastia due to oestrogen therapy. Clin Oncol 5:257–260, 1979.
151. Treves N: Gynecomastia: The origins of mammary swelling in the male: An analysis of 406 patients with breast hypertrophy, 525 with testicular tumors, and 13 with adrenal neoplasms. Cancer 11:1083–1102, 1958.

152. Gupta RK, Naran S, Simpson J: The role of fine needle aspiration cytology (FNAC) in the diagnosis of breast masses in males. Eur J Surg Oncol 14:317–320, 1988.

153. Williams MJ: Gynecomastia: Its incidence, recognition and host characterization in 447 autopsy cases. Am J Med 34:103–112, 1963.

154. Andersen JA, Gram JB: Male breast at autopsy. Acta Pathol Microbiol Immunol Scand [A] 90:191–197, 1982.

155. Jones DJ, Holt SD, Surtees P, Davison DJ, Coptcoat MJ: A comparison of danazol and placebo in the treatment of adult idiopathic gynaecomastia: Results of a prospective study in 55 patients. Ann R Coll Surg Engl 72:296–298, 1990.

156. Plourde PV, Kulin HE, Santner SJ: Clomiphene in the treatment of adolescent gynecomastia: Clinical and endocrine studies. Am J Dis Child 137:1080–1082, 1983.

157. LeRoith D, Sobel R, Glick SM: The effect of clomiphene citrate on pubertal gynaecomastia. Acta Endocrinol (Copenh) 95:177–180, 1980.

158. Parker LN, Gray DR, Lai MK, Levin ER: Treatment of gynecomastia with tamoxifen: A double-blind crossover study. Metabolism 35:705–708, 1986.

159. McDermott MT, Hofeldt FD, Kidd GS: Tamoxifen therapy for painful idiopathic gynecomastia. South Med J 83:1283–1285, 1990.

160. Zachmann M, Eiholzer U, Muritano M, et al: Treatment of pubertal gynaecomastia with testolactone. Acta Endocrinol Suppl (Copenh) 279:218–226, 1986.

161. Alagaratnam TT: Idiopathic gynaecomastia treated with tamoxifen: A preliminary report. Clin Ther 9:483–487, 1987.

162. Webster JP: Mastectomy for gynecomastia through a semicircular intra-areolar incision. Ann Surg 124:557–575, 1946.

163. Ward CM, Khalid K: Surgical treatment of grade III gynaecomastia. Ann R Coll Surg Engl 71:226–228, 1989.

164. Braunstein GD: Gynecomastia. N Engl J Med 357:1229–1237, 2007.

165. Ersöz HO, Önde ME, Terekeci H, et al: Causes of gynaecomastia in young adult males and factors associated with idiopathic gynaecomastia. Int J Androl 25:312–316, 2002.

166. Dejager S, Bry-Gauillard H, Bruckert E, et al: A comprehensive endocrine description of Kennedy's disease revealing androgen insensitivity linked to CAG repeat length. J Clin Endocrinol Metab 87:3893–3901, 2002.

167. Irving LM, Wall M, Neumark-Sztainer D, Story M: Steroid use among adolescents: Findings from Project EAT. J Adolesc Health 30:243–252, 2002.

168. Ley SJ: Cardiac surgery in an era of antiplatelet therapies: Generating new evidence. Reflect Nurs Leadership 28:35–35, 2002.

169. Labrie F, Luu-The V, Labrie C, et al: Endocrine and intracrine sources of androgens in women: Inhibition of breast cancer and other roles of androgens and their precursor dehydroepiandrosterone. Endocr Rev 24:152–182, 2003.

170. Henley DV, Lipson N, Korach KS, Bloch CA: Prepubertal gynecomastia linked to lavender and tea tree oils. N Engl J Med 356:479–485, 2007.

171. Harman SM, Metter EJ, Tobin JD, et al: Longitudinal effects of aging on serum total and free testosterone levels in healthy men. J Clin Endocrinol Metab 86:724–731, 2001.

172. Giordano SH, Buzdar AU, Hortobagyi GN: Breast cancer in men. Ann Intern Med 137:678–687, 2002.

173. Evans GF, Anthony T, Turnage RH, et al: The diagnostic accuracy of mammography in the evaluation of male breast disease. Am J Surg 181:96–100, 2001. [Erratum, Am J Surg 181:579, 2001.]

174. Bowers SP, Pearlman NW, McIntyre RC Jr, et al: Cost-effective management of gynecomastia. Am J Surg 176:638–641, 1998.

175. Brody SA, Loriaux DL: Epidemic of gynecomastia among Haitian refugees: Exposure to an environmental antiandrogen. Endocr Pract 9:370–375, 2003.

176. Rahim S, Ortiz O, Maslow M, Holzman R: A case-control study of gynecomastia in HIV-1-infected patients receiving HAART. AIDS Read 14:23–24, 29, 2004.

177. Di Lorenzo G, Autorino R, Perdonà S, De Placido S: Management of gynaecomastia in patients with prostate cancer: A systematic review. Lancet Oncol 6:972–979, 2005.

178. Satoh T, Fujita KI, Munakata H, et al: Studies on the interactions between drugs and estrogen: Analytical method for prediction system of gynecomastia induced by drugs on the inhibitory metabolism of estradiol using *Escherichia coli* coexpressing human CYP3A4 with human NADPH-cytochrome P450 reductase. Anal Biochem 286:179–186, 2000.

179. Satoh T, Munakata H, Fujita K, et al: Studies on the interactions between drugs and estrogen. II. On the inhibitory effect of 29 drugs reported to induce gynecomastia on the oxidation of estradiol at C-2 or C-17. Biol Pharm Bull 26:695–700, 2003.

180. Satoh T, Tomikawa Y, Takanashi K, et al: Studies on the interactions between drugs and estrogen. III. Inhibitory effects of 29 drugs reported to induce gynecomastia on the glucuronidation of estradiol. Biol Pharm Bull 27:1844–1849, 2004.

181. Rosner W, Auchus RJ, Azziz R, et al: Utility, limitations, and pitfalls in measuring testosterone: An Endocrine Society position statement. J Clin Endocrinol Metab 92:405–413, 2007.

182. Rohrich RJ, Ha RY, Kenkel JM, Adams WP Jr: Classification and management of gynecomastia: Defining the role of ultrasound-assisted liposuction. Plast Reconstr Surg 111:909–923, 2003.

183. Ting ACW, Chow LWC, Leung YF: Comparison of tamoxifen with danazol in the management of idiopathic gynecomastia. Am Surg 66:38–40, 2000.

184. Khan HN, Rampaul R, Blamey RW: Management of physiological gynaecomastia with tamoxifen. Breast 13:61–65, 2004.

185. Lawrence SE, Faught KA, Vethamuthu J, Lawson ML: Beneficial effects of raloxifene and tamoxifen in the treatment of pubertal gynecomastia. J Pediatr 145:71–76, 2004.

186. Hanavadi S, Banerjee D, Monypenny IJ, Mansel RE: The role of tamoxifen in the management of gynaecomastia. Breast 15:276–280, 2006.

187. Boccardo F, Rubagotti A, Battaglia M, et al: Evaluation of tamoxifen and anastrozole in the prevention of gynecomastia and breast pain induced by bicalutamide monotherapy of prostate cancer. J Clin Oncol 23:808–815, 2005.

188. Saltzstein D, Sieber P, Morris T, Gallo J: Prevention and management of bicalutamide-induced gynecomastia and breast pain: Randomized endocrinologic and clinical studies with tamoxifen and anastrozole. Prostate Cancer Prostatic Dis 8:75–83, 2005.

189. Perdonà S, Autorino R, De Placido S, et al: Efficacy of tamoxifen and radiotherapy for prevention and treatment of gynaecomastia and breast pain caused by bicalutamide in prostate cancer: A randomised controlled trial. Lancet Oncol 6:295–300, 2005.

chapter 8

Benign, High-Risk, and Premalignant Lesions of the Breast

STEPHEN R. GROBMYER | EDWARD M. COPELAND III | JEAN F. SIMPSON | DAVID L. PAGE

This chapter presents a classification of the incredible variety of noncancerous lesions presenting in the human female breast, largely as they are identified histopathologically with clinical biopsies. This chapter is stratified into categories that have relevance for the prediction of breast cancer risk in broad terms.[1,2]

The magnitude of risk in these various strata are based on the following assumption: Any changes not reliably indicating an increased risk of subsequent breast cancer greater than 50% above that of similar women controlled for age and length of time at follow-up will be accorded no elevation of risk. The great majorities of these lesions are not associated with seeming cellular increase and are designated as nonproliferative. Nonproliferative lesions occasion biopsy or present clinical symptoms without an association of increased risk. Other lesions that maintain an association with subsequent breast cancer risk are defined as proliferative lesions.

Benign Lesions without Cancer Risk Implications

Benign breast conditions have a diverse array of clinical presentations. The subjective discomfort of mammary pain and clinical signs of lumpiness have little correlation with histologic alterations. Lumpiness on physical examination is common to many benign and malignant situations. The continued use of such broad terms of convenience as *fibrocystic disease* or *fibrocystic change* (FCD or FCC) and *benign breast disease* (BBD) occurs because these terms are deeply embedded in clinical parlance. Despite their imprecision, these terms have utility precisely because of their imprecision, familiarity, and wide reference. In surgical pathology or histopathology, these terms had no precise reference and provided no clear understanding of pathogenesis. The following discussion highlights anatomic pathology while acknowledging that histopathology is an empty exercise without clinical correlates and predictability. Thus, we are highlighting those changes that have clinical implications.

The term *BBD* is an intrinsically imprecise term that refers to all noncancerous lesions of the breast. The use of the term *FCD* has been problematic despite its intent of providing a clinicopathologic correlation between lumpiness and histologic alterations.[3] The difficulty probably arises from the use of the term *disease* without the term *benign*, which has reinforced the widely held belief that cancer risk was elevated in this setting.[4] With the introduction of FCD in the 1940s, an association with cancer was implied by concurrent associations.[5] It was the intent of many recently to remove the cancer implications of FCD by changing the term to *FCC*.[6-8] The need to further define this risk indication has been only partially met through histologic evaluations of breast biopsies.[9] The link between BBD and FCD is made clear with the understanding that most benign biopsies have been termed FCD, and studies of cancer risk have held that the performance of a biopsy constituted BBD with its attendant increased risk of cancer.[10] These broad groupings or associations are referable to the era preceding mammography. It is evident that the introduction of mammography has aided the acceptance of a rigorous reductionist approach in which terms are technique bound (e.g., physical examination, mammogram) and must be individually studied. The net cast by the term BBD may be too broad, and the term FCD inappropriately implicates the presence of disease. All of these terms are in wide and appropriate use, and we prefer FCC.

The aforementioned view that considers FCCs as an imprecise term of convenience is not held uniformly. Many would consider that placing some confines of definition on this condition supports its acceptance as an entity. Bartow and colleagues[11] have studied different ethnic groups and have evidence that supports the idea of FCC or FCD as an entity, because these alterations are uncommon in low-risk cancer groups. All of these fibrous and cystic changes increase rapidly in incidence in the 10 or 15 years before menopause.[12,13] Although it may be difficult to draw sharp borders of definition for these changes, it is certain that they occur in more than 50% of the immediately premenopausal population of high-risk North Americans. The presence of cysts without hyperplasia and other changes noted as proliferative breast disease does not identify a higher-risk group of women when compared with others within the same ethnic or geographically defined risk group.[6] Hyperplastic changes may be more common in breasts that are clinically lumpy, but no formal recent analysis of co-occurrence of these conditions is available. Similarly, reliable mammographic correlates of epithelial hyperplasia are not at hand. Mammograms with increased density have imperfect associations with histologic findings because fibrosis is as common as hyperplasia, although hyperplastic lesions are somewhat more common in dense breasts.[14–16]

HISTOPATHOLOGY OF BENIGN BREAST DISEASE

Foremost of all the benign histologic changes in the breast are cysts and the pink cell apocrine change that so commonly accompanies them. Cysts range in size from approximately 1 mm to many centimeters. It is remarkable that cysts are usually unilocular within the breast. The reason for this configuration is thought to be that they arise as lobular lesions in which the individual acini or terminal ductules dilate, untwist, and unfold to enlarge as a cyst (Fig. 8-1).[17] Whether other lobular units and duct structures are recruited during enlargement is unknown. The small cysts are often inapparent on gross tissue examination. Whether associated fibrosis may make smaller cysts palpable is unclear, but the notion is certainly possible. Haagensen noted that clusters of cysts, each 2 to 3 mm in diameter, were palpable and termed them, along with larger examples, gross cysts.[18,19] In any case, these correlates of palpability have

become less important, particularly when most accept the fact that a biopsy may be appropriate based on clinical or mammographic findings, even if histology demonstrates no determinate abnormality. Understandably, fibrosis is often reported by pathologists in an attempt to explain clinical palpability or mammographic density. The gross appearance of large cysts is often blue, a reflection of the slightly cloudy, brown fluid usually found within. These are accorded the eponymous designation blue-domed cysts of Bloodgood, after Joseph Bloodgood, who studied them and their possible cancer association in the first part of the 20th century.[20]

Many cysts are lined by cells that have characteristic cytologic features of apocrine glands. The cells have many mitochondrial lysosomal and secretory granules that appear pink with eosin staining. The nuclei are also characteristic but less defining in that they are regularly round and often have a prominent round and eosinophilic nucleolus as well. This epithelium is often columnar, with a single protuberance of apical aspect of the cytoplasm appearing as a bleb or snout. Such changes may be prominent in enlarged lobular units and may have minor associations with concurrent atypical lesions.[21,22] Often, the apocrine cells are grouped in tufted or papillary clusters and sometimes produce prominent papillary prolongations from the basement membrane region, which may or may not contain fibrovascular stalks (Figs. 8-2 and 8-3). This papillary apocrine change may demonstrate highly complex patterns but is not associated with a significant increased risk of later cancer development unless there is concurrent atypical hyperplasia (see later discussion).[23] Breast cysts, particularly larger ones, may show no evidence of epithelial lining or may have a simple squamous lining with an extremely flattened and undifferentiated epithelialized surface. Several studies have differentiated these two types of cysts, apocrine and simple, indicating that apocrine cysts have a high potassium content and different steroid hormones.[24] A suggestion of a difference in cancer risk between the two kinds of cysts is unproven.[24,25] Apocrine cysts are probably more commonly associated with multiplicity and recurrence than are nonapocrine cysts.[17,25,26] Whether this alteration of mammary epithelium to

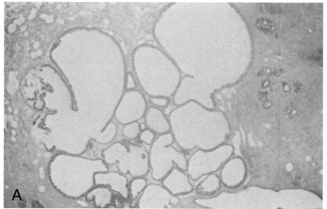
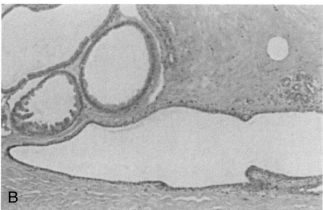

Figure 8-1 A, Apocrine cysts. Acini of this lobular unit have dilated and become distorted. Note entering lobular terminal duct at lower right. Low magnification. (×40.) **B,** Higher power of **A** showing apocrine-like epithelium lining dilated terminal duct and cysts. (×80.)

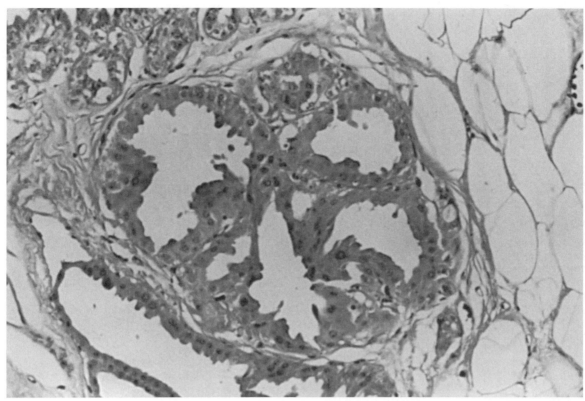

Figure 8-2 These dilated spaces of a lobular unit show prominent coalescent arches. Note prominent apical blebs, or "snouts." (×225.)

resemble that of apocrine sweat glands is a true metaplasia seems a point of practical irrelevance. However, many scholars believe that enzymatic profiles and ultrastructural evidence support a true metaplasia.[27] The frequency of a slight to marked protuberance of cell groups (papillary apocrine change) rather than a smooth, single cell layer is different in the breast compared with the apocrine sweat glands. A protein marker, GCDFP-15, is characteristically present within the cytoplasm and may be a useful marker.[28] Not only is the

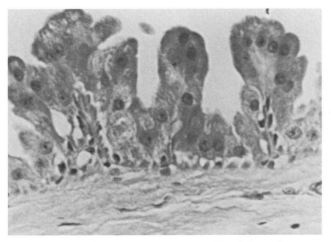

Figure 8-3 Papillary apocrine change. The lining of this cyst shows complex papillary tufts. Note prominent centrally placed nucleoli. (×320.)

characteristic apocrine alteration decorated with this marker, but it is also found in other settings with eosinophilic cytoplasm, such as nondistended lobular units and, less often, sclerosing adenosis (SA).

Intensive studies have not indicated that cysts alone are associated with risk, even when larger ones are separately analyzed.[6,29,30] However, recurrent larger cysts may have a cancer risk indication, as presented by Dixon and associates.[31] Cysts are more common in high-risk geographic groups but are not determinants of cancer risk within geographic groups. Dupont and Page[6] demonstrated a very slight elevation of risk for women with a family history of breast cancer and cysts as opposed to women with a family history of breast cancer alone. This is very mild evidence for premalignant indication of cysts, particularly because this interaction was not present with other indicators and remains an isolated observation. Although epithelial hyperplasia (see later discussion), which is related to increased cancer risk, often coexists with cysts,[30] either change may be present without the other in an individual biopsy specimen or entire breast. The apocrine cytoplasmic alteration is also of no proven importance in breast cancer risk. Apocrine change was found by Wellings and Alpers[32] to be more commonly present concurrently in breasts associated with cancer than those without. However, it is not an indicator of breast cancer risk in a predictive fashion. Moreover, when only cases of papillary apocrine change without concurrent patterns of proliferative disease are considered, the risk of later cancer development is not increased over the expected risk level.[23] In summary, neither cysts nor apocrine change significantly elevate cancer risk in an individual woman in the absence of other considerations.[7,8]

Chronic inflammation, edema, and pigment-laden macrophages are often found around cysts. Pigment-laden macrophages are likely the result of cytochromes from dead cells present at some time in the past. Occasionally, some of the pigment material may represent hemosiderin. Although duct ectasia and cysts have some histologic similarities, they are usually easily separable based on the general contour of the lesions and the greater degree of inflammation and/or scarring associated with duct ectasia.[33] Duct ectasia is usually present adjacent to the nipple, although it may extend a distance into the breast.

Epithelial Hyperplasia and Proliferative Breast Disease

The classification of epithelial hyperplasia in the breast espoused here is based on a large follow-up (cohort) epidemiologic study that sought to link epithelial histologic patterns to magnitudes of risk of breast cancer.[6] The positive relationship of more extensive and complex examples of hyperplasia with carcinoma is supported in many concurrent and, more important, prospective studies.[17,34–42] Although the categories of histologic alteration can be readily compared with many classification systems that have been proposed, a major consideration marks this approach as different.

Rather than supposing a regular stepwise progression or continuum from no change through carcinoma in situ, this approach proposes an absolute separation between carcinoma in situ and other hyperplastic appearances, using several criteria.[43] Furthermore, it recognizes that small examples of lesions with features of carcinoma in situ may be reproducibly recognized because of their small size or their lack of some of the features of well-developed carcinoma in situ. These less than fully developed examples of carcinoma in situ are recognized by the term atypical hyperplasia (AH).[44] This term does not, if it is taken to indicate a moderate increased risk of carcinoma, include all examples of hyperplasia thought to be generically unusual. On the contrary, the specifically defined AH lesions are recognized by a combination of cytologic, histologic, and extent cues,[45] some of which serve to differentiate them from carcinoma in situ and others to differentiate them from "benign."

DEFINITION AND BACKGROUND

Consistent with its definition elsewhere in the body, epithelial hyperplasia of the breast may be understood to mean an increased number of cells relative to a basement membrane. Thus, the increased number of glands without a concomitant increase relative to the basement membrane would not constitute hyperplasia but rather adenosis. Hyperplasia may be considered to represent an increased number of cells above the basement membrane, and because this number is normally two, the presence of three or more cells above the basement membrane constitutes hyperplasia. The discussion that follows is based on the presentations of Wellings and

colleagues,[17] as well as those of our own group.[6] These are a series of concurrent and prospective studies that seek to reproducibly define subgroups of patients and to demonstrate their relationship or lack of relationship to carcinoma present at the same time[17] or developing in the future in a prospective fashion.[6,44]

In most cases, other terms in general usage may be analogized and compared if the same definitions for AH are used. The term papillomatosis, proposed by Foote and Stewart,[46] is still used in North America to indicate the common or usual hyperplasias of moderate and florid degree.

Our approach to the stratification of the hyperplasias is to recognize an atypical lobular type, an apocrine type, and a usual type that includes the remainder of the hyperplastic lesions found in the breast.[47] The three groups recognize patterns regularly found within the breast and do not imply a pathogenetic sequence or a site of origin. The intent of the term usual is to denote that these are the common patterns of cytology and cell relationships seen when cell numbers are increased within the basement membrane–bound spaces within the human breast. The usual type or common patterns of hyperplasia have been termed ductal in the past largely to contrast them with the lobular series. Because these lesions regularly occur within acini of lobular units, the designation of ductal is avoided as an implication for either site of occurrence or site of origin of these cellular populations. Proliferative lesions in true ducts are unusual and are often truly papillary, that is, having branching, fibrous stalks (see later discussion).

The stratification of these hyperplastic lesions of usual type depends largely on quantitative changes. When the alterations begin to approximate patterns seen in carcinoma in situ, these lesions must be differentiated from those termed atypical ductal hyperplasia (ADH). Note that the features of the lesser end of the spectrum, between mild and moderate hyperplasia of usual type, depend on quantity and that the differentiation of the larger lesions from ADH depends on qualitative features of intercellular patterns and cytology (see later discussion).[45] Mild hyperplasia of usual type is characterized by the presence of three or more cells above the basement membrane in a lobular unit or duct and is not associated with any increased risk of cancer. Hyperplastic lesions that reach five or more cells above the basement membrane and tend to cross and distend the space in which they occur are called moderate. Florid is used for more pronounced changes, without any firm definition separating the moderate and the florid categories (Fig. 8-4). The reason for this is not to deny that there are quantitatively lesser and greater phenomena; rather, their reliable separation is not accomplished. Moderate and florid hyperplasia of the usual type is found in more than 20% of biopsies. In follow-up studies, the cancer risk between these two groups was found to be similar (see Chapter 26).

Risk categories may be stratified into slight, moderate, and marked, with slight indicating a risk of 1.5 to 2 times that of the general population and marked indicating about a tenfold increased risk (see Chapter 26). The current status of these assignments of histologic parameters to risk groups is shown in Box 8-1 and has changed little

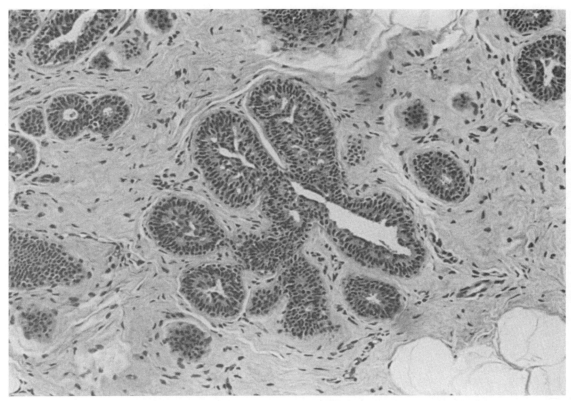

Figure 8-4 Moderate hyperplasia of the usual type. The ductules are partially filled by a heterogeneous population of cells. Note the normally polarized layer of cells just above the basement membrane. (×175.)

BOX 8-1

Relative Risk for Invasive Breast Carcinoma Based on Histologic Examination of Breast Tissue without Carcinoma*

No Increased Risk (No Proliferative Disease)

Apocrine change
Duct ectasia
Mild epithelial hyperplasia of usual type

Slightly Increased Risk (1.5–2 Times)

Hyperplasia of usual type, moderate or florid
Sclerosing adenosis,[†] papilloma

Moderately Increased Risk (4–5 Times)[‡]

Atypical ductal hyperplasia and atypical lobular hyperplasia

High Risk (8–10 Times)[§]

Lobular carcinoma in situ and ductal carcinoma in situ (noncomedo)

*Women in each category are compared with women matched for age who have had no breast biopsy with regard to risk of invasive breast cancer in the ensuing 10 to 20 years. Note: These risks are not lifetime risks.
[†]Jensen and colleagues[48] have shown sclerosing adenosis to be an independent risk factor for subsequent development of invasive breast carcinoma.
[‡]Atypical hyperplasia or borderline lesions
[§]Carcinoma in situ
Modified from Fitzgibbons PL, Henson DE, Hutter RV: Benign breast changes and the risk for subsequent breast cancer: An update of the 1985 consensus statement. Cancer Committee of the College of American Pathologists. Arch Pathol Lab Med 122:1053–1055, 1998.

from that presented by a consensus conference that was supported by the American Cancer Society and the College of American Pathologists.[1,2] The clinical significance of usual hyperplasia of moderate and florid degree rests in the positive demonstration of a slight increased risk (1.5 to 2 times) of subsequent invasive carcinoma. A major change in concept since 1985 is the acceptance of SA as an indicator of slightly increased risk.[48]

The positive histologic features of this group (Figs. 8-5 to 8-7) are as follows:

- There is a mild variation of size, placement, and shape of cells, and more specifically, nuclei. This feature is of great importance in differentiating these lesions from those of AH and noncomedo ductal carcinoma in situ. They are most commonly present within lobular units and terminal ducts.
- The cells often exhibit patterns of swirling or streaming.
- This change in cellular polarity is associated with a redistribution of a structural protein, fodrin, around the cell membrane.[49] As the epithelial cells proliferate, there is a varied shape of secondary lumens, which are often slitlike and are present between the cells within individual spaces.
- The secondary lumens, particularly in larger, more cellular lesions, may be present peripherally, immediately above the cells that surmount the basement membrane of the containing space.

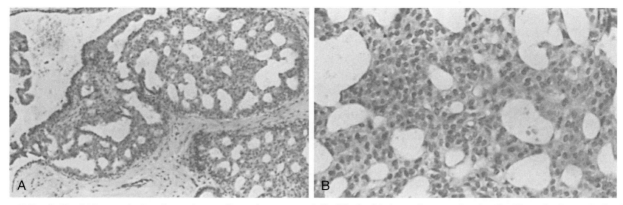

Figure 8-5 **A,** Florid hyperplasia of usual type. Ductules are partially filled with irregular arcade of cells. Note the irregularly shaped secondary lumens. (×150.) **B,** Higher power of **A.** There is mild nuclear variability and irregular placement of cells, features supporting the lack of atypia. (×280.)

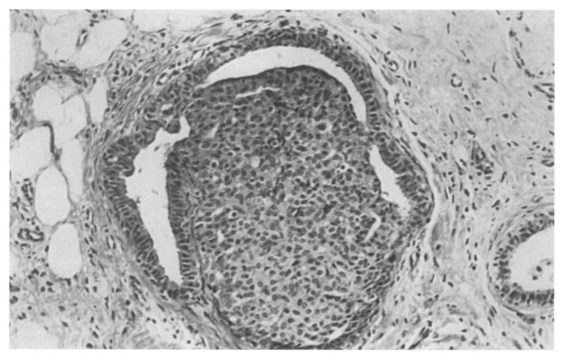

Figure 8-6 Florid hyperplasia of usual type with solid pattern and peripheral placement of secondary spaces. Nuclei are predominantly heterogeneous. (×350.)

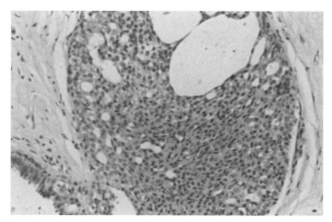

Figure 8-7 Florid hyperplasia of usual type demonstrating prominent nuclear streaming or swirling. (×200.)

- The cells appear to be varied, in cytologic appearance and in placement. Thus nuclei are not evenly separated one from the other. This is concomitant to the swirling or streaming change noted earlier.[50,51]

Atypical Hyperplasia

The intent of the term *AH* is to indicate a group of fairly specific histologic patterns that are not generically "atypical" or "unusual" but whose specific criteria have been shown to implicate an increased risk of later breast cancer development (see Box 8-1 and Chapter 26).[44] The link of specific histologic patterns to a moderate magnitude of risk of breast cancer depends on the use of defined criteria. This link of AH lesions to risk is the result of a group of studies that sought to restrict the term *AH* to a small number of histologic patterns that have some of the same features as the analogous carcinoma in situ lesions. Many other studies[17,52] have supported the link of epithelial hyperplasia to premalignant states in the breast and have led to the current prospective studies.[39,41,42] Basically, the cases of AH seen by the authors are most analogous to the categories termed level 4 (on a scale of 1 to 5, with 5 equal to carcinoma in situ) by Black and Chabon[52] as well as Wellings and associates.[17] Even when diagnostic terms used by hospital pathologists in the 1970s were grouped into analogous categories, a similar but lesser separation of risk groups was accomplished.[34] AH has been shown to be more common in the contralateral breast of women who have breast carcinoma.[53] The atypical hyperplastic lesions have some of the same features as those of carcinomas in situ but either lack a major defining feature of carcinoma in situ or have the features in less developed form.[44,45] The three major defining criteria are cytology, histologic pattern, and lesion extent.[45] These criteria have also been used by others.[27,54-56] Specific histologic features differentiate each of the AHs from lesser categories, as well as from the analogous carcinoma in situ lesions after which they are named: lobular and ductal carcinoma in situ. Thus, the histologic definitions are not viewed as resting within spectra of changes. On the contrary, these histologic categories attempt to accept natural pattern groupings within the complex array of mammary alterations reflected in histologic preparations. However, when no natural grouping is identified, an arbitrary separation is accepted. Arbitrary separation was used to differentiate atypical lobular hyperplasia (ALH) from lobular carcinoma in situ (see later discussion).

Lobular carcinoma in situ (see also Chapter 10) is recognized when there is a well-developed example of filling, distention, and distortion of over half the acini of a lobular unit by a uniform population of characteristic cells. This follows the intent of the original description.[5] The analogous AH lesion, ALH, is recognized when fewer than half of the acini in a lobular unit are completely involved, but the appearance is otherwise similar (Fig. 8-8).[57]

This arbitrary recognition of ALH and lobular carcinoma in situ in a series of changes from a few cells of appropriate appearance within a lobular unit to extreme examples with uniform cellular populations and extreme distortion and filling of acini imposes stratification in what is otherwise an undivided continuum. Many pathologists prefer to use one diagnostic term for this range of histologic appearances (e.g. lobular neoplasia).[58] We espouse this term because it covers both ALH and lobular carcinoma in situ. However, in diagnostic practice, more clinical guidance is given by the use of the separate designations lobular carcinoma in situ and ALH (see Chapter 26 for risk implications).[59]

A specific feature of lobular neoplasia is its tendency to undermine an otherwise normal and certainly different cell population. Because this is the interposition of an abnormal epithelial cell population within another, it has been termed pagetoid spread (because of the obvious analogy to Paget's disease of the nipple). Some have used this phenomenon to indicate diagnostic certainty for lobular carcinoma in situ; however, pagetoid spread does occur when the degree of involvement within lobular units reaches only the diagnostic level of ALH. The histologic patterns produced are usually more subtle in ALH,[60] and the solid pattern of ductal involvement in lobular carcinoma in situ is not seen with ALH. This pattern of involvement of ductal spaces outside of lobular units by the cells of lobular neoplasia in the presence of ALH has been termed ductal involvement in ALH and has been shown to be associated with a slightly higher risk of subsequent breast carcinoma than is found with involvement of the lobular units alone.[61]

The philosophical underpinnings of the diagnostic term *ADH* are the same as those for ALH. Thus, the same features present in the analogous carcinoma in situ lesion are evident but in a less developed form. Because the criteria of ADH are derived from those of ductal carcinoma in situ, histologic criteria for the latter must be understood. Two major criteria are required for the diagnosis of ductal carcinoma in situ (low grade, noncomedo). First, a uniform population of neoplastic cells must populate the entire basement membrane–bound space. Furthermore, this alteration must involve at least

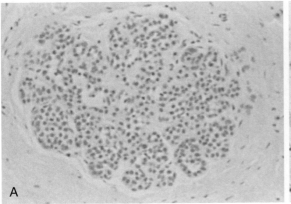
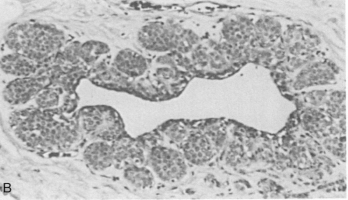

Figure 8-8 **A,** Atypical lobular hyperplasia (ALH). There is a resemblance to lobular carcinoma in situ (LCIS), but fewer than 50% of the individual acini are uniformly distended. (×180.) **B,** ALH undermining a different luminal cellular population. The same appearance may occur in LCIS; the defining diagnostic features must be present in lobular units to distinguish ALH from LCIS. (×180.) (From Page DL, Anderson TJ: Diagnostic histopathology of the breast. Edinburgh, Churchill Livingstone, 1987.)

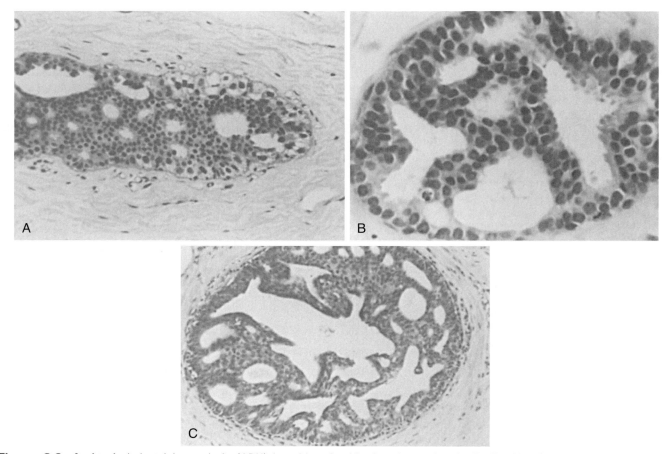

Figure 8-9 A, Atypical ductal hyperplasia (ADH) is evident in this ductule cut longitudinally. Note the regular placement of hyperchromatic nuclei and the regularity of centrally placed secondary lumens. (×190.) **B,** Rigid bar crossing the central portion of the photograph suggests ductal carcinoma in situ (DCIS); however, the cell pattern is not maintained throughout the remainder of the space. Note the polarity of the cells at the lower portion of the space, a finding that indicates ADH rather than DCIS. (×350.) **C,** Although there is some uniformity of some of the intercellular spaces, the cellular prolongations tend to taper and there is a tendency for peripheral placement of secondary spaces. The pattern and cytologic criteria for DCIS are not clearly uniformly met; therefore this is an example of ADH. (×170.) (From Page DL, Anderson TJ: Diagnostic histopathology of the breast. Edinburgh, Churchill Livingstone, 1987.)

two such spaces (Figs. 8-9 and 8-10). An adjunct to assessing the extent of involvement has been put forth by Tavassoli and Norris.[62] They consider lesions smaller than 2 or 3 mm as ADH, with a resulting moderate increase in later cancer development. In addition to extent, an intercellular pattern of rigid arches and even placement of cells must be uniformly present. A helpful secondary criterion is hyperchromatic nuclei, which may not be present in all cases.[45,63] The pattern of comedo ductal carcinoma in situ is not even discussed here because its characteristic extreme nuclear atypia is far beyond the patterns seen in ADH. Without the uniform application of criteria, consistency in diagnosis is unlikely[64]; however, when standardized criteria are applied, concordance is most often ensured.[65]

Some cases of ADH share features with the so-called clinging carcinoma described by Azzopardi.[27] A study from northern Italy indicates a considerable overlap of clinging carcinoma with ADH in histologic patterns and in risk of subsequent cancer development.[37,66,67]

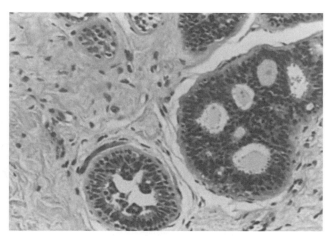

Figure 8-10 Florid hyperplasia of usual type. Although there are hyperchromatism and regularly spaced secondary spaces, there is not a uniform population of evenly spaced cells; this is not diagnostic of atypical ductal hyperplasia. (×225.)

The authors do not believe that the diagnosis of clinging carcinoma as a form of ductal carcinoma in situ is appropriate because it obviously indicates a different behavior from that expected of widely accepted forms of ductal carcinoma in situ (see Chapter 10). Four separate groups[35,39,41,42] have now applied these criteria to large cohorts in long-term follow-up studies, with remarkably similar subsequent risks of cancer development.

Localized Sclerosing Lesions

The classic example of localized sclerosing lesions is SA, which has been long accepted as a gross and histologic mimicker of invasive carcinoma. It is in that capacity that it still has its greatest utility as a recognized diagnostic term and histologic pattern in the armamentarium of histopathologists. In its most usual form, SA is present as a microscopic lesion, probably unrecognized in both clinical and gross examination of tissues. SA is diagnosed only when a clearly lobulocentric change gives rise to enlargement and distortion of lobular units with a combination of increased numbers of acinar structures and a coexistent fibrous alteration (Fig. 8-11). The normal two-cell population is maintained above the basement membrane in most areas, and the glandular units are regularly deformed. The term was proposed by Ewing[68] and further described by Dawson[69] to clearly separate this increase in glands from lesions involving increased numbers of cells within an enclosure of basement membrane (hyperplasia of usual type, epitheliosis).

Enlarged lobular units that appear otherwise normal or with slight gland deformity may not be recognized as SA, but may rather be diagnosed using the noncommittal and appropriately descriptive term *adenosis*. There is a favored association of SA with ALH.[48] Diagnostic patterns of ALH are usually present in nonsclerosed lobules elsewhere in the biopsy and are certainly difficult to recognize when present within a focus of SA. This may be because of the maintenance of relatively small spaces within readily identifiable lesions of SA (see discussion of ALH). The cytologic features of apocrine change may also be seen in adenosis, so-called apocrine adenosis.[70,71] The enlarged nuclei and prominent nucleoli of apocrine cells, when present in a deformed, sclerotic lesion, can occasionally mimic invasive carcinoma. Some have used the appellation *atypical* to describe this setting.[72] We believe that it is not clearly atypical because it is merely apocrine cytology in an unusual site, not a combination of pattern and cytologic atypia. Although it is unusual, we reserve the designation *atypical* for those histopathologic entities that have a proven risk implication for later cancer development.[6]

A palpable mass may be created by aggregations of microscopic foci of SA (aggregate adenosis). This situation has been termed *adenosis tumor*[19] to indicate that a clinically palpable tumor may be produced. SA also commonly contains foci of microcalcification and, when present in this aggregate form, may be detectable with mammography.

The differential diagnosis of these lesions has often been presented as a series or listing of criteria. These most often seek to differentiate SA from infiltrating tubular carcinoma and its variants. In the formation of these listings, little thought has been given to what is done if, for example, three criteria are consistent and the remaining are not. They must, then, be regarded as guidelines and not as hard-and-fast criteria. Fortunately, most of the time, the various criteria are consistent. Such is the variation of the biology of breast disease, or at least the variation of the anatomic expression of breast disease, that occasionally the guidelines will fail or be inconsistent. Usually, careful attention to the fact that SA is lobulocentric will suffice to correctly identify it. It is also true in SA that adjacent tubules tend to take approximately the same or similar shape as their immediate neighbors, although minor variations become marked if one skips to several tubular structures away. Equally true is that occasional ductal structures may be surrounded by a periodic acid–Schiff–positive basement membrane in a benign condition, which tends to be lost in carcinoma. However, many carcinomas have at least an irregular basement membrane and may show immunolocalization of proteins or basement membrane, such as type 4 collagen or laminin.[73,74] Decoration by special stains for myoepithelial markers is also not an absolute indicator of differential diagnosis, largely because these elements are often lost in densely sclerotic foci with glandular atrophy. This is then a helpful but not an absolute criterion. The spaces of a tubular carcinoma tend to be open, occasionally producing an irregular extension of the cluster of cells at one edge, resembling a teardrop. The cells of an infiltrating tubular carcinoma usually are layered singly, and when they are multilayered, the cells appear similar.

A rare condition known as microglandular adenosis (MGA), which may also mimic tubular carcinoma, has been well described.[75-78] In this condition, irregular, nonlobulocentric, small glandular spaces are present in increased numbers and appear to dissect and infiltrate through both stroma and fat, and a clinically palpable mass of several centimeters in diameter may be produced, which may be irregularly demarcated from surrounding

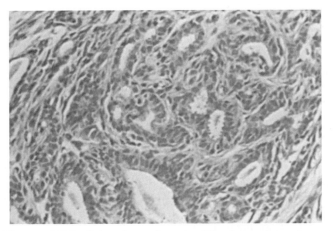

Figure 8-11 Sclerosing adenosis. Glandular elements are deformed and surrounded by stromal fibrous alteration. Two-cell population (basal or myoepithelial and luminal) is focally inapparent. (×240.)

tissue. The importance of this rare lesion is its ability to mimic tubular carcinoma. A similar lesion consisting of myoepithelial cells has been described and may show multiple recurrences.[79] MGA complicated by hyperplastic foci has been documented in two patients in whom carcinoma subsequently developed.[77] An additional 13 cases have been described in which infiltrative carcinoma was present in the background of MGA.[80,81] Because of the rarity of this condition, such associations are not certain. Clinical judgment may suggest various options in this setting, but a conservative stance should be emphasized. In other words, in the differential diagnosis between a benign lesion and cancer of little lethality (tubular carcinoma), one should favor benignancy in enigmatic settings.

RADIAL SCAR AND COMPLEX SCLEROSING LESIONS

Radial scar and complex sclerosing lesions have some similarities to SA: Carcinoma may be mimicked either clinically or histologically; it is with mammography that the mimicry of carcinoma by the larger complex sclerosing lesions is complete. Similar lesions were first described by Fenoglio and Lattes[82] as mimickers of carcinoma. Indeed, the advent of mammography has made the formal recognition of these lesions mandatory. The lesions appear spiculated, hence the term radial scar. The lesions are not lobulocentric but evidently incorporate several very deformed lobular units within their makeup, having as their probable origin a major stem of the duct system. This is particularly true of very large lesions. These are all characterized by a central scar from which elements radiate. The scar may vary through the full range of histologic appearances of the breast, including cystic dilation and units demonstrating hyperplasia and lobulocentric sclerosis like that of SA. Indeed, evaluation of these dense scars with special immune markers may be made difficult by the disappearance of myoepithelial markers in these epithelial elements within the scars. The microscopic features are determined by the degree of maturation, because it is now realized that the classic appearance (Fig. 8-12) represents

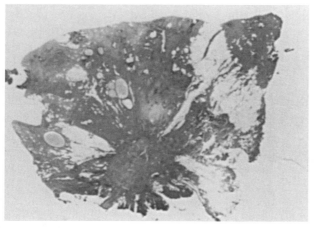

Figure 8-12 Mature radial scar with sclerotic center showing microcystic peripheral parenchyma. (×5.)

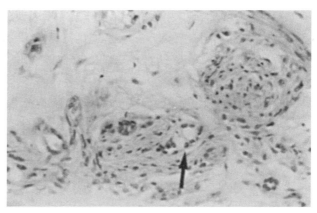

Figure 8-13 Pseudoinfiltration of glandular elements adjacent to a nerve *(arrow)* from a case of radial scar. The entrapped epithelial elements may closely mimic tubular carcinoma. (×300.)

the well-developed stage 2. Lesions at an earlier stage show noticeable spindle cells and chronic inflammatory cells around the central parenchymal components, which are less distorted. The association of hyperplasia and cystic and apocrine change becomes more evident as the lesion matures. There is evidence that the presence of these sclerosing lesions may further elevate cancer risk over other histologic risk indicators when they are present together.[83]

The progressive nature of these lesions was studied ultrastructurally by Battersby and Anderson.[84] A feature associated with early lesions was myofibroblasts in close proximity to degenerating parenchymal structures. Mature radial scars showed relatively few, sparsely distributed stromal myofibroblasts. Within the central scar, there are entrapped epithelial elements that have been appropriately characterized as pseudoinvasive (Fig. 8-13). Although these are the elements that most commonly mimic carcinoma histologically, atypical hyperplastic lesions may be found within the preformed epithelial spaces in the outer portions of the lesion. The entrapped epithelial units may closely mimic tubular carcinoma, and this differential diagnosis may be difficult. However, it should be recalled that tiny tubular carcinomas pose little threat to life and a conservative posture in the diagnosis of these lesions will benefit more patients.

Anderson and Battersby[85] analyzed the qualitative and quantitative features of more than 100 examples of radial scars from cases with and without cancer. Their frequency is similar in both groups and depends heavily on the diligence of search and the amount of tissue assessed. Bilaterality and multifocality were present in both groups, as was the full range of histologic appearance. No premalignant definition of these lesions was supported.

A variety of terms have been proposed for these lesions. However, it is likely that radial scar will maintain dominance. We favor the term complex sclerosing lesion for the larger examples in this series. This is because they do tend to have a variety of appearances, and their complexity with regard to mimicry of carcinoma is clearly portrayed by the term complex. The term radial also is useful to indicate the spiculated nature of the lesions.

Duct Ectasia and Fat Necrosis

DUCT ECTASIA

Duct ectasia is an entity or group of entities that has somewhat unclear confines of definition.[86] Some recognize only dilated ducts, as the term would indicate, as representing this condition. When this approach is taken, the condition is very common but is typically not associated with clinical pain or scarring. The separation of this entity into two large groups affecting different age groups and having different causes is becoming widely recognized.[33]

Most observers reserve the diagnostic term for those conditions in which a clinical presentation includes palpable lumpiness in the region of the breast under the areola. Ducts tend to be involved in a segmental fashion; that is, adjacent ducts extending out into the breast from the nipple are involved. Nipple discharge is a common but not invariable accompaniment of this condition, and undoubtedly the periductal scarring attendant to the later stages of this process is responsible for most cases of benign, acquired nipple inversion.[87] Periductal inflammation is a histologic hallmark of this condition.[27] It is now generally believed that the process begins with such a change and proceeds by destroying the elastic network to ectasia and periductal fibrosis.[24]

Most cases described are found in the perimenopausal age group. There are also younger women who present with inflammation of the ducts in the region of the nipple, which may produce fissures and fistulas with connections from the nipple ducts to the skin at the edges of the areola. The presentation of fistulas in younger women seems to be clearly connected with infection. This so-called periductal mastitis is commonly associated with a history of previous periareolar inflammation.[33] The more classic appearance of duct ectasia in older women may be a more smoldering infection of the larger ducts, and infection as the basis of this condition has been strongly suggested but remains unproven for most cases.[33,88] Very few with duct ectasia have a history of periductal mastitis, suggesting that these two conditions are probably unrelated. There is no association with parity or lactation.[89] As is the case with so many of these benign conditions of the breast, the greatest importance clinically is the mimicry of carcinoma. The plaque-like calcifications that occur within the scarred wall are, of course, visible with mammography (Fig. 8-14). Usually, these calcifications can be differentiated from the more irregular punctate calcifications of comedo carcinoma, but this is not always clear. Besides this frequent approximation to the mammographic appearance of comedo ductal carcinoma in situ, the localized scarring of duct ectasia can produce lumps that are fixed within inflamed scar in the breast. These lumps can very closely mimic carcinoma on occasion. One variant of this condition containing many plasma cells has been termed plasma cell mastitis. This is probably not a separate condition but rather part of the spectrum of duct ectasia. This is known to be a close mimicker of breast carcinoma of lobular infiltrating type, both grossly and microscopically.

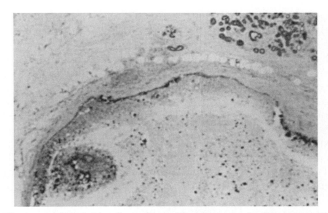

Figure 8-14 Large duct affected by duct ectasia. There is periductal fibrosis and inflammation. Note calcification in the wall of duct. (×50.)

FAT NECROSIS

Fat necrosis is relatively uncommon but may present in a most dramatic fashion, mimicking a well-developed scirrhous carcinoma or even inflammatory carcinoma. In its late, scarred phase, fat necrosis may not have an identifiable preceding traumatic cause; however, the mammographic appearance in the late stages is characteristic.[90] Most cases seen in the more acute phases, with some inflammatory activity still apparent, are associated with an identifiable recent traumatic event.

The histology of fat necrosis in the breast is no different from its appearance in other organs. The characteristic active chronic inflammatory cells are usually evident, with lymphocytes and histiocytes predominating. In the unusual very acute cases presenting within 1 week after an inciting event, polymorphonuclear leukocytes and free, oily, lipid material may be most apparent, particularly on needle aspiration. In this stage, the clinical features of swelling, redness, and warmth are present.

In the later stage, collagenous scar is the predominant finding, with seemingly granular histiocytes surrounding oil cysts of varying size. These "oil cysts" contain the free lipid material released by lipocyte necrosis.[91] The greatest clinical importance of fat necrosis is in its mimicry of carcinoma, as noted earlier. There is no known association with carcinoma or carcinoma risk.

Fibroadenoma and Phyllodes Tumor

FIBROADENOMA

Fibroadenomas (FAs) most often have a characteristic clinical presentation with an easily movable mass, seemingly unfixed to surrounding breast tissue. The gross appearance is usually characteristic. The sharp circumscription and smooth interface with surrounding breast tissue, usually producing an elevation of the FA on cut section, is characteristic. The cut surface is white, although one may identify the epithelial elements, if they are numerous, as light-brown areas. The cut surface is shiny and occasionally may seem to present an almost papillary appearance if the clefts lined by epithelium are larger. There may be slight variation from one area to another, with denser fibrosis in the stroma and, occasionally, calcification. The latter two features are more common in older women.

Although traditionally the risk of subsequent carcinoma in patients with typical FA has not been considered to be higher than that for the general population,[24] one study reported that, overall, FAs were found to be associated with a slight increased relative risk of later cancer.[92] The level of risk varies, depending on the characteristics of the FA itself and the status of the adjacent epithelium. If the adjacent epithelium shows proliferative changes or if the FA is complex, defined as the presence of cysts, SA, epithelial calcifications, or papillary apocrine changes within the FA, the risk is slightly higher than when these changes are absent.[92] Indeed, without these specific features, the women have no increased risk. One of the interesting aspects of this study, also shown by Levi and coworkers,[93] is that the risk identified by FA may not decrease in relative terms in the next 5 or 10 years after identification with biopsy.[92]

Carcinoma arising in FAs is distinctly uncommon. In this setting, lobular carcinoma in situ is the predominant type.[94–96] Risk implications for lobular neoplasia within an FA are not known for certain but probably are no greater than when lobular neoplasia is seen in the usual setting[92]; indeed, a large study indicates that atypical hyperplasia within FAs presents no increased risk of later cancer development.[97] Microscopically, fibrous tissue makes up most of the FA; either the stroma may surround rounded and easily definable ductlike epithelial structures, or the epithelium may be stretched into curvilinear arrangements (Figs. 8-15 and 8-16). This latter pattern has been termed *intracanalicular*, and the former pattern has been termed *pericanalicular*. These two terms are still useful as descriptors but are of no practical or prognostic importance and therefore are not used to define supposed subtypes of FA. Smooth muscle is an extremely rare component of FAs.[98] The epithelium within an FA may have the same appearance as elsewhere in the breast, including apocrine metaplasia.[27] Rarely, squamous metaplasia is present.[99]

FAs that are allowed to grow after initial detection usually cease to grow when they reach 2 to 3 cm in diameter.[19] African Americans more commonly develop FAs than Caucasians, and they develop them at a younger age as well. FAs in African Americans are also more likely to recur.[100] Because FAs are more common in African Americans, related lesions are also probably more common in the African-American population.[101] Infarcts of the breast may occur during pregnancy or lactation with a resultant discrete mass.[102] Approximately 1 of 200 FAs shows infarction.[103,104] Pain and tenderness may occur during pregnancy, and an inflammatory reaction may be accompanied by lymphadenopathy, leading to the clinical impression of carcinoma.

FA may also be regarded as a generic term, referring to any benign, confined tumor of the breast (mass-occupying lesion) that has a mixture of glandular and mesenchymal elements. When it is viewed as a more specific term, special or specific variants of the general pattern are recognized as being separate entities. These include hamartoma, tubular adenoma, lactating adenoma, adenolipoma, juvenile fibroadenoma, and giant adenoma.

Hamartomas of the breast have received greater attention with the introduction of mammography.[105] The series of Hessler and colleagues[106] and Linell and coworkers[107] are important in establishing the notation of hamartomas as first proposed by Arrigoni and coworkers.[108] These are lesions made up of recognizable lobular units, often present at the sharply demarcated margins of these lesions. Fat is rare in FAs, which are also rarely characterized by well-ordered lobular units throughout their substance. Another feature supporting the recognition of hamartomas as separate entities is that their average age of presentation is almost two decades after that for FAs in general. It is the sharp, smooth borders of these lesions and their intermixture with fat that allows mammographic identification in pronounced examples. Duchatelle and associates[109] support the formation of these lesions as more likely to be developmental than neoplastic. A similar lesion is the adenolipoma.[110] These lesions are only one tenth as common as ordinary lipomas.[19]

Other types of FAs, perhaps better regarded as variants rather than as separate entities, are lesions that tend to occur in women in the younger age range; they are characterized by increased cellularity of stroma or epithelium, or both. Duray and colleagues[111] described cellular FAs as being most likely to occur in adolescents and more likely to recur locally as adolescent cellular FA. These lesions bear some resemblance to benign phyllodes tumors of some other classifications. Juvenile FAs are diagnostic terms based on clinical grounds.[112] Oberman[113] initially suggested the use of the term *juvenile adenofibroma* in a review of breast lesions in juveniles. He believed that 5% to 10% of the adenofibromas that occurred in that age group were notable for rapid growth and large size. Pike and Oberman,[114] further elaborating on juvenile adenofibroma, characterized the lesions by their tendency to occur around the time of menarche, the common ductal pattern of epithelial hyperplasia, and the defining stromal hypercellularity. Local recurrence was not believed to be a feature of these lesions. Mies and

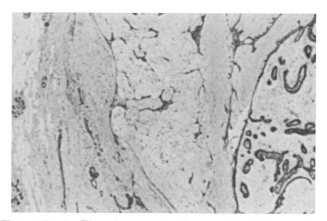

Figure 8-15 Fibroadenoma showing prominent intracanalicular pattern. (×30.)

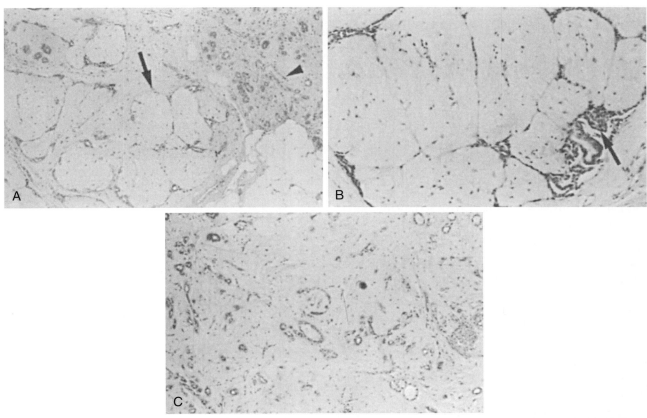

Figure 8-16 A, Fibroadenoma with irregular border. Both intracanalicular *(arrow)* and pericanalicular *(arrowhead)* patterns are well demonstrated. (×30.) **B,** Higher power of **A**. Fixation artifact gives appearance of hyperplastic epithelium *(arrow)*. (×125.) **C,** Same case as **A**. Complex epithelial patterns are evident. (×50.)

Rosen[115] have also described a series of patients with an average age of 26 years who had an unusual and atypical pattern of epithelial hyperplasia within FAs, which is likely to be misinterpreted as carcinoma in situ. No specific clinical feature was suggested. There is certainly no overlap between the latter series of patients and those described by Duray and coworkers,[111] whereas the cases of Pike and Oberman[114] appear to be somewhere intermediate. The practical utility of these interesting approaches to unusual FAs appears to be that rapidly growing lesions in juveniles are usually benign, often have a densely cellular stroma, and less often have prominent epithelial hyperplasia.

The histologic definitions separating FA from phyllodes tumors are even less well defined than are the definitions of benign versus malignant among the phyllodes tumors (see following discussion). It seems clear that the term *phyllodes tumors* are often applied to most large FAs with any suggestion of hypercellularity. As long as the descriptor benign is added to the designation (particularly if the synonymous diagnostic phrase *benign cystosarcoma phyllodes* is used), no harm will come of this usage. Fechner[105] considers up to three mitoses per high-power field as acceptable in FA. Perhaps with the designation of cellular FAs[111] indicating a slightly greater likelihood of local recurrence, the separation of phyllodes tumors from FAs may become more precise. In a carefully reported series of phyllodes tumors, Chua and Thomas[116] recognized 92% as being benign based on the presence of

fewer than five mitoses per 10 high-power fields, only mild stromal pleomorphism, and circumscribed tumor margins. An 18% local recurrence rate for these lesions is within the range of 15% cited for FAs alone, further evidence that clinical terminology for these lesions might be considered a matter of personal choice.

There remains the possibility that FAs may evolve into phyllodes tumors, but that occurrence is not well documented; there are lesions with areas of characteristic FA and other areas with leaflike patterns characteristic of phyllodes tumors.[117] Certainly there has been a recent major change from the prior clinical dictum that any determinate mass had to be surgically removed from the breast. Many surgical groups have noted that characteristic 2- to 3-cm FAs could be watched clinically after careful notation, this being most appropriate in patients younger than 25 years of age and acceptable for those 25 to 30 years of age, although probably not thereafter.[118,119] Also, needle aspiration with characteristic findings should confirm the fact that such lesions are FAs. The natural history of most FAs supports this approach.[120] A condition that may resemble FA is fibromatosis.[121,122] Fibromatosis is benign histologically, and as many as one fourth of these cases may recur after simple excision.[121,122]

Another variant of FA is tubular adenoma. These lesions are uncommon and are recognized as having dominant tubular elements in a circumscribed mass with minimal supporting stroma.[123,124] Grossly tubular adenomas have a fine nodularity.[125] Portions of otherwise characteristic FAs may have the appearance of a tubular adenoma.[126] Uniform tubular structures are seen, and lobular anatomy is usually not evident. Tubular adenomas may have evidence of secretory activity, but when they do not occur in association with pregnancy or lactation, they should not be termed *lactating adenomas*. Lactating adenomas are certainly analogous in some ways to tubular adenomas and may represent a physiologic response of the tubular adenoma to pregnancy.[126] In addition to showing lactational changes, the adenomas presenting in pregnancy have a more evident lobular anatomy than that seen in most tubular adenomas. James and coworkers[127] have supported the notion that the lesions arising in pregnancy, formerly termed lactating adenomas, be termed *breast tumor of pregnancy*. This term is proposed because they are distinct from tubular adenomas and should not be related to lactation (despite histologic changes) because they arise during pregnancy, not during the time of breastfeeding. The microscopic changes seen in the breast tumor of pregnancy are similar to those seen in the normal pregnant breast but are variable in degree and are often out of phase with the normal breast changes resulting from pregnancy.

PHYLLODES TUMOR

The series of mammary tumors known as *phyllodes tumors* continue to pose problems for the physician managing breast disease, largely because of their rarity. Three problems remain incompletely resolved: (1) The confusing terminology of cystosarcoma phyllodes is still in frequent usage; (2) rarity of these lesions has made clear understanding of the borderline between benign and malignant difficult; and (3) there remain a fairly large number of cases, relative to the entire group of lesions, that must continue to be regarded as borderline malignant, presenting obvious problems in patient management, although such "borderline" cases should present a threat of local recurrence only.

First, the replacement of the classic terminology that placed the suffix *sarcoma* on benign and malignant examples of these lesions is a necessary recognition of the evolution of the term sarcoma. When first coined by Müller[128] in 1838, the term meant only a fleshy tumor. The general acceptance of the term to mean predicted malignant behavior did not arise until decades later, and we may regard *cystosarcoma* as a vestigial example of the 19th century descriptive use of that term.[129]

Second, the rarity of these lesions has led them to be misunderstood. Two differential diagnostic problems are represented by this situation: (1) the separation of the benign phyllodes tumors from some similar, and probably closely related, unusual FAs, and (2) the recognition of the truly malignant end of the spectrum of phyllodes tumors.

There is no reliable way to differentiate grossly a giant FA (or the so-called juvenile FA) from a benign phyllodes tumor. Indeed, the tendency to recognize the large size as the dominant characteristic of phyllodes tumor has led to the frequent confusion of these entities. They may be interrelated in any case. A classic gross pattern for a phyllodes tumor includes sharp demarcation from the surrounding normal breast tissue, with the normal tissue obviously compressed. The connective tissue that makes up the greatest bulk of the mass is firm and varies from dense and white to glistening and edematous. Local areas of degeneration lead to cystic and discolored areas. The classic pattern that gave these tumors their name may be evident with smoothly contoured leaf-like areas separated from others by narrow, epithelial-lined spaces.[130]

The histologic appearance of phyllodes tumors may be considered the same as that of large FAs unless some specific guidelines are accepted. Fechner[105] believes that the stroma in phyllodes tumors should have greater cellularity and cell activity but that up to three mitoses per high-power field should be accepted within the definition of FA. Page and colleagues[57] have also accepted that approach and have suggested that the close application of a particularly cellular connective tissue element to the basement membrane region of the epithelial element be the defining factor and that size should have no part in the differential diagnosis of these mixed tumors of the breast (Fig. 8-17). The proliferating stroma is usually rich and cellular, regularly deforming the epithelium into extreme examples of the intracanalicular pattern seen in the more common FAs. The classic paper of Norris and Taylor[131] inaugurated the approach to documenting histologic features as rigorously as possible. Later papers have supported counting mitoses and evaluating the margins with care to determine whether there is an infiltrating focus.[132–134] Evaluated in this way, Chua and Thomas[116] identified five borderline phyllodes tumors, two of which recurred after local excision. A predominantly circumscribed margin, 5 to 10 mitoses per high-power microscopic field, and moderate nuclear pleomorphism were believed to be the defining factors in this group. Thus, borderline lesions are unlikely to reveal evidence of truly malignant behavior and may be more likely to recur locally than the usual phyllodes tumor. Special note should be made of the fact that malignant behavior in phyllodes tumors of young women is extremely rare.[135,136] Most malignant phyllodes tumors reported in the literature that have metastasized have had overgrowth of an obvious sarcomatous element (Fig. 8-18). This malignant element has often been something other than fibrosarcoma (e.g., liposarcoma, rhabdomyosarcoma). Close examination of the stroma with multiple sections is mandatory. The truly malignant phyllodes tumor may be so only in a portion of the tumor where easily

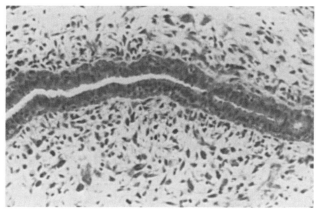

Figure 8-17 Phyllodes tumor. Hypercellular stroma shows nuclear pleomorphism and atypia. (×300.)

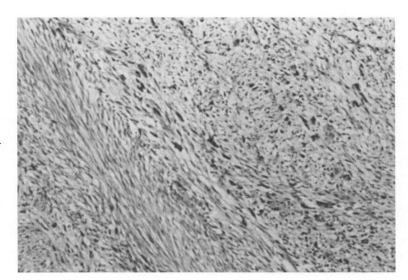

Figure 8-18 Phyllodes tumor. Low-grade fibrosarcomatous element is evident. (×110.)

diagnostic foci of sarcoma may be evident. On the other hand, a richly cellular fibrosarcoma-like stroma present in many foci or diffusely throughout the tumor presents the greatest difficulty in differential diagnosis. This difficulty primarily leads to overdiagnosis of malignancy, as evidenced by the 27 patients reported by Blumencranz and Gray,[137] in which 13 of the phyllodes tumors were diagnosed as malignant because of any combination of increased mitotic activity, invasive borders, or marked pleomorphism. In none of the women in this study did recurrences or metastases develop. Similar experience is reported in other series with patients who had well-sampled, benign phyllodes tumors that were successfully treated with careful excision.[138-140] Incomplete excision of phyllodes tumors has been stressed as a major determinant for local recurrence.[141,142]

Although it is often stated that histologic criteria are not reliable and that lesions appearing to be benign histopathologically may metastasize, these events are poorly characterized or poorly documented. With the use of a borderline category (tumors that usually do not act in a malignant fashion but may be more likely to recur locally), this unpredictability is no longer completely true. Certainly, even tumors with diffuse features of low-grade fibrosarcoma in the stroma rarely act in a malignant fashion. It is not even clear that such borderline tumors reliably recur locally more often than other benign tumors. However, local recurrence has been reported in up to 59% of cases.[143-145] Other series have found that the approximate 15% local recurrence rate accorded FAs was not reliably different from that of phyllodes tumors. Very important, local recurrences are unlikely to evolve into malignancy if this feature was not present in the primary tumor.[146]

PSEUDOANGIOMATOUS STROMAL HYPERPLASIA

Pseudoangiomatous stromal hyperplasia (PASH) is a benign proliferative condition of the breast stromal cells first described by Vuitch and associates.[147] PASH is a member of the family of benign breast lesions thought to be arising from mammary stromal cells.[148] In most cases,

this condition is an incidental finding.[148] Patients with PASH may, however, present with a mass on physical examination or a new finding on imaging studies that may mimic malignancy.[149,150] Historically, PASH has been excised because of uncertainty regarding its natural history and its association with malignancy.[151] Although several reports have described invasive breast cancer coincident with PASH, recent evidence suggests that PASH may be safely clinically observed and not excised in many patients.[149,151] The presence of suspicious findings such as associated microcalcifications should prompt further tissue biopsy or complete excision.[151]

PASH consists predominantly of sheets of benign ductal cells.[147,151] There are "anastomosing slit-like empty spaces lined by spindle cells"[151]; the spaces are separated by dense stroma. PASH has been reported in association with FCC, FAs, and phyllodes tumors.[148,152,153]

PAPILLOMA

The usual and classic solitary papilloma is a mass lesion of the large ducts most often presenting in the subareolar region. In the periphery, papillary lesions are often multiple and continuous with hyperplastic alterations within lobular units, as shown by Ohuchi and colleagues[154] in three-dimensional reconstruction studies of papillomas. Particularly when they are extensive, these lesions may be associated with AH and ductal pattern carcinoma in situ within and adjacent to the peripheral papillomas.

There is an important clinical correlate of these papillary lesions—they commonly present with a hemorrhagic discharge that is usually unilateral from the nipple.[27] This is true for the more central and larger lesions but may be also seen in smaller, more peripheral lesions. A careful follow-up of women with a solitary papilloma showed an increased risk of subsequent carcinoma development.[155] It was suggested that accompanying epithelial hyperplasia was responsible for further elevating the increased risk (see Box 8-1). From the Nashville series of patients, a nested case-control study evaluated the risk of carcinoma development after having a papilloma identified with biopsy.[156] A papilloma with or without ordinary patterns of hyperplasia was associated with only a slight increased risk, similar to other features of proliferative breast disease without atypia.[156] The presence of AH (pattern and extent analogous to ADH) within a papilloma increased the risk of subsequent development of breast cancer, predominantly near the site of the original papilloma. This single study suggests that women who have papillomas with AH may have a similar or higher cancer risk than others who have patterns of AH within breast parenchyma. Other researchers believe that women with multiple papillomas have an increased risk of subsequent development of carcinoma.[19] The co-occurrence of highly atypical hyperplastic lesions (including carcinoma in situ) with these multiple papillomas has been illustrated.[47,157,158]

Histopathology

Papillomas are truly papillary lesions with a branching fibrovascular core surmounted by epithelium (Fig. 8-19). They are most often identified on careful gross examination as lying within dilated ductal sacs. The papillomas may attain several centimeters in size, causing them to appear encysted with the continuity of the duct within which they arose, less apparent than in smaller examples. The texture of papillomas varies from soft to firm with dense sclerotic foci. Focal areas of necrosis and hemorrhage are a natural part of the basic elements of papillomas. Infarction may cause compression and distortion of epithelium, producing the appearance of carcinoma.[159] Squamous metaplasia may also be present.[160] The epithelial lining in benign papillomas varies greatly but is usually easily identified as benign (see Fig. 8-19). A double cell layer with more rounded cells adjacent to the basement membrane and surmounted by more columnar cells is commonly seen. When the cell numbers are increased beyond that, the same rules for atypia (usually ADH) and carcinoma in situ used for hyperplasia may be applied. Thus, there are papillomas with focal atypia that may qualify for AH (see earlier discussion). When the cell proliferation is uniform and attains the features seen in patterns in ductal carcinoma in situ, noninvasive papillary carcinoma is diagnosed (see Chapter 10).

Other lesions bearing resemblance to papilloma are discussed here for convenience, because they remain a portion of the differential diagnosis of those lesions. These include nipple adenoma (florid papillomatosis of the nipple) and nodular adenosis (ductal adenoma).

Nipple adenoma is a term used to describe a variety of appearances that may present in the nipple or immediately adjacent tissues. Patterns of hyperplasia with pseudoinvasion of dense stroma may be taken to be the basic features of these lesions. They may be misinterpreted clinically as Paget's disease because of irregularities of the surface of the nipple. However, they rarely ulcerate and therefore do not have the moist, red appearance of the eczematous features of Paget's disease. These lesions have localized areas of hyperplasia of slightly varying patterns intermixed with fibrous and cystic changes that may suggest atypia. Nipple adenomas or subareolar papillomatosis usually are diagnosed when they are approximately 1 cm or smaller. Patterns of papilloma are also mimicked. Careful histologic sampling and complete excision are important, because foci of carcinoma have been described in such lesions but apparently are rare.[161,162] These lesions often have nuclear hyperchromatism and a relatively high nuclear cytoplasmic ratio, as well as fibrosis—features that may be worrisome.[163] Complex patterns of epithelial hyperplasia enveloped by fibrosis may lead to the mistaken diagnosis of malignancy. Careful attention to these features avoids overdiagnosis of malignancy.[164]

Nodular adenosis and *ductal adenoma* are similar terms for an important group of lesions presenting varied histology. These lesions are most closely related to papillomas with unusual patterns of sclerosis and adenosis.[165] Because these lesions are characteristically surrounded by dense fibrous tissue within which epithelial cells are pseudoinvasive; they may be overdiagnosed as malignancy by the unwary (Fig. 8-20).

An increasingly important and benign lesion comes under many different terms and is often found with mammography because of secretory calcifications which are contained within. It is a favored site for the appearance of ADH and may be associated with other atypical lesions in the area.[21,22] We prefer the descriptive term enlarged *lobular unit with columnar alteration*, adding whatever other features may be present, such as prominent apocrine or secretory change (Fig. 8-21).

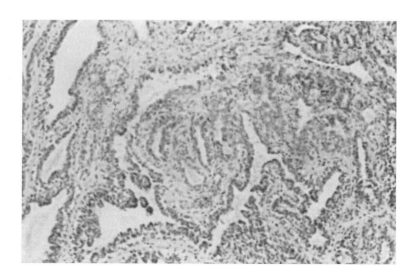

Figure 8-19 Delicate fibrovascular fronds of papilloma covered by single or double epithelial cell layers. (×280.)

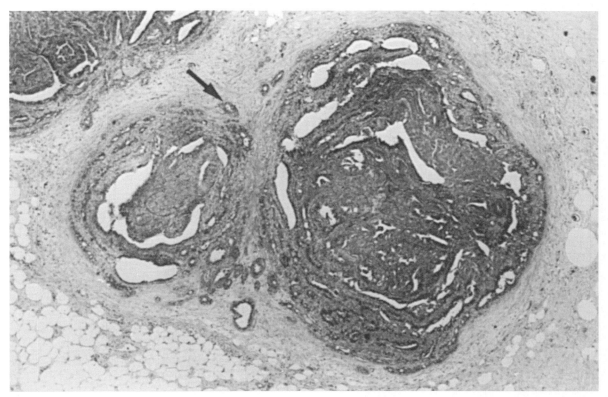

Figure 8-20 Proliferating glandular epithelium of a "ductal adenoma." Irregularities at the interface between adenotic elements and fibrous capsule simulate invasion *(arrow)*. (×70.)

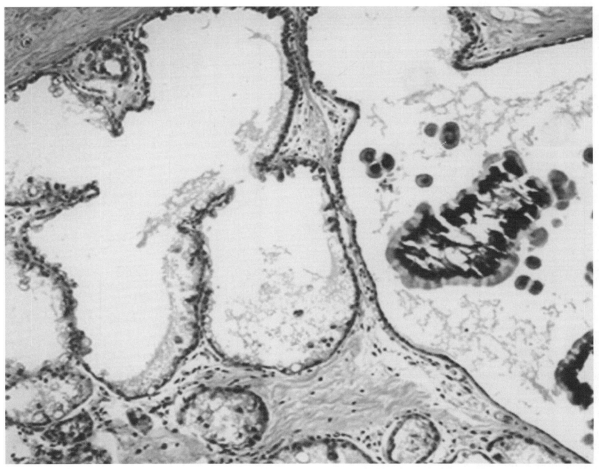

Figure 8-21 Portion of a dilated lobular unit meriting the term *enlarged lobular unit with columnar alteration*. (×200.)

REFERENCES

1. Godfrey SE: Is fibrocystic disease of the breast precancerous? Arch Pathol Lab Med 110:991, 1986.
2. Fitzgibbons PL, Henson DE, Hutter RV: Benign breast changes and the risk for subsequent breast cancer: An update of the 1985 consensus statement. Cancer Committee of the College of American Pathologists. Arch Pathol Lab Med 122:1053–1055, 1998.
3. Bartow SA, Black WC, Waeckerlin RW, Mettler FA: Fibrocystic disease: A continuing enigma. Pathol Annu 17(pt 2):93–111, 1982.
4. Davis HH, Simons M, Davis JB: Cystic disease of the breast: Relationship to carcinoma. Cancer 17:957–978, 1964.
5. Foote FW, Stewart FW: Comparative studies of cancerous versus noncancerous breasts. Ann Surg 121:6–53,1945.
6. Dupont WD, Page DL: Risk factors for breast cancer in women with proliferative breast disease. N Engl J Med 312:146–151, 1985.
7. Hutter RV: Goodbye to "fibrocystic disease." N Engl J Med 312: 179–181, 1985.
8. Love SM, Gelman RS, Silen W: Sounding board. Fibrocystic "disease" of the breast—a nondisease? N Engl J Med 307:1010–1014, 1982.
9. Ernster VL: The epidemiology of benign breast disease. Epidemiol Rev 3:184–202, 1981.
10. Worsham MJ, Raju U, Lu M, et al: Risk factors for breast cancer from benign breast disease in a diverse population. Breast Cancer Res Treat, 2008. [epub ahead of print]
11. Bartow SA, Pathak DR, Black WC, et al: Prevalence of benign, atypical, and malignant breast lesions in populations at different risk for breast cancer. A forensic autopsy study. Cancer 60: 2751–2760, 1987.
12. Frantz VK, Pickren JW, Melcher GW, Auchincloss H Jr: Indicence of chronic cystic disease in so-called "normal breasts": A study based on 225 postmortem examinations. Cancer 4:762–783, 1951.
13. Sandison AT: An autopsy study of the adult human breast: with special reference to proliferative epithelial changes of importance in the pathology of the breast. Natl Cancer Inst Monogr 4:1–145, 1962.
14. Boyd NF, Jensen HM, Cooke G, et al: Mammographic densities and the prevalence and incidence of histological types of benign breast disease. Reference Pathologists of the Canadian National Breast Screening Study. Eur J Cancer Prev 9:15–24, 2000.
15. Martin LJ, Boyd NF: Mammographic density. Potential mechanisms of breast cancer risk associated with mammographic density: Hypotheses based on epidemiological evidence. Breast Cancer Res 10:201–214, 2008.
16. Urbanski S, Jensen HM, Cooke G, et al: The association of histological and radiological indicators of breast cancer risk. Br J Cancer 58:474–479, 1988.
17. Wellings SR, Jensen HM, Marcum RG: An atlas of subgross pathology of the human breast with special reference to possible precancerous lesions. J Natl Cancer Inst 55:231–273, 1975.
18. Haagensen CD: The relationship of gross cystic disease of the breast and carcinoma. Ann Surg 185:375–376, 1977.
19. Haagensen CD (ed): Diseases of the breast, 3rd ed. Philadelphia, WB Saunders, 1986.
20. Bloodgood JC: The pathology of chronic cystic mastitis of the female breast, with special consideration of the blue-domed cyst. Arch Surg 3:445–452, 1921.
21. Shaaban AM, Sloane JP, West CR, et al: Histopathologic types of benign breast lesions and the risk of breast cancer: Case-control study. Am J Surg Pathol 26:421–430, 2002.
22. Fraser JL, Raza S, Chorny K, et al: Columnar alteration with prominent apical snouts and secretions: A spectrum of changes frequently present in breast biopsies performed for microcalcifications. Am J Surg Pathol 22:1521–1527, 1998.
23. Page DL, Dupont WD, Jensen RA: Papillary apocrine change of the breast: Associations with atypical hyperplasia and risk of breast cancer. Cancer Epidemiol Biomarkers Prev 5:29–32, 1996.
24. Dixon JM: Cystic disease and fibroadenoma of the breast: Natural history and relation to breast cancer risk. Br Med Bull 47:258–271, 1991.
25. Dixon JM, Lumsden AB, Miller WR: The relationship of cyst type to risk factors for breast cancer and the subsequent development of breast cancer in patients with breast cystic disease. Eur J Cancer Clin Oncol 21:1047–1050, 1985.
26. Vilanova JR, Simon R, Alvarez J, Rivera-Pomar JM: Early apocrine change in hyperplastic cystic disease. Histopathology 7:693–698, 1983.
27. Azzopardi JG, Ahmed A, Millis RR: Problems in breast pathology. Major Probl Pathol 11:i–xvi, 1–466, 1979.
28. Mazoujian G, Pinkus GS, Davis S, Haagensen DE Jr: Immunohistochemistry of a gross cystic disease fluid protein (GCDFP-15) of the breast. A marker of apocrine epithelium and breast carcinomas with apocrine features. Am J Pathol 110:105–112, 1983.
29. Page DL, Dupont WD: Are breast cysts a premalignant marker? Eur J Cancer Clin Oncol 22:635–636, 1986.
30. Bundred NJ, West RR, Dowd JO, et al: Is there an increased risk of breast cancer in women who have had a breast cyst aspirated? Br J Cancer 64:953–955, 1991.
31. Dixon JM, McDonald C, Elton RA, Miller WR: Risk of breast cancer in women with palpable breast cysts: A prospective study. Edinburgh Breast Group. Lancet 353:1742–1745, 1999.
32. Wellings SR, Alpers CE: Apocrine cystic metaplasia: Subgross pathology and prevalence in cancer-associated versus random autopsy breasts. Hum Pathol 18:381–386, 1987.
33. Dixon JM, Ravisekar O, Chetty U, Anderson TJ: Periductal mastitis and duct ectasia: Different conditions with different aetiologies. Br J Surg 83:820–822, 1996.
34. Carter CL, Corle DK, Micozzi MS, et al: A prospective study of the development of breast cancer in 16,692 women with benign breast disease. Am J Epidemiol 128:467–477, 1988.
35. Dupont WD, Parl FF, Hartmann WH, et al: Breast cancer risk associated with proliferative breast disease and atypical hyperplasia. Cancer 71:1258–1265, 1993.
36. Dupont WD, Rogers LW, Vander Zwaag R, Page DL: The epidemiologic study of anatomic markers for increased risk of mammary cancer. Pathol Res Pract 166:471–480, 1980.
37. Eusebi V, Foschini MP, Cook MG, et al: Long-term follow-up of in situ carcinoma of the breast with special emphasis on clinging carcinoma. Semin Diagn Pathol 6:165–173, 1989.
38. Kodlin D, Winger EE, Morgenstern NL, Chen U: Chronic mastopathy and breast cancer. A follow-up study. Cancer 39:2603–2607, 1977.
39. London SJ, Connolly JL, Schnitt SJ, Colditz GA: A prospective study of benign breast disease and the risk of breast cancer. JAMA 267:941–944, 1992.
40. Moskowitz M, Gartside P, Wirman JA, McLaughlin C: Proliferative disorders of the breast as risk factors for breast cancer in a self-selected screened population: Pathologic markers. Radiology 134:289–291, 1980.
41. Palli D, Rosselli del Turco M, Simoncini R, Bianchi S: Benign breast disease and breast cancer: A case-control study in a cohort in Italy. Int J Cancer 47:703–706, 1991.
42. Marshall LM, Hunter DJ, Connolly JL, et al: Risk of breast cancer associated with atypical hyperplasia of lobular and ductal types. Cancer Epidemiol Biomarkers Prev 6:297–301, 1997.
43. Page DL: Cancer risk assessment in benign breast biopsies. Hum Pathol 17:871–874, 1986.
44. Page DL, Dupont WD, Rogers LW, Rados MS: Atypical hyperplastic lesions of the female breast. A long-term follow-up study. Cancer 55:2698–2708, 1985.
45. Page DL, Rogers LW: Combined histologic and cytologic criteria for the diagnosis of mammary atypical ductal hyperplasia. Hum Pathol 23:1095–1097, 1992.
46. Foote F, Stewart F: Comparative studies of cancerous versus noncancerous breasts. I. Basic morphologic characteristics. Ann Surg 121:6,1945.
47. Page DL: The woman at high risk for breast cancer. Importance of hyperplasia. Surg Clin North Am 76:221–230, 1996.
48. Jensen RA, Page DL, Dupont WD, Rogers LW: Invasive breast cancer risk in women with sclerosing adenosis. Cancer 64:1977–1983, 1989.
49. Simpson JF, Page DL: Altered expression of a structural protein (fodrin) within epithelial proliferative disease of the breast. Am J Pathol 141:285–289, 1992.
50. Bocker W, Bier B, Freytag G, et al: An immunohistochemical study of the breast using antibodies to basal and luminal keratins, alpha-smooth muscle actin, vimentin, collagen IV and laminin.

Part II: Epitheliosis and ductal carcinoma in situ. Virchows Arch A Pathol Anat Histopathol 421:323–330, 1992.

51. Going JJ: Stages on the way to breast cancer. J Pathol 199:1–3, 2003.

52. Black EMC: In-situ carcinoma of the breast. Pathol Annu 4:185–187, 1969.

53. McCarty KS Jr, Kesterson GH, Wilkinson WE, Georgiade N: Histopathologic study of subcutaneous mastectomy specimens from patients with carcinoma of the contralateral breast. Surg Gynecol Obstet 147:682–688, 1978.

54. Ackerman LV, Katzenstein AL: The concept of minimal breast cancer and the pathologist's role in the diagnosis of "early carcinoma." Cancer 39(suppl):2755–2763, 1977.

55. Ashikari R, Huvos AG, Snyder RE, et al: Proceedings: A clinicopathologic study of atypical lesions of the breast. Cancer 33:310–317, 1974.

56. Fisher E: The pathology of breast cancer as it relates to its evolution, prognosis, and treatment. Clin Oncol 1:703–704, 1982.

57. Page DL, Anderson TJ: Diagnostic histopathology of the breast. Edinburgh, Churchill Livingstone, 1987.

58. Haagensen CD, Lane N, Lattes R, Bodian C: Lobular neoplasia (socalled lobular carcinoma in situ) of the breast. Cancer 42:737–769, 1978.

59. Page DL, Kidd TE Jr, Dupont WD, et al: Lobular neoplasia of the breast: Higher risk for subsequent invasive cancer predicted by more extensive disease. Hum Pathol 22:1232–1239, 1991.

60. Fechner RE: Epithelial alterations in the extralobular ducts of breasts with lobular carcinoma. Arch Pathol 93:164–171, 1972.

61. Page DL, Dupont WD, Rogers LW: Ductal involvement by cells of atypical lobular hyperplasia in the breast: A long-term follow-up study of cancer risk. Hum Pathol 19:201–207, 1988.

62. Tavassoli FA, Norris HJ: A comparison of the results of long-term follow-up for atypical intraductal hyperplasia and intraductal hyperplasia of the breast. Cancer 65:518–529, 1990.

63. Jensen HM: Breast pathology, emphasizing precancerous and cancer-associated lesions. In Bulbrook RTD (ed): Comments on breast disease. New York, Liss, 1981.

64. Rosai J: Borderline epithelial lesions of the breast. Am J Surg Pathol 15:209–221, 1991.

65. Schnitt SJ, Connolly JL, Tavassoli FA, et al: Interobserver reproducibility in the diagnosis of ductal proliferative breast lesions using standardized criteria. Am J Surg Pathol 16:1133–1143, 1992.

66. Eusebi V, Feudale E, Foschini MP, et al: Long-term follow-up of in situ carcinoma of the breast. Semin Diagn Pathol 11:223–235, 1994.

67. Bijker N, Peterse JL, Duchateau L, et al: Risk factors for recurrence and metastasis after breast-conserving therapy for ductal carcinoma-in-situ: Analysis of European Organization for Research and Treatment of Cancer Trial 10853. J Clin Oncol 19:2263–2271, 2001.

68. Ewing J: Neoplastic disease. Philadelphia, WB Saunders, 1919.

69. Dawson EK: A histological study of the normal mamma in relation to tumor growth: Early development to maturity. Edinburgh Med J 41:653–682, 1934.

70. Eusebi V, Casadei GP, Bussolati G, Azzopardi JG: Adenomyoepithelioma of the breast with a distinctive type of apocrine adenosis. Histopathology 11:305–315, 1987.

71. Simpson JFP, Page DL, Dupont WD: Apocrine adenosis: A mimic of mammary carcinoma. Surg Pathol 3:289–299, 1990.

72. Carter DJ, Rosen PP: Atypical apocrine metaplasia in sclerosing lesions of the breast: A study of 51 patients. Mod Pathol 4:1–5, 1991.

73. d'Ardenne AJ: Use of basement membrane markers in tumour diagnosis. J Clin Pathol 42:449–457, 1989.

74. Siegal GP, Barsky SH, Terranova VP, Liotta LA: Stages of neoplastic transformation of human breast tissue as monitored by dissolution of basement membrane components. An immunoperoxidase study. Invasion Metastasis 1:54–70, 1981.

75. Clement PB, Azzopardi JG: Microglandular adenosis of the breast—a lesion simulating tubular carcinoma. Histopathology 7:169–180, 1983.

76. McDivitt RW, Stewart FW, Berg JW: Tumors of the breast, 2nd ed. Washington, DC, Armed Forces Institute of Pathology, 1968.

77. Rosen PP: Microglandular adenosis. A benign lesion simulating invasive mammary carcinoma. Am J Surg Pathol 7:137–144, 1983.

78. Tavassoli FA, Norris HJ: Microglandular adenosis of the breast. A clinicopathologic study of 11 cases with ultrastructural observations. Am J Surg Pathol 7:731–737, 1983.

79. Kiaer H, Nielsen B, Paulsen S, et al: Adenomyoepithelial adenosis and low-grade malignant adenomyoepithelioma of the breast. Virchows Arch A Pathol Anat Histopathol 405:55–67, 1984.

80. James BA, Cranor ML, Rosen PP: Carcinoma of the breast arising in microglandular adenosis. Am J Clin Pathol 100:507–513, 1993.

81. Rosenblum MK, Purrazzella R, Rosen PP: Is microglandular adenosis a precancerous disease? A study of carcinoma arising therein. Am J Surg Pathol 10:237–245, 1986.

82. Fenoglio C, Lattes R: Sclerosing papillary proliferations in the female breast. A benign lesion often mistaken for carcinoma. Cancer 33:691–700, 1974.

83. Jacobs TW, Byrne C, Colditz G, et al: Radial scars in benign breast-biopsy specimens and the risk of breast cancer. N Engl J Med 340:430–436, 1999.

84. Battersby S, Anderson TJ: Myofibroblast activity of radial scars. J Pathol 147:33–40, 1985.

85. Anderson TJ, Battersby S: Radial scars of benign and malignant breasts: Comparative features and significance. J Pathol 147:23–32, 1985.

86. Hughes LE: Non-lactational inflammation and duct ectasia. Br Med Bull 47:272–283, 1991.

87. Rees BI, Gravelle IH, Hughes LE: Nipple retraction in duct ectasia. Br J Surg 64:577–580, 1977.

88. Bundred NJ, Dixon JM, Lumsden AB, et al: Are the lesions of duct ectasia sterile? Br J Surg 72:844–845, 1985.

89. Dixon JM, Anderson TJ, Lumsden AB, et al: Mammary duct ectasia. Br J Surg 70:601–603, 1983.

90. Orson LW, Cigtay OS: Fat necrosis of the breast: Characteristic xeromammographic appearance. Radiology 146:35–38, 1983.

91. Bargum K, Nielsen SM: Case report: Fat necrosis of the breast appearing as oil cysts with fat-fluid levels. Br J Radiol 66:718–720, 1993.

92. Dupont WD, Page DL, Parl FF, et al: Long-term risk of breast cancer in women with fibroadenoma. N Engl J Med 331:10–15, 1994.

93. Levi F, Randimbison L, Te VC, La Vecchia C: Incidence of breast cancer in women with fibroadenoma. Int J Cancer 57:681–683, 1994.

94. Diaz NM, Palmer JO, McDivitt RW: Carcinoma arising within fibroadenomas of the breast. A clinicopathologic study of 105 patients. Am J Clin Pathol 95:614–622, 1991.

95. Fondo EY, Rosen PP, Fracchia AA, Urban JA: The problem of carcinoma developing in a fibroadenoma: Recent experience at Memorial Hospital. Cancer 43:563–567, 1979.

96. Pick PW, Iossifides IA: Occurrence of breast carcinoma within a fibroadenoma. A review. Arch Pathol Lab Med 108:590–594, 1984.

97. Carter BA, Page DL, Schuyler P, et al: No elevation in long-term breast carcinoma risk for women with fibroadenomas that contain atypical hyperplasia. Cancer 92:30–36, 2001.

98. Goodman ZD, Taxy JB: Fibroadenomas of the breast with prominent smooth muscle. Am J Surg Pathol 5:99–101, 1981.

99. Salm R: Epidermoid metaplasia in mammary fibroadenoma with formation of keratin cysts. J Pathol Bacteriol 74:221–222, 1957.

100. Organ CH, Jr., Organ BC: Fibroadenoma of the female breast: A critical clinical assessment. J Natl Med Assoc 75:701–704, 1983.

101. Kovi J, Chu HB, Leffall LD Jr: Sclerosing lobular hyperplasia manifesting as a palpable mass of the breast in young black women. Hum Pathol 15:336–340, 1984.

102. Hasson J, Pope CH: Mammary infarcts associated with pregnancy presenting as breast tumors. Surgery 49:313–316, 1961.

103. Majmudar B, Rosales-Quintana S: Infarction of breast fibroadenomas during pregnancy. JAMA 231:963–964, 1975.

104. Wilkinson L, Green WO Jr: Infarction of breast lesions during pregnancy and lactation. Cancer 17:1567–1572, 1964.

105. Fechner RE: Fiberadenoma and related lesions. In Page DL, Anderson TJ (eds): Diagnostic histopathology of the breast. Edinburgh, Churchill Livingstone, 1987.

106. Hessler C, Schnyder P, Ozzello L: Hamartoma of the breast: Diagnostic observation of 16 cases. Radiology 126:95–98, 1978.

107. Linell F, Ostberg G, Soderstrom J, et al: Breast hamartomas. An important entity in mammary pathology. Virchows Arch A Pathol Anat Histol 383:253–264, 1979.

108. Arrigoni MG, Dockerty MB, Judd ES: The identification and treatment of mammary hamartoma. Surg Gynecol Obstet 133:577–582, 1971.

109. Duchatelle V, Auberger E, Amouroux J: Hamartomas of the breast. Apropos of 14 histologically controlled cases. Ann Pathol 6:335–339, 1986.

110. Dyreborg U, Starklint H: Adenolipoma mammae. Acta Radiol Diagn (Stockh) 16:362–366, 1975.

111. Duray PH: Adolescent Cellular fibroadenomas: A clinical and pathologic study. Lab Invest 50:17A, 1984.

112. Ashikari R, Farrow JH, O'Hara J: Fibroadenomas in the breast of juveniles. Surg Gynecol Obstet 132:259–262, 1971.

113. Oberman HA: Breast lesions in the adolescent female. Pathol Annu 14(pt 1):175–201, 1979.

114. Pike AM, Oberman HA: Juvenile (cellular) adenofibromas. A clinicopathologic study. Am J Surg Pathol 9:730–736, 1985.

115. Mies C, Rosen PP: Juvenile fibroadenoma with atypical epithelial hyperplasia. Am J Surg Pathol 11:184–190, 1987.

116. Chua CL, Thomas A: Cystosarcoma phyllodes tumors. Surg Gynecol Obstet 166:302–306, 1988.

117. Maier WP, Rosemond GP, Wittenberg P, Tassoni EM: Cytosarcoma phyllodes mammae. Oncology 22:145–158, 1968.

118. Cant PJ, Madden MV, Close PM, et al: Case for conservative management of selected fibro-adenomas of the breast. Br J Surg 74:857–859, 1987.

119. Cant PJ, Madden MV, Coleman MG, Dent DM: Non-operative management of breast masses diagnosed as fibroadenoma. Br J Surg 82:792–794, 1995.

120. Wilkinson S, Anderson TJ, Rifkind E, et al: Fibroadenoma of the breast: A follow-up of conservative management. Br J Surg 76:390–391, 1989.

121. Rosen PP, Ernsberger D: Mammary fibromatosis. A benign spindle-cell tumor with significant risk for local recurrence. Cancer 63:1363–1369, 1989.

122. Wargotz ES, Norris HJ, Austin RM, Enzinger FM: Fibromatosis of the breast. A clinical and pathological study of 28 cases. Am J Surg Pathol 11:38–45, 1987.

123. Hertel BF, Zaloudek C, Kempson RL: Breast adenomas. Cancer 37:2891–2905, 1976.

124. Persaud V, Talerman A, Jordan R: Pure adenoma of the breast. Arch Pathol 86:481–483, 1968.

125. Moross T, Lang AP, Mahoney L: Tubular adenoma of breast. Arch Pathol Lab Med 107:84–86, 1983.

126. O'Hara MF, Page DL: Adenomas of the breast and ectopic breast under lactational influences. Hum Pathol 16:707–712, 1985.

127. James K, Bridger J, Anthony PP: Breast tumour of pregnancy ("lactating" adenoma). J Pathol 156:37–44, 1988.

128. Muller J: Uber Den Feinern Bau Und Die Formen Der Krankhaften Geschwulste. G Reimer, Berlin, 1838.

129. Hough AJ Jr, Page DL: Perspectives on cartilaginous tumors: Nomenclature, nosology, and neologism. Hum Pathol 20:927–929, 1989.

130. Blichert-Toft M, Hansen JP, Hansen OH, Schiodt T: Clinical course of cystosarcoma phyllodes related to histologic appearance. Surg Gynecol Obstet 140:929–932, 1975.

131. Norris HJ, Taylor HB: Relationship of histologic features to behavior of cystosarcoma phyllodes. Analysis of ninety-four cases. Cancer 20:2090–2099, 1967.

132. Hart WR, Bauer RC, Oberman HA: Cystosarcoma phyllodes. A clinicopathologic study of twenty-six hypercellular periductal stromal tumors of the breast. Am J Clin Pathol 70:211–216, 1978.

133. Murad TM, Hines JR, Beal J, Bauer K: Histopathological and clinical correlations of cystosarcoma phyllodes. Arch Pathol Lab Med 112:752–756, 1988.

134. Pietruszka M, Barnes L: Cystosarcoma phyllodes: A clinicopathologic analysis of 42 cases. Cancer 41:1974–1983, 1978.

135. Briggs RM, Walters M, Rosenthal D: Cystosarcoma phylloides in adolescent female patients. Am J Surg 146:712–714, 1983.

136. Leveque J, Meunier B, Wattier E, et al: Malignant cystosarcomas phyllodes of the breast in adolescent females. Eur J Obstet Gynecol Reprod Biol 54:197–203, 1994.

137. Blumencranz PW, Gray GF: Cystosarcoma phyllodes. Clinical and pathologic study. N Y State J Med 78:623–627, 1978.

138. Chaney AW, Pollack A, McNeese MD, et al: Primary treatment of cystosarcoma phyllodes of the breast. Cancer 89:1502–1511, 2000.

139. Meneses A, Mohar A, de la Garza-Salazar J, Ramirez-Ugalde T: Prognostic factors on 45 cases of phyllodes tumors. J Exp Clin Cancer Res 19:69–73, 2000.

140. Reinfuss M, Mitus J, Duda K, et al: The treatment and prognosis of patients with phyllodes tumor of the breast: An analysis of 170 cases. Cancer 77:910–916, 1996.

141. Moffat CJ, Pinder SE, Dixon AR, et al: Phyllodes tumours of the breast: A clinicopathological review of thirty-two cases. Histopathology 27:205–218, 1995.

142. Abdalla HM, Sakr MA: Predictive factors of local recurrence and survival following primary surgical treatment of phyllodes tumors of the breast. J Egypt Natl Canc Inst 18:125–133, 2006.

143. Hajdu SI, Espinosa MH, Robbins GF: Recurrent cystosarcoma phyllodes: A clinicopathologic study of 32 cases. Cancer 38:1402–1406, 1976.

144. Lindquist KD, van Heerden JA, Weiland LH, Martin JK Jr: Recurrent and metastatic cystosarcoma phyllodes. Am J Surg 144:341–343, 1982.

145. West TL, Weiland LH, Clagett OT: Cystosarcoma phyllodes. Ann Surg 173:520–528, 1971.

146. Martin RG: Sarcomas of the breast. In Gallagher HS (ed): The breast. St. Louis, Mosby, 1978.

147. Vuitch MF, Rosen PP, Erlandson RA: Pseudoangiomatous hyperplasia of mammary stroma. Hum Pathol 17:185–191, 1986.

148. Nassar H, Elieff MP, Kronz JD, Argani P: Pseudoangiomatous stromal hyperplasia (PASH) of the breast with foci of morphologic malignancy: A case of PASH with malignant transformation? Int J Surg Pathol 2008. [epub ahead of print]

149. Ferreira M, Albarracin CT, Resetkova E: Pseudoangiomatous stromal hyperplasia tumor: A clinical, radiologic and pathologic study of 26 cases. Mod Pathol 21:201–207, 2008.

150. Iglesias A, Arias M, Santiago P, et al: Benign breast lesions that simulate malignancy: Magnetic resonance imaging with radiologic-pathologic correlation. Curr Probl Diagn Radiol 36:66–82, 2007.

151. Hargaden GC, Yeh ED, Georgian-Smith D, et al: Analysis of the mammographic and sonographic features of pseudoangiomatous stromal hyperplasia. AJR Am J Roentgenol 191:359–363, 2008.

152. Ibrahim RE, Sciotto CG, Weidner N: Pseudoangiomatous hyperplasia of mammary stroma. Some observations regarding its clinicopathologic spectrum. Cancer 63:1154–1160, 1989.

153. Zanella M, Falconieri G, Lamovec J, Bittesini L: Pseudoangiomatous hyperplasia of the mammary stroma: True entity or phenotype? Pathol Res Pract 194:535–540, 1998.

154. Ohuchi N, Abe R, Takahashi T, Tezuka F: Origin and extension of intraductal papillomas of the breast: A three-dimensional reconstruction study. Breast Cancer Res Treat 4:117–128, 1984.

155. Carter D: Intraductal papillary tumors of the breast: A study of 78 cases. Cancer 39:1689–1692, 1977.

156. Page DL, Salhany KE, Jensen RA, Dupont WD: Subsequent breast carcinoma risk after biopsy with atypia in a breast papilloma. Cancer 78:258–266, 1996.

157. Ohuchi N, Abe R, Kasai M: Possible cancerous change of intraductal papillomas of the breast. A 3-D reconstruction study of 25 cases. Cancer 54:605–611, 1984.

158. Haagensen CD: Breast carcinoma risk and detection. Philadelphia, WB Saunders, 1981.

159. Flint A, Oberman HA: Infarction and squamous metaplasia of intraductal papilloma: A benign breast lesion that may simulate carcinoma. Hum Pathol 15:764–767, 1984.

160. Reddick RL, Jennette JC, Askin FB: Squamous metaplasia of the breast. An ultrastructural and immunologic evaluation. Am J Clin Pathol 4:530–533, 1985.

161. Gudjonsdottir A, Hagerstrand I, Ostberg G: Adenoma of the nipple with carcinomatous development. Acta Pathol Microbiol Scand [A] 79:676–680, 1971.

162. Rosen PP, Caicco JA: Florid papillomatosis of the nipple. A study of 51 patients, including nine with mammary carcinoma. Am J Surg Pathol 10:87–101, 1986.

163. Oberman HA: Benign breast lesions confused with carcinomas. In McDivitt RW (ed): The breast. Baltimore, Williams & Wilkins, 1984.

164. Perzin KH, Lattes R: Papillary adenoma of the nipple (florid papillomatosis, adenoma, adenomatosis). A clinicopathologic study. Cancer 29:996–1009, 1972.

165. Azzopardi JG, Salm R: Ductal adenoma of the breast: A lesion which can mimic carcinoma. J Pathol 144:15–23, 1984.

chapter 9

Congenital and Acquired Disturbances of Breast Development and Growth

KIRBY I. BLAND | J. HARRISON HOWARD |
LYNN J. ROMRELL

Development of the Breast

The mammary glands, or breasts, are considered highly modified sudoriferous glands. The glands develop as ingrowths from the ectoderm, which form the ducts and alveoli. The supporting vascularized connective tissue is derived from mesenchyme. During the fifth or sixth week of development, two ventral bands of thickened ectoderm, called the mammary ridges (or milk lines), are present in the embryo (Fig. 9-1). In many mammals, paired mammary glands develop along these ridges, which extend from the base of the forelimb (future axilla) to the region of the hind limb (inguinal region). The ridges are not prominent in the human embryo and disappear shortly after their formation, except for a small portion that persists in the pectoral region, where a single pair of glands usually develops. Accessory nipples (polythelia) or accessory mammary glands (polymastia) may occur along the original mammary ridges or milk lines (Fig. 9-2) if the structure fails to undergo its normal regression.

Each gland develops as the ingrowth of the ectoderm forms a primary bud of tissue in the underlying mesenchyme (Fig. 9-3A). Each primary bud gives rise to 15 to 20 secondary buds, or outgrowths (see Fig. 9-3B). During the fetal period, epithelial cords develop from the secondary buds and extend into the surrounding connective tissue. By the end of prenatal life, lumens have developed in the outgrowths, forming the lactiferous ducts and their branches (see Fig. 9-3C). At birth, the lactiferous ducts open into a shallow epithelial depression, known as the mammary pit. The pit becomes elevated and transformed into the nipple shortly after birth as a result of proliferation of the mesenchyme underlying the presumptive nipple and areola (see Fig. 9-3D). Failure of elevation of the pit results in a congenital malformation known as inverted nipple.

In newborn infants of both sexes, the breasts often show a transient enlargement and may produce some secretion, often called witch's milk. These transitory changes occur in response to maternal estrogen that crosses the placenta during fetal development. At birth, the breasts appear similar in both sexes, demonstrating the presence of only the main lactiferous ducts. The glands remain underdeveloped until puberty, when in the female the breasts enlarge rapidly in response to estrogen and progesterone secretion by the ovaries. The hormonal stimulation causes proliferation of the glandular tissue as well as fat and other connective tissue elements associated with the breast. The glandular tissue remains incompletely developed until pregnancy occurs. At this time, the intralobular ducts undergo rapid development and form buds that become alveoli.

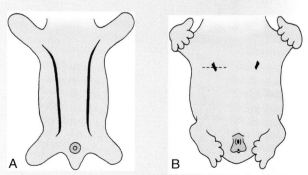

Figure 9-1 The mammary ridges and their regression. **A,** Ventral view of an embryo at the beginning of the fifth week of development (about 28 days), showing the mammary ridges that extend from the forelimb to the hind limb. **B,** A similar view of the ventral embryo at the end of the sixth week, showing the remains of the ridges located in the pectoral region.

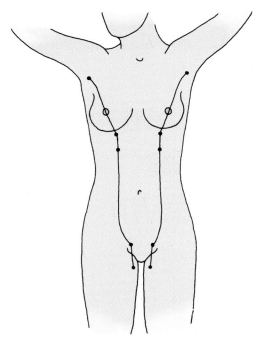

Figure 9-2 Mammary milk line. After development of the milk bud in the pectoral area of ectodermal thickening, the "milk streak" extends from the axilla to the inguinal areas. At week 9 of intrauterine development, atrophy of the bud has occurred except for the presence of the supernumerary nipples or breast.

Russo and Russo[1-3] have shown that the risk of developing breast cancer is heavily affected by endocrine and reproductive influences, especially those created during pregnancy. The risk of breast cancer has long been known to show inverse relationship with early parity (for review, see Russo and colleagues[4]). The risk of breast cancer increases with the age at which a woman bears her first child. This protection appears to be inversely related to

the length of time between menarche and the first pregnancy, as evidenced by the increased risk of cancer if the length of this interval is more than 14 years. Pregnancy has to occur before age 30 to have a protective effect on breast cancer risk. Women who become pregnant after age 30 have a risk above that of nulliparous women. Multiparity does confer additional protection; however, the protective effect is primarily limited to the first birth and persists at all subsequent ages. The mechanism responsible for early first-term pregnancy protection remains largely unknown. Evidence suggests that the differentiation of the mammary gland that is induced by full-term pregnancy inhibits carcinogenic initiation. Studies summarized by Russo and colleagues[4] suggest that the breast of late parous and nulliparous women exhibit characteristics of undifferentiated breast cells that are predisposed to undergo neoplastic differentiation.

The role of genes in both normal development and especially neoplastic changes in the breast is of major interest. Lewis[5] has reviewed the growing literature on the genetic determinants that establish and maintain the integrity of the mammary cells. Recently, there has been a great deal of interest in families of regulatory genes called homeobox genes.[6] These genes encode for proteins that recognize and bind to specific DNA sequences of other genes that control the sequential development of structures and organs. Recent studies of gene expression strongly suggest that homeobox genes may function in the development of the mammary gland and may play a role in the development of breast cancer. Additional genes studied in breast cancer include *EGFR* and *HER2*.[7,8] These genes are part of a tyrosine kinase family involved in cell signaling. *HER2* overexpression has been linked to poor prognosis and early recurrence.[9-11] The advent of trastuzumab has improved survival in patients with metastatic breast cancer with overexpression of *HER2*. Targeting *EGFR* as well as *HER2* has recently shown promise for successfully treating breast cancer.[12] This gene therapy reinforces the importance of genetic studies of normal and pathologic breast development.

Amastia

The congenital absence of one or both breasts (amastia) is a rare clinical anomaly.[13] The first recorded reference to amastia is found in "The Song of Solomon" in the Bible (8:viii): "We have a little sister, and she hath no breast: What shall we do for our sister in the day when she shall be spoken for?" Froriep first described true absence of the breast in 1839.[14] The association of bilateral amastia with other congenital anomalies was described in 1882 by Gilly,[15] who described a 30-year-old woman who presented with absence of the ulna and the ulnar aspect of the right hand. Approximately 50 case reports of amastia were recorded by Deaver and McFarland[16] in their treatise of the breast in 1917. Reports in the literature before the 1960s rarely gave details of amastia.[17] There have been only a few reports of bilateral amastia, defined as complete absence of both breasts and nipples. An extensive review of the literature by Trier[18] documented 43 cases for which data were available. Three presentations were observed: (1) bilateral absence of breasts with congenital ectodermal defects (7 cases), (2) unilateral absence of the breasts

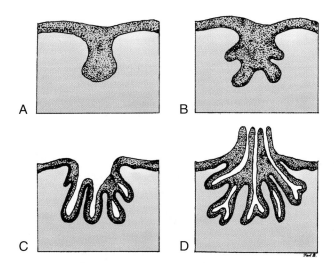

Figure 9-3 Sections through evolutionary development and growth of the mammary bud. **A–C,** Similar sections showing the developing gland at successive stages between the twelfth week and birth. The mammary pit develops, and major lactiferous ducts are present at the end of gestation. **D,** A similar section showing the elevation of the mammary pit by proliferation of the underlying connective tissue forming the nipple soon after birth.

TABLE 9-1		
Congenital Anomalies associated with Bilateral Absence of the Nipples and Breast Tissues		
No. of Patients	**Reported Anomalies**	
1	Atrophy of the right pectoral muscle; absence of the ulna and ulnar side of the hand	
1	Absence of finger on the right hand; deformity of the right foot	
1	Bilateral lobster-claw deformity of the hands and feet; cleft palate	
2	Sparse axillary and pubic hair; saddle nose; hypertelorism; high-arched palate	
1	Short status; short, small nose; broad nasal root; protrusion of the external ear; high-arched palate	
10	No anomalies	

From Trier WC: Complete breast absence. Case report and review of the literature. Plast Reconstr Surg 36:431–439, 1965.

(20 cases), and (3) bilateral absence of the breast (16 cases) with variable associated anomalies (Table 9-1).

Tawil and Najjar[19] reported an additional case of congenital bilateral absence of breasts and nipples in a 12-year-old Arab girl with abnormal ears, macrostomia, and chronic glomerulonephritis. Previously, Goldenring and Crelin[20] described a mother and daughter with similar phenotypes. More recently, Nelson and Cooper[21] documented a family in which the father and two of three daughters were found to have bilateral absence or hypoplasia of the nipples or breast tissue with associated minor defects. The mode of inheritance of this combination of defects is autosomal dominant.[22]

Unilateral absence of the breast (Fig. 9-4) is more common than bilateral amastia, and such subjects are most commonly female. This rare physical defect occurs as a result of complete failure of the development of the mammary ridge at about the sixth week in utero. Most often, abnormalities are not associated with bilateral absence of nipple and breast tissue. However, Trier[18] has observed amastia in association with cleft palate; hypertelorism and saddle nose; and anomalies of the pectoral muscle, ulna, hand, foot, palate, ears, genitourinary tract, and habitus. Occasionally, several members of a family have been affected. At least four reports[18,20,23,24] document the transmission of this anomaly with pedigree penetrance consistent with dominant inheritance.

Triolo and associates[25] observed a case of absence of the nipples (athelia) and amastia in a 28-year-old woman with associated severe dental alterations, nail dystrophies, and irregular cutaneous hyperpigmentation but normal sweating. The diagnosis was hidrotic ectodermal dysplasia, an autosomal dominant hereditary disease. The syndrome was present in the father and two brothers of the patient. The patient also had urinary incontinence due to sphincter urethrae agenesis.

Rich and coworkers[26] described a case of ureteral triplication as a component of an autosomal dominant syndrome consisting of bilateral amastia, pectus excavatum, umbilical hernia, patent ductus arteriosus, dysmorphic low-set ears, ptosis, epicanthic folds with an antimongoloid slant of the eyes, ocular hypertelorism, high-arched palate, flat broad nasal bridge, tapered digits, cubitus valgus, and syndactyly. Nelson and Cooper[21] have also reported the autosomal dominant transmission of breast hypoplasia or athelia in association with webbing of the fingers. Rich and coworkers[26] are the only investigators to report genetically transmitted

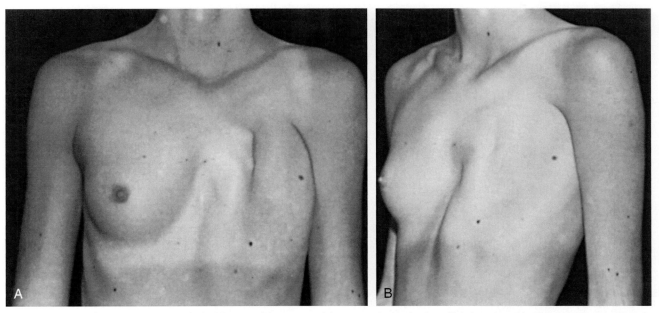

Figure 9-4   A and **B,** Unilateral amastia in 20-year-old woman with concomitant chest wall deformity of ipsilateral ribs 3 to 6 and cartilage. In contrast to those with Poland's syndrome, this patient has accessory musculature of the shoulder, including pectoralis major and minor, latissimus dorsi, and serratus anterior muscles. (Courtesy of Dr. John McCraw, Norfolk, VA.)

ureteral triplication, either alone or in association with bilateral amastia.

Unilateral Congenital Defects of the Breast with associated Defects of the Chest Wall, Ipsilateral Musculature, Subcutaneous Tissues, and Brachysyndactyly (Poland's Syndrome)

In 1841, Alfred Poland[27] published in Guy's Hospital Report the description of a patient who presented with absence of musculature (pectoralis major and minor) of the shoulder girdle and malformations of the ipsilateral upper limb. In this original report of unilateral congenital absence of the pectoralis major and minor muscles, there was associated absence of the external oblique and partial absence of the serratus anterior. Thereafter, numerous authors[28] reported similar findings, with the additional observation of hypoplasia or complete absence of the breast or nipple, costal cartilage and rib defects (ribs 2, 3, and 4 or ribs 3, 4, and 5), hypoplasia of subcutaneous tissues of the chest wall, and brachysyndactyly. This constellation of clinical findings, whether all or partially present, is currently termed

Poland's syndrome. Poland's syndrome is rare with incidence estimated to be 1:20,000 to 1:50,000. The etiology of this malformation is unknown but believed to be related to improper development of the subclavian axis with a resulting impedance of blood flow to the affected structures.[29]

Clinical manifestations of Poland's syndrome are extremely variable, and rarely can all features be recognized in a single individual.[30-33] At least two reports confirm a variant of the disorder associated with large melanotic spots. Because breasts and melanocytes both originate from the ectoderm, abnormalities of breast hypoplasia and hyperpigmentation probably develop from within this germinal layer. Moore and Schosser[34] have reported on Becker's melanosis associated with hypoplasia of the breast and pectoralis major muscle. Zubowicz and Bostwick[35] also have confirmed two patients with areas of diffuse hyperpigmentation overlying a unilaterally hypoplastic breast. Patients often do not request treatment of the pigmented abnormalities, and standard methods used in the therapy of hyperpigmentation often yield unsatisfactory results. Such hyperpigmented areas appear to have no neoplastic risk.

Poland's syndrome is invariably unilateral, with a higher incidence in female than in male patients. When a chest wall defect (ribs, cartilage, or both) is evident, there is usually a deep concavity on expiration and lung herniation with inspiration (Fig. 9-5). The right side is

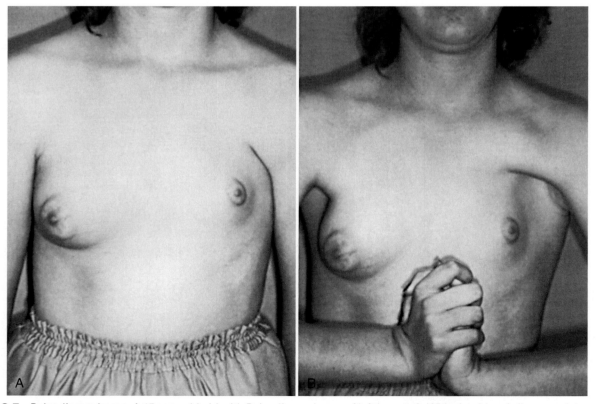

Figure 9-5 Poland's syndrome. A 15-year-old girl with Poland's syndrome of left breast. **A,** With shoulder girdle musculature actively contracted. **B,** There is accentuation of the left hypoplastic breast. There is absence of the sternal head of the pectoralis major although the clavicular head is present. (Courtesy of Dr. Hollis H. Caffee, Division of Plastic and Reconstructive Surgery, University of Florida College of Medicine, Gainesville, FL.)

more commonly affected than the left.[36] The most common defect, breast hypoplasia, is readily recognized, and the rudimentary breast tissue is usually higher on the involved side and medially displaced from its normal anatomic position.

Although the cause is unclear, this syndrome is seldom familial. Despite hypoplastic breast tissue, several cases of breast cancer have been documented on the side affected by Poland's syndrome. Standard techniques for sentinel lymph node biopsy can be used in these patients even though they have altered anatomy.[29,37] Leukemia has been associated with the syndrome, as have other rare congenital anomalies. Similar defects have been noted with exposure to drugs, such as thalidomide.

Treatment of patients with Poland's syndrome varies with the number of anomalies and their physical expression. With the presentation of one or two typical characteristics of Poland's syndrome, patients usually complain only about their appearance. These patients are not functionally embarrassed by their lack of anterior chest wall muscle mass or the small size of their breast. Only in extreme cases, as with total absence of the costal cartilage or segments of the anterior ribs, are patients physically impaired and emotionally disturbed by their deformity. Indications for operative intervention have been discussed by Fokin and Robicsek[38] and include progression of chest depression, lack of protection of the heart and lung, paradoxical chest wall movement. Surgery may also be needed for cosmetic reconstruction of the breast or chest wall musculature. Surgical procedures to correct the deformities of the chest wall have been documented[33] and include (1) subperiosteal grafts from adjacent ribs with free flaps of latissimus dorsi or external oblique,[39] (2) autologous split-rib grafts,[40] (3) split-rib grafts with periosteum that has been detached posteriorly and rotated from the anterior aspect of the defective rib to the sternum,[41] (4) heterologous bone grafts,[42] (5) metallic mesh implants followed by rib grafts from the opposite chest wall,[43] and (6) customized silicon breast and chest wall prostheses to reconstruct both structures in difficult cases.[44] Ravitch[45] popularized the use of split-rib grafts from the opposite chest wall that are placed across the defect and reinforced with Teflon felt. The technique described by Amoroso and Angelats[46] uses autologous tissue of the latissimus dorsi myocutaneous flap to augment the hypoplastic breast and to contour the anterior chest wall while simultaneously augmenting the involved hypoplastic breast. This procedure, initially attempted by Asp and Sulamaa[39] of Finland, was unsuccessful using a free latissimus dorsi flap. Thus, it was abandoned because transplanted muscle atrophied as a result of the omission of the neurovascular pedicle from the transplant, emphasizing the value of preservation of the pedicle when employing this technique. In 1950, Campbell[47] described the use of a latissimus dorsi muscle flap transferred through the axilla for anterior chest wall reconstruction with preservation of the neurovascular bundle. He, too, abandoned this technique because the flap was associated with a cutaneous component or applied over a breast prosthesis unsuccessfully.

Schneider, Hill, and Brown[48] emphasized the value of a single-stage reconstruction. The high success rate and the reliability of this technique, which uses the latissimus dorsi myocutaneous flap, represents remarkable advance over the aforementioned methods. Latissimus dorsi myocutaneous flaps continue to be the most commonly used flap for breast and chest wall reconstruction in patients with Poland's disease. This procedure is now being performed with an endoscopic approach for flap harvest and reconstruction. Additionally, tissue expanders followed by replacement with permanent prosthetic implants is a technique commonly employed for these patients.[49-51]

Computed tomography (CT) provides useful information in planning reconstructive surgery in patients with Poland's syndrome.[52] Hurwitz, Stofman, and Curtin[53] have recently suggested the use of a three-dimensional CT scan as an adjunct for planning chest wall and breast reconstruction in Poland's syndrome. Follow-up with three-dimensional MRI reformation was used to demonstrate the results of the implant reconstruction. The authors suggest that these imaging techniques can be used to accurately portray the three-dimensional tissue deficit and assist in the selection of muscle transposition flaps and reconstructive technique.

Iatrogenic Factors That Initiate Breast Hypoplasia

Failure of complete development of the vestigial male or female breast may occur as a consequence of developmental hypomastia (Fig. 9-6) or may be initiated by therapeutic manipulation or injury of the mammary anlage in infancy or in the prepubertal interval. Rudimentary breast tissue in male and female infants lies beneath the primitive nipple/areola complex at approximately the fourth intercostal space. Thus trauma, incisions, abscess, infectious lesions, or radiation therapy to the breast bud in the infantile or prepubertal era can initiate maldevelopment with hypoplasia of the vestigial breast. The surgeon must be especially aware of the necessity and technique of any incision for drainage of lesions of the areolar complex or masses within the breast bud to avoid subsequent maldevelopment.

Unilateral development of breast tissue in the adolescent female may represent nonisometric growth of breast tissue in precocious or early pubertal states. With this presentation, cautious observation of the contralateral breast is in order. The surgeon should not perform a biopsy on the rudimentary breast structure or the nipple-areola complex using incisional or excisional techniques. The risk of neoplastic lesions is infinitesimally small in this younger age group, whereas the travesty of irreversible damage to the breast bud with subsequent hypoplasia of the breast or amastia is a distinct possibility. The bilaterally symmetric nipple-areola and breast complexes overlie the fourth intercostal space of the infant. In the fully developed breasts of the sexually mature female, the complex may extend to the seventh and eighth intercostal spaces. Thus, excisional biopsies of any chest wall lesions that are initiated before full maturation of the mammae must be approached cautiously.

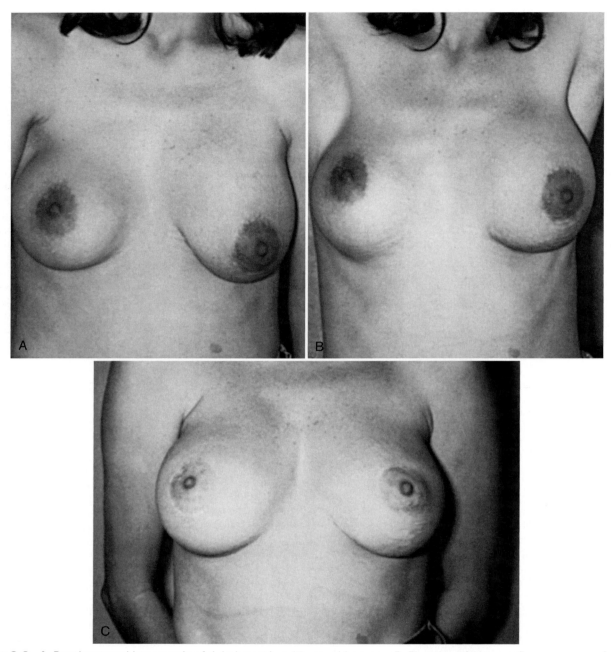

Figure 9-6 **A,** Developmental hypomastia of right breast in a 27-year-old woman. **B,** Elevation of arms confirms presence of pectoralis major and shoulder girdle musculature on side of hypomastia. **C,** Final cosmetic appearance of breasts following augmentation mammaplasty of right breast and reduction mammaplasty with mastopexy of left breast. (Courtesy of Dr. Hal G. Bingham, Division of Plastic and Reconstructive Surgery, University of Florida, College of Medicine, Gainesville, FL.)

Cherup, Siewers, and Futrell[54] documented breast and pectoral muscle maldevelopment after anterolateral and posterolateral thoracotomies in children. Incisions placed through the third and fourth intercostal spaces for repair of congenital heart lesions were evaluated in 28 patients by these authors. In this series, standard anterolateral thoracotomies resulted in a high frequency of breast or pectoral muscular maldevelopment. Using measurements of volumes of the breast and pectoral muscles with plaster molds and linear dimensions of each chest side, the authors concluded that 60% of patients with these incisions had greater than a 20% difference in volume between the two sides. To avoid these maldevelopment syndromes, when the anterolateral or posterolateral thoracotomy must be used, it should be started anteriorly in the seventh or eighth interspace, below the level to which the breast will extend by adulthood, and the incision should be carried no higher than the sixth interspace to avoid the extension of the breast to the axilla. Furthermore, the pectoralis muscles should not be divided but elevated superiorly as a unit from the inferior edge and retracted to avoid subsequent injury to this organ as well.

This technique avoids injury to the neurovascular pedicles of the pectoralis muscles and the breast bud itself.

In 1959 Moss[55] reported that in the prepubertal interval, when the human breast consists mainly of an expanding ductular system, 1500 to 2000 rad delivered through a single portal over an 8-day period initiates striking maldevelopment of this organ. Furthermore, 3000 to 4000 rad administered over 30 days not only permanently arrests growth of glandular epithelium but also concomitantly produces severe fibrosis and hypoplasia of the breast. Following 3000 rad, the result was complete loss of lobules and shrinkage of ductules of breast tissue. Williams and Cunningham,[24] in evaluating the histologic changes of irradiated breasts of women, state that irradiated areas show intense obliterative endarteritis and, in the end stages, marked fragmentation of elastic tissue.

Underwood and Gaul[56] documented severe breast hypoplasia as a consequence of radium therapy implants for a cavernous hemangioma in the region of the left breast of an infant. Subsequently, the contralateral breast matured normally, whereas the ipsilateral involved breast failed to develop. Similar reports of hypoplasia have been recorded by Matthews,[57] who used radium needles applied to the surface of the hemangioma, close to the nipple, when the patient was in her infancy. The report by Weidman, Zimany, and Kopf[58] addresses the necessity of observation of breast hemangiomas and the cautious application of radiotherapy in the treatment of hemangiomas or other lesions of the breast with ionizing radiation. Furthermore, contemporary approaches to the therapy of intrathoracic or chest wall neoplasms dictate modification of irradiation portals that traverse the nipple/areola complex or the breast bud in infantile or prepubertal patients.

Premature Thelarche

The term premature thelarche refers to isolated breast development in the absence of additional signs of sexual maturation in girls younger than 8 years (Fig. 9-7).[59,60] The etiology of premature thelarche is controversial with various hypotheses for actual cause. Wilkins, Blizzard, and Migeon[61] have postulated that an increased sensitivity of breast tissue to low circulating levels of estrogens (estrone, estradiol) secreted during early childhood is the cause of this premature breast development. Several authors have suggested normal or slightly increased plasma estradiol and basal gonadotropin (luteinizing hormone [LH] and follicle-stimulating hormone [FSH]) levels with the presentation.[62] Conflicting results with regard to gonadotropin responsiveness by synthetic gonadotropin-releasing hormone (luteinizing hormone–releasing hormone [LHRH]) have been observed. In premature thelarche, the basal LH and FSH concentrations have been reported as normal or slightly elevated.[63,64] Most recently, Borges and colleagues[65] have confirmed that baseline LH levels are elevated in girls with premature thelarche when compared with normal controls. In a series of 15 patients reported by Caufriez and coworkers,[66] all patients with premature thelarche had normal basal LH and FSH levels

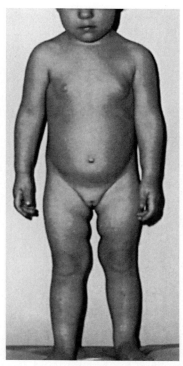

Figure 9-7 Premature thelarche in a 19-month-old girl with isolated breast development in the absence of additional signs of sexual maturation. (Courtesy of Dr. Arlan L. Rosenbloom, Department of Pediatrics, University of Florida College of Medicine, Gainesville, FL.)

for their age and normal responses to LHRH. The observations of these investigators are in agreement with those of Reiter and colleagues[67] and Tenore and associates.[68] These reports suggest that patients with premature thelarche have normal regulation of the hypothalamic-pituitary-gonadal axis.

Caufriez and coworkers[66] confirmed a normal basal prolactin secretion and a normal response to thyrotropin-releasing hormone (TRH) for girls with premature thelarche. Prolactin does not convincingly appear to have a role in the genesis of isolated breast development in prepubertal girls. The endocrinologic relationship of this clinical presentation has been further investigated by Pasquino and associates[69] in nine young girls with premature thelarche who were compared with nine healthy girls and six girls with true precocious puberty. The gonadotropin stimulation test with LHRH was used. Girls with premature thelarche were observed to have LH responses that resemble those of normal girls, and FSH responses were similar to those of patients with precocious puberty. This study suggests that in premature thelarche there is partial activation of the diencephalic-hypophyseal-gonadal axis, which affects FSH alone. The authors conclude that premature thelarche should be considered as one of the disorders that results from altered sensitivity of the hypothalamic receptors that regulate sexual maturation. From a practical point of view, this study emphasizes the utility of the gonadotropin stimulation test with LHRH in girls with premature breast development as a test to distinguish between premature thelarche and true precocious puberty.

Data from Ilicki and coworkers[70] in a long-term follow-up of 68 girls with premature thelarche confirmed that 85% of patients with the disorder had onset before the age of 2 years. In 30.8%, this clinical finding was recognized at birth; in 44%, there was a regression after a standard deviation of 3 (3/12) ± 2 (8/12) years. In this study, basal levels of plasma FSH and response to LHRH were significantly higher ($P < 0.001$) than in prepubertal controls. Of 52 patients, 27 evaluated had increased plasma estradiol, and in 27 of 40 patients tested, urocystograms or vaginal smears confirmed estrogenization. Basal levels of LH and responses to LHRH were prepubertal. In this study, girls with premature thelarche were significantly taller than normal controls of the same age ($P < 0.001$). These investigators suggested that premature thelarche is an incomplete form of precocious sexual development, probably occurring secondary to a derangement in the maturation of the hypothalamic-pituitary-gonadal axis that results in a higher-than-normal secretion of FSH. The authors concluded that the end result appears to be a defect in the peripheral sensitivity to the sexual hormones.

In follow-up of the natural history and endocrine findings of premature thelarche, a longitudinal study from the Institute of Paediatrics, University of Rome, Italy, was completed by Pasquino and associates.[71] This study of 40 girls with premature thelarche confirmed that when the disorder occurred before the age of 2 years, it usually regressed completely, thus representing an isolated and transient phenomenon. Additional studies have shown that girls presenting with premature thelarche after 2 years of age are more likely to progress to precocious puberty, and this may represent the first sign of sexual development, generally leading to early simple puberty.[72] These observations were confirmed by Mills and colleagues,[64] who likewise conducted longitudinal studies of the natural history of the disorder by contacting 46 patients with previously diagnosed cases. These authors observed palpable breast tissue that persisted for 3 to 5 years in 57% of the subjects. Only 11% reported that their breast tissue had continued to enlarge. Patients in whom breast tissue had been present at birth and had persisted were significantly more likely to have progressive enlargement. Comparison of these patients with matched-control subjects showed no relationship between premature thelarche and maternal obstetrical problems, exposure to medications, diet, or prenatal infections. Furthermore, girls with premature thelarche were no more likely than control subjects to have other medical or sexual problems develop during the follow-up interval.

Escobar, Rivarola, and Bergadaá[73] evaluated the plasma concentration of estradiol-17β in premature thelarche and in varying types of sexual precocity. All patients with idiopathic precocious puberty had elevated plasma estradiol concentrations for their ages that showed wide variations. No correlation between the grade of sexual development and the level of estradiol was observed. The plasma estradiol concentrations confirmed good correlation with clinical signs of estrogenic effects in prepubertal and adolescent normal girls (Fig. 9-8). Of their 10 patients with premature thelarche,

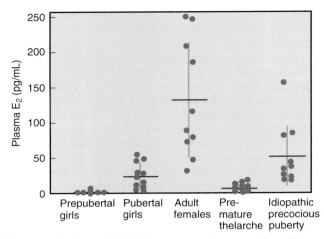

Figure 9-8 Estradiol-17β plasma values in normal females, premature thelarche, and idiopathic precocious puberty. Mean values are indicated by horizontal lines and standard deviations by vertical lines. (From Escobar ME, Rivarola MA, Bergadaá C: Plasma concentration of oestradiol-17β in premature thelarche and in different types of sexual precocity. Acta Endocrinol 81:351–361, 1976.)

7 had prepubertal levels of estradiol. Girls with higher estradiol levels were 7 years older and had urocystograms with moderate estrogenic activity. The findings in these younger girls confirmed the hypothesis that premature thelarche specifically resulted from higher sensitivity of breast tissue to prepubertal estrogen levels, because other estrogen target tissues did not show this stimulatory effect.

Tenore and associates[68] used multivariate analysis (chronologic age, FSH, LH, and bone age-to-chronologic age ratio) to predict the evolution of premature thelarche to central precocious puberty. In a study of 32 girls with premature thelarche, they reported that all subjects with isolated premature thelarche could be sharply distinguished from those who progressed to precocious puberty. In a related long-term study, Pasquino and colleagues[74] retrospectively examined 100 girls with premature thelarche to evaluate whether girls with premature thelarche progress to central precocious puberty. Fourteen of the patients with characteristic premature thelarche progressed during follow-up to precocious or early central precocious puberty. The chronologic age of the 14 girls in this group was 5.1 (standard deviation of 2) years at the onset of premature thelarche and 7.8 (standard deviation of 0.6) years after progression to central precocious puberty. No clinical or hormonal characteristics could be established that separated the 14 girls who progressed to precocious puberty from the 86 girls who did not. The authors concluded that premature thelarche is not always a self-limited condition and that it may sometimes accelerate the timing of puberty. Borges and colleagues[65] have clarified this transition by measuring peak elevation of LH levels after a gonadotropin-releasing hormone stimulation test to help distinguish between premature thelarche and precocious puberty. They confirmed that when LH is elevated above 4.5 IU/L, females do in fact have precocious puberty, not simply premature thelarche. Rosenfield[75] has warned that although premature pubarche, premature thelarche, and precocious puberty are usually simply normal phenomena occurring at an early age, they may sometimes be harbingers of reproductive endocrine disturbances in adulthood. Consequently, girls with these complaints should be followed to ascertain that pubertal reproductive function is eventually normal.

Juvenile (Adolescent, Virginal) Hypertrophy of the Female Breast

Juvenile, or adolescent, hypertrophy of the breast is a commonly observed occurrence in the young adolescent female following a normal puberty. This clinical presentation denotes the adolescent breast that does not cease its rapid pubertal growth and continues to enlarge even into mature years. Most patients with juvenile hypertrophy of the breast have symmetric, bilateral involvement (Fig. 9-9), although unilateral juvenile hypertrophy has been described.[76]

Several conditions may initiate breast asymmetry, including maldevelopment, neoplasms, incisional or excisional biopsies, trauma, and radiotherapy.[77] As noted earlier, developmental abnormalities account for most of these lesions. Mayl, Vasconez, and Jurkiewicz[78] suggested that juvenile hypertrophy, also referred to as macromastia, may occur secondary to a primary defect of the breast or an endocrinologic disorder.[79] The general tenet

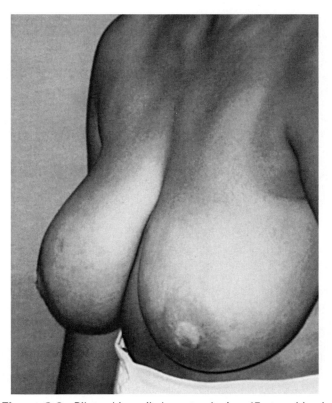

Figure 9-9 Bilateral juvenile hypertrophy in a 17-year-old nulliparous Hispanic girl. The patient presented with mastodynia related to her large breast size. She was not taking any medications known to induce breast gigantism. Therapy consisted of reduction mammaplasty. (Courtesy of Dr. Hollis H. Caffee, Division of Plastic and Reconstructive Surgery, University of Florida College of Medicine, Gainesville, FL.)

has been that an augmented plasma level of estrone or estradiol may induce hypertrophy of the breasts. However, the measurement of various mammotropic hormones as the etiology for the disorder has not yielded precise clinical correlates with breast enlargement. Nonetheless, substantial decreases in plasma progesterone levels have been documented for juvenile hypertrophy in the presence of normal plasma estrogen and growth hormone values. These substantial decreases of progesterone in the hormonal milieu may be causing the abnormality. One could also postulate that target organ tissues (ductal epithelium, collagen and stroma of the adolescent female breast) may have estrogen receptors that are highly responsive to minimal concentrations of the mammotropic steroid hormones (e.g., estrogens, progesterone) that regulate breast growth and development.[80]

Sperling and Gold[81] and Mayl and associates[78] have recommended the use of the antiestrogen drugs dydrogesterone (Gynorest) and medroxyprogesterone acetate (Provera) in the treatment of virginal hypertrophy. Ryan and Pernoll[82] were successful in preventing regrowth of breast parenchyma following reduction mammaplasty in several patients with adolescent hypertrophy by using the drug dydrogesterone. However, a subsequent follow-up report by these investigators suggested its ineffectiveness. Thereafter, partial success for prevention of regrowth was achieved with tamoxifen citrate (Nolvadex). Treatment with tamoxifen may be of value after reduction mammaplasty (subcutaneous mastectomy) in patients with strongly positive estrogen receptor profiles in the removed breast tissue. Using an escalating dose of 10 to 40 mg of tamoxifen citrate per day, these authors were able to achieve reduction of breast bulk with the drug. Theoretically, with the use of this compound, estrogen receptors can be converted to a negative profile status. Bromocriptine has also been used in virginal hypertrophy, similar to treatment of pregnancy-induced gigantomastia, but has been shown to be unsuccessful in juvenile hypertrophy.[83]

The most commonly applied technique for the treatment of adolescent (juvenile) hypertrophy continues to be the subcutaneous mastectomy described by Furnas[84] as a reduction mammaplasty. However, the technique, as reported by De Castro[85] does not represent a panacea for this disorder. Modifications of the subcutaneous mastectomy have subsequently been described by Courtiss and Goldwyn,[86] who used an inferior pedicle technique as an alternative to free nipple and areola grafting for severe macromastia or extreme ptosis. For recurrent adolescent hypertrophy following previously successful reduction mammaplasty, the total glandular mastectomy with subpectoral augmentation may be considered. This aggressive technique, as previously described by Bland and coworkers,[87] should only rarely be necessary in the premenopausal female (Fig. 9-10). The success of this more radical approach depends on the extirpation from the chest wall of all breast tissue that has estrogen hypersensitivity and, thus, the potential for regrowth. Currently, reduction mammaplasty is the definitive therapy for juvenile hypertrophy with the possibility of tamoxifen as an adjunct to surgical treatment.[88]

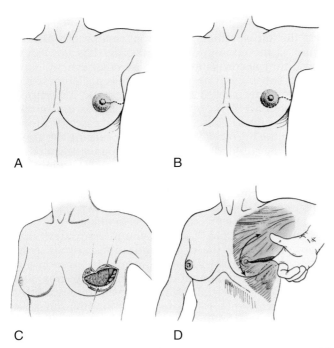

Figure 9-10 Technique for one-stage mastectomy with immediate reconstruction. **A,** Circumferential nipple incision extended transareolarly and in "lazy S" pattern over lateral portion of breast. Nipple and ductal system remain with breast specimen. **B,** When preexisting para-areolar scar is present, or inferior skin envelope must be reduced, circumareolar incision is used. Nipple is circumscribed as in **A. C,** Flap elevation via circumareolar incision with development of skin thickness and extent of dissection identical to modified radical mastectomy technique. **D,** Entering submuscular plane via muscle-splitting incision of serratus anterior at fifth rib level; serratus anterior muscle origins are avulsed from their ribs to beyond sixth rib, and blunt dissection of the subpectoralis major plane is continued superiorly to clavicle and medially to sternum. (From Bland KI, O'Neal B, Weiner LJ, Tobin GR II: One-stage simple mastectomy with immediate reconstruction for high-risk patients. An improved technique: The biologic basis for ductal-glandular mastectomy. Arch Surg 121:221–225, 1986.)

Tuberous Breast Deformity

Tuberous breast deformity was first described in 1976 by Rees and Aston[89] but has been described in many other studies with various names.[90] The malformation causes the affected breasts to resemble the root of a tuberous plant, which was the basis of the original description (Fig. 9-11). The incidence of this condition is unknown. There is a large spectrum of this disease; many women are not likely to seek treatment. It has been documented

that a high percentage of women presenting with asymmetric breast suffer from tuberous deformity.[91] The abnormality can be seen as a unilateral or bilateral phenomenon and is first noticed at puberty with development of the breast tissue.

In an effort to better characterize this deformity, Heimburg and colleagues[92] composed a classification system for the tuberous deformities:

Type I–hypoplasia of the lower medial quadrant

Type II–hypoplasia of the lower medial and lateral quadrants; sufficient skin in the subareolar region

Type III–hypoplasia of the lower medial and lateral quadrants; deficiency of skin in the subareolar region

Type IV–severe breast constriction; minimal breast base

They further describe decreased breast tissue and milk ducts of the lower quadrants, especially the lower medial quadrant. Other modifications of this classification system have been proposed,[93] but most descriptions of the deformity agree that the resulting features are from skin shortage and herniation of breast tissue through the nipple-areolar complex.[91]

Several theories have been proposed for the cause of the tuberous breast defect. The first hypothesis proposed a strong adherence between the dermis and muscular plane along the lower pole of the breast. As the breast develops, it is unable to separate this adherence, and the peripheral expansion of the breast is restricted (Fig. 9-12). The breast tissue then develops forward, enlarging and sometimes herniating into the areola.[93] Mandrekas and associates[94] described a fibrous band at the periphery of the nipple-areola complex, representing a thickening of the superficial fascia that inhibits normal breast development. The fibrous ring does not allow for the growing breast tissue to expand inferiorly. Because there is no superficial fascia underneath the areola, the breast tissue herniates toward the nipple-areola complex.

Along with their early description of this malformation, Rees and Aston[89] were also among the first to describe the principles of treatment for tuberous breast deformity. Many techniques have subsequently been proposed, but the fundamental principles remain correcting breast tissue herniation and lowering of the inframammary fold.[90,91] Single-staged procedures with either reduction mammoplasty or breast augmentation have yielded excellent results in less severe malformations.[92] Simple augmentation of severe deformities has frequently resulted in an unsatisfactory "double bubble" appearance, further accentuating the tuberous deformity.

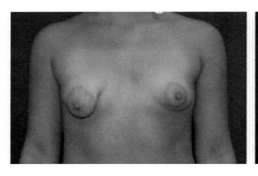

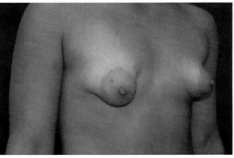

Figure 9-11 A 19-year-old girl with bilateral severe tuberous breast deformity. (From Latham K, Fernandez S, Iteld L, et al: Pediatric breast deformity. J Craniofac Surg 17:454–467, 2006.)

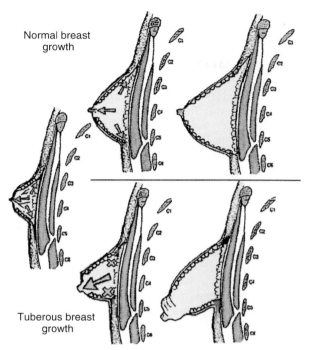

Figure 9-12 Depiction of normal and tuberous breast growth. (From Grolleau JL, Lanfrey E, Lavigne B, et al: Breast base anomalies: Treatment strategy for tuberous breasts, minor deformities, and asymmetry. Plast Reconstr Surg 104:2040–2048, 1999.)

In these patients, multiple procedures with tissue expansion and flaps have been proposed.[90,92] Newer single-staged techniques are now consistently and reproducibly giving satisfactory results, with excellent symmetry of the breasts, conveying a better understanding of the disease process.[91,94]

Drug Induction of Gigantism

Drug-related induction of breast gigantism has been described.[95,96] This disorder may occur in the adolescent or in the fully mature adult breast (Fig. 9-13).

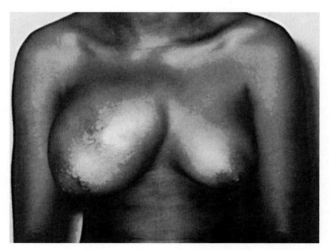

Figure 9-13 Gigantism of drug induction. An 18-year-old black woman with painful unilateral gigantism of the right breast following treatment with ᴅ-penicillamine.

ᴅ-Penicillamine as an etiologic factor in breast enlargement is a poorly understood but well-recognized cause of sudden gigantism. Desai[97] has postulated an effect on sex hormone–binding globulin by ᴅ-penicillamine to increase the amount of circulating free estrogen. Taylor, Cumming, and Corenblum[98] have suggested that ᴅ-penicillamine produces a local effect on the breast, because patients do not show changes in menstrual function while receiving the drug or during the time of maximal breast growth. These authors confirm the effect of danazol (17-α-pregna-2, 4-dien-20-ynol(2,3-d) isoxazol-17β-0; Danocrine) to act by interfering with the sensitivity of the breast parenchymal estrogen receptor, thereby diminishing growth.[99] These studies confirmed both diminution in breast size during the first courses of danazol administration and that these reductions occurred simultaneously with a reduction in plasma circulating estradiol concentrations. Furthermore, the cessation of danazol administration with an increase in breast volume indicated that a reduction in breast size was not simply a coincidental spontaneous remission. This clinical trial did not determine whether the breast shrinkage that resulted with the drug was produced by a reduction in circulating estrogen concentrations or by a local effect. The blocking of estrogen receptors by danazol may mimic the postmenopausal condition and has been successfully applied by Buckle[100] for the treatment of gynecomastia in males.

Breast Hypertrophy with Pregnancy (Gigantomastia)

Massive hypertrophy of the breast with pregnancy is a rare condition of unknown cause. It is often referred to as gigantomastia of pregnancy.[101] The first recorded report of this condition was made by Palmuth in 1648.[102] Moss[103] has revealed that this condition may affect women of all races during the childbearing years but that Caucasian women are more likely to experience this phenomenon than African-American women.[104] The disorder is less common than juvenile (virginal) hypertrophy of the breast, which classically progresses independent of pregnancy and occurs usually between the ages of 11 and 19 years. Gigantomastia of pregnancy usually occurs during the first few months of pregnancy and may progress to necrosis, incapacity, and possibly death.[103] Bilateral breast gigantism is usually observed, although unilateral gigantomastia of pregnancy has been reported.[105]

The typical history is that of a healthy pregnant woman who observes gradual bilateral massive enlargement of her breasts within the first few months of pregnancy. The breasts may enlarge to several times their normal weight and size to become grotesque, huge, and incapacitating. The skin and parenchyma become firm, edematous, and tense and may have prominent subcutaneous veins with a diffuse peau d'orange appearance. As a consequence of rapid breast enlargement and skin pressure, insufficient vascularity of the skin may initiate ulceration, necrosis, infection, or hemorrhage.

In the immediate postpartum period, the hypertrophied breasts recede to approximately their previous volume. With delivery of the fetus, the breasts regress in size but almost always hypertrophy again with succeeding pregnancies. Most authors agree that this condition is hormonal in etiology, but its precise mechanism is unclear. Swelstad and colleagues[104] have proposed multiple inciting factors as possible causes for this problem, including hormonal abnormalities, tissue receptor sensitivity, malignancy, and autoimmune disorders. Whether there is an overproduction of mammotropic hormone from the pituitary or an enhanced sensitivity of breast parenchyma to the hormones of pregnancy (e.g., estriol, estradiol, human chorionic gonadotropin, progestins) has not been firmly established. Parham[106] determined that estrogen and testosterone were of no value in the treatment of gigantism of pregnancy; however, norethindrone may be of value.[107] Hydrocortisone therapy has been attempted without success by Nolan[108]; testosterone has been used with divided results. Moss[103] used fluoxymesterone unsuccessfully, whereas diuretics have been successfully used but with moderate and temporary effect.

Luchsinger[109] was one of the first to suggest that this condition may occur as a consequence of specific individual reactivity of the breast to hormonal stimuli. This author questioned whether in addition to possible hormonal dysfunction, estrogenic placental hormones were sufficiently metabolized in the presence of insufficient liver function. Lewison and colleagues[110] postulated that gigantism of pregnancy may be related to the depression of all steroid hormones and decreased liver function as measured by the salicylate conjugation test. These investigators advocated the use of the progestational agent norethindrone to reduce breast size; however, it was used with mestranol and had to be discontinued when thrombophlebitis occurred. Although liver dysfunction and the inability to metabolize estrogenic hormones have been postulated to be a possible cause for the disorder, it must be noted that many normal pregnancies are accompanied by severe liver failure without the development of gigantomastia. Bromocriptine is the most widely used medical treatment of this problem. It has shown variable results with arrested breast hypertrophy or mild breast size regression; the agent has an inability to return breast to pregestational size.[104] Although the medical approach has variable results, it should be the first line of treatment in an effort to avoid surgical intervention during pregnancy.

In most instances, gigantomastia is self-limiting and does not progress to pyogenic abscesses, skin ulcerations, necrosis, or systemic illness. Breast size will spontaneously regress to its approximate nonpregnant configuration after delivery. The patient should be advised of proper brassiere support, good skin hygiene, and adequate nutrition. Operative intervention may be necessary to relieve severe pain, massive infection, necrosis, slough, and ulceration or hemorrhage if delivery is not imminent. The operative choices include bilateral reduction mammaplasty versus bilateral mastectomies with delayed reconstruction. Gigantomastia is likely to recur with reduction mammaplasty in subsequent pregnancies. Bilateral mastectomies with delayed reconstruction offer the best chance of avoiding recurrence if the patient should become pregnant again. If there is any retained breast tissue, it is likely to hypertrophy with additional pregnancies.[104]

Scott-Conner and Schorr[111] reviewed in detail the diagnosis and management of breast problems during pregnancy and lactation. Furthermore, Howard and Gusterson[112] reviewed the histology of normal physiologic states of the human breast, including prenatal, prepubertal, and pubertal development; adult resting gland; pregnancy; lactation; and postinvolution.

Symmastia: Medial Confluence of the Breast

Symmastia (Greek, *syn*, meaning "together" and *mastos*, meaning "breast") is the contemporary terminology for medial confluence of the breast. This rare clinical anomaly represents a webbing across the midline of breasts that are usually symmetric (Fig. 9-14). More common, however, is the presternal blending (confluence) of the breast tissue that is associated with macromastia. These conditions are most often recognized in individuals who seek reduction mammaplasty.[113]

Like many anomalies of ectodermal origin, a broad spectrum of defects may be observed with this congenital lesion. Cases may range from an empty skin web to those with an apparent confluence of major portions of symmetric breast tissue within the midline. The common denominator is the need for resection of presternal skin to varying degrees. Spence, Feldman, and Ryan[113] recommend correction of the web defect using three methods. The first method is elevation of an inferiorly based triangular skin flap that is advanced superiorly in an inverted Y-V manner following division of excessive medial soft tissue. Thereafter, the divided medial soft tissue is sutured superiorly to the medial pectoralis fascia to create a brassiere-band sling effect. These authors have also used a superiorly based medial flap that contains both skin and soft tissue. Excess skin and soft tissue were excised, and the remaining flap was tailored to fit into a V-shaped defect in the inferior incision. A third option suggested by the authors consists of the vertical division and superior rotation of the excess subcutaneous tissue flaps with elevation of a superiorly based skin flap inserted into a V-shaped defect in the inferior incision. The use of liposuction as an integral part of a surgical correction of symmastia has been reported by Schonegg and associates.[114] Regarding the use of liposuction, McKissock[115] has predicted that the same limitations will apply to the breast as advocates of liposuction have professed exist elsewhere in the body. Thus, the amount of skin involved in the web medially, and its resiliency, will determine the applicability of liposuction techniques for this anomaly. Salgado and Mardini[116] have proposed a periareolar approach to the surgical treatment of symmastia. Dissection is performed superficial to the breast tissue but deep to the subcutaneous tissue. The dermis is then approximated to the periosteum of the sternum with nonabsorbable suture. When used along with liposuction, this technique yields a quite satisfactory result while avoiding a visible midline incision and scar.

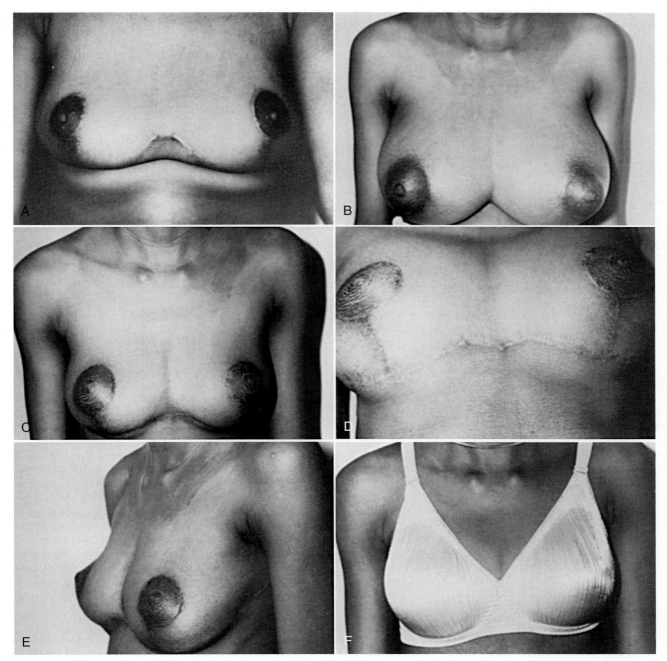

Figure 9-14 Symmastia. **A,** A 24-year-old woman following reduction mammaplasty with persistent central breast web of symmastia. Cosmetic congenital defect was corrected with inserted Y-V advancement flap. **B,** A 19-year-old woman with large, painful breasts and prominent central webbing reportedly present since the beginning of breast development. **C–F,** Postoperative appearance of breasts after correction of symmastia with reduction mammaplasty using the inferior pedicle technique. (From Spence RJ, Feldman JJ, Ryan JJ: Symmastia: The problem of medial confluence of the breasts. Plast Reconstruct Surg 73:261–269, 1984.)

Supernumerary Nipples (Polythelia) and Supernumerary Breast (Polymastia)

In the human embryo, the mammary ridge first becomes apparent in the 7- to 8-mm-long embryo and atrophies before birth. It is the persistence of mammalian tissue along the milk line that results in ectopically displaced or accessory breast tissue (see Figs. 9-1 and 9-2). This congenital anomaly is commonly bilateral and is often unaccompanied by the areola or the nipple (Fig. 9-15). In 1915, Kajava[117] developed a classification system to characterize accessory breast tissue that is still used: (1) the presence of a complete breast with mammary gland tissue and the nipple-areola complex, (2) the presence of gland tissue and nipple, (3) gland tissue and areola, (4) solitary gland tissue, (5) nipple-areola with fat replacement of the mammary gland tissue (pseudomamma), (6) the nipple alone (polythelia), (7) the areola alone (polythelia areolaris), and (8) the presence of a small patch of hair-bearing tissue (polythelia pilosa).

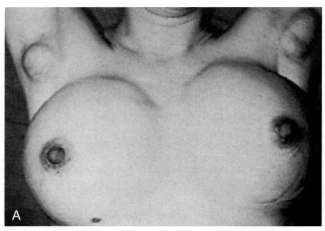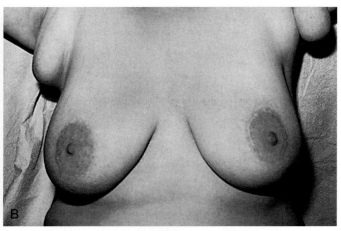

Figure 9-15   A and **B,** Supernumerary breasts presenting as accessory (ectopic) breast tissue bilaterally in the axilla. Note right supernumerary inframammary nipple presenting in the mammary milk line **(A).** (**A,** From Greer KE: Arch Dermatol 109:88, 1974. Copyright © 1974, American Medical Association. All rights reserved. **B,** Courtesy of Dr. Michael M. Meguid, SUNY Health Sciences Center, Syracuse, NY.)

Polythelia represents the most common variant of supernumerary breast components and occurs predominantly between the breast and the umbilicus.[118] However, glandular tissue compatible with complete or variable components of breast parenchyma can occur within the mammary ridge at sites between the axilla and the groin. Velanovich[119] has reviewed the embryology, clinical presentation, diagnosis, treatment, and clinical significance of supernumerary nipples, supernumerary breasts, and ectopic breast tissue. Important considerations concerning these common anomalies include the following:

- Supernumerary nipples, supernumerary breasts, and ectopic breast tissue most commonly develop along the milk lines.
- Whereas polythelia is evident at birth, supernumerary and ectopic breast tissue is evident only after hormonal stimulation that occurs at puberty or during pregnancy.
- Ectopic breast tissue is subject to the same pathologic changes that occur in normally positioned breasts.
- Axillary ectopic breast tissue may be confused with other malignant and benign lesions occurring in the area.
- Polythelia may indicate associated conditions, most notably urologic malformations or urogenital malignancies.

The presence of supernumerary or accessory nipples (Fig. 9-16) is a relatively common, minor congenital anomaly that occurs in both sexes, with an estimated frequency of 1 in 100 to 1 in 500 persons.[120] Mehes[121,122] and Mehes and associates[123] have reported the frequency of supernumerary nipples as 0.22% in a white European population, which is significantly lower than the incidence of 1.63% found by Rahbar[124] in black American neonates. This represents a 7.4-fold increase for the anomaly in blacks. In the newborn Jewish population reported by Mimouni and associates,[125] the higher incidence of 2.5% for polythelia was observed. This high frequency of supernumerary nipples could possibly be related to ethnic differences but, as acknowledged by

some authors, may be related to a systematic technique for examination of the newborn.

Congenital supernumerary nipples may occur in any size or configuration along the mammary milk line extending from the nipple to the symphysis pubis. As noted earlier, the supernumerary nipple anomaly may be easily overlooked in young infants, in whom these ectopic lesions often appear only as a small spot with a diameter of 2 to 3 mm. Moore and Schosser[34] observed that supernumerary nipples usually develop just below the normal breast in the white population, with less common occurrence in abdominal or inguinal sites.[126] Abramson[127] observed bilateral supernumerary nipples in approximately half of patients with polythelia. In the ectopic sites, polythelia takes origin from the extramammary buds that are present along the ventral embryonic mammary ridges (see Fig. 9-3A). Only a minority of persons with this clinical anomaly have more than two extra nipples.[34]

Polythelia should be searched for in the routine physical examination of every newborn, and the presence of the condition should be reported to the parents. This is important for the following reasons, as reported by Mimouni and associates[125]:

- Supernumerary breasts in females may respond to fluctuations in hormones in a physiologic manner such that pubertal enlargement, premenstrual swelling, tenderness, and lactation during pregnancy and parturition may occur.
- Patients with polythelia may be subject to the same spectrum of pathologic diseases observed in normal breasts (e.g., neoplasms, fibroadenomas, papillary adenomas, cysts, or carcinomas).[128–131]
- The supernumerary nipples may be associated with other congenital diseases such as vertebral anomalies,[132,133] cardiac arrhythmias, or renal anomalies.[128,134–139]

In embryogenesis, polythelia occurs during the third month of gestation, when the embryonic mammary ridge fails to regress normally—an event coincident with the development of the urogenital and other organ systems. Although various malformations have been associated with polythelia (Table 9-2), attention has

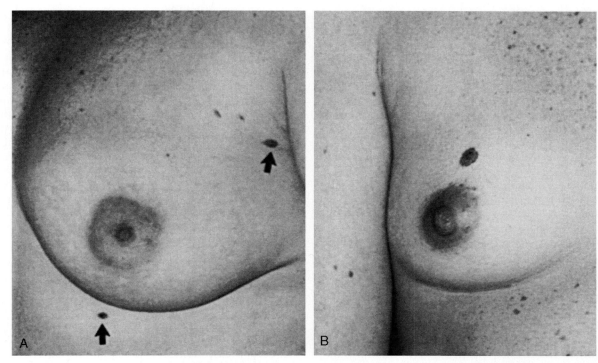

Figure 9-16 Supernumerary nipple. **A,** A 38-year-old woman with supernumerary nipples *(arrows)* above (in axilla) and below the normal left breast in the mammary milk line. **B,** Supernumerary nipple and areolar complex (rudimentary) in upper right breast of a 22-year-old woman. Excisional biopsy was the preferred treatment.

been drawn to the high incidence of renal anomalies and malignancies in children with supernumerary nipples.[140] The association between supernumerary nipples and occult anomalies of the urogenital system has been reported in at least two non–U.S. pediatric populations. These studies from Hungary[55] and Israel[141] have reported that 23% and 40%, respectively, of children with polythelia had obstructive renal abnormalities or duplications of the excretory system. Studies in Hungarian children have shown no link between polythelia and renal anomalies. Jojart and Seres[142] have found the prevalence of supernumerary nipples to be

4.29% among healthy newborns and 5.86% among healthy schoolchildren. Ultrasound was used to examine the urogenital system of 496 children with supernumerary nipples and 2367 control patients. The prevalence of renal anomalies was 3.74% in children with supernumerary nipples and 3.17% in the control group; 2.86% in newborns with supernumerary nipples and 1.89% in control newborns. The differences were not significant. The association of polythelia with urogenital malformations continues to be controversial. Recommendations vary from no screening to the screening of all children with polythelia. The true association of these two entities likely has not been elucidated completely.[143,144]

Polythelia has also been associated with cancers of the testis and kidney.[123,145-147] Familial as well as sporadic occurrences of polythelia with renal cancer, urogenital anomalies, and germ cell tumors have been reported.[133,147-149] Goedert and associates[146] evaluated 299 medical students, of whom 8 (2.7%) had polythelia. This frequency of the anomaly yielded an estimated relative risk of testicular cancer for men with polythelia of 4.5 (95% confidence interval, 1.6 to 12.4). Goedert and coworkers[145] also linked renal adenocarcinoma with polythelia. In a cohort of 32 patients with renal adenocarcinoma, a disproportionate number of patients exhibited polythelia. The authors suggest that this may represent a genetic or developmental link between renal adenocarcinoma and polythelia.

Intra-areolar polythelia represents a nipple-areola unit within the mammary ridge such that a dichotomy of the vestigial breast and nipple-areola complex exists. Only a few cases of bilateral intra-areolar polythelia have been

TABLE 9-2

Polythelia and associated Conditions

Urinary Tract Abnormalities	Cardiac Abnormalities	Miscellaneous Abnormalities
Renal agenesis	Cardiac conduction disturbances, especially left bundle branch block	Pyloric stenosis
Renal cell carcinoma		Epilepsy
Obstructive disease		Ear abnormalities
Supernumerary kidney(s)	Hypertension Congenital heart anomalies	Arthrogryposis multiplex congenita

From Pellegrini JR, Wagner RF Jr: Polythelia and associated conditions. Am Fam Physician 28:129–132, 1983.

recorded. Multiplicity of nipples is not uncommon, and they are bilateral in approximately half of patients so affected. As many as 10 nipples have been recorded in a single patient.[150] Atypical locations have been noted secondary to the displaced embryonal primordium.[151]

The presence of supernumerary nipples may necessitate operative therapy in instances in which discharge, tumor, or cyst formation is evident. Simple elliptical excision placed in lines of cleavage or skin folds is preferred to achieve maximum cosmesis. Primary closure is usually possible and allows the surgeon to achieve a superior cosmetic result.

Polymastia also results from the embryonic mammary ridge (see Fig. 9-1A) failing to undergo normal regression (see Fig. 9-1B). Causal factors are as yet unknown. The prevalence of polymastia was 0.1% in the Collaborative Perinatal Project reported by Chung and Myrianthopoulos,[152] although Orti and Oazi[153] suggested a frequency approaching 1%. In a longitudinal survey of minor congenital defects, Mehes[121,122] and Mehes and associates[123] observed that supernumerary breasts were present in 0.2% of children; 8 of the 20 affected children in the study also had major renal anomalies. Similar to polythelia, reports on polymastia suggest an association between renal adenocarcinoma and renal malformations.[140,154]

A familial occurrence of the polymastia anomaly has been observed.[98,153] DeGrouchy and Turleau[155] document the association of polymastia with congenital cytogenetic syndromes, especially those involved with chromosomes 3 and 8. Furthermore, other congenital anomalies, notably Turner's syndrome (ovarian agenesis and dysgenesis with chromosomal karyotypes of 45,X, but mosaic patterns [45,X/46,XX or 45,X/46,XX/47, XXX] are seen) and Fleisher's syndrome (lateral displacement of the nipples to the midclavicular lines with bilateral renal hypoplasia[156]), may have polymastia as a component of the syndrome (Fig. 9-17).

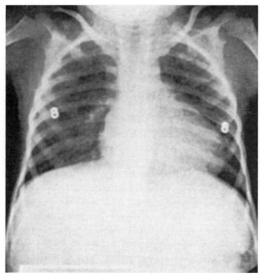

Figure 9-17 Fleisher's syndrome. Posteroanterior chest roentgenogram of a 5-year-old with bilateral renal hypoplasia. Although the clavicles are not horizontal, the lateral displacement of the nipples (designated by the lead markers 8) is apparent. (From Fleisher DS: Lateral displacement of the nipples, a sign of bilateral renal hypoplasia. J Pediatr 69:806–809, 1966.)

In a 1995 case presentation and review of the literature regarding carcinoma of ectopic breast tissue, Evans and Guyton[157] reported that of a total of 90 cases of carcinoma of ectopic breast tissue, 64 occurred in the axilla. The combined survival beyond the 4-year post-treatment period was 9.4%. No survival advantage was found for radical or modified radical mastectomy over local excision combined with axillary dissection or radiation. The researchers found that the correct preoperative diagnosis was rarely made, and they suggested that improved prognosis requires diagnostic suspicion and early biopsy of suspicious ectopic masses that occur along the embryonic milk lines. In related studies, fine-needle biopsy has been found to be useful in the diagnosis and management of ectopic breast tissue.[150,158,159]

Accessory (Ectopic) Axillary Breast Tissue

Ectopic axillary breast tissue is a relatively uncommon occurrence but is a relatively common variant of polymastia.[160] Greer[118] noted the presence of accessory axillary breast tissue to be apparent only at or after puberty, with the most rapid growth observed during pregnancy. Jeffcoate[161] has suggested that axillary breast tissue may represent true ectopic tissue not contiguous with the breast but more commonly represents an enlargement of the axillary tail of Spence. Thus, to determine the presence or absence of accessory axillary breast tissue, one must distinguish between an enlargement of the axillary tail and ectopically displaced mammary tissues of the milk line. The occurrence of ectopic breast tissue *outside the axilla* is exceedingly rare. Dworak and associates[162] and Reck and colleagues[163] were the first to report a hamartoma of ectopic breast tissue in the inguinal region. The finding, confirmed with histopathologic examination, occurred in a 50-year-old woman suspected of having a chronic incarcerated hernia.

The discovery of accessory axillary breast tissue usually occurs during the first pregnancy as a consequence of the secondary changes initiated with hormonal stimulation by ovarian estradiol and placental estriol. The symptomatic axillary breast tissue becomes painfully enlarged and, on rare occasion, may develop galactoceles with milk secretion via contiguous skin pores.[164] Although these anomalies may not become evident until the first pregnancy, once the lesions are recognized, they continue to recur with subsequent pregnancies and may undergo cyclical changes during menstruation. De Cholnoky[151] noted pathologic findings in 26 cases of axillary breast tissue that included normal breast tissue (9), cystic disease (10), fibroadenoma (3), mastitis (4), and atypical ductal hyperplasia (1) or carcinoma (2). Often, the clinician identifies the lesion as excess axillary fat, although lymphadenitis, lymphoma, metastatic carcinoma, and hidradenitis suppurativa are common misdiagnoses. After identification of the hormonal dependency with pregnancy or menstruation, the clinician can often establish the diagnosis, especially if a history of lactation during the puerperium is confirmed.

Management consists of reassuring the patient of its common benignity and its embryologic origin. However, accessory axillary tissue may be misdiagnosed as the symptomatic alterations inherent with pathologic changes of breast tissue (e.g., carcinoma and the benign breast tissue spectrum). Treatment of symptomatic accessory breast tissue during the puerperium and pregnancy involves conservative management for most clinical presentations. The presence of dense, nodular masses suggestive of malignant transformation necessitates aggressive approaches to rule out carcinoma.[165] As this hormonally dependent accessory breast tissue rapidly regresses when lactation ceases, the patient can be reassured but should be admonished that enlargement and painful, lactating, accessory tissue may recur with subsequent pregnancy. Elliptically placed incisions in skin folds of the axilla allow complete dissection and removal of the breast tissue beneath the skin and over the underlying fascia. The cosmetically oriented resections of the accessory tissue are usually curative, although the lesion may recur if excision is incomplete.

Acknowledgments

The authors gratefully acknowledge the photographs and technical assistance supplied by Dr. Arlan L. Rosenbloom, Department of Pediatrics, and Drs. Hal G. Bingham and H. Hollis Caffee, Division of Plastic Surgery, University of Florida.

REFERENCES

1. Russo IH, Russo J: Mammary gland neoplasia in long-term rodent studies. Environ Health Perspect 104:938–967, 1996.
2. Russo J, Russo I: Development of the human mammary gland. New York, Plenum Press, 1987.
3. Russo J, Russo IH: Biological and molecular bases of mammary carcinogenesis. Lab Invest 57:112–137, 1987.
4. Russo J, Hu YF, Silva ID, Russo IH: Cancer risk related to mammary gland structure and development. Microsc Res Tech 52:204–223, 2001.
5. Lewis MT: Homeobox genes in mammary gland development and neoplasia. Breast Cancer Res 2:158–169, 2000.
6. Chen H, Sukumar S: Role of homeobox genes in normal mammary gland development and breast tumorigenesis. J Mammary Gland Biol Neoplasia 8:159–175, 2003.
7. Chan SK, Hill ME, Gullick WJ: The role of the epidermal growth factor receptor in breast cancer. J Mammary Gland Biol Neoplasia 11:3–11, 2006.
8. Slamon DJ, Leyland-Jones B, Shak S, et al: Use of chemotherapy plus a monoclonal antibody against HER2 for metastatic breast cancer that overexpresses HER2. N Engl J Med 344: 783–792, 2001.
9. Hynes NE, Stern DF: The biology of erbB-2/neu/HER-2 and its role in cancer. Biochim Biophys Acta 1198:165–184, 1994.
10. Ravdin PM, Chamness GC: The c-erbB-2 proto-oncogene as a prognostic and predictive marker in breast cancer: a paradigm for the development of other macromolecular markers—a review. Gene 159:19–27,1995.
11. Slamon DJ, Godolphin W, Jones LA, et al: Studies of the HER-2/neu proto-oncogene in human breast and ovarian cancer. Science 244:707–712, 1989.
12. Konecny GE, Pegram MD, Venkatesan N, et al. Activity of the dual kinase inhibitor lapatinib (GW572016) against HER-2-overexpressing and trastuzumab-treated breast cancer cells. Cancer Res 66:1630–1639, 2006.
13. Hubert C: Etude sur l'amastic, thesis. Paris, 1907.
14. Froriep L: Beobachtung eines Falles von Mangel der Brustdruse. Notizen aus dem Gebiete der Natur and Heilkunst 1, 1839.
15. Gilly E: Absence complete de mamelles chez une femme mère: Atrophie de membre supéarieur droit. Courrier Med 32,1882.
16. Deaver J, McFarland J: The breast: Anomalies, diseases and treatment. Philadelphia, P Blakiston's & Sons, 1917.
17. Weinberg W: Zur vererbung des zwergwuchses. Arch Rass Ges Biol 9:710–718, 1912.
18. Trier WC: Complete breast absence. Case report and review of the literature. Plast Reconstr Surg 36:431–439, 1965.
19. Tawil HM, Najjar SS: Congenital absence of the breasts. J Pediatr 73:751–753, 1968.
20. Goldenring H, Crelin ES: Mother and daughter with bilateral congenital amastia. Yale J Biol Med 33:466–467, 1961.
21. Nelson MM, Cooper CK: Congenital defects of the breast—an autosomal dominant trait. S Afr Med J 61:434–436, 1982.
22. Wilson MG, Hall EB, Ebbin AJ: Dominant inheritance of absence of the breast. Humangenetik 15:268–270, 1972.
23. Fraser F: Dominant inheritance of absent nipples and breasts. Roma, Istituto Gregorio Mendel, 1956.
24. Williams IG, Cunningham GJ: Histological changes in irradiated carcinoma of the breast. Br J Radiol 24:123–133, 1951.
25. Triolo O, Allegra A, Stella Brienza L, et al: Familial ectodermal dysplasia with agenesis of the breasts and the external urethral sphincter. Description of a case. Minerva Ginecol 45:139–142, 1993.
26. Rich MA, Heimler A, Waber L, Brock WA: Autosomal dominant transmission of ureteral triplication and bilateral amastia. J Urol 137:102–105, 1987.
27. Poland A: Deficiency of the pectoral muscles. Guys Hosp Rep 6, 1841.
28. Pers M: Aplasias of the anterior thoracic wall, the pectoral muscles, and the breast. Scand J Plast Reconstr Surg 2:125–135, 1968.
29. Una J, Vega V, Gutierrez I, et al: Breast cancer, Poland's syndrome, and sentinel lymph node involvement. Clin Nucl Med 32: 613–615, 2007.
30. Fabian MC, Fischer JD: A variant of Poland's syndrome. Can J Surg 37:67–69, 1994.
31. Mace JW, Kaplan JM, Schanberger JE, Gotlin RW: Poland's syndrome. Report of seven cases and review of the literature. Clin Pediatr (Phila) 11:98–102, 1972.
32. Martin LW, Helmsworth JA: The management of congenital deformities of the sternum. JAMA 179:82–84, 1962.
33. Urschel HC Jr, Byrd HS, Sethi SM, Razzuk MA: Poland's syndrome: Improved surgical management. Ann Thorac Surg 37:204–211, 1984.
34. Moore JA, Schosser RH: Becker's melanosis and hypoplasia of the breast and pectoralis major muscle. Pediatr Dermatol 3:34–37, 1985.
35. Zubowicz V, Bostwick J III: Congenital unilateral hypoplasia of the female breast associated with a large melanotic spot: report of two cases. Ann Plast Surg 12:204–206, 1984.
36. David TJ: Nature and etiology of the Poland anomaly. N Engl J Med 287:487–489, 1972.
37. Okamo H, Miura K, Yamane T, Fujii H, Matsumoto Y: Invasive ductal carcinoma of the breast associated with Poland's syndrome: Report of a case. Surg Today 32:257–2560, 2002.
38. Fokin AA, Robicsek F: Poland's syndrome revisited. Ann Thorac Surg 74:2218–2225, 2002.
39. Asp K, Sulamaa M: On rare congenital deformities of the thoracic wall. Acta Chir Scand 118:392–404, 1960.
40. Ravitch MM: Operative treatment of congenital deformities of the chest. Am J Surg 101:588–597, 1961.
41. Ravitch M: Congenital deformities of the chest wall and their operative correction. Philadelphia, WB Saunders, 1977.
42. Heeker W, Daum R: Chirurgishces vorgchen bei kongenitalen brustwanddefekten. Chirurg 11, 1964.
43. Fevre M, Hannouche D: Thoracic breach due to aplasia or costal anomalies. Ann Chir Infant 9:153–166,1968.
44. Hochberg J, Ardenghy M, Graeber GM, Murray GF: Complex reconstruction of the chest wall and breast utilizing a customized silicone implant. Ann Plast Surg 32:524–528, 1994.
45. Ravitch MM: Disorders of the sternum and the thoracic wall, 3rd ed. Philadelphia, WB Saunders, 1976.
46. Amoroso PJ, Angelats J: Latissimus dorsi myocutaneous flap in Poland syndrome. Ann Plast Surg 6:287–290, 1981.

47. Campbell DA: Reconstruction of the anterior thoracic wall. J Thorac Surg 19:456–461, 1950.
48. Schneider WJ, Hill HL Jr, Brown RG: Latissimus dorsi myocutaneous flap for breast reconstruction. Br J Plast Surg 30:277–281, 1977.
49. Freitas Rda S, o Tolazzi AR, Martins VD, et al: Poland's syndrome: Different clinical presentations and surgical reconstructions in 18 cases. Aesthetic Plast Surg 31:140–146, 2007.
50. Gravvanis AI, Panayotou PN, Tsoutsos DA: Poland syndrome in a female patient reconstructed by endoscopically assisted technique. Acta Chir Plast 49:37–39, 2007.
51. Martinez-Ferro M, Fraire C, Saldana L, et al: Complete videoendoscopic harvest and transposition of latissimus dorsi muscle for the treatment of Poland syndrome: A first report. J Laparoendosc Adv Surg Tech A 17:108–113, 2007.
52. Bainbridge LC, Wright AR, Kanthan R: Computed tomography in the preoperative assessment of Poland's syndrome. Br J Plast Surg 44:604–607, 1991.
53. Hurwitz DJ, Stofman G, Curtin H: Three-dimensional imaging of Poland's syndrome. Plast Reconstr Surg 94:719–723, 1994.
54. Cherup LL, Siewers RD, Futrell JW: Breast and pectoral muscle maldevelopment after anterolateral and posterolateral thoracotomies in children. Ann Thorac Surg 41:492–497, 1986.
55. Moss T: Therapeutic radiology. St Louis, Mosby, 1959.
56. Underwood G, Gaul L: Disfiguring sequelae from radium therapy: Results of treatment of a birthmark adjacent to the breast of a female infant. Arch Dermatol 57:918, 1948.
57. Matthews DN: Treatment of haemangiomata. Br J Plast Surg 6:83–88, 1953.
58. Weidman AI, Zimany A, Kopf AW: Underdevelopment of the human breast after radiotherapy. Arch Dermatol 93:708–710, 1966.
59. Job J: Le deáveloppement preámatureá isoleá des seins chez les fillettes. Arch Fr Peádiatr 32, 1975.
60. Nelson KG: Premature thelarche in children born prematurely. J Pediatr 103:756–758, 1983.
61. Wilkins L, Blizzard RM, Migeon CJ: The diagnosis and treatment of endocrine disorders in childhood and adolescence. Springfield, IL, Charles C Thomas, 1965.
62. Guyda HJ, Johanson AJ, Migeon CJ, Blizzard RM: Determination of serum luteinizing hormone (SLH) by radioimmunoassay in disorders of adolescent sexual development. Pediatr Res 3: 538–544, 1969.
63. Kenny FM, Midgley AR Jr, Jaffe RB, et al: Radioimmunoassayable serum LH and FSH in girls with sexual precocity, premature thelarche and adrenarche. J Clin Endocrinol Metab 29:1272–1275, 1969.
64. Mills JL, Stolley PD, Davies J, Moshang T Jr: Premature thelarche. Natural history and etiologic investigation. Am J Dis Child 135: 743–745, 1981.
65. Borges MF, Pacheco KD, Oliveira AA, et al: Premature thelarche: Clinical and laboratorial assessment by immunochemiluminescent assay. Arq Bras Endocrinol Metabol 52:93–100, 2008.
66. Caufriez A, Wolter R, Govaerts M, et al: Gonadotropins and prolactin pituitary reserve in premature thelarche. J Pediatr 91: 751–753, 1977.
67. Reiter EO, Kaplan SL, Conte FA, Grumbach MM: Responsivity of pituitary gonadotropes to luteinizing hormone-releasing factor in idiopathic precocious puberty, precocious thelarche, precocious adrenarche, and in patients treated with medroxyprogesterone acetate. Pediatr Res 9:111–116, 1975.
68. Tenore A, Franzese A, Quattrin T, Sandomenico ML, et al: Prognostic signs in the evolution of premature thelarche by discriminant analysis. J Endocrinol Invest 14:375–381, 1991.
69. Pasquino AM, Piccolo F, Scalamandre A, Malvaso M, et al: Hypothalamic-pituitary-gonadotropic function in girls with premature thelarche. Arch Dis Child 55:941–944, 1980.
70. Ilicki A, Prager Lewin R, Kauli R, et al: Premature thelarche—natural history and sex hormone secretion in 68 girls. Acta Paediatr Scand 73:756–762, 1984.
71. Pasquino AM, Tebaldi L, Cioschi L, et al: Premature thelarche: A follow up study of 40 girls. Natural history and endocrine findings. Arch Dis Child 60:1180–1182, 1985.
72. Verrotti A, Ferrari M, Morgese G, Chiarelli F: Premature thelarche: A long-term follow-up. Gynecol Endocrinol 10:241–247, 1996.
73. Escobar ME, Rivarola MA, Bergadaá C: Plasma concentration of oestradiol-17β in premature thelarche and in different types of sexual precocity. Acta Endocrinol (Copenh) 81:351–361, 1976.
74. Pasquino AM, Pucarelli I, Passeri F, et al: Progression of premature thelarche to central precocious puberty. J Pediatr 126: 11–14, 1995.
75. Rosenfield RL: Normal and almost normal precocious variations in pubertal development premature pubarche and premature thelarche revisited. Horm Res 41(suppl 2):7–13, 1994.
76. Lorino CO, Finn M: Unilateral juvenile hypertrophy of the breast. Br J Radiol 60:193–195, 1987.
77. Martin J: Treatment of cystic hygromas. Tex State J Med 50, 1954.
78. Mayl N, Vasconez LO, Jurkiewicz MJ: Treatment of macromastia in the actively enlarging breast. Plast Reconstr Surg 54:6–12, 1974.
79. Li ZH, Tong ZH, Luo GY, Cai HM: Congenital hypertrichosis universalis associated with gingival hyperplasia and macromastia. Chin Med J (Engl) 99:916–917, 1986.
80. Bland KI, III CE: Breast disease: Physiologic considerations. St Louis, Mosby, 1988.
81. Sperling RL, Gold JJ: Use of an anti-estrogen after a reduction mammaplasty to prevent recurrence of virginal hypertrophy of breasts. Case report. Plast Reconstr Surg 52:439–442, 1973.
82. Ryan RF, Pernoll ML: Virginal hypertrophy. Plast Reconstr Surg 75:737–742, 1985.
83. Arscott GD, Craig HR, Gabay L: Failure of bromocriptine therapy to control juvenile mammary hypertrophy. Br J Plast Surg 54: 720–723, 2001.
84. Furnas DW: Subcutaneous mastectomy for juvenile hypertrophy of the breast: report of a case. Br J Plast Surg 35:367–370, 1982.
85. De Castro CC: Subcutaneous mastectomy for gigantomastia in an adolescent girl. Case report. Plast Reconstr Surg 1977;59: 575–578.
86. Courtiss EH, Goldwyn RM: Reduction mammaplasty by the inferior pedicle technique. An alternative to free nipple and areola grafting for severe macromastia or extreme ptosis. Plast Reconstr Surg 59:500–507, 1977.
87. Bland KI, O'Neal B, Weiner LJ, Tobin GR II: One-stage simple mastectomy with immediate reconstruction for high-risk patients. An improved technique: the biologic basis for ductal-glandular mastectomy. Arch Surg 121:221–225, 1986.
88. Baker SB, Burkey BA, Thornton P, LaRossa D: Juvenile gigantomastia: Presentation of four cases and review of the literature. Ann Plast Surg 46:517–525, discussion 525–526, 2001.
89. Rees TD, Aston SJ: The tuberous breast. Clin Plast Surg 3: 339–347, 1976.
90. Latham K, Fernandez S, Iteld L, et al: Pediatric breast deformity. J Craniofac Surg 17:454–467, 2006.
91. Pacifico MD, Kang NV: The tuberous breast revisited. J Plast Reconstr Aesthet Surg 60:455–64, 2007.
92. von Heimburg D, Exner K, Kruft S, Lemperle G: The tuberous breast deformity: Classification and treatment. Br J Plast Surg 49:339–345, 1996.
93. Grolleau JL, Lanfrey E, Lavigne B, et al: Breast base anomalies: Treatment strategy for tuberous breasts, minor deformities, and asymmetry. Plast Reconstr Surg 104:2040–2048, 1999.
94. Mandrekas AD, Zambacos GJ, Anastasopoulos A, et al: Aesthetic reconstruction of the tuberous breast deformity. Plast Reconstr Surg 112:1099–1108; discussion 1109, 2003.
95. Desautels JE: Breast gigantism due to d-penicillamine. Can Assoc Radiol J 45:143–144, 1994.
96. Finer N, Emery P, Hicks BH: Mammary gigantism and D-penicillamine. Clin Endocrinol (Oxf) 21:219–222, 1984.
97. Desai SN: Sudden gigantism of breasts: drug induced? Br J Plast Surg 26:371–372, 1973.
98. Taylor PJ, Cumming DC, Corenblum B: Successful treatment of D-penicillamine-induced breast gigantism with danazol. Br Med J (Clin Res Ed) 282:362–363, 1981.
99. Guillebaud J, Fraser IS, Thorburn GD, Jenken G: Endocrine effects of danazol in menstruating women. J Int Med Res 1977;5 Suppl 3:57–66.
100. Buckle R: Studies on the treatment of gynaecomastia with danazol (Danol). J Int Med Res 5(suppl 3):114–123, 1977.
101. Blaydes RM, Kinnebrew CA: Massive breast hyperplasia complicating pregnancy; report of a case. Obstet Gynecol 12:601–602, 1958.
102. Palmuth P: Observationem medicarum centuriae tres poshumae. Braunschweig, cent ii OBS, 1648.

103. Moss WM: Gigantomastia with pregnancy. A case report with review of the literature. Arch Surg 96:27–32, 1968.

104. Swelstad MR, Swelstad BB, Rao VK, Gutowski KA: Management of gestational gigantomastia. Plast Reconstr Surg 118:840–848, 2006.

105. Sharma K, Nigam S, Khurana N, Chaturvedi KU: Unilateral gestational macromastia—a rare disorder. Malays J Pathol 26:125–128, 2004.

106. Parham KJ: Gigantomastia. Report of a case. Obstet Gynecol 18:375–379, 1961.

107. Jessing A: Excessive mammary hypertrophy in pregnancy treated with androgenic hormones. Nord Med 63:237–239, 1960.

108. Nolan JJ: Gigantomastia: report of a case. Obstet Gynecol 19:526–529, 1962.

109. Luchsinger J: Bilateral mammary hypertrophy during pregnancy. Rev Obstet Ginecol Venez 20:707–710, 1960.

110. Lewison EF, Jones GS, Trimble FH, da LL: Gigantomastia complicating pregnancy. Surg Gynecol Obstet 110:215–223, 1960.

111. Scott-Conner CE, Schorr SJ: The diagnosis and management of breast problems during pregnancy and lactation. Am J Surg 170:401–405, 1995.

112. Howard BA, Gusterson BA: Human breast development. J Mammary Gland Biol Neoplasia 5:119–137, 2000.

113. Spence RJ, Feldman JJ, Ryan JJ: Symmastia: The problem of medial confluence of the breasts. Plast Reconstr Surg 73:261–269, 1984.

114. Schonegg WD, Peters U, Schonleber G, et al: Reduction-plasty of the breast in symmastia. Geburtshilfe Frauenheilkd 51:853–855, 1991.

115. McKissock P: Discussion of symmastia: the problem of medial confluence of the breast. Plast Reconstr Surg 73, 1984.

116. Salgado CJ, Mardini S: Periareolar approach for the correction of congenital symmastia. Plast Reconstr Surg 113:992–994, 2004.

117. Kajava Y: The proportions of supernumerary nipples in the Finnish population. Duodecim 31:143–170, 1915.

118. Greer KE: Accessory axillary breast tissue. Arch Dermatol 109:88–89, 174.

119. Velanovich V: Ectopic breast tissue, supernumerary breasts, and supernumerary nipples. South Med J 88:903–906, 1995.

120. Cohen AJ, Li FP, Berg S, et al: Hereditary renal-cell carcinoma associated with a chromosomal translocation. N Engl J Med 301:592–595, 1979.

121. Mehes K: Association of supernumerary nipples with other anomalies. J Pediatr 95:274–275, 1979.

122. Mehes K: Association of supernumerary nipples with other anomalies. J Pediatr 102:161, 1983.

123. Mehes K, Szule E, Torzsok F, Meggyessy V: Supernumerary nipples and urologic malignancies. Cancer Genet Cytogenet 24:185–188, 1987.

124. Rahbar F: Clinical significance of supernumerary nipples in black neonates. Clin Pediatr (Phila) 21:46–47, 1982.

125. Mimouni F, Merlob P, Reisner SH: Occurrence of supernumerary nipples in newborns. Am J Dis Child 137:952–953, 1983.

126. Camisa C: Accessory breast on the posterior thigh of a man. J Am Acad Dermatol 3:467–469, 1980.

127. Abramson DJ: Bilateral intra-areolar polythelia. Arch Surg 110:1255, 1975.

128. Kumar S, Cederbaum AI, Pletka PG: Renal cell carcinoma in polycystic kidneys: Case report and review of literature. J Urol 124:708–709, 1980.

129. Mate K, Horvath J, Schmidt J: Simultaneous occurrence of polythelia and heart conduction disorders. Orv Hetil 117: 2863–2866, 1976.

130. Mate K, Horvath J, Schmidt J, et al: Polythelia associated with disturbances of cardiac conduction. Cor Vasa 21:112–116, 1979.

131. Miller G, Bernir I: Adenomatose erosive du mamelon. Can J Surg 8, 1965.

132. Carella A, Barnaba A, Mossa A, Spadetta V: Case report on supernumerary breast associated with multiple vertebral malformations. Acta Neurol (Napoli) 26:136–142, 1971.

133. Cellini A, Offidani A: Familial supernumerary nipples and breasts. Dermatology 185:56–58, 1992.

134. Brightmore TG: Cystic lesion of a dorsal supernumerary breast in a male. Proc R Soc Med 64:662–663, 1971.

135. Kenney RD, Flippo JL, Black EB: Supernumerary nipples and renal anomalies in neonates. Am J Dis Child 141:987–988, 1987.

136. Lau F, Henline R: Ureteral anomalies: Report of a case manifesting three ureters on one side with one ending blindly in an aplastic kidney and a bifid pelvis with a single ureter on the other side. JAMA 96:587–591, 1931.

137. McFarland WL, Wallace S, Johnson DE: Renal carcinoma and polycystic disease. J Urol 107:530–532, 1972.

138. Ng RC, Suki WN: Renal cell carcinoma occurring in a polycystic kidney of a transplant recipient. J Urol 124:710–712, 1980.

139. Goeminne L: Synopsis of mammo-renal syndromes. Humangenetik 14:170–171, 1972.

140. Blackard CE, Mellinger GT: Cancer in a horseshoe kidney. A report of two cases. Arch Surg 97:616–627, 1968.

141. Varsano IB, Jaber L, Garty BZ, Mukamel MM, Grunebaum M: Urinary tract abnormalities in children with supernumerary nipples. Pediatrics 73:103–105, 1984.

142. Jojart G, Seres E: Supernumerary nipples and renal anomalies. Int Urol Nephrol 26:141–144, 1994.

143. Grotto I, Browner-Elhanan K, Mimouni D, et al: Occurrence of supernumerary nipples in children with kidney and urinary tract malformations. Pediatr Dermatol 18:291–294, 2001.

144. Leung AK, Robson WL: Renal anomalies in familial polythelia. Am J Dis Child 144:619–620, 1990.

145. Goedert JJ, McKeen EA, Fraumeni JF Jr: Polymastia and renal adenocarcinoma. Ann Intern Med 95:182–184, 1981.

146. Goedert JJ, McKeen EA, Javadpour N, et al: Polythelia and testicular cancer. Ann Intern Med 101:646–647, 1984.

147. Mehes K: Familial association of supernumerary nipple with renal cancer. Cancer Genet Cytogenet 86:129–130, 1996.

148. Tollerud DJ, Blattner WA, Fraser MC, et al: Familial testicular cancer and urogenital developmental anomalies. Cancer 55: 1849–1854, 1985.

149. Urbani CE, Betti R: Familial aberrant mammary tissue: a clinico-epidemiological survey of 18 cases. Dermatology 190:207–209, 1995.

150. Das DK, Gupta SK, Mathew SV, et al: Fine needle aspiration cytologic diagnosis of axillary accessory breast tissue, including its physiologic changes and pathologic lesions. Acta Cytol 38:130–135, 1994.

151. De Cholnoky T: Accessory breast tissue in the axilla. N Y State J Med 51:2245–2248, 1951.

152. Chung CS, Myrianthopoulos NC: Factors affecting risks of congenital malformations. I. Analysis of epidemiologic factors in congenital malformations. Report from the Collaborative Perinatal Project. Birth Defects Orig Artic Ser 11:1–22, 1975.

153. Orti E, Qazi Q: Polymastia. New York, Alan R Liss, 1979.

154. Lorbek W: A case of trifid ureter. Wien Med Wochenschr 102:222–224, 1952.

155. DeGrouchy J, Turleau C: Clinical atlas of human chromosomes. New York, John Wiley & Sons, 1977.

156. Fleisher DS: Lateral displacement of the nipples, a sign of bilateral renal hypoplasia. J Pediatr 69:806–809, 1966.

157. Evans DM, Guyton DP: Carcinoma of the axillary breast. J Surg Oncol 59:190–195, 1995.

158. Vargas J, Nevado M, Rodriguez-Peralto JL, De Agustin PP: Fine needle aspiration diagnosis of carcinoma arising in an ectopic breast. A case report. Acta Cytol 39:941–944, 1995.

159. Velanovich V: Fine needle aspiration cytology in the diagnosis and management of ectopic breast tissue. Am Surg 61:277–278, 1995.

160. John C: Uber akzessorische Milchdrüsenaand Warzen, insbesondere über milchdrüsemähnliche Bildungen in der Achselhoêe. Arch Gynakol 126, 1925.

161. Jeffcoate T: Principles of gynecology. London, Butterworth, 1967.

162. Dworak O, Reck T, Greskotter KR, Kockerling F: Hamartoma of an ectopic breast arising in the inguinal region. Histopathology 24:169–171, 1994.

163. Reck T, Dworak O, Thaler KH, Kockerling F: Hamartoma of aberrant breast tissue in the inguinal region. Chirurg 66:923–926, 1995.

164. Roux J: Lactation from axillary tail of breast. BMJ 1, 4904, 28, 1955.

165. Guerry RL, Pratt-Thomas HR: Carcinoma of supernumerary breast of vulva with bilateral mammary cancer. Cancer 38:2570–2574, 1976.

SECTION IV

Pathology of Malignant Lesions

In Situ Carcinomas of the Breast: Ductal Carcinoma in Situ and Lobular Carcinoma in Situ

STEPHEN P. POVOSKI | SANFORD H. BARSKY

Over the past several decades, the widespread adoption of mammographic screening has had a significant impact on the incidence, diagnosis, classification, and treatment of all breast diseases. These changes have been particularly profound for in situ carcinoma of the breast. As a result, there has been a vast increase in the number of publications in the literature with regard to the definition, diagnostic criteria, and both short-term and long-term risks associated with specific histologic variants or types of in situ carcinoma of the breast.

In situ carcinomas of the breast were first recognized in the early 20th century and were identified morphologically as cells cytologically similar to those of invasive carcinomas but confined to ductal structures within the breast parenchyma. Such lesions were generally found to be located adjacent to areas of invasive carcinoma. The original definitions given to in situ carcinomas of the breast were arbitrary. Opportunities to study the natural history and behavior of such in situ lesions independent of an invasive component of disease or after a surgical procedure less than that of mastectomy were previously rarely encountered.[1-3] Since that time, several studies relying on the review of archival slide material have demonstrated basic differences between distinct histologic patterns of in situ carcinomas. This subsequently resulted in the distinction between those lesions representing purely markers of increased risk (e.g., lobular carcinoma in situ [LCIS] and atypical hyperplasia, with increased breast cancer risk that was essentially equally distributed to either breast) and committed premalignant lesions (e.g., ductal carcinoma in situ [DCIS], with increased breast cancer risk that was more often reported to be confined to the ipsilateral breast[4-6]).

The classical studies of Wellings and Jensen focused attention on the terminal ductal-lobular unit as a common anatomic site for the development of hyperplastic changes of both the ductal and the lobular type as well as corresponding neoplastic lesions.[7] The terms *DCIS* and *LCIS* were once meant to signify separate anatomic origins, with one originating within the ductal structures and the other originating within the lobular structures. However, this anachronous concept is now recognized to be inaccurate. Unfortunately, the idea of distinct lobular and ductal origins for breast neoplasms continues to persist despite our current understanding of neoplastic development within the breast. Currently, the term *DCIS* refers to patterns of abnormal epithelial cell proliferation associated with a prominent involvement of true ducts within the in situ carcinoma category and has a high risk of local recurrence without adequate local treatment. Thus, DCIS is essentially a diagnosis of exclusion, including in its broad sweep any lesion deemed in situ carcinoma that does not exhibit the cytologic features of lobular neoplasia cells.[8-10] In part, this distinction remains important because the distribution of DCIS and LCIS within a breast as well as between the breasts represents a recognized difference between these two in situ carcinoma entities. In that regard, those studies that have specifically addressed the incidence rate or relative risk of developing a subsequent ipsilateral and contralateral invasive breast cancer in women with in situ carcinoma have traditionally shown a higher incidence rate or relative risk of contralateral invasive breast cancer for those women with LCIS compared with those women with DCIS.[11-14] Although these differences between DCIS and LCIS have persisted within the literature, the most recently reported series demonstrate that this difference is likely much smaller than previously thought.[13,14]

Recent Insights into the Unique Biology of Ductal Carcinoma in Situ and Lobular Carcinoma in Situ

DCIS, in many respects, should be regarded as carcinoma of the ductal system for it possesses all of the molecular and biological abnormalities as frankly invasive carcinoma.[15–18] DCIS is clonal and frequently expresses abnormal p53 and *HER2/neu*. It has the same loss of heterozygosity patterns as its invasive counterpart. Using comparative genomic hybridization studies, DCIS exhibits no gains or losses of chromosomal regions compared with its invasive counterpart. Rather, DCIS is held in check by a surrounding layer of myoepithelial cells that exert paracrine suppressive effects on invasion.[19–23] Because of this, the histopathologic patterns of DCIS usually strongly correlate with its invasive counterpart, when present in individual cases. For example, papillary DCIS (Fig. 10-1) tends to invade as papillary adenocarcinoma. Cribriform DCIS (Fig. 10-2) and solid DCIS (Fig. 10-3) of intermediate nuclear grades tend to invade as a moderately differentiated adenocarcinoma. Comedo DCIS of high nuclear grade (Fig. 10-4) tends to invade as a poorly differentiated adenocarcinoma. The precursor lesion of DCIS is thought to be atypical ductal hyperplasia (ADH) for the DCIS of low or intermediate nuclear grades. Simple ductal hyperplasia, based on loss of heterozygosity and genomic hybridization studies, is no longer thought to be a precursor lesion of either ADH or DCIS. A recently described lesion, flat epithelial atypia or columnar cell atypia (Figs. 10-5 and 10-6), based on its abnormal nuclear features and its presence juxtaposed to DCIS, especially high-grade DCIS, is thought to be a possible precursor lesion. However, this has not yet been proved in prospective studies. Clearly the evidence is incontrovertible that DCIS can and often progresses to frank invasive adenocarcinoma, and clearly the same clone is involved.

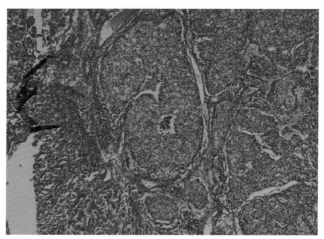

Figure 10-2 The cribriform type of noncomedo ductal carcinoma in situ, in contrast, consists of intraductal proliferations showing bridging and "Roman arch" formation.

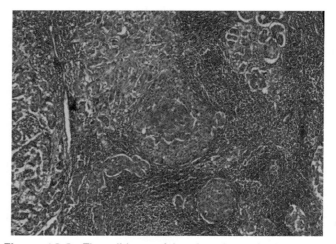

Figure 10-3 The solid type of ductal carcinoma in situ exhibits a solid sheet of intraluminal cells.

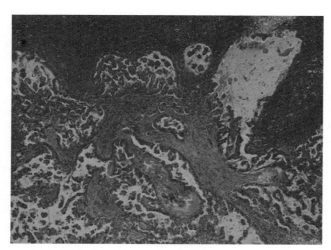

Figure 10-1 The micropapillary type of noncomedo ductal carcinoma in situ is characterized by intraductal papillations projecting into a central lumen.

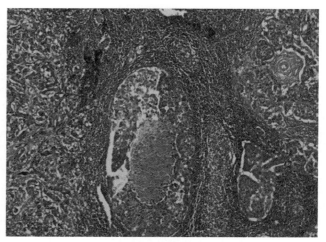

Figure 10-4 The comedo type of ductal carcinoma in situ exhibits a solid pattern of intraluminal proliferation with high nuclear grade and central necrosis.

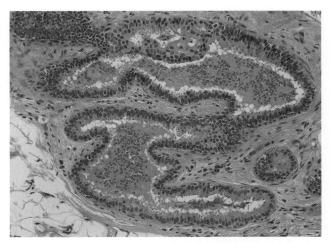

Figure 10-5 The lesion of flat columnar epithelial atypia is characterized by dilated ducts lined by a single luminal cell layer.

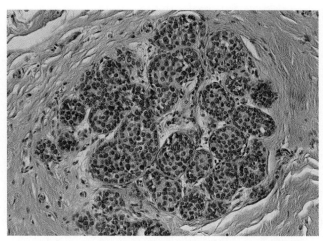

Figure 10-7 Lobular carcinoma in situ of the classic type fills and distends acini.

With LCIS, the story is both similar as well as different. Emerging evidence has suggested that LCIS is a heterogeneous disease.[24] Some types of LCIS are associated with a 4- to 10-fold increased risk of invasive breast carcinoma (Fig. 10-7). The increased risk can be associated with any type of infiltrating breast carcinoma, including both ductal as well as lobular carcinoma. Other forms of LCIS may be more innocuous. Still others, for example, those that express more nuclear pleomorphism, such as pleomorphic LCIS (Fig. 10-8), may actually progress to invasive lobular carcinoma (Fig. 10-9). This latter type of LCIS resembles DCIS in its biology. Still other types of LCIS can mimic other features of DCIS. Some LCIS spreads laterally through the ductal system analogous to Paget's disease (Fig. 10-10). This spread of LCIS is aptly termed pagetoid spread. Preliminary molecular studies of LCIS by loss of heterozygosity and genomic hybridization confirm the molecular heterogeneity of LCIS. Some LCIS has few, if any, obvious chromosomal abnormalities. Other types of LCIS exhibit evidence of genomic instability. Still other types of LCIS exhibit the same clonal abnormalities as its invasive lobular counterpart. This molecular heterogeneity suggests that some forms of LCIS may be innocuous; others may confer increased risk for the development of breast cancer; and still others can directly progress to invasive lobular breast cancer. This latter type of LCIS is therefore analogous to DCIS. Clearly, the appropriate therapy would depend on the type of LCIS present. So-called innocuous LCIS could be treated by "watchful waiting," genomically unstable LCIS with an increased risk of breast cancer could be treated with tamoxifen, and the LCIS that directly progresses to invasive carcinoma could be treated with surgical extirpation. Obviously, prospective randomized studies and not just historical controls are needed to resolve the LCIS question.

One consistent molecular difference between LCIS and DCIS is the loss of E-cadherin expression by either mutation, promoter methylation or cis/trans promoter silencing in LCIS but the maintenance of expression of E-cadherin in DCIS. This observation can be extended to invasive lobular versus invasive ductal carcinoma as well.

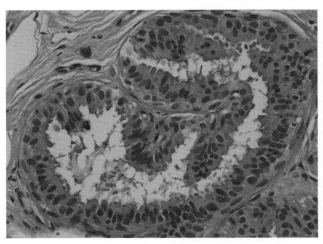

Figure 10-6 At higher magnification, the single luminal cell layer is columnar in shape and manifests marked nuclear atypia.

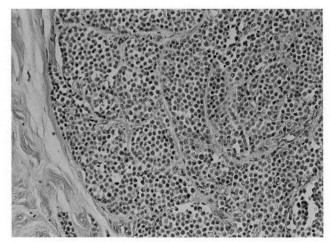

Figure 10-8 Lobular carcinoma in situ of the pleomorphic type exhibits individual cells that are larger and more individually defined.

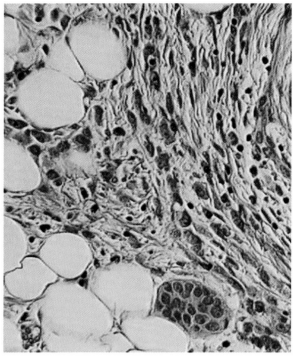

Figure 10-9 Lobular carcinoma in situ, especially of the pleomorphic type *(bottom)*, can directly progress to invasion *(central and top)*.

Pathology of Ductal Carcinoma in Situ

DCIS comprises a heterogeneous group of noninvasive neoplastic proliferations with diverse morphologies and risks of subsequent recurrence and invasive transformation (Figs. 10-11 to 10-17). Although DCIS probably arises predominantly in the terminal ductal-lobular unit, it often extends out to involve extralobular ducts. Compared with LCIS, DCIS is generally more variable histologically and cytologically, with larger and more pleomorphic nuclei and a tendency to form microacini, cribriform spaces, or papillary structures. In some cases,

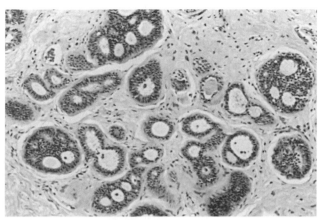

Figure 10-11 Low-power photograph demonstrating the full extent of the evidence supporting a diagnosis of atypical ductal hyperplasia (ADH). Note that there are only three or four spaces in which a central population of uniform cells may be seen. In the others, only narrow bars cross from one side to the other. Thus, there are pattern and cell population features of ductal carcinoma in situ (DCIS). However, in the three largest spaces involved, there are cells adjacent to the basement membrane that appear different; thus a diagnosis of ADH rather than DCIS is made. (×75.)

the periphery of these lesions may include patterns overlapping with atypical hyperplasia.[25] Pathologists do not agree whether or not small lesions should be considered atypical hyperplasia or in situ carcinoma. In general, lesions that involve only a few membrane-bound spaces and that measure less than 2 to 3 mm in greatest dimension should be regarded as hyperplastic lesions (with or without atypia) and not in situ carcinoma. There is a greater degree of concordance in larger lesions, however.[26] Pathologists tend to agree about the diagnosis of difficult, smaller, borderline lesions if they have agreed on criteria[27] (Table 10-1). Occasionally, it may be difficult to distinguish DCIS and LCIS histologically, with some forms of DCIS characterized by small uniform cells with a solid growth pattern simulating LCIS. In rare instances, in situ neoplastic proliferations are indeterminate. In such cases, they are presumed to

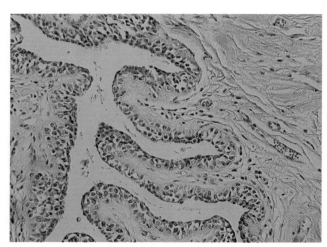

Figure 10-10 Lobular carcinoma in situ can also exhibit pagetoid spread into adjacent ducts.

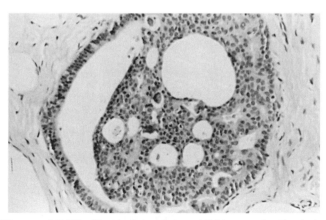

Figure 10-12 Photomicrograph exhibiting a detail of the polarization of luminal cells near the basement membrane that are quite different from the evenly placed and "suspicious" cells present in the central proliferation. This is atypical ductal hyperplasia. (×200.)

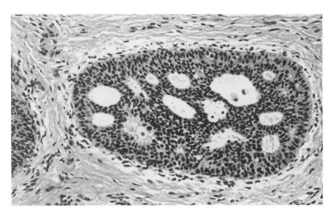

Figure 10-13 This central cribriform pattern of similar cells with outer cells normally polarized (above basement membrane) is probably the most common pattern of atypical ductal hyperplasia. (×150.) (From Anderson TJ, Page DL: Risk assessment in breast cancer. In Anthony PP, MacSween RNM, Lowe DG [eds]: Recent advances in histopathology, vol 17. Edinburgh, Churchill Livingstone, 1997.)

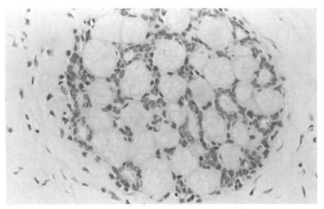

Figure 10-14 Collagenous spherulosis, a pattern sometimes confused with atypical ductal hyperplasia or ductal carcinoma in situ.[95] Note that the spaces are defined by a secreted material that may be seen faintly. The spaces are surrounded by a sparse population of cells that everywhere is tapered or thinned in its extent. Such a pattern is not recognized as atypical. (×150.)

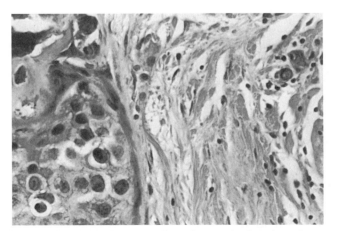

Figure 10-15 High-power view of comedo ductal carcinoma in situ demonstrating necrosis in the upper left-hand corner. Note also that the stroma is altered about this area, which occurs frequently in this type of carcinoma in situ. (×700.)

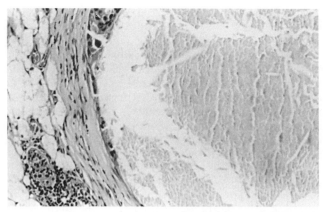

Figure 10-16 Occasionally cellular necrosis in comedo ductal carcinoma in situ is so extensive that very few atypical cells remain. Indeed, the necrosis may appear to extend to the basement membrane. (×125.)

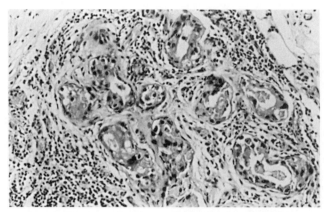

Figure 10-17 Characteristic of more advanced and comedo carcinoma–type examples of ductal carcinoma in situ is the spread of highly atypical cells into lobular units. Here this phenomenon of so-called cancerization of lobules is demonstrated. (×200.)

have the prognostic implications of both diagnoses (e.g., local evolution to invasion for DCIS and increased general risk in each breast for LCIS).[9] It has been proposed that E-cadherin stains are useful in such overlap cases,[28,29] but it should be pointed out that no long-term follow-up study has examined the implications of E-cadherin staining or absence thereof for regional breast cancer risk. It has been our approach to diagnose such

TABLE 10-1
Classification Schema for Ductal Carcinoma in Situ

1. Differentiation, mainly based on nuclear morphology and cell polarization[46]
2. Nuclear grade and necrosis[47]
3. Intersection of nuclear grade and extent of necrosis similar to Silverstein, but with separate identification of special types[59]

It is evident that the classification scheme should promote consistency.

cases as in situ carcinoma, mixed pattern, and to indicate that a regional risk for local recurrence should be assumed.

Terminology is an important consideration here, and as noted earlier, there are distinct clinical implications concerning the terms *lobular* and *ductal*. Although the inherited terms have a historical legacy that may carry other significance, they have the impelling merit of familiarity. It is for us to develop more specific criteria for subtypes and to accept that it is the criteria linked to clinical end point analysis that guides clinical practice.[26] One significant problem is the wonderfully earthy word *comedo*. It refers to the lowly comedones (e.g., acne) of common experience from our teen years, an unfailing image of the gross appearance of these lesions. Bloodgood coined the term *comedo-adenoma* because when treated with mastectomy in the Halstedian era, it was associated with long-term survival.[30] For Bloodgood, the alternative to carcinoma was adenoma, a lesion capable of cure when adequately excised. The term *comedo* remains descriptive and is now somewhat confusingly used to indicate both a type of DCIS with a coagulation-type necrosis and frequent nuclear debris, as well as merely the evidence of necrosis alone (comedo necrosis). Now, most students of DCIS use comedo as a modifier for DCIS, signifying high-grade lesions that exhibit necrosis.

A major transition in our thinking regarding DCIS was the idea that perhaps not all DCIS cases were the same and that the different histologic appearances of DCIS might in fact have important clinical implications. Translating this concept into practical terms, it was suggested that if comedo-type DCIS did have a more menacing clinical import, then one should err on the side of including any questionable case within this category.[9] Thus in 1989, the critically important concept of further stratification was introduced[31] as a part of the inception of the modern era of understanding of DCIS. Because minor amounts of necrosis may be seen in the common hyperplasias without features of atypia, specific guidelines are necessary to make appropriate stratifications. Thus, inclusion of an intermediate-grade category has been adopted by the majority of DCIS classifications put forth since the early 1990s (Table 10-2) to recognize examples with minimal necrosis and a moderate degree of nuclear pleomorphism.

Conventionally, DCIS has been classified on the basis of architectural features, such as comedo, cribriform, papillary, solid, and micropapillary.[32,33] Although comedo-type DCIS includes advanced nuclear abnormalities within the neoplastic proliferation as part of the definition, the diagnosis of other patterns of DCIS were based on architecture alone. These patterns were accepted to be overlapping when DCIS was considered one entity and not held to have separate clinical or biologic implications.[33,34] The first indication that distinguishing among comedo, noncomedo, and micropapillary subtypes,[35] as well as separation by grade,[31] was of clinical utility certainly inaugurated the modern era of DCIS in 1989.

The increasing use of breast-conserving therapy (BCT) in the treatment of mammographically detected DCIS has permitted studies on factors that predict local

TABLE 10-2
Ductal Carcinoma in Situ Classifications*

	Necrosis	Nuclear Grade I	Nuclear Grade II	Nuclear Grade III
Lagios[31]	+		Intermediate	High
	−	Low		
Silverstein[47]	−		Group 2	Group 3
	−		Group 1	Group 3
Solin[49]	+			Comedo
	−		Noncomedo	

High, intermediate, or low indicates respective nuclear grade.
*Based on nuclear grade and necrosis.
Modified from Lagios MD: Ductal carcinoma in situ: Controversies in diagnosis, biology, and treatment. Breast J 1:67–78, 1995.

recurrences and invasive events in the remaining breast after excisional biopsy. Before a large number of small mammographically detected DCIS cases were found with screening, mastectomy was the only acceptable treatment for DCIS, and still remains a standard treatment for multifocal and multicentric disease.[36,37]

Three prognostic factors have been shown to be important in local control of DCIS after attempts at BCT.[38] These are (1) the extent (size) of disease in the breast (and its corollary, the residuum after an attempt at excision), (2) the status of margins (also reflecting residual disease in the breast), and (3) the grade of the DCIS (and possibly pure subtype, particularly micropapillary). The most significant of these factors appears to be margin status, followed by histologic grade.[39-46] High nuclear grade and necrosis together define forms of DCIS at much higher risk of local recurrence and invasive transformation. The grade of a DCIS is largely independent of the conventional pattern classification. For example, lesions of high nuclear grade can exhibit any architectural pattern (although lack of precise patterns is most common).[31,46] However, as recognized in the classification system of Holland and associates[46] (see Table 10-1), ordered intercellular relationships are most common in lesions of low nuclear grade. There is a growing consensus that classifications based on nuclear grade and necrosis can identify the majority of patients with DCIS who are at risk for short-term local recurrence and invasive transformation after excision[21,47-50] with or without irradiation. Most of these short-term recurrences are associated with DCIS exhibiting high (3/3 or grade III) nuclear grade morphology and significant coagulative necrosis. Such lesions would be conventionally classified as comedo DCIS. Studies using conventional classification schemes have shown that most short-term failures are associated with comedo-type DCIS.[50-53] It should be recalled that the term comedo-type DCIS is not synonymous with high nuclear grade when it is used to indicate necrosis only. Some lesions exhibiting comedo-type necrosis and a solid growth pattern are composed of intermediate-grade and, in rare cases, borderline low-grade nuclei (Figs. 10-18 to 10-27).

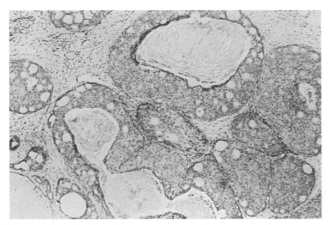

Figure 10-18   This low-power view of a common form of ductal carcinoma in situ shows solid cellular masses distending basement membrane–bound spaces. Within these cellular masses are sharply defined, rounded secondary lumens. There are central areas of necrosis as well as evident distention and distortion of the involved spaces. (×75.)

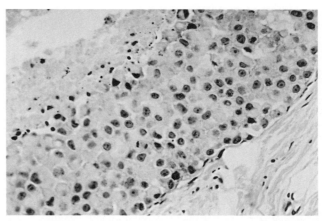

Figure 10-21   This example of intermediate-grade ductal carcinoma in situ (DCIS) presents highly atypical nuclei but not the most advanced, bizarre, and varied cytologic patterns often seen in comedo DCIS. Although one might debate whether these represent intermediate-grade nuclei, the limited luminal necrosis (here at upper left and elsewhere in this case) indicate an intermediate-grade designation. (×350.)

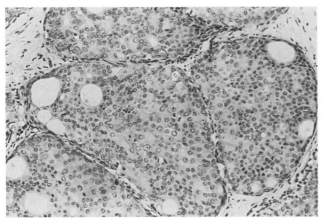

Figure 10-19   This high-power view of Figure 10-11 demonstrates that the nuclei are of low grade, being similar one to another and without demonstrated irregularity. The presence of necrosis and low-grade nuclei is indicative of a condition intermediate between well-developed comedo ductal carcinoma in situ (DCIS) and the usual noncomedo DCIS. (×200.)

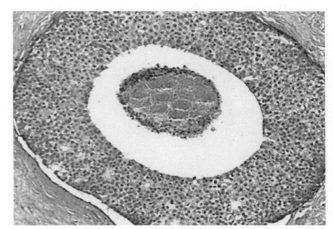

Figure 10-22   In this example of intermediate-grade ductal carcinoma in situ, the presence of necroses helps define the category. Low- to intermediate-grade nuclei are present. (×200.) (From Anderson TJ, Page DL: Risk assessment in breast cancer. In Anthony PP, MacSween RNM, Lowe DG [eds]: Recent advances in histopathology, vol 17. Edinburgh, Churchill Livingstone, 1997.)

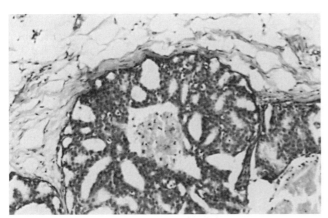

Figure 10-20   This example of ductal carcinoma in situ is characterized by sinuous, interconnecting strands of hyperchromatic cells. Note the few necrotic cells centrally. (×100.)

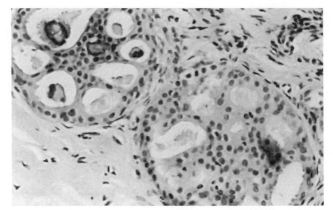

Figure 10-23   Rigid arches of a cribriform pattern variant of ductal carcinoma in situ. Note: Calcified material in central spaces is not indicative of cellular necrosis. (×225.)

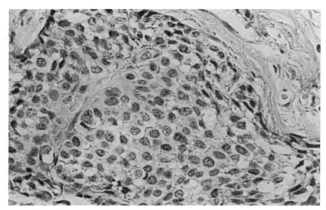

Figure 10-24 An example of a solid pattern variant of ductal carcinoma in situ. There are no evident intercellular spaces, and the slightly irregular placement of cells and sharply defined intercellular contours are not consistent with lobular carcinoma in situ. (×450.)

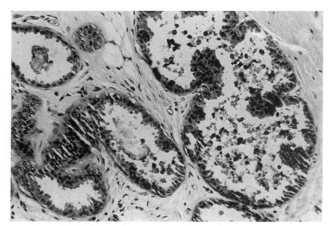

Figure 10-25 Micropapillary ductal carcinoma in situ with necrosis. Although some cells have lighter cytoplasm, the nuclear pattern is similar throughout. (×400.)

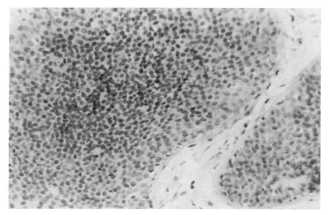

Figure 10-26 This solid variant of atypical ductal hyperplasia (ADH) is diagnostically very similar to solid ductal carcinoma in situ. The more vesicular nuclei in the second population of cells render a diagnosis of ADH. (×150.)

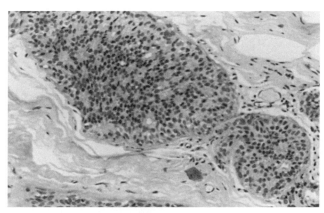

Figure 10-27 The microglandular or "endocrine" pattern of solid ductal carcinoma in situ. (×150.)

Information regarding the potential for recurrence of low-grade (noncomedo-type) DCIS after biopsy or BCT resides in a small number of published studies. It is clear that in the short-term (5 to 10 years), few local recurrences or invasive transformations occur. However, a recent update of the only study of low-grade DCIS present at biopsy (without planned excision[5]) and with extended follow-up[6,54] noted a substantial delayed recurrence rate of invasive lesions (e.g., approximately 37% and 50% at 25 years and more than 40 years of follow-up, respectively). Although the sample is small, it is significant that recurrences were generally in the same quadrant and, in some women, in the site of the prior biopsy, thus representing a biology identical to that of higher-grade DCIS and a risk that does not diminish after menopause. This biology of DCIS should be contrasted with that of risk marker lesions (e.g., ADH and atypical lobular hyperplasia [ALH]), which do not predict the side of involvement and in which risk diminishes postmenopausally (at least for ALH and LCIS).[26,55–57]

There are several published classifications of DCIS,[58] many of which use nuclear grade and necrosis as the major distinguishing features in a general classification applying to most cases of specific subtypes. The separations achieved by these classifications are different and in part may affect the interpretation of outcome results (Table 10-3). DCIS characterized by nuclear morphology (high grade III; e.g., advanced atypia) and necrosis is uniformly classified as high grade.[25,31,47–49,51,59] The European Organization for Research and Treatment of Cancer (EORTC) classification,[46] although it does not use conventional nuclear grade or necrosis as major discriminates, would also regard this as a high grade or, in their terminology, a poorly differentiated DCIS. Fisher and colleagues[60] summarized the pathology analysis from the National Surgical Adjuvant Breast Project (NSABP) studies on DCIS and noted that DCIS with grade III nuclei and DCIS that exhibited larger areas of necrosis (greater than one third of ducts involved) had a higher local recurrence rate. The authors reported these results separately, not analyzing the risk associated with

TABLE 10-3

Subclassification of Ductal Carcinoma in Situ of the Breast*

Histology	Nuclear Grade	Necrosis	Final DCIS Grade
Comedo	High	Extensive	High
Intermediate[†]	Intermediate	Focal or absent	Intermediate
Noncomedo[‡]	Low	Absent	Low

DCIS, ductal carcinoma in situ.
*Common presentation.
[†]Often a mixture of noncomedo patterns.
[‡]Solid, cribriform, papillary, or focal micropapillary.

the two features in concert. Despite the differences in classification,[58] it would appear that high-grade DCIS can be recognized uniformly, with all investigators showing that the high-grade subtype, so defined, has the highest risk of local recurrence and invasive transformation.

The recognition that necrosis and high nuclear grade usually cluster together[61] may foster agreement between observers by using limited necrosis as a way of defining an intermediate grade category.[31,59,62] The separate classifications are less consistent with regard to the remainder of the heterogeneous noncomedo-type group (see Table 10-2). DCIS with grade III nuclei but without necrosis, an uncommon situation, is classified as high grade by Silverstein and coworkers,[47] but "noncomedo" (a lower grade) by Solin and associates.[49] Lagios and colleagues[31] and Silverstein and coworkers[47] use nuclear grade to separate the remaining DCIS groups. However, Lagios and colleagues[31] classify low-grade DCIS as grade I nuclei without necrosis and intermediate-grade DCIS as grade II with or without necrosis. Silverstein and coworkers[47] separate DCIS with nuclear grades I and II on the basis of necrosis. Group I (low grade) may exhibit grade I or II nuclei but no necrosis, whereas DCIS with grade I or II nuclei but with any necrosis is classified as intermediate (group II). Solin and associates[49] regard all DCIS without grade III nuclei and necrosis as noncomedo-type DCIS. Despite these differences in classification, all investigators have shown a substantially diminished local recurrence rate for DCIS that is not characterized by grade III nuclei and necrosis. Moreover, in those studies in which DCIS is divided into three groups, as opposed to the dichotomous comedo/ noncomedo structure, there is a recognizable intermediate group (intermediate grade, group II, intermediately differentiated) that exhibits a morphology and a risk intermediate between low-grade and high-grade DCIS.

Classification of Ductal Carcinoma in Situ

Although nuclear grade and necrosis would appear to define most of the risk associated with DCIS, certain architectural patterns appear to bear clinical significance

independent of the nuclear grade. For example, DCIS with almost pure micropapillary architectural features is strongly associated with extensive disease, that is, within seemingly separate foci of different quadrants.[35,51] This growth pattern makes adequate excision extremely difficult. In some cases, mammographic and histopathologic evidence of disease is present in all four quadrants of the breast. As a result, most clinical studies that define DCIS with micropapillary features and low nuclear grade were based on excisions without theoretically adequate margins of resection.

Conventional classification of DCIS covers perhaps 85% of what is recognized as noninvasive ductal carcinoma. A number of less common subtypes remains to be fully defined morphologically and with regard to risk. Proliferations with apocrine features, bridging the spectrum from minimal atypia to frank DCIS, were the subject of a proposed classification by O'Malley and associates.[63] Because of the difficulty of applying traditional rules regarding cellular atypia and architecture to apocrine lesions, this schema proposed that definitive diagnoses of low-grade apocrine DCIS be limited to cases measuring at least 8 mm in size. In addition, a borderline category was proposed for lesions measuring 4 to 8 mm, with the suggestion that these lesions had the relative risk implications of at least ADH. Furthermore, apocrine DCIS, which is characteristically estrogen receptor negative, progesterone receptor negative, and androgen receptor positive and represents a heterogeneous group of lesions ranging from low-grade lesion (which should be differentiated from atypical hyperplastic apocrine lesions) to obvious malignant, high-grade tumors (which are difficult to recognize as apocrine), was more recently classified into three histologic grades based on nuclear grade and necrosis by Leal and colleagues,[64] similar to schema for classical DCIS. Confirmation of the utility of any of these approaches to classifying such apocrine lesions awaits long-term follow-up analysis of cases treated with conservative surgery.

Another contender for special-type status is the so-called endocrine type of DCIS,[65,66] which presents a particularly low-grade pattern of disease. Similarly, a possible special type characterized by hypersecretory features is discussed subsequently. In all of these less common special types of DCIS, a major limitation is the lack of precise confines of histologic definition that specifically and reproducibly describes the entire spectrum of changes with a linkage to clinical implications corroborated by long-term follow-up studies. With this background of remaining uncertainty, it is generally recommended that all the traditional rules for characterization and classification be applied to these less common entities, so as not to misdiagnose or mistreat such in situ lesions.

The classification of DCIS has been subjected to different approaches, each with advantages and disadvantages. The purpose of any classification scheme for DCIS is to predict the likelihood of recurrences and the likelihood of progression to invasion, and no classification scheme is ideal from these perspectives. For these reasons, newer classification schemes are continually evolving. The classification scheme proposed by Page and Lagios is summarized (see Tables 10-2 and 10-3).[31,59,62] Several other DCIS classifications are presented (see Table 10-1), providing a basis from which to understand the slightly varied approaches. The major differences between Page's classification and most of the other schemes is that Page's uses the intersection of two variables—necrosis and nuclear grade—to foster agreement. It is common to debate between adjacent nuclear grades, viz, 1 or 2, and 2 or 3. The extensiveness of the necrosis is to be used to aid in the resolution of these issues. In a test set, agreement was fostered by this approach.[59] The second feature of Page's scheme is to separate some special types of DCIS because they present patterns not readily allowing grading. In the special case of pure (not intermixed with solid or cribriform) micropapillary DCIS, Page believes that the usual extensiveness of disease is independent of the nuclear grade. It should be noted that separating special types from the majority of cases is precisely what we do with invasive disease.

Extent of Disease

Clinical concern with the evaluation of size or extent of the area of the breast occupied by DCIS was an early focus during the development of BCT for this disease entity. By using a serial subgross sectioning technique correlated with specimen radiography, developed by Egan and associates,[67,68] a clear association was shown between the likelihood of invasive growth and the extent of disease.[34] Egan's technique permitted correlative studies of radiographic images and pathologic mapping of areas of involvement by DCIS in mastectomy specimens. The initial concern was whether occult invasion might exist in the breast separate from an adequately excised focus of DCIS. This has not generally been shown to be the case. DCIS cases measuring 25 mm or less, completely excised, were not associated with demonstrable occult areas of invasion in those cases that subsequently went to mastectomy and standard pathologic assessment. Silverstein[69] demonstrated a similar correlation between the extent of disease and the likelihood of invasion, as did Patchefsky and coworkers.[35] What was not clearly described at the time was that the invasive focus always occurred within the area occupied by DCIS and that the area occupied by DCIS had a segmental distribution, as clearly noted subsequently.[70,71] Using the same serial subgross technique but applying it to radial segments of the breast, which more closely approximate the true anatomy of the ductal system, Holland and colleagues[71] were able to define more clearly the relationships of DCIS to mammographic microcalcification and to the remaining breast. They identified different distribution patterns among DCIS of different subtypes. High-grade DCIS (poorly differentiated) was more closely defined by the extent of mammographic microcalcifications. Therefore, its extent could be estimated with more certainty preoperatively. It was also associated with

fewer discontinuities or "skip areas" in its distribution. In contrast, DCIS of lower grades (intermediate and well differentiated) were poorly associated with microcalcification and often exhibited a discontinuous distribution. However, Faverly and associates[70] note that 85% of low-grade (well-differentiated) DCIS would be excised with a 10–mm margin. Despite the greater likelihood of residual disease, lower grades of DCIS have a much lower frequency of local recurrence after attempts at BCT, at least in the first 10 years of follow-up.[43,53]

Extensiveness, Multicentricity, and Multifocality

The literature on the multicentricity and multifocality of DCIS remains confusing because of the different definitions, methods of tissue processing, and sampling techniques used, as well as differences in the perspective of the investigators. Two groups of investigators, both of which used Egan's serial subgross technique of examination,[67,68] exemplify useful approaches to resolving this problem. The focus of Lagios and coworkers was on the question of residual disease after segmental mastectomy (or lumpectomy), a new and radical direction for American surgeons at the time.[34] They defined as multicentric any focus lying beyond 5 cm of the border of the resection. In most cases, this feature defined involvement in another quadrant. Holland and colleagues[71] and Faverly and associates[70] (although clearly concerned about the success of a surgical resection) were focused more on the distribution of the disease. Multicentric DCIS, by very definition, required a 4–cm zone of uninvolved breast tissue between the primary and any potential multicentric site. Discontinuous foci of DCIS within 4 cm were defined as multifocal. Holland and colleagues noted that only 5% of cases of DCIS were multicentric using this definition.[71] To what extent these data reflect the large size of DCIS in their patient population remains unknown. However, Faverly and associates[70] reported that 63% of the cases of DCIS studied at mastectomy had an extent greater than 5 cm (50 mm), whereas Lagios and coworkers,[34] in a similar mastectomy series, noted that 52% were 25 mm or less and 25% were 50 mm or more. Irrespectively, it is most prudent to clearly describe the extent and distribution of disease within the breast in unequivocal terms that cannot be misinterpreted.

Distribution

The considerations of the extent of DCIS are discussed primarily in Chapter 12. It is generally accepted that there is a somewhat segmental anatomy of the breast. Although these segmental lobes are not precisely placed or sized, they are generally viewed as subtending regions drained by major ducts and are somewhat overlapping in distribution (see Chapter 12). The hallmark of DCIS is its somewhat orderly spread through the large duct system. The segmental lobes are not precisely demarcated anatomically, but rather, the major spread in any given case of DCIS appears to be within the same segmental lobe toward and away from the nipple and in adjacent segmental lobes as well. This clinical situation may be varied in that a major lesion deep within the breast may involve many lobular units, and then a single duct may seem to ascend toward the nipple with few other lobular elements involved. This is demonstrated by Ohtake and colleagues[72] and also illustrated by the three-dimensional reconstruction studies of Moffat and Going.[73]

Mammographic Correlation

The distribution of DCIS within the breast, its association with microcalcification, the types of microcalcification, and the likelihood that DCIS may exhibit an extensive growth pattern with a substantial risk of residual disease after attempts at excision are also correlated with grade and subtype. High-grade DCIS with comedo necrosis exhibits a greater extent, is often segmental[71,73,74] (see Chapter 12) and contiguous in distribution, is more closely associated with microcalcifications, and is less likely to show an intermittent or discontinuous distribution in the breast.[70,75] In contrast, DCIS of intermediate and low grades is less likely to exhibit a contiguous growth pattern, especially on mammography, even if its distribution can be understood to lie within a segmental duct system. DCIS of these lower grades is more likely to exhibit discontinuous but regional growth and to show less association with microcalcification, although many cases are continuous on three-dimensional reconstruction studies. From a clinical and mammographic point of view, high-grade comedo-type DCIS is more likely to be adequately excised, given its association with microcalcification and contiguous growth pattern. Nonetheless, it is associated with the greatest risk of local recurrence and invasive transformation. An important study of the growth pattern of DCIS in time has come from the group in Nottingham.[76] Rates of change and direction of change in mammographic calcifications was correlated with DCIS histology. Growth rates increased with increasing nuclear grade of DCIS, and the DCIS growth rate was greatest along an axis toward and away from the nipple. The latter finding demonstrated preferential growth of DCIS along the radiating anatomy of the ducts from the nipple to the end of the breast disk. There may be a special form of DCIS that demonstrates discontinuous spread histologically within ducts[77] and that is associated with recurrence despite performance of an extensive quadrantectomy. Low-grade DCIS is more likely to be inadequately excised unless surgical resection margins are carefully assessed with means other than mammography for residual disease in the same quadrant. Nonetheless, it is associated with a lower risk of subsequent recurrence and invasive transformation.

Margin Status

Assessment of the adequacy of surgical resection margins during BCT for DCIS has been a major focus of attention since the inception of BCT in the mid-1970s. The most common method of margin assessment is based on the use of India ink or some other permanent dye or pigment and selective sampling. This method works well for invasive carcinomas in which a likely area of involved margins can be estimated with palpation in most cases and confirmed with a few appropriate sections. This method, although still applicable, is more problematic for DCIS, in which the lesion is generally not palpable, is not grossly visible, may not be uniformly associated with microcalcification, and may have a discontinuous distribution. In these circumstances, margins must be examined more comprehensively. This often substantially increases the number of tissue samples or cassettes (blocks) prepared. However, neither margin involvement nor occult microinvasion can be entirely excluded without more complete tissue processing. Differences in the kind of tissue processing used can contribute significantly to outcome results in BCT for DCIS.[10,78] This is a major limitation of large multicenter clinical trials in which the patients may be randomized but the pathologists and their technique for specimen processing are not.

Considering that careful and precise assessment of surgical resection margin status is likely the most critical variable in determining the recurrence rate for DCIS (e.g., theoretically if the lesion has been completely removed, then further therapy should not make a difference), it is little wonder that carefully designed single-institution studies with consistent and rigorous pathologic assessment of the specimens have proved so useful. Ideally, breast specimens should be oriented by the surgeon in reference to the nipple and axilla and processed such that the extent of the lesion and its proximity to margins in all three dimensions can be determined. Multicolor inking protocols considerably facilitate analysis, along with uniform sectioning of the specimen at 2- to 3-mm intervals. In addition, specimen radiography to aid in lesion identification and in the focused submission of blocks on larger specimens is advocated. However, the histologic appearance of the lesion should never be compromised by compression of the submitted specimen during specimen radiography.

The adequacy of surgical resection margins for DCIS has long been and continues to be an area of ongoing debate. This debate has been fueled by the propensity of DCIS to exhibit a discontinuous distribution within the breast tissue. Early on, the NSABP defined "margins as free when the tumor is not transected."[60,79] As a result, an arbitrary assignment of 1 mm or greater has been considered by many as an acceptable standard.[80] However, many have challenged this minimalistic view to the adequacy of surgical resection margins. Previous work by Holland and colleagues[71,81] and Silverstein and associates[42,82] has suggested that a 1–mm margin may not be adequate for DCIS. In analyzing the results of initial attempts at excision biopsy, Silverstein and associates noted that 45% of cases of DCIS that were thought to be adequately excised had residual disease, either at re-excision or on mastectomy, and that, all other factors being equal, the distance of the free margin was directly related to the probability of local recurrence.[42] However, even using a definition of 1 mm as an adequate margin achieves a better local recurrence-free survival than did the NSABP-B-17 criterion of non-transsection of DCIS (e.g., 16% of local recurrence at 124 months' mean follow-up[39] vs. 22% local recurrence rate at 43 months' mean follow-up[79]). There are those that strongly advocate extremely wide margins ($\geq$10 mm) based on the classical findings of Silverstein and associates[42] in which they demonstrated that DCIS patients with margins greater than 10 mm had the lowest local recurrence rate. Conversely, those same particular patients did not receive added benefit from whole-breast radiation therapy compared with those DCIS patients with closer margins who did benefit from whole-breast radiation therapy.[42] Most recently, a more moderate viewpoint has been portrayed in the literature with recommendations of margins in the range of greater than 2 mm to up to 5 mm.[83,84] Despite all these differing opinions, there has yet to be a consensus reached or any consensus statements published on setting finite criteria for defining the adequacy of surgical resection margins during BCT for DCIS. Lastly, the contribution of specimen handling (e.g., compressive vs. noncompressive specimen mammogram) as well as specimen and tissue pathology processing to creating artifactually close or positive margins has been long suggested[38] but has never been systematically evaluated. Although such handling and processing variables likely have a significant impact on cases of invasive carcinomas because of the obvious contrast in tissue quality between the invasive cancer "mass" and surrounding fibrofatty tissue within the excised breast tissue, their contribution on cases of DCIS is less likely as a result of the general lack of a masslike quality of DCIS within the excised breast tissue.

Risks of Evolution and Recurrence from Ductal Carcinoma in Situ

On one hand, it is evident that high-grade, comedo/high-grade DCIS lesions are not easily cured, that recurrences are common even after radiation therapy, and that such lesions have a high risk of evolution to invasive carcinoma.[42,82] In contrast, small, noncomedo DCIS are nonobligate precursor lesions, and it is estimated that only 25% to 50% of such lesions will eventually evolve into invasive carcinomas if left untreated for several decades.[4,6,54] They may be regarded as lesions of increased risk because their relative risk of later invasive cancer development is about 10 times that of the general population. There is strong evidence that DCIS of small size and low histologic grade is easily cured with local

excision without radiation therapy.[42,82] This is certainly true of lesions that are smaller than 1 cm in largest dimension. Thus, the best estimate of the size of a DCIS lesion should be stated even for core biopsy specimens to help facilitate clinical management. The greatest extent of a lesion is assessed most easily with careful pathologic-mammographic correlation, which is essential in such instances. Precisely which concurrence of histologic grade, size, and margin clearance is to be the determinant of therapeutic decision making is an area under ongoing investigation. However, it should be understood that local recurrence in the setting of a low-grade lesion is unlikely to be a life-threatening event and that a woman's desire for breast conservation with a willingness to accept the possibility of local recurrence may be as important with regard to therapeutic decision making as any other consideration. In contrast, local recurrence in the setting of a high-grade DCIS lesion is much more likely to be associated with invasion, high-grade histology, and development of metastases.[5,50] Thus, careful pathologic assessment of DCIS lesions that includes histologic pattern, grade, size, and margin status is essential for optimal clinical management and should be considered an essential part of any breast biopsy report for DCIS.[83-85]

Receptor Proteins, Oncogenes, Tumor Suppressor Genes, and Ploidy

A wealth of information in the literature describes the presence and distribution of specific oncogenes, receptor proteins, and measures of ploidy and proliferative activity in DCIS. Initially, there was an expectation that such investigations would be able to identify DCIS subgroups that are at increased risk for invasive transformation or local recurrence after BCT, particularly among patients at highest risk. In part, these expectations were met, but largely by demonstrating a correlation between specific oncogenes or gene products and DCIS subtypes recognized with conventional morphologic analysis as being a high risk for recurrence (e.g., high-grade [poorly differentiated], comedo-type DCIS, or both).

The clearest association between an oncogene and a DCIS subtype is seen with *HER2/neu* oncogene and its *erbB2* product, which is largely restricted to DCIS subtypes characterized by large cell type and higher nuclear grade.[86-91] Bartkova and colleagues[92] have shown that among those cases of DCIS that are of mixed subtypes, *HER2/neu* expression is seen only in the large cell component, and this factor is dramatically evident in cases in which the mixed cell population occurs within single ductules (Fig. 10-28).

DePotter and associates[87] demonstrated a significant association between *HER2/neu*-positive large cell–type DCIS and the extent of disease in the breast, which was independent of mitotic index, and hypothesized that *HER2/neu/erbB2* has a role in motility of in situ carcinomas within the ductal epithelium. Gupta and

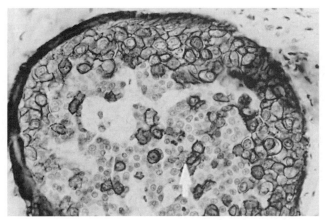

Figure 10-28 Immunocytochemical stain for *erbB2* with strong membrane staining of large cells in a higher-grade ductal carcinoma in situ. Note the presence of a negative, small-cell population. (×200.)

coworkers[93] have shown that E-cadherin expression is associated with the apparent degree of differentiation or orderliness. The cadherins are related to lateral complex integrity, polarity, and probably cell-to-cell communication.

p53, largely studied with immunoperoxidase techniques in noninvasive lesions, is also correlated with high nuclear grade subtypes.[5,86,91,94] O'Malley and colleagues,[63] among others, have noted that p53 protein over-expression is largely limited to high-grade, comedo-type DCIS. Immunohistochemical studies have shown over-expression in some cases in which p53 mutations were not detected by sequencing in the most highly conserved portion of the gene. Poller and coworkers[94] concluded that there was no relationship between *p53* and *HER2/neu* status; they nonetheless noted that almost all cases of *p53*-positive DCIS were large cell, with 35.8% of large cell DCIS being *p53* positive and only 4.1% of small cell DCIS being *p53* positive.[63] Others have documented similar relationships between high-grade DCIS, *HER2/neu*, and *p53*.[46,86,90,95]

Estrogen receptor and progesterone receptor protein expression, as demonstrated with immunohistochemistry, shows consistent, but not absolute, correlation with DCIS subtypes.[96] Bobrow and coworkers[86] noted an association between cytonuclear differentiation and progesterone status. DCIS with "poor" cytonuclear differentiation, as opposed to "good" differentiation, tended to lack demonstrable progesterone receptors. Similarly, Poller and associates[97] noted that estrogen receptor expression is related to noncomedo architecture, negative *HER2/neu* status, small cell size, and surprisingly higher S-phase fraction on flow cytometry. Wilbur and Barrows[96] noted a similar trend between grade (i.e., cytonuclear differentiation) and receptor status. They noted that 75% of estrogen receptor–negative DCIS exhibited nuclear grade III morphology (high grade), whereas only 14% of estrogen receptor–positive DCIS were nuclear grade III. Leal and colleagues[88] and Zafrani and co-workers[91] noted no relationship between DCIS subtype

and receptor status. These studies suggest that there is a weak association between high nuclear grade and negative receptor status similar to that noted in many high-grade invasive carcinomas.

Despite the fact that some investigators used two-tiered classification and others used three-tiered classifications, agreement between the studies has been substantial. DCIS subtypes characterized by large cell type and high nuclear grade tend to be *HER2/neu* positive, are more likely *p53* positive[94,95] and estrogen receptor negative,[96] are aneuploid, and are more likely to exhibit a higher S-phase fraction or other measurement of proliferation. They are also more likely to exhibit significant comedo-type necrosis, periductal stromal desmoplasia, and a diffuse increase in microvessel density.[48,98,99] In contrast, DCIS of small cell size, and of intermediate or low nuclear grade, or of noncomedo-type architecture tend to be *erbB2* and *p53* negative and diploid and, in most studies, exhibit a lower S-phase fraction and a tendency toward positive receptor status.[100] They also tend to lack significant necrosis and stromal reaction.

Despite concerted efforts using immunohistochemical demonstration of oncogenes and determination of ploidy and S-phase fraction with flow and image cytometry, identification of a subset of morphologically defined high-grade DCIS at even greater risk of invasive transformation remains elusive. Somewhat surprisingly, cyclin D expression was found to be similar and high in all grades of DCIS, with low levels in most ADH lesions.[101] In contrast, most genetic and molecular analyses have shown that the low-grade DCIS lesions are more similar to ADH than they are to high-grade DCIS lesions. The cyclins D, especially cyclin D1, control important transitional events in the cell cycle, especially entrance into DNA synthesis. Morphologic grading achieves as much separation as do numerous ancillary tests. Susnik and associates,[102] using a classification based on nuclear texture features quantified with high-resolution image cytometry, were able to identify 100% of high-grade comedo-type DCIS concurrently associated with invasion and 80% of noncomedo-type lesions associated with invasion. The study design was necessarily retrospective, but the results are suggestive. If further validated, automated quantitative analysis of nuclear texture features in DCIS may be able to identify patients at different levels of risk. However, prospective studies are needed to certify the prospective utility of these approaches.

Simpson and associates[103] compared NM23 expression in situ carcinoma associated with an invasive component with those not associated concurrently with an invasive component and found there was a higher expression of NM23 in comedo-type DCIS unassociated with an invasive component, suggesting that NM23 expression within comedo-type lesions might identify lesions with a lesser risk of evolution to invasion and metastatic capacity. Goldstein and Murphy[104] evaluated nuclear grade in a three-scale system and found grades of invasive and in situ components to agree most of the time.

Special Types of Ductal Carcinoma in Situ with Special Implications

HYPERSECRETORY DUCTAL CARCINOMA IN SITU

Hypersecretory changes in the breast represent a type of cellular presentation and cytoplasmic differentiation. Although they are poorly understood at present, these histologic elements coexisting with atypia appear to be associated with special features in the distribution and perhaps evolution of in situ disease toward malignancy. These lesions tend not to produce a lump within the breast and often have benign-appearing, lobular-type calcifications because it is the central secretion that calcifies. Often, the mammogram produces patterns that outline the lobules in an area of the breast. The presentation of the disease is commonly regional but does not have the uniformity of continuity seen in most forms of DCIS.

This entity was first described by Rosen and Scott in 1984.[105] The original paper and the follow-up presentation by the same group in 1988[106] emphasized the cystic dilation of the spaces involved and allowed for a category of atypia without the designation of DCIS. The association with the development of clinically evident malignancy in most of these cases was inapparent or unproved.[107] Often these cases present striking patterns of hugely enlarged nuclei abutting into the lumen, as seen in hypersecretory changes in the endometrium.[108,109]

The approach to these extremely difficult cases is generally to recognize atypicality in a biopsy and recommend careful continued mammographic surveillance. Unfortunately, calcifications may be present in clearly benign secretory alterations in the same region, representing a challenge for mammographic follow-up.[75]

However, there are a certain number of cases in which the diagnosis of DCIS is mandatory, and this diagnostic plateau is reached definitively when true ducts are involved. The recognition of DCIS status is particularly evident when patterns of micropapillary DCIS are reached.[110] It is indeed this favorite association with micropapillary DCIS that may be one of the more interesting elements in this complex of newly recognized diseases.[111] Because of the regional presentation of this disease, it has occasionally been suggested segmentectomy or quadrantectomy, although again the regionality of this disease appears to be not as precise as that seen in more typical cases of DCIS. It is clearly different from ALH and does not often coexist with ALH.

PAGET'S DISEASE OF THE NIPPLE

Paget's disease of the breast has been recognized as a specific clinical entity for more than 100 years, but it does not inherently imply any extension of the disease process beyond the nipple.[112] Thus, the diversity of disease from within the breast after presentation of Paget's disease of the nipple is what needs to be emphasized, and Paget's disease of the breast should no longer be viewed as a type of breast cancer. Rather, Paget's disease of the nipple should be viewed as a type of initial presentation of a breast cancer. After complete evaluation of the presentation, the overall disease process may be local or extensive within the breast.[113-116]

The classical and still relevant presentation is with an eczematous area of the nipple. This feature may be subtle or evolve to an obviously eroded, weeping lesion. The underlying process is population of the epidermis of the nipple surface with a scattering of neoplastic breast epithelial cells. Often, but not uniformly, these cells are identical with a DCIS lesion in the underlying ducts.[106,107] In advanced cases, the process may extend from the nipple to the pigmented skin of the areolar region and even to the adjacent surrounding, nonpigmented skin of the breast. The terms *pagetoid change* and *pagetoid features* are used for the interspersion of one cell type within another anywhere within the ducts and lobules of the breast. Immunohistochemical stains for *erbB2* (see Fig. 10-28) are useful in demonstrating these cells and are often helpful in the differential diagnosis, because *erbB2* expression is common to virtually all examples of Paget's disease of the nipple.[87,117]

Paget's disease is usually associated with extensive DCIS within the breast.[118] In the early mammographic era, Paget's disease of the nipple was associated with invasive carcinoma and DCIS in 50% of cases. The practical importance with regard to accepting conservation, when possible, is that at present about only 10% of cases are associated with disease confined to the immediate area of the nipple and are amenable to excision of the nipple-areola complex for cure.[119,120] Because of the importance of Paget's disease and recently emerging information concerning this disease, there is a separate chapter (see Chapter 14) exclusively devoted to Paget's disease of the breast.

ENCYSTED, NONINVASIVE PAPILLARY CARCINOMA

Encysted, noninvasive papillary carcinoma is an entity with features that are otherwise diagnostic for DCIS. These lesions are essentially anatomically confined and probably represent DCIS arising in and overtaking the residual aspects of an intraductal papilloma. The DCIS component usually is low grade, but it can be intermediate. The clinical importance of these lesions was originally clarified by Carter, Orr, and Merino,[121] who introduced the concept of an encysted lesion and reached a conclusion that in the absence of adjacent DCIS in neighboring ducts, local excision of these lesions is curative.[122,123] This valuable study has not been improved on. It is consistent with all the information we have at present about the importance of the extensiveness of regional DCIS with regard to the likelihood of local recurrence. It is widely recognized that a pattern of these lesions has very tall cells similar to those seen in villous adenoma of the colon with enlarged hyperchromatic nuclei. These nuclei are present without an increased cell number above fibrovascular stalks. Such an entity is considered as an encysted, noninvasive lesion within this category (Fig. 10-29).

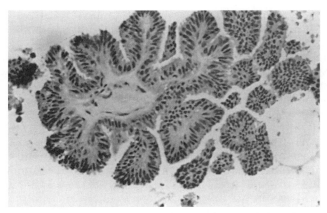

Figure 10-29 The presence of tall and hyperchromatic cells surmounting these papillary fronds supports the possibility of a diagnosis of encysted papillary carcinoma. Usually the epithelium is much more atypical and closely mimics that found in other ductal carcinoma in situ patterns. (×125.)

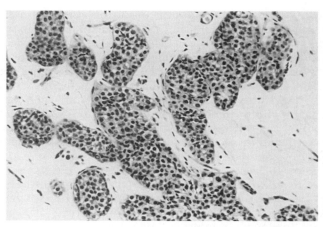

Figure 10-30 An example of lobular carcinoma in situ showing complete distention and filling of the majority of spaces in this area by characteristic population of cells. (×200.)

It should be noted that the cutoff point between papillomas with atypia (analogous to ADH), encysted or otherwise, from the nonencysted and encysted papillary carcinoma lesions is unclear. Reports by Raju and Vertes[124] and Page and coworkers[125] have stated that some degree of atypia similar to that of ADH present within papillomas may increase the likelihood of later cancer occurrence, but the two studies are in disagreement. There is an indication from the study by Page and coworkers[125] that well-developed atypical hyperplasia within papillomas of any size indicates increased likelihood of local occurrence of carcinoma, or at least regional occurrence of carcinoma after local excision for biopsy alone. There is no certainty at this time that wider excision after such a finding is necessary. However, it is recommended that careful mammographic surveillance of the area continue until this situation is better determined.

Pathology of Lobular Carcinoma in Situ

Epithelial proliferative lesions (noninvasive or in situ) of the human breast termed lobular were inaugurated by the introduction of the term LCIS in 1941 by Foote and Stewart.[126] Critical to the definition and concept was the distinctive caricature of lobular units produced by the diagnostic clustering of three major criteria: distention, distortion, and filling by a population of characteristic cells (Figs. 10-30 to 10-32). Also important to the definition, in all probability, was that more than 60% of invasive cancers presenting with single filing of cancer cells with similar cytology have such in situ lesions present in the same breast. Through the 1970s and 1980s, an important general acceptance of LCIS as an elevated cancer risk marker was established.[33,127] The two important papers of 1978 by Haagensen and colleagues[128] and Rosen and associates[129] concluded that there was generally no difference in risk between more well-developed and less well-developed histologic examples, and the reports included minor

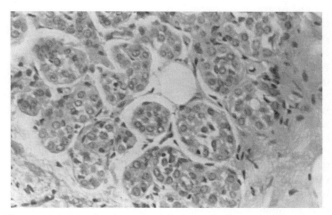

Figure 10-31 Portion of a lobular unit demonstrating some distention and little filling of the involved acini. This is atypical lobular hyperplasia. (×300.)

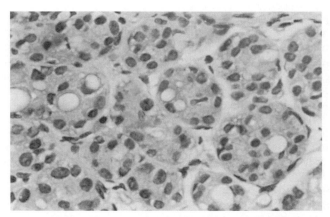

Figure 10-32 The vacuoles or globules in the cytoplasm are characteristic of lobular neoplasia. Note that some of the cells have the appearance of signet ring cells. (×400.)

histologic examples with little distortion of lobular units in their overall analysis. The Haagensen paper introduced the term *lobular neoplasia* (LN).[128] Page and coworkers in a large Nashville cohort of benign breast biopsies separated lesser lesions, reported lesser risk for such lesser lesions, and continued to vehemently stress the distinguishing features between ALH and LCIS (considering both these two entities to represent stages of LN).[57,130] These distinctions were later further discussed within the work of both Bodian, Perzin, and Lattes[131] and Fisher and associates.[132]

Bodian, Perzin, and Lattes continued to use the term LN to describe the full range of changes from ALH to LCIS.[131] Page and coworkers continued to use separate and different terminology, describing histologically less well-developed examples as ALH, because they demonstrated that such lesser entities were associated with a lower risk of cancer.[56,57] Of importance, Bodian, Perzin, and Lattes[131] and the work of the NSABP[132] have divided the LN spectrum into well-developed examples and less well-developed examples on a numeric basis. It has been suggested by Page and coworkers[130] that the NSABP series by Fisher and associates[132] is a biased series based on the fact that the cases were originally diagnosed by study pathologists as DCIS. Both of these recent studies[131,132] found a lower risk for less well-developed examples, whether it is called ALH or LN numbers 1 and 2, as opposed to LN 3. In the report by Bodian, Perzin, and Lattes,[131] the incidence of LN in a group of 2134 biopsies was more than 10%. Page and coworkers[130] have suggested that this is a highly selected series and that what the researchers classified as ALH included most of the cases within the broad range of cases in LN. Contrary, using their own restricted criteria for LCIS, Page and coworkers found an incidence of only 0.5% of LCIS in an unselected series of just over 10,000 biopsies.[57,130] In this regard, Page and coworkers continue to stress the point that the term LN should apply to a very wide range of changes from maximal to minimal, with LCIS referring to maximal changes, and that ALH refers to the rest of such lesions.[130] Furthermore, in addition to the fact that the work of both Bodian, Perzin, and Lattes[131] and Page and associates[57,130] supported the belief that less extensive histologic disease has less cancer risk, both series also have recognized that LN identified in patients older than 55 years of age was of less clinical significance. Lastly, although the work of Bodian, Perzin, and Lattes[131] did not indicate that ductal involvement by LN incurs a greater risk, Page and colleagues (using their own criteria[57]) found that ductal involvement conferred a somewhat increased risk when present in cases of ALH within the lobular units.[133]

Thus, the terminology used for ALH, LCIS, and LN continues to signify an increased risk of later cancer development in either breast, and other useful interactive associations remain to be further evaluated. Although the usual and common examples of LN are clearly multifocal with sparing of scattered lobular units, there is a suggestion by Page and associates that the risk of later breast cancer favors the breast that had ALH on biopsy,[134,135] with about 65% of later cancer occurring in the ipsilateral breast. Whatever the terminology, it is clear that lesser examples of histologic involvement (e.g., ALH) are associated with lower risk than more classic and more extensive examples recognized as fully developed LCIS, and most findings are best regarded as ALH.[134-136] The LN spectrum, with LCIS representing the fully developed example, is clearly very different from that of DCIS, although rare examples of local proliferation share features of each category and may be best regarded as exemplifying each lesion for patient care purposes.

With the more recent advent of minimally invasive breast biopsy technology, a developing theme within the literature has been seen with regard to the importance of finding LN (e.g., either ALH and/or LCIS) in such core breast biopsy specimens. There is certainly a wide range of opinions that have been given with regard to the necessity of subsequent formal surgical excision.[137-148] Nevertheless, it is apparent that there is little agreement; no obvious consensus has yet been reached. It is likely that the extent of LN found within the submitted core breast biopsy specimen, as well as the type of minimally invasive breast biopsy device used (e.g., smaller 14-gauge to 18-gauge automated spring-loaded core biopsy devices vs. larger 8-gauge to 11-gauge vacuum-assisted core biopsy devices) and the volume of the sampled tissue that is extracted with such devices, may become important variables in the decision making process concerning whether a formal surgical excision is subsequently warranted.

REFERENCES

1. Dean L, Geschickter CF: Comedo carcinoma of the breast. Arch Surg 36:225–232, 1938.
2. Geschickter CF: Diseases of the breast. Philadelphia, JB Lippincott, 1993.
3. Gillis DA, Dockerty MB, Clagett OT: Preinvasive intraductal carcinoma of the breast. Surg Gynecol Obstet 110:555, 1960.
4. Betsill WL Jr, Rosen PP, Lieberman PH, Robbins GFI: Intraductal carcinoma: long-term follow-up after treatment by biopsy alone. JAMA 239:1863–1867, 1978.
5. Page DL, et al: Intraductal carcinoma of the breast: follow-up after biopsy only. Cancer 49:751–758, 1982.
6. Page DL, et al: Continued local recurrence of carcinoma 15–25 years after a diagnosis of low grade ductal carcinoma in situ of the breast treated by biopsy only. Cancer 76:1197, 1995.
7. Wellings SR, Jensen HM: On the origin and progression of ductal carcinoma in the human breast. J Natl Cancer Inst 50:1111–1118, 1973.
8. Page DL, Anderson TJ: How should we categorize breast cancer? Breast 2:217–219, 1993.
9. Page DL, Anderson TJ, Rogers LWCarcinoma in situ (CIS). In Page DL, Anderson TJ (eds): Diagnostic histopathology of the breast. Edinburgh, Churchill Livingstone, 1987, pp 157–192.
10. Page DL, Lagios MD: Pathology and clinical evolution of ductal carcinoma in situ (DCIS) of the breast. Cancer Lett 86:1–4, 1994.
11. Webber BL, Heise H, Neifeld JP, Costa J: Risk of subsequent contralateral breast carcinoma in a population of patients with in-situ breast carcinoma. Cancer 47:2928–2932, 1981.
12. Habel LA, Moe RE, Daling JR, et al: Risk of contralateral breast cancer among women with carcinoma in situ of the breast. Ann Surg 225:69–75, 1997.
13. Rawal R, Lorenzo Bermejo J, Hemminki K: Risk of subsequent invasive breast carcinoma after in situ breast carcinoma in a population covered by national mammographic screening. Br J Cancer 92:162–166, 2005.
14. Li CI, Malone KE, Saltzman BS, Daling JR: Risk of invasive breast carcinoma among women diagnosed with ductal carcinoma in situ and lobular carcinoma in situ, 1988–2001. Cancer 106:2104–2112, 2006.

15. Barsky SH, Shao ZM, Bose S: Should DCIS be renamed carcinoma of the ductal system? Breast J 5:70–72, 1999.
16. Chang HR, Soo C, Barsky SH: In situ breast cancer. In Haskell C (ed): Cancer treatment. Philadelphia, WB Saunders, 2000.
17. Barsky SH, Sternlicht M, Safarians S, et al: Evidence of a dominant transcriptional pathway which regulates an undifferentiated and complete metastatic phenotype. Oncogene 15:2077–2091, 1997.
18. Barsky SH, Doberneck SA, Sternlicht M, et al: "Revertant" DCIS in human axillary breast carcinoma metastasis. J Pathol 183:188–194, 1997.
19. Sternlicht M, Kedeshian P, Shao ZM, et al: The human myoepithelial cell is a natural tumor suppressor. Clin Cancer Res 3:1949–1958, 1997.
20. Sternlicht M, Barsky SH: The myoepithelial defense: A host defense against cancer. Med Hypotheses 48:37–46, 1997.
21. Nguyen M, Lee MC, Wang JL, et al: The human myoepithelial cell displays a multifaceted anti-angiogenic phenotype. Oncogene 19:3449–3459, 2000.
22. Barsky SH, Kedeshian P, Alpaugh ML: Maspin and myoepithelial cells. In Hendrix MJC (ed): Maspin. Georgetown, TX, Landes Bioscience, 2002.
23. Barsky SH, Sternlicht M: The myoepithelial cell in DCIS. In Silverstein MJ (ed): Ductal carcinoma in situ of the breast. Baltimore, Williams & Wilkins, 1997.
24. Barsky SH, Bose S: Should LCIS be regarded as a heterogeneous disease? Breast J 5:407–412, 1999.
25. Lennington WJ, Jensen RA, Dalton LW, Page DL: Ductal carcinoma in situ of the breast: Heterogeneity of individual lesions. Cancer 73:118–124, 1994.
26. Page DL, Rogers LW: Combined histologic and cytologic criteria for the diagnosis of mammary atypical ductal hyperplasia. Hum Pathol 23:1095–1097, 1992.
27. Schnitt SJ, Connolly JL, Tavassoli FA, et al: Interobserver reproducibility in the diagnosis of ductal proliferative breast lesions using standardized criteria. Am J Surg Pathol 16:1133–1143, 1992.
28. Acs G, Lawton TJ, Rebbeck TR, et al: Differential expression of E-cadherin in lobular and ductal neoplasms of the breast and its biologic and diagnostic implications. Am J Clin Pathol 115:85–98, 2001.
29. Jacobs TW, Pliss N, Kouria, Schnitt SJ: Carcinomas in situ of the breast with indeterminate features: Role of E-cadherin staining in categorization. Am J Surg Pathol 25:229–236, 2001.
30. Bloodgood JC: Comedo carcinoma (or comedo-adenoma) of the female breast. Am J Cancer 22:842–849, 1934.
31. Lagios MD, Margolin FR, Westdahl PR, Rose MR: Mammographically detected duct carcinoma in situ: Frequency of local recurrence following tylectomy and prognostic effect of nuclear grade on local recurrence. Cancer 63:618–624, 1989.
32. Azzopardi JG: Problems in breast pathology. Philadelphia, WB Saunders, 1979.
33. McDivitt RW, Stewart FW, Berg JW: Tumors of the breast. Washington, DC, Armed Forces Institute of Pathology, 1968.
34. Lagios MD, Westdahl PR, Margolin FR, Rose MR: Duct carcinoma in situ: Relationship of extent of noninvasive disease to the frequency of occult invasion, multicentricity, lymph node metastases, and short-term treatment failures. Cancer 50:1309–1314, 1982.
35. Patchefsky AS, Schwartz GF, Finkelstein SD, et al: Heterogeneity of intraductal carcinoma of the breast. Cancer 63:731–741, 1989.
36. Ernster VL, Barclay J, Kerlikowske K, et al: Incidence of and treatment for ductal carcinoma in situ of the breast. JAMA 275:913–918, 1996.
37. Winchester DP, Amench HR, Osteen RT, et al: Treatment trends for ductal carcinoma in situ of the breast. Ann Surg Oncol 2:207–213, 1995.
38. Schnitt SJ, Abner A, Gelman R, et al: The relationship between microscopic margins of resection and the risk of local recurrence in patients with breast cancer treated with breast-conserving surgery and radiation therapy. Cancer 74:1746–1751, 1994.
39. Lagios MD: Ductal carcinoma in situ: controversies in diagnosis, biology and treatment. Breast J 1:67–78, 1995.
40. Silverstein MJ, Barth, Poller DN, et al: Ten-year results comparing mastectomy to excision and radiation therapy for ductal carcinoma in situ of the breast. Eur J Cancer 9:1425–1427, 1995.
41. Silverstein MJ, Lagios MD, Craig PH, et al: A prognostic index for ductal carcinoma in situ. Cancer 77:2267–2274, 1996.
42. Silverstein MJ, Lagios MD, Groshen S, et al: The influence of margin width on local control of ductal carcinoma in situ of the breast. N Engl J Med 340:1455–1461, 1999.
43. Chan KC, Knox WF, Sinha G, et al: Extent of excision margin width required in breast conserving surgery for ductal carcinoma in situ. Cancer 91:9–16, 2001.
44. Kerlikowske K, Molinaro A, Cha I, et al: Characteristics associated with recurrence among women with ductal carcinoma in situ treated by lumpectomy. J Natl Cancer Inst 95:1692–1702, 2003.
45. Macdonald HR, Silverstein MJ, Lee LA, et al: Margin width as a sole determinant of local recurrence after breast conservation in patients with ductal carcinoma in situ of the breast. Am J Surg 192:420–422, 2006.
46. Holland R, Peterse JL, Millis RR, et al: Ductal carcinoma in situ, a proposal for a new classification. Semin Diagn Pathol 11:167–180, 1994.
47. Silverstein MJ, Poller DN, Waisman, et al: Prognostic classification of breast ductal carcinoma-in-situ. Lancet 345:1154–1157, 1995.
48. Sneige N, McNeese MD, Atkinson EN, et al: Ductal carcinoma in situ treated with lumpectomy and irradiation: Histopathological analysis of 49 specimens with emphasis on risk factors and long term results. Hum Pathol 26:642–649, 1995.
49. Solin LJ, Yeh IT, Kurtz J, et al: Ductal carcinoma in situ (intraductal carcinoma) of the breast treated with breast-conserving surgery and definitive irradiation: Correlation of pathologic parameters with outcome of treatment. Cancer 71:2532–2542, 1993.
50. Bijker N, Peterse JL, Duchateau L, et al: Risk factors for recurrence and metastasis after breast-conserving therapy for ductal carcinoma-in-situ: Analysis of European Organisation for Research and Treatment of Cancer Trial 10853. J Clin Oncol 19:2263–2271, 2001.
51. Bellamy CO, McDonald, Salter DM, et al: Noninvasive ductal carcinoma of the breast: The relevance of histologic categorization. Hum Pathol 24:16–23, 1993.
52. Bornstein BA, Recht A, Connolly JL, et al: Results of treating ductal carcinoma in situ of the breast with conservative surgery and radiation therapy. Cancer 67:7–13, 1991.
53. Schwartz GF, Finkel GC, Garcia JC, et al: Subclinical ductal carcinoma in situ of the breast: Treatment by local excision and surveillance alone. Cancer 70:2468–2474, 1992.
54. Sanders ME, Schuyler PA, Dupont WD, Page DL: The natural history of low-grade ductal carcinoma in situ of the breast in women treated by biopsy only revealed over 30 years of long-term follow-up. Cancer 103:2481–2484, 2005.
55. London SJ, Connolly JL, Schnitt SJ, Colditz GA: A prospective study of benign breast disease and risk of breast cancer. JAMA 267:941–944, 1992.
56. Page DL, Dupont WD, Rogers LW, Rados MS: Atypical hyperplastic lesions of the female breast: A long-follow-up study. Cancer 55:2698–2708, 1985.
57. Page DL, Kidd TE, Dupont WD, et al: Lobular neoplasia of the breast: Higher risk for subsequent invasive cancer predicted by more extensive disease. Hum Pathol 22:1232–1239, 1991.
58. Douglas-Jones AG, Gupta SK, Attanoos RI, et al: A critical appraisal of six modern classifications of ductal carcinoma in situ of the breast (DCIS): Correlation with grade of associated invasive carcinoma. Histopathology 29:397–409, 1996.
59. Scott MA, Lagios MD, Axelsson K, et al: Ductal carcinoma in situ of the breast: Reproducibility of histological subtype analysis. Hum Pathol 28:967–973, 1997.
60. Fisher ER, Costantino J, Fisher B, et al: Pathologic findings from the National Surgical Adjuvant Breast Project (NSABP) protocol B-17: Intraductal carcinoma (ductal carcinoma in situ). Cancer 75:1310–1319, 1995.
61. Harrison M, Coyne JD, Gorey T, Dervan PA: Comparison of cytomorphological and architectural heterogeneity in mammographically detected ductal carcinoma in situ. Histopathology 28:445–450, 1996.
62. Lagios MD: Duct carcinoma in situ: Pathology and treatment. Surg Clin North Am 70:853–871, 1990.
63. O'Malley FP, Page DL, Nelson EH, Dupont WD: Ductal carcinoma in situ of the breast with apocrine cytology: Definition of a borderline category. Hum Pathol 25:164–168, 1994.
64. Leal C, Henrique R, Monteiro P, et al: Aprocrine ductal carcinoma in situ of the breast: Histologic classification and expression of biological markers. Hum Pathol 32:487–493, 2001.

65. Ashworth MT, Haqqani MT: Endocrine variant of ductal carcinoma in situ of breast: Ultrastructural and light microscopical study. J Clin Pathol 39:1355–1359, 1986.

66. Tsang WY, Chan JK: Endocrine ductal carcinoma in situ (E-DCIS) of the breast: A form of low-grade DCIS with distinctive clinicopathologic and biologic characteristics. Am J Surg Pathol 20:921–943, 1996.

67. Egan RL: Multicentric breast carcinomas: Clinical-radiographic pathologic whole organ studies and 10–year survival. Cancer 49:1123–1130, 1982.

68. Egan RL, Ellis JR, Powell RW: Team approach to the study of disease of the breast. Cancer 71:847–854, 1971.

69. Silverstein MJ: Intraductal breast carcinoma: Two decades of progress? Am J Clin Pathol 14:534, 1991.

70. Faverly DR, Burgers L, Bult P, Holland R: Three dimensional imaging of mammary ductal carcinoma in situ: clinical implications. Semin Diagn Pathol 11:193–198, 1994.

71. Holland R, Hendriks J, Verbeek AL, et al: Extent, distribution, and mammographic/histological correlations of breast ductal carcinoma in situ. Lancet 335:519–522, 1990.

72. Ohtake T, Abe R, Kimijima I, et al: Intraductal extension of primary invasive breast carcinoma treated by breast-conservative surgery: Computer graphic three-dimensional reconstruction of the mammary duct–lobular systems. Cancer 76:32–45, 1995.

73. Moffat DF, Going JJ: Three dimensional anatomy of complete duct systems in human breast: pathological and developmental implications. J Clin Pathol 49:48–52, 1996.

74. Johnson JE, Page DL, Winfield AC, et al: Recurrent mammary carcinoma after local excision: a segmental problem. Cancer 75:1612–1618, 1995.

75. Liberman L, Van Zee KJ, Dershaw DD, et al: Mammographic features of local recurrence in women who have undergone breast-conserving therapy for ductal carcinoma in situ. AJR Am J Roentgenol 168:489–493, 1997.

76. Thomson JZ, Evans AJ, Pinder SE, et al: Growth pattern of ductal carcinoma in situ (DCIS): A retrospective analysis based on mammographic findings. Br J Cancer 85:225–227, 2001.

77. Ohuchi N, Furuta A, Mori S: Management of ductal carcinoma in situ with nipple discharge: Intraductal spreading of carcinoma is an unfavorable pathologic factor for breast-conserving surgery. Cancer 74:1294–1302, 1994.

78. Page DL, Lagios MD: Pathologic analysis of the National Surgical Adjuvant Breast Project (NSABP) B-17 trial: Unanswered questions remaining unanswered considering current concepts of ductal carcinoma in situ. Cancer 75:1219–1222, 1995.

79. Fisher B, Constantino J, Redmond C, et al: Lumpectomy compared with lumpectomy and radiation therapy for the treatment of intraductal breast cancer. N Engl J Med 328:1581–1586, 1993.

80. Cheng L, Al-Kaisi NK, Gordon NH, et al: Relationship between the size and margin status of ductal carcinoma in situ of the breast and residual disease. J Natl Cancer Inst 89:1356–1360, 1997.

81. Holland R, Connolly JL, Gelman R, et al: The presence of an extensive intraductal component following a limited excision correlates with prominent residual disease in the remainder of the breast. J Clin Oncol 8:113–118, 1990.

82. Silverstein MJ, Waisman JR, Gamagami P, et al: Intraductal carcinoma of the breast (208 cases): Clinical factors influencing treatment choice. Cancer 66:102–108, 1990.

83. Neuschatz AC, DiPetrillo T, Steinhoff M, et al: The value of breast lumpectomy margin assessment as a predictor of residual tumor burden in ductal carcinoma in situ of the breast. Cancer 94:1917–1924, 2002.

84. Dillon MF, McDermott EW, O'Doherty A, et al: Factors affecting successful breast conservation for ductal carcinoma in situ. Ann Surg Oncol 14:1618–1628, 2007.

85. Bijker N, Peterse JL, Duchateau L, et al: Histological type and marker expression of the primary tumour compared with its local recurrence after breast-conserving therapy for ductal carcinoma in situ. Br J Cancer 84:539–544, 2001.

86. Bobrow LG, Happerfield LC, Gregory WM, et al: The classification of ductal carcinoma in situ and its association with biological markers. Semin Diagn Pathol 11:199–207, 1994.

87. De Potter CR, Schelfhout AM, Verbeeck P, et al: Neu overexpression correlates with extent of disease in large cell ductal carcinoma in situ of the breast. Hum Pathol 26:601–606, 1995.

88. Leal CB, Schmitt FC, Bento MJ, et al: Ductal carcinoma in situ of the breast: Histologic categorization and its relationship to ploidy and immunohistochemical expression of hormone receptors, p53, and c-erb B-2 protein. Cancer 75:2123–2131, 1995.

89. Simpson JF, Page DL: Pathology of preinvasive and excellent-prognosis breast cancer. Curr Opin Oncol 7:501–505, 1995.

90. Steeg PS, Clare SE, Lawrence JA, Zhou Q: Molecular analysis of premalignant and carcinoma in situ lesions of the human breast. Am J Pathol 149:733–738, 1996.

91. Zafrani B, Leroyer A, Fourquet A, et al: Mammographically-detected ductal in situ carcinoma of the breast analyzed with a new classification: A study of 127 cases: correlation with estrogen and progesterone receptors, p53 and c-erB-2 proteins, and proliferative activity. Semin Diagn Pathol 11:199–207, 1994.

92. Bartkova J, Barnes DM, Millis RR, Gullick WJ: Immunohistochemical demonstration of c-erbB-2 protein in mammary ductal carcinoma in situ. Hum Pathol 21:1164–1167, 1990.

93. Gupta SK, Douglas-Jones AG, Jasani B, et al: E-cadherin (E-cad) expression in duct carcinoma in situ (DCIS) of the breast. Virchows Arch 430:23–28, 1997.

94. Poller DN, Roberts EC, Bell JA, et al: p53 protein expression in mammary ductal carcinoma in situ: Relationship to immunohistochemical expression of estrogen receptor and c-erbB-2 protein. Hum Pathol 24:463–468, 1993.

95. Barnes DM, Bartkova J, Camplejohn RS, et al: Overexpression of the c-erb B-2 oncoprotein: Why does this occur more frequently in ductal carcinoma in situ than in invasive mammary carcinoma and is this of prognostic significance? Eur J Cancer 28:644–648, 1992.

96. Wilbur DC, Barrows GH: Estrogen and progesterone receptor and c-erbB-2 oncoprotein analysis in pure in situ breast carcinoma: An immunohistochemical study. Mod Pathol 6:114–120, 1993.

97. Poller DN, Snead DR, Roberts EC, et al: Oestrogen receptor expression in ductal carcinoma in situ of the breast: Relationship to flow cytometric analysis of DNA and expression of the c-erbB-2 oncoprotein. Br J Cancer 68:156–161, 1993.

98. Guidi AJ, Fischer L, Harris JR, Schnitt SJ: Microvessel density and distribution in ductal carcinoma in situ of the breast. J Natl Cancer Inst 86:614–619, 1994.

99. Sasano H, Miyazaki S, Gooukon Y, et al: Expression of p53 in human esophageal carcinoma: An immunohistochemical study with correlation to proliferating cell nuclear antigen expression. Hum Pathol 23:1238–1243, 1992.

100. Zafrani B, Vielh P, Fourquet A, et al: Conservative treatment of early breast cancer: Prognostic value of the ductal in situ component and other pathological variables on local control and survival: long-term results. Eur J Cancer Clin Oncol 25:1645–1650, 1989.

101. Weinstat-Saslow D, Merino MJ, Manrow RE, et al: Overexpression of cyclin D mRNA distinguishes invasive and in situ breast carcinomas from nonmalignant lesions. Nat Med 1:1257–1260, 1995.

102. Susnik B, Worth A, Palcic B, et al: Differences in quantitative nuclear features between ductal carcinoma in situ (DCIS) with and without accompanying invasive carcinoma in the surrounding breast. Anal Cell Pathol 8:39–52, 1995.

103. Simpson JF, O'Malley FP, Dupont WD, Page DL: Heterogeneous expression of nm23 gene product in noninvasive breast carcinoma. Cancer 73:2352–2358, 1994.

104. Goldstein NS, Murphy T: Intraductal carcinoma associated with invasive carcinoma of the breast: A comparison of the two lesions with implications for intraductal carcinoma classification systems. Am J Clin Pathol 106:312–318, 1996.

105. Rosen PP, Scott M: Cystic hypersecretory duct carcinoma of the breast. Am J Surg Pathol 8:31–41, 1984.

106. Guerry P, Erlandson RA, Rosen PP: Cystic hypersecretory hyperplasia and cystic hypersecretory duct carcinoma of the breast: Pathology, therapy, and follow-up of 39 patients. Cancer 61:1611–1620, 1988.

107. Jensen RA, Page DL: Cystic hypersecretory carcinoma: What's in a name? Arch Pathol Lab Med 112:1179, 1988.

108. Arias-Stella J: Atypical endometrial changes associated with the presence of chorionic tissue. Arch Pathol 58:112–128, 1954.

109. Arias-Stella J: Atypical endometrial changes produced by chorionic tissue. Hum Pathol 3:450–453, 1972.

110. Anderson TJ, Page DL: Risk assessment in breast cancer. In Anthony PP, MacSween RN, Lowe DG (eds): Recent advances in histopathology, vol 17. Edinburgh, Churchill Livingstone, 1997, pp 69–91.

111. Page DL, Kasami M, Jensen RA: Hypersecretory hyperplasia with atypia in breast biopsies. Pathol Case Rev 1:36–40, 1996.

112. Fechner RE: One century of mammary carcinoma in situ: What have we learned? Am J Clin Pathol 100:654–661, 1993.

113. Bulens P, Vanuytsel L, Rijnders A, Van der Schueren E: Breast conserving treatment of Paget's disease. Radiother Oncol 17: 305–309, 1990.

114. Salvadori B, Fariselli G, Saccozzi R: Analysis of 100 cases of Paget's disease of the breast. Tumori 62:529–536, 1976.

115. Chaudary MA, Millis RR, Lane EB, Miller NA: Paget's disease of the nipple: A ten year review including clinical, pathological, and immuno-histochemical findings. Breast Cancer Res Treat 8:139–146, 1986.

116. Dixon AR, Galea MH, Ellis IO, et al: Paget's disease of the nipple. Br J Surg 78:722–723, 1991.

117. Ramachandra S, Machin L, Ashley S, et al: Immunohistochemical distribution of c-erbB-2 in in situ breast carcinoma—a detailed morphological analysis. J Pathol 161:7–14, 1990.

118. Page DL, Steel CM, Dixon JM: ABC of breast diseases: Carcinoma in situ and patients at high risk of breast cancer. BMJ 310: 39–42, 1995.

119. Lagios MD, Westdahl PR, Rose MR, Concannon SI: Paget's disease of the nipple: Alternative management in cases without or with minimal extent of underlying breast carcinoma. Cancer 54: 545–551, 1984.

120. Bijker N, Rutgers EJ, Duchateau L, et al: Breast-conserving therapy for Paget disease of the nipple: A prospective European Organization for Research and Treatment of Cancer study of 61 patients. Cancer 91:472–477, 2001.

121. Carter D, Orr SL, Merino MJ: Intracystic papillary carcinoma of the breast: After mastectomy, radiotherapy or excisional biopsy alone. Cancer 52:14–19, 1983.

122. Corkill ME, Sneige N, Fanning T: Fine-needle aspiration cytology and flow cytometry of intracystic papillary carcinoma of breast. Am J Clin Pathol 94:673–680, 1990.

123. Estabrook A, Asch T, Gump F, et al: Mammographic features of intracystic papillary lesions. Surg Gynecol Obstet 170:113–116, 1990.

124. Raju U, Vertes D: Breast papillomas with atypical ductal hyperplasia: A clinicopathologic study. Hum Pathol 27:1231–1238, 1996.

125. Page DL, Salhany KE, Jensen RA, Dupont WD: Subsequent breast carcinoma risk after biopsy with atypia in a breast papilloma. Cancer 78:258–266, 1996.

126. Foote FW, Stewart FW: Lobular carcinoma in situ. Am J Pathol 17:491, 1941.

127. McDivitt RW, Hutter RV, Foote FW, Stewart FW: In situ lobular carcinoma: A prospective follow-up study indicating cumulative patient risks. JAMA 201:96–100, 1967.

128. Haagensen CD, Lane N, Lattes, Bodian C: Lobular neoplasia (so-called lobular carcinoma in situ) of the breast. Cancer 42: 737–769, 1978.

129. Rosen PP, Lieberman PH, Braun DW, et al: Lobular carcinoma in situ of the breast: Detailed analysis of 99 patients with average follow-up of 24 years. Am J Surg Pathol 2:225–251, 1978.

130. Page DL, Lagios MD, Jensen RA: In situ carcinomas of the breast: Ductal carcinoma in situ, Paget's disease, lobular carcinoma in situ. In Bland KI, Copeland EM (eds): The breast: Comprehensive management of benign and malignant disorders, 3rd ed. New York, Elsevier, 2003, pp 255–277.

131. Bodian CA, Perzin KH, Lattes R: Lobular neoplasia: Long term risk of breast cancer in relation to other factors. Cancer 78: 1024–1034, 1996.

132. Fisher ER, Costantino J, Fisher B, et al: Pathologic findings from the National Surgical Adjuvant Breast Project (NSABP) protocol B-17: Five-year observations concerning lobular carcinoma in situ. Cancer 78:1403–1416, 1996.

133. Page DL, Dupont WD, Rogers LW: Ductal involvement by cells of atypical lobular hyperplasia in the breast: A long-term follow-up study of cancer risk. Hum Pathol 19:201–207, 1988.

134. Page DL, Dupont WD, Rogers LW, Rados MS: Atypical hyperplastic lesions of the female breast: A long-term follow-up study. Cancer 55:2698–2708, 1985.

135. Marshall LM, Hunter DJ, Connolly JL, et al: Risk of breast cancer associated with atypical hyperplasia of lobular and ductal types. Cancer Epidemiol Biomarkers Prev 6:297–301, 1997.

136. Fitzgibbons PL: Atypical lobular hyperplasia of the breast: A study of pathologists' responses in the College of American Pathologists Performance Improvement Program in Surgical Pathology. Arch Pathol Lab Med 124:463–464, 2000.

137. Liberman L, Sama M, Susnik B, et al: Lobular carcinoma in situ at percutaneous breast biopsy: Surgical biopsy findings. AJR Am J Roentgenol 173:291–299, 1999.

138. Berg WA, Mrose HE, Ioffe OB: Atypical lobular hyperplasia or lobular carcinoma in situ at core-needle breast biopsy. Radiology 218:503–509, 2001.

139. Jacobs TW, Connolly JL, Schnitt SJ: Nonmalignant lesions in breast core needle biopsies: To excise or not to excise? Am J Surg Pathol 26:1095–1100, 2002.

140. Renshaw AA, Cartagena N, Derhagopian RP, Gould EW: Lobular neoplasia in breast core needle biopsy specimens is not associated with an increased risk of ductal carcinoma in situ or invasive carcinoma. Am J Clin Pathol 117:797–799, 2002.

141. Shin SJ, Rosen PP: Excisional biopsy should be performed if lobular carcinoma in situ is seen on needle core biopsy. Arch Pathol Lab Med 126:697–701, 2002.

142. Middleton LP, Grant S, Stephens T, Stelling CB, et al: Lobular carcinoma in situ diagnosed by core needle biopsy: When should it be excised? Mod Pathol 16:120–129, 2003.

143. Bauer VP, Ditkoff BA, Schnabel F, Brenin D, et al: The management of lobular neoplasia identified on percutaneous core breast biopsy. Breast J 9:4–9, 2003.

144. Foster MC, Helvie MA, Gregory NE, et al: Lobular carcinoma in situ or atypical lobular hyperplasia at core-needle biopsy: Is excisional biopsy necessary? Radiology 231:813–819, 2004.

145. Elsheikh TM, Silverman JF: Follow-up surgical excision is indicated when breast core needle biopsies show atypical lobular hyperplasia or lobular carcinoma in situ: A correlative study of 33 patients with review of the literature. Am J Surg Pathol 29:534–543, 2005.

146. Mahoney MC, Robinson-Smith TM, Shaughnessy EA: Lobular neoplasia at 11–gauge vacuum-assisted stereotactic biopsy: Correlation with surgical excisional biopsy and mammographic follow-up. AJR Am J Roentgenol 187:949–954, 2006.

147. Karabakhtsian RG, Johnson R, Sumkin J, Dabbs DJ: The clinical significance of lobular neoplasia on breast core biopsy. Am J Surg Pathol 31:717–723, 2007.

148. Brem RF, Lechner MC, Jackman RJ, et al: Lobular neoplasia at percutaneous breast biopsy: Variables associated with carcinoma at surgical excision. AJR Am J Roentgenol 190:637–641, 2008.

Infiltrating Carcinomas of the Breast: Not One Disease

CHARLES SHAPIRO | SANFORD H. BARSKY

Overview

In this emerging era of personalized medicine, we have begun to think of breast cancer as not one disease, although for decades the disease was really regarded as a singular entity. Although pathologists were one of the first groups to recognize that morphologically breast cancer was a heterogeneous group of diseases, it was not until the evolution of recent molecular classifications, the availability of targeted therapies, and the emerging observations provided by pharmacogenomics that made us all realize that breast cancer could not be treated as one disease. This chapter reviews the historical pathologic observations of breast cancer, merges this historical perspective with emerging molecular insights, and offers a vision for where the field is heading in the first decades of the 21st century.

Historical Pathologic Classification

Understanding the histopathologic features of breast cancer has been recognized anew as a necessary element for appropriate management of breast carcinoma.[1-10] Standard staging procedures recognize the extremes of the prognostic spectrum, and many therapeutic decisions are based on the tumor, node, metastasis (TNM) system; however, additional prognostic information is available through careful, focused histopathologic examination. The use of chemotherapy in an adjuvant setting has raised the question of whether such therapy will be beneficial—either because the patient already has an excellent prognosis or because the prognosis is so poor that high-dose chemotherapy is indicated. This chapter reviews the histopathology of invasive breast carcinoma, emphasizing the proven and potential settings in which it provides prognostic information.

There have been two general approaches to prognostication via histopathologic analysis. The first categorizes carcinomas based on specific features, recognizing the so-called special-type carcinomas. The second approach evaluates individual characteristics of the carcinoma, such as nuclear pleomorphism or gland formation (grading). Recognizing the special-type carcinomas makes it possible to identify a group of patients with an extremely good prognosis, often approaching or equaling that of the general population. In contrast, a subset of patients who have a very poor prognosis can be identified (representing about 25% of invasive breast carcinomas) with careful histologic grading. We endorse both of these approaches to histopathologic analysis for most cases, as described in the following sections.

HISTOLOGIC TYPES OF INVASIVE CARCINOMA

Much of the terminology of breast lesions is divided into lobular and ductal, based principally on historical perspectives. Early classifications of breast carcinomas used the term lobular for tumors commonly associated with lobular carcinoma in situ. Because ducts were the other source of epithelium within the breast, lesions that did not have a lobular pattern were referred to as ductal. In fact, most breast lesions, both benign and malignant, originate in the terminal duct lobular unit,[4] but the terms lobular and ductal continue to be used because they are so deeply ingrained in clinical parlance. Because fewer than 10% of invasive carcinomas are of the lobular type, the term ductal has no specific meaning.

We support the histologic classification that recognizes special types of mammary carcinoma defined in terms of specific histologic criteria (Table 11-1). In general, these special types are associated with less malignant potential than ordinary carcinomas that lack these special features. Terminology varies, but in general the frequency of these special types in different series is comparable. The special-type carcinomas make up about 20% to 30% of all invasive carcinomas (this figure is higher for carcinomas detected in screening programs),

TABLE 11-1					
Incidence (%) of Special-Type Carcinomas in Different Series					
Series	Lobular	Tubular	Medullary	Mucinous	Total
Rosen[5]	10	1	10	2	23
Fisher[6]	5	1	6	2	14
Fu[7]	11	7	15	2	35
Wallgren[8]	14	7	6	0	27
Page[9]	10	7*	5	2	24
Ellis[10]	16	3*	3	1	23
Anderson[11]	7	10	0	0.5	22

*Includes tubular and invasive cribriform carcinoma.

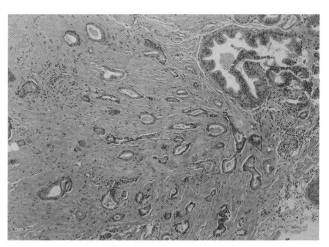

Figure 11-1 Infiltrating tubular carcinoma is an example of a well-differentiated ductal carcinoma that strongly correlates with the luminal A molecular subtype, discussed later in the chapter.

the remainder being invasive ductal or no special type (NST) carcinomas.[11-14] Fisher and colleagues[15] have termed these latter carcinomas not otherwise specified; however, we prefer the designation NST, to be consistent with the special-type terminology and to serve as a reminder to look for the features of special type in every case.[6] To qualify as a special-type carcinoma, at least 90% of the tumor should contain the defining histologic features; if the features are present in 75% to 90% of the tumor (variant), the prognosis is often better than that for a carcinoma that contains no special features.[9,16] The variant patterns are less powerful indicators of prognosis than their pure counterparts, however. Obviously, it is essential to sample the carcinoma thoroughly, paying attention to the possibility of heterogeneity. Although we stress the precise histopathologic criteria that qualify a carcinoma as a special type, an analysis of outcome from the Surveillance, Epidemiology, and End Results (SEER) programs shows that even without central slide review, an improved survival is seen with these special types of carcinoma.[17]

Tubular Carcinoma

Probably the most important special type is tubular carcinoma[18-20] because distant metastatic potential is highly unlikely when this tumor is present in pure form.[21,22] The diagnosis is made when characteristic angulated tubules, composed of cells with low-grade nuclei, comprise at least 90% of the carcinoma (Fig. 11-1). These neoplastic tubules are haphazardly arranged and are often found infiltrating between existing benign structures. Low-grade ductal carcinoma in situ and atypical ductal hyperplasia are common findings.[9] Tubular carcinoma has also been termed well-differentiated carcinoma, but this designation lacks precision, because carcinomas of no special type can also be well differentiated.

The prognosis for patients with tubular carcinoma depends on the purity of the histologic pattern.[18,21,23] In the classic series of 54 cases reported by Cooper, Patchefsky, and Krall,[18] all 12 patients whose carcinoma was composed purely of the characteristic low-grade, angulated tubules survived 15 years, regardless of tumor size.

In screening programs, tubular carcinoma represents 9% of detected carcinomas,[11,13] whereas in mammographic series, this special type of carcinoma is responsible for as many as 27% of detected carcinomas.[14] Mammographic features include a spiculated mass, with or without associated microcalcifications, or, less commonly, asymmetric density and architectural distortion with associated calcifications.[24] Diagnostic features of tubular carcinoma seen in fine-needle aspiration specimens have been described.[25]

Tubular carcinoma represents only about 3% to 5% of all invasive carcinomas; thus, the significance may be lost when cases are grouped and analyzed only by stage. The importance of tubular carcinoma lies with therapeutic decisions for individual patients. Tubular carcinoma has the biologic correlates of a low-grade cancer (estrogen receptor [ER] positive, diploid, low S-phase, no expression of c-erbB2 or epidermal growth factor receptor) and is more likely to occur in older patients. The survival of patients with tubular carcinoma is generally similar to that of the general population, and systemic adjuvant therapy may be avoided in these patients.[26] A review of surgical therapy states that for cases of pure tubular carcinoma with an adequate negative margin, mastectomy, radiation, or even axillary lymph node dissection may be unnecessary.[27,28]

Invasive Cribriform Carcinoma

Closely related, histologically and biologically, to tubular carcinoma is invasive cribriform carcinoma (ICC).[29,30] Histopathologically, these carcinomas infiltrate the stroma as islands of cells that have the same appearance as cribriform-type ductal carcinoma in situ (Fig. 11-2). Differentiating cribriform in situ from ICC may be difficult because of distortion and scarring. If tumor nests can be demonstrated within fat, beyond the confines of lobular units, the distinction is less difficult. Without this feature, irregular clustering of cellular islands signifies an invasive process. Another helpful feature is that the invasive islands in ICC are usually evenly spaced and often of

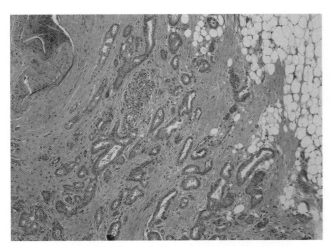

Figure 11-2 Infiltrating cribriform carcinoma is another example of a well-differentiated ductal carcinoma that also strongly correlates with the luminal A molecular subtype. Often, tubular and cribriform carcinomas coexist.

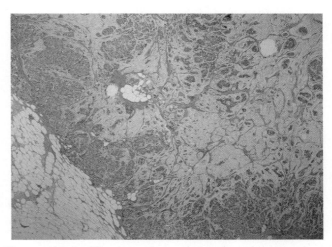

Figure 11-4 Mixed mucinous (*central*) and nonmucinous (*bottom*) carcinomas do not exhibit such an excellent prognosis probably because of the contribution of the nonmucinous areas.

uniform size.[9] About one fourth of cases have intermixed areas of tubular carcinoma. Because both tubular carcinoma and ICC have equally excellent prognoses, this feature has no bearing on an otherwise excellent prognosis.

In studies of pure tubular carcinoma[18] and ICC,[29,30] the presence of one or two positive low axillary lymph nodes did not adversely affect survival. The importance of pattern purity is emphasized, because the presence of carcinoma that does not conform to special-type criteria increases the likelihood not only of nodal involvement but also of shorter survival.[18,21,29,30]

Mucinous Carcinoma

Mucinous (colloid) carcinoma, when present in its pure form, is also associated with an excellent prognosis. Its defining histologic characteristic is extracellular pools of mucin in which low-grade tumor aggregates appear to be suspended (Fig. 11-3). As with tubular carcinoma,

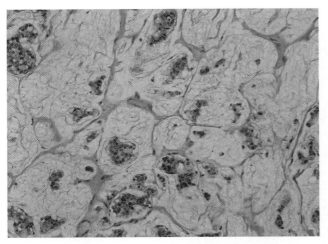

Figure 11-3 Mucinous and mixed (colloid) carcinomas consist of tumor cells embedded within an abundant mucinous extracellular matrix. Their prognosis is excellent, probably because their overall tumor burden is less than 1% of an equivalent nonmucinous breast cancer.

the importance of pure patterns is essential to ensure an excellent prognosis (90% 10-year survival)[31] in the absence of adjuvant chemotherapy.[26] Other studies confirm that the excellent prognosis of mucinous carcinoma is confined to pure examples of this special type of breast carcinoma.[32-37]

Pure and mixed mucinous carcinomas (Fig. 11-4) also have different mammographic appearances. On mammograms, whereas pure mucinous carcinoma has a circumscribed, lobular contour (corresponding histologically to pools of extracellular mucin), mixed carcinomas have an ill-defined, irregular contour. This lack of circumscription corresponds histologically to the interface between invasive carcinoma and the often-fibrotic stroma.[38]

Infiltrating Lobular Carcinoma

Infiltrating lobular carcinoma (ILC) has important clinical correlates, but there has been disagreement about prognostic implications. The different histologic definitions of this entity, whose incidence ranges from 1% to 20%, reflect this disagreement.[39,40] The two defining features of ILC are cytology and pattern of infiltration. The classic ILC is composed of small cells with cytologic features identical to those of lobular carcinoma in situ: regular, round, bland nuclei and cytoplasm with occasional intracytoplasmic lumina.[41,42] Morphometric analysis of the nuclei in classic ILC shows small nuclear volume, adding a quantitative measure to the cytologic criteria.[43] These cells infiltrate in single-file, frequently encircling existing structures (so-called targetoid pattern). When these two features are found in combination, the classic (or pure) pattern of ILC is diagnosed (Fig. 11-5). It is this form of ILC that is most often associated with lobular carcinoma in situ. Variant patterns have been described in which either the cytologic features or infiltrative pattern is present.[9,44-48] These include the solid, alveolar, mixed, and pleomorphic variants of ILC.

Part of the controversy surrounding the prognostic implications of ILC relates to the inconsistent application

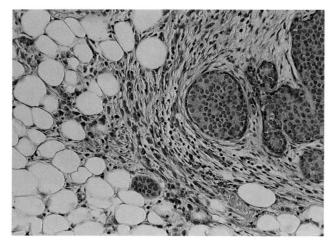

Figure 11-5 Infiltrating lobular carcinomas exhibit the classic areas of "Indian filing" and targetoid growth.

of histologic definition. Whereas some experts require at least 80%[44,49] of the carcinoma to have the appropriate ILC features, others have accepted as little as 5% as defining of ILC.[50] Studies that have shown an improved prognosis associated with ILC limit this prediction to the classic form of the disease.[44,49,51,52] The prognosis is intermediate (70% to 80% 5-year survival), falling between the excellent prognosis of tubular and related carcinomas and the often poor prognosis of carcinomas of no special type.[9] The importance of low-grade cytologic examination in diagnosing classic ILC is emphasized by two studies of so-called pleomorphic lobular carcinoma. Although the pattern of infiltration (single-file growth pattern) is similar to that of classic ILC, cytologic features are too pleomorphic for that diagnosis, and in both series, pleomorphic lobular carcinoma was associated with aggressive behavior.[45,48] The solid variant of ILC also appears to have a poor prognosis.[53] A molecular correlate of the dyshesive growth pattern that defines ILC has been described in mutations in the cell adhesion molecule E-cadherin.[54]

ILC is notorious for presenting diagnostic difficulties, clinically and radiographically. Although ILC is often associated with a discrete mass, a large proportion of these lesions are difficult to detect because of their insidious growth pattern. When compared with cancers of no special type but of similar size, patients with ILC have a better survival.[55]

ILC is often multifocal and bilateral, especially the pleomorphic variant.[56] These features have little bearing on outcome, either overall survival[56] or disease-free survival after conservative therapy.[52,57]

Medullary Carcinoma

Medullary carcinoma has characteristic mammographic, clinical, and pathologic correlates. Medullary carcinoma is a common phenotype of hereditary breast cancer and is found in women who are at risk for cancer because of mutations in the tumor suppressor gene *BRCA1*.[58] This genetic characteristic is in large part attributable to the young age of the patients.[59]

The distinctive smooth, pushing border of medullary carcinoma is reflected mammographically as a sharply circumscribed mass. Grossly, medullary carcinoma has a uniform, soft consistency. The essential histologic features include islands of tumor cells having irregular borders, without sharp edges, that are often connected (Fig. 11-6). These islands do not invade the adjacent breast tissue, but they appear to push against it instead, resulting in a smooth interface with the adjacent normal breast tissue.[9] Unlike the special-type carcinomas discussed earlier, medullary carcinoma is characterized by nuclei that have pronounced anaplastic features. The nuclei are large and pleomorphic, with clumped chromatin, frequent nucleoli, and readily identifiable mitotic figures. The other required histologic feature is a prominent infiltrate of lymphocytes and plasma cells in the loose connective tissue between the cellular islands. Multifactorial analysis has shown that high mitotic count, pushing tumor margins, and a lymphocytic infiltrate are independently associated with *BRCA1* mutations.[60]

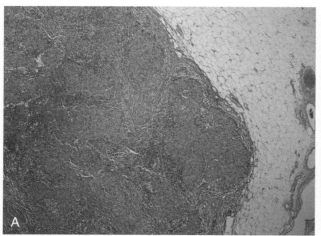 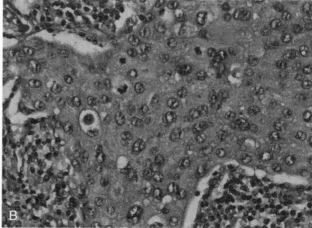

Figure 11-6 **A,** Medullary carcinomas tend to be well-circumscribed but paradoxically very anaplastic. **B,** The malignant cells of medullary carcinomas are embedded in a lymphocytic and plasma cell rich syncytium. This histologic type tends to be triple negative as well as associated with *BRCA1* inherited breast cancer.

Unlike medullary carcinoma in other organs, medullary carcinoma of the breast is rarely associated with microsatellite instability.[61]

The special prognostic features of medullary carcinoma have received considerable attention. The need for adhering to careful histologic guidelines is evident, because currently this entity is overdiagnosed,[62] despite the availability of specific histopathologic criteria.[63] When these histologic guidelines are followed, node-negative medullary carcinoma predicts a good prognosis; otherwise, the predictive utility is not clear.[64,65] A better prognosis for the so-called medullary variant, or atypical medullary carcinoma, is not predicted beyond what would be expected for an ordinary intermediate-grade NST carcinoma.[65]

Invasive Mammary Carcinomas of No Special Type

Approximately three fourths of invasive breast carcinomas do not have histopathologic features that would allow their inclusion into the aforementioned categories. These have been referred to as ductal because they do not have the lobular pattern described previously. Regardless of this common usage, these carcinomas have not been proved to arise in ducts, and in practice, they are diagnosed through exclusion because they do not fit into any of the special-type categories. For these reasons, we support the designation NST carcinomas, which is equivalent to the descriptor used by Fisher's group, ductal without special features or otherwise not specified type.[6]

No specific histopathologic features are consistently associated with infiltrating mammary carcinoma NST. These NST carcinomas are characterized by a variety of patterns, from solid to small tightly cohesive nests to single-cell infiltrative patterns (Figs. 11-7 and 11-8). Gland formation may be present, and often a mixture of these patterns is found in an individual carcinoma. Moreover, any of the patterns described for special-type carcinomas can be found focally.

These infiltrating NST carcinomas have the worst prognosis. Unlike the special-type carcinomas, limited

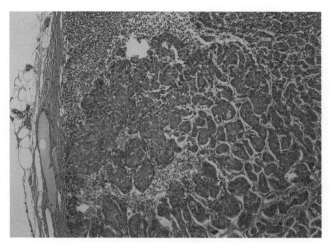

Figure 11-8   The presence of tumor infiltrating lymphocytes in infiltrating ductal carcinomas can be variable, but in general correlate with increasing grade.

prognostic information is obtained from the histologic patterns, because these are quite variable. Instead, prognosis is largely based on tumor stage.[66]

Despite the availability of well-defined histologic criteria for the different types of mammary carcinoma, the terminology used by surgical pathologists to report breast cancers is often inconsistent, as shown by the report from the SEER program of the National Cancer Institute. This update listed more than 20 histologic types of invasive carcinomas based on pathology reports.[67] Despite the lack of consistency in reporting, the 5-year survival for the special-type carcinomas was nevertheless better than that for those of NST.[67]

Unusual Types of Invasive Carcinoma

The preceding discussion of types of invasive carcinomas includes those commonly encountered. Several types of carcinomas are only occasionally encountered, representing in total less than 2% of all breast carcinomas.[9] Despite their rarity, specific diagnostic terms should be used in pathology reporting because of inherent clinical correlates.[9]

Micropapillary carcinoma is a particular type of invasive ductal carcinoma where islands of tumor cells fall within tissue spaces (Fig. 11-9). Many of these spaces are not lined by endothelial cells, but some spaces are. This suggests that micropapillary carcinomas may manifest florid but early lymphovascular invasion.

Then there is, of course, inflammatory breast carcinoma (IBC) characterized by florid lymphovascular tumor emboli especially within dermal lymphatics (Fig. 11-10). Because of the importance of IBC, an entire chapter has been devoted to this entity (see Chapter 87).

Secretory carcinoma is usually small and well circumscribed. The characteristic histologic feature is the presence of abundant intracellular and extracellular clear areas that contain secretions. Most examples are associated with discontinuous fibrous tissue that is often prominent within the lesion. The secretory material stains with periodic acid–Schiff stain and other mucosubstance

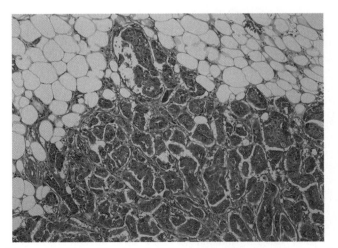

Figure 11-7   Infiltrating ductal carcinomas previously termed carcinomas of no special type display ductal structures invading adjacent breast adipose tissue.

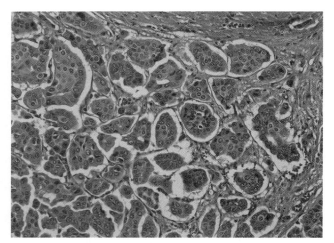

Figure 11-9 Micropapillary carcinomas exhibit lymphovascular emboli within spaces, many of which lack an endothelial lining. However, some spaces are endothelial-lined.

stains. Originally described in juveniles, secretory carcinoma can also affect older women.[68] Features that ensure an excellent prognosis include young age, tumor diameter less than 2 cm, and no stromal invasion at the periphery of the lesion.[9,69,70]

Whereas squamous metaplasia may be a feature of NST carcinomas, squamous cell carcinoma as a pure pattern of breast carcinoma is distinctly unusual. Often cystic, squamous cell carcinoma of the breast may also assume a solid pattern with keratinization. The prognosis of squamous cell carcinoma of the breast is probably the same as that for ordinary intermediate- to high-grade carcinoma NST.[71] The importance in its recognition lies with better understanding in the event of later metastases.[9]

Rarely, breast carcinoma displays the same pattern as well-accepted salivary gland tumors. The most important salivary gland type of tumor in the breast is adenoid cystic carcinoma because of potential confusion in progno-

sis. In the salivary gland proper, this tumor is infiltrative and, despite a long clinical course, may be lethal. In contrast, adenoid cystic carcinoma of the breast is associated with an excellent prognosis, and death from distant metastases is not recorded.[72–74] The histologic, cytologic, and immunohistochemical features of this unusual breast tumor have been presented.[72,73,75] Adenoid cystic carcinoma regularly lacks ER and shows increased cellular proliferation[76,77]; however, these features do not negate the excellent prognosis associated with adenoid cystic carcinoma. The lack of ER likely reflects derivation from ER myoepithelial cells, rather than lack of differentiation. Mucoepidermoid carcinoma of the breast has the same histopathologic features as the salivary gland counterpart. The salient features—mucin production and squamous differentiation—can, however, be a nonspecific feature of mammary carcinoma NST. The identification of mucoepidermoid carcinoma is probably important only when it is a low-grade tumor.[78,79] Case reports of high-grade mucoepidermoid carcinoma have demonstrated an aggressive course.[80,81] The histogenesis of this unusual neoplasm has been studied ultrastructurally,[82] immunohistochemically,[82,83] and biochemically.[83]

The term *metaplastic carcinoma* encompasses a group of tumors that show both epithelial and mesenchymal features. The mesenchymal component may show squamous, spindled, cartilaginous, or osseous differentiation (Fig. 11-11). With ultrastructural and immunohistochemical analysis, the sarcomatoid areas have been demonstrated to be of epithelial origin.[84,85] Despite the unusual appearance of these heterogeneous tumors,[86,87] the prognosis is similar to that for stage-matched invasive mammary carcinomas NST.[84,88] A subset of metaplastic carcinoma has been recognized as having distinct clinicopathologic correlates.[89] Tumors with growth patterns resembling fibromatosis were found to be associated with local but not distant recurrence. This is important because such lesions were previously classified with other metaplastic carcinomas.

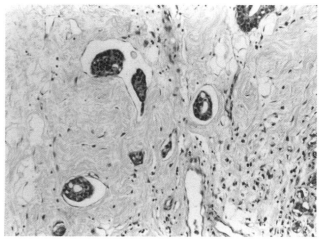

Figure 11-10 Inflammatory breast carcinoma exhibits florid lymphovascular emboli which extend away from the main mass and can involve dermal lymphatics.

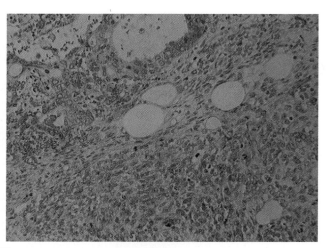

Figure 11-11 Metaplastic carcinomas exhibit "epithelial-mesenchymal transition" in that a prominent spindle cell component is present adjacent to the epithelial component suggesting that the former is derived from the latter.

PROGNOSIS OF INVASIVE BREAST CARCINOMA

Predicting outcome for patients with breast carcinoma, especially those whose carcinoma is confined to the breast, is of critical importance. Enormous efforts have been expended to identify predictors of prognosis. Evaluating which of these factors gives significant independent information is difficult because available studies have differences in the end points being evaluated, patient groups, length of follow-up, and treatments, as well as inconsistent inclusion of known prognostic factors to test for independent significance in the final analysis.[2,90,91]

The College of American Pathologists (CAP) Cancer Committee continues to address the clinical relevance of prognostic markers for solid tumors.[1,92] Previous CAP conferences have classified prognostic factors into three general categories based on their clinical utility and results of clinical investigation.[1] The most recent CAP conference refined these classifications; the clinically important category includes factors that are well supported by the literature and are in general use in patient management, including TNM staging information, histologic tumor type, histologic grade, mitotic figure count, and hormone receptor status.[92]

Tumor Stage

Tumor stage is the most useful means for predicting survival. The TNM staging system, the mainstay for prognostication for breast cancer, considers three variables[90]: diameter of the primary tumor (T), lymph node metastasis (N), and distant metastasis (M). The primary tumor is categorized as T_1 if it is 2 cm or smaller in diameter, T_2 if greater than 2 but not greater than 5 cm, and T_3 if larger than 5 cm. The size of the primary tumor and the status of axillary lymph nodes are independent and additive in predicting survival.[66] Both parameters reflect the tumor's ability to spread distantly.[66,93]

As important as the tumor size is, it is important to distinguish the invasive component in establishing the T stage, because the in situ component does not have metastatic capacity.[94,95] Staging is especially useful at the extremes of the scale. Clearly, the prognosis associated with a small carcinoma (1 cm) that does not involve axillary lymph nodes is so good that adjunctive measures are unlikely to have any impact.[96,97] On the other hand, most experts would agree that patients with 3-cm carcinomas should receive adjuvant therapy. However, pure special-type carcinomas, such as tubular and mucinous carcinomas, have an excellent long-term prognosis, even if they attain this size.[16] The challenge for surgical pathologists is to apply the specific histologic criteria that would allow their recognition consistently, thus ensuring good prognosis.

There have been some recent changes in the TNM staging system[98] that address the status of lymph nodes. These changes are especially timely considering the current emphasis placed on sentinel lymph node examination. A category of pN_1mi is created for micrometastasis (>0.2 mm and <2 mm). The category of pN_0 is subcategorized to address the identification of isolated tumor cells detected with ancillary methods, such as immunohistochemical or molecular methods, but verified on routine hematoxylin and eosin (H&E) stained slides.[98] Other changes include the classification of metastases into the infraclavicular lymph nodes (now N_3) and the supraclavicular lymph nodes (now N_3 rather than M_1).

The status of axillary lymph nodes continues to be essential in the staging and prognostication of breast cancer, especially in small tumors. Sentinel lymph node biopsy is an increasingly accepted staging procedure. However, with this procedure comes the opportunity to detect occult disease, the significance of which is still under investigation. The sixth edition of the American Joint Commission for Cancer (AJCC) staging manual allows for the separate reporting of these foci, with clarification of the method of detection. This approach should allow the separate analysis of the impact that occult metastatic cells may have on a patient's outcome. A careful review of this topic has been presented.[99] The CAP has recommended that immunohistochemical evidence of metastases to lymph nodes unsupported by documentation with routine H&E stains not be regarded as evidence of regional metastases.[92]

Histologic Grading

Although the prognosis for small or special-type carcinomas is favorable, prognostication for the remainder of patients, especially those with negative lymph nodes, is uncertain. Histologic grading of breast carcinomas may help stratify this group of patients. Unfortunately, careful grading of breast carcinoma has not been carried out consistently, despite the requirement for grading other malignancies.

Grading systems may be based on architectural or cytologic features. We endorse the grading system of Scarff, Bloom, and Richardson (SBR), as modified by Elston and Ellis.[100] The most recent CAP consensus conference endorses this system,[92] as well as the sixth edition of the AJCC Cancer Staging Manual. Also known as the combined histologic grade, this system is a composite of degrees of glandular formation, nuclear pleomorphism, and mitotic activity. Each of these parameters is assigned a numerical score based on specific criteria (Table 11-2). The scores from each category are then summed:

- 3 (lowest score possible), 4, or 5—equivalent to grade 1
- 6 or 7—equivalent to grade 2
- 8 or 9—equivalent to grade 3

The grader who uses this system is required to evaluate each parameter, with the result that interobserver agreement is fostered.

Although the Scarff, Bloom, and Richardson system has been used for many years, modification and extensive application to more than 2000 cases of primary operable breast cancer by Elston and Ellis[100] have clarified criteria, strengthening predictive power and reproducibility. Elston and Ellis have shown a highly significant correlation between grade and both relapse-free and overall survival. The distribution of cases within

TABLE 11-2

Combined Histologic Grading System

Tubule Formation (%)	Nuclear Pleomorphism	Mitotic Activity*
>75% = 1	Mild = 1	<10 per 10 hpf = 1
10%–75% = 2	Moderate = 2	10–19 per 10 hpf = 2
<10% = 3	Marked = 3	≥20 per 10 hpf = 3

*Based on high-power field (hpf) area of 0.274 mm^2.
Modified from Elston CW, Ellis IO: Pathologic prognostic factors in breast cancer. I. The value of histologic grade in breast cancer: Experience from a large study with long-term follow-up. Histopathology 19:403, 1991.

the three grades is also interesting: 19% were grade 1; 34%, grade 2; and 47%, grade 3. This contrasts with other grading schemes that place approximately two thirds of cases into the poorly differentiated category, thus reducing predictive power.[15] Others have shown that grading is predictive of outcome,[101] being second only to lymph node involvement as an independent prognostic factor.[102] Histologic grade of small carcinomas is especially important in prognostication.[103] In general, the special-type carcinomas have low nuclear grade, as determined both histologically and with cell cycle analysis.[104]

Although histologic grading of breast carcinoma has not been accepted as widely in North America as in Europe, there is a recent trend toward increased use of histologic grading.[105] The reproducibility of histologic grading using the combined histologic grading system has been demonstrated.[106,107] The Nottingham Prognostic Index (NPI) incorporates tumor size, lymph node status, and the combined histologic grade with independent prediction of outcome, including small (<1 cm) tumors.[101,108]

Proliferative Activity

An assessment of proliferative activity is an important factor in breast cancer prognosis, although it has not been as widely verified as the parameters described previously. Cellular proliferation may be assessed in several ways, most practically through quantification of mitotic figures. The latter method is endorsed by the most recent CAP consensus conference.[92] As a component of the combined histologic grade, a high mitotic rate is the strongest indicator of a poor prognosis[109] for both node-negative[110] and node-positive breast cancer.[111] By itself, the mitotic count has been shown to be a powerful predictor of recurrence and survival.[112,113]

Proliferation is commonly analyzed through flow cytometric analysis of DNA, from which the percentage of cells in S phase may be calculated. Correlation is also seen between an elevated S-phase fraction and high histologic grade. Although an elevated S-phase fraction appears to be an important predictor of poor disease-free and overall survival, in multivariate analysis the

prognostic power of S phase may lose its independent significance if histologic grade is included in the analysis.[114] Standardization of methods and the establishment of meaningful divisions of S phase continue to be investigated.[115]

Disadvantages of flow cytometric analysis relate to the requirement for tissue beyond that necessary for the histopathologic diagnosis and the inability to be sure which cells are being analyzed. These drawbacks are not unique to flow cytometry but relate to any process that requires a tissue homogenate. Another approach for assessing growth fraction is immunohistochemical analysis for nuclear antigens associated with cell proliferation. The most widely studied of these is the Ki-67 antigen, which is present in all phases of the cell cycle except G_0. Expression of Ki-67 correlates with other measures of cell proliferation (thymidine labeling,[116] mitotic count,[117] and S-phase fraction[118]) and is an independent prognostic indicator when present in high levels.[119]

Immunohistochemical methods of determining cell proliferation are attractive because they circumvent the disadvantages described for flow cytometry. The proliferation antigen Ki-67 is easily detected by using antibody MIB1 and antigen retrieval techniques, which allow assessment of routinely processed tissue.[120] Reactivity of this antibody correlates with mitotic activity and tumor grade[121] and, compared with other markers of proliferation, may have the greatest predictive value.[122,123] Along with lymph node status, tumor size, and grade, MIB1 reactivity is an independent prognostic indicator.[121]

Estrogen Receptor

The immunohistochemical determination of ER in paraffin-embedded tissue yields results that closely parallel biochemical determinations. These tissue section analyses are advantageous for several reasons. One, the same tissue that is used for making the diagnosis is used for the ER analysis. Thus, tissue is conserved, which is especially important with smaller cancers. Two, the presence of ERs is detected in the context of histopathology. Thus, the physician is ensured that the positive signal detected is emanating from carcinoma instead of benign epithelium. The biochemical assay is based on a tissue homogenate, so it is impossible to know which cells are responsible for a positive signal. This is also an issue if carcinoma in situ, rather than the invasive component, is assayed biochemically. Three, greater sensitivity is achievable with the immunohistochemical assay. If a carcinoma is not very cellular or if there are many contaminating stromal or inflammatory cells, a resulting dilutional effect may be encountered in the biochemical assay. In contrast, positive cells, even if very rare, are easily recognized immunohistochemically.

Several studies have shown the benefits of immunohistochemical analysis for ERs.[124,125] Although the clinical predictive power of the biochemical method has been well established,[126] the immunohistochemical method for determining ER status is superior in predicting response to adjuvant endocrine therapy[127] and adoption of the immunohistochemical method of ER determination has been supported.[128]

Additional Elements Occasionally Helpful in Prognostication

The prognostic significance of vascular invasion has not been completely straightforward. In general, lymphatics are the vessels most often involved in breast carcinoma, although blood vessels sometimes contain carcinoma. Misinterpreting carcinoma in soft tissue spaces or intraductal carcinoma as tumor in lymphatic spaces is often responsible for the overdiagnosis of lymphatic invasion. However emerging evidence has suggested that these "space artifacts" may not be true artifacts but may be indicative of early stage true lymphovascular invasion (LVI; see Figs. 11-9 and 11-10). These mistakes may be avoided if the physician requires the presence of tumor cell emboli in a space lined by endothelial cells to make the histologic determination of vascular invasion (see Fig. 11-10).

Studies that have adhered to this criterion for vascular space involvement have found that peritumoral lymphatic invasion portends a worse prognosis. This has been found in lymph node–positive cases[129] and in node-negative cases.[130,131] Moreover, for primary carcinomas that are smaller than 2 cm in greatest diameter, lymphatic involvement was an independent predictor of the presence of axillary lymph node metastasis.[132]

Carcinoma involving the lymphatic spaces of the dermis often results in the distinctive clinical entity IBC, as has been mentioned. This diagnosis is made when a breast containing carcinoma is red, edematous, and warm. Dermal lymphatic invasion can be demonstrated in most patients so affected (see Fig. 11-10). The presence of one feature and not the other (clinical signs versus histologic demonstration of dermal lymphatic invasion) has resulted in some controversy about outcome. It is rare for patients with inflammatory carcinoma to survive 5 years, although a multimodality approach—multiagent chemotherapy, surgery, and irradiation—may improve survival.[133] As has been stated, because of the importance of IBC, a separate chapter is devoted exclusively to this disease (see Chapter 87).

In summary, prognostication based on tumor stage, histologic recognition of special types of carcinomas, and careful histologic grading are proven predictive factors. Surgical pathology reporting is incomplete without them. Likewise, studies of new prognostic factors should include these proven factors in the final analysis of independent significance.[134]

Emerging Molecular Classification

Emerging molecular classifications have also contributed to the paradigm shift that human breast cancer is not one disease. Breast cancer is now considered as consisting of at least five different molecular subtypes, which are each characterized by distinct gene expression profiles.[135-137] This is of paramount importance because the patients with varying subtypes have different clinical outcomes and each responds differently to treatment (Table 11-3). For example, the luminal A and B subtypes are phenotypically characterized by the expression of estrogen receptors; however, the overall survival of patients with luminal A cancers is significantly greater then patients with luminal B cancers.[138] The HER2 overexpressing subtype occurs in about 10% to 20% of breast cancers, and these patients respond to trastuzumab, a humanized monoclonal antibody directed to the external domain of HER2 (or erbB2) transmembrane tyrosine kinase,[139-142] and lapatinib, a small molecule inhibitor of HER1 (epidermal growth factor receptor) and HER2 that inhibits homo- and heterodimerization of the internal domains HER1,2, and 3 required for receptor activation.[143,144] Likewise, the HER2 overexpressing and basal subtypes have higher initial responses to anthracycline-based chemotherapy then the luminal subtypes but poorer disease-free survival.[145]

Another emerging molecular subtype is the luminal C subtype, which corresponds to the histopathologic subtype of infiltrating lobular carcinoma. The subtypes

---

TABLE 11-3

Major Subtypes of Breast Cancer Defined by Gene Profiles

Subtype	Percent[146,147]	Outcome[138,*] DDS	Outcome[138,*] OS	Standard IHC[145,146]
Luminal A	51–61	75	90	ER+, PR+, HER2−
Luminal B	14–16	47	40	ER+ and/or PR+, HER2+
HER2	7–9	34	31	ER and PR−, HER2+
Basal	11–20	18	0	ER, PR, and HER2− Cytokeratin 5/6 and EGFR+
Unclassified	2–6	NA	NA	Negative for all markers

DDS, distant-disease free survival; EGFR, epidermal growth factor receptor; ER, estrogen receptor; IHC, immunohistochemistry; OS, overall survival; PR, progesterone receptor.
*Percent of patients without distant metastases or alive with systemic therapy at 5 years.
From Perou CM, Sorlie T, Eisen MB, et al: Molecular portraits of human breast tumours. Nature 406:747–752, 2000; and Sorlie T, Perou CM, Tibshirani R, et al: Gene expression patterns of breast carcinomas distinguish tumour subclasses with clinical implications. Proc Natl Acad Sci USA 98:10869–10874, 2001.

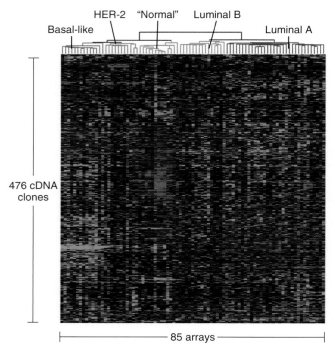

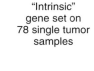

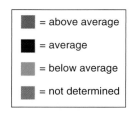

Figure 11-12 The major molecular subclassification for breast cancer based on gene expression profiling. (Sorlie T, Perou CM, Tibshirani R, et al: Gene expression patterns of breast carcinomas distinguish tumor subclasses with clinical implications. Proc Natl Acad Sci USA 98:10869–10874, 2001. Copyright 2001 National Academy of Sciences, USA.)

defined by gene expression arrays also can be approximated by standard immunohistochemical stains (see Table 11-3).[146,147]

Increasingly, clinical trials are being designed for the different subtypes, particularly with respect to *HER2* overexpressing and basal subtypes. In contrast, prior clinical trials required that the patient have only histologic confirmation of breast cancer. As new targeted and biologically based therapies are developed, it is critical that they be evaluated in the context of the subtypes of breast cancer. Clearly, the molecular subtypes based on gene expression profiling (Fig. 11-12) dictate prognosis (Fig. 11-13).

PROGNOSTIC PROFILES IN BREAST CANCER

The disease-free and overall survival and the benefits of systemic antiestrogen therapy and chemotherapy had been garnered from the results of randomized trials. Over the past 20 years, an international collaboration resulted in meta-analyses that were updated every 5 years.[148,149] An online decision tool (www.adjuvantonline.com) developed by Ravdin and others was useful in making treatment decisions regarding the benefits of systemic therapies.[150] Characteristics of the breast cancer such as size, grade, ER, and nodal status are input into the model, and results are interpreted as the 10-year absolute benefits on disease-free and overall survival with or without systemic therapy. The results predicted by the decision tool were highly concordant with the long-term follow-up in the British Columbia Breast Cancer Outcomes database of more than 4000 breast cancer patients,[151] and in clinical practice it was easy to use by both patients and physicians and both informed and affected decisions about adjuvant chemotherapy.[152]

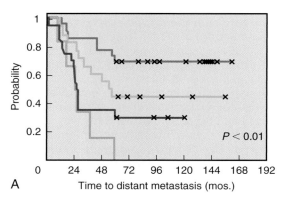

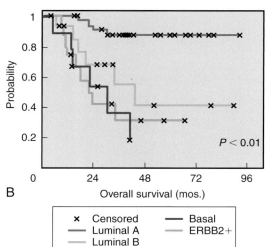

Figure 11-13 Metastasis-free survival **(A)** and overall survival **(B)** in the various molecular subtypes of human breast cancer. (Brenton JD, Carey LA, Ahmed AA, et al: Molecular classification and molecular forecasting of breast cancer: Ready for clinical application? J Clin Oncol 23:7350–7360, 2005.)

The molecular subclassification discussed previously indicated the global gene expression profile could predict biology of breast cancer and from this subclassification emerged attempts to refine or focus on selected gene expression profiles that could predict response to hormonal therapy, the need for chemotherapy and type required, and other predictive information.

PREDICTIVE PROFILES IN BREAST CANCER

Recently, three different approaches based on gene profiling of breast cancers have been introduced. These are the 21-gene, the 70-gene, and the 76-gene profiles (Oncotype DX, Mammoprint, and multicenter profile).[153-169] See also the findings of G Gulnur, K Huebner, and CL Shapiro (unpublished data). The 21-gene profile was first developed by selecting 16 genes, which were apportioned into groups that were associated with proliferation, invasiveness, ER, and *HER2*, plus five reference genes, and determining their expression by reverse transcription polymerase chain reaction (Fig. 11-14). These expression profiles were transformed into a continuous variable termed the *recurrence score*. This score was used as a prognostic factor for adjuvant tamoxifen in patients with ER-positive, lymph node–negative breast cancers and as a predictor factor in identifying those patients who would benefit most by receiving adjuvant chemotherapy.[155,156] Six 10-micron sections and one H&E slide from the standard formalin-fixed paraffin-embedded tissue block was the source material for this assay (www.genomichealth.com). The Oncotype DX test is being prospectively validated in a large ongoing clinical trial (The Trial Assigning Individualized Options for Treatment, or TAILOR X or PACCT trial; www.cancer.gov/clinicaltrials).[157,158]

The Mammoprint test (Fig. 11-15) was based on the work of van de Vijver and others at the Netherlands Cancer Institute in Amsterdam.[159,160] This test segregated patients with lymph node–negative breast cancers into "good" versus "poor" prognostic groups based on a 70-gene expression profile.[161] This test required a sample of breast cancer be either fresh frozen or placed in RNA stabilization solution and a kit provided by the manufacturer (www.agendia.com). The 70-gene profile is also being prospectively validated in a large ongoing trial (Microarray in Node-Negative Disease May Avoid Chemotherapy, or MINDACT).[162]

The 76-gene profile (Fig. 11-16) was developed and validated in a multicenter study to show a good versus a poor signature (Fig. 11-17).

The 21-gene, 70-gene, and 76-gene profiles all show reasonably high concordance (about 80%) despite containing different genes.[163] In addition, studies demonstrate that they function as independent prognostic factors adding additional information to the standard prognostic profiles.[161,164] Preliminary reports show that these tests influence oncologists' decisions concerning adjuvant chemotherapy recommendations[158] and that they are cost-effective because they identify patients who may not benefit from chemotherapy.[165,166] Other molecular testing is emerging, such as the breast cancer wound signature thought to confer a poor prognosis (Fig. 11-18).

However, there are limitations with each test. No test has been independently and prospectively validated, and there is no evidence that their findings can be extrapolated to patients that fall outside of the original "training set." Furthermore, U.S. Food and Drug Administration (FDA) approval has been slow in coming. Still, these tests illustrate a "proof of principle" that molecular profiling can predict response to therapy and guide proper therapy. Over the next decade, more molecular tests will emerge that will provide better predictive information as we attempt to personalize breast cancer therapy under the axiom that "one size does not fit all."

Emerging Pharmacogenomic Classification

Still other molecular testing aimed not at the tumor but at the patient is taking center stage in providing predictive information. This is within the exciting field of pharmacogenomics. For example, the efficacy of tamoxifen in treating ER-positive breast cancer may be related to the ability of the patient to metabolize this drug. The ratio of HOXB13 to IL17BR is thought to predict tamoxifen resistance in terms of progression-free survival.[170] In another study, the influence of the CYP2D6 genotype, which in turn governs the rate of conversion of tamoxifen to endoxifen, its active metabolite,[169,171,172] influenced time to relapse, relapse-free survival, disease-free survival, and overall survival (Fig. 11-19). On October 18, 2006, an FDA advisory panel recommended that the labeling for tamoxifen should be revised to alert prescribers that patients with breast cancer who poorly metabolize the drug have an increased risk of recurrence of the disease. The FDA's Clinical Pharmacology Subcommittee of the Advisory Committee for Pharmaceutical Science also said that the cancer drug's labeling should warn that certain antidepressants can inhibit the body's ability to metabolize tamoxifen. Commercial tests for measuring 2D6 genotyping are available on both whole blood as well as on a buccal swab. The question can be asked: Should we perform routine 2D6 testing? The evidence to date has

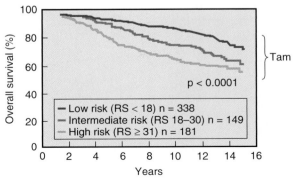

Figure 11-14 Overall survival based on the Oncotype DX score. (Data from Paik S, Shak S, Tang G, et al: A multigene assay to predict recurrence of tamoxifen-treated, node-negative breast cancer. N Engl J Med 351:2817–2826, 2004. Copyright © 2004 Massachusetts Medical Society. All rights reserved.)

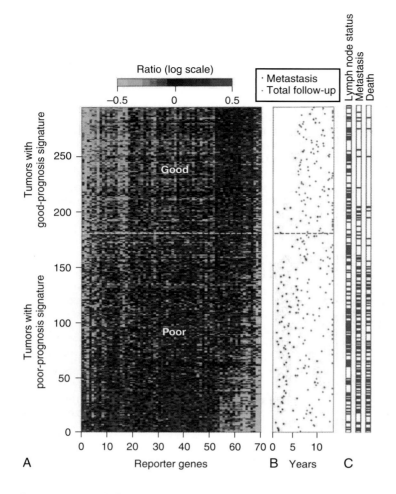

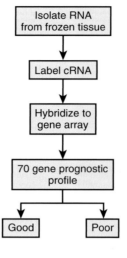

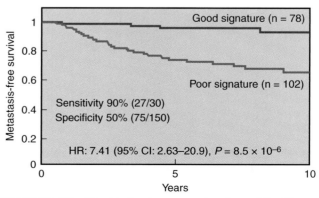

Figure 11-15 The 70-gene prognostic profile. (van de Vijver MJ, He YD, van 't Veer LJ, et al: A gene-expression signature as a predictor of survival in breast cancer. N Engl J Med 347:1999–2009, 2002. Copyright © 2004 Massachusetts Medical Society. All rights reserved.)

been generated from relatively small retrospective trials. There have been no prospective validations that testing will affect outcome. In summary, although molecular profiling of both tumor and patient will eventually lead to better prognostic and predictive factors and identification of new drug and pathway targets with improvement of the therapeutic ratio (efficacy/toxicity), molecular profiling is still not ready for "prime time."

Molecular profiling is still not ready for use in clinical decision making because for such profiling to be used in such a role, it must be demonstrated to have independent prognostic as well as predictive value above standard prognostic factors. Molecular profiling must be genuinely validated prospectively by validation sets that go beyond the original training sets. Molecular profiling needs to show a demonstrative benefit to routine practice and must be cost-effective. That day when these requirements will be met is coming.

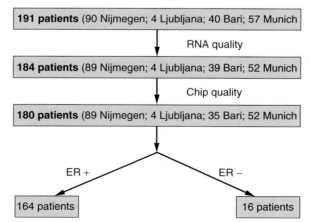

Figure 11-16 The 76-gene prognostic profile: multicenter. ER, estrogen receptor. (Data from Foekens JA, Atkins D, Zhang Y, et al: Multicenter validation of a gene expression-based signature in lymph node-negative primary breast cancer. J Clin Oncol 24:1665–1671, 2006.)

Figure 11-17 The good versus poor signature of the 76-gene profile. (Data from Foekens JA, Atkins D, Zhang Y, et al: Multicenter validation of a gene expression-based signature in lymph node-negative primary breast cancer. J Clin Oncol 24:1665–1671, 2006.)

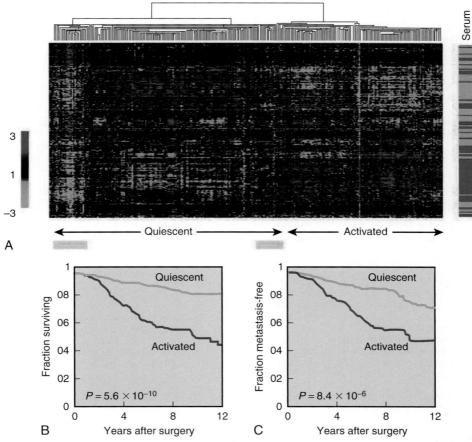

Figure 11-18 A–C, The "wound signature" gene profile of human breast cancer and its influence on metastasis-free survival and overall survival. (Chang HY, Nuyten DS, Sneddon JB, et al: Robustness, scalability, and integration of a wound-response gene expression signature in predicting breast cancer survival. Proc Natl Acad Sci USA; 102: 3738–3743, 2005. Copyright 2005 National Academy of Sciences, USA.)

Figure 11-19 A–D, Influence of CYP2D6 genotypes on time to relapse (TTR), relapse-free survival (RFS), disease-free survival (DFS), and overall survival (OS). This is an example where the patient's pharmacogenomic profile may be predictive independent of tumoral profile. (Data from Goetz MP, Knox SK, Suman VJ, et al: The impact of cytochrome P4502D6 metabolism in women receiving adjuvant tamoxifen. Breast Cancer Res Treat 101:113–121, 2007; Rae JM, Goetz MP, Hayes DF, et al: CYP2D6 genotype and tamoxifen response. Breast Cancer Res Treat 7:E6, 2005; and Goetz MP, Suman VJ, Ingle JN, et al: A two-gene expression ratio of homeobox 13 and interleukin-17B receptor for prediction of recurrence and survival in women receiving adjuvant tamoxifen. Clin Cancer Res 12[Pt 1]: 2080–2087, 2006.)

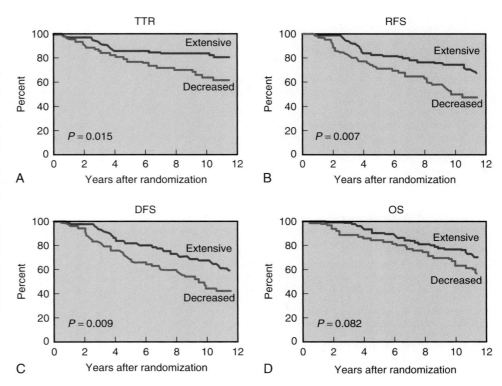

REFERENCES

1. Henson DE, et al: College of American Pathologists Conference XXVI on clinical relevance of prognostic markers in solid tumors: Summary. Arch Pathol Lab Med 119:1109, 1995.
2. Page DL: Prognosis and breast cancer: recognition of lethal and favorable prognostic types. Am J Surg Pathol 15:334, 1991.
3. Reynolds T: Breast cancer prognostic factors: the search goes on. J Natl Cancer Inst 86:480, 1994.
4. Wellings SR, Jensen HM, Marcum RG: An atlas of subgross pathology of the human breast with special reference to possible precancerous lesions. J Natl Cancer Inst 55:231, 1975.
5. Rosen PP: The pathologic classification of human mammary carcinoma: Past, present, and future. Ann Clin Lab Sci 9:144, 1979.
6. Fisher B, Redmond C, Fisher ER, and participating NSABP investigators: The contribution of recent NSABP clinical trials of primary breast cancer therapy to aid understand of tumor biology: An overview of findings. Cancer 46:1009, 1980.
7. Fu Y, et al: The relationship of breast cancer morphology and estrogen receptor protein status. Progr Surg Pathol 51:1, 1981.
8. Wallgren A, Silverward S, Eklund G: Prognostic factors in mammary carcinoma. Acta Radiol 5:1, 1976.
9. Page DL, Anderson TJ, Sakamoto G: Infiltrating carcinoma: Major histological types. In Page DL, Anderson TJ (eds): Diagnostic histopathology of the breast. Edinburgh, Churchill Livingstone, 1987.
10. Ellis IO, et al: Pathologic prognostic factors in breast cancer. II. Histologic type. Relationship with survival in a large study with long term follow-up. Histopathology 20:479, 1992.
11. Anderson TJ, et al: Comparative pathology of breast cancer in a randomised trial of screening. Br J Cancer 64:108, 1991.
12. Anderson TJ, et al Comparative pathology of prevalent and incident cancers detected by breast screening. Lancet 1:519–523, 1986.
13. Patchefsky AS, et al: The pathology of breast cancer detected by mass population screening. Cancer 40:1659, 1977.
14. Rajakariar R, Walker RA: Pathological and biological features of mammographically detected invasive breast carcinomas. Br J Cancer 71:150, 1995.
15. Fisher ER, Sass R, Fisher B, and participating NSABP investigators: Pathologic findings from the National Surgical Adjuvant Project for breast cancer (protocol no. 4). Discriminates for tenth year treatment failure. Cancer 53:712, 1984.
16. Dixon JM, et al: Long term survivors after breast cancer. Br J Surg 72:445, 1985.
17. Gamel JW, et al: The impact of stage and histology on the long-term clinical course of 163,808 patients with breast carcinoma. Cancer 77:1459, 1996.
18. Cooper HS, Patchefsky AS, Krall RA: Tubular carcinoma of the breast. Cancer 42:2334, 1978.
19. McDivitt RW, Boyce W, Gersell D: Tubular carcinoma of the breast: Clinical and pathological observations concerning 135 cases. Am J Surg Pathol 6:401, 1982.
20. Parl FF, Richardson LD: The histological and biological spectrum of tubular carcinoma of the breast. Hum Pathol 14:694, 1983.
21. Winchester DJ, et al: Tubular carcinoma of the breast: Predicting axillary nodal metastases and recurrence. Ann Surg 223:342, 1996.
22. Anderson TJ, et al: Pathology characteristics that optimize outcome prediction of a breast screening trial. Br J Cancer 83:487, 2000.
23. Stalsberg H, Hartmann WH: The delimitation of tubular carcinoma of the breast. Hum Pathol 31:601, 2000.
24. Elson BC, et al: Tubular carcinoma of the breast: Mode of presentation, mammographic appearance, and frequency of nodal metastases. AJR Am J Roentgenol 161:1173, 1993.
25. Dawson AE, Logan-Young W, Mulford DK: Aspiration cytology of tubular carcinoma: Diagnostic features with mammographic correlation. Am J Clin Pathol 101:488, 1994.
26. Diab SG, et al: Tumor characteristics and clinical outcome of tubular and mucinous carcinomas. J Clin Oncol 17:1442, 1999.
27. Baker RR: Unusual lesions and their management. Surg Clin North Am 70:963, 1990.
28. Mailbenco DC, et al: Axillary lymph node metastases associated with small invasive breast carcinomas. Cancer 85:1530, 1999.
29. Page DL, et al: Invasive cribriform carcinoma of the breast. Histopathology 7:525, 1983.
30. Venable JG, Schwartz AM, Silverberg SG: Infiltrating cribriform carcinoma of the breast: A distinctive clinicopathologic entity. Hum Pathol 21:333, 1990.
31. Komari K, et al: Mucinous carcinoma of the breast in Japan: A prognostic analysis based on morphologic features. Cancer 61:989, 1988.
32. Andre S, et al: Mucinous carcinoma of the breast: A pathologic study of 82 cases. J Surg Oncol 58:162, 1995.
33. Clayton F: Pure mucinous carcinomas of the breast: Morphologic features and prognostic correlates. Hum Pathol 17:34, 1986.
34. Rasmussen BB, Rose C, Christensen IB: Prognostic factors in primary mucinous breast carcinoma. Am J Clin Pathol 87:155, 1987.
35. Fentiman IS, et al: Mucoid breast carcinomas: Histology and prognosis. Br J Cancer 75:1061, 1997.
36. Northridge ME, et al: The importance of histologic type on breast cancer survival. J Clin Epidemiol 50:283, 1997.
37. Avisar E, et al: Pure mucinous carcinoma of the breast: A clinicopathologic correlation study. Ann Surg Oncol 5:447, 1998.
38. Wilson TE, et al: Pure and mixed mucinous carcinoma of the breast: Pathologic basis for differences in mammographic appearance. AJR Am J Roentgenol 165:285, 1995.
39. Haagensen CD (ed): Diseases of the breast, 2nd ed. Philadelphia, WB Saunders, 1971.
40. Donegan WL, Perez-Mesa CM: Lobular carcinoma—an indication for elective biopsy of the second breast. Ann Surg 176:178, 1972.
41. Battifora H: Intracytoplasmic lumina in breast carcinoma: A helpful histopathologic feature. Arch Pathol 99:614, 1975.
42. Quincy C, et al: Intracytoplasmic lumina: A useful diagnostic feature of adenocarcinomas. Histopathology 19:83, 1991.
43. Ladekarl M, Sorensen FB: Prognostic, quantitative histopathologic variables in lobular carcinoma of the breast. Cancer 72:2602, 1993.
44. Dixon JM, et al: Infiltrating lobular carcinoma of the breast. Histopathology 6:149, 1982.
45. Eusebi V, Magalhaes F, Azzopardi JG: Pleomorphic lobular carcinoma of the breast: An aggressive tumor showing apocrine differentiation. Hum Pathol 23:655, 1992.
46. Fechner RE: Histologic variants of infiltrating lobular carcinoma of the breast. Hum Pathol 6:373, 1975.
47. Martinez V, Azzopardi JG: Invasive lobular carcinoma of the breast: Incidence and variants. Histopathology 3:47, 1979.
48. Weidner N, Semple JP: Pleomorphic variant of invasive lobular carcinoma of the breast. Hum Pathol 23:1167, 1992.
49. DiCostanzo D, et al: Prognosis in infiltrating lobular carcinoma: An analysis of "classical" and variant tumors. Am J Surg Pathol 14:12, 1990.
50. Wheeler JE, Enterline HT: Lobular carcinoma of the breast in situ and infiltrating. Pathol Annu 2:161, 1976.
51. Haagensen CD, et al: Lobular neoplasia (so-called lobular carcinoma in situ) of the breast. Cancer 42:737, 1978.
52. Silverstein MJ, et al: Infiltrating lobular carcinoma: Is it different from infiltrating duct carcinoma? Cancer 73:1673, 1994.
53. du Toit RS, et al: Invasive lobular carcinomas of the breast: The prognosis of histopathological subtypes. Br J Cancer 60:605, 1989.
54. Berx G, et al: E-cadherin is inactivated in a majority of invasion human lobular breast cancers by truncation mutations throughout its extracellular domain. Oncogene 13:1919, 1996.
55. Toikkanen S, Pylkkanen L, Joensuu H: Invasive lobular carcinoma of the breast has better short- and long-term survival than invasive ductal carcinoma. Br J Cancer 76:1234, 1997.
56. Dixon JM, et al: Infiltrating lobular carcinoma of the breast: An evaluation of the incidence and consequence of bilateral disease. Br J Surg 70:513, 1983.
57. Schnitt SJ, et al: Influence of infiltrating lobular histology on local tumor control in breast cancer patients treated with conservative surgery and radiotherapy. Cancer 64:448, 1989.
58. Eisinger F, et al: Mutations at BRCA1: The medullary breast carcinoma revisited. Cancer Res 58:1588, 1998.
59. Marcus JN, et al: Hereditary breast cancer: Pathobiology, prognosis, and BRCA1 and BRCA2 gene linkage. Cancer 77:697, 1996.
60. Lakhani SR: The pathology of familial breast cancer: Morphologic aspects. Breast Cancer Res 1:31, 1991.

61. Lee SC, et al: Microsatellite instability is infrequent in medullary breast cancer. Am J Clin Pathol 115:823, 2001.

62. Rubens JR, et al: Medullary carcinoma of the breast: Overdiagnosis of a prognostically favorable neoplasm. Arch Surg 125:601, 1990.

63. Ridolphi RL, et al: Medullary carcinoma of the breast: A clinical pathological study with 10 year follow-up. Cancer 40:1365, 1977.

64. Pedersen L, et al: Medullary carcinoma of the breast: Prevalence and prognostic importance of classical risk factors in breast cancer. Eur J Cancer 31A:2289, 1995.

65. Rapin V, et al: Medullary breast carcinoma: A reevaluation of 95 cases of breast cancer with inflammatory stroma. Cancer 61:2503, 1988.

66. Carter CL, Allen C, Henson DE: Relation of tumor size, lymph node status, and survival in 24,740 breast cancer cases. Cancer 63:181, 1989.

67. Berg JW, Hutter RVP: Breast cancer. Cancer 75:257, 1995.

68. Oberman HA: Secretory carcinoma of the breast in adults. Am J Surg Pathol 4:465, 1980.

69. Akhtar M, et al: Secretory carcinoma of the breast in adults: Light and electron microscopic study of three cases with review of the literature. Cancer 51:2245, 1983.

70. Tavassoli FA, Norris HJ: Secretory carcinoma of the breast. Cancer 45:2404, 1980.

71. Azzopardi JG: Problems in breast pathology. Philadelphia, WB Saunders, 1979.

72. Lamovec J, et al: Adenoid cystic carcinoma of the breast: A histologic, cytologic, and immunohistochemical study. Semin Diag Pathol 6:153, 1989.

73. Pastolero G, et al: Proliferative activity and p53 expression in adenoid cystic carcinoma of the breast. Mod Pathol 9:215, 1996.

74. Peters GM, Wolff M: Adenoid cystic carcinoma of the breast Report of 11 new cases, review of the literature and discussion of biological behavior. Cancer 52:680, 1982.

75. Kasami M, et al: Maintenance of polarity and a dual cell population in adenoid cystic carcinoma of the breast: An immunohistochemical study. Histopathology 32:232, 1998.

76. Trendell-Smtih NJ, Peston D, Shousha S: Adenoid cystic carcinoma of the breast: A tumor commonly devoid of estrogen receptors and related proteins. Histopathology 35:241, 1999.

77. Kleer CG, Oberman HA: Adenoid cystic carcinoma of the breast: Value of histologic grading and proliferative activity. Am J Surg Pathol 22:569, 1998.

78. Fisher ER, et al: Mucoepidermoid and squamous cell carcinomas of the breast with reference to squamous metaplasia and giant cell tumors. Am J Surg Pathol 7:15, 1983.

79. Patchefsky AS, et al: Low-grade mucoepidermoid carcinoma of the breast. Arch Path Lab Med 103:196, 1979.

80. Hastrup N, Sehested M: High-grade mucoepidermoid carcinoma of the breast. Histopathology 9:887, 1985.

81. Kovi J, Duong HD, Leffall LS Jr: High-grade mucoepidermoid carcinoma of the breast. Arch Pathol Lab Med 105:612, 1981.

82. Hanna W, Kahn HJ: Ultrastructural and immunohistochemical characteristics of mucoepidermoid carcinoma of the breast. Hum Pathol 16:941, 1985.

83. Lüchtrath H, Moll R: Mucoepidermoid mammary carcinoma: Immunohistochemical and biochemical analyses of intermediate filaments. Virchows Arch A Patho Anat Histopathol 416:105–113, 1989.

84. Gersell D, Katzenstein AL: Spindle cell carcinoma of the breast: A clinicopathologic and ultrastructural study. Hum Pathol 12:550, 1981.

85. Santeusanio G, et al: Metaplastic breast carcinoma with epithelial phenotype of pseudosarcomatous components. Arch Pathol Lab Med 112:82, 1988.

86. Wargotz ES, Deos PH, Norris HJ: Metaplastic carcinomas of the breast. II. Spindle cell carcinoma. Hum Pathol 20:732, 1989.

87. Wargotz ES, Norris HJ: Metaplastic carcinomas of the breast. V. Metaplastic carcinoma with osteoclastic giant cells. Hum Pathol 21:1142, 1990.

88. Bauer TW, et al: Spindle cell carcinoma of the breast: four cases and review of the literature. Hum Pathol 15:147, 1984.

89. Gobbi H, et al: Metaplastic breast tumors with a dominant fibromatosis-like phenotype have a high rate of local recurrence. Cancer 85:2170, 1999.

90. Burke H, Henson DE: Criteria for prognostic factors and for an enhanced prognostic system. Cancer 72:3131, 1993.

91. McGuire WL: Breast cancer prognostic factors: evaluation guidelines. J Natl Cancer Inst 83:154, 1991 (editorial).

92. Fitzgibbons PL, et al: Prognostic factors in breast cancer: College of American Pathologists consensus statement 1999. Arch Pathol Lab Med 124:966, 2000.

93. Veronesi U, et al: Local recurrences and distant metastases after conservative breast cancer treatments: partly independent events. J Natl Cancer Inst 87:19, 1995.

94. Abner AL, et al: Correlation of tumor size and axillary lymph node involvement with prognosis in patients with T1 breast carcinoma. Cancer 83:2502, 1998.

95. Fentiman IH, et al: Prognosis of patients with breast cancers up to 1 cm in diameter. Eur J Cancer 32:417, 1996.

96. McGuire WL, Clark GM: Prognostic factors and treatment decision in axillary-node negative breast cancer. N Engl J Med 326:1756, 1992.

97. Osborne CK: Prognostic factors for breast cancer: have they met their promise? J Clin Oncol10:679, 1992.

98. Greene FL, (eds): AJCC cancer staging manual, 6th ed. New York, Springer-Verlag, 2002.

99. Weaver DL, et al: Pathologic analysis of sentinel and non-sentinel lymph nodes in breast carcinoma: A multicenter study. Cancer 88:1099, 2000.

100. Elston CW, Ellis IO: Pathological prognostic factors in breast cancer. I. The value of histologic grade in breast cancer: Experience from a large study with long-term follow-up. Histopathology 19:403, 1991.

101. Arnesson LG, et al: Histopathology grading in small breast cancers <10 mm: Results from an area with mammography screening. Breast Cancer Res Treat 44:39, 1997.

102. Contesso G, et al: The importance of histologic grade in long-term prognosis of breast cancer: A study of 1,010 patients, uniformly treated at the Institut Gustave-Roussy. J Clin Oncol 5:1378, 1987.

103. Joensuu H, Pylkkanen L, Toikkanen S: Late mortality from pT1N0M0 breast carcinoma. Cancer 85:2183, 1999.

104. Bergers E, et al: Prognostic implications of different cell cycle analysis models of flow cytometric DNA histograms of 1,301 breast cancer patients: Results from the Multicenter Morphometric Mammary Carcinoma Project (MMMCP). Int J Cancer 74:260, 1997.

105. Henson EE, et al: Relationship among outcome, stage of disease, and histologic grade for 22,616 cases of breast cancer: The basis for a prognostic index. Cancer 68:2142, 1991.

106. Dalton LW, Page DL, Dupont WD: Histological grading of breast cancer: A reproducibility study. Cancer 73:2765, 1994.

107. Frierson HFJ, et al: Interobserver reproducibility of the Nottingham modification of the Bloom and Richardson histologic grading scheme for infiltrating ductal carcinoma. Am J Clin Pathol 103:195, 1995.

108. Kollias J, et al: The prognosis of small primary breast cancers. Eur J Cancer 35:908, 1999.

109. Parl F, Dupont WD: A retrospective cohort study of histologic risk factors in breast cancer patients. Cancer 50:2410, 1982.

110. Page DL, et al: Prediction of node-negative breast cancer outcome by histologic grading and S-phase analysis by flow cytometry: An Eastern Cooperative Oncology Group Study (2192). Am J Clin Oncol 24:10, 2001.

111. Simpson JF, et al: Prognostic value of histologic grade and proliferative activity in axillary node-positive breast cancer: results from the Eastern Cooperative Oncology Group companion study, EST 4189. J Clin Oncol 18:2059, 2000.

112. Clayton F: Pathologic correlates of survival in 378 lymph node negative infiltrating ductal breast carcinomas: Mitotic count is the best single predictor. Cancer 68:1309, 1991.

113. Van Diest PJ, Baak JPA: The morphometric prognostic index is the strongest prognosticator in premenopausal lymph node-negative and lymph node-positive breast cancer patients. Hum Pathol 22:326, 1990.

114. O'Reilly SM, et al: Node-negative breast cancer: Prognostic subgroups defined by tumor size and flow cytometry. J Clin Oncol 8:2040, 1990.

115. Hedley DW, et al: Consensus review of the clinical utility of DNA cytometry in carcinoma of the breast. Cytometry 14:482, 1993.

116. Kamel OW, et al: Thymidine labeling index and Ki-67 growth fractions in lesions of the breast. Am J Pathol 134:107, 1989.

117. Isola J, et al: Evaluation of cell proliferation in breast carcinoma: Comparison of Ki-67 immunohistochemical study, DNA flow cytometric analysis, and mitotic count. Cancer 65:1180, 1990.

118. Dettmar P, et al: Prognostic impact of proliferation-associated factors MIB-1 (Ki-67) and S phase in node negative breast cancer. Br J Cancer 75:1525, 1997.

119. Wintzer H-O, et al: Ki-67 immunostaining in human breast tumors and its relationship to prognosis. Cancer 67:421, 1991.

120. Cattoretti G, et al: Monoclonal antibodies against recombinant parts of the Ki-67 antigen (MIB 1 and MIB 3) detect proliferating cells in microwave-processed formalin-fixed paraffin sections. J Pathol 168:357, 1992.

121. Pinder SE, et al: Assessment of the new proliferation marker MIB1 in breast carcinoma using image analysis: Association with other prognostic factors and survival. Br J Cancer 71:146, 1995.

122. Keshgegian AA, Cnaan A: Proliferation markers in breast carcinoma: Mitotic figure count, S-phase fraction, proliferation cell nuclear antigen, Ki-67, and MIB-1. Am J Clin Pathol 104:42, 1995.

123. Clahsen PC, et al: The utility of mitotic index, oestrogen receptor and Ki-67 measurements in the creation of novel prognostic indices for node-negative breast cancer. Eur J Surg Oncol 25:356, 1999.

124. Allred DC, et al: Immunocytochemical analysis of estrogen receptors in human breast carcinomas: Evaluation of 130 cases and a review of the literature regarding concordance with the biochemical assay and clinical relevance. Arch Surg 125:107, 1990.

125. Pertschuk LP, et al: Estrogen receptor immunocytochemistry in paraffin embedded tissues with ER1D5 predicts breast cancer endocrine response more accurately than H222Sp gamma in frozen sections or cytosol-based ligand-binding assays. Cancer 77:2514, 1996.

126. Allred DC: Should immunohistochemical examination replace biochemical hormone receptor assays in breast cancer? Am J Clin Pathol 99:1, 1993.

127. Harvey JM, et al: Estrogen receptor status by immunohistochemistry is superior to the ligand-binding assay for predicting response to adjuvant endocrine therapy in breast cancer. J Clin Oncol 17:1474, 1999.

128. Taylor CR: Paraffin section immunocytochemistry for estrogen receptor: The time has come. Cancer 77:2419, 1996.

129. Davis BW, et al, and the Ludwig Breast Cancer Study Group: Prognostic significance of peritumoral vessel invasion in clinical trials of adjuvant therapy for breast cancer with axillary lymph node metastasis. Hum Pathol 16:1212, 1985.

130. Clemente CG, et al: Peritumoral lymphatic invasion in patients with node-negative mammary duct carcinoma. Cancer 69:1396, 1992.

131. De Mascarel I, et al: Obvious peritumoral emboli: An elusive prognostic factor reappraised: Multivariate analysis of 1320 node-negative breast cancers. Eur J Cancer 34:58, 1998.

132. Chadha M, et al: Predictors of axillary lymph node metastases in patients with T1 breast cancer: a multivariate analysis. Cancer 73:350, 1994.

133. Perez CA, et al: Management of locally advanced carcinoma of the breast. II. Inflammatory carcinoma. Cancer 74:466, 1994.

134. Page DL: Special types of invasive breast cancer, with clinical implications. Am J Surg Pathol 27:832, 2003.

135. Perou CM, Sorlie T, Eisen MB, et al: Molecular portraits of human breast tumours. Nature 406:747–752, 2000.

136. Sorlie T, Perou CM, Tibshirani R, et al: Gene expression patterns of breast carcinomas distinguish tumor subclasses with clinical implications. Proc Natl Acad Sci USA 98:10869–10874, 2001.

137. Sorlie T, Tibshirani R, Parker J, et al: Repeated observation of breast tumor subtypes in independent gene expression data sets. Proc Natl Acad Sci USA 100:8418–8423, 2003.

138. Brenton JD, Carey LA, Ahmed AA, et al: Molecular classification and molecular forecasting of breast cancer: Ready for clinical application. J Clin Oncol 23:7350–7360, 2005.

139. Hudis CA: Trastuzumab—mechanism of action and use in clinical practice. N Engl J Med 357:39–51, 2007.

140. Piccart-Gebhart MJ, Procter M, Leyland-Jones B, et al: Trastuzumab after adjuvant chemotherapy in HER2-positive breast cancer. N Engl J Med 353:1659–1672, 2005.

141. Romond EH, Perez EA, Bryant J, et al: Trastuzumab plus adjuvant chemotherapy for operable HER2-positive breast cancer. N Engl J Med 353:1673–1684, 2005.

142. Slamon DJ, Leyland-Jones B, Shak S, et al: Use of chemotherapy plus a monoclonal antibody against HER2 for metastatic breast cancer that overexpresses HER2. N Engl J Med 344:783–792, 2001.

143. Montemurro F, Valabrega G, Aglietta M: Lapatinib: A dual inhibitor of EGFR and HER2 tyrosine kinase activity. Expert Opin Biol Ther 7:257–268, 2007.

144. Geyer CE, Forster J, Lindquist D, et al: Lapatinib plus capecitabine for HER2-positive advanced breast cancer. N Engl J Med 355:2733–2743, 2006.

145. Carey LA, Dees EC, Sawyer L, et al: The triple negative paradox: Primary tumor chemosensitivity of breast cancer subtypes. Clin Cancer Res 13:2329–2334, 2007.

146. Carey LA, Perou CM, Livasy CA, et al: Race, breast cancer subtypes, and survival in the Carolina Breast Cancer Study. JAMA 295:2492–2502, 2006.

147. Cheang MCU, Voduc D, Bajdik C, et al: Basal-like breast cancer defined by five biomarkers has superior prognostic value than triple-negative phenotype. Clin Cancer Res 14:1368–1376, 2008.

148. Early Breast Cancer Trialists' Collaborative Group: Effects of chemotherapy and hormonal therapy for early breast cancer on recurrence and 15-year survival: An overview of the randomised trials. Lancet 365:1687–1717, 2005.

149. Clarke M, Collins R, Darby S, et al: Effects of radiotherapy and of differences in the extent of surgery for early breast cancer on local recurrence and 15-year survival: An overview of the randomised trials. Lancet 366:2087–2106, 2005.

150. Ravdin PM, Siminoff LA, Davis GJ, et al: Computer program to assist in making decisions about adjuvant therapy for women with early breast cancer. J Clin Oncol 19:980–991, 2001.

151. Olivotto IA, Bajdik CD, Ravdin PM, et al: Population-based validation of the prognostic model ADJUVANT! for early breast cancer. J Clin Oncol 23:2716–2725, 2005.

152. Siminoff LA, Gordon NH, Silverman P, et al: A decision aid to assist in adjuvant therapy choices for breast cancer. Psycho-oncology 15:1001–1013, 2006.

153. Cheang MCU, van de Rijn M, Nielsen TO: Gene expression profiling of breast cancer. Annu Rev Pathology: Mechanisms of Disease 3:67–97, 2008.

154. Marchionni L, Wilson RF, Wolff AC, et al: Systematic review: Gene expression profiling assays in early-stage breast cancer. Ann Intern Med 148:358–369, 2008.

155. Paik S, Shak S, Tang G, et al: A multigene assay to predict recurrence of tamoxifen-treated, node-negative breast cancer. N Engl J Med 351:2817–2826, 2004.

156. Paik S, Tang G, Shak S, et al: Gene expression and benefit of chemotherapy in women with node-negative, estrogen receptor-positive breast cancer. J Clin Oncol 24:3726–3734, 2006.

157. Taube SE, Jacobson JW, Lively TG: Cancer diagnostics: Decision criteria for marker utilization in the clinic. Am J Pharmacogenomics 5:357–364, 2005.

158. Sparano JA, Paik S: Development of the 21-gene assay and its application in clinical practice and clinical trials. J Clin Oncol 26:721–728, 2008.

159. van 't Veer LJ, Dai H, van de Vijver MJ, et al: Gene expression profiling predicts clinical outcome of breast cancer. Nature 415:530, 2002.

160. van de Vijver MJ, He YD, van't Veer LJ, et al: A gene-expression signature as a predictor of survival in breast cancer. N Engl J Med 347:1999–2009, 2002.

161. Buyse M, Loi S, van't Veer L, et al: Validation and clinical utility of a 70-gene prognostic signature for women with node-negative breast cancer. J Natl Cancer Inst 98:1183–1192, 2006.

162. Cardoso F, van't Veer L, Rutgers E, et al: Clinical application of the 70-gene profile: The MINDACT Trial. J Clin Oncol 26:729–735, 2008.

163. Fan C, Oh DS, Wessels L, et al: Concordance among gene-expression-based predictors for breast cancer. N Engl J Med 355:560–569, 2006.

164. Sun Y, Goodison S, Li J, et al: Improved breast cancer prognosis through the combination of clinical and genetic markers. Bioinformatics 23:30–37, 2007.

165. Dobbe E, Gurney K, Kiekow S, et al: Gene-expression assays: New tools to individualize treatment of early-stage breast cancer. Am J Health Syst Pharm 65:23–28, 2008.

166. Lyman GH, Cosler LE, Kuderer NM, et al: Impact of a 21-gene RT-PCR assay on treatment decisions in early-stage breast cancer: An economic analysis based on prognostic and predictive validation studies. Cancer 109:1011–8, 2007.

167. Foekens JA, Atkins D, Zhang Y, et al: Multicenter validation of a gene expression-based prognostic signature in lymph node-negative primary breast cancer. J Clin Oncol 24:1665–1671, 2006.

168. Chang HY, Nuyten DS, Sneddon JB, et al: Robustness, scalability, and integration of a wound-response gene expression signature in predicting breast cancer survival. Proc Natl Acad Sci USA 102:3738–3743, 2005.

169. Goetz MP, Suman VJ, Ingle JN, et al: A two-gene expression ratio of homeobox 13 and interleukin-17B receptor for prediction of recurrence and survival in women receiving adjuvant tamoxifen. Clin Cancer Res 12(Pt 1):2080–2087, 2006.

170. Jansen MP, Sieuwerts AM, Look MP, et al: HOXB13-to-IL17BR expression ratio is related with tumor aggressiveness and response to tamoxifen of recurrent breast cancer: A retrospective study. J Clin Oncol 25:662–668, 2007.

171. Jin Y, Destra Z, Stearns V, et al: CYP2D6 genotype, antidepressant use, and tamoxifen metabolism during adjuvant breast cancer treatment. J Natl Cancer Inst 97:30–39, 2005.

172. Caraco Y: Genes and the response to drugs. N Engl J Med 351:2867–2869, 2004.

Extent and Multicentricity of in Situ and Invasive Carcinoma

WILLIAM B. FARRAR | DOREEN AGNESE |
MARY EDGERTON | JOYCE E. JOHNSON |
PHILIP L. DUTT | DAVID L. PAGE

The terms *multicentricity* and *multifocality* have been used for decades to indicate seeming or real multiplicity of cancer within an individual breast. The terms have no intrinsically different meaning but have recently been interpreted as follows: *Multicentricity* indicates multiple but independent sites of origin usually in a separate duct system or relatively remote from one another; *multifocality* indicates multiple foci of the same tumor, relatively close to each other, usually in the same quadrant. Multicentricity has been considered an important factor when planning breast-conserving surgery. However, many cases that would have previously been deemed multicentric in the past are now recognized as multiple lesions within a breast segment that result from spread of intraductal carcinoma within the three-dimensional duct system. Although multicentricity is important in planning surgical therapy, its true prevalence is much less than originally estimated. Indeed, extent of disease, in situ or invasive, is a concept that has essentially replaced that of multifocality and multicentricity, particularly in the planning of surgical therapy. Bilaterality, the occurrence of carcinoma in the contralateral breast is excluded by definition and is discussed separately in Chapters 81 and 83. Also, excluded is concurrence of breast carcinoma and sarcoma, which is reviewed in Chapters 11 and 13. Multicentricity associated with lobular carcinoma in situ (LCIS) is discussed separately in Chapter 10. The studies of intraductal carcinoma referenced in this chapter largely apply to ductal carcinoma in situ (DCIS) only, either by exclusion of LCIS or because of the greater proportion of cases with DCIS included in the studies.

The prevalence of true multicentricity is difficult to estimate from the literature. In 1957, Qualheim and Gall[1] published one of the first studies to distinguish between cancerous foci in the vicinity of a primary mass and those that might be regarded as distant. In their study, they referred to 157 cases of cancer and by looking at large sections of the breast, they noted an incidence of 17% independent cancers in the vicinity of the dominant mass and 35% in other areas of the breast. In another study by Gallagher and Martin,[2] areas of atypical hyperplasia or intraductal cancer were found near or remote from the dominant lesion in 75% of 34 cancers and 50% were invasive cancers. In a 1962 study by Tellem and associates,[3] the researchers found an incidence of microscopic cancer in 26.5% of 64 cases in quadrants different than the index lesion.

With the advent of conservative breast surgery, a number of other published studies addressed the extent of disease. They looked especially at the question of local recurrences in patients who underwent a lumpectomy with or without radiation.

The standard definition of multicentricity applied in studies published by Fisher and colleagues as part of the National Surgical Adjuvant Breast Project (NSABP) required that a second cancer be present in a separate quadrant from the dominant mass. In their 1975 publication,[4] they detected multicentric cancer in 121 of 904 breasts surgically removed for a clinical overt invasive cancer. This incidence of 13.4% was regarded to be conservative because the probability of identifying such a lesion appeared to increase as the number of samples per patient increased.

In 1985, Holland and associates[5] published a study of multiple foci of tumor using distance from the primary mass to predict recurrence, thereby bypassing the issue of defining multicentricity. Of the 282 invasive cancers, 105 (37%) showed no tumor foci in the mastectomy specimen around the reference lesion. In 56 (20%), tumor foci were present within 2 cm, in 121 (43%), tumors were present more than 2 cm from the noninvasive cancers, and in 46 cases (16%), they contained invasive cancers as well. If the 264 invasive cancers in the series that were 4 cm or less in diameter had been removed with a margin of 3 to 4 cm, 7% to 9% of the patients would have had invasive cancer left in the removed breast tissue and 4% to 9% would have had foci of noninvasive cancer left in the remaining breast tissue. This study did provide an estimate of the amount of invasive and noninvasive tumor that can be expected to remain in the breast after breast conserving surgery.

In 1994, Faverly, with Holland and associates,[6] applied three-dimensional imaging to study the distribution of intraductal carcinoma as constrained by the anatomy of the breast duct system. Since then, Ohtake and associates[7,8] and Mai and colleagues[9] have used computer-generated reconstructions of the mammary duct system in three dimensions to study the pattern of distribution of intraductal and invasive carcinoma in relation to the duct system. They discovered that apparent multicentricity is often the result of intraductal spread of the tumor. This finding has highlighted the intraductal problem of formulating a useful definition of multicentricity based on distance or quadrant.

Other studies have added the elements of time and biology (natural history) by observing the evaluation (or lack of it) of clinical disease in the living breast after partial mastectomy. The results of breast-conserving surgery show that recurrent disease most often occurs locally, within the spatial constraints that the geometry of the duct system places on the spread of in situ carcinoma. Simply put, more than 90% of local recurrences of breast carcinoma in many women treated with breast-conserving surgery are in the immediate vicinity of the primary tumor.[10] This implies that the extensiveness of in situ carcinoma within a duct system and margin status are the more relevant issues for predicting outcome in most cases.[5,11]

A perfect definition of multicentricity referable to all settings is essentially impractical because of the difficulties inherent in visualizing the three-dimensional micro-anatomy of the breast. Distinguishing independently originating breast carcinomas from multiple foci of invasion resulting from intramammary spread of carcinoma along ducts is difficult. Therefore, multicentricity as a descriptor is necessarily arbitrary and becomes a function of the method used for detection. Consider here the anatomy of the breast. The breast is a branching (racemose) gland with 15 to 20 collecting (lactiferous) ducts exiting at the nipple. Each of these ductal systems or lobes subserves hundreds of lobular units, which are collections of acinar elements.[12] In a three-dimensional reconstruction based on one patient, Ohtake and colleagues[8] noted that only 2 of the duct systems actually communicated with one another, and the remaining 14 were anatomically independent. Although the ductal systems are not grossly definable anatomic units separated by septa, only immediately adjacent radiating ductal systems overlap (Fig. 12-1), with limited opportunity for communication.[12] Quadrants represent an attempt to divide the breast into independent duct systems; however, the boundaries are drawn arbitrarily, and true duct systems may overlap into an adjacent quadrant at the periphery.

Given this anatomy, apparent multicentricity resulting from spread along a single duct system would be expected

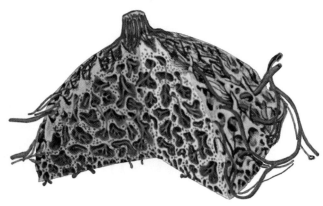

Figure 12-1 Proposed anatomy of the breast with partial lobar oriented ductal system. However, recent studies have shown that the human ductal system is more complex than simple radiating anatomy. Although anastomoses between ductal systems may not occur, individual ductal systems may overlap with each other with respect to the area of the breast they serve much like venous drainage networks. One ductal system may not be confined to a single breast quadrant. (Redrawn from Love SM, Barsky SH: Anatomy of the nipple and breast ducts revisited. Cancer 101:1947, 2004.)

to appear in a radial distribution from nipple to periphery. This radial distribution, combined with the irregular branching system of duct systems that exists in three-dimensions, explains the fact that a single intraductal breast cancer may appear as separate foci in the two-dimensional slides routinely used for diagnosis. Mai and colleagues,[9] who performed computer-assisted three-dimensional reconstruction of intraductal and invasive mammary carcinoma (lobular carcinoma was excluded) from 30 mastectomy specimens, found that intraductal carcinoma presented with radial distribution corresponding to the geometry of each ductal system. They also noted that multiple foci of invasive carcinoma were connected by intervening intraductal carcinoma within a single duct system. Ohtake and colleagues[7] have taken the viewpoint that multicentricity requires demonstration of histologic non-continuity of intraductal tumor through the mammary ductal tree. Of note, there are no cases of lobular carcinoma in their series. As stringent as this requirement appears, even it may allow an overestimate of true multicentricity. Both Mai and associates[9] and Faverly and colleagues[6] report that discontinuities of intraductal tumor within a single mammary duct tree, detected at a subgross level, are not uncommon. Recent studies indicate that the phenomenon of "pagetoid spread" of intraductal carcinoma[13] may lead to apparent discontinuities in intraductal tumor that originate from the same "index" carcinoma.

Studies using molecular biology to differentiate independent sources for multicentric carcinoma (discussed later) also support the concept of a single index case that spreads through the duct system.[14–16] As such, the true definition of multicentric should require demonstration of independent molecular events that result in the local occurrence of carcinoma in independent duct systems. This definition would require three-dimensional reconstruction of the duct systems along with molecular profiling studies, procedures that are not a part of routine processing of breast specimens. Therefore, multicentricity is likely to remain arbitrarily defined. Extent of disease is more amenable to measurement in routine pathologic examination of specimens. Given that the prevalence of true multicentricity is overestimated, extent of disease (discussed in more detail later) may be more relevant in the majority of cases when planning breast-conserving surgical therapy.

Cheatle and Cutler[17] first defined multicentricity as two lesions separated by normal breast tissue. Since then, most authors have adhered to the quadrant rule, which defines multicentric lesions as second tumors lying in a different quadrant from that in which the primary or dominant lesion is located. Some authors regard the subareolar region as a fifth mammary region, separate from the four quadrants. Others place subareolar lesions in the most closely associated quadrant.

In addition to the quadrant rule, some authors have used a distance rule, with specific distances applied ranging from 5 to 2 cm. It should be noted that Lagios[18] uses the 5-cm distance rule because such a distance generally places a second lesion in a different quadrant. European guidelines define the criteria for multicentricity as the presence of two or more distinct tumor foci either at a distance of at least 4 cm and/or present in different quadrants.[19]

All of these definitions have shortcomings. Egan and McSweeney[20] offered a possible solution to the problem by using multiple criteria; (1) wide separation of foci grossly, radiographically, and microscopically; (2) a pattern of multiple areas scattered throughout much of the breast; or (3) sharp delineation of different histologic types. In their early work, Holland and associates[5] cleverly avoided the problems of both the rule of quadrants and the arbitrary distance definitions of multicentricity by measuring the distance from the secondary foci to the dominant lesion and graphing the frequencies at which invasive and noninvasive foci were located at various distances from the edge of the dominant lesion. Their approach has important therapeutic implications with regard to how generous the margins around tumors should be in lumpectomy specimens.

On balance, it should be remembered that the quadrants rule has been the most commonly used definition. The following cases demonstrate the difficulties encountered with identifying multicentric breast carcinoma based on information obtained from standard pathology procedures. The lesion that attracted attention clinically or mammographically and led to diagnostic procedures is called the primary or dominant lesion, and other malignant lesions are called secondary lesions. Pathology reports in which multiple simultaneous lesions are grossly identifiable and separately measurable should emphasize the largest lesion.[21]

    Case 1. A 46-year-old woman underwent a modified radical right mastectomy for a 2 × 1.7 × 1.3 cm mass in the lower inner quadrant. Histologically, this was an infiltrating mammary carcinoma of predominantly lobular type with an extensive intraductal component (EIC; Fig. 12-2). Sampling of the upper inner quadrant revealed a separate 0.7 × 0.5 × 0.5 cm focus of infiltrative lobular carcinoma with extensive LCIS.

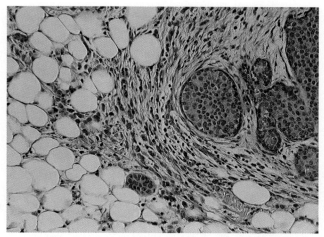

Figure 12-2 Extension of prominent intraductal component *(right)* beyond border of invasive lobular carcinoma *(left)*.

    Case 2. An 87-year-old woman had two clinically apparent masses in her left breast. The decision to perform mastectomy was based on a diagnosis of carcinoma made on material obtained with fine-needle aspiration of a mass in the upper inner quadrant. The left mastectomy specimen contained an 8 × 5 × 4 cm mass in the upper inner quadrant that histologically was invasive mammary carcinoma of no special type adjacent to DCIS (Fig. 12-3). The upper outer quadrant contained a separate, smaller 3.5 × 3 × 2.2 cm mass with a similar histologic appearance. Biopsy of a lesion in the right breast at the time of mastectomy revealed DCIS.

    Case 3. A 47-year-old woman underwent mastectomy. The mastectomy specimen contained invasive mammary carcinoma of no specific type. Elsewhere in the most remote sites were extensive areas of invasive carcinoma with mucinous features (Fig. 12-4).

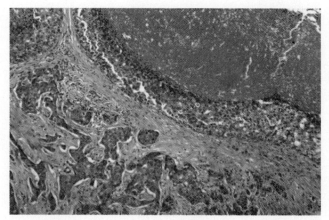

Figure 12-3 Infiltrating mammary carcinoma (invasive ductal carcinoma) found in the large mass in the upper inner quadrant in Case 2. Loss of heterozygosity studies and comparative genomic hybridization studies from microdissected areas of ductal carcinoma in situ (DCIS) and invasive carcinoma from the same case show clonal identity between the two regions, proof positive that the DCIS clone gives rise to the invasive carcinoma.

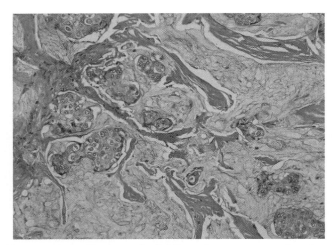

Figure 12-4 Mucinous (colloid) carcinoma present elsewhere in the breast of the patient described in Case 3.

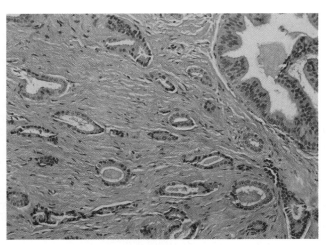

Figure 12-6 Invasive carcinoma is seen juxtaposed with ductal carcinoma in situ (DCIS). In this case (Case 4) the DCIS was extensive DCIS (extensive intraductal component) and united the three foci of invasive carcinoma.

Case 4. A mammogram revealed three lesions in a single quadrant in a 43-year-old woman (Fig. 12-5). All three were invasive carcinomas with EICs (Fig. 12-6). As is often the case, each invasive focus appeared histologically similar. Tissue sampled between each of the lesions demonstrated in situ carcinoma only. This case demonstrates the important association of DCIS with the occurrence of multiple carcinomas within one breast.

Case 5. A 30-year-old woman had a palpable mass in the left upper outer quadrant, a few centimeters from the nipple. A biopsy revealed a 15-mm intermediate-grade carcinoma of no special type, with intratumoral and adjacent extensive DCIS of solid, cribriform, and focal comedo types. A quadrantectomy contained two additional foci of invasive carcinoma of similar histology, 8 and 6 mm in size, in addition to a 1-mm focus of residual carcinoma in

the wall of the biopsy cavity. Tissue taken from between each of the three invasive foci showed high-grade (comedo) carcinoma in situ (Fig. 12-7). The distribution of the DCIS and multiple foci of invasive carcinoma are depicted schematically (Fig. 12-8).

The exact prevalence of multicentricity is uncertain. Using either the quadrant rule or a minimum distance rule, the reported prevalence has ranged from 4% to 75%.[22,23] This variation is attributable to many variables, the most obvious of which are (1) a lack of consistency in the definition of multicentricity and (2) the method for examining specimens. In the 20 specimens examined in three dimensions by Ohtake and collaborators,[7] there were no occurrences of multiple carcinoma foci, either invasive or in situ, without intervening

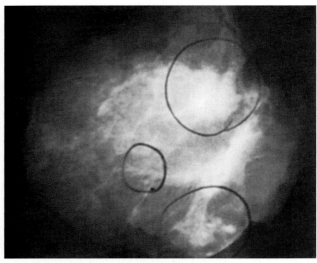

Figure 12-5 Mammogram described in Case 4 showing three radiographic lesions within the circles. Each contained invasive carcinomas of similar histologic pattern with extensive intraductal components. Note that all three are linked by connective tissue strands that histologically contained ductal carcinoma in situ. (Courtesy of L. Ming Hang, MD, Escondido, CA.)

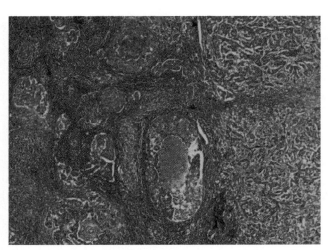

Figure 12-7 High-grade comedo ductal carcinoma in situ (DCIS) from Case 5 is depicted in the left and central portion. On the right the DCIS progresses into invasive poorly differentiated ductal carcinoma centrally. In general, there is a strong correlation between nuclear grade, DNA ploidy, proliferation markers, and other biomarkers expressed by the DCIS portion and the invasive carcinoma portion, suggesting that the latter originates from the former.

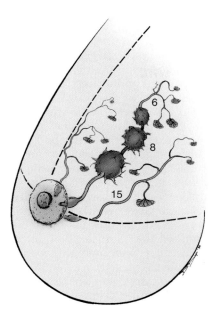

Figure 12-8 Lateral aspect of left breast in Case 5. Three histologically similar foci of invasive carcinoma present in the upper outer quadrant with intervening in situ carcinoma (hatching). The numbers indicate the size of the invasive foci in millimeters.

intraductal carcinoma. In the three cases of patients each with multiple breast carcinomas that were examined for clonality by Noguchi and colleagues,[15] there were also no cases in the carcinomas that could be attributed to independent molecular events. In any series studying multicentricity, one should be aware of the method used to examine the breast. The most thorough methods involve three-dimensional imaging of the breast and/or molecular techniques. This would require examination of breast tissue using a combination of radiographs, a dissecting microscope, and microscopic examination of whole tissue sections from the breast that have been frozen and serially sectioned at 2- to 5-mm intervals[7–9],[18,22] and/or using molecular techniques to evaluate for clonality.[5–16,24]

In Situ Lesions

The reported prevalence of multicentricity has varied, depending on whether the primary lesion is an in situ or an invasive lesion and on the histologic type of the primary lesions. The risk of multicentricity associated with LCIS is discussed in Chapter 10 and is not repeated here.

DCIS is rarely present without some connection in three dimensions if one considers DCIS with apparent gaps and confined to a single ductal system as connected. As such, it is more likely to be multifocal disease rather than multicentric disease. The frequency with which DCIS has been reported as multicentric has ranged from 0% to 78%.[25–30] The difficulty in assessing true multicentricity (i.e., arising form independent index tumors in separate duct systems) and the variability in pathology procedures to detect multicentricity can explain the broad

range in estimates of its prevalence. Faverly and coworkers[6] examined 60 mastectomy specimens in the most detailed study of DCIS to date, using three-dimensional reconstruction of the site, extent, and growth pattern of tumor foci. Only one of these had what they defined as a multicentric occurrence of DCIS (i.e., a separate focus of DCIS present with at least 4 cm of uninvolved glandular structures between it and the primary focus).

Faverly and coworkers[6] determined that 50% of cases of DCIS in their series demonstrated gaps, of which 83% were smaller than 1 cm. Mai and colleagues[9] found that 21% of their 28 cases of invasive carcinoma with associated DCIS also exhibited skip areas in the DCIS. These results were obtained with subgross level imagining. Faverly's group predicted that breast-conserving surgery with an intraductal-free margin of 1 cm should eradicate approximately 90% of DCIS. Interestingly, the three-dimensional reconstruction of duct systems performed by Ohtake and colleagues[8] has suggested that removal of a single duct system is adequate therapy in nearly 90% of cases, based on the number of anastomoses connecting otherwise independent duct systems in their reconstruction. This prediction has been borne out in studies by Silverstein and associates,[11] who published a study of recurrences as a function of margin. They concluded that breast-conserving surgery with a 1-cm tumor-free margin for DCIS was successful in patients more than 98% of the time.

Invasive Lesions

Although invasive ductal carcinoma is the most common type of invasive mammary carcinoma, it is fortunately associated with one of the lowest rates of multicentricity. Gump and colleagues[31] found that it was the least likely to be multicentric with a 19% rate of multicentricity, compared with a rate of 27% for all types. The rate of multicentricity increases when other factors are present. For example, the rate of multicentricity associated with minimally invasive ductal carcinoma is apparently greater than that associated with usual invasive ductal carcinoma.[32] This increase may not be related to the small size of the invasive component per se but rather to its regular presence in cases of extensive DCIS. The rate of multicentricity is increased approximately twofold when infiltrating ductal carcinoma is associated with LCIS.[33]

Infiltrating lobular carcinoma is associated with elevated rates of multicentricity.[33] Fisher and associates[4] showed that invasive lobular carcinoma was more frequently associated with invasive secondary lesions but not with noninvasive secondary lesions. Some authors have pointed out that most of the secondary lesions lie near the primary and probably represent recurrences or spread of the original invasive lobular carcinoma rather that true multicentricity.[34]

Ascertaining accurate rates of multicentricity for special types of invasive mammary carcinoma is difficult because of small sample sizes. Lagios, Rose, and Margolin[35] reported that 56% of tubular carcinoma was multicentric. In a study of minimal invasive carcinoma (lesions = 10 mm in diameter), 59% of small tubular carcinomas were multicentric,[4] although other studies have shown lower rates of multicentricity compared with the average for all cancers.[36] In studies with both large[33] and small[37] numbers of examples, medullary carcinoma has been shown to have one of the lowest rates of multicentricity. It is difficult to draw conclusions about the rate of multicentricity associated with colloid or mucinous carcinoma because of the small numbers of cases studied.[22,37]

Combined Invasive and in Situ Carcinoma

Several authors have noted that multicentricity is more likely if invasive carcinoma coexists with a significant amount of intraductal carcinoma.[4,23,38] Middleton and colleagues[23] have recently studied a series of 32 patients diagnosed with multicentric invasive carcinoma who underwent a mastectomy. Only one patient did not exhibit essentially identical histology across the multiple foci of tumor. Twenty-four of the patients had invasive mammary carcinoma of no specific type (invasive ductal carcinoma). Of these, 20 had DCIS that was associated with at least one of the foci of invasion. There were eight cases of infiltrating lobular carcinoma, only four of which were associated with LCIS. The remaining patient with LCIS had mixed DCIS and LCIS, with two foci of invasive mammary carcinoma (ductal). The nipple was involved in 10 of the patients. Spread of intraductal tumor into separate duct systems via communication at the nipple may explain an apparent association with multicentricity.

Mai and coworkers[9] performed three-dimensional reconstructions from 30 mastectomy specimens with invasive mammary carcinoma (ductal). Infiltrating lobular carcinoma was excluded from the study. Of the 30 cases, 28 had coexistent DCIS. Only 1 of 28 cases with combined invasive and in situ carcinoma had multiple invasive tumor foci, each present in a separate quadrant. These three foci had similar histology, and there was extensive DCIS at the nipple associated with invasion. This finding again supports the argument that multicentricity, defined as multiple independent carcinogenesis events, is not as common as previously thought and suggests that the nipple may be associated with apparent multicentricity because of local duct convergence.

BIOLOGIC STUDIES

Evaluation of multicentric tumors using subcellular and molecular technologies has expanded current understanding of the true biologic nature of multicentric tumors and may allow more precise definitions of multicentric and extensive. Two different hypotheses, excluding intramammary metastases, have been introduced to explain the etiology of multicentric disease. One of these suggests that the multiple sites develop by intraductal spread, which may appear discontinuous at the subgross level, from an "index" case. The other hypothesis supports the concept of a genetic alteration that occurs during development and distributes extensively or locally in the breast depending on the stage of development at which it occurs. This first hit predisposes the affected region, and a second, localized genetic event results in carcinoma.[39] If the latter hypothesis is correct, there will be a combination of shared and distinct molecular events that define the separate foci of carcinoma.

Noguchi and associates,[15] in a study of 30 patients with invasive mammary carcinoma (ductal), demonstrated that clonality within a tumor could be established by measuring the restriction fragment length polymorphism (RFLP) of the tumor using the X-linked phosphoglycerate kinase gene (*PGK*). They then evaluated individual foci of invasive mammary carcinoma (ductal) in each of three women with two, three, and four separate ipsilateral lesions. They found that the separate foci exhibited the identical RFLP for each patient, strong evidence that seemingly independent foci of cancer are likely to be related.

A study applying cytogenetic analysis[16] to multicentric tumors ("macroscopically distinct," 5 to 15 mm apart) also supports the hypothesis of intraductal spread of tumor as the major mechanism for apparent multifocality. However, the presence of cytogenetically unrelated clones within a single focus suggests that breast cancer may in fact be polyclonal. Thus, diverging molecular evolution of a single focus may make it difficult to differentiate between independent "index" cases and evolution of tumor that has spread from a single "index" case. In fact, molecular evolution may in part explain histologic heterogeneity in DCIS within independent duct systems.

Fujii and colleagues[14] studied invasive tumors for allelic losses at seven different chromosomal loci and compared the alterations in these tumors with those present in DCIS within the same breast. A high degree of concordance of specific losses between the in situ and invasive lesions supports the concept of multifocal rather than truly multicentric carcinoma. A variable degree of heterogeneity in allelic losses at one or more loci in 8 of the 20 cases examined is again attributed to some degree of clonal divergence in the evolution of breast cancer.

Early protein-based immunocytochemical techniques,[40] certainly the least reliable of these methodologies, generated conflicting results in a study of 24 cases of "separate" tumors. More recently a study of morphology combined with immunohistochemistry for estrogen receptor, progesterone receptor, *HER2/neu*, and *Ki-67* in 32 patients who had undergone modified radical mastectomy supported the hypothesis that multicentric mammary carcinoma results from intraductal spread.[23] As noted earlier, all but one (97%) of the patients in that study had identical histology in the separate tumor foci.

Associated Factors

Numerous authors have proposed various factors to be associated with increased risk of multicentricity, defined by occurrence in multiple quadrants or within a minimum distance. The problem with interpreting these studies is the inherently arbitrary definition of multicentricity in standard pathology reports. As described earlier, many of the lesions called multicentric are likely multifocal manifestations of DCIS or multiple foci of invasion with intervening intraductal carcinoma. The presence of a lesion in the nipple or subareolar area is perhaps the most clearly and consistently demonstrated factor for multicentricity.[4,23,37,41,42] Mai and coworkers[9] discovered that DCIS exhibited a pyramidal shape, "fanning out" from the nipple to the posterior of the breast. As described earlier, it is possible that the convergence of the duct systems at the nipple explains the seemingly increased multicentricity in the subareolar tissue.

Studies looking for a relationship between multicentricity and tumor size,[4,5,18,22,31,33,43–46] patient age,[4,33,44,46] family history,[37,44] or nodal status[4,33,44–49] have generated mixed results. Lagios, Westdahl, and Rose[22] found an association of multicentricity with tubular carcinoma. Among other factors studied and shown to have no relationship to receptor status are height, weight, parity,[24] specific breast or quadrant involved, amount of necrosis,[4] nuclear grade, expression of the adhesion molecule CD44v6,[50] preexisting or concurrent benign breast disease,[4,46] and bilaterality.[46]

CLINICAL FOLLOW-UP STUDIES

The primary relevance of multicentric disease is essentially for patients who desire or undergo breast-conserving therapy. Middleton and coworkers,[23] who studied multicentricity in patients who had undergone mastectomies, found no difference in disease-free survival for women with apparently multicentric versus unicentric invasive carcinoma. In their earlier study, 75% of the cases were invasive mammary carcinoma and 25% had infiltrating lobular carcinoma. The authors were unable to determine whether the equivalence in survival rates was a result of the type of treatment the women received.

The recent studies described earlier in this chapter with extensive three-dimensional reconstruction suggest that multicentricity of carcinoma, either DCIS or an invasive (not lobular) carcinoma associated with DCIS, defined as independent sources of tumor located in separate duct systems, is actually an unlikely event, whereas multifocality of either invasive or in situ carcinoma is not uncommon. Given the near-complete independence of the ductal systems, breast-conserving surgery may be adequate therapy when disease is localized and, if based on a segmental anatomy, may also be adequate when extensive or invasive or multifocal DCIS is present. The latter may also present with foci of invasive carcinoma, but these will originate within the same duct system nearly 90% of the time.

As such, the phenomenon of extensive intraductal carcinoma with multifocal invasive or in situ tumor is the more commonly encountered issue than true multicentricity when planning surgical therapy for a patient with breast carcinoma. The collaborative study between medical schools at Nijmegen and Harvard represent one of the early comprehensive studies to address an EIC as a clinically relevant factor in the study of breast carcinoma.[21] The definition of an EIC for this study was similar to that in a previous study by Schnitt and associates[51] and consisted of two criteria: (1) DCIS was present prominently (≥25%) within the infiltrating tumor, and (2) DCIS was present clearly extending beyond the infiltrating margin of the tumor. Mastectomy specimens from 214 patients were studied with a three-dimensional reconstructive technique; the study design was predicated on a practical clinical question: Can the findings in an excisional biopsy predict residual tumor within the remaining breast? Excisional biopsies with extensive in situ carcinoma were in fact far more likely (74% vs. 42%) to be associated with residual carcinoma, primarily in situ disease, in the mastectomy specimen. The EIC-positive patients were also more likely to have additional foci of invasive carcinoma within the breast at the time of mastectomy. However, this difference was small and reached statistical significance only within the immediate vicinity of the primary tumor (within 2 cm of the margin of the primary tumor). The major difference, then, between the EIC-positive and EIC-negative tumors was in the extent of the in situ disease of ductal type within the remainder of the breast (Fig. 12-9).[5] Intralymphatic channel tumor involvement was not different between the two tumor types.

The Holland study on the predictive capability of EIC produced results compatible with other studies on this phenomenon.[51–53] It has been confirmed in studies from Amsterdam[54,55] and London.[56] Other earlier studies did not support the predictive usefulness of EIC with regard to local treatment failure. This disparity may be explained by the fact that one of these studies used a large resection[57] and the other required histologic documentation of tumor-free margins.[58]

The more recent studies with three-dimensional reconstruction by Ohtake and coworkers[8] along with Mai and coworkers,[9] described earlier in this chapter, also support the concept of extensive intraductal carcinoma as an important factor in determining the effectiveness of breast-conserving therapy. However, this does not necessarily imply that breast-conserving therapy will not be successful. Mai and coworkers attribute the success of segmental resection in treating breast carcinoma to the

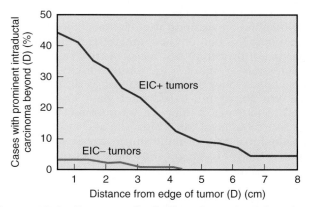

Figure 12-9 Frequency distribution of prominent intraductal carcinoma at various distances from the edge of the primary tumor. (From Holland R, Connolly JL, Gelman R, et al: The presence of an extensive intraductal component (EIC) following a limited excision correlates with prominent residual disease in the remainder of the breast. J Clin Oncol 8:113, 1990.)

high prevalence of DCIS restricted to a single duct system. They go even further and suggest that failures using segmental resection for small carcinomas may in part be related to the pyramidal shape of the distribution of the DCIS. Supportive of this hypotheses is a small study of mastectomy specimens obtained following local failure after lumpectomy, which found that recurrences were located in the same quadrant as the primary lesion and were present radial to the initial tumor (either closer to the nipple or toward the axilla).[59] Mai and coworkers also suggest involvement of the nipple and lack of recognition of an EIC associated with a small, palpable invasive lesion as possible causes for failures in segmental resections.

Other approaches to local therapy may abrogate the negative effect of clinically occult multicentricity on the rate of local recurrence,[10,60–62] even in the setting of a subareolar lesion.[63]

We have seen the concept of multicentricity evolve from merely an observed phenomenon to a more specific model-based definition using a three-dimensional reconstruction of the breast mammary tree and molecular profiles of the tumor. Observed multicentricity in cases of invasive mammary carcinoma has been strongly associated with involvement of the nipple and the presence of an EIC. Discovery of a focus of invasive carcinoma more than 4 cm from the edge of a definable invasive carcinoma is uncommon, and the rate of this occurrence is approximately that of development of a second primary in the opposite breast. Multicentricity and bilaterality have sometimes been considered related in some respects. Considering that true multicentricity occurs as a result of independent molecular events, one would expect the rates of multicentricity and bilaterality to be similar. The published rates and circumstances of multiple occurrence of ipsilateral and contralateral breast carcinoma are in fact quite different. Most "secondary" lesions in the ipsilateral breast, therefore, likely represent (multifocal) evolution from intraductal extension of the primary lesion. This model is supported by imaging and molecular studies of seemingly multicentric tumors,[6–9,15,16] with confirmation in the clinical finding that more than 90% of occurrences after local removal of a carcinoma from a breast are found in the same segment as the original carcinoma[59] (see Chapter 22).

Difficulties in defining the relationships of multiple tumors should not obscure the recognition that it is important only insofar as it has predictive value for treatment success or failure. True multicentricity, defined as independent index sources of tumor, is difficult to estimate and occurs much less often than has been published. Therefore, it may be appropriate to consider extensive intraductal carcinoma, the likely cause of most published instances of multicentric disease, as the more important factor in prognosticating success of treatment.

Clinical Implications of Multicentricity

A number of prospective, randomized clinical trials have demonstrated equivalent survival for in situ and invasive breast cancers treated with mastectomy or breast conservation.[64–66] Therefore, the current standard of care for the management of both invasive and in situ breast cancers is a breast-conserving approach. One of the major contraindications to a breast-conserving approach is the presence of multicentric disease.[67] In addition, the presence of an EIC coexistent with an invasive breast carcinoma predicts an increased risk of local failure with a breast-conserving approach. Two large European randomized trials [the Breast Cancer Cooperative Group of the European Organization for Research and Treatment of Cancer (EORTC) and the Danish Breast Cancer Cooperative Group (DBCG)] compared breast-conserving therapy and mastectomy in stage I and stage II breast cancer. In their analysis, Voogd and colleagues reported that the risk of local recurrence after breast-conserving therapy for women with infiltrating ductal carcinomas with EIC was 2.52 times higher that that in those without EIC. The 10-year actuarial rates were 21% and 9%, respectively.[68] Therefore, it is critical to accurately assess the extent of disease so that the appropriate surgical intervention can be planned. The consideration of partial breast irradiation only amplifies the importance of accurately determining whether or not multicentric disease is present.

Magnetic resonance imaging (MRI) is being used with increasing frequency in an effort to assess extent of disease more accurately, although its exact role is still in evolution. Recently, the American Cancer Society published guidelines for the use of MRI in conjunction with mammography in women at high risk for breast cancer; however, there was thought to be insufficient evidence to recommend for or against the addition of MRI in women with a personal history of intraductal or invasive carcinoma.[69] A number of studies have demonstrated that the addition of MRI to the preoperative workup for localized breast cancer will identify additional foci of tumor in 10% to 27% of cases, and some have also reported that the addition of MRI had a significant impact on the surgical management in these women.[70–77]

Bilimoria and colleagues evaluated 155 women with breast cancer diagnosed by mammography, ultrasonography, and needle biopsy who underwent preoperative bilateral breast MRI.[70] A total of 124 additional suspicious lesions were identified in 73 patients, and there was a change in surgical management in 36 patients. In 10 patients, lumpectomy was converted to mastectomy (8 beneficial, 2 unnecessary) and wider excision was performed in 21 patients (10 beneficial, 11 unnecessary). Five patients underwent contralateral surgery. Overall, these investigators determined that breast MRI resulted in a beneficial change in surgical management in 9.7% of these newly diagnosed breast cancer cases. In a retrospective review of 267 patients with primary breast tumors who had undergone MRI prior to definitive surgery, Bedrosian and colleagues found that planned surgical management was altered in 26% of the patients.[75] Pathologic verification of malignancy in the surgical specimen confirmed the need for wider or separate excision or mastectomy in 71% of cases. Berg and associates evaluated 121 breast cancer cases and found that MRI resulted in conversion to mastectomy in 25% and wider excision in 3%.[76] Deurloo and colleagues evaluated 116 breast cancer cases and determined that 6% underwent wider excision and 15.5% underwent mastectomy as a result of preoperative MRI.[77]

Of course, all of the previously cited studies make the assumption that the identification of the additional tumor detected by MRI is beneficial to the patient. It is not known whether these additional foci of tumor detected by MRI are biologically important. Whether these foci would result in recurrence after breast conservation and radiation therapy with or without chemotherapy and/or hormonal therapy is unknown.

Another important clinical question raised by the presence of multicentric invasive breast cancer is the appropriate method for nodal assessment. Sentinel lymph node biopsy has become the standard of care for evaluating the nodal status in patients with clinically node-negative breast cancer. The presence of multicentric disease was initially thought to be a contraindication to the performance of sentinel lymph node biopsy because of concerns that these tumors might involve more than one dominant lymphatic drainage pattern. This might result in inaccurate nodal staging and high false-negative rates.[78,79] A number of investigators have addressed this issue and demonstrated that the technique appears to be valid in multicentric disease as well.[80-83]

Tousimis and colleagues at Memorial Sloan-Kettering Cancer Center reviewed their single institution prospective sentinel lymph node database and identified 70 patients with multifocal or multicentric breast cancer who had undergone sentinel lymph node biopsy followed by a planned axillary node dissection in which at least 10 axillary nodes were excised.[80] The sentinel lymph node biopsy accuracy was 96%; the sensitivity, 92%; and the false-negative rate, 8%. There was no statistically significant difference between these results and those of published sentinel lymph node biopsy validation studies. The results of this retrospective study suggested that sentinel lymph node biopsy may be a reliable alternative to complete nodal dissection in the setting of multicentric disease.

Knauer and coworkers published the results of a multi-institutional validation trial in which 3730 patients underwent sentinel lymph node biopsy in 15 hospitals; 142 of these patients had multicentric disease.[81] Compared with the patients with unicentric cancer, there was a significantly higher rate of sentinel lymph node metastases in the multicentric cancer cases, but there was no difference in detection and false-negative rates. Ferrari and colleagues performed a prospective study to evaluate the accuracy of sentinel lymph node biopsy in multifocal and multicentric breast cancer.[82] In this study, 31 patients with a preoperative diagnosis of multifocal[75] or multicentric[82] invasive and clinically node-negative breast cancer underwent sentinel lymph node assessment followed by subsequent axillary node dissection regardless of sentinel node status. Patients received either a periareolar injection or two intradermal injections over the site of the two dominant tumors and lymphoscintigraphy was performed. In the majority of cases, (approximately 93%, regardless of injection route), lymphoscintigraphy demonstrated convergence to a single pathway. Sentinel lymph node accuracy in this study was 96.8%; the

sensitivity, 92.8%; and the false-negative rate, 7.1%. In the single false-negative case, the lymph node had been identified by the surgeon as strongly suspicious for skip metastasis. The authors concluded that sentinel lymph node biopsy was highly accurate in multifocal and multicentric disease and should no longer be considered a contraindication.

In conclusion, multicentricity-extent of disease continues to be a controversial topic. As you have read in this short chapter, defining extent of disease is difficult. As technology improves with MRI and possibly positron emission tomography (PET) scans, we are able to better define extent of disease in a patient prior to surgical decisions. Will the new technology add to better survival or to more aggressive management without any proven benefit?

REFERENCES

1. Qualheim RE, Gall EA: Breast carcinoma with multiple sites of origin. Cancer 10:460–468, 1957.
2. Gallager HS, Martin JE: The study of mammary carcinoma by mammography and whole organ section. Cancer 23:855–878, 1969.
3. Tellem M, Prive L, Meranze D: Four quadrant study of breast removed for carcinoma. Cancer 15:10–17, 1962.
4. Fisher ER, Fisher B, Sass R, et al: Pathologic findings from the National Surgical Adjuvant Breast Project (Protocol No. 4). I. Observations concerning the multicentricity of mammary cancer. Cancer 35:247–253, 1975.
5. Holland R, Veling S, Mravunac M, Hendriks J: Histologic multifocality of Tis, T1-2 breast carcinomas: Implications for clinical trials of breast conserving surgery. Cancer 56:979–990, 1985.
6. Faverly DR, Burgers L, Bult P, Holland R: Three dimensional imaging of mammary duct carcinoma in situ: Clinical implications. Semin Diagn Pathol 11: 193–198, 1994.
7. Ohtake T, Rikiya A, Kimijima I, et al: Intraductal extension of primary invasive breast carcinoma treated by breast-conserving surgery: Computer graphic three dimensional reconstruction of the mammary duct-lobular system. Cancer 73:32–45, 1995.
8. Ohtake T, Kimijima I, Fukushima T, et al: Computer-assisted complete three dimensional reconstruction of the mammary ductal-lobular systems: Implications of ductal anastomoses for breast-conserving surgery. Cancer 91:2263–2272, 2001.
9. Mai KT, Yazdi H, Burns B, Perkins D: Pattern of distribution of intraductal and infiltrating ductal carcinoma: A three dimensional study using serial coronal giant sections of the breast. Hum Pathol 31:464–474, 2000.
10. Harris EE, Solin LJ: The diagnosis and treatment of ductal carcinoma in situ of the breast. Breast J 6:78–95, 2000.
11. Silverstein MJ, Lagios M, Groshen S, et al: The influence of margin width on local control of ductal carcinoma in situ of the breast. N Engl J Med 340:1455–1461, 1999.
12. Moffat DF, Going JJ: Three dimensional anatomy of complete duct systems in human breast: Pathological and developmental implications. J Clin Pathol 49:48–52, 1996.
13. Mannes KD, Edgerton M, Simpson JF, et al: Pagetoid spread in ductal carcinoma in situ: Characterization and computer simulation. Abstract 164. U.S. and Canadian Academy of Pathology 91st Annual Meeting Chicago, Feb 23–Mar 1, 2002.
14. Fujii H, Marsh C, Cairns P, et al: Genetic divergence in the clonal evolution of breast cancer. Cancer Res 56:1493–1497, 1996.
15. Noguchi S, Aihara T, Motomura K, et al: Discrimination between multicentric and multifocal carcinomas of the breast through clonal analysis. Cancer 74:872–877, 1994.
16. Teixeira MR, Pandis N, Barrdi G, et al: Cytogenetic analysis of multifocal breast carcinomas: Detection of karyotypically unrelated clones as well as clonal similarities between tumor foci. Br J Cancer 70:922–927, 1994.
17. Cheatle GL, Cutler M: Tumors of the breast: Their pathology, symptoms, diagnosis and treatment. Philadelphia, JB Lippincott, 1931.

18. Lagios MD: Multicentricity of breast carcinoma demonstrated by routine correlated serial subgross and radiographic examination. Cancer 40:1726–1734, 1977.
19. European Commission: European guidelines for quality assurance in mammography screening, 2nd ed. Luxembourg, Office of Official Publications of the European Communities, 1996, II-C-15–II-C-16.
20. Egan RL, McSweeney MB: Multicentric breast carcinoma. Recent Results Cancer Res 90:28–35, 1984.
21. Holland R, Connolly JL, Gelman R, et al: The presence of an extensive intraductal component (EIC) following a limited excision correlates with prominent residual disease in the remainder of the breast. J Clin Oncol 8:113–118, 1990.
22. Lagios MD, Westdahl PR, Rose MR: The concept and implications of multicentricity in breast carcinoma. Pathol Annu 16:83–102, 1981.
23. Middleton LP, Vlastos G, Mirza N, et al: Multicentric mammary carcinoma. Cancer 94:1910–1916, 2002.
24. Fisher ER, Sass R, Fisher B, et al: Pathologic findings from the National Surgical Adjuvant Breast Project (Protocol No. 6). I. Intraductal carcinoma (DCIS). Cancer 57:197–208, 1986.
25. Patchefsky AS, Schwartz G, Finkelstein S, et al: Heterogeneity of intraductal carcinoma of the breast. Cancer 63:731–741, 1989.
26. Simpson T, Thirlby RC, Dail DH: Surgical treatment of ductal carcinoma in situ of the breast: 10- to 20-year follow-up. Arch Surg 127:468–472, 1992.
27. Ashikari R, Hajdu SI, Robbins GF: Intraductal carcinoma of the breast. Cancer 28:1182–1187, 1971.
28. Alpers CE, Wellings SR: The prevalence of carcinoma in situ in normal and cancer associated breast. Hum Pathol 16:796–807, 1985.
29. Posner MC, Wolmark N: Noninvasive breast carcinoma. Breast Cancer Res Treat 21:155–164, 1992.
30. Ringberg A, Palmer B, Linell F, et al: Bilateral and multifocal breast carcinoma: A clinical and autopsy study with special emphasis on carcinoma in situ. Eur J Surg Oncol 17:20–29, 1991.
31. Gump FE, Shikora S, Habif D, et al: The extent and distribution of cancer in breasts with palpable primary tumors. Ann Surg 204:384–390, 1986.
32. Schwartz GF, Patchesfsky A, Feig S, et al: Multicentricity of non-palpable breast cancer. Cancer 45:2913–2916, 1980.
33. Lesser ML, Rosen PP, Kinne DW: Multicentricity and bilaterality in invasive breast carcinoma. Sugery 91:234–240, 1982.
34. Schnitt SJ, Connolly J, Recht A, et al: Influence of infiltrating lobular histology on local tumor control in breast cancer patients treated with conservative surgery and radiotherapy. Cancer 64:448–454, 1989.
35. Lagios MD, Rose MR, Margolin FR: Tubular carcinoma of the breast: Association with multicentricity, bilaterally, and family history of mammary carcinoma. Am J Clin Pathol 73:25–30, 1980.
36. McDivitt RW, Boyce W, Gersell D: Tubular carcinoma of the breast: Clinical and pathological observations concerning 135 cases. Am J Surg Pathol 6:401–411, 1982.
37. Rosen PP, Fraccia AA, Urban JA, et al: "Residual" mammary carcinoma following simulated partial mastectomy. Cancer 35:739–747, 1975.
38. Arbutina DR, Cruz B, Harding C, Cornwell M: Multifocality in the earliest detectable breast cancers. Arch Surg 127:421–423, 1992.
39. Sharpe CR: A developmental hypothesis to explain the multicentricity of breast cancer. CMAJ 159:55–59, 1998.
40. Dawson PJ, Baekey PA, Clark RA: Mechanism of multifocal breast cancer: An immunocytochemical study. Hum Pathol 26:965–969, 1995.
41. Anderson JA, Pallesen RM: Spread to the nipple and areola in carcinoma of the breast. Ann Surg 189:367–372, 1979.
42. Luttges J, Kalbfleisch H, Prinz P: Nipple involvement and multicentricity in breast cancer: A study on whole organ sections. J Cancer Res Clin Oncol 113:481–487, 1987.
43. Morgenstern L, Kaufman PA, Friedeman NB: The case against tylectomy for carcinoma of the breast. Am J Surg 130:251–258, 1975.
44. Sarnelli R, Squartini F: Multicentricity in breast cancer: A submicroscopic study. Pathol Annu 21:143–158, 1986.
45. Sarnelli R, Squartini F: Structure, functional changes, and proliferative pathology of the human mammary lobule in cancerous breasts. J Natl Cancer Inst 67:33–46, 1975.
46. Westman-Naeser S, Bengtsson E, Eriksson O, et al: Multifocal breast carcinoma. Am J Surg 142:255–257, 1981.
47. De Laruentiis M, Gallo C, De Placido S, et al: A predictive index of axillary nodal involvement in operable breast cancer. Br J Cancer 73:1241–1247, 1996.
48. Arisio R, Salino A, Cassoni P, et al: What modifies the relation between tumor size and lymph node metastases in T1 breast carcinomas? J Clin Pathol 53:846–850, 2000.
49. Chua B, Dng O, Taylor R, Boyages J: Frequency and predictors of axillary lymph node metastases in invasive breast cancer. ANZ J Surg 71:723–728, 2001.
50. Ruibal A, Schneider J, del Rio MC, et al: Expression of the adhesion molecule CD44v6 in infiltrating ductal carcinomas of the breast is associated with hormone dependence: Our experience with 168 cases. Rev Esp Med Nucl 19:350–355, 2000.
51. Schnitt SJ, Connolly JL, Harris JR, et al: Pathologic predictors of early local recurrence in stage I and II breast cancer treated by primary radiation therapy. Cancer 53:1049–1057, 1984.
52. Harris JR, Connolly J, Schnitt S, et al: Clinical-pathologic study of early breast cancer treated by primary radiation therapy. J Clin Oncol 1:184–189, 1983.
53. Schnitt SJ, Connolly JL, Khettry U: Pathologic findings on reexcision of the primary site in breast cancer patients considered for treatment by primary radiation therapy. Cancer 59:675–681, 1987.
54. Bartelink JH, Borger JH, van Dongen JA, Peterse JL: The impact of tumor size and histology on local control after breast-conserving therapy. Radiother Oncol 11:279–303, 1988.
55. Voogd AC, Neilsen M, Peterse JL, et al: Differences in risk factors for local and distant recurrence after breast-conserving therapy or mastectomy for stage I and II breast cancer: Pooled results of two large European randomized trials. J Clin Oncol 19:1688–1697, 2001.
56. Lindley R, Bulman A, Parsons P: Histologic features predictive of an increased risk of early recurrence after treatment of breast cancer by local tumor excision and radical radiotherapy. Surgery 105:13–20, 1989.
57. Van Limbergen E, van den Bogaert W, van der Schueren E, Rijnders A: Tumor excision and radiotherapy as primary treatment of breast cancer: Analysis of patient and treatment parameters and local control. Radiother Oncol 8:1–9, 1987.
58. Fisher B, Redmond C, Poisson R, et al: Eight-year results of a randomized clinical trial comparing total mastectomy and lumpectomy with or without irradiation in the treatment of breast cancer. N Engl J Med 320:822–828, 1989.
59. Johnson JE, Page DL, Winfield AC, et al: Recurrent mammary carcinoma after local excision: A segmental problem. Cancer 75:1612–1618, 1995.
60. Veronesi U, Salvadori B, Luini A, et al: Breast conservation is a safe method in patients with small cancer of the breast: Long term results of three randomized trials on 1,973 patients. Eur J Cancer 31A:1574–1579, 1995.
61. Weng EY, Juillard GJ, Parker RG, et al: Outcomes and factors impacting local recurrence of ductal carcinoma in situ. Cancer 88:1643–1649, 200.
62. Skinner KA, Silverstein MJ: The management of ductal carcinoma in situ of the breast. Endocr Relat Cancer 8:33–45, 2001.
63. Haffty BG, Wilson L, Smith R, et al: Subareolar breast cancer: Long-term results with conservative surgery and radiation therapy. Int J Radiat Oncol Biol Phys 33:53–57, 1995.
64. Fisher B, Anderson S, Bryant J, et al: Twenty-year follow-up of a randomized trial comparing total mastectomy, lumpectomy, and lumpectomy plus irradiation for the treatment of invasive breast cancer. N Engl J Med 347:1233–1241, 2002.
65. Poggi MM, Danforth DN, Sciuto LC, et al: Eighteen-year results in the treatment of early breast carcinoma with mastectomy versus breast conservation therapy: The National Cancer Institute randomized trial. Cancer 98:697–702, 2003.
66. Nakamura S, Woo C, Silberman H, et al: Breast-conserving therapy for ductal carcinoma in situ. A 20-year experience with excision plus radiation therapy. Am J Surg 184:403–409, 2002.
67. Morrow M, Harris JR: Practice guidelines for breast conservation therapy in the management of invasive breast cancer. J Am Coll Surg 205:362–376, 2007.
68. Voogd AC, Nielsen M, Peterse JL, et al: Differences in risk factors for local and distant recurrence after breast-conserving therapy or mastectomy for stage I and II breast cancer. Pooled results of two large European randomized trials. J Clin Oncol 19:1688–1697, 2001.

69. Saslow D, Boetes C, Burke W, et al: American Cancer Society guidelines for breast screening with MRI as an adjunct to mammography. CA Cancer J Clin 57:75–89, 2007.
70. Bilimoria KY, Cambric A, Hansen NM, et al: Evaluating the impact of preoperative breast magnetic resonance imaging on the surgical management of newly diagnosed breast cancers. Arch Surg 142:441–447, 2007.
71. Lee JM, Orel SG, Czerniecki BJ, et al: MRI before re-excision surgery in patients with breast cancer. AJR Am J Roentgenol 182:473–480, 2004.
72. Liberman L, Morris EA, Dershaw DD, et al: MRI imaging of the ipsilateral breast in women with percutaneously proven breast cancer. AJR Am J Roentgenol 180:901–910, 2003.
73. Fischer U, Kopka L, Grabbe E: Breast carcinoma: Effect of preoperative contrast-enhanced MR imaging on the therapeutic approach. Radiology 213:881–888, 1999.
74. Drew PJ, Chatterjee S, Turnbull LW, et al: Dynamic contrast enhanced magnetic resonance imaging of the breast is superior to triple assessment for the preoperative detection of multifocal breast cancer. Ann Surg Oncol 6:599–603, 1999.
75. Bedrosian I, Mick R, Orel SG, et al: Changes in the surgical management of patients with breast carcinoma based on preoperative magnetic resonance imaging. Cancer 2003;98:468–473.
76. Berg WA, Gutierrez L, NessAiver MS, et al: Diagnostic accuracy of mammography, clinical examination, US, and MRI imaging in preoperative assessment of breast cancer. Radiology 233:830–849, 2004.
77. Deurloo EE, Peterse JL, Rutgers EJ, et al: Additional breast lesions in patients eligible for breast-conserving therapy by MRI: Impact on preoperative management and potential benefit of computerized analysis. Eur J Cancer 41:1393–1401, 2005.
78. Veronesi U, Paganelli G, Viale G, et al: Sentinel lymph node biopsy and axillary dissection in breast cancer: Results in a large series. J Natl Cancer Inst 91:368–373, 1999.
79. Hsueh EC, Turner RR, Glass EC, et al: Sentinel node biopsy in breast cancer. J Am Coll Surg 1999; 189: 207–213.
80. Tousimis E, Van Zee KJ, Fey JV, et al: The accuracy of sentinel lymph node biopsy in multicentric and multifocal invasive breast cancers. J Am Coll Surg 197:529–535, 2003.
81. Knauer M, Konstantiniuk P, Haid A, et al: Multicentric breast cancer: A new indication for sentinel node biopsy—a multi-institutional validation study. J Clin Oncol 24:3374–3380, 2006.
82. Ferrari A, Dionigi P, Rovera F, et al: Multifocality and multicentricity are not contraindications for sentinel lymph node biopsy in breast cancer surgery. World J Surg Oncol 4:79–86, 2006.
83. Kim HJ, Lee SL, Park EH, et al: Sentinel node biopsy in patients with multiple breast cancer. Breast Cancer Res Treat 109:503–506, 2008.

chapter 13

Mesenchymal Neoplasms of the Breast

PAUL E. WAKELY JR

With the exception of fibroepithelial tumors, mesenchymal neoplasms, particularly sarcoma of the breast, are rare. Primary breast sarcoma accounts for less than 1% of all breast malignancies and less than 5% of all soft tissue sarcomas.[1] Estimated annual incidence is 17 new cases per 1,000,000 women.[2] Other than radiation-induced angiosarcoma (AS), no definitive etiologic relationship exists between sarcomatous and nonsarcomatous mesenchymal neoplasms including silicone prosthesis or augmentation mammoplasty.[3] A 90-year search of the Mayo Clinic database revealed that primary breast sarcoma accounted for 0.06% of all breast cancers.[4] AS, fibrosarcoma, and pleomorphic sarcoma were the most frequent subtypes. Tumor size was the most valuable prognostic factor, with 91% overall survival for women with sarcomas less than or equal to 5 cm and 50% for those with sarcomas greater than 5 cm. The generic term *stromal sarcoma* should be discouraged because most sarcomas can be more specifically subtyped. Unlike carcinoma, mammary sarcoma of any type rarely metastasizes to lymph nodes, thus negating the need for axillary dissection or sentinel lymph node biopsy. With few exceptions, sarcomas require total mastectomy.

Fibroepithelial Neoplasms

FIBROADENOMA

Fibroadenoma (FA) is a common cause of breast masses that are prone to affect women younger than 30 years of age. FA is a painless, mobile lump(s) that is unilateral, bilateral, or infrequently multifocal. The cut surface has a distinctive bulging, firm, off-white nodular look, which is sharply delimited from surrounding breast tissue. Calcification may be present. A homogeneous increase in stromal connective tissue distorts ductal epithelium into long, thin intersecting compressed strands (intracanalicular pattern) or surrounds ductules in a circumferential manner (pericanalicular pattern).[5] Both patterns may occur in the same mass; neither have biologic significance. Stromal nuclei are spindle-shaped and euchromatic with smooth nuclear contours. Ductal

epithelium may exhibit a wide range of proliferative and nonproliferative changes.[6] In situ or invasive carcinoma is only rarely reported and occurs mostly in older patients. "Juvenile FA" is a diagnosis reserved for tumors that have a rapid growth rate, are very large (>10 cm), and arise in adolescence.

PHYLLODES TUMOR

Phyllodes tumor (PT) is an exceptionally uncommon, rarely bilateral breast neoplasm representing less than 1% of all primary breast tumors.[7,8] The incidence may be higher in Asian women.[9] After it was first described, it was not known to have malignant potential for almost 100 years.[8] Mean age at diagnosis is 45 years, although a broad age range exists, and average tumor size is 4 to 5 cm. Grossly, PT has a whorled pattern with visible cracks or fissures. Cystic change is common in large neoplasms. The biphasic nature involves a benign epithelial component and an abnormally cellular stromal/mesenchymal component. Although the stroma is generally more cellular than that seen in FA, a more important distinguishing feature is that stromal cellularity is heterogeneous. Frond-like stromal overgrowth (accounting for the term *phyllodes*) produces an exaggerated intracanalicular pattern and is also a more reliable feature of PT (Fig. 13-1). Like FA, benign PT has a circumscribed edge, cytologically uniform stromal cells, and few mitoses.

Histologic grading into benign, borderline, and malignant categories is recommended. This classification is based on a constellation of features, including cellularity, mitotic count, pleomorphism, degree of stromal overgrowth (defined as lack of any epithelial component in at least 1 low-power/40× field), and whether the border is infiltrative or circumscribed.[5] Different authors use different mitotic counts to subdivide PT into various grades ranging from 1 to 2 per 10 high-power fields (hpf) for benign PT[5,10] up to 10 per 10 hpf (Fig. 13-2).[11] The World Health Organization (WHO) avoids a strict numerical count because of the variability of hpf among microscopes. Instead, a semiquantitative method of few if any mitoses, intermediate number of mitoses, and numerous mitoses (>10 mitoses per 10 hpf) is used to

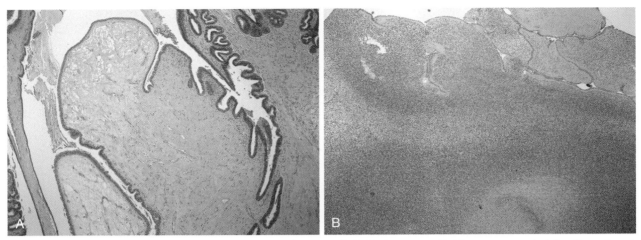

Figure 13-1 A, Leaflike fronds define the low-power architecture of phyllodes tumor. **B,** The stroma underlying these fronds has increased cellularity with varying numbers of mitosis.

help subclassify PT into benign, borderline, and malignant categories, respectively (see Fig. 13-2).[12] Along with stromal heterogeneity, hyalinization and myxoid change are common.[5] Isolated bizarre giant cells have no behavioral significance.[13] Benign heterologous elements, including chondroid, osseous, squamous and lipomatous metaplasia, may be seen in benign PT, whereas malignant PT may contain foci of liposarcoma, osteosarcoma, and rhabdomyosarcoma. Distinction between benign PT and FA is imprecise, and it is particularly problematic with core needle biopsy specimens. Lee and colleagues found higher stromal cellularity (compared with FA in >50% of the cores), stromal overgrowth, fragmentation (defined as stromal fragments with epithelium at one or both ends), and adipose tissue within stroma to be four statistically significant features useful in separating PT from FA in needle biopsies.[14]

Malignant PT accounts for 10% to 30% of all cases. It is recognizable by its cellular pleomorphism, stromal overgrowth, atypical heterologous elements, and mitotic count (Fig. 13-3A). *Ki-67* staining has been used as a proliferation marker but adds little to mitosis counting. Size alone is not a predictor of malignancy. Overexpression of *p53*[15] and epidermal growth factor receptor gene[16] seems to correlate with progression in grade from benign to malignant, but the prognostic significance is currently unclear. Estrogen receptor and progesterone receptor expression appear to be inversely related to histologic grade.[17] Recurrence correlates primarily with completeness of resection; however, it is not certain even with positive margins. Locally recurrent tumors are usually of same grade as the original. Pseudoangiomatous stromal hyperplasia (PASH) within PT correlates with a decreased risk of recurrence in one study.[9] Metastases occur in less than 10% of cases and consist of sarcomatous stroma.[18,19] Lung, pleura and bone are the most common metastatic sites (see Fig. 13-3B). Lymph node metastasis is rare and seen only in advanced cases. The presence of visceral metastasis of malignant PT confirms its malignant sarcomatous nature.

MAMMARY HAMARTOMA

Hamartoma is a well-delimited mass that occurs in perimenopausal women as an incidental mammographic finding. It is composed of benign breast lobules, adipose

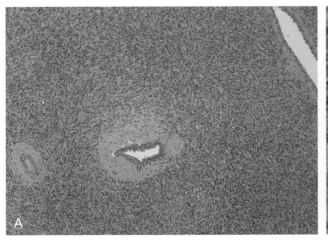
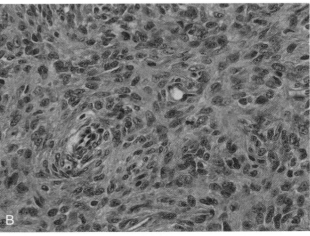

Figure 13-2 A, A borderline phyllodes tumor with increased stromal cellularity. **B,** This tumor also exhibits prominent mitoses.

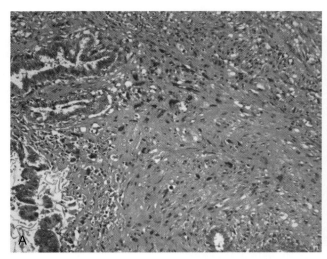 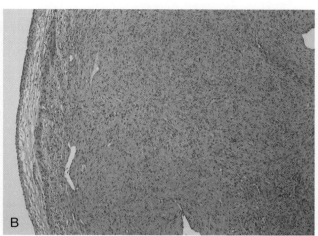

Figure 13-3 A, Malignant phyllodes tumor (PT). Pleomorphic and spindle-shaped enlarged nuclei concentrate just beneath the hyperplastic ductal epithelium, which is at the left of the field. **B,** Metastasis of malignant PT to bronchus confirms its malignant nature.

tissue, and fibrous tissue in varying quantity without the lobular structure of FA and is outlined by a pseudocapsule of compressed breast tissue.

Fibroblastic and Myofibroblastic Neoplasms

FIBROMATOSIS

Fibromatosis is a proliferation of fibroblasts that comprises less than 0.2% of breast lesions.[20,21] Women of a wide age range (15 to 80 years of age; median, 40 years) are affected. A unilateral painless, firm mass that is mammographically indistinguishable from carcinoma is typical. Grossly, this is a firm, off-white lesion averaging 2 to 3 cm that deceptively appears to be circumscribed; some cases show irregular stellate borders. Even with circumscribed lesions, radially oriented extensions of tumor subtly infiltrate adjacent tissue, creating difficulty in

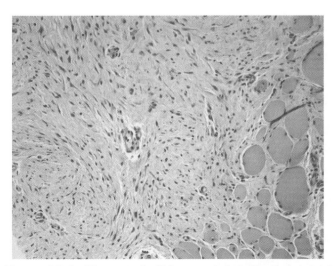

Figure 13-4 Fibromatosis. This example is infiltrating skeletal muscle (*right edge*) of the chest wall. Note the abundant stromal collagen and slender cell nuclei.

judging adequacy of resection. Light microscopy reveals banal-appearing fibroblasts with oval to spindle-shaped pale nuclei arranged in interlacing fascicles set in a variably dense collagenous matrix (Fig. 13-4). Lymphocyte clusters are common. Fibromatoses are vimentin and β-catenin (80%) positive, and they are cytokeratin, estrogen receptor, and progesterone receptor negative.[22] Although fibromatosis carries no metastatic potential, it is locally aggressive, with a risk that ranges from 14% to 38%. Complete surgical excision with negative margins remains standard treatment.

MYOFIBROBLASTOMA

Mammary-type myofibroblastoma (MYB) is an uncommon neoplasm that affects men almost as much as women. A unilateral circumscribed mass occurs in patients in their fifth to ninth decades. MYB ranges from 1 to 10 cm and has a homogeneous bulging pink cut surface. Multilobulation and myxoid foci may be seen. Microscopically, a spindle cell proliferation with very few mitoses set in a fibrous stroma is apparent.[23] Collagen bundles are typically thick and ropy, with cells laid down in short, randomly intersecting fascicles rather than the long, sweeping fascicles of fibromatosis (Fig. 13-5). Cells have small oval/elongated nuclei, small nucleoli, and occasional grooves. Mitoses are rare, but mast cells are usually numerous. Morphologic variations include an infiltrative rather than circumscribed border; myxoid change; multinucleated giant cells; and cartilaginous, osseous, or fatty metaplasia (so-called lipomatous MYB).[24–26] The myofibroblastic nature is demonstrated by reactivity with desmin, α-smooth muscle actin, and variable staining with CD34, bcl-2, and estrogen and progesterone receptors.[27] Complete excision is curative.

SOLITARY FIBROUS TUMOR AND HEMANGIOPERICYTOMA

So-called hemangiopericytoma is an older term used for a benign spindle cell neoplasm where the branching vascular pattern is its most conspicuous feature.

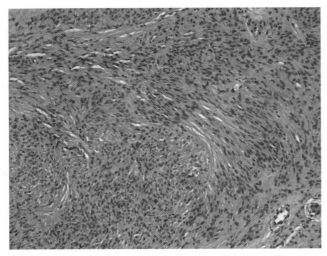

Figure 13-5 Myofibroblastoma. More cellular than fibromatosis, the cells have a short fascicular pattern.

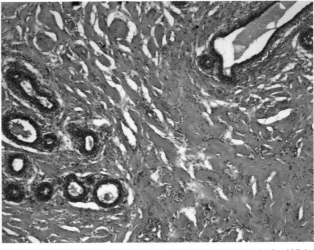

Figure 13-6 Pseudoangiomatous stromal hyperplasia. Widely patent, empty slits partially obscure the proliferating spindle cells as they surround benign lobules.

Its occurrence in the breast is rare.[28] Most of these neoplasms are currently classified as solitary fibrous tumor. They range from 1 to 19 cm and exhibit a firm grey-white cut surface. Proliferating plump oval to spindle cells focally entrap ducts and ductules at the lesion's edge. A thin-walled "staghorn" type branching vascular pattern is seen throughout the tumor. Differences between solitary fibrous tumor and MYB include a haphazard mixture of hyper- and hypocellular regions in solitary fibrous tumor in contrast to a sharper separation of cellular foci by hypocellular zones, resulting in a multilobular pattern in MYB.[29] Although both tumors are CD34 positive, solitary fibrous tumor does not express myogenic markers.

PSEUDOANGIOMATOUS STROMAL HYPERPLASIA

PASH is not a true vascular lesion but a peculiar proliferation of cytologically bland stromal fibroblasts/myofibroblasts that creates empty slitlike spaces mimicking a vasoformative neoplasm.[30,31] On average, patients are diagnosed in the fourth decade, but a wide continuum exists. The clinical spectrum of PASH ranges from an incidental microscopic finding (most common), to a palpable/nodular mass (rare), to diffuse breast involvement. Nodular forms resemble FA or mammary hamartoma on imaging and grossly. Tissue spaces formed by separation of densely hyalinized collagen fibers may or may not be lined by cells (Fig. 13-6). This proliferation may create a concentric perilobular pattern.[32,33] Fibroblasts lack cytologic atypia or mitoses; necrosis and effacement of normal breast tissue are absent. Gynecomastia-like changes include apocrine metaplasia, ductal hyperplasia and cystic change.[34] Cells show staining with CD34, muscle specific actin, calponin, and progesterone receptor[35]; CD31 and cytokeratin stains are negative.

FIBROSARCOMA–PLEOMORPHIC SARCOMA (MALIGNANT FIBROUS HISTIOCYTOMA)

Pleomorphic sarcoma, not otherwise specified, is also still known as malignant fibrous histiocytoma (MFH). With the advent of routine immunohistochemistry, MFH is a rare tumor. Thirty cases were reported in a recent review.[36] Thorough tissue sampling is required to exclude a sarcoma arising in malignant PT, and immunohistology is necessary to exclude a high-grade sarcoma showing specific mesenchymal differentiation. Jones and colleagues divided 32 sarcomas that fit the spectrum of fibrosarcoma (FS)/MFH into low-grade (FS) and high-grade (MFH) forms.[37] Median age of patients was 45 and 69 years, respectively. Low-grade FS showed an interlacing "herringbone" pattern of relatively monotonous spindle cells, whereas MFH tumors showed a greater degree of cell pleomorphism with many mitoses. In addition, most had a classic "storiform" pattern of intersecting fascicles of cells. No low-grade FS had distant metastases (mean follow-up = 8 years), whereas almost one third of high-grade patients died of disease.

Vascular Neoplasms

HEMANGIOMA

Vascular neoplasms occur either within breast parenchyma proper or in the overlying skin/subcutis. Endothelial markers CD34 and CD31 are nearly always positive; rarely required for benign vascular tumors, they are important in the recognition of malignant neoplasms. CD31 is the most sensitive and specific marker; variable staining is seen with factor VIII–related antigen. Mammary hemangioma has been described from infancy to the elderly. All hemangiomas lack anastomosing connections, endothelial tufting, and atypical mitoses, and they are often incidental findings. Of the various subtypes, cavernous hemangioma is most common, consisting of large, widely dilated vessels separated by thin fibrous septa and lined by flattened endothelial cells. Intraluminal thrombi are not uncommon. Capillary hemangioma consists of numerous small, closely packed vascular channels with a lobular pattern, which often lack luminal red cells. Venous hemangioma is rare, ranges from 1 to 5 cm, and is composed of large venous channels lined by flattened endothelial cells surrounded by a wall of smooth muscle.[38] Perilobular hemangioma consists of a lobular expansion of small to medium-sized blood-filled vessels within the intralobular stroma. Many examples also extend into extralobular stroma and adipose tissue.[39] It is not particularly rare, being encountered in 11% of 210 forensic autopsies.[40]

Atypical vascular lesions following radiation therapy are usually restricted to the dermis, and in contrast to AS are well circumscribed and generally less than 1 cm. They present as erythematous/bluish papules, nodules, or vesicles. There is a median latency of 3.5 years postradiation.[41] Atypical vascular lesions have a lymphangiomatous quality, with thin-walled irregular vascular spaces that are empty or filled with proteinaceous material. Focal dissection into dermal collagen is seen. Endothelial cell nuclei are hyperchromatic, with some displaying a hobnail projection into the lumen, but lacking the necrosis, mitoses, and dissection into the subcutis typical of AS. Their clinical behavior is benign.[41-43] Some experts have proposed that atypical vascular lesions and cutaneous AS represent a morphologic continuum.[41]

Intravascular papillary endothelial hyperplasia, a benign vascular lesion commonly associated with thrombus formation, is rarely reported in the breast. The largest series of 17 patients spanned adolescents to elderly.[44] Most presented with a circumscribed unilateral subcutaneous or superficial intraparenchymal mass. Papillary endothelial hyperplasia is sometimes surrounded by smooth muscle of a vessel wall and contains fresh and clotted blood, cystic spaces, and small fibrinous papillae covered by plump or flattened nuclei. The combination of focal nuclear tufting, papillae, and vascular anastomosis serves to create confusion with AS. Unlike AS, papillary endothelial hyperplasia is circumscribed, rarely larger than 2 cm, and does not infiltrate adjacent breast lobules.

ANGIOMATOSIS

Angiomatosis (diffuse hemangioma) of the breast is rare. It affects patients from infancy to the sixth decade. A diffuse network of sinusoidal small and large anastomosing vessels affects a large area of the breast. Vessels proliferate around but not into terminal duct lobular units.[45] In contrast to AS, vessels have a uniform distribution; a heterogeneous appearance of large venous, cavernous, and capillary type channels; and endothelial cells that lack cytologic atypia or tufting.

HEMANGIOENDOTHELIOMA

Epithelioid hemangioendothelioma is an exceedingly rare primary breast tumor.[46] Like its soft tissue equivalent, an infiltrative population of epithelioid cells is arranged in nests or short cords and has rounded enlarged nuclei and eosinophilic or singly vacuolated cytoplasm. It is set in a chondromyxoid or hyaline matrix. A possible association with breast implants has been reported.[47] Dissimilar to hemangioma, epithelioid hemangioendothelioma can be misinterpreted as a carcinoma because of its epithelioid morphology and positive staining with pan-cytokeratin markers in addition to endothelial markers.

ANGIOSARCOMA AND RELATED SYNDROMES

AS has a disproportionate propensity for the breast because it accounts for 15% to 34% of all breast sarcomas.[48] However, it is responsible for only 5% of soft tissue sarcomas.[49] AS is the most common *symptomatic* intraparenchymal vascular lesion of the breast[50] and the most common nonphyllodes sarcoma of the breast.[48] Even so, it remains a rare entity, comprising less than 1% of all breast tumors. The WHO subdivides AS into four clinical categories: (1) primary AS; (2) secondary AS following radical mastectomy and ipsilateral lymphedema, also known as Stewart-Treves (S-T) syndrome; (3) secondary AS following radical mastectomy and radiotherapy; and (4) secondary AS following conservative management and radiotherapy.[51] Light microscopy is similar in these different clinical subtypes.

Primary AS affects premenopausal women primarily (range, 14 to 82 years of age; mean = 35 years). A large review showed that 13% occurred in pregnant women and that 21% involved the contralateral breast.[52] Tumors range from 1 to 20 cm, averaging 4 to 5 cm, and they typically present as a painless mass. Macroscopically, the cut surface varies from hemorrhagic and spongy (low-grade AS) to a firm, dull-white variably necrotic mass (high-grade AS). The most widely recognized histologic classification subdivides AS into low, intermediate, and high grades, with 5-year overall survival rates of 91%, 68%, and 14%, respectively.[50] Histologic grading is the most important predictor of recurrence[53] but should be avoided on a core needle biopsy specimen because of inherent sampling bias. High-grade (grade III) AS is most common in younger patients and consists of more than 50% solid and spindle cell areas. These foci exhibit pleomorphism, hyperchromatic nuclei, macronucleoli, numerous mitoses, endothelial tufting, and papillary formation. A characteristic of AS is infiltration and destruction of preexisting terminal duct lobular units. CD31 stain is nearly always positive in grade III AS; CD34 and factor VIII–related antigen may be negative. FLI-1 has been reported as a sensitive, although not specific, marker of AS.[54]

Low-grade (grade I) AS is deceptively bland and potentially misdiagnosed as hemangioma. It has widely patent interanastomosing vascular channels that dissect

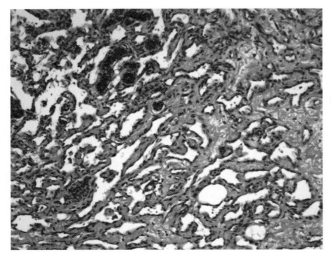

Figure 13-7 Angiosarcoma. A small lobule (*upper left*) is being infiltrated by anastomosing vascular channels lined by hyperchromatic nuclei.

within stroma but are lined by hyperchromatic nuclei with very few or no mitoses (Fig. 13-7). Solid foci, papillary formations, and blood lakes are absent. Intermediate-grade tumors have less than 25% solid foci and occasional endothelial tufting, but they lack necrosis. A diagnostic pitfall is the bland, almost hemangioma-like appearance at the periphery of low- and intermediate-grade AS. This is particularly challenging in a small biopsy or incompletely sampled tumor. The epithelioid variant of AS mimics carcinoma and not uncommonly expresses cytokeratin along with CD31. Bone, liver, lung, and brain are common metastatic sites. Because AS has a predilection for microscopic extension beyond the main mass, wide margins are required, thereby necessitating mastectomy in most patients. Prognosis is grade-related, with 10-year survival of 81% and 14% for grade I and grade III AS, respectively.[55]

AS developing in the ipsilateral arm following radical mastectomy with axillary dissection as described by Stewart and Treves (S-T syndrome) is secondary to long-standing lymphedema.[56] The incidence is 0.1% to 0.5%, and it develops, on average, 10 years after mastectomy. Pulmonary metastases are common, with a median survival of 19 months.[57] Increased use of breast-conservation surgery and sentinel node biopsy will lead to a reduction in this clinical form of AS.

Postradiation AS is a cancer of postmenopausal women. On average, affected patients are in their sixth to seventh decades.[58,59] It can arise either in the chest wall postmastectomy, or currently, it is more apt to occur in the breast after conservative treatment. Unlike primary AS, it is primarily a dermal/subcutaneous tumor, with patients commonly complaining of cutaneous violaceous or nonpigmented nodules, plaques, vesicles, and macules.[60] The incidence of AS, which is five to nine times higher in patients with breast cancer who receive radiotherapy,[61,62] is estimated to be 0.09% to 0.16%.[63] Relative risk assessments range from 11 to 15.9,[64] with a latency period of 6 months to 17 years (median; 5 to 6 years).[58,59,65] Light microscopy reveals an ill-defined

infiltrative neoplasm dissecting within dermal collagen and involving subcutaneous fat. Cells lining slitlike spaces show moderate nucleomegaly, hyperchromasia, and distinct nucleoli. Mitotic figures and papillary tufting are commonplace. Similar to primary AS, these may be subdivided into low-, intermediate-, and high-grade sarcoma. Most patients suffer multiple local recurrences; thus, the mainstay of treatment is wide local excision.[60]

Lipomatous Neoplasms

LIPOMA

Intramammary lipoma is uncommon, with most appearing in perimenopausal women. They are well demarcated and thinly encapsulated, showing identical morphology as the surrounding mature adipose tissue. Degenerative changes such as focal fat necrosis, calcification, hyalinization, or myxoid change are possible. Angiolipoma is typically a subcutaneous lesion composed of small capillary sized vessels within a lipoma. Intraluminal thrombi are commonly seen.[66,67] Chondrolipoma contains plates of hyaline-type cartilage randomly distributed within a nodule of adipose tissue.

LIPOSARCOMA

Primary pure liposarcoma of the breast is exceedingly rare. Purported examples require sufficient tumor sampling to exclude an underlying malignant phyllodes tumor with secondary liposarcomatous differentiation.[68] There are no distinguishing clinical features. Patients range from young adults to elderly individuals. They present with a slow growing, sometimes painful mass. Most are larger than 5 cm, firm, and well demarcated. All major histologic subtypes (well-differentiated, myxoid/round cell, dedifferentiated, and pleomorphic) have been reported.[69] Like their soft tissue equivalent, mammary liposarcoma shows lipogenic differentiation (Fig. 13-8) and has the potential to locally recur and metastasize.

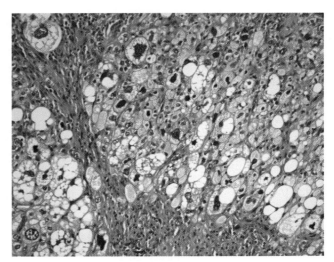

Figure 13-8 Liposarcoma. Cells with monstrously large nuclei contain micro- and macrovacuolated lipid-filled cytoplasm.

Neural Neoplasms

GRANULAR CELL TUMOR

Granular cell tumor is an uncommon lesion prone to arise in African-American women. It can be confused with carcinoma both clinically (very firm to palpation, skin retraction) and radiologically (irregular spiculated mass).[70,71] Peak age is the fourth decade. Less than 5% of lesions are multifocal. The cut surface shows a spiculated scirrhous grey white/yellow lesion. Microscopically, large cells with an enormous amount of coarsely granular cytoplasm infiltrate a densely collagen matrix. Nuclei are slightly enlarged and rarely display any mitoses. S-100 staining is present in nearly all cases. Rare malignant forms are characterized by high cellularity, large nuclei, mitoses, and spindling.[72]

Myogenic Neoplasms

LEIOMYOSARCOMA

Leiomyosarcoma is a rare breast malignancy that develops in women who are in their fourth to eighth decades.[73] Smooth muscle in the nipple-areolar complex may be a source for it to arise in this site.[74] It consists of a spindle cell proliferation with elongated blunt-ended nuclei and merging cytoplasmic processes, which create fascicles and whorled patterns. As in other sarcomas, histologic grade is dependent on cellularity, mitotic count, necrosis, and cellular atypia. Immunohistology shows expression of actin, smooth muscle actin, desmin (focal), and occasionally cytokeratin (focal). Local recurrence and distant metastases are common, sometimes developing as long as 15 years after surgery.[75]

RHABDOMYOSARCOMA

Rhabdomyosarcoma (RMS) of the breast mostly represents a metastasis from an extramammary site. A 25-year review found that only 2% of nonphyllodes primary breast sarcomas were RMS, whereas AS was the most common type.[48] RMS differentiation may develop in malignant PT or metaplastic carcinoma. Patients with both primary and metastatic pure RMS are adolescent females, and the overwhelming histology (>90%) shows an alveolar subtype, which is known as ARMS.[76] Classic ARMS has loosely cohesive cells, producing spaces surrounded by fibrous septa. Solid type ARMS consists of a solid sheet of cells. Both contain small rounded cells with minimal cytoplasm. Immunohistology is required to confidently diagnose RMS. Myogenin is the most sensitive and specific stain; desmin, myoglobin, and muscle-specific actin are also useful. ARMS has a unique cytogenetic abnormality; t(2;13)(q35;q14) allows distinction from other sarcomas using fluorescence in situ hybridization.[77] Five-year survival with resected RMS and without metastatic disease is greater than 90% for stage I disease and falls to 80%, 70%, and 30%, for stages II, III, and IV, respectively.[78]

Osseous Neoplasms

Pure osteosarcoma can account for as many as 12% of primary breast sarcomas. Mean age in a large study was 64 years.[79] Coarse calcification is seen mammographically and produces a gritty sensation when sectioned. Osteosarcoma is often well demarcated and varies from hard to somewhat firm depending on the amount of osseous differentiation. Microscopy shows malignant spindle, stellate, and variably pleomorphic cells intimately associated with osteoid production.[79,80] Osteoid varies from thin, lacelike eosinophilic stroma to thick, bony trabeculae. Five-year survival is 38%, with the lungs a favored metastatic site. Metaplastic carcinoma or malignant PT with heterologous chondro-osseous differentiation must be excluded.

REFERENCES

1. Moore MP, Kinne DW: Breast sarcoma. Surg Clin North Am 76: 383–392, 1996.
2. May D, Stroup N: The incidence of sarcomas of the breast among women in the US 1973–1986. Plast Reconstr Surg 87:193–194, 1991.
3. Engel A, Lamm S, Lai S: Human breast sarcoma and human breast implantation: a time trend analysis based on SEER data (1973–1990). J Clin Epidemiol 48:539–544, 1995.
4. Adem C, Reynolds C, Ingle JN, et al: Primary breast sarcoma: Clinicopathologic series from the Mayo clinic and review of the literature. Br J Cancer 91:237–241, 2004.
5. Rosen PP (ed): Fibroepithelial lesions. In Rosen's breast pathology, 2nd ed. Philadelphia, Lippincott Williams & Wilkins, 2001, pp 163–200.
6. Kuijper A, Mommers ECM, van der Wall E, et al: Histopathology of fibroadenoma of the breast. Am J Clin Pathol 115:736–742, 2001.
7. Rowell MD, Perry RR, Hsiu JG, et al: Phyllodes tumor. Am J Surg 165:376–379, 1993.
8. Grabowski J, Salzstein SL, Sadler GR, et al: Malignant phyllodes tumors: A review of 752 cases. Am Surg 73:967–969, 2007.
9. Tan PH, Jayabaskar T, Chuah KL, et al: Phyllodes tumor of the breast: The role of pathologic parameters. Am J Clin Pathol 123: 529–540, 2005.
10. Kleer CG, Giordano TJ, Braun T, et al: Pathologic, immunohistochemical, and molecular features of benign and malignant phyllodes tumors of the breast. Mod Pathol 14:185–190, 2001.
11. Moffatt CJC, Pinder SE, Dixon AR, et al: Phyllodes tumours of the breast: A clinicopathological review of 32 cases. Histopathology 27:205–218, 1995.
12. Bellocq JP, Magro G: Fibroepithelial tumours. In Tavassoli FA, Devilee P (eds): World Health Organization classification of tumours. Pathology and genetics of tumours of the breast and female genital organs. Lyon, France, IARC Press, 2003, pp 100–103.
13. Powell CM, Cranor ML, Rosen PP: Multinucleated stromal giant cells in mammary fibroepithelial neoplasms: A study of 11 patients. Arch Pathol Lab Med 118:912–916, 1994.
14. Lee AH, Hodi Z, Ellis IO, et al: Histological features useful in the distinction of phyllodes tumour and fibroadenoma on needle core biopsy of the breast. Histopathology 51:336–344, 2007.
15. Tse GMK, Putti TC, Kung FYL, et al: Increased p53 protein expression in malignant mammary phyllodes tumors. Mod Pathol 15:734–740, 2002.
16. Kersting C, Kuijper A, Schmidt H, et al: Amplifications of the epidermal growth factor receptor gene (EGFR) are common in phyllodes tumors of the breast and are associated with tumor progression. Lab Invest 86:54–61, 2006.
17. Tse GMK, Lee CS, Kung FYL, et al: Hormonal receptors expression in epithelial cells of mammary phyllodes tumors correlates with pathologic grade of the tumor: A multicenter study of 143 cases. Am J Clin Pathol 118:522–526, 2002.

18. Chen WH, Cheng SP, Tzen CY, et al: Surgical treatment of phyllodes tumors of the breast: Retrospective review of 172 cases. J Surg Oncol 91:185–194, 2005.

19. Ben Hassouna J, Damak T, Gamoudi A, et al: Phyllodes tumors of the breast: A case series of 106 patients. Am J Surg 192:141–147, 2006.

20. Wargotz E, Norris HJ, Austin RM, et al: Fibromatosis of the breast. A clinical and pathological study of 28 cases. Am J Surg Pathol 11:38–45, 1987.

21. Devouassoux-Shisheboran M, Schammel MD, Man YG, et al: Fibromatosis of the breast: Age-correlated morphofunctional features of 33 cases. Arch Pathol Lab Med 124:276–80, 2000.

22. Deyrup AT, Tretikova M, Montag AG: Estrogen receptor-β expression in extraabdominal fibromatoses; an analysis of 40 cases. Cancer 106:208–213, 2006.

23. Wargotz ES, Weiss SW, Norris HJ: Myofibroblastoma of the breast: Sixteen cases of a distinctive benign mesenchymal tumor. Am J Surg Pathol 11:493–502, 1987.

24. Fukunaga M, Ushigome S: Myofibroblastoma of the breast with diverse differentiations. Arch Pathol Lab Med 121:599–603, 1997.

25. Magro G, Michal M, Bisceglia M: Benign spindle cell tumors of the mammary stroma: Diagnostic criteria, classification, and histogenesis. Pathol Res Pract 197:453–466, 2001.

26. Hamele-Bena D, Cranor ML, Sciotto C, et al: Uncommon presentation of mammary myofibroblastoma. Mod Pathol 9:786–790, 1996.

27. Magro G, Bisceglia M, Michal M: Expression of steroid hormone receptors, their regulated proteins, and bcl-2 protein in myofibroblastoma of the breast. Histopathology 36:515–521, 2000.

28. Arias-Stella J, Rosen PP: Hemangiopericytoma of the breast. Mod Pathol 1:98–103, 1988.

29. Salomao DR, Crotty TB, Nascimento AG: Myofibroblastoma and solitary fibrous tumor of the breast: Histopathologic and immunohistochemical studies. Breast 10:49–54, 2001.

30. Rosen PP (ed): Benign mesenchymal neoplasms. In Rosen's breast pathology, 2nd ed. Philadelphia, Lippincott Williams & Wilkins, 2001, pp 757–766.

31. Drijkoningen M, Tavassoli FA, Magro G, et al: In Tavassoli FA, Devilee P (eds): World Health Organization classification of tumours. Pathology and genetics of tumours of the breast and female genital organs. Lyon, France, IARC Press, 2003, pp 90–91.

32. Vuitch MF, Rosen PP, Erlandson RA: Pseudoangiomatous hyperplasia of mammary stroma. Hum Pathol 17:185–191, 1986.

33. Powell CM, Cramer ML, Rosen PP: Pseudoangiomatous stromal hyperplasia (PASH). A mammary stromal tumor with myofibroblastic differentiation. Am J Surg Pathol 19:270–277, 1995.

34. Ferreira M, Albarracin CT, Resetkova E: Pseudoangiomatous stromal hyperplasia tumor: A clinical radiologic and pathologic study of 26 cases. Mod Pathol 21:201–207, 2008.

35. Anderson C, Ricci A Jr, Pedersen CA, et al: Immunocytochemical analysis of estrogen and progesterone receptors in benign stromal lesions of the breast. Evidence for hormonal etiology in pseudoangiomatous hyperplasia of mammary stroma. Am J Surg Pathol 15:145–149, 1991.

36. Kijima Y, Umekita Y, Yoshinaka H, et al: Stromal sarcoma with features of giant cell malignant fibrous histiocytoma. Breast Cancer 14:239–244, 2007.

37. Jones MW, Norris HJ, Wargotz ES, et al: Fibrosarcoma-malignant fibrous histiocytoma of the breast. A clinicopathologic study of 32 cases. Am J Surg Pathol 16:667–674, 1992.

38. Rosen PP, Jozefczyk MA, Boram LH: Vascular tumors of the breast. IV. Venous hemangioma. Am J Surg Pathol 9:659–665, 1985.

39. Jozefczyk MA, Rosen PP: Vascular tumors of the breast. II. Perilobular hemangiomas and hemangiomas. Am J Surg Pathol 9:491–503, 1985.

40. Lesueur GC, Brown RW, Bhathal PS: Incidence of perilobular hemangioma in the female breast. Arch Pathol Lab Med 107:308–10, 1983.

41. Brenn T, Fletcher CDM: Radiation-associated cutaneous atypical vascular lesions and angiosarcoma: Clinicopathologic analysis of 42 cases. Am J Surg Pathol 29:983–996, 2005.

42. Fineberg S, Rosen PP: Cutaneous angiosarcoma and atypical vascular lesions of the skin and breast after radiation therapy for breast carcinoma. Am J Clin Pathol 102:757–763, 1994.

43. Gengler C, Coindre J-M, Leroux A, et al: Vascular proliferations of the skin after radiation therapy for breast cancer: clinicopathologic analysis of a series in favor of a benign process. A study from the French sarcoma group. Cancer 109:1584–1598, 2007.

44. Branton PA, Lininger R, Tavassoli FA: Papillary endothelial hyperplasia of the breast: the great impostor for angiosarcoma. Int J Surg Pathol 11:83–87, 2003.

45. Rosen PP: Vascular tumors of the breast: III. Angiomatosis. Am J Surg Pathol 9:652–658, 1985.

46. Insabato L, DiVizio D, Terracciano LM, et al: Epithelioid hemangioendothelioma of the breast. Breast 8:295–297, 1999.

47. Marsh Rde W, Walker MH, Jacob G, Liu C: Breast implants as a possible etiology of epithelioid hemangioendothelioma and successful therapy with interferon-alpha2. Breast J 11:257–261, 2005.

48. Blanchard DK, Reynolds CA, Grant CS, et al: Primary nonphyllodes breast sarcomas. Am J Surg 186:357–361, 2003.

49. Callery C, Rosen PP, Kinne D: Sarcoma of the breast: A study of 32 patients with reappraisal of classification and therapy. Ann Surg 201:527–532, 1985.

50. Donnell RM, Rosen PP, Lieberman PH, et al: Angiosarcoma and other vascular tumors of the breast. Pathologic analysis as a guide to prognosis. Am J Surg Pathol 5:629–642, 1981.

51. Drijkoningen M, Tavassoli FA, Magro G, et al: In Tavassoli FA, Devilee P (eds): World Health Organization classification of tumours. Pathology and genetics of tumours of the breast and female genital organs. Lyon, France IARC Press, 2003, pp 94–96.

52. Chen KTK, Kirkegaard DD, Bocian JJ: Angiosarcoma of the breast. Cancer 46:368–371, 1980.

53. Merino MJ, Carter D, Berman M: Angiosarcoma of the breast. Am J Surg Pathol 7:53–60, 1983.

54. Rossi S, Orvieto E, Furlanetto A, et al: Utility of the immunohistochemical detection of FLI-1 expression in round cell and vascular neoplasm using a monoclonal antibody. Mod Pathol 17:547–552, 2004.

55. Rosen PP, Kimmel M, Ernsberger D: Mammary angiosarcoma. The prognostic significance of tumor differentiation. Cancer 62:2145–2151, 1988.

56. Stewart FW, Treves N: Lymphangiosarcoma in postmastectomy lymphedema. A report of 6 cases in elephantiasis chirurgica. Cancer 1:64–81, 1948.

57. Woodward AH, Ivins JC, Soule EH: Lymphangiosarcoma arising in chronic lymphedematous extremities. Cancer 30:562–572, 1972.

58. Strobbe LJ, Peterse HL, van Tinteren H, et al: Angiosarcoma of the breast after conservation therapy for invasive cancer, the incidence and outcome. An unforeseen sequela. Breast Cancer Res Treat 47:101–109, 1998.

59. Cafiero F, Gipponi M, Peressini A, et al: Radiation associated angiosarcoma: Diagnostic and therapeutic implications—two case reports and review of the literature. Cancer 77:2496–2505, 1996.

60. Monroe AT, Fiegenberg S, Mendenhall N: Angiosarcoma after breast-conserving therapy. Cancer 97:1832–1840, 2003.

61. Yap J, Chuba PJ, Thomas R, et al: Sarcoma as a second malignancy after treatment for breast cancer. Int J Radiat Oncol Biol Phys 52:1231–1237, 2002.

62. Karlsson P, Holmberg E, Samuelsson A, et al: Soft tissue sarcoma after treatment for breast cancer—a Swedish population based study. Eur J Cancer 34:2068–2075, 1998.

63. West JG, Qureshi A, West JE, et al: Risk of angiosarcoma following breast conservation: A clinical alert. Breast J 11:115–123, 2005.

64. Huang J, Mackillop WJ: Increased risk of soft tissue sarcoma after radiotherapy in women with breast carcinoma. Cancer 92:172–180, 2001.

65. Billings SD, McKenney JK, Folpe AL, et al: Cutaneous angiosarcoma following breast-conserving surgery and radiation: An analysis of 27 cases. Am J Surg Pathol 28:781–788, 2004.

66. Rosen PP: Vascular tumors of the breast. V. Nonparenchymal hemangiomas of mammary subcutaneous tissues. Am J Surg Pathol 9:723–729, 1985.

67. Yu GH, Fishman SJ, Brooks JS: Cellular angiolipoma of the breast. Mod Pathol 6:497–499, 1993.

68. Powell CM, Rosen PP: Adipose differentiation in cystosarcoma phyllodes. Am J Surg Pathol 18:720–727, 1994.

69. Austin RM, Dupree WB: Liposarcoma of the breast: a clinicopathologic study of 20 cases. Hum Pathol 17:906–913, 1986.

70. Adeniran A, Al-Ahmadie H, Mahoney MC, et al: Granular cell tumor of the breast: A series of 17 cases and review of the literature. Breast J 10:528–531, 2004.

71. Gibbons D, Leitch M, Coscia J, et al: Fine needle aspiration cytology and histologic findings of granular cell tumor of the breast: Review of 19 cases with clinical radiologic correlation. Breast J 6:27–30, 2000.

72. Fanburg-Smith JC, Meis-Kindblom JM, Fante R, et al: Malignant granular cell tumor of soft tissue: Diagnostic criteria and clinicopathologic correlation. Am J Surg Pathol 22:779–794, 1998.

73. Falconieri G, Della D, Zanconati F, et al: Leiomyosarcoma of the female breast: Report of two new cases and review of the literature. Am J Clin Pathol 108:19–25, 1997.

74. Parham DM, Robertson AJ, Hussein KA, et al: Leiomyosarcoma of the breast: Cytological and histological features with a review of the literature. Cytopathology 3:245–252, 1992.

75. Chen KTK, Kuo T-T, Hoffman KD: Leiomyosarcoma of the breast: A case of long survival and late hepatic metastases. Cancer 47:1883–1886, 1981.

76. Hays DM, Donaldson SS, Shimada H, et al: Primary and metastatic rhabdomyosarcoma in the breast: Neoplasms of adolescent females, a report from the Intergroup Rhabdomyosarcoma Study. Med Pediatr Oncol 29:181–189, 1997.

77. Nishio J, Althof PA, Bailey JM, et al: Use of a novel FISH assay on paraffin-embedded tissues as an adjunct to diagnosis of alveolar rhabdomyosarcoma. Lab Invest 86:547–556, 2006.

78. Crist WM, Anderson JR, Meza JL, et al: Intergroup rhabdomyosarcoma study. IV: Results for patients with nonmetastatic disease. J Clin Oncol 19:3091–3102, 2001.

79. Silver SA, Tavassoli FA: Primary osteogenic sarcoma of the breast: A clinicopathologic analysis of 50 cases. Am J Surg Pathol 22:925–933, 1998.

80. Bahrami A, Resetkova E, Ro JY, et al: Primary osteosarcoma of the breast: Report of 2 cases. Arch Pathol Lab Med 131:792–795, 2007.

chapter 14

Paget's Disease of the Breast

RAFAEL E. JIMENEZ

Paget's disease (PD) of the breast or nipple is an eczematous condition in the nipple and areolar skin, which is histologically characterized by the presence of neoplastic cells of glandular differentiation interspersed within the keratinocytes of the epidermis. In approximately 90% of cases, the condition is associated with an in situ or invasive breast carcinoma, whether detected previously, simultaneously, or subsequently to its diagnosis. PD constitutes approximately 1% of the cases of breast carcinoma diagnosed in the United States.[1,2]

PD was described in 1874 by Sir James Paget, who considered it a preneoplastic or paraneoplastic process preceding the appearance of breast carcinoma.[3] Not until 1904 did Jacobaeus describe the histopathology of PD and propose that it represented spread of carcinoma cells into the epidermis of the nipple from an underlying preexisting neoplasm.[4] Today, this is the most accepted theory regarding the pathogenesis of this entity, although alternative mechanisms are still defended by some.

According to recently published data from the Surveillance, Epidemiology, and End Results (SEER) registry of the National Cancer Institute,[1] despite an increase of 10% in the incidence of both invasive and in situ ductal carcinomas of the breast from 1988 to 2002, the incidence of PD decreased by 45% in the same period. Eighty-six percent of cases were associated with an underlying invasive or in situ carcinoma. The median age of presentation was 62 years, although it was reported as 70 in a Scandinavian study.[2]

Clinical Presentation

PD usually presents as a chronic eczematous lesion in the nipple or—in more advanced cases—also involves the adjacent areolar skin (Fig. 14-1). This finding is present in 25% to 98% of cases, depending on the series.[2,5–10] Rare cases of involvement of the chest skin beyond the breast have been reported.[11] Nipple erythema or ulceration is also fairly common. As many as 20% of patients may have symptoms lasting for more than a year before seeking medical attention.[2] Even then, diagnosis may be delayed, because some symptoms may improve with topical medication. Nipple inversion can be present in as many as 20% of cases, and nipple discharge has been reported in as many as 36% of patients.[5] Other symptoms centered in the nipple include pruritus, pain, and induration.[6] As many as 40% of women have a palpable mass on presentation, and some may present with enlarged axillary lymph nodes.[6] A case associated with surrounding ipsilateral eruptive seborrheic keratoses (Leser Trélat sign) has been reported.[12] Asymptomatic cases may occur in 22% to 67% of cases, depending on the series.[7–10] In these cases, the patient usually has undergone surgery for a clinically detected breast cancer, and histologic changes of PD are found in the resection specimen.

Radiologic Findings

Only about 35% to 50% of patients with PD have a mammographic abnormality suggestive of malignancy.[8,9] Of the patients who present with PD without an underlying palpable breast mass, about 50% have negative mammographies; about 30% have abnormalities limited to the nipple-areolar-subareolar region, including nipple thickening, retroareolar mass, nipple retraction, or calcifications; and 20% have abnormalities in the breast parenchyma, including calcifications or suspicious masses.[9] In contrast, more than 90% of patients who present primarily with a palpable mass in which PD was detected subsequently to the excision of the mass have an abnormal mammogram. Most patients with a normal mammogram are associated with ductal carcinoma in situ (DCIS).[9] In the series of Ikeda and colleagues, invasive carcinoma was present in 5.5% of patients with negative mammograms, 60% of patients with microcalcifications, and 82% of patients with mammographic findings of a mass.[9] Ultrasound demonstrates a primary tumor in as many as 67% of cases,[8] including those in which the mammography is negative. Most commonly, ultrasonography reveals an image of a mass or, occasionally, more subtle changes such as parenchymal heterogeneity and hypoechogenic areas. Magnetic resonance imaging (MRI) is increasingly being used,

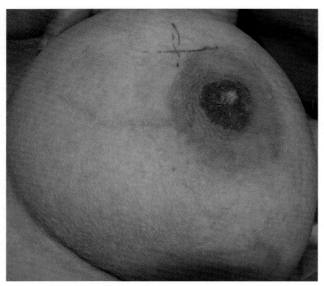

Figure 14-1 Classic presentation of Paget's disease, with scaling and crusting of nipple and areolar and periareolar skin. (Courtesy of Dr. Doreen Agnese, MD, The Ohio State University Department of Surgery.)

particularly in cases without a palpable mass, ultrasonographic, or mammographic findings.[13] It may reveal thickening and enhancement of the nipple, and may detect underlying foci of DCIS when is not otherwise evident. In the series of Frei and associates, eight of nine cases of PD and underlying DCIS were associated with abnormal findings on MRI.[14] MRI may be particularly useful to establish extent of disease in patients in which breast-conserving surgery is being contemplated.[14]

Histopathology

The hallmark of PD is the presence of neoplastic cells within the epidermis that show abundant clear cytoplasm and tend to spread individually in between the native keratinocytes (Fig. 14-2). These cells can be present in any layer of the epidermis; they are usually more numerous in the basal strata and can form intraepidermal aggregates and even glandular structures.[15,16] They are also pleomorphic and display prominent nucleoli and frequent mitoses. In addition, they commonly show intracytoplasmic mucin-filled vacuoles in as many as 25% to 50% of cases,[17,18] which are highlighted with a periodic-acid-Schiff or mucicarmine stain. The epidermis can show hyperkeratosis, hyperplasia, or ulceration, with frequent crusting. The underlying dermis shows reactive changes, including frequent lymphoplasmacytic infiltrate and hypervascularity.

The neoplastic cells (commonly referred to as Paget cells) often extend into the underlying lactiferous ducts. Involvement of the deeper portions of these is denser and can merge imperceptively with underlying DCIS, which is more often high nuclear grade, and of solid or comedo type. Association with lobular carcinoma in situ has been reported, although it is extremely rare.[19,20] In these cases, bilateral PD may be present.[20]

When an invasive component is present, it is usually of ductal type and high histologic grade. Most often it is located in the central portion of the breast, occasionally abutting the dermis. However, relatively distant or even peripheral tumors can be seen, connected to the PD through ducts involved by DCIS.

Paget cells are usually positive for markers of breast epithelium differentiation. As opposed to the surrounding epidermis they are frequently positive for cytokeratin 7, CAM 5.2, and other low-molecular-weight cytokeratins, and negative for high-molecular-weight cytokeratins.[21,22] They usually show expression of MUC1, carcinoembryonic antigen, epithelial membrane antigen, and occasionally gross fluid cystic disease protein. The vast majority of cases show strong overexpression of the HER2/neu protein[23] and amplification of the gene.[24] This is not surprising, because the majority of underlying in situ or invasive tumors are high grade and frequently overexpress HER2/neu. This would also explain the relatively low frequency of estrogen or progesterone receptor expression in PD.[23]

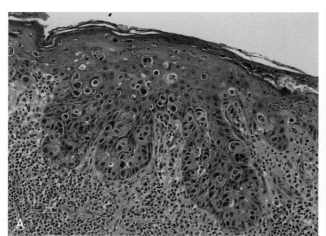
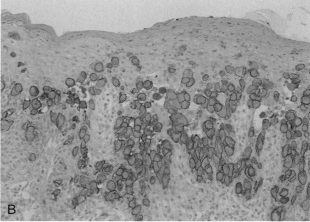

Figure 14-2 **A,** Classic histologic picture of Paget's disease, with neoplastic cells with clear cytoplasm and pleomorphic nuclei interspersed within native keratinocytes. Notice the concentration of the neoplastic cells in the basal layers of the epidermis. **B,** Tumor cells are positive for *HER2/neu* overexpression.

As many as 18% of Paget's cells express S100 protein,[25] in keeping with the occasional expression of this marker by breast carcinomas. However, contrary to melanoma cells, HMB45 is consistently negative.

Pathogenesis

The most accepted explanation for the development of PD is that Paget cells result from the migration of cells from the underlying adenocarcinoma through the epidermis, the so-called epidermotropic theory. This theory is supported by the existence of an underlying carcinoma in about 90% of cases of PD, which usually shares phenotypic similarities with Paget cells.[26] Further support for this theory comes from the recently reported decrease in incidence of PD despite an increase in breast cancer incidence, suggesting that the former is a result of earlier detection of tumors at a point prior to the spread of malignant cells into the epidermis.[1] The occurrence of secondary PD also supports an epidermotropic mechanism for this phenomenon. In these cases, PD is seen surrounding an area in the skin that has been directly invaded by a tumor,[17] not necessarily in the proximity of the nipple, suggesting a tumoral origin of the Paget cells. Recently, a molecular mechanism has been proposed to explain the migration capabilities of Paget cells.[27] According to this model, heregulin-α is produced by keratinocytes, as demonstrated by the presence of heregulin-α messenger RNA in skin keratinocytes. This factor induces spreading, motility, and chemotaxis of cultured breast cancer cells, a phenomenon likely mediated through its binding to HER3 or HER4 receptors, which in turn are dimerized to highly overexpressed HER2. Migration capability of cultured cells was inhibited when they were previously exposed to monoclonal antibody AB2 directed against the extracellular domain of HER2/neu.[27] Vimentin expression in breast cancer cell lines has also been associated with increased motility and invasiveness in vitro.[28,29] In one study,[30] vimentin expression was found in 44.7% of cases of mammary PD, suggesting a potential role of this intermediate filament in cell motility and migration.

On the other hand, approximately 10% of cases of PD are not associated with an underlying breast cancer. Some studies have shown genotypic differences between Paget cells and underlying carcinoma cells.[31] Furthermore, some cases of PD associated with underlying DCIS show large portions of the ducts between both processes uninvolved by neoplastic changes (i.e., skipped areas).[32] These findings have prompted an alternative explanation of PD histogenesis, which is commonly referred to as the intraepidermal transformation theory. This hypothesis maintains that Paget cells arise in situ from transformation of multipotential cells in the epidermis or from the terminal portion of the lactiferous duct at its junction with the epidermis.[32,33] The occurrence of extramammary PD (i.e., presence of similar histologic findings in other sites of the body) gives further support to this theory, particularly because extramammary PD is much less often associated with an underlying malignancy.

At the core of this theory are Toker cells, which are considered by some to be precursors of PD. Toker cells are inconspicuous clear cells that are predominantly located immediately above the opening of the lactiferous sinuses.[34] They are detected in 10% of nipples with routine histology but in as many as 83% of cases when immunohistochemical stains are used.[35] They are distributed in a dispersed fashion within the epidermis, mainly as scattered individual cells. Their cytomorphologic features are bland, without suggestion of malignancy (Fig. 14-3). Ultrastructurally they are globoid with dendritic cytoplasmic projections, and they are distinct from surrounding keratinocytes, Langerhans cells, melanocytes, and Merkel cells.[36] Toker cells are immunophenotypically similar to Paget cells, sharing expression of cytokeratin 7 and CAM 5.2, absence of high-molecular-weight cytokeratin expression, and negative S100- and HMB45-expression.[35–37] They differ in the negative expression of mucin, HER2/neu, and epithelial membrane antigen.[36,38] The similarities between Toker and Paget cells have suggested that the former may represent the cell that undergoes malignant transformation in the initial phases of PD.[36] A case reported of PD confined to the areola associated with multifocal Toker cell hyperplasia suggests that indeed Toker cells play a significant role in the pathogenesis of PD.[39] Whether Toker cells themselves are the result of upward migration of ductal cells into the epidermis, or on the contrary represent an in situ transformation of keratinocytes, is still unresolved.[35,38,40] Other authors have suggested that Paget cells derive directly from altered keratinocytes, a suggestion that has been supported by the finding of desmosomes between Paget cells and adjacent keratinocytes.[33] Chen and colleagues reported that despite steadily decreasing incidence rates of PD with an underlying tumor between 1988 and 2002, the incidence rates of PD without an underlying tumor remained unchanged.[1] These data suggest that although a majority of cases of PD originate by epidermotropic extension of preexisting tumor cells, a smaller proportion (i.e., those without an underlying malignancy) do appear to arise from intraepidermal transformation.

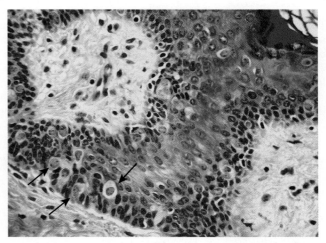

Figure 14-3 Toker cells are seen in a large proportion of normal nipples *(arrows)*. They are believed to be cells of lactiferous duct origin, migrating into the epidermis of the nipple. Notice the similarities with Paget cells, except for their bland cytologic features.

Differential Diagnosis

CLINICAL

PD of the nipple presents as a chronic eczematous condition involving the nipple and the areola. As such, other eczematous conditions are necessarily in the differential diagnosis and are probably more often considered before PD, particularly when a breast mass is not detected. These conditions include dermatophyte infection, psoriasis, contact dermatitis, and erosive nipple adenoma (see later discussion).[41,42] A case of pemphigus vulgaris mimicking PD has been reported.[43] A thorough clinical examination may be valuable in differentiating these conditions; it may reveal systemic changes that could orient the diagnosis. The finding of a palpable breast mass is an ominous sign that points to the diagnosis of PD. Ultimately, tissue examination may be necessary to reach a conclusive diagnosis.

Primary malignant melanoma of the nipple is an infrequent event, and in most reported cases PD was a strong consideration in the differential diagnosis; it could not be disproved until a biopsy was performed.[44,45] Similarly, PD can mimic malignant melanoma, because not infrequently Paget cells can be hyperpigmented.[46] Tissue diagnosis is mandatory to exclude these two entities.

Clinicians have several options to obtain tissue to exclude a diagnosis of PD. A wedge biopsy of the skin and underlying breast tissue renders the most diagnostic material, because it includes a well-represented epidermis and usually underlying lactiferous ducts. A punch biopsy may have a lower diagnostic yield because of the discontinuous nature of Paget cells. A shave biopsy frequently is unsuccessful, because the abundance of keratinized debris and exudate usually predominates over diagnostic material. Scraping or imprint of the nipple surface is an affordable and accessible method for rapid diagnosis, although data on sensitivity and specificity of the technique is limited.[47–49]

PATHOLOGIC

The histopathologic differential diagnosis of PD includes a series of conditions that may display intraepidermal clear cells, a histologic picture also known as a pagetoid pattern. These include non-neoplastic conditions, benign pathologic processes, and other malignancies[37] (Table 14-1).

Glycogenated squamous cells are frequently seen in the nipple epidermis. They constitute keratinocytes with accumulated glycogen within their cytoplasm, giving them the appearance of clear cells interspersed within more classic keratinocytes. These cells usually show a pyknotic angulated nucleus, and the surrounding cytoplasm appears empty on routine histology. They are predominantly located in the midepidermis.[17] Some authors consider them to be reactive in nature and refer to them as pagetoid dyskeratosis.[50,51] Toker cells, as described previously, are benign clear cells seen normally in the nipple epidermis. As discussed, they are immunoreactive with cytokeratin 7 and likely represent benign ductal cells extending into the epidermis. They differ from Paget cells in that they do not show cytologic features of malignancy and are consistently negative for HER2/neu and epithelial membrane antigen.

Nipple adenoma is part of the differential diagnosis not only because it may clinically present as an eczematous lesion in the nipple, but also because it is usually associated with Toker cell hyperplasia, mimicking PD.[38,41] Nipple adenomas are localized lesions characterized by an adenomatous proliferation of ducts and tubules and associated with florid epithelial and myoepithelial cell hyperplasia, usually within a desmoplastic stroma. The architectural complexity of the lesion may be confused with invasive or in situ carcinoma, leading to the erroneous interpretation of the associated Toker cell hyperplasia as PD. If in doubt, a HER2/neu stain can help in determining the exact nature of these cells.

Squamous cell carcinoma in situ or Bowen's disease can present with a pagetoid pattern. This variant shows isolated atypical keratinocytes dispersed in the epidermis, usually on a background of normally maturing cells. Contrary to Paget cells, these cells can show single cell keratinization, intercellular bridges and cytoplasmic keratohyaline granules. Frequently, also, the lesion is associated with classic Bowen disease nearby. In difficult cases, immunophenotyping resolves the issue, because these cells are negative for cytokeratin 7 and CAM 5.2 and positive for high-molecular-eight cytokeratin.[21]

Malignant melanoma is, as stated, not only a seriously considered differential diagnosis clinically but also pathologically. Paget cells frequently incorporate melanin from adjacent epidermal cells, further complicating the histologic picture. However, as stated, primary malignant melanoma of the nipple is a very infrequent disease that should not be diagnosed before thoroughly excluding the possibility of PD. Immunohistochemistry is usually helpful, because Paget cells are negative for HMB45 negative and positive for cytokeratin 7, whereas melanoma

TABLE 14-1

Differential Expression of Immunohistochemical Markers in Entities Potentially Confused with Paget's Disease

	Cytokeratin 7	CAM 5.2	HMWCK	S100	HMB-45	HER2/neu
Paget's disease	+++	+++	−	+/−	−	+++
Toker cells	+++	+++	−	−	−	−
Malignant melanoma	−	−	−	+++	+++	−
Bowens disease	−	−	+++	−	−	−

+++, consistently expressed; −, consistently nonexpressed; +/−, variable expression; HMWCK, high-molecular-weight cytokeratin.

cells show the opposite immunophenotype. As mentioned, S100 protein is not useful in this differential diagnosis, because some cases of PD may show positivity for this marker.

Other diagnoses that enter in the differential algorithm of a pagetoid histologic pattern include more exotic entities, such as pagetoid Spitz nevus, clear cell papulosis, sebaceous carcinoma, Merkel cell carcinoma, eccrine porocarcinoma, cutaneous T-cell lymphoma, and histiocytosis X.[37] Adequate histologic sampling and judicious use of immunohistochemistry usually suffice to arrive to the correct diagnosis.

Management

Surgical management for PD has traditionally consisted of radical mastectomy.[19,52] Although this is most likely a reflection of the historical management of breast cancer, other arguments have been mentioned to support maintaining this treatment modality, despite the general trend to offer a more conservative treatment for other forms of breast cancer. Arguments favoring a more radical approach to the surgical management of PD include the difficulty in establishing preoperatively the extent of the underlying malignancy in patients with PD and a higher aggressive behavior of tumors associated with PD. Zakaria and associates reported a series of cases of PD, in which 48.7% were associated with no clinically palpable mass and a benign mammography, implying that preoperative assessment may significantly underestimate the presence and extent of underlying disease.[53] Similarly, in the series of Kothari and coworkers, only 25% of cases had disease confined to the retroareolar region, and the true extent of disease was underestimated by mammography in 43% of cases.[5] Furthermore, 63% of cases with only clinical nipple abnormalities and no breast mass—a population that should benefit from less aggressive therapy—had multifocal or multicentric tumors, limiting the probabilities of performing breast-conserving surgery. In this same study, 60% of all underlying tumors were histologic grade III, and 82.5% were positive for HER2/neu overexpression, implying an aggressive phenotype that theoretically would require aggressive therapy.

Despite this reasoning, however, several studies have demonstrated the feasibility of breast-conserving therapy in patients with PD. Pierce and colleagues reported their experience with 30 cases from several collaborative institutions treated with local surgery and radiotherapy.[54] Of these, 29 patients had noninvasive disease. They found a 5- and 8-year local recurrence rate of 9% and 16%, respectively; these rates were very similar to those reported for cases of DCIS treated with radiotherapy in other parts of the breast. Seven years later, this group updated their data to report recurrence rates at 10 and 15 years post-treatment, which were 17% and 24%, respectively, and they reported 5-, 10-, and 15-year disease-free survival of 97%, 93%, and 93%, respectively.[55] A 2001 report of the European Organization for Research and Treatment of Cancer (EORTC) on a prospective study of 61 patients with PD treated with breast-conserving surgery and radiotherapy showed a 5.2% local recurrence rate at 5 years.[56] In all patients in this study, margins were required to be confirmed free by histologic analysis after surgery. Singh and associates reported a similar outcome in patients treated with mastectomy and patients treated with breast-conserving surgery.[57] Similarly, Kawase and coworkers reported no significant differences in overall, disease-specific, or recurrence-free survival between patients with PD treated with mastectomy and with breast-conserving surgery.[58] Joseph and colleagues also reported no difference in overall recurrence and mortality rates between patients treated with mastectomy and with breast conservation.[59] Radiotherapy, however, seems to be a mandatory adjuvant therapy in cases treated with breast-conserving surgery, to ensure adequate control rates. Dixon and associates reported that 4 of 10 patients treated with cone excision had local recurrences, with 2 patients developing metastatic disease eventually.[60] None of these patients received postoperative radiotherapy. More recently, Polgar and coworkers reported on 33 patients treated with cone excision without radiotherapy. The local recurrence rate was 33.3%, a much higher rate than that reported in series where adjuvant radiotherapy was used.[61]

Despite the data suggesting that breast-conserving surgery plus radiotherapy is an effective method of treating PD, mastectomy continues to be the most popular method of treatment. In recent data from SEER on 1642 women with PD who underwent surgery between 1988 and 2002,[1] 18% underwent central lumpectomy and 82% underwent mastectomy. Eighty-four percent of women with PD and invasive, centrally located tumors smaller than 2 cm underwent mastectomy rather than central lumpectomy, compared with 52% of those without PD that had similarly centrally located, small tumors. Similarly, 64% of women with centrally located DCIS associated with PD underwent mastectomy, compared with 37% of those with centrally located DCIS without PD during this same period. These data suggest a significant bias to perform mastectomy in PD, even in presence of tumors that would likely be managed more conservatively had they not presented with PD. In this analysis, the 15-year breast cancer-specific survival rate was 92% and 94% for patients who underwent central lumpectomy and mastectomy, respectively, for PD associated with noninvasive tumors. Similarly, the 15-year breast cancer-specific survival rate in patients who had PD with an underlying invasive tumor was 87% for patients who underwent central lumpectomy and 60% for patients who underwent mastectomy.

Evaluation of the axilla in patients with PD is determined by the type and stage of associated tumor. Thus, some groups have studied the feasibility of performing sentinel lymph node (SLN) biopsy in patients with PD. Sukumvanich and associates studied a cohort of patients with PD, which they divided into those presenting with PD alone (only nipple skin changes) versus those presenting as PD with associated findings (skin changes plus palpable mass or abnormal mammographic findings). They found a success rate of SLN biopsy of 98%, with a mean number of SLN removed of three. In the first group, 27% of patients had invasive ductal carcinoma, despite the absence of associated findings. In 11% of these, the SLN contained metastatic carcinoma.[62] Laronga and colleagues studied 54 patients with PD, 36 of which had been managed with SLN biopsy. In four of five patients with metastatic carcinoma, the metastasis was detected through SLN biopsy. In three of these, the SLN was the only lymph node positive for tumor, suggesting that SLN biopsy is an equally useful technique in this setting.[63] Thus, the limited published data suggest that SLN biopsy is a viable alternative in the management of patients with PD and should be used according to guidelines established for regular breast cancers.

Prognosis

Prognosis in PD is largely determined by the underlying breast tumor. Relatively little data exist on outcome of PD without an underlying breast carcinoma. In the previously mentioned SEER data report, the 15-year cancer-specific survival for PD without underlying tumors was 88%, compared with 94% for PD associated only with DCIS and 61% for PD associated with invasive ductal carcinoma.[1] It is known that tumors associated with PD usually have aggressive histologic features. In the same series, patients with PD were more likely to have histologically high-grade tumors, positive lymph nodes, negative estrogen receptor status, and negative progesterone receptor status, but only size of tumor and lymph node status were independent prognostic factors for survival on multivariate analysis.[1] Similarly, in the series of Kothari and coworkers, 60% of underlying invasive tumors were histologic grade III, 96.5% of the in situ tumors were high grade, and HER2/neu overexpression was present in 82.5% and 96.5 of invasive and in situ tumors, respectively.[5] This is not unexpected, considering the pivotal role that HER2/neu may have in the pathogenesis of PD.[27] However, the development of PD itself does not appear to confer additional prognostic impact to these tumors. In the same series,[5] patients with PD did not have a different overall survival rates than controls, when matched for age, tumor size, grade, nodal status, and HER2/neu status. Differences in survival based on the presence or absence of a palpable mass are explained by the fact that patients without a palpable mass are more likely to have noninvasive tumors, compared with patients with a palpable mass, which overwhelmingly have invasive tumors.[10,53] In one study, patients who presented without a palpable mass had a 5-year overall survival of 94%; 73% of them had only DCIS with no invasive component, and 84% had an N_0 nodal status. In contrast, patients who presented with a palpable mass had a 19% 5-year overall survival; only 8% of them had only DCIS with no invasive component, and only 50% had a N_0 nodal status.[10]

REFERENCES

1. Chen CY, Sun LM, Anderson BO: Paget disease of the breast: Changing patterns of incidence, clinical presentation, and treatment in the U.S. Cancer 107:1448–1458, 2006.
2. Dalberg K, Hellborg H, Warnberg F: Paget's disease of the nipple in a population based cohort. Breast Cancer Res Treat 111:313–319, 2008.
3. Paget J: On disease of the mammary areola preceding cancer of the mammary gland. St Bartholomew's Hosp Rep 10:87–89, 1874.
4. Jacobaeus H: Paget's disease und sein Verhültniss zum Milchdrüsenkarzinom. Virchows Arch 178:124–142, 1904.
5. Kothari AS, Beechey-Newman N, Hamed H, et al: Paget disease of the nipple: A multifocal manifestation of higher-risk disease. Cancer 95:1–7, 2002.
6. Jamali FR, Ricci A Jr, Deckers PJ: Paget's disease of the nipple-areola complex. Surg Clin North Am 76:365–381, 1996.
7. Fu W, Mittel VK, Young SC: Paget disease of the breast: Analysis of 41 patients. Am J Clin Oncol 24:397–400, 2001.
8. Gunhan-Bilgen I, Oktay A: Paget's disease of the breast: Clinical, mammographic, sonographic and pathologic findings in 52 cases. Eur J Radiol 60:256–263, 2006.
9. Ikeda DM, Helvie MA, Frank TS, et al: Paget disease of the nipple: Radiologic-pathologic correlation. Radiology 189:89–94, 1993.
10. Sheen-Chen SM, Chen HS, Chen WJ, et al: Paget disease of the breast—an easily overlooked disease? J Surg Oncol 76:261–265, 2001.
11. Kanwar AJ, De D, Vaiphei K, et al: Extensive mammary Paget's disease. Clin Exp Dermatol 32:326–327, 2007.
12. Shamsadini S, Wadji MB, Shamsadini A: Surrounding ipsilateral eruptive seborrheic keratosis as a warning sign of intraductal breast carcinoma and Paget's disease (Leser Trélat sign). Dermatol Online J 12:27, 2006.
13. Capobianco G, Spaliviero B, Dessole S, et al: Paget's disease of the nipple diagnosed by MRI. Arch Gynecol Obstet 274:316–318, 2006.
14. Frei KA, Bonel HM, Pelte MF, et al: Paget disease of the breast: Findings at magnetic resonance imaging and histopathologic correlation. Invest Radiol 40:363–367, 2005.
15. Barnes PJ, Dumont RJ, Higgins HG: Acinar pattern of mammary Paget's disease: A case report. Breast J 13:520–526, 2007.
16. Shousha S: Glandular Paget's disease of the nipple. Histopathology 50:812–814, 2007.
17. Rosen P: Rosen's breast pathology, 2nd ed. Philadelphia, Lippincott Williams & Wilkins, 2001.
18. Tavassoli F: Pathology of the breast, 2nd ed. New York, McGraw-Hill, 1999.
19. Ashikari R, Park K, Huvos AG, et al: Paget's disease of the breast. Cancer 26:680–685, 1970.
20. Sahoo S, Green I, Rosen PP: Bilateral Paget disease of the nipple associated with lobular carcinoma in situ. Arch Pathol Lab Med 126:90–92, 2002.
21. Lau J, Kohler S: Keratin profile of intraepidermal cells in Paget's disease, extramammary Paget's disease, and pagetoid squamous cell carcinoma in situ. J Cutan Pathol 30:449–454, 2003.
22. Liegl B, Leibl S, Gogg-Kamerer M, et al: Mammary and extramammary Paget's disease: An immunohistochemical study of 83 cases. Histopathology 50:439–447, 2007.
23. Fu W, Lobocki CA, Silberberg BK, et al: Molecular markers in Paget disease of the breast. J Surg Oncol 77:171–178, 2001.
24. Bianco MK, Vasef MA: HER-2 gene amplification in Paget disease of the nipple and extramammary site: A chromogenic in situ hybridization study. Diagn Mol Pathol 15:131–135, 2006.
25. Gillett CE, Bobrow LG, Millis RR: S100 protein in human mammary tissue—immunoreactivity in breast carcinoma, including Paget's disease of the nipple, and value as a marker of myoepithelial cells. J Pathol 160:19–24, 1990.
26. Cohen C, Guarner J, DeRose PB: Mammary Paget's disease and associated carcinoma. An immunohistochemical study. Arch Pathol Lab Med 117:291–294, 1993.
27. Schelfhout VR, Coene ED, Delaey B, et al: Pathogenesis of Paget's disease: Epidermal heregulin-alpha, motility factor, and the HER receptor family. J Natl Cancer Inst 92:622–628, 2000.
28. Hendrix MJ, Seftor EA, Chu YW, et al: Role of intermediate filaments in migration, invasion and metastasis. Cancer Metastasis Rev 15:507–525, 1996.
29. Hendrix MJ, Seftor EA, Seftor RE, et al: Experimental co-expression of vimentin and keratin intermediate filaments in human breast cancer cells results in phenotypic interconversion and increased invasive behavior. Am J Pathol 150:483–495, 1997.
30. Hanna W, Alowami S, Malik A: The role of HER-2/neu oncogene and vimentin filaments in the production of the Paget's phenotype. Breast J 9:485–490, 2003.

31. Morandi L, Pession A, Marucci GL, et al: Intraepidermal cells of Paget's carcinoma of the breast can be genetically different from those of the underlying carcinoma. Hum Pathol 34:1321–1330, 2003.

32. Mai KT, Yazdi HM, Perkins DG: Mammary Paget's disease: Evidence of diverse origin of the disease with a subgroup of Paget's disease developing from the superficial portion of lactiferous duct and a discontinuous pattern of tumor spread. Pathol Int 49:956–961, 1999.

33. Mai KT: Morphological evidence for field effect as a mechanism for tumour spread in mammary Paget's disease. Histopathology 35:567–576, 1999.

34. Toker C: Clear cells of the nipple epidermis. Cancer 25:601–610, 1970.

35. Lundquist K, Kohler S, Rouse RV: Intraepidermal cytokeratin 7 expression is not restricted to Paget cells but is also seen in Toker cells and Merkel cells. Am J Surg Pathol 23:212–219, 1999.

36. Marucci G, Betts CM, Golouh R, et al: Toker cells are probably precursors of Paget cell carcinoma: A morphological and ultrastructural description. Virchows Arch 441:117–123, 2002.

37. Kohler S, Rouse RV, Smoller BR: The differential diagnosis of pagetoid cells in the epidermis. Mod Pathol 11:79–92, 1998.

38. Zeng Z, Melamed J, Symmans PJ, et al: Benign proliferative nipple duct lesions frequently contain CAM 5.2 and anti-cytokeratin 7 immunoreactive cells in the overlying epidermis. Am J Surg Pathol 23:1349–1355, 1999.

39. van der Putte SC, Toonstra J, Hennipman A: Mammary Paget's disease confined to the areola and associated with multifocal Toker cell hyperplasia. Am J Dermatopathol 17:487–493, 1995.

40. Yao DX, Hoda SA, Chiu A, et al: Intraepidermal cytokeratin 7 immunoreactive cells in the non-neoplastic nipple may represent interepithelial extension of lactiferous duct cells. Histopathology 40:230–236, 2002.

41. Healy CE, Dijkstra B, Walsh M, et al: Nipple adenoma: A differential diagnosis for Paget's disease. Breast J 9:325–326, 2003.

42. Rolz-Cruz G, Kim CC: Tumor invasion of the skin. Dermatol Clin 26:89–102, 2008.

43. Guyton DP, Sloan Stakleff K, Regula E: Pemphigus vulgaris mimicking Paget's disease of the breast. Breast J 9:319–322, 2003.

44. Kinoshita S, Yoshimoto K, Kyoda S, et al: Malignant melanoma originating on the female nipple: A case report. Breast Cancer 14:105–108, 2007.

45. Lin CH, Lee HS, Yu JC: Melanoma of the nipple mimicking Paget's disease. Dermatol Online J 13:18, 2007.

46. Mitchell S, Lachica R, Randall MB, et al: Paget's disease of the breast areola mimicking cutaneous melanoma. Breast J 12:233–236, 2006.

47. Gupta RK, Simpson J, Dowle C: The role of cytology in the diagnosis of Paget's disease of the nipple. Pathology 28:248–250, 1996.

48. Lucarotti ME, Dunn JM, Webb AJ: Scrape cytology in the diagnosis of Paget's disease of the breast. Cytopathology 5:301–305, 1994.

49. Samarasinghe D, Frost F, Sterrett G, et al: Cytological diagnosis of Paget's disease of the nipple by scrape smears: a report of five cases. Diagn Cytopathol 9:291–295, 1993.

50. Garijo MF, Val D, Val-Bernal JF: Pagetoid dyskeratosis of the nipple epidermis: An incidental finding mimicking Paget's disease of the nipple. APMIS 116:139–146, 2008.

51. Tschen JA, McGavran MH, Kettler AH: Pagetoid dyskeratosis: A selective keratinocytic response. J Am Acad Dermatol 19:891–894, 1988.

52. Paone JF, Baker RR: Pathogenesis and treatment of Paget's disease of the breast. Cancer 48:825–829, 1981.

53. Zakaria S, Pantvaidya G, Ghosh K, et al: Paget's disease of the breast: Accuracy of preoperative assessment. Breast Cancer Res Treat 102:137–142, 2007.

54. Pierce LJ, Haffty BG, Solin LJ, et al: The conservative management of Paget's disease of the breast with radiotherapy. Cancer 80:1065–1072, 1997.

55. Marshall JK, Griffith KA, Haffty BG, et al: Conservative management of Paget disease of the breast with radiotherapy: 10- and 15-year results. Cancer 97:2142–2149, 2003.

56. Bijker N, Meijnen P, Peterse JL, et al: Breast-conserving treatment with or without radiotherapy in ductal carcinoma-in-situ: Ten-year results of European Organisation for Research and Treatment of Cancer randomized phase III trial 10853—a study by the EORTC Breast Cancer Cooperative Group and EORTC Radiotherapy Group. J Clin Oncol 24:3381–3387, 2006.

57. Singh A, Sutton RJ, Baker CB, et al: Is mastectomy overtreatment for Paget's disease of the nipple? Breast 8:191–194, 1999.

58. Kawase K, Dimaio DJ, Tucker SL, et al: Paget's disease of the breast: There is a role for breast-conserving therapy. Ann Surg Oncol 12:391–397, 2005.

59. Joseph KA, Ditkoff BA, Estabrook A, et al: Therapeutic options for Paget's disease: A single institution long-term follow-up study. Breast J 13:110–111, 2007.

60. Dixon AR, Galea MH, Ellis IO, et al: Paget's disease of the nipple. Br J Surg 78:722–723, 1991.

61. Polgar C, Orosz Z, Kovacs T, et al: Breast-conserving therapy for Paget disease of the nipple: A prospective European Organization for Research and Treatment of Cancer study of 61 patients. Cancer 94:1904–1905, 2002.

62. Sukumvanich P, Bentrem DJ, Cody HS III, et al: The role of sentinel lymph node biopsy in Paget's disease of the breast. Ann Surg Oncol 14:1020–1023, 2007.

63. Laronga C, Hasson D, Hoover S, et al: Paget's disease in the era of sentinel lymph node biopsy. Am J Surg 192:481–483, 2006.

Primary and Secondary Dermatologic Disorders of the Breast

MOHAMMAD S. DIAB | ANGELA SHEN |
JOHN DUNG HOANG PHAM | SARA B. PETERS

Overview

The skin of the breast, similar to other truncal skin, consists of keratinizing stratified squamous epithelium overlying a relatively thick dermis. Adnexal structures, primarily hair follicles and eccrine glands, blood vessels, lymphatics, and cutaneous nerves, reside within the dermis. The subcutaneous fatty tissue that envelops the mammary ducts and glands proliferates as a result of hormonal influences, especially at puberty and during pregnancy. The highly specialized skin of the nipple has a papillomatous surface and numerous openings for lactiferous ducts, sebaceous glands, and apocrine glands. Areolar skin is similar but may have a few vellus or terminal hairs and clusters of large sebaceous glands (the tubercles of Montgomery). These units also contain lactation ductlike foci that produce milklike substances.[1,2]

Numerous dermal disorders, including congenital anomalies, benign and malignant neoplasms, and manifestations of localized and systemic dermatoses, may involve the skin of the breast. In reviewing the dermatologic disorders of the breast, one useful approach is to divide these diverse disease entities into those primary diseases that are specific, nearly specific, or common for the skin of the breast and those secondary disorders that predominantly affect other dermatologic areas of the body but affect the breast incidentally or less commonly. Sometimes our decision to classify a disease as a primary versus a secondary breast disorder is arbitrary. Both types of dermatologic disorders also mimic primary or secondary diseases of the breast parenchyma. For all these reasons, it is important for both the breast generalist as well as the breast specialist to be versed in these primary and secondary dermatologic disorders of the breast.

Primary Breast Dermatologic Disorders

PRIMARY CONGENITAL AND DEVELOPMENTAL DISORDERS

Hypoplasia and associated Conditions

Bilateral hypoplasia of the breast may occur in Turner's (XO) syndrome. Hypomastia, defined as breast size of 200 mg (mL) or less in an adult female, may occur in otherwise healthy women or in association with mitral valve prolapse.[3] Acquired hypoplasia is associated with wasting diseases such as human immunodeficiency virus (HIV) infection, anorexia nervosa, and tuberculosis. Unilateral hypoplasia has been described in the Poland anomaly—unilateral absence of the sternocostal portion of the pectoralis major muscle, ipsilateral syndactyly, absence of axillary hair, and abnormal fingerprint patterns.[4] Unilateral hypoplasia has also been described in association with large, irregularly shaped melanotic macules that cover the hypoplastic breast and wrap laterally onto the back. Basilar hyperpigmentation of melanocytes without significant melanocytic hyperplasia or atypia is seen on histologic examination.[5] Morphea (localized scleroderma) of the chest wall in a prepubertal child may lead to deformity and hypoplasia of the breast in later years.[6] Other congenital neural syndromes may be associated with breast hypoplasia.[7–10]

Rudimentary (absent or maldeveloped) nipples may be present as an isolated congenital defect or as a component of the scalp-ears-nipple (SEN) syndrome.[11–13] This disorder is inherited in an autosomal dominant fashion. Cutaneous manifestations include aplasia cutis congenita of the scalp, protuberant cupped or folded external ears, and sparse axillary hair. The malformed nipple appears as a small dimple without pigmentation or recognizable structure; the breast may also fail to develop.

Hyperplasias and Hamartomas and associated Conditions

Polythelia (supernumerary nipples; Fig. 15-1) or polymastia (supernumerary breasts) develops along embryonic lines that stretch from the axillas to the inner thighs. Notably, vulvar lesions that previously were termed *supernumerary nipples* actually represent adenomas of vulvar apocrine—or mammary-like glands; the so-called milk lines do not cross the vulva. Most supernumerary breast tissue takes the form of insignificant, gently raised, pigmented papules. Histologically, these accessory structures may consist of nipple, areola, or glandular tissue in any combination. Microscopic sections of accessory mammary tissue are very similar to those of normal breast. The epidermis displays acanthosis with undulating papillomatosis and basal layer hyperpigmentation. In the dermis, smooth muscle bundles, mammary glands, and ducts are noted.

Becker's nevus is a hamartoma of pigmented epidermis, terminal hairs, and erector pili muscles usually found on the chest, shoulder, upper back, or upper arm. It is an androgen-dependent lesion that typically appears in males in the second and third decades but occasionally affects females. Rarely, this benign pigmented lesion is often mistaken clinically for a giant pigmented hairy melanocytic nevus. It is associated with abnormalities of the underlying musculoskeletal system, including spina bifida, scoliosis, localized lipoatrophy, and hypoplasia of the pectoralis muscle, which can lead to hypoplasia or compensatory hyperplasia of the breast.

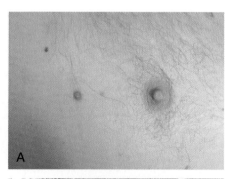
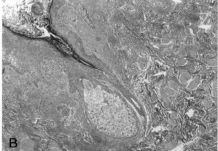

Figure 15-1 **A,** Accessory nipple is observed inferior to main nipple. **B,** Histologically the accessory nipple may consist of a ductal orifice as well as areolar-type smooth muscle fascicles.

Hyperplasia, adenomas, and rarely carcinomas can involve these tissues, as they do the breast proper. In a study from Japan, small benign adnexal polyps of the areola were reported to involve 4% of neonates. These small (1-mm), firm, pink papules contain hair follicles, eccrine glands, and vestigial sebaceous glands. Most wither rapidly and fall off shortly after birth.[14] The rare familial syndrome of hereditary acrolabial telangiectasia, a type of hamartoma, consists of an extensive network of superficial, thin-walled vessels and variable proliferation of vessels in the deeper soft tissues. These superficial vessels impart a bluish hue to the lips, areolas, nipples, and nail beds, which may be mistaken for cyanosis at birth. Varicose veins and migraine headaches may develop in adulthood. No serious vascular or coagulative sequelae have been reported in these cases.[15]

Gynecomastia

Gynecomastia occurs in males and refers to inappropriate enlargement of the breasts. Drugs such as estrogen and marijuana can cause gynecomastia. Congenital anomalies such as Klinefelter's syndrome can also cause this condition. Gynecomastia is not associated with malignant transformation, although in Klinefelter's syndrome, the incidence of both gynecomastia and breast cancer are increased.

The histologic appearance of gynecomastia moves from an early active phase into an inactive quiescent phase. In the active phase, there is ductal proliferation and hyperplasia of stromal parenchyma accompanied by a periductal or diffuse mixed lymphoplasmacytic and mononuclear infiltrate. The ducts may develop papillary and cribriform patterns with a prominent myoepithelial layer. As the lesion develops, the inactive phase is attained; this phase is characterized by ductal epithelial atrophy and stromal fibrosis.

PRIMARY INFLAMMATORY DISORDERS

Dermatoses of the Nipple

Nipple Eczematous Dermatitis (Nummular Eczema). Nipple eczematous dermatitis (nummular eczema; Fig. 15-2) clinically presents as ill-defined, erythematous, scaly patches or plaques with lichenification when it is chronic. Nipple eczema is the most common presentation of atopic dermatitis (AD) of the breast. It had been considered as a minor criterion in the diagnosis of AD.[16-21] At present, it is not included in the diagnostic minor criteria for AD.[17] But it is an important diagnostic sign of AD, especially during prepuberty[22] and breastfeeding.[23] Nipple eczema may present as erythema, scale, crusting, fissures, vesicles, erosions, or lichenification.[18,19] Both nipples are commonly involved. Nummular eczema may also present as single or multiple erythematous, slightly raised plaques with fine to moderate scale, slight oozing, and pruritus. Involvement of the nipple (nipple eczema) may mimic Paget's disease or Bowen's disease. Nipple eczema may also mimic a number of other inflammatory or infectious etiologies. In fact, all these disorders often present as a scaly nipple–areola complex (Table 15-1). Involvement localized to a

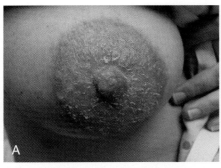

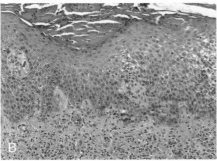

Figure 15-2 **A,** Nipple eczema can mimic the appearance of contact dermatitis as well as Paget's disease or Bowen's disease. **B,** Histologically, epidermal hyperproliferation and spongiosis is observed together with a lymphocytic infiltrate.

TABLE 15-1
Differential Diagnosis of Common Scaly Disorders of the Skin of the Breast

Inflammatory Dermatoses

Seborrheic dermatitis

Psoriasis

Pityriasis rosea

Chronic contact dermatitis

Discoid lupus erythematosus

Darier's disease

Nummular eczema

Nipple eczema

Jogger's nipples

Infections

Erythrasma

Tinea corporis

Tinea versicolor

Neoplasms

Lichen planus-like keratosis

Actinic keratosis

Superficial basal cell carcinoma

Bowen's disease

Paget's disease

Mycosis fungoides

mastectomy scar may also raise suspicion of breast carcinoma recurrence but may just be eczema. A punch biopsy specimen of eczema shows spongiotic dermatitis with variable features of chronicity and rules out malignancy (see Fig. 15-2B). During an acute flare, the predominant histologic finding is spongiosis with intraepidermal edema manifesting as microvesicles or frank bullae. Neutrophilic collections in the stratum corneum and focal parakeratosis, along with serum and crust, can occasionally be observed as lesions become irritated and impetiginized. In the dermis, a superficial perivascular lymphocytic infiltrate with occasional eosinophils accompanies the acute changes. As the lesion progresses, the degree of spongiosis and inflammation diminishes, and epidermal hyperproliferation becomes more prominent, manifesting as either regular psoriasiform acanthosis or irregular epidermal thickening. Lymphocytes persist but in fewer numbers. The differential diagnosis includes allergic contact dermatitis,[24–26] irritant dermatitis ("jogger's nipple"),[27] lichen simplex chronicus, candidal infection (during lactation),[23] and Paget's disease.[28] Nummular eczema may be difficult to distinguish from chronic allergic contact dermatitis; patch testing may identify an offending allergen. Nummular eczema may also be difficult to distinguish from jogger's nipples. Finally, the human mite *Sarcoptes scabiei* can infest the nipple, areola, and inframammary creases. Patients present with extreme pruritus and excoriation. Scrapings mixed on a slide with a drop of oil topped with a coverslip reveal the organism's eggs and feces. Topical scabicides usually eradicate the mite.

Nipple Allergic Contact Dermatitis. Allergic contact dermatitis of the nipple (Fig. 15-3) is a type of nipple dermatitis of the breast but is less common. Contact dermatitis to lanolin, beeswax emollients, chamomile ointments, and nail polish has been reported.[22,24,25] Contact dermatitis most often results from a nickel allergy, and the lesions appear under bra straps and hooks in the shape of the offending metal part. Other common causes of contact dermatitis are topical medications, perfumes, latex, and airborne allergens. A careful history of environmental exposures and the use of patch tests usually identify the offending agent. Histologic examination of a biopsy specimen shows a spongiotic dermatitis with eosinophils (see Fig. 15-3). Changes resulting from chronic rubbing

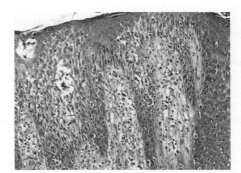

Figure 15-3 Allergic contact dermatitis. Allergic contact dermatitis of the nipple can mimic nipple eczema histologically but shows more spongiosis and more eosinophilic infiltrate.

(lichen simplex chronicus) may also be present if the exposure is a long-standing one.

Nipple Irritant Dermatitis. Nipple irritant dermatitis or so-called jogger's nipple usually develops in active adults and is secondary to friction with clothing.

Treatment of nipple dermatitis is tailored to cause. For AD, treatment consist of gentle cleansing, moisturizers, and topical corticosteroids as needed, and topical calcineurin inhibitors may be used for maintenance. In cases of allergic contact dermatitis, identification and subsequent avoidance of the triggering factor is the treatment of choice. Symptomatic relief may be obtained with topical corticosteroids. In cases of irritant dermatitis, relief may be achieved via wearing soft clothing or applying adhesive tape to protect the nipple.

The most important issue with respect to nipple dermatitis is to distinguish it from Paget's disease of the nipple. If a nipple dermatitis does not resolve with topical therapy, the diagnosis of Paget's disease should be more seriously considered. A biopsy may prove necessary for definitive diagnosis.

Dermatoses of the Areola and Adjacent Dermis

Radiation Dermatitis. Three forms of radiation dermatitis can involve the skin of the breast. The first and most common type is erythema with fine scales that develops during the course of radiotherapy. This is uncomfortable but self-limited and generally can be managed with soothing topical treatments. Months to years later, scarring, atrophy, telangiectasia, and scaling may overlie old radiation portals. This form of radiodermatitis is rare but chronic and may progress to tissue necrosis, ulceration, and de novo cutaneous malignancies (usually squamous cell carcinoma or basal cell carcinoma). Finally, patients who have previously received radiation therapy may develop radiation recall dermatitis when exposed to subsequent chemotherapy agents; a painful, erythematous macular papular rash erupts over the previous radiation port site.[29-33] Vitiligo has also been reported following radiotherapy.[34]

Hidradenitis Suppurativa. A heavy mixed inflammatory infiltrate extending deep into the dermis usually predominates. In active lesions, collections of abscesses are noted along with follicular plugging and sinus tract formation. While the skin attempts to heal, granulation tissue, broken hair shafts, keratin debris, and ensuing foreign body giant cells may be evident. With burned out lesions, extensive fibrosis along with eradication of normal adnexal structures represents the end stage.

Subareolar Abscess. Repeated abscess formation (Fig. 15-4) in the subareolar region results in squamous metaplasia of the terminal ends of lactiferous ducts, further sequestering and propagating abscess pockets.

Ruptured Epidermal or Sebaceous Inclusion Cyst. A ruptured epidermal inclusion or sebaceous cyst can be characterized by intense inflammation and abscess formation as well. Common sites include the subareolar tissues. Often, a ruptured cyst can mimic the appearance of infiltrative carcinomas on palpation and physical examination.

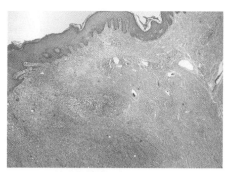

Figure 15-4 Subareolar abscess. The subareolar region is susceptible to abscess formation, sometimes mimicking the appearance of infiltrating carcinoma.

Dermatoses of the Underlying Subcutaneous Tissue

Mastitis. There are a number of different types of mastitis, all of which produce the classic symptoms of mastodynia. Mastitis is defined as inflammation of the breast, irrespective of cause; it can be infectious or noninfectious (Fig. 15-5). Health care providers define mastitis as "a constellation of symptoms that include, fever, malaise, and the classic wedge-shaped infected area of the lactating breast." The incidence of mastitis is approximately 10% in mothers by 3 months postpartum.[35] Reported rates range from 2% to 33%,[36] and the condition can occur in nonlactating patients. Abscesses also occur and are more likely to occur within the first 6 weeks postpartum.[36] Abscesses occur in about 3% of women who experience breast inflammation.[37,38] A prevalence of 23% has been reported for *Candida albicans* colonization at 2 weeks postpartum, but not all of these women develop an infection.[39] However, ductal infections are also caused by *Staphylococcus aureus*,[40,41] and mixed infections[41] have been documented.

Infectious mastitis is most frequently caused by *S. aureus* and coagulase-negative staphylococci.[36,42-45] Another known cause is streptococci, and this should be suspected whenever bilateral mastitis presents early postpartum. Other causes include *Bacteroides* spp., *Escherichia coli*, or other gram-negative bacteria, group A and group B hemolytic streptococci, *Peptostreptococcus* spp., *Mycobacterium tuberculosis* (rare), and *Candida* spp. (rare).[36,44,45] In the case of infectious mastitis, especially *Candida* mastitis during breastfeeding, both mother and infant need to be treated simultaneously.

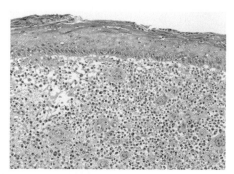

Figure 15-5 Mastitis. This example of mastitis was infectious in nature and caused by *Staphylococcus aureus*.

Noninfectious mastitis may occur and should be considered as "milk stasis" secondary to ineffective or obstructed milk removal.[42] When breast milk is obstructed, the paracellular pathways open, resulting in increased levels of sodium and chloride,[42-44] decreased levels of lactose and potassium, and leakage of inflammatory cytokines, which can provoke fever, chills, and muscle aches, clinically mimicking an infectious process.[36,42]

Mastitis can present with no significant redness, fever, or systemic symptoms, or may be so severe as to require intravenous antibiotics and hospitalization. Infectious mastitis typically presents with a fever greater than 38.5°C, flulike symptoms, and a wedge-shaped area of localized tenderness.

Treatment is focused on reversing milk stasis, maintaining milk supply, and continuing breastfeeding, along with providing maternal comfort. Patients with acute pain, severe symptoms, systemic symptoms, and/or fever need prompt medical attention with the appropriate antibiotics and incision and drainage of an abscess.

There are also special types of mastitis, all of which may have either an infectious, inflammatory or "milk stasis" etiology: puerperal mastitis, plasma cell mastitis, lymphocytic mastitis, and foreign body mastitis.

- Puerperal mastitis. Histologic appearance is dependent on chronicity of lesions. Although acute involvement shows neutrophilic influx along with focal necrosis, chronic lesions often display organized abscess formation with variable degree of fibrosis and fistula formation.
- Plasma cell mastitis. Microscopic sections of lesions exemplify an extreme periductal mastitis characterized by an impressive plasma cell reaction to retained ductal secretions. Key features for diagnosis include ductal epithelial hyperplasia accompanied by an intense surrounding lymphoplasmacytic infiltrate. Often, xanthomatous features can be observed as lymphocytes and plasma cells surround zones of histiocytes engulfing disrupted ductal material. Rarely observed are neutrophils and periductal fibrosis.
- Lymphocytic mastitis. This is also known as sclerosing lymphocytic lobulitis, which characterizes the histologic appearance. There are circumscribed aggregates of lymphocytes within and surrounding terminal ducts and lobules associated with surrounding stromal fibrosis. Perivascular lymphocytic inflammation and germinal centers are also noted.
- Foreign body mastitis. Paraffin or silicon injections for cosmetic purposes induce a foreign body reaction with a characteristic histologic appearance. The exogenous deposits are often removed during tissue processing, revealing a residual "swiss cheese" appearance to the biopsy specimen. Microscopic examination reveals characteristic vacuoles of variable size surrounded by macrophages and foreign body giant cells. When the reaction is severe, cutaneous ulceration, capsule formation, and sinus tracts can develop. The same histopathology can be produced by ruptured or "bleeding" silicone breast implants. Breast implants are discussed in Chapter 18.

Fat Necrosis. Although fat necrosis may occur anywhere in the body, its common presence in the breast, especially within the subcutaneous tissues of the breast (Fig. 15-6), makes us classify it as a primary inflammatory disorder of the breast. Fat necrosis is a benign nonsuppurative sterile inflammatory disease of adipose tissue initially described in the breast in 1920.[46,47] The incidence is estimated to be 0.6% in the breast, representing 2.75% of all benign lesions.[46-49] It is found in 0.8% of breast tumors and 1% of cases of surgical breast reduction.[50] The average age of patients is 50 years.[46-49] Causes include trauma,[46-49] radiotherapy[51-53] anticoagulation (warfarin),[54] cyst aspiration, biopsy, lumpectomy, reduction mammoplasty, implant removal, breast reconstruction with tissue transfer,[55] duct ectasia, and breast infection. Less common causes include polyarteritis nodosa, Weber-Christian disease, and granulomatous angiopanniculitis. In some patients, the cause is unknown.[56]

Fat necrosis is a sterile, inflammatory process resulting from aseptic saponification of fat by means of blood and tissue lipase.[57] It is recognized histologically as fat-filled macrophages and foreign body giant cells surrounded by interstitial infiltration of plasma cells.[58] Apoptosis and necrosis prevail in fat necrosis of the breast. Healing occurs by fibrosis, which begins at the periphery of the cystlike areas. Depending on the degree of fibrosis, these areas are either replaced completely by fibrous tissue or remain as cavities.[55,59] Calcification occurs in the area of fibrosis and is a relatively late finding.[60] Clinical presentations range from an incidental benign finding to a lump.[59,61] In most cases fat necrosis is clinically occult; however, it may be a single or multiple smooth, round, firm nodules or irregular masses and can also be associated with ecchymosis, erythema, inflammation, pain, skin retraction or thickening, nipple retraction, and lymphadenopathy.[55,59,62,63]

Fat necrosis can present as a mass on palpation and as a hypoechoic area on ultrasound imaging. Clinically, therefore, it can mimic the appearance of invasive carcinoma. It is obviously important to distinguish fat necrosis from invasive carcinoma, and thus biopsy is sometimes warranted. Diagnosis can be made via fine needle aspiration cytology (FNAC) or core biopsy. Core biopsy of breast lesions has been shown to be more sensitive than FNAC.[57] Ironically, one of the side effects of biopsy is iatrogenic fat necrosis, which contributes

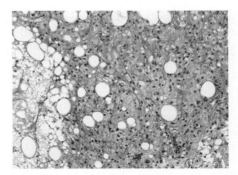

Figure 15-6 Fat necrosis. In the breast, fat necrosis characterized by foamy macrophages and fat digestion can be an insidious and progressive lesion.

to an additional enlarging mass. Unfortunately, some patients experience biopsy after biopsy only to reveal a diagnosis of ongoing fat necrosis.

Other Forms of Panniculitis. Panniculitis (inflammation of the subcutaneous tissue) may be encountered in the breast from many different causes. Ruptured or bleeding implants may also cause extensive panniculitis. Silicone granulomas appear as painful, irregularly shaped lumps or plaques in patients who have received injections of free silicone or whose silicone implants have ruptured. Microscopic examination of this tissue shows a characteristic "swiss cheese" granulomatous inflammatory pattern where the silicone has dissolved out of multinucleate giant cells and extracellular areas during histologic processing. Factitial panniculitis is also a possibility. It arises from repetitive attempts by the patient at self-harm. Possible presentations may mimic virtually any dermatosis and include excoriation, ulceration, puncture wounds and embedded foreign bodies, eczema, vesiculobullous lesions, and nipple discharge. Factitial disease should be considered when an unusual pattern or presentation is not consistent with established clinicopathologic entities or when the patient exhibits an unusual or strange affect or response to the problem. Careful clinical evaluation with mammography and biopsy, if necessary, should be taken to rule out primary organic disease of the breast. Psychiatric evaluation is recommended in cases of suspected factitial panniculitis.

PRIMARY NEOPLASTIC DISORDERS

Primary Benign Neoplastic Disorders

Seborrheic Keratosis. The most common epithelial neoplasm of the breast is seborrheic keratosis. The lesions are unattractive, warty, waxy papules and small plaques that sit on the surface of the skin. Their color generally ranges from tan to brown to shades of gray, but shades of red may also be seen. Bleeding and crusting are common, particularly in lesions that the patient manipulates or that are constantly irritated by clothing. A patient may have only a few or a hundred or more keratoses, which develop synchronously or metachronously. The Leser-Trélat sign is the sudden appearance of numerous seborrheic keratoses in a patient with an internal malignancy and is related to high levels of circulating epidermal growth factor, presumably produced by the tumor. Although many histologic variants of seborrheic keratoses have been described, all exhibit hyperkeratosis, papillomatosis, acanthosis, horn cysts, and variable inflammation. Treatment consists of ablation of bothersome lesions.

Lichen Planus–Like Keratoses. Lichen planus–like keratoses, also called benign lichenoid keratoses, are solitary (rarely multiple) 5- to 20-mm, bright red, violaceous, or brown plaques on the chest and upper back. Clinically, they can mimic lentigo and other pigmented lesions, superficial basal cell carcinoma, or squamous cell carcinoma in situ. The histologic features are virtually identical to those of lichen planus with hyperkeratosis, hypergranulosis, acanthosis, and a dense bandlike lymphocytic inflammatory infiltrate at the base of the lesion; site and clinical presentation distinguish these two disorders.

Benign Adnexal Tumors. Adnexal tumors of pilosebaceous origin[64-69] that occur on the breast are usually cystic and include the epidermoid cyst, trichilemmal cyst (pilar cyst), pilomatrixoma, eruptive vellus hair cyst, and steatocystoma. Eruptive vellus hair cysts are asymptomatic 1- to 2-mm follicular papules that appear suddenly late in childhood or in early adulthood and have an autosomal dominant inheritance pattern. Histologic examination reveals a cyst lined by stratified, squamous keratinizing epithelium filled with laminated keratin debris and one to many small, vellus hairs. Rupture with accompanying granulomatous inflammation is common. Some hypothesize that eruptive vellus hair cysts and steatocystomas are variants of one disorder. Steatocystomas are small, solitary (steatocystoma simplex) or multiple (steatocystoma multiplex), 1- to 5-mm yellowish papules containing a creamy or oily fluid.

Steatocystoma multiplex is inherited in an autosomal dominant fashion. These cysts are lined by thin, stratified squamous epithelium with a prominent homogeneous, eosinophilic, folded cuticle, mimicking a sebaceous duct. Flattened sebaceous lobules may be seen in contiguity with the epithelial lining. The cysts usually appear empty, because the oily substance within them is dissolved during processing. Steatocystoma multiplex (Fig. 15-7) is an uncommon, sporadic, or more commonly autosomal dominant inherited disorder usually present as multiple asymptomatic cysts on the trunk and proximal extremities.[70-72] Solitary steatocystoma simplex has no hereditary tendency. The condition begins in adolescence or young adulthood and affects both sexes equally. It usually lacks surface punctum but may exude a creamy or oily fluid when punctured. The condition has been associated with pachyonychia, acrokeratosis verruciformis, hypertrophic lichen planus, hypohidrosis, hidradenitis suppurativa, and natal teeth. A relationship between steatocystomas and vellus hair cysts has been reported. Hybrid lesions with histologic features of both conditions have been described. Steatocystoma multiplex express keratins 10 and 17 in contrast to eruptive vellus hair cysts, which express only keratin 17. Treatment usually is not required for these benign conditions; however, treatment may be attempted for scarring inflammatory lesions and may include oral tetracycline antibiotics. Isotretinoin therapy also has been shown to be effective in some

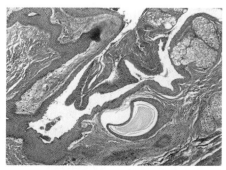

Figure 15-7 Steatocystoma multiplex. This lesion can occur in the breast and consists of a cyst lined by stratified squamous epithelium with mature sebaceous glands in the wall.

patients. Surgical treatment may include aspiration, surgical excision, or destruction with the carbon dioxide laser.

Eccrine tumors that have been reported to occur on the breast include eccrine poromas (a tumor of the intraepithelial portion of the eccrine duct), hidradenomas (a tumor of the straight portion of the eccrine duct), and spiradenomas (a tumor of the deep coiled gland). Eccrine poromas appear clinically as solitary, pedunculated, red or flesh-colored lesions that are often mistaken for pyogenic granulomas. Histologic examination shows a proliferation of broad, anastomosing bands of small, cuboidal cells beneath a flattened epidermis. Within these broad bands of epithelium are small, often slitlike, duct spaces. The absence of peripheral palisading is an important distinguishing feature from basal cell carcinoma. The intervening stroma is edematous and richly vascular.

Hidradenomas are solitary intradermal tumors, 0.5 to 2 cm in diameter, with intact overlying skin. Microscopically within the dermis they are well-circumscribed, sometimes encapsulated, lobules of polygonal and cuboidal cells in which are embedded simple tubular ducts. The polygonal cells have round nuclei with basophilic cytoplasm and indistinct cell borders. The cuboidal cells have clear or pale cytoplasm; when clear cells are numerous, the tumor may be termed clear cell hidradenoma. Reduplicated basement membrane material, appearing as homogeneous, dull, eosinophilic masses, are often present within or surrounding the tumor. Mitoses may be present and, unless atypical in appearance, should not be taken as a sign of malignancy.

Spiradenomas present as solitary, markedly tender, deep dermal or subcutaneous masses. Microscopic examination reveals deeply basophilic, sharply demarcated lobules of small cuboidal cells within the dermis and subcutaneous tissue. Two types of epithelial cells are present. One cell type consists of cells with relatively large, centrally placed clear nuclei and scant cytoplasm that forms ductular structures. The second cell type—smaller, with small, dark nuclei and wispy basophilic cytoplasm—is found primarily at the periphery of the lobules. As in hidradenomas, abundant hyaline-like, reduplicated basement material may be found. Simple but complete excision of eccrine tumors is the appropriate management.

The adenomas of sweat, apocrine, and sebaceous glands that occur as primary dermatologic neoplasms must be distinguished from invasive breast cancer, which can involve the skin of the breast. Adenomas of sweat, apocrine, and sebaceous glands usually consist of well-differentiated appearing tubular and glandular structures that can mimic the appearance of tubular carcinomas or well-differentiated carcinomas of the breast. The presence of the expression of estrogen and progesterone receptors by immunohistochemistry in the latter and the absence in the former is the definitive way of distinguishing benign adnexal adenomas from infiltrating breast cancers.

Erosive Adenomatosis of the Nipple. Erosive adenomatosis of the nipple (Fig. 15-8) is a rare, benign neoplasm of breast lactiferous ducts.[73-77] Its peak incidence is in the fifth decade. This condition usually presents clinically with a unilateral erythematous crusting lesion with induration of the nipple that may be accompanied by ulceration. Clinically, it may be mistaken for Paget's

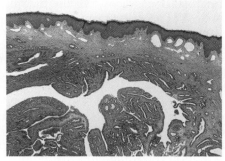

Figure 15-8 Erosive adenomatosis of the nipple, which consists of a benign proliferation of glands within the lactiferous sinuses that is important to distinguish from carcinoma.

disease or nipple eczema, and histologically, it may be mistaken for carcinoma. Therefore, it is important to exclude an underlying infiltrating carcinoma. Excisional biopsy is most helpful in establishing the diagnosis. Management is by complete excision.

Erosive adenomatosis of the nipple presents most often in a perimenopausal woman with crusting or oozing of one nipple. The affected nipple appears eroded or ulcerated, and a serous discharge is common; a subareolar mass may be present. On histologic examination, two patterns of growth are evident. The first pattern associated with erosive lesions is adenomatous; a proliferation of round, oval, or irregularly shaped ducts is embedded in a fibrovascular or hyalinized stroma. The ducts are lined by cuboidal to columnar epithelium with an outer myoepithelial layer. The second pattern associated with a mass effect is papillomatous; papillary proliferations of columnar epithelial and surrounding cuboidal myoepithelial cells fill and distend the ducts. In both patterns, the overlying or adjacent epithelium is acanthotic, and numerous plasma cells may be seen in the stroma. Important differences from breast ductal carcinoma in situ include absence of atypia and mitotic figures. True cribriform intraductal patterns are not seen, and myoepithelial cells are ubiquitously present. This lesion is benign, and simple resection is adequate.

Primary Malignant Neoplastic Disorders

Paget's Disease of the Breast. Paget's disease of the nipple (Fig. 15-9) is mentioned here because it is a very

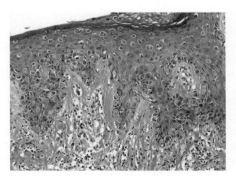

Figure 15-9 Paget's disease of the breast. Paget's disease consists of malignant Paget's cells percolating through the nipple. This disease can mimic nipple eczema or contact dermatitis. Often, with Paget's disease, there is an underlying malignancy.

important dermatologic disease of the breast. Although extramammary Paget's disease can occur anywhere along the milk line, the disease is mainly characterized by being localized to the breast and hence it is included as a primary breast neoplasm. Paget's disease was first described in 1856 by Velpeau,[78] and it was then described by Sir James Paget in 1874 as a syndrome in which ulceration of the nipple was associated with an underlying cancer.[79] Paget's disease of the breast is an uncommon neoplasm, accounting for 1% to 3% of all breast tumors.[80–82] Clinically, it presents as erythema, eczema, ulceration, bleeding, and itching of the nipple or areola. The most frequently reported symptoms are nipple discharge and scaling or eczematous changes such as erythema, eczema, or ulceration. Most patients have two or more symptoms. The eczematous reaction almost always appears first on the nipple, subsequently spreading to the areola.[83,84] The diagnosis of Paget's disease is often delayed for months.

The pathogenesis of Paget's disease still remains unclear and debatable. The transformation theory speculates that Paget's cells are transformed in situ keratinocytes of the epidermis.[85] However, the most widely accepted theory speculates that Paget's cells are ductal carcinoma cells that have migrated from the underlying mammary ducts to the epidermis.[86,87] The latter theory is supported by the presence of associated underlying breast carcinoma in a majority of patients.[80,81,88]

Paget's disease of the breast often presents in association with an underlying invasive or noninvasive carcinoma, or with no underlying neoplasm. The rate of associated underlying carcinoma or ductal carcinoma in situ in Paget's disease of the breast is approximately 80%.[80,87,89–91] The underlying carcinoma can be located in any part of the breast. The underlying carcinoma that is associated with Paget's disease is multifocal or multicentric in 32% to 41% of cases.[89,90] It is characterized histologically by the infiltration of the epidermis with large round and ovoid tumor cells with abundant pale cytoplasm and vesicular nuclei.[91]

In one series, the most associated underlying noninvasive carcinoma (ductal carcinoma in situ) is the "comedo" type.[80,81] Others have reported that the "solid" type (33%) was higher than the "comedo" type (23%).[92] Invasive carcinoma associated with Paget's disease was more commonly estrogen and progesterone negative, with a higher pathologic grade.[92,93] A high positivity for c-erbB-2 in Paget's breast disease with underlying invasive and noninvasive carcinoma was reported.[92,94–96] Overexpression by c-erbB-2 is associated with aggressive disease and with worse prognosis.[97–99]

Diagnosis is via histologic examination, followed by imaging with magnetic resonance, ultrasound, or mammography. In case of noninvasive breast cancer, magnetic resonance imaging has a sensitivity of 95% compared to a value of 70% for mammography.[100]

Treatment with breast-conserving surgery has demonstrated similar long-term survival rates to those of mastectomy.[91,101–103] Sentinel lymph node biopsy should be considered to evaluate the axillary lymph nodes in all patients with Paget's disease.[104,105] The prognosis depends on the presence or absence of an invasive underlying

cancer. Because of the importance of Paget's disease and its wider significance in the breast than just as a dermatologic disease, it is discussed extensively in Chapter 14.

Inflammatory Breast Cancer. Inflammatory breast carcinoma (Fig. 15-10) is included as a primary breast dermatologic malignancy because it presents as red, warm, slightly indurated, and tender skin overlying the breast. Dermal and subcutaneous lymphatics contain numerous tumor emboli that are similar in appearance to the primary carcinoma. Vascular congestion and tissue edema accompany the lymphatic blockage. Congested, dilated capillaries and lymphatics in the superficial dermis are permeated with tumor. Recurrent metastatic carcinoma, most often found in mastectomy scars, also manifests as florid lymphovascular tumor emboli, so-called secondary inflammatory breast carcinoma. Because of the importance of this condition, it is discussed in detail in Chapter 87.

Angiosarcoma. Angiosarcoma can occur elsewhere in the body, but its unique clinicopathologic presentation in the breast, association with prior breast irradiation, and usual superficial location within the mammary dermis make it appropriate to classify angiosarcoma as a primary breast neoplastic disorder (Fig. 15-11). Angiosarcoma of the breast is, however, uncommon. It was first reported by Schmidt in 1887.[106] The frequency of this rare tumor is 0.04% of primary mammary tumors[107] and approximately 8% of mammary sarcomas.[108] Angiosarcomas have been labeled under different names such as hemangioendothelioma,[109] hemangioblastoma,[110] hemangiosarcoma,[111,112] hemangiosarcoma,[107] and metastasizing angioma.[113–115] It carries a very poor prognosis, with a 5-year survival of 8% to 50%.[116] Metastases from mammary angiosarcomas have been reported in the lung, skin, liver, bone, central nervous system, spleen, ovary, lymph nodes, and heart.[117,118]

Angiosarcomas can also occur within the axilla or arm as a result of long-standing lymphedema. These angiosarcomas are referred to as the Stewart-Treves syndrome. These angiosarcomas arise as a result of chronic lymphedema (swelling resulting from lymphatic obstruction), although it is not clear exactly what the pathogenic mechanism is. Chronic lymphedema occurs as a complication of mastectomy and/or radiotherapy for breast cancer.

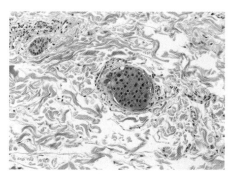

Figure 15-10 Inflammatory breast carcinoma, which consists of lymphovascular tumor emboli within the dermis. This condition often mimics the appearance of mastitis, and dermal biopsy may prove necessary.

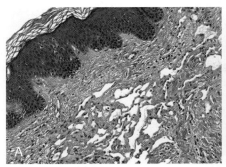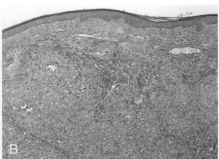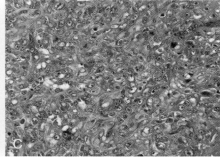

Figure 15-11 Angiosarcoma, its precursors and mimics. **A,** Atypical vascular ectasia from irradiation. This lesion may be a possible precursor of angiosarcoma or a mimic, but it is not angiosarcoma. **B,** Example of solid vascular proliferation in the breast dermis indicative of angiosarcoma. **C,** Higher-power view of angiosarcoma indicating nuclear and cellular anaplasia.

Irradiation of the breast can produce a vascular ectasia within the superficial dermis that can exhibit atypical features (see Fig. 15-11A). This histology falls short of angiosarcoma. However, when the vascular proliferation progresses to invade the breast lobules or becomes solid (see Fig. 15-11B), it is considered to represent angiosarcoma. Higher magnification confirms its highly anaplastic cellular and nuclear features (see Fig. 15-11C).

Both primary angiosarcomas of the breast postirradiation and primary angiosarcomas of the axilla secondary to lymphedema show dermal infiltration by ill-defined vascular spaces lined with atypical endothelial cells. Well-differentiated lesions show an anastomosing network of vessels lined by a single layer of endothelial cells with mild to moderate nuclear atypia. Less well-differentiated areas show more endothelial nuclear pleomorphism, with increasing necrosis and mitotic activity. Focal papillary protrusions can be observed. Although most lesions are well differentiated, poorly differentiated lesions exhibit sheets of dedifferentiated cells with no clearly visible vascular lumen. There is associated high nuclear atypia, necrosis, mitoses, and hemorrhage. Angiosarcomas are positive for CD31 and CD34.

Prior to the use of radiation therapy for breast cancer, angiosarcomas of the breast used to occur during the third and fourth decades of life.[119] About 6% to 12% of the cases were diagnosed during pregnancy.[117,118] Angiosarcomas of the breast have increasingly been associated with radiation therapy and lymphedema that occurs after surgical and radiation treatment for breast cancer.[119-123] They account for more than 50% of all sarcomas identified in patients who had prior radiation therapy but only 20% of sarcomas in those who had no prior radiation therapy.[119] With the increasing use of breast-conserving therapy and adjuvant irradiation, it is expected that the incidence of angiosarcomas will increase in the future.

Preoperative diagnosis of angiosarcomas of the breast using aspiration cytology and biopsy is often difficult.[117] Diagnosis is best established via incisional biopsy. Ultrastructural examination can reveal the vascular nature of angiosarcomas and demonstrate Weibel-Palade bodies and pinocytic vesicles. Immunostaining for factor VIII–related antigen is also helpful for the diagnosis.[124]

Treatment involves a multidisciplinary approach because angiosarcomas of the breast are quite resistant to classic chemotherapy. Doxorubicin-based neoadjuvant therapy is reserved for unresectable tumors and tumors larger than 5 cm in diameter or those invading the chest wall. Breast angiosarcomas are best treated with a combination of radiotherapy and chemotherapy for local control. In some cases, mastectomy may be part of the treatment protocol. Chemotherapy and radiation may be first attempted to down-stage the tumor and/or render it resectable.

Surgical treatment of nonbreast angiosarcomas is usually contraindicated in tumors that extend to vital structures, in those of massive size, or in multicentric tumors. Angiosarcomas of the breast, however, can be treated with early and complete surgical excision of the mass with tumor-free margins, if achievable. However, angiosarcomas often extend microscopically beyond their gross margins, and therefore, simple excision is unacceptable because of its high rate of local recurrence. Radical mastectomy is used only if the tumor extends to the deep fascia. Axillary dissection is not indicated because nodal involvement is rare. The decision for mastectomy is hence dictated by the following:

- The size and location of the tumor
- The multicentricity of the disease
- The ability to follow the breast mammographically and by physical examination for evidence of recurrence postoperatively
- The preference of the patient

Unlike angiosarcomas, other sarcomas of the breast rarely occur predominately in the skin. Those that occur deeper in the breast are covered in Chapter 13.

Malignant Adnexal Tumors. Malignant neoplasms of eccrine and apocrine glands[64-69] can occur in the breast, and when they occur at these sites, they must be distinguished from breast cancer. Breast neoplasms of eccrine and apocrine glands are rare, accounting for less than 0.001% of all primary breast cancers. Although most are categorized as primary "sweat gland carcinomas," apocrine lesions are much more common than eccrine lesions (Fig. 15-12). They usually present clinically as indurated, slowly growing plaques with irregular outlines. Histologically, lesions may consist of cylindrocarcinoma, spiradenocarcinoma, or malignant apocrine mixed tumors. Malignant adnexal tumors may evolve from benign adnexal tumors. Lesions frequently affect young adults. A whole range of adnexal malignancies

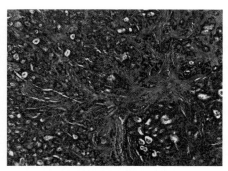

Figure 15-12 Apocrine adenocarcinoma, a malignant adnexal tumor of the breast, can resemble infiltrating ductal breast carcinoma, from which it must be distinguished.

may occur. Adnexal carcinomas, like adenomas, may mimic the appearance of breast carcinomas. The presence of the expression of estrogen and progesterone receptors in the latter by immunohistochemistry and the absence in the former is the definitive way of distinguishing adnexal adenocarcinomas from breast cancer. The treatment for adnexal carcinomas is surgical therapy with wide margins. Metastatic potential, however, is very real.

Secondary Breast Dermatologic Disorders

SECONDARY INFLAMMATORY DISORDERS

Infectious Disorders

Erythrasma. Erythrasma (Fig. 15-13) is a superficial cutaneous bacterial infection caused by the organism *Corynebacterium minutissimum*. Although usually intertriginous, disciform erythrasma presents as a well-demarcated, oval, reddish brown patch with fine scaling. Both clinical forms may be diagnosed by the characteristic coral-red fluorescence under Wood's light. Biopsies often appear normal under hematoxylin and eosin staining. Small coccobacilli in the superficial stratum corneum can be highlighted with Gram stains, as well as periodic acid–Schiff and methenamine silver preparations. Treatment consists of oral or topical erythromycin.[125]

Candidiasis. Candidiasis on routine histology is subtle. The characteristic histologic clue to the diagnosis is the presence of neutrophils in the stratum corneum, initially resembling impetigo. The underlying epidermis may show variable degree of spongiosis and mild acanthosis. Spores and hyphae elements can be better visualized with periodic acid–Schiff staining.

Dermatophytosis (Tinea). One useful clue to the microscopic diagnosis of tinea is the "sandwich sign," which is the presence of orthokeratosis or parakeratosis interspersed within normal basket-weave stratum corneum. In addition, some degree of spongiosis or psoriasiform hyperplasia may be present along with a variable inflammatory response. Fungal hyphae are usually observed in the stratum corneum or within follicles, and can be best highlighted with periodic acid–Schiff or Gomori methenamine silver stains (Fig. 15-14).

Noninfectious Disorders

Blistering or Bullous Cutaneous Eruptions. Blistering or bullous cutaneous eruptions limited to the breast are rare; when they occur in the breast, they are usually part of a secondary manifestation. Of these, the most common is herpes zoster (shingles), which manifests as severe stinging, burning pain in a dermatomal distribution, followed within a few days by a papulovesicular eruption with small, grouped vesicles on an erythematous base. Constitutional symptoms such as fever, headache, and malaise may precede or accompany a severe outbreak. Postherpetic neuralgia persists in as many as 15% of patients. The Tzanck smear shows multinucleate keratinocytes with nuclear molding. A biopsy usually is not necessary; however, when obtained, it shows characteristic viral cytopathologic features of ballooning and reticular degeneration of keratinocytes, multinucleate keratinocytes with ground-glass nuclei and nuclear molding, and leukocytoclastic vasculitis in the underlying small dermal capillaries. Prompt administration of antiviral drugs (e.g., famciclovir) leads to resolution of the initial lesion, with a marked decrease in the incidence, severity, and duration of postherpetic neuralgia. Topical capsaicin may also be used to control the pain of postherpetic neuralgia. Rarely, cutaneous herpes simplex with axillary adenopathy infects the nipple of a mother who is breastfeeding, producing herpetic

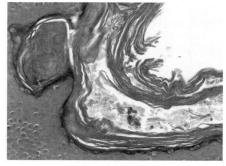

Figure 15-13 Erythrasma. Erythrasma is a secondary infectious disease of the breast resulting from a cutaneous superficial bacterial infection, as evidenced by the appearances of small coccobacilli in the superficial stratum corneum.

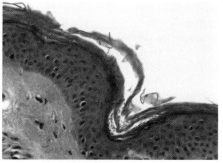

Figure 15-14 In contrast to erythrasma, dermatophytosis (tinea) is caused by a fungus, and fungal hyphae are observed within the stratum corneum.

gingivostomatitis. Viral cultures of mother and infant establish the diagnosis.[126]

Another type of blistering disease is traumatic in nature and caused by improper or prolonged breastfeeding. This may result in exquisitely painful, small (1- to 3-mm), translucent vesicles, or sore, cracked, fissured nipples. Viral and bacterial cultures are predictably negative. Soothing topical treatments applied immediately after nursing and gently washed off before the next feeding may be helpful.

Lichen Sclerosis et Atrophicus. Lichen sclerosis et atrophicus (LS) is an inflammatory disease of unknown cause and incompletely elicited pathogenesis. Clinically the entity was first described by Hallopeau in 1887.[127] Extragenital LS is most common on the neck and shoulders but can occur in the breast. It is usually asymptomatic or can be accompanied by pruritus. In the breast it may present in the inframammary area. Typically, the eruption of LS begins as white, polygonal papules that coalesce into plaques with comedo-like plugs or evenly spaced dells. The dells may disappear, leaving a smooth, often porcelain-white plaque. LS may exhibit the isomorphic or "Koebner" phenomenon.[128] LS is not, itself, a premalignant condition and the association is more "casual than causal."[129–133] However, it is associated with squamous cell cancer in the genital area. A possible explanation for this is that the association of LS with cancer involves infection with human papillomavirus.[134,135] It is generally accepted, however, that cancer does not develop within pediatric or extragenital LS, including LS of the breast.[136] There are many reports of a possible link of LS with autoimmune disorders or with the presence of autoantibodies.[137,138] Vitiligo and alopecia areata have been reported in association with genital and extragenital LS, including breast LS.[139–143] Thyroid disease, especially Graves' disease[144–146] and both type 1 and type 2 diabetes, have been reported in association with LS.[141,147–151]

Initial lesions of LS show epidermal atrophy along with superficial dermal edema associated with an underlying bandlike lymphocytic infiltrate. As the lesions become more sclerotic, the papillary dermis becomes homogenized and the epidermis is attenuated with flattening of the rete ridges. Treatment is with topical steroids.

Seborrheic Dermatitis. Acute seborrheic dermatitis (Fig. 15-15) involving the breast skin is histologically nonspecific and is similar to seborrheic dermatitis elsewhere. Microscopic examination reveals spongiosis associated with a mild superficial, perivascular, and perifollicular lymphocytic infiltrate. More chronic lesions are often psoriasiform with focal parakeratosis, most prominent around follicular openings. The main histologic differential diagnosis is psoriasis, but in seborrheic dermatitis, neutrophilic exocytosis, Munro microabscesses, and confluent parakeratosis are absent.

Seborrheic dermatitis is marked clinically by its characteristic distribution in the scalp, eyebrows, eyelid margins, cheeks, nasolabial folds and paranasal areas, external ear canals, beard (men), presternal area or when it occurs in the breast, within the inframammary folds. Although generally a dry, powdery scale, when there is extensive presternal or inframammary involvement, the lesions may have coarser scales on an erythematous base with follicular pustules. The clinical course is chronic, with remissions and exacerbations. Low-potency topical steroids are the treatment of choice. Topical antifungal treatment (ketoconazole [Nizoral]) has also shown efficacy; therefore, the yeast *Pityrosporum ovale* is believed to play a role.[152] The differential diagnosis includes psoriasis, tinea corporis, tinea versicolor, erythrasma, and contact dermatitis.

Psoriasis. Psoriasis (Fig. 15-16) is distinguished by characteristic lesions on the elbows, knees, and other extensor body surfaces, but it can also occur on the breast. Psoriasis, especially when it involves the areola or nipple, may be difficult to distinguish clinically from Bowen's disease (squamous cell carcinoma in situ). A biopsy readily distinguishes the two entities. There are other entities in the differential diagnosis. The expanding oval lesions of tinea corporis and tinea versicolor have a peripheral collarette of scale and more haphazard distribution, and fungal hyphae may be identified on potassium hydroxide preparation in the office or in biopsy specimens.

Chronic plaque-type psoriasis of the breast is characterized by hyperkeratosis with confluent parakeratosis, hypogranulosis, regular acanthosis, suprapapillary epidermal thinning, and neutrophilic exocytosis within the stratum corneum (Munro microabscesses) and the spinous layer (spongiform pustules of Kogoj). In the dermis, a mild perivascular lymphocytic infiltrate can be observed along with tortuous dilated capillaries extending upward into the suprapapillary plate, accounting

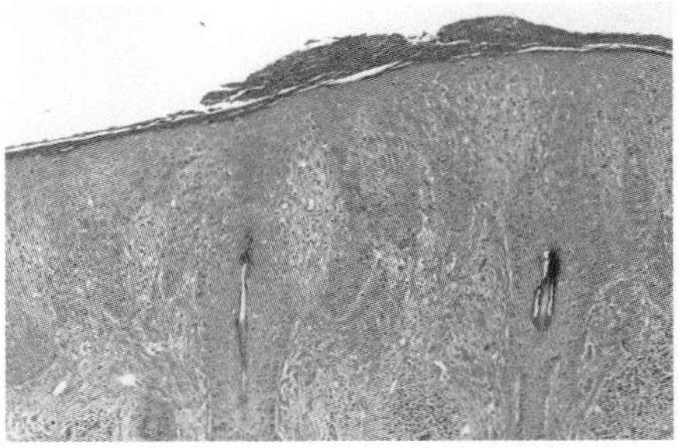

Figure 15-15 Seborrheic dermatitis. Seborrheic dermatitis may secondarily affect the breast and is characterized by parakeratosis, spongiosis, acanthosis, and lymphocytic infiltration.

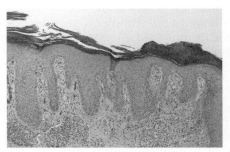

Figure 15-16 Psoriasis. Psoriasis may also secondarily affect the breast and can be similar in appearance to seborrheic dermatitis. However, in psoriasis, confluent parakeratosis and neutrophilic exocytosis are present.

for the Auspitz phenomenon. Guttate psoriasis differs histologically from chronic plaque-type psoriasis by showing more focal parakeratosis and less acanthosis. Inverse or flexural psoriasis involving the intertriginous folds of the breast tends to be more spongiotic and less classic than the chronic stable plaque type. The characteristic feature in pustular psoriasis is the aggregation of neutrophils between keratinocytes and within the stratum corneum.

Drug Hypersensitivity Reactions. Drug hypersensitivity reactions can occur anywhere in the body, including the breast. As with the myriad of clinical manifestations of drug hypersensitivity, pathologic findings are equally diverse. Patterns range from interface dermatitis with perivascular inflammation and minimal epidermal change, to lichenoid dermatitis, to intraepidermal pustular aggregates. All can be seen with variable degree of keratinocyte necrosis. Although presence of eosinophils is a vital clue to a drug reaction, clinicopathologic correlation is absolutely essential.

Coumarin Necrosis. Coumarin necrosis occurs in patients with inborn or acquired abnormalities of the coagulation cascade, particularly deficiencies of protein C or protein S. These patients develop seemingly paradoxical intravascular coagulation with initiation of warfarin anticoagulant therapy because of depletion of vitamin K–dependent antithrombosis factors. The intravascular thrombi form preferentially in relatively cool, fatty areas of the body such as the breasts, buttocks, and abdominal panniculus, and they are exquisitely painful. Widespread ischemic tissue necrosis is the usual outcome. Prevention through prior anticoagulation with heparin before initiation of warfarin therapy is recommended.[153]

Biopsy specimens reveal hemorrhagic necrosis of the epidermis and breast parenchyma along with characteristic noninflammatory fibrin thrombi formation in the dermal vasculature. As the skin attempts to heal, scar tissue and granulomatous inflammation can appear.

Pyoderma Gangrenosum. Pyoderma gangrenosum–like ulcerative lesions on the breast have been reported in patients with lupus anticoagulant syndrome.[154]

Mondor's Disease. Mondor's disease is a superficial thrombophlebitis of the thoracoepigastric, lateral thoracic, or superior epigastric vein and can present on the breast. The usual presentation is a tender, firm, linear cord. Affected patients are usually in the third to fifth decade, and women outnumber men 3 to 1. Most cases are idiopathic; a few may be related to trauma, surgery, illness, or another skin condition near the involved vessel.[155] One historic case of breast carcinoma presenting as Mondor's disease has been reported; inflammatory breast carcinoma should always be considered.[156] Treatment is symptomatic, and most cases resolve in several weeks.

Granuloma Annulare. Granuloma annulare, a disease of collagen necrobiosis, can occur anywhere in the body, including the breast. Microscopic examinations of classic palisading granuloma annulare reveal collections of epithelioid histiocytes and giant cells surrounding a central zone of necrobiosis consisting of degenerated connective tissue and mucin. Epidermal

changes are usually minimal. Perivascular lymphocytes and eosinophils are sometimes noted.

In the less overt interstitial form of granuloma annulare, the histologic changes are more subtle. The dermis appears "busy" and more cellular from an initial low-power assessment. Higher magnification reveals strands of lymphocytes and histiocytes along with mucin, separating collagen bundles. Definitive formed areas of necrobiosis are absent.

Sarcoidosis. Systemic sarcoidosis can affect any organ, including the breast. Biopsy specimens display epithelioid non-necrotizing granulomas with a variably surrounding lymphoplasmacytic reaction. Occasionally, asteroid or Schaumann bodies can be present within the multinucleated giant cells that accompany the granulomas. This finding is suggestive and supportive of, but not pathognomonic, for sarcoidosis.

Miscellaneous Papulosquamous Disorders. Other papulosquamous disorders that affect other areas of the body more often than the breast can still present on the breast occasionally. These include pityriasis rosea, with its oval, finely scaling, salmon-colored patches, and lupus erythematosus (Fig. 15-17). Darier's disease (keratosis follicularis) is an uncommon, autosomal dominant papulosquamous disorder with a seborrheic dermatitis–like distribution that can infrequently occur on the breast. The affected skin develops firm, discrete, 2- to 3-mm, red to brown spiny papules that make the skin look dirty and that may coalesce to form large plaques. The disease can be exacerbated by heat, high humidity, exposure to ultraviolet or ionizing radiation, or trauma. Secondary bacterial or fungal infection is common. This disorder has a characteristic, although not pathognomonic, histologic appearance. Individual keratinocytes in the suprabasal layer dissociate from their adjacent keratinocytes because of loss of intercellular bridges (acantholysis). These acantholytic cells undergo premature keratinization (dyskeratosis) and are shed as shrunken, round, or flattened cells (corp ronds and grains). Oral synthetic retinoids may be used to control the primary lesions, although the disease recurs when retinoids are discontinued. Case reports suggest topical 5-fluorouracil and adapalene 0.1% gel are successful and more easily tolerated alternatives.[157,158] Avoiding or minimizing exposure to exacerbating factors

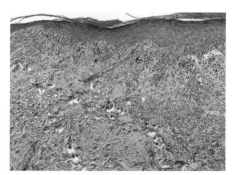

Figure 15-17 Systemic lupus erythematosus can manifest itself in the skin of the breast and exhibit the characteristic lymphocytic infiltrate with epidermal atrophy and hydropic degeneration of the epidermal basal layer.

is a mainstay of therapy. Appropriate topical or oral antibiotics may be used to combat documented secondary infections. Grover's disease, or transient acantholytic dermatosis, exhibits a nearly identical histologic picture but is characterized clinically by an eruption of itchy papules and macules on the upper chest and back of adults. It can also occasionally affect the breast. There is no familial predisposition, and the disease is self-limited.

Miscellaneous Connective Tissue Disorders. Systemic scleroderma appears as firm, indurated, white plaques with a central depression and faintly violaceous borders that can occur anywhere on the body, including the breast. If scleroderma is localized, it is called morphea (Fig. 15-18). Scleroderma can either be localized (also called localized scleroderma or linear scleroderma as well as morphea) or may be associated with systemic sclerosis or calcinosis cutis, Raynaud's phenomenon, esophageal involvement, sclerodactyly, and telangiectasia (CREST syndrome). The differential diagnosis includes scar, sclerotic carcinoma, sclerodermoid graft-versus-host disease, and dermatomyofibroma.[159,160] Biopsy shows thickened sclerotic collagen (see Fig. 15-18), particularly at the interface of the reticular dermis and the subcutaneous tissue with a sparse to mild lymphoplasmacytic inflammatory infiltrate. Therapy consists of potent topical steroids or steroids under occlusion, but although progression of the lesion may be inhibited, the plaque generally does not resolve.

Lupus panniculitis is a systemic disease that can affect the breast. It consists of a predominantly lobular process with characteristic hyaline necrosis of fat lobules associated with variable degree of fibrosis, mucin, and calcium deposition. Nodular lymphocytic aggregates that resemble lymphoid follicles can often be seen. Epidermal changes may or may not be present.

Dermatomyositis (Fig. 15-19) is also a systemic disease that can affect the breast. Microscopic features of dermatomyositis can be very subtle and consists of interface changes including basal vacuolar liquefactive degeneration, thickened basement membrane, epidermal atrophy, and presence of dermal mucin. The inflammation is sparse with few scattered interface and perivascular

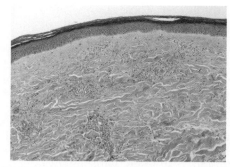

Figure 15-19 Dermatomyositis. This systemic disorder can present in the breast as epidermal atrophy and perivascular lymphocytic infiltration.

lymphocytes. The histology of dermatomyositis is almost indistinguishable from lupus erythematosus. Occasionally, dermal or subcutaneous calcification can be noted.

SECONDARY NEOPLASTIC DISORDERS

Benign Disorders

Galactoceles. Microscopically, galactoceles are lined by cuboidal or flattened epithelium with cytoplasmic vacuolization resulting from lipid accumulation. Fibrosis usually surrounds intact cysts, whereas chronic inflammation can be seen with rupture. The lumen contains inspissated secretions.

Solitary Steatocystomas. Steatocystoma multiplex has been discussed previously, but solitary steatocystoma can also occur within the breast. Biopsies show cysts within the dermis lined by stratified squamous epithelium associated with a corrugated eosinophilic cuticle layer. Flattened lobules of mature sebaceous glands are usually found focally within the cyst wall. The lumen usually contains keratin, vellus hairs, or sebum.

Vellus Hair Cysts. Histologically, vellus hair cysts are lined by a thin stratified squamous epithelial layer. The lumen contains small vellus hairs arranged in a haphazard manner admixed with loose laminated keratin debris.

Benign Melanocytic Neoplasms. Although pigmented melanocytic lesions can occur anywhere in the body, pigmented lesions of the breast are common (Fig. 15-20); the average white adult has 40 to 100 benign melanocytic nevi scattered over all body surfaces,

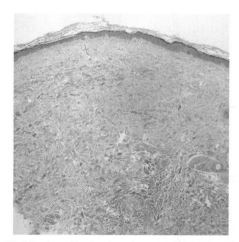

Figure 15-18 Localized scleroderma or morphea is seen as dense collagenous bundles forming a nodule in the breast dermis.

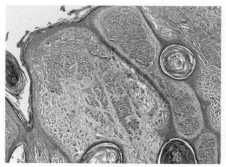

Figure 15-20 Intradermal nevus. Intradermal nevi are common in the breast.

including the breast. These lesions range from simple lentigos (basilar hyperpigmentation of keratinocytes with little or no increase in melanocytes) to junctional, compound, and intradermal melanocytic nevi. Nevi are generally smaller than 0.5 cm, oval to round, tan to brown, evenly pigmented, macular or papular lesions with relatively smooth borders; congenital nevi may be larger, darker, and slightly asymmetrical.

Dermatofibromas. Solitary dermatofibromas (Fig. 15-21) can occur in the breast. Histology reveals dermal proliferation of short interlacing fascicles of spindled fibroblasts and histiocytes with intervening entrapped dense hyalinized collagen bundles. The overlying epidermis may show variable degree of hyperplasia and hyperpigmentation.

Nevoid Hyperkeratosis. Nevoid hyperkeratosis of the nipple or areola is histologically characterized by orthokeratotic hyperkeratosis, acanthosis, and papillomatosis with occasional keratotic plugging and mild papillary dermal fibrosis. Microscopic differential diagnoses include seborrheic keratosis and epidermal nevus.

Connective Tissue Neoplasms. Cherry angiomas are extremely common, red to violaceous papules measuring a few millimeters in diameter that appear mainly on the trunk and proximal extremities of adults but can also occur on the breasts. Histologic examination shows a cluster of dilated thin-walled vessels in the superficial dermis. Angiokeratomas, similar vascular lesions that extend up into the squamous epithelium, may be markers for Fabry's disease (α-galactosidase deficiency) and should prompt a search for clusters of angiokeratomas around the navel and on the genitals, corneal opacities, and symptoms of anhidrosis or hypohydrosis.[161] Enzyme assays establish the diagnosis. Sinusoidal hemangioma, a variant of cavernous hemangioma,[162] and progressive lymphangioma, a rare benign proliferation of lymph channels,[163,164] have both been reported to involve the breast. Piloleiomyomas are benign proliferations of erector pili muscles—the smooth muscle attached to hair follicles that produces "goose bumps." Erector pili are especially prominent in the nipple-areolar area, and hence this lesion can also occur in this region. Piloleiomyomas are often exquisitely painful and respond to light touch, stroking, or chilling with painful contraction. Bilateral smooth muscle tumors arising in the areola and nipple have been reported.[165] Calcium channel blockers have been used to control activation of these muscles when excision is not feasible. Piloleiomyomas are also a feature of Becker's nevus (discussed at the beginning of the chapter) but in this setting are not painful. Sometimes these

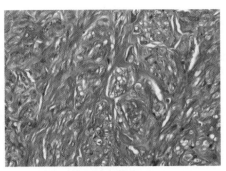

Figure 15-22 Leiomyoma. Leiomyomas or pilileiomyomas are uncommon in the nipple-areola area but can occur and must be distinguished from infiltrating breast carcinomas.

piloleiomyomas can grow large and present as a nipple or areolar mass. Gross leiomyoma of the nipple (Fig. 15-22) is a rare lesion, with only about 30 published cases[166-170] since it was first described by Virchow.[171]

Although rare examples of smooth muscle tumors of the breast parenchyma have been reported,[168,172,173] most leiomyomas of the breast occur in a subareolar location. The etiology of these benign tumors is unclear, and a family history or genetic linkage has not been reported.[174] Nipple leiomyomas may be asymptomatic for long periods or present with a mass or recurrent attacks of severe pain that occur spontaneously, after application of pressure, or after exposure to cold.[166,167,175,176] The pain is thought to be related to contractions of the neoplastic smooth muscle.[177,178] Examination may reveal a single, small, firm subdermal papule that enlarges the nipple. The differential diagnosis includes papilloma, adenoma, and Paget's disease. In contrast to Paget's disease, leiomyomas show characteristic pain without inflammation.[167,170] Cytologic atypia and mitotic figures are not seen.[170,174,176,179] Surgical excision may be helpful for symptomatic tumors.

Dermatomyofibroma (fibrohistiocytic tumor)[159,160] and granular cell tumor (a tumor of neural origin) are both rare and benign. Simple excision is curative. The occurrence of myxomas, spotty pigmentation, endocrine overactivity, and schwannomas define Carney's complex, a multisystem connective tissue tumor syndrome inherited in an autosomal dominant fashion. Typical sites for the myxomas include eyelids and the external ear canal. However, they can also occur in the breast, especially in the nipple. Histologic examination of these rare tumors shows a hypocellular tumor with stellate fibroblasts embedded in an abundant gelatinous blue-gray matrix.[180] The identification of a myxoma on biopsy of a mass lesion of the nipple should prompt a search for skin stigmata and metabolic abnormalities.

Malignant Disorders

Actinic Keratosis and Bowen's Disease. These precursor lesions usually occur on sun-exposed areas but can occur on the skin of the breast. These precursor lesions can give rise to invasive squamous cell carcinomas. Squamous cell carcinomas arising from foci of Bowen's disease or foci of actinic keratosis can be

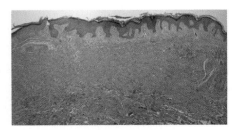

Figure 15-21 Dermatofibroma. Common skin lesions also commonly occur in the breast dermis.

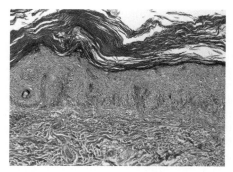

Figure 15-23 Bowen's disease. Bowen's disease or carcinoma in situ, characterized by crowded atypical squamous epithelium, can occur on the breast, may be related to prior irradiation and most importantly, may progress to invasive squamous cell carcinoma.

caused by therapeutic irradiation exposure. Individuals differ in their sensitivity to irradiation. Carriers of the ataxia-telangiectasia gene may be more sensitive to the effects of ionizing radiation. Other individual sensitivities and susceptibilities may also exist in the DNA repair enzymes. Generally, scaly, rough intraepithelial proliferations of atypical keratinocytes, so-called actinic keratoses, precede the development of invasive carcinoma. Squamous cell carcinoma in situ, also called Bowen's disease, clinically appears as a velvety red patch that is sharply demarcated from the adjacent skin (Fig. 15-23). The risk of developing invasive carcinoma from Bowen's disease is estimated at 5%.[181]

Squamous Cell Carcinoma. Squamous cell carcinomas, although an uncommon diagnosis on the breast, can occur on any mucocutaneous surface, including the breast, and display similar microscopic findings. Lesions range from well-differentiated to poorly differentiated carcinomas. Well-differentiated squamous cell carcinomas are characterized by a downward lobular growth of atypical keratinocytes with some degree of pleomorphism and mitosis (Fig. 15-24). Scattered detached islands are evident along with intercellular bridges, keratin pearls, and apoptotic cells. Poorly differentiated squamous cell carcinomas, on the other hand, are highly infiltrative and lack overt features of their epithelial origin such as keratinization and intercellular bridges. Perineural invasion and sclerotic changes are more common as the tumor becomes more aggressive.

Basal Cell Carcinoma. Basal cell carcinoma (BCC) is the most common malignancy both in men and women, especially in whites, and is more prevalent than all other malignancies combined. Fortunately, this tumor usually remains confined to the skin, and metastases rarely occur, although local recurrence can be a problem. BCC arises most frequently on sun-damaged skin but also can occur on protected skin also, as well as on the breast (Fig. 15-25). The most common type of BCC is the noduloulcerative variant, which presents as a pearly nodule with overlying and adjacent telangiectasia. Ulceration may be present. Histologically, the tumor consists of nests of small, basaloid epithelial cells in continuity with the overlying epithelium. Peripheral palisading (the picket fence–like arrangement of the cells at the rim of the nests) distinguishes BCC from adnexal tumors. Two variants of BCC are of special interest in the breast: superficial multifocal basal cell carcinoma and fibroepithelioma of Pinkus. Superficial multifocal BCC presents clinically as a sharply marginated erythematous patch or plaque with slight scale. Histologic examination shows widely spaced nests of basaloid cells budding off the base of the overlying epithelium, surrounded by a loose, myxomatous inflamed stroma. Spontaneous regression, which is common, leaves a nonspecific superficial scar, and the lesion may be missed on a small punch biopsy. Levels through the submitted tissue or repeat biopsy may be necessary to establish the diagnosis. Fibroepithelioma of Pinkus is a pink or tan, sessile nodule that on histologic examination shows thin, anastomosing strands of basaloid cells embedded in abundant stroma. Careful searching reveals foci of peripheral palisading. This tumor is thought to be a BCC that proliferates along the framework provided by preexisting benign eccrine ducts. There is a common proliferation of basaloid keratinocytes with large, fairly uniform nuclei and scant cytoplasm. Tumor cells are usually embedded within a fibromyxoid stroma associated with inflammation. A characteristic feature of BCC is retraction of the stroma around the tumor islands, creating clefts. Histologic subtypes of BCC include superficial, nodular, pigmented, morpheaform, and with squamous differentiation.

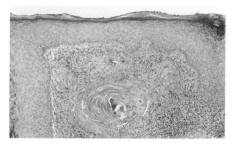

Figure 15-24 Squamous cell carcinoma. Invasive squamous cell carcinoma exhibits keratin pearl formation and an invasive growth pattern and can occur in the breast.

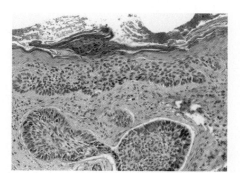

Figure 15-25 Basal cell carcinoma. Basal cell carcinoma, the most common cancer of men and women, can also occur in the breast and is characterized by islands of cells with peripheral palisading.

Malignant Melanoma. Malignant melanomas, like BCCs and squamous cell carcinomas, are more commonly observed in sun-exposed areas and are related to sun exposure. However, they can and do occur in the skin of the breast (Fig. 15-26). Pigmented lesions that change, grow, ulcerate, itch, bleed, show significant color variation, or develop border irregularities should be excised to rule out melanoma. Primary melanoma of the skin of the breast accounts for 1.8% to 5% of melanomas.[182,183] A properly performed excisional biopsy that includes a narrow rim of clinically normal skin and completely removes the melanocytic lesion is necessary for accurate histologic evaluation and diagnosis. Wood's lamp examination enhances the pigmentary variation between normal and involved skin and may help delineate the borders of suspect lesions. For lesions larger than 2 cm or if total excision poses problems with closure (e.g., in the nipple or areola), an incisional biopsy can be performed from the thickest or darkest portion of the lesion. The initial evaluation of a patient with a suspected melanoma includes a personal history, family history, and appropriate physical examination that includes a whole-body skin examination and palpation of the regional lymph nodes. The focus of this evaluation is to identify risk factors, signs, or symptoms of metastases, atypical moles, and additional melanomas.[184]

Any of the major types of malignant melanoma can occur on the breast. Superficial spreading melanomas demonstrate atypical proliferation of nested, often epithelioid appearing, melanocytes associated with prominent pagetoid spread. A bandlike inflammatory infiltrate is often noted in the superficial dermis. Lentigo maligna melanomas show epidermal atrophy and prominent solar elastosis associated with subtle proliferation of melanocytes, commonly with fusiform cytology, along the basal layer with invasion into the superficial dermis. Pagetoid spread is less likely to be found, but often there is extension of tumor cells down along adnexal elements. Nodular melanomas are predominantly thick dermal lesions with limited intraepidermal spread, usually bridging across no more than three rete ridges. The cytology is epithelioid, similar to that of superficial spreading

melanoma. Desmoplastic melanomas show spindled melanocytes embedded within a fibrotic stroma, suggesting the presence of a scar from initial glances. Further examination reveals spindled cells arranged in haphazard, fascicular, or storiform growth patterns. Melanin pigmentation is often scant or absent. Unlike the immunohistochemical profile of other types of melanomas where S100 and HMB-45 are usually strongly positive, HMB-45 is either weak or absent in desmoplastic melanomas.

Of these types, however, the most common subtype of melanoma that arises on the breast is the superficial spreading type. Clinically, the lesions are large, asymmetrical plaques of variable color (from white—indicating areas of regression—to black, brown, blue, or red). Nodules within the plaque indicate areas of dermal invasion. Histologic evaluation shows a proliferation of atypical, single and nested melanocytes within the epidermis, often exhibiting pagetoid upward spread. Individual melanocytes are large, with dusty to chunky pigmentation and large, prominent nucleoli. In situ melanomas are confined to the epidermis and skin appendages. Invasive melanomas invade into the dermis and provoke a variable inflammatory host response. Depth of invasion is generally reported both by Clark's level, which reflects the functional level of invasion, and Breslow's thickness, which is the depth of invasion as measured by a calibrated ocular micrometer. Tumor staging described in the sixth edition of the American Joint Committee on Cancer Manual has undergone some significant revisions.[185-187] Any invasive melanoma 1 mm or smaller in thickness is tumor stage I. Without ulceration, such thin melanomas are stage T_{1a} if also only level II or III. Stage T_{1b} lesions have ulceration and/or are level IV. Approximately 25% of melanomas arise in preexisting melanocytic nevi. Attempts to identify which patients are at risk for malignant transformation have led to recognition of the familial melanoma syndromes. These patients have family or personal histories of melanoma and often have large, atypical nevi by both clinical and histologic criteria.[188-192]

Standard therapy for melanoma is surgical excision. For melanoma in situ, excision of the lesion or biopsy site with a 0.5-cm border of clinically normal skin and a layer of the subcutaneous tissue is sufficient. The surgical margin should be histologically free of tumor. Elective (i.e., prophylactic) regional lymph node dissection is not indicated for patients with thin melanomas. Removal and microscopic examination of the sentinel lymph node identified by dye or lymphoscintigraphy for micrometastatic melanoma has emerged as an important management tool for intermediate-thickness (1- to 4-mm) melanomas. Extensive diagnostic studies (e.g., computed tomography, magnetic resonance imaging, scintigraphy) are not indicated and should not be performed when staging asymptomatic patients[182]; however, origin of the melanoma from the skin of the breast is an independent but significant negative prognostic factor.[185-187] An exception is primary melanomas of the nipple and areola, which are exceedingly rare and

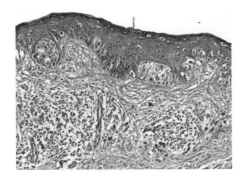

Figure 15-26 Malignant melanoma. Malignant melanoma can also occur in the breast. Although overall its biology is similar to melanomas elsewhere, melanomas of the nipple and areola are thought to have a better prognosis than nonbreast melanomas; the reasons for this are not understood.

overall have a better prognosis and lower incidence of metastasis than other melanomas of the breast.[185-187] Other negative prognostic factors include measured thickness of the melanoma from the granular layer of the epidermis to the deepest tumor cell greater than 1.5 mm, ulceration, angioinvasion, neural invasion, and male sex. Obviously, regional or distant lymphadenopathy or symptoms suggesting distant organ metastases are grave prognostic indicators. The clinical management of melanoma is no different just because it occurs on the skin of the breast.

Dermatofibrosarcoma Protuberans. Dermatofibrosarcoma protuberans (DFSP) is a low-grade skin sarcoma that usually occurs at nonmammary sites but can occur in the breast. DFSP has cytology similar to dermatofibroma, with dermal proliferation of spindled cells arranged in a storiform or herringbone pattern, interlaced with collagen bundles. Little nuclear atypia and mitoses are noted. Architecturally, however, the tumor is found to infiltrate deep into the subcutis in a honeycomb pattern. DFSPs are positive for CD34, whereas dermatofibromas are positive for factor 13a. Recent chromosomal studies and array comparative genomic hybridization (CGH) have defined characteristic amplifications and rearrangements.

Lymphomas and Pseudolymphomas. Cutaneous lymphoid infiltrates, both pseudolymphomas and lymphomas, may involve the skin of the breast (Fig. 15-27). Rosai-Dorfman disease (sinus histiocytosis with massive lymphadenopathy), an uncommon benign lymphoproliferative disorder, was reported masquerading as a

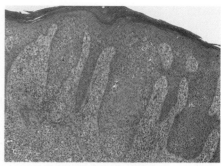

Figure 15-28 Mycosis fungoides. Mycosis fungoides is characterized by atypical dermal lymphocytes showing epidermotropism. It can similarly either arise in the breast or secondarily involve the breast.

clinically malignant left breast mass in a male patient.[193] A cutaneous lymphocytoma associated with Lyme disease manifested as a nodule in the areola of a child and resolved after treatment with ceftriaxone.[194] Mycosis fungoides, a form of cutaneous T-cell lymphoma (Fig. 15-28), which usually appears as brownish red patches with fine scale and delicate wrinkling on the skin of the trunk, can present in intertriginous areas such as inframammary folds and axillae.

Careful clinical evaluation of the patient and ancillary studies, including biopsy tissue submitted for routine processing and for molecular and genetic analysis, allow accurate categorization of most lymphoproliferative disorders. The subject of primary and secondary breast lymphoma is discussed extensively in Chapter 17.

Satellite Skin Metastasis. One should keep in mind at all times that the skin of the breast is a potential site of metastases of breast carcinoma. When the skin is involved, the breast cancer is staged as a T_4, which confers a poor prognosis. Four clinical patterns are observed: inflammatory carcinoma, telangiectatic carcinoma, nodular carcinoma, and carcinoma en cuirasse. One or more types may be present in the same patient. Sometimes, the clinical presentation, with a swollen, hard, or inflamed breast or an inverted nipple, strongly suggests skin involvement by cancer (Fig. 15-29). Other times, a biopsy is necessary (Fig. 15-30).

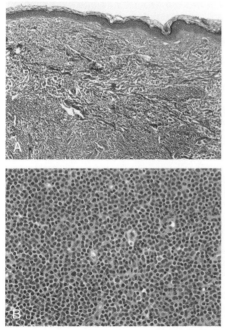

Figure 15-27 Small lymphocytic lymphoma. A small lymphocytic lymphoma can either arise in the breast or secondarily involve the breast. **A,** Here a small lymphocytic infiltrate is observed to infiltrate the dermis of the breast. **B,** At higher magnification, the cells consist of relatively mature lymphocytes.

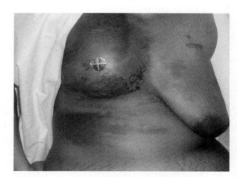

Figure 15-29 Carcinoma erysipeloids. Carcinoma erysipeloids of the breast can be obvious as a hard plaque appearance of the breast due to infiltration of the breast dermis by carcinoma cells.

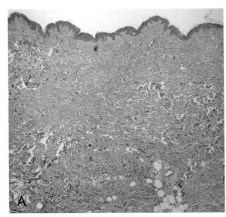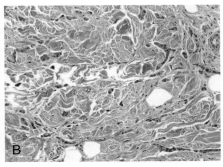

Figure 15-30 A, Breast carcinoma cells directly infiltrating the dermis of the breast. **B,** Higher magnification shows the carcinoma cells percolating through the collagen and adipose tissue. This biology, when present, uniformly confers a poor prognosis.

REFERENCES

1. Smith DM Jr, Peters TG, Donegan WL: Montgomery's areolar tubercle: A light microscopic study. Arch Pathol Lab Med 106:60, 1982.
2. Watkins F, Giacomantonio M, Salibury S: Nipple discharge and breast lump related to Montgomery's tubercles in adolescent females. J Pediatr Surg 23:718, 1988.
3. Rosenberg CA, Derman C, Grabb WC: Hypomastia and mitral valve prolapse: Evidence of a linked embryologic and mesenchymal dysplasia. N Engl J Med 309:1230, 1983.
4. David TJ: Nature and etiology of the Poland anomaly. N Engl J Med 287:487, 1972.
5. Zubowicz V, Bostwick J: Congenital unilateral hypoplasia of the female breast associated with a large melanotic spot: Report of two cases. Ann Plast Surg 12:204, 1984.
6. Treiber ES, Goldberg NS, Levy H: Breast deformity produced by morphea in a young girl. Cutis 54:267, 1994.
7. Glinick SE, et al: Becker's melanosis: Associated abnormalities. J Am Acad Dermatol 9:509, 1983.
8. Happle R: Epidermal nevus syndromes. Semin Dermatol 14:111, 1995.
9. Moore JA, Schosser RH: Becker's melanosis and hypoplasia of the breast and pectoralis major muscle. Pediatr Dermatol 3:34, 1985.
10. Van Gerwen HJ, et al: Becker's nevus with localized lipoatrophy and ipsilateral breast hypoplasia. Br J Dermatol 129:213, 1993.
11. Edwards MJ, et al: Scalp-ear-nipple syndrome: Additional manifestations. Am J Med Genet 50:247, 1994.
12. Finlay AY, Marks R: An hereditary syndrome of lumpy scalp, odd ears, and rudimentary nipples. Br J Dermatol 99:423, 1978.
13. Wilson MG: Absent nipples. Humangenetik 15:268, 1972.
14. Hindano A, Kobayishi T: Adnexal polyp of neonatal skin. Br J Dermatol 92:659, 1975.
15. Millns JL, Dickin CH: Hereditary acrolabial telangiectasia. Arch Dermatol 115:474, 1979.
16. Hanifin JM, Rajka G: Diagnostic features of atopic dermatitis. Acta Dermatol Venereol 92: S44–S47, 1980.
17. Girolomoni G, Abeni D, Masini C, et al: The epidemiology of atopic dermatitis in Italian schoolchildren. Allergy 58:420–425, 2003.
18. Whitaker-Worth DL, Carlone V, Susser WS, et al: Dermatologic disease of the breast and nipple. J Am Acad Dermatol 2000; 43:733–751, 2000.
19. Mevorah B, Frenk E, Wietlisbach V, et al: Minor clinical features of atopic dermatitis: Evaluation of their diagnostic significance. Dermatologica 177:360–364, 1988.
20. Nagaraja Kanwar AJ, Dhar S, et al: Frequency and significance of minor clinical features in various age-related subgroup atopic dermatitis in children. Pediatr Dermatol 13:10–13, 1996.
21. Rudzki E, Samuchucki Z, Litewska D, et al: Clinical features of atopic dermatitis and a family history of atopy. Allergy 46:125–128, 1991.
22. Ward KA, Burton JL: Dermatologic diseases of the breast in young women. Clin Dermatol 15:45–52, 1997.
23. Amir L: Eczema of nipple and breast: A case report. J Hum Lact 9:173–175, 1993.
24. Garcia M, del Pozo MD, Diez J, et al. Allergic contact dermatitis from a beeswax nipple-protective. Contact Dermatitis 33:440–441, 1995.
25. McGeorge BC, Steele MC: Allergic contact dermatitis of the nipple from Roman chamomile ointment. Contact Dermatitis 24:139–140, 1991.
26. Kapur N, Goldsmith PC: Nipple dermatitis—not all what it "seams." Contact Dermatitis 45:44–45, 2001.
27. Bergfeld WM, Taylor JS: Trauma, sports and the skin. Am J Ind Med 8:403–413, 1985.
28. Gibbons C, Harvey L: The clinical presentation of intraductal carcinoma of the breast. Br J Clin Pract 41:694–696, 1987.
29. Perez EA, Campbell DL, Ryu JK: Radiation recall dermatitis induced by edatreate in a patient with breast carcinoma. Cancer Invest 13:604, 1995.
30. Phillips KA, Urch M, Bishop JF: Radiation recall dermatitis in a patient treated with paclitaxel. J Clin Oncol 13:305, 1995 (letter).
31. Polgar C, Orosz Z, Fodor J: Is postirradiation angiosarcoma of the breast so rare and does breast lymphedema contribute to its development? J Surg Oncol 76:239, 2001.
32. Raghavan VT, Bloomer WD, Merkel DE: Taxol and radiation recall dermatitis. Lancet 341:1354, 1993 (letter).
33. Burstein HJ: Side effects of chemotherapy: Radiation recall dermatitis from gemcitabine. J Clin Oncol 18:693, 2000.
34. Levine EL, Ribeiro GG: Vitiligo and radiotherapy: The Koebner phenomenon demonstrated in patients with vitiligo undergoing radiotherapy for carcinoma of the breast. Clin Oncol R Coll Radiol 6:133, 1994.
35. Foxman B, D'Arcy H, Gillespie B, et al: Lactation mastitis: Occurrence and medical management among 946 breastfeeding women in the United States. Am J Epidemiol 155:103–114, 2002.
36. World Health Organization 2000 Website. Mastitis: Causes and management. Department of Child and Adolescent Health and Development, Geneva, Switzerland, 2000.
37. Kvist LJ, Hall-Lord ML, Larsson BW: A descriptive study of Swedish women with symptoms of breast inflammation during lactation and their perceptions of the quality of the care given at a breastfeeding clinic. Int Breastfeed J 2:2, 2007.
38. Amir L, Forester D, McLachlan H, Lumley J: Incidence of breast abscess in lactation women: Report from an Australian cohort. BJOG 111:1378–1381, 2004.
39. Francis-Morrill J, Heinig MJ, Pappagianis D, Dewey K: Diagnostic value of signs and symptoms of mammary candidosis among lactating women. J Hum Lact 20:288–295, 2004.
40. Thomasson P, Johansson VA, Wassberg C, Petrini B: Breastfeeding, pain and infection. Gynecol Obstet Invest 46:73–74, 1998.
41. Betzold C: Infections of the mammary ducts in the breastfeeding mother. J Nurs Pract 1:15–21, 2005.
42. Fetherston C: Mastitis in lactating women: Physiology or pathology? Breastfeed Rev 9:5–12, 2001.

43. Riordan J: Breastfeeding and human lactation, 3rd ed. Sudbury, MA, Jones and Bartlett, 2005.

44. Fetherston C, Lai C, Hartmann P: Relationships between symptoms and changes in breast physiology during lactation mastitis. Breastfeed Med 1:136–145, 2006.

45. Lawrence RA, Lawrence RM: Breastfeeding: A guide for the medical profession, 6th ed. St. Louis, Mosby, 2005.

46. Lee BJ, Adair F: Traumatic fat necrosis of the female breast. Ann Surg 72:188–195, 1920.

47. Adair FE, Munzer JT: Fat necrosis of the female breast: Report of one hundred test cases. Am J Surg 74:117–128, 1947.

48. Hadfield G: Fat necrosis of the breast. Br J Surg 17:673–682, 1930.

49. Pullyblank AM, Davies JD, Basten J, Rayter Z: Fat necrosis of the female breast—Hadfield re-visited. Breast 10:388–391, 2001.

50. Pui MH, Movson I: Fatty tissue breast lesions. Clin Imag 27:150–155, 2003.

51. Stefanik DF, Brereton HD, Lee TC, et al: Fat necrosis following breast irradiation for carcinoma: Clinical presentation and diagnosis. Breast 8:4–6, 1982.

52. Clarke D, Curtis JL, Martinez A, et al: Fat necrosis of the breast simulating recurrent carcinoma after primary radiotherapy in the management of early stage breast carcinoma. Cancer 52:442–445, 1983.

53. Rostom AY, El-Sayed ME: Fat necrosis of the breast: An unusual complication of lumpectomy and radiotherapy in breast cancer. Clin Radiol 38:31, 1987.

54. Lopez Valle CA, Hebert G: Warfarin-induced complete bilateral breast necrosis. Br J Plast Surg 45:606–609, 1992.

55. Hogge JP, Robinson RE, Magnant CM, Zuurbier RA: The mammographic spectrum of fat necrosis of the breast. Radiographics 15:1347–1356, 1995.

56. Chala LF, de Barros N, de Carmargo Moraes P, et al: Fat necrosis of the breast: Mammographic, sonographic, computed tomography, and magnetic resonance imaging findings. Curr Probl Diagn Radiol 33:106–126, 2004.

57. Frates MC, Homer MJ, Robert NJ, Smith TJ: Noniatrogenic breast trauma. Breast Dis 5:11–19, 1992.

58. Youssefzadeh S, Wolf G, Imhof H: MR findings of a breast oil cyst containing a fat-fluid level. A case report. Acta Radiol 35:492–494, 1994.

59. Evers K, Troupin RH: Lipid cyst: Classic and atypical appearances. AJR Am J Roentgenol 157:271–273, 1991.

60. Cyrlak D, Caepenter PM: Breast imaging case of the day. Radiographics 19:S80–S83, 1999.

61. Soo MS, Kornguth PJ, Hertzberg BS: Fat necrosis in the breast: Sonographic features. Radiology 206:261–269, 1998.

62. Bassett LW, Gold RH, Cove HC: Mammographic spectrum of traumatic fat necrosis: The fallibility of "pathognomonic" signs of carcinoma. AJR Am J Roentgenol 130:119–122, 1978.

63. Orson LW, Cigtay OS: Fat necrosis of the breast: Characteristic xeromammographic appearance. Radiology 146:35–38, 1983.

64. Abenoza P, Ackerman AB: Neoplasms with eccrine differentiation—Ackerman's histologic diagnosis of neoplastic skin diseases: A method by pattern analysis. Philadelphia, Lea & Febiger, 1989.

65. Requena L, Kiryu H, Ackerman AB: Neoplasms with apocrine differentiation—Ackerman's histologic diagnosis of neoplastic skin disease: A method by pattern analysis. Philadelphia, Lippincott-Raven, 1998.

66. Gulmen S, Pullon PA: Sweat gland carcinoma of the lips. Oral Surg Oral Med Oral Pathol 41:643, 1976.

67. Kelly DE, Klein KM, Harrigan WF: Lip reconstruction following resection for an unusual basal-cell carcinoma. Oral Surg Oral Med Oral Pathol 40:19, 1975.

68. Chamberlain RS, Huber K, White JC, et al: Apocrine gland carcinoma of the axilla: Review of the literature and recommendations for treatment. Am J Clin Oncol 22:1, 1999.

69. Urso C, Bondi R, Paglierani M, et al: Carcinomas of sweat glands. Arch Pathol Lab Med 125:498, 2001.

70. Ahn SK, Chung J, Lee WS, et al: Hybrid cysts showing alternate combination of eruptive vellus hair cyst, steatocystoma multiplex, and epidermoid cyst, and an association among the three conditions. Am J Dermatopathol 18:645, 1996.

71. Hurlimann AF, Panizzon RG, Burg G: Eruptive vellus hair cyst and steatocystoma multiplex: Hybrid cysts. Dermatology 192:64, 1996.

72. Tomkova H, Fujimoto W, Arata J: Expression of keratins (K 10 and K 17) in steatocystoma multiplex, eruptive vellus hair cysts, and epidermoid and trichilemmal cysts. Am J Dermatopathol 19:250, 1997.

73. Albers SE, Barnard M, Thorner P, et al: Erosive adenomatosis of the nipple in an eight-year-old girl. J Am Acad Dermatol 40:834–837, 1999.

74. Jones DV: Florid papillomatosis of the nipple duct. Cancer 8:315–319, 1955.

75. Burdick C, Rinehart RM, Matsumoto T, et al: Nipple adenoma and Paget's disease in a man. Arch Surg 91:835–838, 1965.

76. Bourlond J, Bourlond-Reinert L: Erosive adenomatosis of the nipple. Dermatology 1992;185:319–324.

77. Diaz NM, Palmer JO, Wick MR: Erosive adenomatosis of the nipple: Histology, immunohistology, and differential diagnosis. Mod Pathol 5:179–184, 1992.

78. Velpeau A: On disease of the mammary areola preceding cancer of the mammary region (trans: Mitchell H). Sydenham Society, London, 1856.

79. Paget J: On disease of the mammary areola preceding carcinoma of the mammary gland. St Bartholomews Hosp Rep 10:87–89, 1874.

80. Ashikari R, Park K, Huvos AG, Urban JA: Paget's disease of the breast. Cancer 26:680–685, 1970.

81. Chaudary MA, Millis RR, Lane EB, Miller NA: Paget's disease of the nipple: A ten-year review including clinical, pathological, and immunohistochemical findings. Breast Cancer Res Treat 8:139–146, 1986.

82. Dixon AR, Galea MH, Ellis IO, et al: Paget's disease of the nipple. Br J Surg 78:722–723, 1991.

83. Osther PJ, Balslev E, Blichert-Toft M: Paget's disease of the nipple. Acta Chir Scand 156:343–352, 1990.

84. Jamali FR, Ricci A, Deckers PJ: Paget's disease of the breast. Am J Surg 76:365–381, 1970.

85. Muir R: Pathogenesis of Paget's disease of the nipple and associated lesions. Br J Surg 22:728–737, 1935.

86. Inglis K: Paget's disease of the nipple, with special reference to changes in the ducts. Am J Pathol 22:1–33, 1946.

87. Yim JH, Wick MR, Philpott GW, et al: Underlying pathology in mammary Paget's disease. Ann Surg Oncol 4:287–292, 1997.

88. Kollmorgen DR, Varanasi JS, Edge SB, Carson WE III: Paget's disease of the breast: A 33-year experience. J Am Coll Surg 187:171–177, 1998.

89. Kothari AS, Beechey-Newman N, Hamed H, et al: Paget disease of the nipple: A multifocal manifestation of higher-risk disease. Cancer 95:1–7, 2002.

90. Fu W, Mittel VK, Young SC: Paget disease of the breast: Analysis of 41 patients. Am J Clin Oncol 24:397–400, 2001.

91. Bijker N, Rutgers EJ, Duchateau L, et al: Breast-conserving therapy for Paget's disease of the nipple. Cancer 91:472–477, 2001.

92. Caliskan M, Gatti G, Sosnovskikh I, et al: Paget's disease of the breast: The experience of the European Institute of Oncology and review of the literature. Breast Cancer Res Treat 112:513–521, 2008.

93. Chen C, Sun L, Anderson B: Paget disease of the breast: Changing patterns of incidence, clinical presentation, and treatment in the U.S. Cancer 107:1448–1458, 2006.

94. Haerslev T, Krag JG: Expression of citokeratin and erbB-2 oncoprotein in Paget's disease of the nipple. An immunohistochemical study. APMIS 100:1041–1047, 1992.

95. Wolber RA, Dupuis BA, Wick MR: Expression of c-erb-B2 oncoprotein in mammary and extrammamary Paget's disease. Am J Clin Pathol 96:243–247, 1991.

96. Lammie GA, Barnes DM, Millis RR, Gullick WJ: An immunohistochemical study of the presence of c-erbB-2 protein in Paget's disease of the nipple. Histopathology 15:505–514, 1989.

97. Winstanley J, Cooke T, Murray GD, et al: The long term significance of c-erB-2 in primary breast cancer. Br J Cancer 63:447–450, 1991.

98. McCann AH, Dervan PA, O'Regan M, et al: Prognostic significance of c-erbB-2 and oestrogen receptor status in human breast cancer. Cancer Res 51:3296–3303, 1991.

99. Lovekin C, Ellis IO, Locker A, et al: c-erbB-2 oncoprotein expression in primary and advanced breast cancer. Br J Cancer 63:439–443, 1991.

100. Soderstrom CE, Harms SE, Copit DS, et al: 3D RODEO breast MRI of lesions containing ductal carcinoma in situ. Radiology 201:427–432, 1996.

101. Kawase K, Dimaio DJ, Tucker SL, et al: Paget's disease of the breast: There is a role for breast-conserving therapy. Ann Surg Oncol 1:21–27, 2005.

102. Chen C, Sun L, Anderson B: Paget disease of the breast: Changing patterns of incidence, clinical presentation, and treatment in the U.S. Cancer 107:1448–1458, 2006.

103. Pierce LJ, Haffty BG, Solin LJ, et al: The conservative management of Paget's disease of the breast with radiotherapy. Cancer 80:1065–1072, 1997.

104. Sukumvanich P, Bentrem DJ, Cody HS, et al: The role of sentinel lymph node biopsy in Paget's disease of the breast. Ann Surg Oncol 14:1020–1023, 2007.

105. Laronga C, Nasson D, Hoover S, et al: Paget's disease in the era of sentinel lymph node biopsy. Am J Surg 192:481–483, 2006.

106. Schmidt GB: Ueber das Angiosarkom der Mamma. Arch Klin Chir 36:421–427, 1887.

107. Agarwal PK, Mehrotra R: Haemangiosarcoma of the breast. Ind J Cancer 14:182–185, 1977.

108. Alvarez-Fernandez E, Salinero-Paniagua E: Vascular tumors of the mammary gland. Virchows Arch (Pathol Anat) 394:31–47, 1981.

109. Stout AP: Hemangio-endothelioma: A tumor of blood vessels featuring vascular endothelial cells. Ann Surg 118:445–464, 1943.

110. Batchelor GB: Haemangioblastoma of the breast associated with pregnancy. Br J Surg 46:647–649, 1959.

111. Hamazaki M, Tanaka T: Hemangiosarcoma of the breast: Case report with scanning electron microscopic study. Acta Pathol Jpn 28:605–613, 1978.

112. Steingaszner LC, Enzinger FM, Taylor HB: Hemangiosarcoma of the breast. Cancer 18:352–360, 1965.

113. Borrmann R: Metastasenbildung bei histologisch gutartigen Geschwülsten: Fall von metastasierendem Angiom. Beitr Pathol Anat 40:372–393, 1907.

114. Ewing J: Neoplastic diseases, a textbook on tumors. Philadelphia, WB Saunders, 1919, pp 223–224.

115. Tibbs D: Metastasizing hemangioma: A case of malignant hemangioendothelioma. Br J Surg 40:465–470, 1953.

116. Merino MJ, Berman M, Carter D: Angiosarcoma of the breast. Am J Surg Pathol 1:53–60, 1983.

117. Chen KT, Kirkegaard DD, Bocian JJ: Angiosarcoma of the breast. Cancer 46:268–271, 1980.

118. Rosen PR, Kimmel M, Ernsberger D: Mammary angiosarcoma. Cancer 62:2145–2151, 1988.

119. Hacking EA Jr, Tiltman AJ, Dent MA: Angiosarcoma of the breast. Clin Oncol 10:177–180, 1984.

120. Yap J, Chuba PJ, Thomas R, et al: Sarcoma as a second malignancy after treatment for breast cancer. Int J Radiat Oncol Biol Phys 52:1231–1237, 2002.

121. Pendlebury SC, Bilous M, Langlands AO: Sarcomas following radiation therapy for breast cancer: A report of three cases and a review of the literature. Int J Radiat Oncol Biol Phys 31:405–410, 1995.

122. Hatfield PM, Schulz MD: Postirradiation sarcoma. Including 5 cases after X-ray therapy of breast carcinoma. Radiology 96:593–602, 1970.

123. Taghian A, de Vathaire F, Terrier P, et al: Long-term risk of sarcoma following radiation treatment for breast cancer. Int J Radiat Oncol Biol Phys 21:361–367, 1991.

124. Gupta RK, Naran S, Dowle C: Needle aspiration cytology and immunohistochemical study in a case of angiosarcoma of the breast. Diagn Cytopathol 1991;7:363–365, 1991.

125. Tschen JA, Ramsdell WM: Disciform erythrasma. Cutis 31:541, 1983.

126. Dekio S, Kawasaki Y, Jidoi J: Herpes simplex on nipples inoculated from herpetic gingivostomatitis of a baby. Clin Exp Dermatol 11:664, 1986.

127. Hallopeau H: Leçons cliniques sur les maladées cutanées et syphiliques. Union Med Can 43:472, 1887.

128. Stühmer A: Balanitis xerotica obliterans (post operationem) und ihre beziehungem zur Kraurosis glandis et preaeputii Penis. Arch Derm Syph (Berlin) 156:613–623, 1928.

129. Woodruff JD, Baens JS: Interpretation of atrophic and hydrothrophic alterations in the vulvar epithelium. Am J Obstet Gynecol 86:713–723, 1963.

130. Oberfield RA: Lichen sclerosus et atrophicus and kraurosis vulvae. Arch Dermatol 83:144–153, 1962.

131. Ackerman AB: The lives of lesions. Philadelphia, Lea & Febiger, 1984, pp 131–137, 194–201.

132. Wallace HJ: Lichen sclerosus et atrophicus. Trans St Johns Hosp Derm Soc 57:9–30, 1971.

133. Cario GM, House MJ, Paradinas FJ: Squamous cell carcinoma of the vulva in association with mixed vulvar dystrophy in an 18-year-old girl. Br J Obstet Gynaecol 91:87–90, 1984.

134. Woodruff JD: Carcinoma in situ of the vulva. Clin Obstet Gynecol 28:230–239, 1985.

135. Buscema J, Stern J, Woodruff JD: The significance of the histologic alterations adjacent to invasive vulvar carcinoma. Am J Obstet Gynecol 137:902–909, 1980.

136. Shirer JA, Ray MC: Familial occurrence of lichen sclerosus et atrophicus. Arch Dermatol 123:485–488, 1987.

137. Tremaine RDL, Miller RA: Lichen sclerosus et atrophicus. Int J Dermatol 28:10–16, 1989.

138. Nomland R: Lichen sclerosus et atrophicus (Hallopeau) and related cutaneous atrophies. Arch Dermatol Syph 21P:575–594, 1930.

139. Herzberg JJ, Meyer-Rohr J, Unna PJ: Sclerolichen Gougerot. Arch Klin Exp Dermatol 216:246–259, 1963.

140. Wallace HJ: Lichen sclerosus et atrophicus. Trans St Johns Hosp Derm Soc 57:9–30, 1971.

141. Helm KF, Gibson LE, Muller SA: Lichen sclerosus et atrophicus in children and young adults. Pediatr Dermatol 8:97–101, 1991.

142. Murphy FR, Lipa M, Haberman HF: Familial vulvar dystrophy of lichen sclerosus type. Arch Dermatol 118:329–331, 1982.

143. Williams GA, Richardson AC, Hatchcock EW: Topical testosterone in dystrophic diseases of the vulva. Am J Obstet Gynecol 96:21–30, 1966.

144. Foulds IS: Lichen sclerosus et atrophicus of the scalp. Br J Dermatol 103:197–200, 1980.

145. Ayhan A, Urman B, Yuece K, et al: Topical testotosterone for lichen sclerosus. Int J Gynaecol Obstet 30:253–255, 1989.

146. Poskitt L, Wojnarowska F: Lichen sclerosus as a cutaneous manifestation of thyroid disease [letter]. J Am Acad Dermatol 28:665, 1993.

147. Garcia-Bravo B, Sánchez-Pedreno P, Rodríguez-Pichardo A, et al: Lichen sclerosus et atrophicus. J Am Acad Dermatol 19:482–485, 1988.

148. Pasieczny TAH: The treatment of balanitis xerotica obliterans with testosterone propionate ointment. Acta Derm Venereol (Stockh) 57:275–277, 1977.

149. Suurmond D: Lichen sclerosus et atrophicus of the vulva. Arch Dermatol 90:143–152, 1964.

150. Tremaine R, Adam JE, Orizaga M: Morphea coexisting with lichen sclerosus et atrophicus. Int J Dermatol 29:486–489, 1990.

151. Aberer E, Neumann R, Lubec G: Acrodermatitis chronica atrophicans in association with lichen sclerosus et atrophicans: Tubulointersititial nephritis and urinary excretion of spirochete-like organisms. Acta Derm Venereol (Stockh) 67:62–65, 1987.

152. Bergbrant IM: Seborrhoeic dermatitis and Pityrosporum yeasts. Curr Top Med Mycol 6:95, 1995.

153. DeFranzo AJ, Marasco P, Argenta LC: Warfarin-induced necrosis of the skin. Ann Plast Surg 34:203, 1995.

154. Selva A, et al: Pyoderma gangrenosum-like ulcers associated with lupus anticoagulant. Dermatology 189:182, 1994.

155. Green RA, Dowden RV: Mondor's disease in plastic surgery patients. Ann Plast Surg 20:231, 1988.

156. Finkel LJ, Griffiths CE: Inflammatory breast carcinoma (carcinoma erysipeloides): An easily overlooked diagnosis. Br J Dermatol 129:324, 1993.

157. Cianchini G, et al: Acral Darier's disease successfully treated with adapalene. Acta Derm Venereol 81:57, 2001.

158. Knulst AC, De La Faille HB, Van Vloten WA: Topical 5-fluorouracil in the treatment of Darier's disease. Br J Dermatol 133:463, 1995.

159. Colome MI, Sanchez RL: Dermatomyofibroma: Report of two cases. J Cutan Pathol 21:371, 1994.

160. Mentzel T, Calonje E, Fletcher CD: Dermatomyofibroma: Additional observations on a distinctive cutaneous myofibroblastic tumour with emphasis on differential diagnosis. Br J Dermatol 129:69, 1993.

161. Shelley ED, Shelley WB, Kurczynski TW: Painful fingers, heat intolerance, and telangiectases of the ear: Easily ignored childhood signs of Fabry disease. Pediatr Dermatol 12:215, 1995.

162. Calonje E, Fletcher CD: Sinusoidal hemangioma: A distinctive benign vascular neoplasm within the group of cavernous hemangiomas. Am J Surg Pathol 15:1130, 1991.

163. Meunier L, Barneon G, Meynadier J: Acquired progressive lymphangioma. Br J Dermatol 131:706, 1994.

164. Rosso R, Gianelli U, Carnevali L: Acquired progressive lymphangioma of the skin following radiotherapy for breast carcinoma. J Cutan Pathol 22:164, 1995.

165. Dawn G, et al: Bilateral symmetrical pilar leiomyomas on the breasts. Br J Dermatol 133:331, 1995.

166. Nascimento AG, Karas M, Rosen PP, et al: Leiomyoma of the nipple. Am J Surg Pathol 3:151–154, 1979.

167. Tsujioka K, Kashihara M, Imamura S: Cutaneous leiomyoma of the male nipple. Dermatologica 170:98–100, 1985.

168. Diaz-Arias AA, Hurt MA, Loy TS, et al: Leiomyoma of the breast. Hum Pathol 20:396–399, 1989.

169. Webber J: Leiomyoma of the nipple. S Afr J Surg 13:117–120, 1975.

170. Haier J, Haensh W, Schon M: Leiomyoma as a rare differential diagnosis of Paget's disease of the nipple. Acta Obstet Gynecol Scand 76:490–491, 1997.

171. Virchow R: Uber cavernose (erektile) Geschwulste und Teleangiektasien. Virchows Arch Pathol Anat 6:525–554, 1854.

172. Nazario ACP, Tanaka CI, Lima GR, et al: Leiomyoma of the breast. A case report. Sao Paulo Med J 113:992–994, 1995.

173. Tamir G, Yampolsky I, Sandbank J: Parenchymal leiomyoma of the breast. Report of a case and clinicopathological review. Eur J Surg Oncol 21:88–89, 1995.

174. Howard LK, Hirsch EF: Leiomyoma of the breast. J Surg Oncol 62:62–64, 1996.

175. Pujol RM, Fernandez MT: A solitary papule on the nipple. Arch Dermatol 127:571–576, 1991.

176. Nasemann T, Schmidt KU: Solitary leiomyoma of the nipple. Aktuel Dermatol 11:134–135, 1985.

177. Stout AP: Solitary cutaneous and subcutaneous leiomyoma. Am J Cancer 24:435–464, 1937.

178. Webber B: Leiomyoma of the nipple. S Afr J Surg 13: 117–120, 1975.

179. Velasco M, Ubeda B, Autonell F, Serra C: Leiomyoma of the male areola infiltrating the breast tissue [letter]. AJR Am J Roentgenol 164:511–512, 1995.

180. Carney JA: Carney complex: The complex of myxomas, spotty pigmentation, endocrine overactivity and schwannomas. Semin Dermatol 14:90, 1995.

181. Thomas JM: Premalignant and malignant epithelial tumors. In Sams WM, Lynch J (eds): Principles and practice of dermatology. New York, Churchill Livingstone, 1990.

182. Lee YN, Sparks FC, Morton DL: Primary melanoma of the skin of the breast region. Ann Surg 185:17, 1977.

183. Roses DF, et al: Cutaneous melanoma of the breast. Ann Surg 189:112, 1979.

184. National Institutes of Health Consensus Development Conference: Diagnosis and treatment of early melanoma. Bethesda, MD, National Institutes of Health, 1992.

185. Garbe C, et al: Primary cutaneous melanoma: Prognostic classification of anatomic location. Cancer 75:2492, 1995.

186. Papachristou DN, et al: Melanoma of the nipple and areola. Br J Surg 66:287, 1979.

187. Balch CM, et al: Melanoma of the skin. In Greene FL, et al (eds): AJCC staging manual, 6th ed. New York, Springer-Verlag, 2002.

188. Carey WP Jr, et al: Dysplastic nevi as a melanoma risk factor in patients with familial melanoma. Cancer 74:3118, 1994.

189. Goldstein AM, Tucker MA: Genetic epidemiology of familial melanoma. Dermatol Clin 13:605, 1995.

190. Lucchina LC, et al: Familial cutaneous melanoma. Melanoma Res 5:413, 1995.

191. Newton JA: Genetics of melanoma. Br Med Bull 50:677, 1994.

192. Newton JA: Familial melanoma. Clin Exp Dermatol 18:5, 1993.

193. Mac Moune Lai F, et al: Cutaneous Rosai-Dorfman disease presenting as a suspicious breast mass. J Cutan Pathol 21:377, 1994.

194. Gautier C, Vignolly B, Taieb A: Benign cutaneous lymphocytoma of the breast areola and erythema chronicum migrans. Arch Pediatr 2:343, 1995.

chapter 16

Digital Automation of Breast Biomarker Immunocytochemistry

SANFORD H. BARSKY | MOHAN UTTARWAR

The digital revolution has taken center stage in both clinical medicine and biomedical research. Digital telemedicine, radiology, and cardiology have replaced traditional subjective diagnostic modalities in their respective specialties. Pathology, the interpretation of disease patterns under the microscope, has not until recently begun to embrace this digital revolution. For more than 150 years since the time of Virchow, pathologists have diagnosed diseases based on their subjective interpretations of visual patterns produced by passing light through translucent tissue sections. Because the interpretation of these patterns is subjective, interobserver variability (variance among different pathologists' interpretation of the same slide set), intraobserver variability (variance among the same pathologist's interpretation of the same slide set over time), and fatigue variability often confound accurate disease interpretation. Two recent technologic developments, however, have begun to catalyze progress and wider acceptance of digital pathology. The first was the creation of a high throughput microscopic slide scanner, which can convert traditional glass microscopic slides to digital images that can be stored, retrieved, shared via the Internet, and most importantly, algorithmically analyzed. The second was the creation of epithelial-recognition algorithms (ERAs) and specific-recognition algorithms (SRAs) that could identify and quantitate immunocytochemical staining patterns[1,2] and specific histologic features such as nuclear size and mitosis. These initial approaches to digital pathology had to be first explored in a research setting, because routine clinical applications would require stringent U.S. Food and Drug Administration approval. However, numerous research applications were soon discovered where the power of virtual microscopy and digital imaging algorithms could be realized.

High Throughput Approaches to Tissue Microarrays

These ERAs and SRAs could be applied to digital images of both whole microscopic slides as well as tissue microarrays (TMAs). TMAs are a form of high throughput screening where numerous tissue biopsies from hundreds of patients can be analyzed on a single microscopic slide and resulting image. High throughput screening is taking center stage in biomedical research; high throughput screening methods such as cDNA and "oligospotted" microarrays, proteomic blots, and TMAs allow biomedical researchers to analyze patient biospecimens (tissues and fluids) for DNA, RNA and protein content.[3-5] To achieve the goal of personalized medicine within the next decade where patients' treatments are individualized, physicians must discover predictive markers that guide individualized therapy. The final and ultimate proof of any putative biomarker discovered by genomic or proteomic approaches lies in an evaluation of its pattern of in situ tissue expression that only TMAs can provide. The advent of digital pathology approaches and imaging technology that can scan TMAs into "virtual slides" with high resolution and analyze their images algorithmically will accelerate the discovery of predictive biomarkers.

In recent studies, we have applied our algorithms (ERAs and SRAs) to whole slides and TMAs from human cases of breast, colon, and lung cancer and analyzed each case for two nuclear, cytoplasmic, and membrane immunocytochemical markers that were either homogeneously or heterogeneously expressed and compared the algorithmic measurements with the subjective ones.[1,2] We were able to report the successful creation of both ERAs based on selective imaging properties (Gaussian kernel and elongation ratio) and SRAs based on pixel colors (red, green, and blue; RGB) and gray scale intensities that can analyze both immunocytochemical staining and specific histologic features. Compared with traditional subjective pathologic interpretation, these digital imaging algorithms were better able to identify cancer cells in a background of stroma (Fig. 16-1); successfully compartmentalize the cancer cells into nucleus, cytoplasm, and membrane; and accurately and rapidly quantitate the degree of immunocytochemical staining (Fig. 16-2). These illustrations depict one

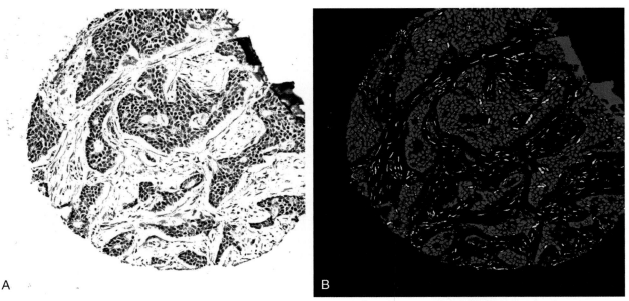

Figure 16-1 Breast cancer tissue sample **(A)** is subjected to image processing and the application of the epithelial-recognition algorithms that could image the carcinoma cells red and the stromal cells yellow **(B)**. An applied filter could remove the noncarcinomatous areas, allowing the application of the subsequent immunocytochemical specific-recognition algorithms to only the carcinoma cells.

of the many immunocytochemical markers that were studied—in this case, the estrogen receptor (ER) in human breast cancer. These initial algorithmic approaches established a proof of principle that diverse tissue patterns of disease could be studied and analyzed using artificial intelligence.

Clinical Applications

Life science information technology has begun to revolutionize all aspects of medicine.[6-10] Anatomical pathology has, however, lagged behind this life science information technology revolution. Anatomical pathology is a field of

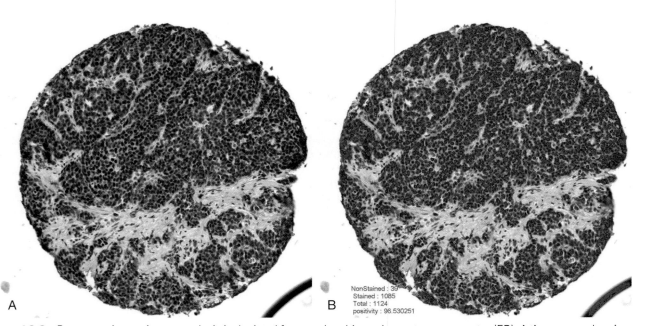

Figure 16-2 Breast carcinoma image analysis is depicted for a nuclear biomarker, estrogen receptor (ER). A tissue core showing positive ER immunoreactivity **(A)** was preprocessed by mask removal and contrast enhancement followed by epithelial area identification. Only in this epithelial area were the tumoral nuclei imaged and then based on their more red than blue pixel values; the ER-positive nuclei were imaged red as distinguished from the ER-negative nuclei, which were imaged green **(B)**. The epithelial area was calculated at 80.376%, percent ER positivity at 96.530%, and median nuclear intensity of the positive nuclei at 94 (0, most intense; 255, least intense).

medicine that relies on the visual interpretation of tissues patterns of disease. The interpretation of these patterns is subjective. Even though immunocytochemistry has added a targeted and more objective approach to disease pattern interpretation,[7] interobserver, intraobserver, and fatigue variability are still issues that confound successful disease interpretation.

Because immunocytochemical staining patterns measure specific single targets rather than the relatively complex and intricate disease patterns seen on hematoxylin and eosin (H&E) staining, immunocytochemical studies would inherently be more amenable to digital image algorithm design and implementation.[8,9] In the present study, we have created, implemented and validated novel imaging algorithms for estrogen and progesterone receptors, as well as HER2/neu, three important prognostic and predictive biomarkers of human breast cancer. Unlike other commercial and public imaging systems,[11,12] these algorithms were independent of proprietary hardware and were based on not just luminosity and color but also many other imaging properties, including epithelial pattern recognition and nuclear morphology.

STEPS IN VIRTUAL SLIDE CREATION AND ANALYSIS

Image Acquisition

Image acquisition used either a scanner (Aperio Scan-Scope T2 System, Vista, California; or iSCAN, BioImagene, Inc., Cupertino, California) or microscope with attached digital camera (Paxcam, MIS, Villa Park, Illinois) or analog camera (Hitachi HVD30, Hitachi, San Francisco, California), all capable of producing images with a resolution of 20 pixels/10μ. Areas of each image were screened, and the area of interest richest in tumor cells was manually selected for image processing. Images were processed initially by "jpg" conversion of scanned virtual slides or direct "jpg" photomicrograph capture. Following image acquisition, images were screened for quality, enhanced, and processed.

Software for Image Analysis

For our overall approach of writing the software for image processing and analysis, we used Visual C++. Visual C++ has many features which are required for the development of core image processing algorithms. With Visual C++, we have created imaging algorithms that enhance and process the imported images so that ultimately we can recognize and quantitate nuclear ER and progesterone receptor (PR) immunoreactivity and membrane HER2/neu immunoreactivity.

Quality of Image Evaluation

Every acquired image was not of sufficient quality to be further evaluated. Several criteria determined image quality. These included luminosity, sharpness, and contrast. Poor image quality could be a function of several factors: variation in staining, nonuniform illumination of the sample, or nonlinear quantitation of the image

capturing device. A number of techniques could be used to improve image quality and normalize image variations. With these techniques, some inferior images could be improved to the point that they could be evaluated. Still, some images could not be improved sufficiently and had to be discarded. Roughly 5% of the imported images needed to be discarded. Preprocessing algorithms attempted to reduce the effect of variations in staining intensity and the effects of colored masks and other anomalies. These preprocessing algorithms had four distinct steps: verifying the image content, mask removal, contrast enhancement, and background removal.

Verifying the Content of the Image

The cell detection process could be simplified if processing fields or areas of slides that did not have tissue were skipped. This could be detected by computing the mean and standard deviations of the red, blue, and green planes of the image. In the case of the areas without tissue, there were little or no variations in colors. Standard deviations, which reflected variation, were low.

Mask Removal

The mask or background in an image was represented by determining the mean of pixel values. By mapping the mean of pixel values to the mid-value of the pixel value range, we achieved a mask removal effect or normalization of the background to a standard value. To accomplish mask removal, the contrast was stretched. The contrast stretching could be applied on the gray image as well as in each color plane separately.

Let us consider the gray image. If X_{min} is the minimum gray value in the image and X_{max} is the maximum gray value in the image where $X_{min} = 0, \ldots 255$, then if x was the original gray value of any pixel, its contrast stretch value was:

$$T(x) = 255 * \left(\left(\frac{X - X_{min}}{X_{max} - X_{min}} \right) \right)$$

Contrast Enhancement

For contrast enhancement, the algorithms first differentiated the objects of interest from the background. At this point, we were not considering the finer details within the object. Therefore, we transformed the image in such a manner that objects that were darker than the background became even darker. If the background was bright (which normally was the case), using the preprocessing algorithms, the background became even brighter. Contrast in a digital image referred to the difference in color values between any two given pixels. Color values at a given pixel were independently computed from the RGB components of the given color image.

The first step in this preprocessing was the determination of the active range of intensities in each of the colors. We computed the histogram of all color planes (RGB) of the input image. We used these histograms to compute a minimum intensity such that, starting from lowest intensity, the cumulative pixels up to minimum intensity was equal to 0.5% of total pixels in the image. Next, we mapped the active range to (0, 255). All pixels with values less than minimum intensity were discarded (Fig. 16-3). In each color plane, we computed the probability density function from the histogram as follows:

$$T(\mathbf{r}_k) = 255 * \sum \left(\frac{n_i}{n}\right)$$
$$j = 0, \ldots k; k = 0, \ldots, 255$$

Brightness was a subjective descriptor that was almost impossible to measure. Here, we increased or decreased the brightness using the control function that follows:

$$x^1 = x^0 + (\text{control value}) * x^0$$

High contrast images were visually appealing. However, the linear contrast enhancement had one serious limitation; it led to saturation at both the high and low end of the intensity range. To avoid this, we used a nonlinear contrast adjustment scheme known as the gamma correction.

The transformation function we used can be expressed as follows:

$$T(r) = r^\gamma$$

where $\gamma < 1$ reduced the contrast, and $\gamma > 1$ increased the contrast.

Background Removal

The region of interest could be detected based on two distinctive features of the epithelial area. The epithelial area was darker compared with the stromal area, and the epithelial cells were more densely packed than the stromal cells. We computed the minimum background intensity using mean and standard deviation. The minimum background intensity was computed independently for each color plane. If any color component of a pixel was greater than the respective minimum background intensity, then the pixel was treated as a background pixel. All background pixels were given 255 values in RGB planes.

PRINCIPLES OF IMAGE ALGORITHMS

Once the image had been optimized using the various preprocessing algorithms, the image was analyzed with a combination of epithelial and nuclear recognition algorithms that use both colorimetric (RGB) as well as intensity (gray scale) values. A flow chart of these algorithms is depicted in Figure 16-3.

Epithelial Recognition Algorithms

Epithelial cell detection used the Gaussian kernel. The Gaussian kernel was a well-known imaging concept for weighted averaging of pixels in a small window centered around a given pixel. The region of interest could be detected based on two distinctive features of the epithelial area. The epithelial area was darker compared to the stromal area, and the epithelial cells were more densely packed than the stromal cells.

Specific-Nuclear Recognition Algorithms

The nuclear recognition algorithms and the determination of positive versus negative staining were initially predicated on the colorimetric differences between stained and unstained nuclei. Positive nuclei demonstrating brown staining consist of pixels with more red than blue. These algorithms then used the gray scale (0 to 255) to quantitate intensity of staining. So, for example, the mean, median, and modal intensities of staining of all positive nuclei could easily be determined.

Specific Membrane Recognition Algorithms

For the membrane recognition algorithms to correctly identify the membrane of the cancer cell, the cancer cell first had to be compartmentalized into nucleus, cytoplasm, and membrane. The membrane was defined as a peripheral structure oriented around the nucleus in a 360-degree fashion. After defining the membrane, the algorithm detected the pixels on the basis of RGB colors with brown defined as pixels with more red than blue. Positive staining membranes were detected in this manner. For each membrane, the exact extent and degree of immunoreactivity was determined, and the overall percentage of cancer cells and the percent membrane circumference showing positivity was determined. From this determination, an ordinal score of HER2/neu immunoreactivity was assigned. The intent of the algorithmic ordinal value measurement was to imitate or duplicate what the pathologist sees subjectively. The power of any imaging algorithm was that it could actually quantitate what was imaged.

In this case, the membrane immunoreactivity could be defined as the product of the median staining intensity (calculated on a gray scale [0 to 255, with 0 being the darkest or most intense and 255 being the lightest or least intense]) and the membrane thickness (calculated on the basis of RGB colors, with brown defined as pixels with red > blue). The details of this calculation are summarized. Because we needed to express the median membrane intensity on a continuous scale that reflected increased staining, the 0 to 255 gray scale of membrane intensity had to be compressed and inverted to a 0 to 100 scale, with 0 being least intense and 100 most intense. The product of this median membrane intensity and membrane thickness was also expressed on a 0 to 100 scale.

VALIDATION OF ALGORITHM MEASUREMENTS OF ESTROGEN AND PROGESTERONE RECEPTORS BY COMPARISON WITH SUBJECTIVE MEASUREMENTS

The overall measurements provided by the algorithms were compared with the subjective scores for both ER and PR. A total of 67 cases was studied for ER and a total of 54 cases for PR. For these comparisons, standard tests of statistical analysis were used. Intraclass correlations were calculated to assess the level of agreement among percent positivity scores collectively for ER and PR. One

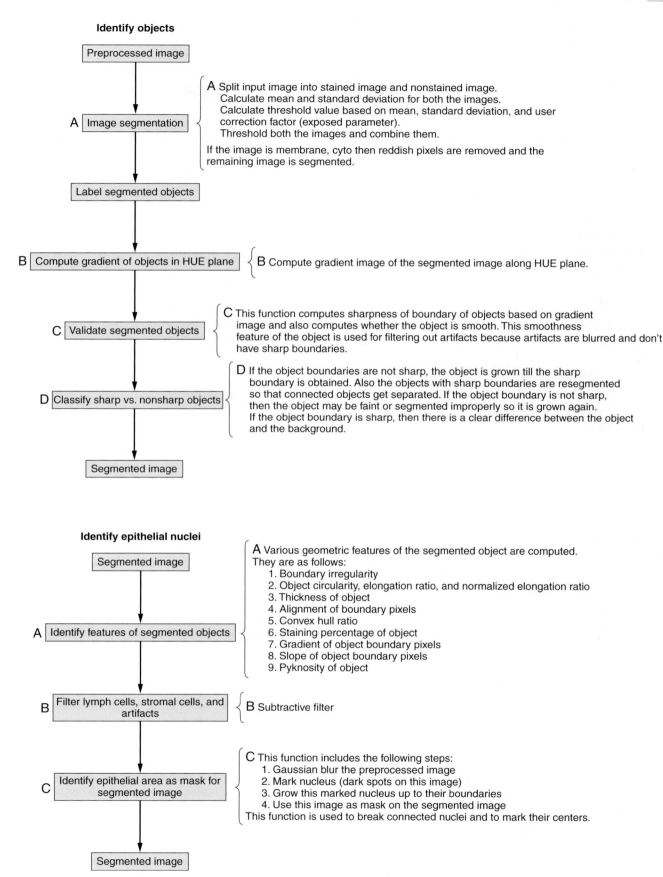

Identify objects

Preprocessed image

A Image segmentation

A Split input image into stained image and nonstained image. Calculate mean and standard deviation for both the images. Calculate threshold value based on mean, standard deviation, and user correction factor (exposed parameter). Threshold both the images and combine them.

If the image is membrane, cyto then reddish pixels are removed and the remaining image is segmented.

Label segmented objects

B Compute gradient of objects in HUE plane

B Compute gradient image of the segmented image along HUE plane.

C Validate segmented objects

C This function computes sharpness of boundary of objects based on gradient image and also computes whether the object is smooth. This smoothness feature of the object is used for filtering out artifacts because artifacts are blurred and don't have sharp boundaries.

D Classify sharp vs. nonsharp objects

D If the object boundaries are not sharp, the object is grown till the sharp boundary is obtained. Also the objects with sharp boundaries are resegmented so that connected objects get separated. If the object boundary is not sharp, then the object may be faint or segmented improperly so it is grown again. If the object boundary is sharp, then there is a clear difference between the object and the background.

Segmented image

Identify epithelial nuclei

Segmented image

A Identify features of segmented objects

A Various geometric features of the segmented object are computed. They are as follows:
1. Boundary irregularity
2. Object circularity, elongation ratio, and normalized elongation ratio
3. Thickness of object
4. Alignment of boundary pixels
5. Convex hull ratio
6. Staining percentage of object
7. Gradient of object boundary pixels
8. Slope of object boundary pixels
9. Pyknosity of object

B Filter lymph cells, stromal cells, and artifacts

B Subtractive filter

C Identify epithelial area as mask for segmented image

C This function includes the following steps:
1. Gaussian blur the preprocessed image
2. Mark nucleus (dark spots on this image)
3. Grow this marked nucleus up to their boundaries
4. Use this image as mask on the segmented image
This function is used to break connected nuclei and to mark their centers.

Segmented image

Figure 16-3 Summary of preprocessing and epithelial-recognition algorithms.

intraclass correlation was calculated for the agreement among three subjective raters. Separate intraclass correlations were calculated for agreement between the algorithm and each subjective rater. Intercept-only random effects models were fit to the ER/PR data, with random effect variance components for slides, raters, and error variance. The intraclass correlation was calculated as the variance component for the individual slides divided by the sum of the three variance components. Confidence intervals for the intraclass correlations were calculated using the delta method.

VALIDATION OF ALGORITHM MEASUREMENTS OF HER2/neu BY COMPARISON WITH SUBJECTIVE MEASUREMENTS AND HER2/neu FLUORESCENCE IN SITU HYBRIDIZATION

To assess interrater agreement, weighted kappa statistics were calculated for each pair of HER2/neu scores (each pair of subjective raters and also the ordinal algorithm score paired with each subjective rater). The number of agreements and disagreements between the algorithm and each subjective rater were then tabulated, with disagreements categorized based on whether the algorithm gave a higher or lower score than the subjective rater. The data were summarized in this way in order to characterize tendencies regarding the direction of the disagreements.

We separately analyzed all subjective 0, 1+, 2+, and 3+ cases and, within each group, correlated the subjective and algorithmic measurements with HER2/neu fluorescent in situ hybridization (FISH) specifically to see whether the algorithmic measurements helped resolve the usually ambiguous HER2/neu 2+ group. We analyzed not only the algorithmic continuous scale measurements but also the algorithmic ordinal scale measurements from this perspective. Using HER2/neu FISH as the gold standard and a HER2/Cep17 ratio greater than 2.2 as positive, we calculated the positive predictive value (true positives/[true positives + false positives]) and the negative predictive value (true negatives/[true negatives + false negatives]) for each of the subjective, algorithmic ordinal, and algorithmic continuous score measurements.

RESULTS OF DIGITAL IMAGE ANALYSIS

Estrogen and Progesterone Receptors

For over a decade, the semiquantitative immunohistochemistry of ER and PR has been the "standard of care," replacing the more quantitative but cumbersome dextran charcoal method. However, the subjective and ordinal nature of ER and PR immunohistochemistry might benefit from more objectivity and reproducibility. This is provided with digital pathology.

Image acquisition by using a scanner or an analog or digital camera with microscope uniformly produced sharp images with high contrast. For approximately 10% of the images, mask removal and contrast enhancement improved image quality. For approximately 5% of the acquired images, image quality was below the standard where the algorithms were not interpretable. A typical processed and enhanced image from a representative ER-positive case (Fig. 16-4) and a representative ER-negative case (Fig. 16-5) is depicted.

For both ER and PR, an arbitrary cutoff of greater than or equal to 10% positivity has been historically interpreted as positive. Using this value, the subjective interpretations revealed 51 cases interpreted as positive and 16 cases as negative for ER, and 31 cases interpreted as positive and 23 cases negative for PR. The positive ER cases exhibited a range of a values of 35% to 90% and the negative ER cases a range of values of 0% to 9%. The positive PR cases exhibited a range of values of 30% to 90% and the negative PR cases a range of values of 0% to 9%.

The algorithmic measurements showed a 85% agreement with the subjective measurements as far as a determination of positivity/negativity of ER and a 81% agreement with PR. For ER, there were eight cases where the subjective interpretation was negative and the algorithms recorded a positive score. In two cases, the subjective interpretation was positive, whereas the algorithms recorded a negative score. For PR, there were ten cases where the subjective interpretation was negative and the algorithms recorded a positive score. In three cases, the subjective interpretation was positive, whereas the algorithms recorded a negative score.

The algorithm-based actual values for ER and PR percentage nuclear positivity strongly correlated with the subjective measurements (intraclass correlation: 0.77; 95% confidence interval: 0.59, 0.95) yet exhibited no interobserver, intraobserver, or fatigue variability. The intraclass correlation was very high among the subjective raters. The intraclass correlations between the algorithm and the subjective raters were lower but still in the range generally considered good to excellent. Because the algorithm recorded percent positivity on a true continuous scale, there were few instances where the score given by a subjective rater matched the algorithm score exactly. Among those cases not matching exactly, the algorithm tended to record a higher percent positivity than the subjective raters. In the three subjective raters, the algorithm recorded a higher percent positivity in 84% of the cases not matching exactly. The algorithmic image detection of ER and PR immunoreactivity appeared to be more sensitive than subjective interpretation.

In addition, the algorithms provided measurements of nuclear ER and PR staining intensity (mean, mode and median staining intensity of positive staining nuclei), clinically important parameters that subjective measurements could not assess (Fig. 16-6). These measurements of intensity of ER and PR nuclear staining did not necessarily correlate with either subjective or algorithmic measurements of percent positivity.

HER2/neu

Similar image acquisition and application of the specific membrane algorithms were highly effective in identifying the membrane region of the breast carcinoma cell and distinguishing it from the nucleus and cytoplasm.

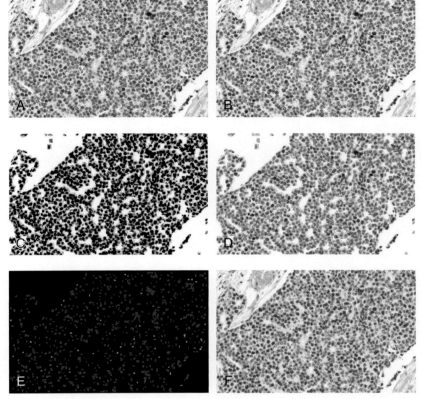

Figure 16-4 Estrogen receptor (ER)–positive case. Immunocytochemical image of ER–positive lesion showing brown-staining of positive nuclei **(A)**, with the image preprocessed by mask removal **(B)** and contrast enhancement **(C)** followed by epithelial area identification **(D)**. In this epithelial area, all tumoral nuclei (*blue*) are imaged **(E)** and then based on more red than blue pixel values, and the ER-positive nuclei (red) are distinguished from the ER-negative nuclei (*green*) and imaged appropriately **(F)**.

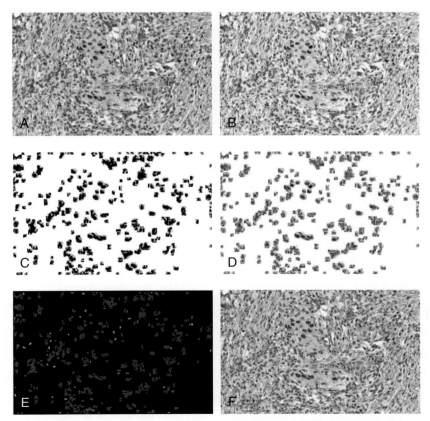

Figure 16-5 Estrogen receptor (ER)–negative case. Immunocytochemical image of ER showing relative absence of brown-staining of nuclei **(A)**, with the image preprocessed by mask removal **(B)** and contrast enhancement **(C)** followed by epithelial area identification **(D)**. In this epithelial area, all tumoral nuclei (*blue*) are imaged **(E)** and then based on more red than blue pixel values, and the ER-positive nuclei (red) are distinguished from the ER-negative nuclei (*green*) and imaged appropriately **(F)**.

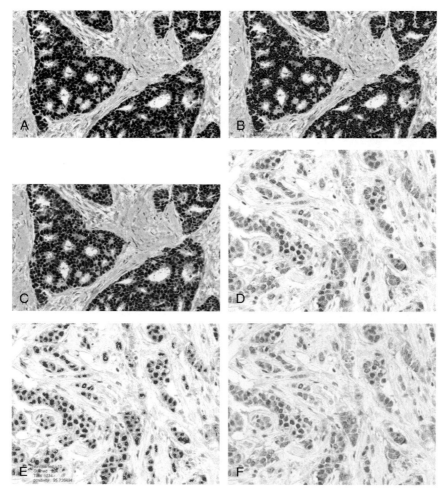

Figure 16-6 Median nuclear intensity is an independent parameter distinct from percent positivity. In estrogen receptor (ER)-positive cases **(A)**, not only can percentage positivity be measured by the algorithm **(B)**, but the median intensity of ER positivity among the positive nuclei can also be measured **(C)**. Results are expressed as relative gray scale values, with 0 being most intense and 255 least intense. This case demonstrates high median nuclear intensity. In another case, even when the percentage positivity measured by the algorithm is high **(D)**, the median intensity of ER positivity among the positive nuclei can be low **(E)**. Results are expressed as relative gray scale values **(F)**.

Subsequent algorithms were able to calculate both an ordinal value of HER2/neu membrane immunoreactivity analogous to the subjective interpretation as well as a value of HER2/neu immunoreactivity based on an expanded continuous scale that subjective review could not assess. The algorithm-based measurements of HER2/neu both on the ordinal scale and on the continuous scale exhibited no interobserver, intraobserver, or fatigue variability. Typical images from both whole slides as well as TMA cores exhibiting a gamut of HER2/neu immunoreactivity are depicted (Figs. 16-7 to 16-9).

There was a generally good correlation between the algorithmic ordinal scale measurements and the subjective scores (intraclass correlation: 0.84; 95% confidence interval: 0.79, 0.89). For both whole slides as well as the TMA measurements for the majority of comparisons, the weighted kappa statistic between algorithm and rater was greater than between raters. This suggested that the degree of interobserver variability was greater than the level of agreement/disagreement between algorithm and rater. With both whole slides as well as TMA cores,

when the algorithm and the subjective rater gave different scores, the algorithm score tended to be higher. The algorithm gave a higher score than the subjective rater in 50.7% of cases. The algorithm score was lower than the subjective rater in only 9.8% of cases. Most of these score discrepancies were between scores of 0 and 1+ and between scores of 1+ and 2+.

The HER2/neu FISH scores were obtained as a gold standard to which the subjective, the ordinal algorithmic values, and the continuous scale algorithmic values could be compared. The methodology described earlier was used to calculate the ratio of error variance to total variance for each rater. Lower ratios indicated stronger association with the FISH score. The ratio of error variance to total variance was smallest in the continuous algorithm score (0.46), indicating that this score had the strongest association with the FISH score. Among the ordinal scores (subjective vs. algorithmic), the algorithm-derived scores had the stronger association with the FISH scores (ratio = 0.59).

With respect to their predictive values, the algorithmic continuous score was better able to discriminate true

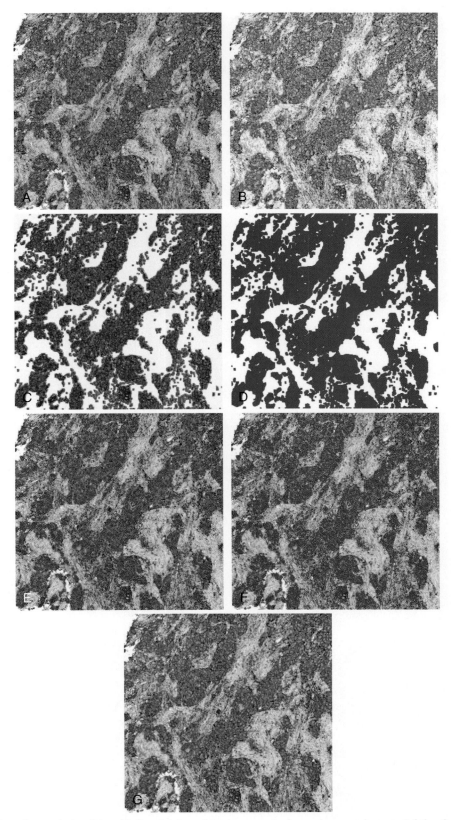

Figure 16-7 HER2/neu from whole slide with 3+ staining. A high amount of membranous brown staining is evident **(A)**; the image was preprocessed by mask removal **(B)** and contrast enhancement **(C)** followed by epithelial area identification **(D)**. In this epithelial area, all tumoral nuclei (*blue*) are imaged **(E)** and then based on more red than blue pixel values, and the prominent membrane positive area (*red*) is distinguished from the unstained area and imaged appropriately **(F)**; the thickness of this membrane is calculated based on more red than blue pixel values and then the median membrane intensity is calculated using the modified and inverted gray scale **(G)**. In addition to the assignment of an ordinal score, the product of membrane thickness and median intensity is used to assign a continuous score value of Her2/neu immunoreactivity.

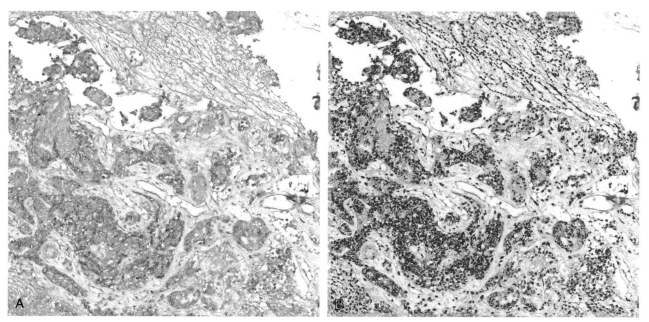

Figure 16-8 HER2/neu from whole slide with 1+ staining. A low amount of membranous brown staining is evident **(A)**; the image was preprocessed and the degree of membrane immunoreactivity in only the epithelial area determined. The weak membrane positive area (*red*) is distinguished from the unstained area and imaged appropriately **(B)**. Results are expressed as both an ordinal as well as continuous score.

positives from true negatives (Table 16-1). Both the subjective and the algorithmic ordinal scores had a relatively low positive predictive value (38%–39% vs. 44–45%) in the 2+ group. The continuous algorithm scores, on the other hand, when stratified between 11- to 19-year-olds and 20- to 29-year-olds (groups that generally corresponded to the 2+ ordinal classification), were able to produce a high negative predictive value (90%–94%) in the former group and a relatively high positive predictive value (75%–78%) in the latter group (see Table 16-1). Furthermore, the algorithmic continuous scale measurements were better able to determine the true degree of gene amplification.

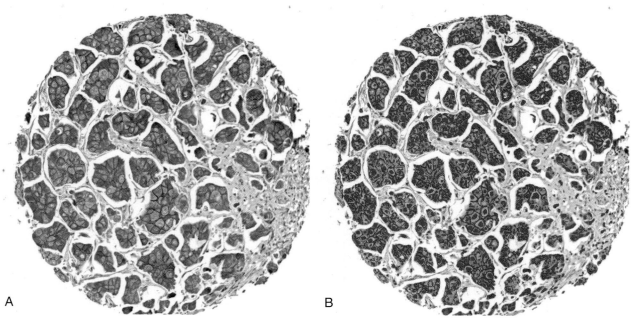

Figure 16-9 HER2/neu from tissue microarray core with 2+ staining. Moderate membranous brown staining is evident **(A)**; the image was preprocessed and the degree of immunoreactivity in only the epithelial area determined. The membrane positive area (*red*) is distinguished from the unstained area and imaged appropriately **(B)**; results are expressed as both an ordinal as well as continuous score.

TABLE 16-1

Predictive Values of Subjective versus Algorithmic Immunocytochemical Measurements Using *Her2/Neu* Fluorescence in Situ Hybridization as the Gold Standard

Subjective (ordinal)	0	Negative predictive value	+1	Negative predictive value	+2	Positive predictive value	+3	Positive predictive value		
Whole slide (n = 150)	60	100%	32	78%	36	39%	22	96%		
TMA core (n = 300)	130	100%	70	88%	60	38%	40	95%		
Algorithm (ordinal)	0	Negative predictive value	+1	Negative predictive value	+2	Positive predictive value	+3	Positive predictive value		
Whole slide (n = 150)	60	100%	26	96%	40	45%	24	96%		
TMA core (n = 300)	130	100%	62	100%	66	44%	42	95%		
Algorithm (continuous)	0–5	Negative predictive value	6–10	Negative predictive value	11–19	Negative predictive value	20–29	Positive predictive value	30–100	Positive predictive value
Whole slide (n = 150)	60	100%	25	100%	20	90%	20	75%	25	100%
TMA core (n = 300)	130	100%	62	100%	34	94%	32	78%	42	100%

Significance and Future Importance of Digital Image Analysis

A number of different commercial and public imaging systems have been used or could be used to measure ER and PR immunoreactivity in human breast cancer.[11–13] The limits of any immunocytochemical study are three-fold: specificity, affinity, avidity, and sensitivity of the antibody being used[7]; the antigenic target within the tissues being studied[13–17]; and the imaging system used for analysis. Algorithmic-based image analysis eliminates some of the limitations of subjective interpretations, namely interobserver, intraobserver, and fatigue variability. In addition, algorithmic-based image analysis can provide a continuous mathematically quantifiable measurement of immunoreactivity instead of the arbitrary ordinal values provided by subjective measurements. Once the field of view is selected by the pathologist, algorithmic analysis is almost instantaneous, objective, and reproducible. In our opinion, this adds value.

ER and PR immunocytochemical staining produce colorimetric differences in nuclear staining that conventionally have been interpreted manually by pathologists and expressed as percentage of positive tumoral nuclei. The ER and PR status of human breast cancer represents important prognostic and predictive markers of this cancer that dictate therapeutic decisions, but their subjective interpretation result in interobserver, intraobserver, and fatigue variability.[13,18–20] Subjective measurements are traditionally limited to a determination of percentage of tumoral nuclei that show positive immunoreactivity.

Digital imaging algorithms, in addition to providing precise measurements of percent nuclear positivity, provide measurements of nuclear ER and PR staining intensity (mean, mode, and median staining intensity of positive-staining nuclei), parameters that subjective review does not usually assess. Although some subjective studies of ER and PR have evaluated intensity of nuclear staining on an ordinal scale of 0, weak, intermediate, and strong intensity and have combined these measurements with percentage of nuclear positivity,[15] the imprecise and largely subjective nature of these measurements confound meaningful interpretations. Currently, clinical trials are in progress examining the effects of tamoxifen, aromatase inhibitors, and chemotherapy on breast cancer in both an adjuvant and neoadjuvant setting.[21, 22] Their effects on the expression of ER, PR, and other nuclear markers mandate accurate, objective, and reproducible quantification of both percentage and intensity of receptor expression and not just a subjective determination of positive versus negative staining. The automated algorithms that precisely quantitate the percentage of staining and measure intensity on a continuous scale are better suited to provide this important data than traditional subjective review.

For HER2/neu, algorithmic-based image analysis eliminates most of the limitations of subjective interpretations. This analysis can also provide a mathematically quantifiable and highly reproducible measurement of immunoreactivity not provided by subjective measurements. In addition, algorithmic-based image analysis can offer measurements that simply cannot be measured subjectively. The expanded algorithms used in the present study were able to quantitate HER2/neu immunostaining on a continuous scale, which correlated much more strongly with HER2/neu FISH, the gold standard in HER2/neu measurements. Furthermore, these continuous scale algorithms were able to provide better positive and negative predictive values by better "resolving" the somewhat ambiguous 2+ ordinal grouping of HER2/neu immunoreactivity. Furthermore, the continuous scale algorithms allowed for more precise quantification of the degree of HER2/neu expression. With the ordinal scale, anywhere from 2.2- to 60-gene amplification is reflected by the same 3+ level of expression, yet with the continuous scale, the range of expression can vary from 20 to as much as 100. Clearly, all 3+ cases are not the same. This ability to further refine measurements of the exact degree of immunostaining based on quantitative image characteristics improves on our assessment of overall HER2/neu immunoreactivity. Just as our measurements of HER2/neu immunoreactivity need not be limited to traditional ordinal values, our measurements of HER2/neu FISH need not be limited also to only the interval ratios (0.8 – 1.2; 1.2 – 2.1; ≥2.2) that are usually reported. There is no reason why HER2/neu FISH cannot be measured and reported on a continuous scale. In fact, even HER2/neu FISH can be analyzed by algorithmic image analysis rather than just subjectively. We are in the process of developing algorithms that can analyze HER2/neu FISH.

Therefore, the algorithmic measurements of HER2/neu on a continuous scale might be expected to provide a better biomarker of prognosis and response to therapy. Cases all identified as 3+ may, in fact, be quite heterogeneous and biologically diverse in terms of their degree of gene amplification, their behavior, and their response to therapy. The algorithmic continuous scale measurements may better define this heterogeneity. Future clinical trials examining the effects of targeted therapies against the HER2/neu receptor mandate accurate, objective, and reproducible quantification of HER2/neu expression.[23,24] The automated algorithms that precisely quantitate HER2/neu immunoreactivity on a continuous scale are better suited to provide this important data than traditional subjective review. Outcome data on HER2/neu status and the efficacy of trastuzumab (Herceptin) has been limited outside of clinical trials. Trastuzumab was only recently approved in an adjuvant setting, and many of the patients in our retrospective study did not receive trastuzumab treatment. A retrospective study comparing our digital algorithmic classifications would need to be stratified to those patients who received trastuzumab and those who did not. In other words, we would need to compare our measurements of HER2/neu as a prognostic marker separately from our measurements of HER2/neu as a predictive marker. We presently are accruing cases to address these questions.

Image analysis continues to develop, and it is being used as methods for improved pathologic detection[25] and analysis.[26] The real power of the present algorithms lies in their untapped potential for full automation. The present algorithms lack discriminatory power to recognize tumor cell density or to discriminate tumor cells from normal epithelial cells. Subjective evaluations of ER, PR or HER2/neu immunocytochemical staining tacitly use a subjective step of selection of the area of the slide containing the most tumor cells. Pathologists do this routinely and somewhat subconsciously. Recognition of the region of interest or field of view containing the highest density of tumor cells is certainly within the potential of algorithmic analysis and, if we can create such algorithms, image analysis of ER, PR, and HER2/neu can be fully automated in the not-too-distant future.

Conflict (Duality) of Interests

Sanford H. Barsky, MD, is the Donald A. Senhauser Endowed Chair of Pathology at Ohio State and a founder of BioImagene, Inc. Dr. Barsky currently serves as the Medical Director of BioImagene, Inc. (uncompensated) but is a minority share holder. Mohan Uttarwar is the Chief Executive Officer of BioImagene, Inc.

REFERENCES

1. Sharangpani GM, Joshi AS, Porter K, et al: Semi-automated imaging system to quantitate estrogen and progesterone receptor immunoreactivity in human breast cancer. J Microsc 226:244–255, 2007.
2. Joshi AS, Sharangpani GM, Porter K, et al: Semi-automated imaging system to quantitate Her-2/neu membrane receptor immunoreactivity in human breast cancer. Cytometry A 71:273–285, 2007.
3. Torhorst J, Bucher C, Kononen J, et al: Tissue microarrays for rapid linking of molecular changes to clinical endpoints. Am J Path 159:2249–2256, 2001.
4. Kononen J, Bubendorf L, Kallioniemi A, et al: Tissue microarray for high-throughput molecular profiling of tumor specimens. Nat Med 4:844–847, 1998.
5. Mobasheri R, Airley CS, Foster GS, Shakibaei M: Post-genomic applications of tissue microarrays: Basic research, prognostic oncology, clinical genomics and drug discovery. Histopathology 19:325–355, 2004.
6. Acharyya S, Lawrence B, Baum JK, et al: Diagnostic performance of digital versus film mammography for breast-cancer screening, New Eng J Med 353:1773–1783, 2005.
7. Adams GP, Tai MS, McCartney JE, et al: Avidity-mediated enhancement of in vivo tumor targeting by single-chain Fv dimers. Clin Cancer Res 12:1599–1605, 2006.
8. Castelli, F, Frith C, Frith U, et al: Movement and mind: A functional imaging study of perception and interpretation of complex intentional movement patterns. NeuroImage 12:314–325, 2000.
9. Chen JH, Chuang KH: Image-based physiological artifacts estimation and correction technique for functional MRI. Magn Reson Med 46:344–353, 2001.
10. Cox RE, Flagle C, Hooper FJ, et al: Effect of filmless imaging on the utilization of radiologic services. Radiology 215:163–167, 2000.
11. Ellis B, Decker WJ, McLaren G: Histological reconstruction and automated image analysis. ChromaVision Medical Systems, Inc. U.S. Patent 6,631,203, 2003.
12. Ellis, B, Decker WJ, McLaren G: Histological reconstruction and automated image analysis. Clarient, Inc., U.S. Patent 6,947,583, 2005.
13. Goldhirsch A, Glick JH, Gelber RD, et al: Seventh international conference on adjuvant therapy of primary breast cancer. J Clin Oncol 19:3817–3827, 2001.
14. Gonzalez RC, Woods RE: Digital image processing. Boston, Addison-Wesley, 1992, p 174.
15. Harvey JM, Clark GM, Osborne CK, Allred DC: Estrogen receptor status by immunohistochemistry is superior to the ligand-binding assay for predicting response to adjuvant endocrine therapy in breast cancer. J Clin Oncol 17:1474–1481, 1999.
16. Jain AK: Fundamentals of digital image processing. Englewood Cliffs, NJ, Prentice-Hall, 1989, pp 241–243.
17. Neves JI, Begnami MD, Arias, V, Santos GC: Antigen retrieval methods and estrogen receptor immunoexpression using 1D5 antibody: A comparative study. Int J Surg Pathol 13:353–357, 2005.

18. Osborne CK: Tamoxifen in the treatment of breast cancer. N Engl J Med 339:1609–1618, 1998.

19. Pal SK, Ghosh A: Image segmentation using fuzzy correlation. Inf Sci 62:223–250, 1992.

20. Ravdin PM, Green S, Dorr TM, et al: Prognostic significance of progesterone receptor levels in estrogen receptor-positive patients with metastatic breast cancer treated with tamoxifen: Results of a prospective Southwest oncology group study. J Clin Oncol 10: 1284–1291, 1992.

21. Shao ZM, Li J, Wu J, Han QX, et al: Neo-adjuvant chemotherapy for operable breast cancer induces apoptosis. Breast Can Res Treat 53:263–269, 1999.

22. Wu J, Shen ZZ, Lu JS, et al: Prognostic role of p27 and apoptosis in human breast cancer. Br J Cancer 79:1572–1578, 1999.

23. Slamon DJ, Romond EH, Perez EA: Advances in adjuvant therapy for breast cancer. Clin Adv Hemotol Oncol 4:4–9, 2006.

24. Finn RS, Slamon DJ: Monoclonal antibody therapy for breast cancer: Herceptin. Cancer Chemother Biol Response Modif 21: 223–33, 2003.

25. Van Driel-Kulker AMJ, Eysackers MJ, Dessing MTM, et al: A simple method to select specific tumor areas in paraffin blocks for cytometry using incident fluorescence microscopy. Cytometry 7:601–604, 1986.

26. Mehes G, Lorch T, Ambros PR: Quantitative analysis of disseminated tumor cells in the bone marrow by automated fluorescence image analysis. Cytometry 42:357–362, 2000.

chapter 17

Breast Lymphoma

NINA J. KARLIN

Primary extranodal involvement has been described for several organs that contain lymphoid tissue, including skin, bone, brain, gastrointestinal tract, thyroid, testis, Waldeyer's ring, and breast. Primary lymphoma of the breast is not a common entity and is usually a non-Hodgkin's type. In fact, the majority is B-cell lymphomas, and the most common histologic type is diffuse large B-cell lymphoma (DLBCL; Fig. 17-1). The T-cell phenotype is extremely rare. Intermediate- and high-grade histologies predominate, including mantle cell lymphomas (Fig. 17-2), but follicular lymphomas, mucosa-associated lymphoid tissue (MALT) lymphomas, and marginal zone lymphomas (Fig. 17-3) have also been described. Rare instances of breast involvement by Hodgkin's lymphoma have also been described in the literature.[1]

Only a few hundred cases of primary breast lymphoma have been reported in small retrospective series,[2-15] and only one prospective study has been identified.[16] Primary breast lymphoma arises from resident stromal lymphocytes and accounts for 2.2% of extranodal lymphomas.[17] Approximately 1% of patients with extranodal disease have breast involvement, and only 0.1% of breast tumors are lymphomas.[18] It most frequently occurs in women between 50 and 60 years of age, although it can also occur in men[19] and in younger women. In fact, when it occurs in younger women or pregnant women, it is more often bilateral, and more often exhibits features of a Burkitt's or Burkitt's-like lymphoma[20] (Fig. 17-4). Furthermore, contralateral relapse occurs in up to 15% of cases, which suggests a possible malignant clone or a homing mechanism.

Primary breast lymphoma may be accurately diagnosed when the breast is the first major site of lymphomatous manifestation and there is no evidence of concurrent, systemic disease. Morphologically, there are no differences between primary and secondary breast lymphoma, but it is important to distinguish between the two. Wiseman and Liao reported that primary breast lymphoma must satisfy several criteria: adequate pathologic evaluation, mammary tissue and lymphomatous infiltrate must be in close association, and exclusion of either systemic lymphoma or previous extramammary lymphoma.[21] Importantly, ipsilateral axillary lymph node involvement is accepted as part of the definition of primary breast lymphoma.[21] Breast lymphoma may be considered secondary when the breast is involved, in addition to widespread systemic lymphomatous involvement. Such would be the case in chronic lymphocytic leukemia (CLL) or in small lymphocytic lymphoma with secondary involvement of the breast (Fig. 17-5). Although in many situations where there is both breast as well as systemic involvement, it is impossible to determine which came first.

Clinical Features

Most breast lymphomas present as a painless, mobile, enlarging mass. They tend to be larger than epithelial breast cancers, and the average size is 4 cm. Interestingly, the right breast is more frequently involved than the left breast. Patients may also present with respiratory symptoms, bulky lymphadenopathy, "B" symptoms, and central nervous system (CNS) disease.

Spontaneous regression of primary breast lymphoma has also been reported but remains quite infrequent.[22] Primary non-Hodgkin's lymphoma has also been reported to have arisen from an intramammary lymph node (thus, in this case, it may be considered nodal).[23] Intravascular large B-cell lymphoma of the breast has also been described.[24] Finally, six cases of anaplastic large cell lymphoma (T-cell variant) have been described in association with silicone breast implants.[25]

The epidemiology, natural history, appropriate treatment, and prognosis of primary breast lymphoma is somewhat controversial, and a firm consensus has not been fully established. The majority of information on this entity is culled from case reports and retrospective reviews. Some series suggest that the breast is an unfavorable primary site and carries a worse prognosis than that of other extranodal lymphomas of the same stage. The overall survival rate of primary breast lymphoma with a B-cell phenotype is 43% at 5 years.[26] This is worse than that reported for extranodal lymphoma of the thyroid (79%)[27] and Waldeyer's ring (70%).[28] Some studies also suggest a higher rate of contralateral organ and CNS relapse (in similar fashion to primary testicular lymphoma).[29,30] Contralateral involvement can be either synchronous or metachronous up to 10 years after the first lesion. Whether primary breast lymphoma exhibits tropism for the CNS remains a contentious and unresolved issue.

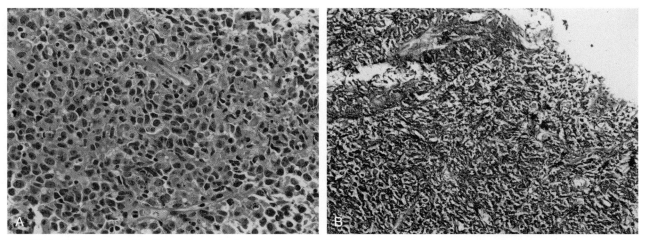

Figure 17-1   Diffuse large B cell lymphoma is the most common histologic type of primary breast lymphoma **(A)**, confirmed immunohistochemically by positive CD20 **(B)**.

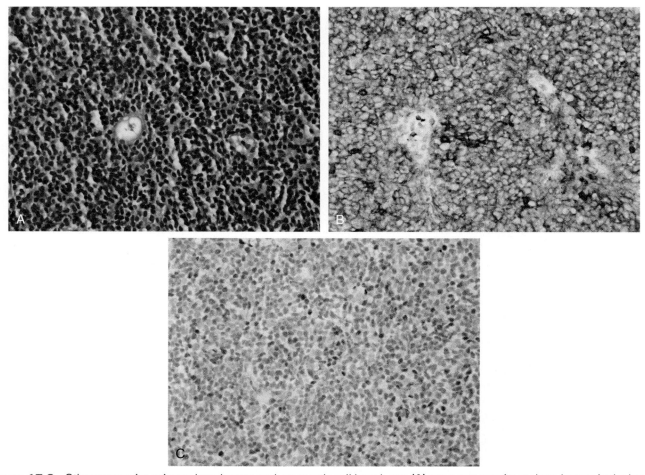

Figure 17-2   Other aggressive primary lymphomas such as mantle cell lymphoma **(A)** can occur as primary lymphomas in the breast, confirmed immunohistochemically by positive CD5 **(B)** and bcl-1 **(C)** staining.

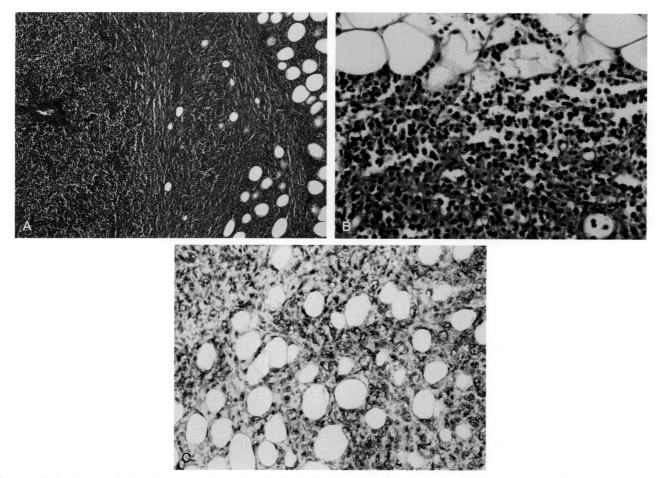

Figure 17-3 Low-grade lymphomas, such as marginal zone lymphomas, can likewise occur as primary breast lymphoma. At low magnification, a "marginal" zone of lymphocytes is seen **(A)**, illustrated at higher magnification as a monotonous sheet of cells **(B)**, and confirmed by intense CD20 immunoreactivity **(C)**.

Radiologic Features

Malignant lymphoma of the breast is frequently well defined and circumscribed and difficult to distinguish from other types of tumor by mammography. A typical radiographic appearance is a well-circumscribed, oval-shaped mass without calcification. However, mammographic findings may range from a discrete, well-circumscribed nodule with benign features to a lesion with speculated borders. Patients with primary breast lymphoma may even have normal mammography. Sonographic features also can vary, and quite often they reveal hypoechogenicity with well-defined borders that lack significant acoustic shadowing. It should be stressed, however, that a wide spectrum of appearances can be found on ultrasound with primary breast lymphoma. Fluoro(^{18}F)-2-deoxyglucose positron emission tomography (FDG-PET) maintains a sensitivity and specificity of 89% and 100% for non-Hodgkin's lymphoma.[31]

Pathologic Features

Diagnosis of breast lymphoma is based on cytologic and histopathologic features of this unique neoplasm. Histologically, breast lymphoma typically resembles other anatomic site lymphomas. A uniform population of malignant lymphoid cells densely infiltrates mammary lobules and effaces normal parenchymal architecture (see Figs. 17-1 to 17-5). Distinction of breast lymphoma from poorly differentiated breast carcinomas and pseudolymphoma is important. Fine needle aspiration cytologic examination is a useful but limited tool for primary breast lymphoma. It can be difficult to distinguish lymphoid cells from reactive lymphocytes. Studies of clonality may be useful. Adequate tissue biopsy for histopathologic evaluation and immunophenotyping remains a key step. However, even after pathologic review of tissue, primary breast lymphoma may be difficult to diagnose. Immunohistochemical markers can aid conventional histologic examination. Some authors

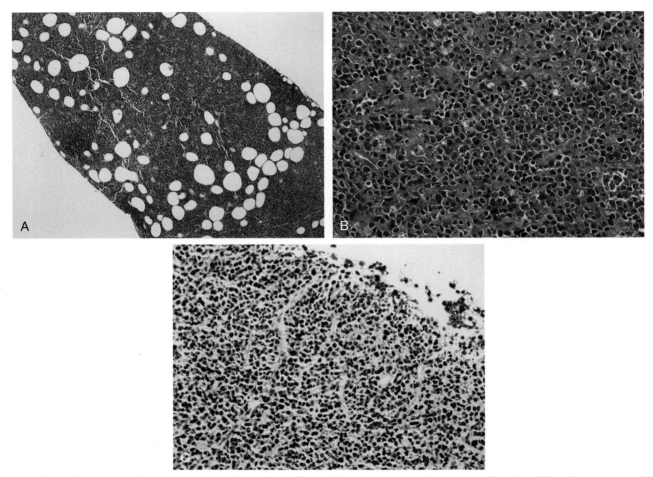

Figure 17-4 High-grade primary breast lymphomas (e.g., Burkitt's) can also occur. At low magnification, diffuse involvement of the breast is observed **(A)**, confirmed at higher magnification as a highly infiltrative process **(B)**, and marked by a very high (>98%) Ki-67 proliferative index **(C)**.

suggest that BOB.1 and Oct2 are overexpressed in primary breast lymphoma and may be useful immunohistochemical markers for DLBCL of the breast.[32] Other investigators have shown that primary breast DLBCLs have high proliferative rates and characteristics of a nongerminal center phenotype[26] (see Fig. 17-1). They postulate that these characteristics may contribute to a poorer prognosis. In addition, molecular analysis techniques using (cDNA) microarrays may facilitate identification of different molecular "signatures" in lymphomas with identical morphology (as has been the case with nodal DLBCLs).

Staging

Most of our knowledge of primary breast lymphoma, because of the rareness of the disease, comes from isolated case reports or a limited series of cases.[33-55] Primary breast lymphomas are staged similarly to other non-Hodgkin's lymphomas, and the Ann Arbor staging system is used. Minimum recommended studies include computed tomography of the chest, abdomen, and pelvis; bone marrow biopsy; and laboratory data (complete blood count with differential, serum chemistry, liver function tests, and lactate dehydrogenase). Furthermore, assessment of the contralateral breast is mandatory, because primary breast lymphoma can be bilateral.[48]

Treatment and Prognosis

Treatment for primary breast lymphoma varies widely and is guided by the subtype and stage of lymphoma. Mastectomy generally is not recommended,[33] because these malignancies are extremely sensitive to both multiagent chemotherapy combined with Rituxan and/or radiation therapy. For aggressive lymphoma limited to the breast, as well as for indolent lymphoma that is stage IIE or higher, systemic chemotherapy remains the treatment of choice. Radiotherapy, which may also be incorporated into the treatment schema, is the treatment of choice for indolent lymphoma limited to the breast. It is used as sole treatment for stage IE indolent lymphoma and follow-up chemotherapy for aggressive stage IE and IIE non-Hodgkin's lymphoma.

CNS intrathecal prophylaxis may be considered for patients with primary DLBCL or Burkitt's lymphoma of

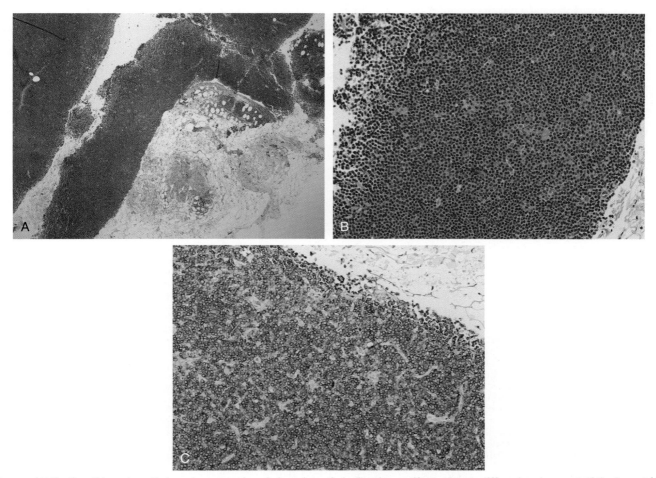

Figure 17-5 Small lymphocytic lymphoma or chronic lymphocytic leukemia manifests also as diffuse involvement of the breast **(A)**, seen at higher magnification as an infiltrate of small round lymphocytes **(B)**, and confirmed by bcl-2 immunoreactivity **(C)**.

the breast due to a high incidence of CNS relapse with these histologic subtypes.[34,56,57] However, this remains something of a contentious issue.

The histologic subtype of primary breast lymphoma (as categorized in the World Health Organization classification) and the clinical stage (as determined by the Ann Arbor staging system) seem to be the most important prognostic factors. Clearly, further studies regarding the biology and patterns of spread of extranodal, primary breast lymphoma are needed.

REFERENCES

1. Dixon JM, Lumsden AB, Krajewski A, et al: Primary lymphoma of the breast. Br J Surg 74:214–216, 1987.
2. DeBlasio D, McCormick B, Straus D, et al: Definitive irradiation for localized non-Hodgkin's lymphoma of breast. Int J Radiat Oncol Biol Phys 17:843–846, 1989.
3. Giardini R, Piccolo C, Rilke F: Primary non-Hodgkin's lymphomas of the female breast. Cancer 69:725–735, 1992.
4. Abbondanzo SL, Seidman JD, Lefkowitz M, et al: Primary diffuse large B-cell lymphoma of the breast. A clinicopathologic study of 31 cases. Pathol Res Pract 192:37–43, 1996.
5. Au WY, Chan AC, Chow LW, et al: Lymphoma of the breast in Hong Kong Chinese. Hematol Oncol 15:33–38, 1997.
6. Ha CS, Dubey P, Goyal LK, et al: Localized primary non-Hodgkin's lymphoma of the breast. Am J Clin Oncol 21:376–380, 1998.
7. Lyons JA, Myles J, Pohlman B, et al: Treatment and prognosis of primary breast lymphoma: A review of 13 cases. Am J Clin Oncol 23:334–336, 2000.
8. Wong WW, Schild WE, Halyard MY, et al: Primary non-Hodgkin lymphoma of the breast: The Mayo Clinic experience. J Surg Oncol 80:9–25, 2002.
9. Domchek SM, Hecht JL, Fleming MD, et al: Lymphomas of the breast: Primary and secondary involvement. Cancer 94:6–13, 2002.
10. Kuper-Hommel MJ, Snijder S, Janssen-Heijnen ML, et al: Treatment and survival of 38 female breast lymphomas: A population-based study with clinical and pathological reviews. Ann Hematol 82: 397–404, 2003.
11. Gholam D, Bibeau F, El Weshi A, et al: Primary breast lymphoma. Leuk Lymphoma 44:1173–1178, 2003.
12. Vignot S, Ledoussal V, Nodio P, et al: Non-Hodgkin's lymphoma of the breast: A report of 19 cases and a review of the literature. Clin Lymphoma 6:37–42, 2005.
13. Liu MT, Hsieh CY, Wang AY, et al: Primary breast lymphoma: A pooled analysis of prognostic factors and survival in 93 cases. Ann Saudi Med 25:288–293, 2005.
14. Choo SP, Lim ST, Wong EH, et al: Breast lymphoma: Favorable prognosis after treatment with standard combination chemotherapy. Onkologie 29:4–18, 2006.
15. Ryan GF, Roos DR, Seymour JF: Primary non-Hodgkin's lymphoma of the breast: Retrospective analysis of prognosis and patterns of failure in two Australian centers. Clin Lymphoma Myeloma 6:337–341, 2006.
16. Aviles A, Delgado S, Nambo MJ, et al: Primary breast lymphoma: Results of a controlled clinical trial. Oncology 69:256–260, 2005.

17. Fruchart C, Denoux Y, Chaste J, et al: High grade primary breast lymphoma: Is it a different clinical entity? Breast Cancer Res Treat 93:91–98, 2005.

18. Ganjoo K, Advani R, Mariappan M, et al: Non-Hodgkin lymphoma of the breast. Cancer 110:25–30, 2007.

19. Mpallas G, Simatos G, Tasidou A, et al: Primary breast lymphoma in a male patient. Breast 13:436–438, 2004.

20. Vasilakaki T, Zizi-Sermpetzoglou A, Katsamagkou E, et al: Bilateral primary breast lymphoma, a case report. Eur J Gynaec Oncol 27: 623–624, 2006.

21. Wiseman C, Liao KT: Primary lymphoma of the breast. Cancer 29: 1705–1712, 1972.

22. Iihara K, Yamaguchi K, Nishimura Y, et al: Spontaneous regression of malignant lymphoma of the breast. Pathol Int 54:537–542, 2004.

23. Venizelos ID, Tatsiou ZA, Vakalopoulos S, et al: Primary non-Hodgkin's lymphoma arising in an intramammary node. Leuk Lymphoma 46:451–455, 2005.

24. Monteiro M, Duarte I, Cabecadas J: Intravascular large B-cell lymphoma of the breast. Breast 14:75–78, 2005.

25. Newman MK, Zemmel NJ, Bandak AZ, et al: Primary breast lymphoma in a patient with silicone breast implants: A case report and review of the literature. J Plast Reconstr Aesthet Surg 61:822–825, 2008.

26. Yoshida S, Nakamura N, Sasaki Y, et al: Primary breast diffuse large B-cell lymphoma shows a non-germinal center B-cell phenotype. Mod Pathol 18:398–405, 2005.

27. Derringer GA, Thompson LD, Frommelt RA, et al: Malignant lymphoma of the thyroid gland: A clinicopathologic study of 108 cases. Am J Surg Pathol 24:623–639, 2000.

28. Yong W, Zhang Y, Zheng W, et al: Prognostic factors and therapeutic efficacy of combined radio-chemotherapy in Waldeyer's ring non-Hodgkin lymphoma. Chin Med J (Engl) 113:148–150, 2000.

29. Seymour JF, Solomon B, Wolf MM, et al: Primary large-cell non-Hodgkin's lymphoma of the testis. A retrospective analysis of patterns of failure and prognostic factors. Clin Lymphoma 2: 109–115, 2001.

30. Zucca E, Conconi A, Mughal T, et al: Patterns of outcome and prognostic factors in primary large-cell lymphoma of the testis in a survey by the International Extranodal Lymphoma Study Group. J Clin Oncol 21:20–27, 2003.

31. Kim MJ, Kim E-K, Park SY: Multiple nodular adenosis concurrent with primary breast lymphoma. Clin Radiol 60:126–129, 2005.

32. Kuroda H, Tamaru J, Takeuchi I, et al: Primary diffuse large B-cell lymphoma of the breast. Breast Cancer 14:317–322, 2007.

33. Jennings WC, Baker RS, Murray SS, et al: Primary breast lymphoma: The role of mastectomy and the importance of lymph node status. Ann Surg 245:784–789, 2007.

34. Fruchart C, Denoux Y, et al: High grade primary breast lymphoma: Is it a different clinical entity? Breast Cancer Res Treat 93:191–198, 2005.

35. Yaqoob N, Pervez S, Kayani N, et al: Frequency and characteristics of breast lymphomas presenting to a tertiary care hospital, Pakistan. J Pak Med Assoc 56:441–443, 2006.

36. Anuradha, Sinha A, Ramrakhiani D: Primary non-Hodgkin's lymphoma of the breast. Acta Cytologica 49:661–665, 2005.

37. Pisani F, Romano A, Borza P, et al: Diffuse large B-cell lymphoma involving the breast. A report of four cases. J Exp Clin Cancer Res 25:277–281, 2006.

38. Chakraborty J, Paul R, Sarkar R, et al: Primary non-Hodgkin's lymphoma of breast: A case report. Indian J Pathol Microbiol 50:315–317, 2007.

39. Ryan G, Roos D, Seymour J: Primary non-Hodgkin's lymphoma of the breast: Retrospective analysis of prognosis and patterns of failure in two Australian centers. Clin Lymphoma Myeloma 6:337–341, 2006.

40. Brogi E, Harris N: Lymphomas of the breast: Pathology and clinical behavior. Semin Oncol 26:357–364, 1999.

41. Pasta V, Midulla C, Monti M, et al: Unusual breast tumors: Primary lymphoma, a case report. Tumori 90:507–509, 2004.

42. Suzuki Y, Tokuda Y, Okumura A, et al: Three cases of malignant lymphoma of the breast. Jpn J Clin Oncol 30:33–36, 2000.

43. Ribrag V, Bibeau F, Weshi A, et al: Primary breast lymphoma: A report of 20 cases. Br J Haematol 115:253–256, 2001.

44. Ogawa T, Mizutani M, Yabana T, et al: A case of Burkitt's lymphoma involving both breasts. Breast Cancer 12:234–237, 2005.

45. Uesato M, Miyazawa Y, Gunji Y, et al: Primary non-Hodgkin's lymphoma of the breast: report of a case with special reference to 380 cases in the Japanese literature. Breast Cancer 12:154–158, 2005.

46. Vardar E, Ozkok G, Cetinel M, et al: Primary breast lymphoma cytologic diagnosis. Arch Path Lab Med 129:694–696, 2005.

47. Mason H, Johari V, March D, et al: Primary breast lymphoma: Radiologic and pathologic findings. Breast J 11:495–505, 2005.

48. Woo O, Yong H, Shin B, et al: Synchronous bilateral primary breast lymphoma: MRI and pathologic findings. Breast J 13:429–430, 2007.

49. Ma Sy, Shek TW, Au WY: Pagetiform relapse of primary breast lymphoma. Haematologica 89:e28, 2004.

50. Jennings W, Baker R, Murray S, et al: Primary breast lymphoma: The role of mastectomy and the importance of lymph node status. Ann Surg 245:784–789, 2007.

51. Kuroda H, Tamaru J, Takeuchi I, et al: Primary diffuse large B-cell lymphoma of the breast. Breast Cancer 14:317–322, 2007.

52. Lin Y, Guo X, Shen K, et al: Primary breast lymphoma: Long-term treatment outcome and prognosis. Leuk Lymphoma 47: 2102–2109, 2006.

53. Aviles A, Castaneda C, Neri N, et al: Rituximab and dose dense chemotherapy in primary breast lymphoma. Haematologica 92: 1147–1148, 2007.

54. Nagata S, Nishimura A, Iwashita Y: Primary breast lymphoma in the right breast during treatment for left breast cancer. World J Surg Oncol 5:689–698, 2007.

55. Fritzsche F, Pahl S, Petersen I, et al: Anaplastic large-cell non-Hodgkin's lymphoma of the breast in periprosthetic localization 32 years after treatment for primary breast cancer—a case report. Virchows Arch 449:561–564, 2006.

56. Hill Q, Qwen R: CNS prophylaxis in lymphoma: Who to target and what therapy to use. Blood Rev 20:319–322, 2006.

57. Yamazki H, Hanada M, Kitada M, et al: Four cases of central nervous system involvement of breast malignant lymphoma. Jpn J Clin Oncol 33:399–403, 2003.

chapter 18

Breast Implants and Related Methods of Breast-Modifying Surgery

MICHAEL J. MILLER

Overview

Breast implants are medical devices used to alter the size and shape of breasts for aesthetic and reconstructive purposes. Millions of women have undergone breast implant surgery since silicone gel–filled implants were introduced more than 40 years ago, and implantation surgery continues to be one of the most popular procedures in plastic surgery. In the 1990s, controversy arose regarding the safety of breast implants. Given this fact and wide clinical use, it is inevitable that clinicians practicing in specialties related to women's health will encounter patients who are considering implants or have already had them and are asking questions about the contemporary use of breast implants. This chapter reviews the history of breast implants and current techniques for breast-modifying surgery. Silicone chemistry, clinical applications, and current knowledge about safety are reviewed to enable the practitioner to answer commonly asked questions about breast implants.

Historical Background

The modern history of surgery to modify breast appearance began in the late 1800s. Early techniques included autologous tissue transfers from a variety of donor sites. The complexities of tissue transfer led to attempts to implant a variety of synthetic and naturally occurring substances (Table 18-1). Direct injections became popular because of simplicity. Practitioners, who were often unlicensed, injected different liquids and particulate suspensions into the breast parenchyma, which often resulted in adverse outcomes as severe as complete loss of the breasts and death.

Medical-grade silicone appeared to be associated with the fewest complications and to hold the most promise as an injectable material. In the early 1960s, the U.S. Food and Drug Administration (FDA) approved a trial of liquid silicone injection for soft tissue augmentation. Nevertheless, up to 50% of patients who had this procedure performed experienced adverse long-term results,[1] and the practice has since been discontinued. Although it is unlikely that direct injection of foreign substances will be revived, injection of autologous fat that is processed from tissue aspirated during liposuction procedures is a new clinical technique that has recently been reported.[2] Long-term results and best practices of these techniques are still under study, but they appear to be promising, particularly for localized deformities.

Difficulties encountered with direct injection provided incentive to develop formed alloplastic implants for modifying breast volume. These had the disadvantage of requiring open surgery but they afforded more controlled localization of the material within the breast. In the early to mid-1900s devices fashioned from a

TABLE 18-1

Synthetic and Natural Substances Historically Used for Breast Augmentation

Paraffin
Ivory
Glass balls
Ground rubber
Ox cartilage
Terylene wool
Gutta percha
Dicora
Polyethylene chips
Ivalon sponge (polyvinyl alcohol–formaldehyde)
Ivalon in polyethylene sac
Polyether foam sponge (Etheron)
Polyethylene (Polystan) tape or strips wound into a ball
Polyurethane foam sponge
Teflon-silicone prosthesis

number of substances were tried including ivory, glass, and synthetic polymers (see Table 18-1). Most led to contracting scar and a firm, unnatural appearance. The exceptions were devices made of silicone polymers. Silicone had already demonstrated favorable performance in other medical applications such as urethral reconstruction, joint replacement, and implanted shunts, and these observations led to the development of silicone breast implants. In 1963, in Houston, Texas, Cronin and Gerow reported the first use of silicone breast implants.[3] Over the next 25 years, an estimated 1.27 million women received silicone gel–filled implants for either aesthetic breast surgery or reconstruction,[4] with numbers steadily increasing to more than 2 million by the year 2000. It is estimated that as many as 100,000 women undergo placement of breast implants each year in the United States.

Breast implants that are currently available are made of a silicone shell filled with either physiologic saline solution or silicone gel (Figs. 18-1 to 18-3). Each has advantages and disadvantages. Saline-filled implants can be adjusted to optimum size at the time of insertion. They also avoid concerns raised by the past controversy about the safety of silicone gel. However, they have a tendency to be firmer, form visible wrinkles in the breast skin, and cause less natural changes in breast contour with physical manipulation or changes in body position (see Fig. 18-1). Silicone gel–filled implants are designed to simulate the density of natural human tissue and therefore tend to yield a more natural result (see Figs. 18-2 and 18-3).

Despite the superior performance of silicone gel–filled implants, they became the topic of intense controversy in the 1990s and early 2000s because of concern about the devices being linked to systemic disease. Unanswered questions related to autoimmune disorders, arthritis, collagen vascular disease, pregnancy, and lactation caused the FDA to reclassify the devices and restrict their use

in the United States pending comprehensive studies to confirm safety and efficacy. These devices, which had been used for nearly 30 years and placed into hundreds of thousands of women, were suddenly no longer available for general use, spawning intense public debate and numerous law suits against manufacturers and clinicians. One of the catalysts behind the FDA ruling was the observation that high titers of antisilicone antibodies were observed in uncontrolled cohorts of women with silicone implants, possibly providing a biologic basis for systemic disease. It was suggested that silicone gel diffused across the elastomer shell, so-called "gel bleed," exposing the patient to liquid silicone, which acted as a hapten and gave rise to autoimmune disease. When controls (women with no implants) were examined, similar titers of antisilicone antibodies were observed. This observation confirmed the fact that silicone exposure is ubiquitous in modern culture. Sources of silicone exposure consist of food, medications, and cosmetics, as well as most invasive medical procedures, including common interventions such as percutaneous injections and intravenous catheters. Needles and catheters are generally coated with silicone-containing compounds and can generate silicone antibodies. Nevertheless, because of the level of concern and broad base of unanswered questions, the silicone gel–filled breast implants were removed from the general market in the United States while clinical studies mandated by the FDA were completed.[5] Throughout this period, the devices continued to be available in Europe and South America. Ultimately, concerns about systemic disease related to breast implants proved unfounded, and in 2006, the devices were made available again for general use in the United States. To understand the nature of the controversy and the clinical performance of breast implants, it is important to review the fundamentals of silicone chemistry and medical device application.

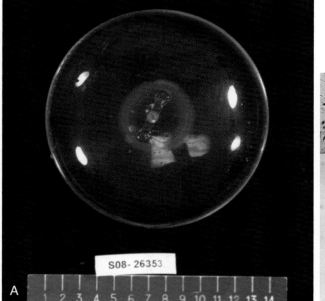

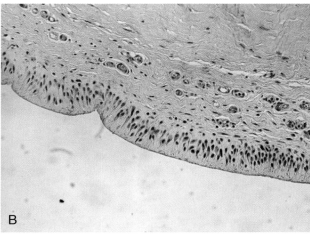

Figure 18-1 **A,** Typical gross appearance of intact saline implant. **B,** The implant capsule of saline implants can show "synovialization" of surrounding fibroblasts where they palisade and give the histologic appearance of synovium. This is a normal response by the host to wall off the implant.

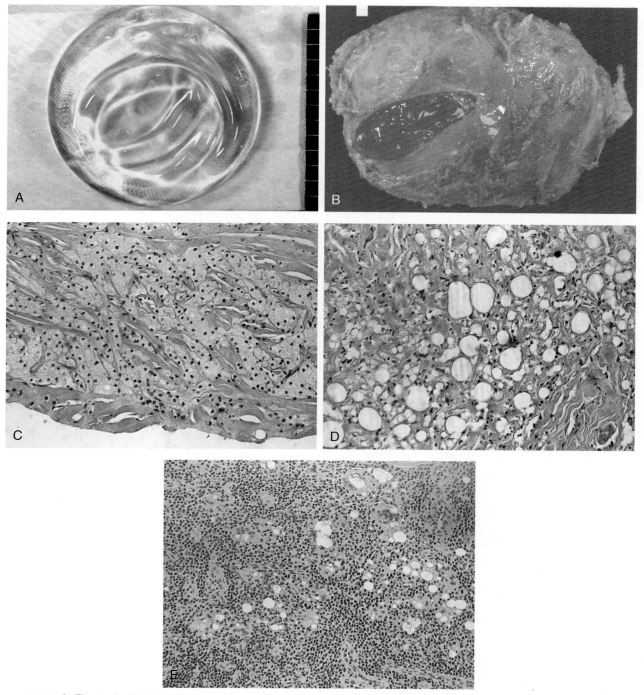

Figure 18-2   A, The typical intact silicone implant exhibits a firmer consistency but well-contained silicone. **B,** A ruptured silicone implant, in contrast, exudes free silicone. **C,** Often, even intact implants leak silicone that would exist as deposits within the implant capsule even when there was no overt rupture. The silicone deposits could exist free or be phagocytosed by macrophages (depicted). **D,** Silicone implants, when overtly ruptured, exhibit massive deposits of silicone with significant chronic and foreign body giant cell inflammation, the so-called silicone granuloma. **E,** Some free silicone, in the case of extracapsular rupture, could migrate to the axillary lymph nodes.

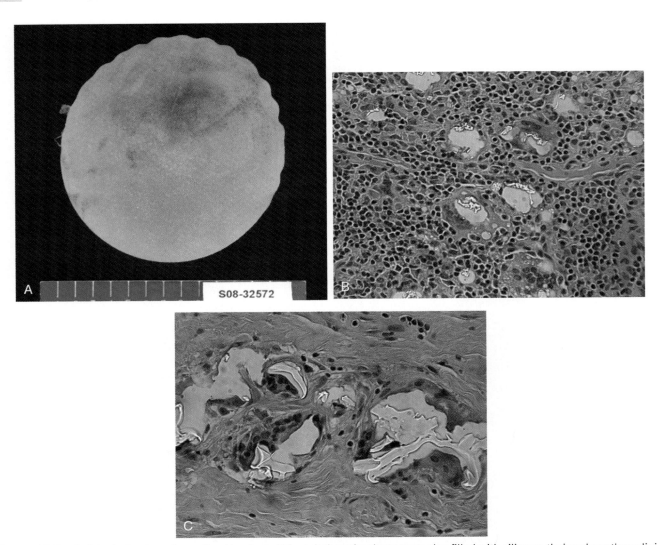

Figure 18-3 A, A typical polyurethane-lined implant. Although these implants were also filled with silicone, their polyurethane lining resulted in a rough texture to their surface, which was designed to integrate better with adjacent tissues. **B,** Polyurethane tends to degrade after implantation. Here, fragments of its polyurethane fibroelastomer shell are observed within foreign body giant cells as birefringent deposits. **C,** Polyurethane crystals could migrate from the implant surface and integrate within host tissues often engulfed by foreign body giant cells.

Silicone and Breast Implants

Given the common use and the history of controversy related to silicone devices in plastic surgery, it is especially important for the clinician to be familiar with the fundamentals of silicone chemistry and nomenclature (Table 18-2). *Silicone* refers to a family of polymers with a molecular backbone of alternating silicon (Si) and oxygen (O) atoms. *Silicon* is a semimetallic element found in nature as silica (SiO_2), the most common substance on earth. It is located just below carbon on the periodic table and thus has a similar chemical behavior, most notably the ability to form long chain molecules. The basic repeating unit silicone polymer is *siloxane* (R_2SiO), named because it contains silicon, oxygen, and alkane (saturated hydrocarbon) side groups. The most common formation used in medicine is *poly(dimethylsiloxane; PDMS)*, in which the siloxane monomer carries two methyl ($-CH_3$) groups. Modifying the length and molecular weight of PDMS affects the mechanical properties of silicone polymers. Low-molecular-weight formulations (<30 monomers) short chains yield materials with viscosity similar to mineral oil, and high-molecular-weight formulations ($\geq$3000 monomers) are solids.[6] Other factors used to control material properties are the degree of cross-linking between polymer chains, additives such as fine silica particles, and the curing process. Soft silicone used for filling breast implants is cured in a hydrosilation reaction. This involves siloxane chains with some methyl groups replaced with vinyl groups ($CH_2=CH-$) that bond to receptive hydride groups ($H-$) in other chains in a reaction catalyzed by platinum, yielding a lightly cross-linked elastomer with softness similar to breast tissue. Small amounts of residual platinum from this reaction may be detected in silicone gel breast implants, and some forms of platinum have immunogenic potential, raising concern about possible adverse reactions. Nevertheless, there have been no reports that positively relate the trace amounts of platinum found

TABLE 18-2

Silicone Nomenclature and Chemistry

Term	Symbol	Definition
Silicon	Si	Element on periodic table
Silica	SiO_2	Most abundant substance on earth
Siloxane	R_2SiO	Monomer containing silicon, oxygen, and alkane side groups
Silicone	$[R_2SiO]_n$	Polymer of siloxane
Poly (dimethylsiloxane) (PDMS)	$[(CH_3)_2SiO]_n$	Silicone formulation for medical applications

$$\left[-\underset{\underset{CH_3}{|}}{\overset{\overset{CH_3}{|}}{Si}} - O - \right]_n$$

Siloxane

$$CH_3 - \underset{\underset{CH_3}{|}}{\overset{\overset{CH_3}{|}}{Si}} - O - \underset{\underset{CH_3}{|}}{\overset{\overset{CH_3}{|}}{Si}} - O - \underset{\underset{CH_3}{|}}{\overset{\overset{CH_3}{|}}{Si}} - O - \underset{\underset{CH_3}{|}}{\overset{\overset{CH_3}{|}}{Si}} - O - \underset{\underset{CH_3}{|}}{\overset{\overset{CH_3}{|}}{Si}} - O - \underset{\underset{CH_3}{|}}{\overset{\overset{CH_3}{|}}{Si}} - O - \underset{\underset{CH_3}{|}}{\overset{\overset{CH_3}{|}}{Si}} - O$$

Silicone
Poly(dimethylsiloxane)

in breast implants to human disease, and based on the type and quantity of platinum used in manufacturing, there exists no biologically plausible rationale for health problems from this cause.

Silicone-based medical devices have been in use since the late 1950s when a silicone product was first used to replace the urethra.[6] Excellent biocompatibility and versatile properties have led to many medical applications of silicone. Low-molecular-weight formulations are used as lubricants for syringes, needles, hand creams, facial cosmetics, food additives, and symptomatic treatments for gastrointestinal disorders. Higher-molecular-weight formulations are used to fabricate many shunts and catheters, infusion ports, laryngeal implants, intraocular lenses, and coatings on the tissue interface of implantable devices such as cardiac pacemakers and implantable infusion pumps. In plastic surgery, silicone implants have been used in craniofacial surgery for malar, nasal, and chin augmentation and to reconstruct the orbital floor. In hand surgery, they have been used for arthroplasty, flexor tendon replacement, and bone block spacers.

Clinical Use of Breast Implants

Breast implants are devices intended to increase the volume or alter the shape of the breast. The principle indications are aesthetic breast enlargement and reconstruction of deformities related to breast cancer, trauma, or congenital abnormalities.

AESTHETIC SURGERY

Aesthetic breast surgery is performed on women with breasts that are anatomically normal but of undesirable size and/or shape. Typical candidates are women between 30 and 35 years of age. Surgical techniques vary based on the choice of surgical incisions and location of the device beneath the breast. Incisions must be as inconspicuous as possible, in keeping with the aesthetic purpose of the procedure. They may be placed in the inframammary fold, around the areola (i.e., circumareolar), or in the axilla, depending on the size of the breast and preferences of the patient and surgeon. An endoscopic approach through the umbilicus has been described, but this is not widely performed and is the subject of some controversy.[7] The implant may be placed superficial to the pectoralis major muscle, deep to the muscle, or partially in both positions using a technique that releases the muscle from the insertions of the chest wall to allow the implant to be covered by muscle on the superior portion but rest directly beneath the breast parenchyma inferiorly. At times insertion of a breast implant is accompanied by other procedures that modify the shape of the breast. The most common adjunctive procedure is a mastopexy, or breast lift, in which the nipple–areola complex is repositioned higher on the breast mound and a portion of the breast skin is removed from the inferior breast between the areola and the inframammary fold.

RECONSTRUCTIVE SURGERY

Reconstructive breast surgery is performed on women with deformities caused by trauma, congenital abnormalities, or tumors. Chest wall trauma, particularly soft tissue injuries in prepubescent females, can cause breast deformities that can be improved with reconstructive surgery using breast implants. Congenital breast deformities may create unilateral breast volume deficiencies with breast asymmetry. The best example is Poland's syndrome, which is characterized by unilateral underdevelopment of the chest wall and sometimes associated with webbing of the fingers of the hand on the affected side. The most common indication for breast reconstruction is to repair deformities caused by breast cancer treatment.

The concept of breast reconstruction for cancer dates from 1906 when Obredanne described a procedure to restore the breast using a pectoralis muscle flap. His procedures, developed in France, were never adopted in the United States, primarily because of the influence of William Halsted. He strongly opposed these procedures and was so influential in American surgery that postmastectomy reconstruction was not considered for most of this century.[8] During the past 20 years, however, improved understanding of breast tumor biology has rendered much of Halsted's principles for breast cancer surgery obsolete. This understanding, combined with technical advances in reconstructive surgery, has resulted in greater acceptance of postmastectomy reconstruction.

The modern movement toward immediate breast reconstruction began in the 1970s with procedures designed to restore the breast after mastectomy for nonmalignant disease.[9,10] Reports of immediate reconstruction for malignant disease followed.[11] Georgiade and colleagues reported the first large series (62 patients) in 1982, concluding that immediate reconstruction offered advantages over delayed reconstruction including excellent technical results, less expense and morbidity, and no apparent adverse affect on the natural course of the malignancy.[12]

Throughout the 1980s, immediate reconstruction became increasingly adopted. Most procedures were based on the use of tissue expanders and breast implants.[13–15] Inflatable saline breast implants with single or double lumens as well as immediate subcutaneous placement of polyurethane-covered implants[16,17] were introduced to avoid the need for a second operation to place a permanent breast implant after tissue expansion. Procedures using surgical flaps such as the latissimus dorsi musculocutaneous flap[18] and the transverse rectus abdominis musculocutaneous (TRAM) flap[19] were also advocated for immediate reconstruction. Finally, microsurgical free tissue transfer procedures were introduced as the most advanced form of immediate breast reconstruction.[20] During the 1990s, further refinements resulted in more reliable techniques, improved patient selection, and greater cooperation between reconstructive and ablative surgeons to yield the highest quality results.

Immediate breast reconstruction based entirely on the use of implanted devices is initially the most expedient technique. Sometimes it is possible to insert a full-size implant at the time of mastectomy when the breasts are small (volume, <400 mL) and the patient is a young nonsmoker with good chest wall musculature.[21,22] In most patients, however, a period of tissue expansion is required. This is accomplished using an inflatable device called a tissue expander, which is inserted beneath the pectoralis major and serratus anterior muscles. Full expansion usually requires 6 to 8 weeks to complete, and an implant exchange is performed 4 to 6 months later. The advantages of this technique are that it involves minimum additional surgery at the time of the mastectomy, has a recovery period essentially the same as that of the mastectomy alone, and creates no additional scarring. The disadvantages of this technique are the length of time necessary to complete the entire reconstruction (up to 1 year), the requirement for a minimum of two operative procedures, and a less predictable cosmetic result. Although the final shape of the breast may be satisfactory, it may lack a natural consistency because of the thin soft tissue covering the device, especially when saline-filled implants are used. This method is ideal for a slender, small-breasted woman with minimal ptosis who wishes to avoid additional scarring and time for convalescence. It may also be suitable for women undergoing bilateral reconstruction because symmetry is more easily achieved if both breasts are restored using the same technique.

Breast implants can be combined with soft tissue flaps for reconstruction. The latissimus dorsi musculocutaneous flap is the most common transfer used in combination with breast implants. Other flaps may also be used depending on patient preference and tissue availability.[23] The principal advantage in using a tissue flap is immediate replacement of missing skin and soft tissue. The implant allows the final breast volume to be accurately reproduced to match the contralateral breast or, in bilateral reconstruction, adjust the breast size according to the patient's desires. The advantages of this technique are that the implant is protected by abundant tissue, a period of tissue expansion is avoided, and the full benefit of preserving the breast skin is realized to achieve a natural-appearing breast. The disadvantage of this technique compared with implants alone is that it results in additional scarring and requires a longer period of recovery. For many patients, this approach represents an acceptable compromise between implant-only reconstruction and autologous tissue reconstruction, incorporating some of the advantages and disadvantages of each.

Complications of Breast Implants

Local complications and adverse events are well characterized because of years of clinical use (Table 18-3). Tissue does not attach to silicone, and implants are prone to migrate and deform. The biologic response to the implant depends on the size, shape, surface texture, and porosity (see Figs. 18-1 to 18-3). Local complications are the primary indication for reoperation after breast implant surgery. Reoperation is one gauge of the frequency of local and perioperative complications, and it has been reported in several studies with cohorts up to 7000 women. Gabriel and associates[24] reported a reoperation rate of 23.8% in 749 women implanted at the Mayo Clinic, with indications ranging from implant removal to drainage of hematoma over an average period of 7.8 years follow-up after implantation.

The principle adverse outcomes of breast implant surgery include capsule contracture, infection, pain syndrome, and device rupture.

TABLE 18-3

Reported Local and Perioperative Complications

Axillary adenopathy

Acute and chronic breast and chest wall pain

Chest wall skeletal changes

Gel implant rupture (intra- and extracapsular)

Gel migration

Hemorrhage at the operative site

Implant extrusion

Implant fibrous capsular contracture

Implant filler port or valve leakage

Implant misplacement

Implant shifting or displacement

Infection with toxic shock syndrome

Intra-implant infection

Lactation and galactocele

Loss or change in sensation of the breast or nipple

Nipple or flap necrosis

Operative wound infection

Peri-implant calcification

Peri-implant hematoma or seroma

Peri-implant infection

Pneumothorax

Saline implant deflation

Silicone exudation through skin or nipple

Silicone granuloma

Skin blistering, cysts, and necrosis

Skin rashes

Swelling of the breast

CAPSULE CONTRACTURE

The mature response to silicone implants is generally fibrous capsule formation (see Figs. 18-1 and 18-2), which facilitates maintaining implant position and, if necessary, eases subsequent removal. This capsule can undergo contraction similar to hypertrophic scar formation and lead to discomfort and disfigurement.[6] This contraction is the most frequent adverse reaction reported in the use of these devices.

An early effort to eliminate the problem of capsule contracture around breast implants involved applying a porous coating made of polyurethane produced by a polymerization process using polydiethylene glycol and toluene diisocyanate to the implant's smooth surface. This resulted in a textured surface that facilitated tissue invasion (see Fig. 18-3) and significantly reduced the rate of early capsule contracture.[25,26] These devices were quite popular until concerns arose regarding the fate of the polyurethane coating. The coating was found to undergo partial degradation under physiologic conditions, evidenced in part by clinical studies in which fragmentation could be observed on histology of tissue removed from around the polyurethane-coated implants (see Fig. 18-3). The degradation was possibly releasing a compound called 2,4-toluenediamine (2,4-TDA),[27] which is a known carcinogen in animals but not in humans. Epidemiologic and animal experimental data did not support an association between polyurethane and human disease such as cancer, and the weight of existing evidence suggests that there is no association. Nevertheless, polyurethane-coated implants were removed from the market in the United States in 1991.

INFECTION

As with any implanted alloplastic device, absence of tissue incorporation by breast implants contributes to the risk of infection. Infection is one of the most common reasons for clinical implant failure. It has long been recognized that implanted foreign bodies are more susceptible to infection compared with undamaged tissues, allowing transformation of usually typically non-pathogenic or opportunistic organisms into virulent pathogens. Biomaterial-associated infections occur with smaller inoculums of bacteria, resist antibiotic treatment, and tend to persist until the foreign material is removed. Even low-level contamination without frank infection can have undesirable effects, such as fibrous capsule contracture around breast implants.[28] Treating biomaterial-related infections causes additional patient morbidity and can cost five to ten times more than the original procedure. The risk of infection can be minimized by the clinician guided by a good understanding of the biologic mechanisms involved.

The pathogenesis of biomaterial infections follows a well-characterized sequence of events. Infection begins with bacterial adherence to the biomaterial surface with strong chemical bonds. Organisms rapidly proliferate, forming colonies up to hundreds of organisms thick. They secrete polysaccharides and proteins that combine with devitalized cellular material, environmental adsorbates, and microscopic debris on the surface of the material to form a nutritive and protective extracellular matrix called a *biofilm*, an almost universal feature of bacterial surface colonization. Most of the organisms reside in the three-dimensional space of the biofilm rather than on the actual surface of the material. The biofilm creates an avascular microenvironment wherein optimal conditions exist for bacterial proliferation. The organisms are protected from circulating antibodies, macrophages, and other components of the host defenses. Surface adherent microorganisms require at least 100 times higher antibiotic levels to achieve minimal inhibitory or bactericidal effects demonstrated in standard susceptibility testing. Some medical devices are surface treated with antimicrobials to reduce the risk of infection. These are mostly devices intended to reside in normally sterile cavities or spaces while traversing potentially contaminated locations outside the patient's body (e.g., central venous and urinary catheters). Antibiotic-coated devices intended for permanent implantation in plastic surgery are still experimental.

The risk of infection and associated morbidity mandates meticulous surgical technique when handling and using biomaterials in a clinical setting. The device surface must not be damaged, extra care is required to avoid incidental contamination, and precise surgical technique must be used that minimizes adjacent tissue damage.

PAIN SYNDROME

Localized pain can occur after breast implant surgery, but the literature is conflicting about its incidence and significance. Pain as a reported indication for breast implant removal occurs in 1%[24] to 36% of cases.[29] It appears to be related to location of the implant (i.e., submuscular or subglandular placement), indication for use (i.e., aesthetic augmentation or postmastectomy breast reconstruction) and implant filling material (saline or silicone gel). The greatest incidence of pain seems associated with saline-filled devices used for reconstruction, but this is clouded by an underlying incidence of postmastectomy chest wall pain in as many as 20% of patients regardless of whether reconstruction was performed.[30] The cause of pain is unclear, but it is speculated that nerve, muscle, or soft tissue compression or distortion may play a role. Implant removal may improve symptoms.

DEVICE RUPTURE

As with any medical device, breast implants are subject to failure caused by defects of manufacturing, use, or wear. The most significant consequence of device failure is implant rupture (see Figs. 18-2 and 18-3). Failure of the implant shell can occur because of inadvertent damage caused by the surgeon during placement of the device or by fatigue failure with repetitive loading after placement. Silicone rubber subjected to repetitive loading and deformation can fragment, resulting in a breach of the shell with extravasation of the filling material. With saline-filled devices, this usually leads to complete deflation and harmless absorption of the fluid (see Fig. 18-1). Clinically this is manifested by rapid loss of breast volume (i.e., deflation) and is obvious to the patient. On the other hand, if the device is filled with silicone gel, a rupture event might not be detected because the fibrous capsule surrounding the implant tends to contain the extravasated material. The patient exhibits minimal or no clinical signs. This is called an intracapsular rupture (see Fig. 18-2). If the gel appears outside of the fibrous capsule it is referred to as extracapsular rupture. These patients appear more likely to have physical findings, including loss of breast volume, nodules, asymmetry, tenderness, and changes in breast consistency. According to various studies, this occurs in 12% to 35% of patients.[31,32] The most reliable way to detect a rupture event is by magnetic resonance imaging (MRI). MRI exploits difference in silicone, water, and fat resonance frequencies to deliver high-resolution images of silicone gel breast implants. It can be used to detect implant rupture with a sensitivity and specificity of greater than 90%.[33] A rupture is identified by the presence of multiple curvilinear lines of low-intensity signal seen within the high-intensity signal silicone gel, the so-called "linguine sign." The most recent generation of silicone gel implants contains a highly cohesive siloxane polymer that is not liquid and tends to remain contained within the silicone elastomer shell even when a rupture occurs. If these implants rupture, the characteristic appearance on MRI is of a noncollapsed shell that assumes a tear-drop shape rather than the totally collapsed appearance of the linguine sign. Although no systemic disorders have been linked to ruptured silicone gel implants, local symptoms can occur and the recommended treatment is total capsulectomy and removal of the ruptured implant.[34]

SYSTEMIC COMPLICATIONS

The possibility of systemic diseases caused by breast implants caused controversy throughout the 1990s and early 2000s regarding the safety of these devices. Officials of the FDA decided to restrict the use of silicone gel implants, allowing them only through participation in a carefully monitored safety study.[5,35] In countries outside of the United States, silicone gel breast implants remained available and in common use. Subsequent clinical, epidemiologic, and basic research provided no evidence for increased risk of systemic disorders such as connective tissue diseases, cancer, or neurologic disorders associated with silicone gel breast implants. The most comprehensive study confirming the absence of a link between silicone gel breast implants and systemic disease was published in June, 1999, by the Institute of Medicine. A complete review of all available literature up to that point was examined and failed to support any association based on epidemiologic data or confirm any biologically plausible basis for an association between silicone exposure and systemic disorders. In 2006, silicone gel breast implants became generally available once again in the United States under conditions requiring completion of ongoing studies, device tracking, age restrictions, and specific clinician training prior to use.

REFERENCES

1. Vinnik CA: The hazards of silicone injections [editorial]. JAMA 236:959, 1976.
2. Yoshimura K, Sato K, Aoi N, et al: Cell-assisted lipotransfer for cosmetic breast augmentation: Supportive use of adipose-derived stem/stromal cells. Aesthetic Plast Surg 32:48–55, discussion 56–57, 2008.
3. Cronin TD, Gerow FJ: Augmentation mammoplasty: A new "natural feel" prothesis. Transactions of the Third International Congress of Plastic Surgery, October 13–18, 1963.
4. Terry MB, Skovron ML, Garbers S: The estimated frequency of cosmetic breast augmentation among US women, 1963 through 1988. Am J Public Health 85(Pt 1):1122–1124, 1995, comment in Am J Public Health 86:891–892, 1996.
5. Kessler DA: The basis of the FDA's decision on breast implants. N Engl J Med 326:1713–1715, 1992.
6. Costantino PD: Synthetic biomaterials for soft-tissue augmentation and replacement in the head and neck. Otolaryngol Clin North Am 27:223–262, 1994.
7. Brennan WA, Haiavy J: Transumbilical breast augmentation: A practical review of a growing technique. Ann Plast Surg 59: 243–249, 2007.
8. Teimourian B, Adham MN: Louis Ombredanne and the origin of muscle flap use for immediate breast mound reconstruction. Plast Reconstr Surg 72:905–910, 1983.
9. Lessa S, Carreirão S: Subcutaneous mastectomy and immediate breast reconstruction by local dermofat flap. Ann Plast Surg 3:330–337, 1979.

10. Pennisi VR: Subcutaneous mastectomy and fibrocystic disease of the breast. Clin Plast Surg 3:205–216, 1976.
11. Albo RJ, Gruber R, Kahn R: Immediate breast reconstruction after modified mastectomy for carcinoma of the breast. Am J Surg 140:131–136, 1980.
12. Georgiade G, Georgiade N, McCarty KS Jr, Seigler HF: Rationale for immediate reconstruction of the breast following modified radical mastectomy. Ann Plast Surg 8:20–28, 1982.
13. van Heerden JA, Jackson IT, Martin JK Jr, Fisher J: Surgical technique and pitfalls of breast reconstruction immediately after mastectomy for carcinoma: Initial experience. Mayo Clin Proc 62:185–191, 1987.
14. Cohen IK, Turner D: Immediate breast reconstruction with tissue expanders. Clin Plast Surg 14:491–498, 1987.
15. Ward J, Cohen IK, Knaysi GA, Brown PW: Immediate breast reconstruction with tissue expansion. Plast Reconstr Surg 80:559–566, 1987.
16. Artz JS, Dinner MI, Foglietti MA, Sampliner J: Breast reconstruction utilizing subcutaneous tissue expansion followed by polyurethane-covered silicone implants: A 6-year experience. Plast Reconstr Surg 88:635–639, discussion 640–641, 1991.
17. Artz JS, Dinner MI, Sampliner J: Breast reconstruction with a subcutaneous tissue expander followed with a polyurethane-covered silicone breast implant. Ann Plast Surg 20:517–521, 1988.
18. Mendelson BC: Breast conservation and breast reconstruction. Med J Aust 20;2:156–157, 1983.
19. Drever JM, Hodson-Walker NJ: Immediate breast reconstruction after mastectomy using a rectus abdominis myodermal flap without an implant. Can J Surg 25:429–431, 1982.
20. Grotting JC, Urist MM, Maddox WA, Vasconez LO: Conventional TRAM flap versus free microsurgical TRAM flap for immediate breast reconstruction. Plast Reconstr Surg 83:828–841, discussion 842–844, 1989 [comment in Plast Reconstr Surg 84:1005–1006, 1989].
21. Paulson RL, Chang FC, Helmer SD: Kansas surgeons' attitudes toward immediate breast reconstruction: A statewide survey. Am J Surg 168:543–546, 1994.
22. Bailey MH, Smith JW, Casas L, et al: Immediate breast reconstruction: Reducing the risks. Plast Reconstr Surg 83:845–851, 1989 [comment in Plast Reconstr Surg 84:1015–1016, 1989].
23. Miller MJ, Rock CS, Robb GL: Aesthetic breast reconstruction using a combination of free transverse rectus abdominis musculocutaneous flaps and breast implants. Ann Plast Surg 37:258–264, 1996.
24. Gabriel SE, Woods JE, O'Fallon WM, et al: Complications leading to surgery after breast implantation. N Engl J Med 6;336:677–682, 1997 [comment in N Engl J Med 6;336:718–719, 1997].
25. Herman S: The Meme implant. Plast Reconstr Surg 73:411–414, 1984.
26. Capozzi A, Pennisi VR: Clinical experience with polyurethane-covered gel-filled mammary prostheses. Plast Reconstr Surg 68:512–520, 1981.
27. Benoit FM. Degradation of polyurethane foams used in the Meme breast implant. J Biomed Mat Res 27:1341–1318, 1993.
28. Pajkos A, Deva AK, Vickery K, et al: Detection of subclinical infection in significant breast implant capsules. Plast Reconstr Surg 111:1605–1611, 2003.
29. Peters W, Smith D, Fornasier V, et al: An outcome analysis of 100 women after explantation of silicone gel breast implants. Ann Plast Surg 39:9–19, 1997.
30. Stevens PE, Dibble SL, Miaskowski C: Prevalence, characteristics, and impact of postmastectomy pain syndrome: An investigation of women's experience. Pain 61:61–68, 1995.
31. Ahn CY, DeBruhl ND, Gorczyca DP, et al: Comparative silicone breast implant evaluation using mammography, sonography, and magnetic resonance imaging: Experience with 59 implants. Plast Reconstr Surg 94:620–627, 1994.
32. Anderson B, Hawtof D, Alani H, Kapetansky D: The diagnosis of ruptured breast implants. Plast Reconstr Surg 84:903–907, 1989.
33. Gorczyca DP, Gorczyca SM, Gorczyca KL, et al: The diagnosis of silicone breast implant rupture. Plast Reconstr Surg 120:49S–61S, 2007.
34. Rohrich RJ, Beran SJ, Restifo RJ, Copit SE: Aesthetic management of the breast following explantation: Evaluation and mastopexy options. Plast Reconstr Surg 101:827–837, 1995.
35. Kilpadi DV, Feldman DS: Biocompatibility of silicone gel breast implants. In Wise DL, Trantolo DJ, Lewandrowski KU, et al (eds): Biomaterials engineering and devices: Human applications. Totowa, NJ, Humana Press, 2000.

SECTION V

Natural History, Epidemiology, Genetics, and Syndromes of Breast Cancer

chapter 19

Epidemiology of Breast Cancer

**KATHERINE W. REEVES | ALANA G. HUDSON |
VICTOR G. VOGEL**

It is predicted that 182,460 American women will be diagnosed with invasive breast cancer in 2008 alone.[1] Breast cancer is the most commonly diagnosed cancer in women in the United States and accounts for 26% of all female cancers (excluding nonmelanoma skin cancers and in situ cancers).[1] Although breast cancer may occur in men, it is rare; the American Cancer Society estimates that 1990 new cases of male breast cancer will be diagnosed in 2008.[1] In U.S. women, breast cancer ranks second to lung cancer in terms of cancer mortality, with 40,480 female breast cancer deaths predicted for 2008.[1] Breast cancer deaths account for 15% of the burden of cancer mortality in U.S. females.[1] Mortality from breast cancer has decreased in recent years because of early detection and improved treatment of the disease. Data from the National Cancer Institute's Surveillance Epidemiology and End Results (SEER) program show that the breast cancer mortality rate declined 2.3% each year between 1990 and 2003.[2] The percentage of women surviving at least 5 years after diagnosis has risen to 88%, and the 5-year survival is 98% for women diagnosed with localized disease.[2]

Traditional Risk Factors for Breast Cancer

Breast cancer incidence rises sharply with age (Fig. 19-1). The overall incidence rate of breast cancer is low at younger ages (e.g., 1.4 per 100,000 in women 20 to 24 years of age).[3] As women begin to transition through menopause, the rates of breast cancer increase substantially; data from SEER show that between 1999 and 2003 the incidence rate of breast cancer was 119.3 per 100,000 for women 40 to 44 years of age, 249 per 100,000 for women 50 to 54 years of age, and 388.3 for women 60 to 64 years of age. The highest rate of breast cancer was observed in women 75 to 79 years of age, in whom 490.4 incident cases of breast cancer were diagnosed for every 100,000 women.[3]

Breast cancer rates differ by race and ethnicity. Although African-American women have a lower overall incidence of breast cancer compared with Caucasian women (rates of 118.9 per 100,000 vs. 137.6 per 100,000, respectively, for 1999–2003),[3] African Americans have a higher incidence of breast cancer before 35 years of age.[2] Breast cancer mortality was substantially greater at all ages in African Americans (34.4 deaths per 100,000) than it was in Caucasians (25.4 deaths per 100,000) for the years 1999–2003.[4]

The reasons for these disparities are not well understood, although a number of possible explanations have been suggested and investigated. These include (1) differential utilization of mammographic screening and stage at diagnosis, (2) differential effect and/or distribution of breast cancer risk factors, (3) differences in inherent genetic susceptibility, (4) differences in tumor characteristics, (5) differential access to treatment, and (6) differences in prevalence of comorbidities in women diagnosed with breast cancer. Each of the six hypothesized explanations for the racial disparities in breast cancer incidence and mortality has some merit. Mammography use is generally similar between African Americans and Caucasians,[2] and differences in stage at diagnosis can be at least partially explained by differences in obesity.[5] Therefore, screening and differences in stage at diagnosis are likely not the most important factors. Likewise, access to treatment is important, but disparities in mortality exist even in systems in which African Americans and Caucasians have equal access.[6,7] Genetic susceptibility may also be important, yet the impact of such factors is not well understood.[8-10] It appears that the differential distribution of risk factors, especially obesity,[11-13] differences in tumor characteristics,[14-17] and differences in comorbid conditions[18,19] between African-American and Caucasian patients with breast cancer are largely responsible for the racial disparity observed in breast cancer.

As shown in Figure 19-2, breast cancer incidence and mortality are higher in African-American and Caucasian women than in women of other races and ethnicities. Breast cancer incidence in Asians and Pacific Islanders was 93.5 per 100,000 in 1999–2003. Incidence in Hispanics was 87.1 per 100,000 for the same period.

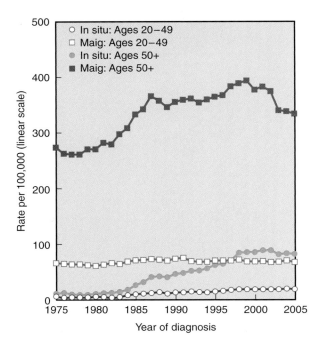

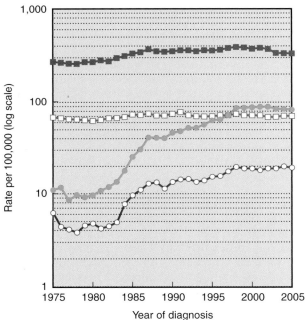

Figure 19-1 Breast cancer incidence rates by age among U.S. women, 1975–2005. (From Ries LAG, Melbert D, Krapcho M, et al [eds]: Surveillance Epidemiology and End Results [SEER] Cancer Statistics Review, 1975–2005. National Cancer Institute, Bethesda, MD, http://seer.cancer.gov/csr/1975_2005. Based on November 2007 SEER data submission, posted to the SEER website 2008.)

Incidence in Native Americans and Alaskan Natives was 74.4 per 100,000 for 1999–2002.[3] Mortality rates (per 100,000) for these time periods were 12.6 for Asians and Pacific Islanders, 16.3 for Hispanics, and 13.8 for Native Americans and Alaskan Natives.[4]

Epidemiologists often use statistics such as the relative risk (RR) or the odds ratio (OR) to determine if a given factor (e.g., age, weight, smoking status) is associated with disease (Table 19-1). The RR is defined as the risk of disease in those exposed to the factor in question divided by the risk of disease in those not exposed to the factor. A hazard ratio is conceptually similar to the RR but is calculated using survival analysis. The OR is an indirect measure of the RR, calculated as the odds of exposure to a given factor in those with disease divided by the odds of exposure in those without disease. For both measures, values above 1 indicate a positive association between the factor and disease, a value of 1 indicates no association, and values below 1 indicate a negative association.

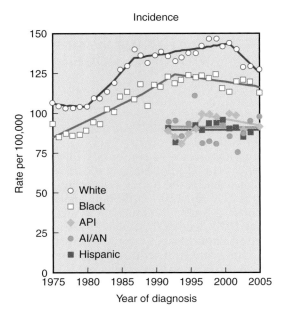

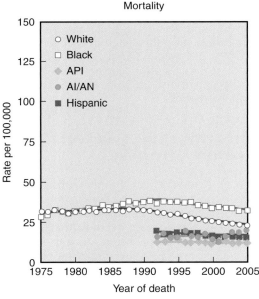

Figure 19-2 Breast cancer incidence and mortality among U.S. women by race, 1975–2005. API, Asian/Pacific Islander; AI/AN, American Indian/Alaska native. (From Ries LAG, Melbert D, Krapcho M, et al [eds]: Surveillance Epidemiology and End Results [SEER] Cancer Statistics Review, 1975–2005. National Cancer Institute, Bethesda, MD, http://seer.cancer.gov/csr/1975_2005. Based on November 2007 SEER data submission, posted to the SEER website 2008.)

TABLE 19-1

Traditional Risk Factors for Breast Cancer, Relative Risks, and associated Population Attributable Risks

Risk Factor	Comparison Category	Risk Category	Relative Risk	Prevalence (%)	Population Attributable Risk*
Age at menarche	16 years	Younger than 12 years	1.3	16	0.05
Age at menopause	45 to 54 years	After 55 years	1.5	6	0.03
Age when first child born alive	Before 20 years	Nulliparous or older than 30 years	1.9	21	0.16
Benign breast disease	No biopsy or fine needle aspiration	Any benign disease	1.5	15	0.07
		Proliferative disease	2	4	0.04
		Atypical hyperplasia	4	1	0.03
Family history of breast cancer	No first-degree relative affected	Mother affected	1.7	8	0.05
		Two first-degree relatives affected	5	4	0.14

*Population attributable risk = [prevalence × (relative risk − 1)]/{[prevalence × (relative risk−1)] + 1}.
Adapted from Harris JR, Lippman ME, Veronesi U, Willet W: Breast cancer (1). N Engl J Med 327:319–328, 1992. Copyright © 1992 Massachusetts Medical Society. All rights reserved.

A variety of genetic, environmental, and behavioral factors may explain the racial differences in the incidence of breast cancer. Migration studies have documented that the risk of breast cancer is higher in Asian-American women born in the west compared with those born in Asia (RR 1.6; 95% confidence interval [CI]: 1.2–2.1).[20] Risk of breast cancer is further increased with the number of the woman's grandparents born in the west (RR 1.89; 95% CI 1.2–3 for a woman with one to two grandparents born in the west compared with a woman with all grandparents born in Asia). Risk is decreased in more recent immigrants (RR 0.32; 95% CI 0.18–0.57 for 2–4 years lived in the west) compared to those who have lived in the west their entire lives.[20] A recent study also reported that incidence rates for breast cancer in Asian Americans in Los Angeles County rose substantially between 1993 and 1997.[21] Most notably, the incidence rate for breast cancer in Japanese-American women in this county is rapidly approaching that of non-Hispanic white women.[21] Factors such as acculturation and adoption of a Western diet may at least partially explain these recent trends.[21]

BENIGN BREAST DISEASE

One accepted hypothesis about the origin of breast cancer is that cells progress through sequential changes over a period of years. In some women, ductal cells proliferate, resulting in intraductal hyperplasia, and proliferative hyperplasia progresses to atypia. In a smaller number of women, lobular or ductal carcinoma in situ develops. Some, but not all, of these women eventually develop invasive malignancy.

Benign breast lesions can be classified according to their histologic appearance (Table 19-2). Benign breast lesions thought to impart no increased risk of breast cancer include adenosis, duct ectasia, simple fibroadenoma, fibrosis, mastitis, mild hyperplasia, cysts, and metaplasia of the apocrine or squamous types.[22,23] Lesions associated with a slight increase in the subsequent risk of developing invasive breast cancer include complex fibroadenoma, moderate or florid hyperplasia with or without atypia, sclerosing adenosis, and papilloma. Atypical hyperplasia of the ductal or lobular type is associated with a 4- to 5-fold increased risk of developing subsequent breast cancer, and this risk increases to approximately 10-fold if it is also associated with a family history of invasive breast cancer in a first-degree relative.

Substantially increased risk of developing subsequent invasive breast cancer is seen in premenopausal women (as compared with postmenopausal women) with atypical lobular hyperplasia. In premenopausal women, the effect of atypical lobular hyperplasia is nearly twice as great as that of atypical ductal hyperplasia.[24,25]

FAMILY HISTORY

Women who have a first-degree relative with a history of breast cancer are at increased risk of the disease themselves.[26] The risk conferred by family history is further increased if the affected family member was diagnosed with the disease at a younger age. For example, a woman with a first-degree relative diagnosed with breast cancer before 40 years of age has a 5.7 times increased risk (99% CI 2.7–11.8) of being diagnosed with breast cancer before she is 40 compared with a woman of the same age but without a family history of breast cancer.[27] Two genes, *BRCA1* and *BRCA2*, have been implicated in familial breast cancer but account for less than 10% of all breast cancer cases.[28] *BRCA* mutations are most strongly related to breast cancer occurring in younger, premenopausal women. In women diagnosed with breast cancer before age 40, 9% have a *BRCA* mutation, compared with only 2% of women of any age diagnosed with breast cancer.[29]

REPRODUCTIVE FACTORS

Early age at menarche and late age at menopause have been found to increase the risk of breast cancer, whereas premenopausal oophorectomy reduces risk. Late age at first and possibly last full-term pregnancy have been

TABLE 19-2

Classification of Benign Breast Disease and the Risk of Subsequent Breast Cancer

Benign Lesion	Description	Associated Relative Risk of Breast Cancer*	
		With Family History of Breast Cancer	**Without Family History of Breast Cancer**
Proliferative Disease without Atypia		2.4–2.7	1.7–1.9
Moderate and florid ductal hyperplasia of the usual type	Most common type of hyperplasia; cells do not have the cytologic appearance of lobular or apocrine-like lesions; florid lesions have a proliferation of cells that fill more than 70% of the involved space		
Additional lesions	Intraductal papilloma, radial scar, sclerosing adenosis, apocrine metaplasia		
Atypical Hyperplasia		11	4.2–4.3
Atypical ductal hyperplasia	Has features similar to ductal carcinoma in situ but lacks the complete criteria for that diagnosis		
Atypical lobular hyperplasia	Defined by changes that are similar to lobular carcinoma in situ but lack the complete criteria for that diagnosis		
Nonproliferative	Normal, cysts, duct, ectasia, mild hyperplasia, fibroadenoma	1.2–2.6	0.9–1

*Relative risks represent the range of values reported in the published literature.
Adapted from Vogel VG: Breast cancer risk factors and preventive approaches to breast cancer. In Kavanagh JS, Einhorn N, DePetrillo AD (eds): Cancer in women. Cambridge, MA, Blackwell Scientific Publications, 1998, pp 58–91; and Fitzgibbons PL, Henson DE, Hutter RV: Benign breast changes and the risk for subsequent breast cancer: An update of the 1985 consensus statement. Cancer Committee of the College of American Pathologists. Arch Pathol Lab Med 122:1053–1055, 1998.

associated with an elevated risk; risk decreases with increasing parity.[30] Breastfeeding has also been shown to decrease the risk of breast cancer.[28,31] The timing of the initiation of the carcinogenic process is an important consideration when studying the effect of reproductive factors on the risk of breast cancer.[32] Risk of premenopausal breast cancer decreases about 9% (95% CI 7–11%) for each one-year increase in age at menarche, whereas risk of postmenopausal breast cancer decreases only about 4% (95% CI 2–5%) for each one-year increase in age at menarche. Risk of breast cancer increases with increasing age at first full-term pregnancy by 5% (95% CI 5–6%) per year for breast cancer diagnosed before menopause, and by 3% (95% CI 2%–4%) for cancers diagnosed after

menopause. Each full-term pregnancy is associated with a 3% (95% CI 1%–6%) reduction in risk of breast cancer diagnosed before menopause, whereas the reduction was 12% (95% CI 10–14%) for breast cancer diagnosed later.

Newer Risk Factors for Breast Cancer

The field of breast cancer epidemiology is a vibrant and evolving body of knowledge. Newer and more recently identified risk factors (Table 19-3) and protective factors (Table 19-4) for breast cancer are discussed individually in the sections that follow.

TABLE 19-3

Newer Epidemiologic Risk Factors for Breast Cancer

Characteristic	Menopausal Status*	Comparison Category	Risk Category	Estimate of Effect†
Genetic Factors				
BRCA1 mutation[a]	Both	No mutation	Mutation present in gene	Lifetime risk 50%–73% by age 50 and 65%–87% by age 70
BRCA2 mutation[a]	Both	No mutation	Mutation present in gene	Lifetime risk 59% by age 50 and 82% by age 70
Hormonal Factors				
Oral contraceptive use[b]	Both	Never users	Current users	RR 1.24 (1.15–1.33)
	Both	Never users	≥10 years since last use	RR 1.01 (0.96–1.05)
Postmenopausal hormone therapy use	Postmenopausal[c]	Nonusers with an intact uterus	Estrogen + progestin users	HR 1.24 (1.01–1.54)
	Postmenopausal[d]	Nonusers with a hysterectomy	Estrogen users	HR 0.80 (0.62–1.04)

TABLE 19-3—Cont.

Newer Epidemiologic Risk Factors for Breast Cancer

Characteristic	Menopausal Status*	Comparison Category	Risk Category	Estimate of Effect[†]
Circulating estradiol	Premenopausal[e]	Lowest quartile	Highest quartile	OR 1 (0.66–1.52)
	Postmenopausal[f]	Lowest quintile	Highest quintile	RR 2 (1.47–2.71)
Circulating estrone	Premenopausal[e]	Lowest quartile	Highest quartile	OR 1.16 (1.48–3.22)
	Postmenopausal[f]	Lowest quintile	Highest quintile	RR 2.19 (1.48–3.22)
Testosterone	Premenopausal[e]	<1.13 nmol/L	≥2.04 nmol/L	OR 1.73 (1.16–2.57)
	Postmenopausal[f]	Lowest quintile	Highest quintile	RR 2.22 (1.59–3.10)
Other Biological Factors				
Mammographic breast density[g]	Both	<5% density	≥75% density	RR 4.64 (3.64–5.91)
Bone mineral density[h]	Postmenopausal	Lowest quartile at each of three skeletal sites	Highest quartile at each of three skeletal sites	RR 2.70 (1.4–5.3)
Circulating IGF-I[i]	Premenopausal	25th percentile	75th percentile	OR 1.93 (1.38–2.69)
	Postmenopausal	25th percentile	75th percentile	OR 0.95 (0.62–1.33)
Circulating IGFBP-III[i]	Premenopausal	25th percentile	75th percentile	OR 1.96 (1.28–2.99)
	Postmenopausal	25th percentile	75th percentile	OR 0.97 (0.53–1.77)
Behavioral Factors				
Body mass index[j]	Postmenopausal	<21 kg/m²	≥33 kg/m²	RR 1.27 (1.03–1.55)
Height[j]	Premenopausal	<1.60 cm	≥1.75 cm	RR 1.42 (0.95–2.12)
	Postmenopausal	<1.60 cm	≥1.75 cm	RR 1.28 (0.94–1.76)
Weight[j]	Postmenopausal	<60 kg	≥80 kg	RR 1.25 (1.02–1.52)
Alcohol use[j]	Both	Never drinkers	>12 g/day	RR 1.10 (1.06–1.14)
Smoking[k]	Postmenopausal	Never smokers	Smoked > 40 years	RR 1.5 (1.2–1.9)
Night work[l]	Both	No nightshift work	Any nightshift work	OR 1.48 (1.36–1.61)
Dietary Factors				
Total fat intake[m]	Both	Lowest quantile	Highest quantile	OR 1.13 (1.03–1.25)
Saturated fat intake[m]	Both	Lowest quantile	Highest quantile	OR 1.19 (1.06–1.35)
Meat intake[m]	Both	Lowest quantile	Highest quantile	OR 1.17 (1.06–1.29)
Environmental Factors				
Ionizing radiation[n]	Both	0–0.09 Gy exposure to Nagasaki or Hiroshima atomic bomb	≥0.50 Gy exposure to Nagasaki or Hiroshima atomic bomb	RR varies depending on age at exposure: RR = 9 at age 0–4; RR = 2 at age 35–39

IRR, incidence rate ratio; OR, odds ratio; RR, relative risk.

*Refers to menopausal status at the time of diagnosis.

[†]95% confidence intervals are given in parentheses.

[a]From National Cancer Institute.[29]

[b]From Collaborative Group on Hormonal Factors in Breast Cancer.[88]

[c]From Chlebowski RT, Hendrix SL, Langer RD, et al.[94]

[d]From Stefanick ML, Anderson GL, Margolis KL, et al.[95]

[e]From Kaaks R, Berrino F, Key T, et al.[66]

[f]From Key T, Appleby P, Barnes I, et al.[62]

[g]From McCormack VA, dos Santos Silva I.[99]

[h]From Zmuda JM, Cauley JA, Ljung BM, et al.[60]

[i]From Renehan AG, Zwahlen M, Minder C, et al: Insulin-like growth factor (IGF)-I, IGF binding protein-3, and cancer risk: Systematic review and meta-regression analysis. Lancet 363:1346–1353, 2004.

[j]From Ellison RC, Zhang Y, McLennan CE, et al.[124]

[k]From Cui Y, Miller AB, Rohan TE: Cigarette smoking and breast cancer risk: Update of a prospective cohort study. Breast Cancer Res Treat 100:293–299, 2006.

[l]From Megdal SP, Kroenke CH, Laden F, et al: Night work and breast cancer risk: A systematic review and meta-analysis. Eur J Cancer 41:2023–2032, 2005.

[m]From Boyd NF, Stone J, Vogt KN, et al: Dietary fat and breast cancer risk revisited: A meta-analysis of the published literature. Br J Cancer 89:1672–1685, 2003.

[n]From Tokunaga M, Land CE, Yamamoto T, et al.[133]

TABLE 19-4

Possible Protective Factors for Breast Cancer

Characteristic	Menopausal Status*	Reference Group	Comparison Group	Estimate of Effect[†]
Reproductive Factors				
Parity[a]	Both	Nulliparous	2 live births	OR 0.91 (0.85–0.97)
Breastfeeding[b]	Premenopausal	Never breastfed	Ever breastfed	RR 0.78 (0.66–0.91)
	Postmenopausal	Never breastfed	Ever breastfed	RR 1.04 (0.95–1.14)
Preeclampsia[c]	Both	No preeclampsia	Ever preeclampsia	ORs range from 0.27 (0.08–0.63) to 0.81 (0.61–1.1)
Hormonal Factors				
Estrogen metabolite ratio[d]	Premenopausal	2:16-OH ratio ≤1.80	2:16-OH ratio ≥3.29	OR 0.55 (0.23–1.32)
	Postmenopausal	2:16-OH ratio ≤1.77	2.16-OH ratio ≥3.66	OR 1.31 (0.53–3.18)
Circulating sex hormone–binding globulin	Premenopausal[l]	<31.1 nmol/L	≥64.5 nmol/L	OR 0.95 (0.65–1.40)
	Postmenopausal[m]	Lowest quintile	Highest quintile	RR 0.66 (0.43–1)
Other Biological Factors				
Bone fracture[e]	Postmenopausal	No fracture in past 5 years	History of fracture	OR 0.80 (0.68–0.94)
Behavioral Factors				
Body mass index[f]	Premenopausal	<21 kg/m^2	≥33 kg/m^2	RR 0.58 (0.34–1)
Physical activity	Premenopausal[n]	<9.1 hours/week	≥20.8 hours/week	OR 0.74 (0.52–1.05)
	Postmenopausal[o]	Not currently active	>40 metabolic-equivalent hours per week	RR 0.78 (0.62–1)
Nonsteroidal anti-inflammatory drug (NSAID) use[g]	Both	Nonusers	Current user of any NSAID	OR 0.80 (0.73–0.87)
Dietary Factors				
Calcium (dietary)[h]	Postmenopausal	≤500 mg/day	>1250 mg/day	RR 0.80 (0.67–0.95)
Folate (total)[i]	Both	150–299 µg/day	≥600 µg/day	RR 0.93 (0.83–1.03)
Soy[j]	Premenopausal	Low intake	High intake	OR 0.70 (0.58–0.85)
	Postmenopausal	Low intake	High intake	OR 0.77 (0.60–0.98)
Vitamin D (total)[k]	Postmenopausal	<400 IU	≥800 IU	RR 0.89 (0.77–1.03)

IRR, incidence rate ratio; OR, odds ratio; RR, relative risk.
*Refers to menopausal status at the time of diagnosis.
[†]95% confidence intervals are given in parentheses.
[a]From Lambe M, Hsieh CC, Chan HW, et al: Parity, age at first and last birth, and risk of breast cancer: A population-based study in Sweden. Breast Cancer Res Treat 38:305–311, 1996.
[b]From Newcomb PA, Storer BE, Longnecker MP, et al.[31]
[c]From Innes KE, Byers TE.[97]
[d]From Muti P, Bradlow HL, Micheli A, et al.[84]
[e]From Newcomb PA, Trentham-Dietz A, Egan KM, et al: Fracture history and risk of breast and endometrial cancer. Am J Epidemiol 153:1071–1078, 2001.
[f]From van den Brandt PA, Spiegelman D, Yaun SS, et al.[36]
[g]From Khuder SA, Mutgi AB: Breast cancer and NSAID use: A meta-analysis. Br J Cancer 84:1188–1192, 2001.
[h]From McCullough ML, Rodriguez C, Diver WR, et al: Dairy, calcium, and vitamin D intake and postmenopausal breast cancer risk in the Cancer Prevention Study II Nutrition Cohort. Cancer Epidemiol Biomarkers Prev 14:2898–2904, 2005.
[i]From Zhang S, Hunter DJ, Hankinson SE, et al: A prospective study of folate intake and the risk of breast cancer. JAMA 281:1632–1637, 1999.
[j]From Trock BJ, Hilakivi-Clarke L, Clarke R: Meta-analysis of soy intake and breast cancer risk. J Natl Cancer Inst 98:459–471, 2006.
[k]From Robien K, Cutler GJ, Lazovich D: Vitamin D intake and breast cancer risk in postmenopausal women: The Iowa Women's Health Study. Cancer Causes Control 18:775–782, 2007.
[l]From Kaaks R, Berrino F, Key T, et al.[66]
[m]From Key T, Appleby P, Barnes I, et al.[62]
[n]From John EM, Horn-Ross PL, Koo J: Lifetime physical activity and breast cancer risk in a multiethnic population: The San Francisco Bay area breast cancer study. Cancer Epidemiol Biomarkers Prev 12:1143–1152, 2003.
[o]From McTiernan A, Kooperberg C, White E, et al: Recreational physical activity and the risk of breast cancer in postmenopausal women: The Women's Health Initiative Cohort Study. JAMA 290:1331–1336, 2003.

ANTHROPOMETRY

Obesity has emerged as a significant risk factor for postmenopausal breast cancer and is possibly a protective factor for premenopausal breast cancer. Further, adjustment for measures of obesity attenuates, but does not eliminate, the racial difference in stage at breast cancer diagnosis.[33,34] The most frequently used measure of obesity is the body mass index (BMI). BMI is a measure of weight for height and is calculated as weight in kilograms divided by the square of height in meters. In postmenopausal women, some studies report either no association or only a weak association between BMI and risk of breast cancer,[12,35] whereas the vast majority report that increased BMI significantly raises the risk of breast cancer[36–38] (e.g., a 4% increase in the odds of postmenopausal breast cancer for every 1 kg/m^2 increase in current BMI[37]). A meta-analysis of prospective studies found that the risk of breast cancer increased 7% with each 4 kg/m^2 increase in BMI in postmenopausal women.[36] Some studies have reported that the positive association between BMI and risk of postmenopausal breast cancer occurs only or more strongly in women with certain other risk factors, such as a family history of breast cancer[39] or older age.[40] A consistent finding is that elevated BMI increases the risk of postmenopausal breast cancer only in women who have never used postmenopausal hormone therapy (HT).[38,41–43]

Central adiposity, commonly measured by waist circumference or waist-to-hip ratio, has been positively associated with postmenopausal breast cancer,[44,45] and this effect is stronger in women who never used HT.[44] Finally, multiple studies have reported that weight gain during adulthood increases the risk of postmenopausal breast cancer[46] and that weight loss can reduce this risk.[47,48]

Obesity appears to have an opposite effect on the risk of breast cancer in premenopausal women. Few studies report either a positive association[49] or no association[46] between BMI and premenopausal breast cancer. Many studies, however, have reported that BMI is inversely associated with risk of premenopausal or early-age breast cancer.[36,50,51] For example, the same meta-analysis that reported a positive association between BMI and the risk of postmenopausal breast cancer reported a significant negative association between BMI and risk of premenopausal breast cancer, with an 11% reduction in risk for every 4 kg/m^2 increase in BMI (RR 0.89; 95% CI 0.81–0.97).[36] The effect of BMI on the risk of premenopausal breast cancer may vary by race, with one study reporting a negative association in Caucasian women but no association in African-American women.[12]

Similar relationships between obesity and risk of premenopausal breast cancer are observed when other anthropometric measures are considered. Weight has been reported to be either negatively associated[36,46] or not associated[52,53] with premenopausal breast cancer. One study reported a positive association between waist-to-hip ratio and risk of premenopausal breast cancer,[45] whereas another reported no association.[44] The effect of weight gain on premenopausal breast cancer may also vary by race, with studies of Caucasian women reporting either no[54,55] or a negative association,[43] whereas a study

of Hispanic women reported a nonsignificant positive association.[55] Overall, the totality of the current evidence suggests that obesity reduces the risk of premenopausal breast cancer.

ENDOGENOUS HORMONES

Exposure to estrogen is closely linked to the etiology of breast cancer. Estrogen is a female sex hormone that is required for a number of processes in the body. The mechanisms through which estrogens contribute to the carcinogenic process are complex; however, evidence exists confirming that estrogens cause both normal and malignant breast cell proliferation.[56] Many established risk factors for breast cancer can be attributed to either some means of elevated estrogen exposure or cyclical ovarian function. For example, both an early age of menarche and a late age of menopause are related to prolonged exposure to the high levels of estrogen that occur during the menstrual cycle, and both are associated with increased risk of breast cancer.[57,58] Surgical menopause, which results in an abrupt arrest of estrogen secretion by the ovaries, is protective against breast cancer.[59] Moreover, the rate of age-specific breast cancer slows around the time of menopause, a time when estrogen levels decline.[3] Increased bone mineral density, a potential reflection of cumulative estrogen exposure, is associated with increased breast cancer development in menopausal women.[60] Obesity, which is positively correlated with circulating estrogen levels, is associated with risk of postmenopausal breast cancer.[36,60]

Numerous studies have consistently demonstrated that increased levels of endogenous estrogen are related to increased risk of breast cancer in postmenopausal women.[61,62] For example, a meta-analysis of nine prospective studies examining hormone levels in relation to postmenopausal breast cancer reported a twofold increase (RR 2; 95% CI 1.47–2.71; P trend < 0.001) in risk of breast cancer for women in the highest quintile of estradiol compared with those in the lowest quintile.[62]

The association between estradiol and premenopausal breast cancer, however, is far less clear. Estradiol levels fluctuate throughout the menstrual cycle, with peaks occurring toward the ends of both the follicular and luteal phases.[63] Some studies have reported similar positive associations between estradiol and breast cancer in premenopausal women,[64,65] whereas others have reported no association.[66–68] Studies of estradiol and premenopausal breast cancer have been limited by a number of factors, however, including small numbers,[65] failure to control for phase of the menstrual cycle,[65,68] and inclusion of cases that were premenopausal at the time of the blood sample but not at the time of breast cancer diagnosis.[65,66] The largest and most recent study, a nested case-control study of 197 cases and 394 matched controls from the Nurses' Health Study II, reported that free estradiol (RR 2.4; 95% CI 1.3–4.5 for fourth vs. first quartile) and total estradiol (RR 2.1; 95% CI 1.1–4.1 for fourth vs. first quartile) levels during the follicular phase were positively associated with breast cancer, whereas free and total estradiol levels during the luteal phase were not.[64] Although this study was prospective, carefully controlled for phase of the menstrual cycle, and used large numbers, the menopausal status of the cases at the time of diagnosis was unclear.

In addition to the observational studies linking circulating estradiol concentration and risk of breast cancer, convincing data from large clinical trials show that drugs blocking the action of estrogen reduce breast cancer incidence. The risk reduction is more pronounced in women with higher estrogen levels than in those with lower levels, thus further strengthening the evidence that estrogen exposure is associated with the development of breast cancer.[69,70] In the Multiple Outcomes of Raloxifene Evaluation (MORE) trial, it was found that postmenopausal women with the highest estradiol levels had a 2.1-fold risk of breast cancer compared with women with the lowest estradiol levels.[71] Women in the placebo arm of the trial had nearly seven times the risk of developing breast cancer than women with estradiol levels lower (0.6% per year) than the assay's detection limit, and women with circulating levels of estradiol greater than 10 pmol/L in the raloxifene group had a breast cancer rate 76% lower than women with similar levels of estradiol in the placebo group. Thus, inhibiting the action of estrogen plays an obvious role in reducing the risk of breast cancer.[69]

DIETARY FAT AND SERUM ESTRADIOL

Varying levels of fat consumption may influence incidence of hormonally dependent breast cancer by modifying levels of circulating estrogens.[72-74] In fact, free fatty acids added to plasma can significantly increase levels of estradiol in vitro.[75,76] A meta-analysis of 13 intervention trials found serum estradiol levels to be 23% (95% CI −27.7%, −18.1%) lower in healthy postmenopausal women consuming the least amount of dietary fat when compared to women with the highest fat intake.[72] The Diet and Androgens (DIANA) Randomized Trial found a nonsignificant reduction in serum estradiol (−18% in intervention group vs. −5.5% in control group; $P = 0.13$) in postmenopausal women consuming a low animal fat and high omega-3 diet.[73] However, not all studies evaluating dietary fat and estrogen levels have observed reductions in circulating estradiol levels; it has been hypothesized that inadequate dietary assessment may be one cause of this contradiction.

ESTROGEN METABOLISM

There is growing evidence that the way estrogen is metabolized is associated with the risk of breast cancer.[77,78] Estradiol metabolism is predominantly oxidative; it is first (reversibly) converted to estrone, which is irreversibly converted to either 2- or 16-α-hydroxy (2-OH and 16-OH, respectively) estrone in order to eliminate it from the body. Both 16-OH estrone and 16-OH estradiol strongly activate the classical estrogen receptor and, like estradiol, can stimulate uterine tissue growth.[79] On the other hand, the 2-OH metabolites do not appear to promote cellular proliferation and may even have antiestrogenic effects.[80] Because the 2-OH and 16-OH metabolites compete for a limited substrate pool, a rise in one pathway will reduce the amount of product in the competing pathway. Thus, the relative activity of these two metabolic pathways (2:16-OH) may be an endocrine biomarker for risk of breast cancer.

Despite the biologic evidence, epidemiologic support is lacking. Only a handful of studies have explored the association between the risk of breast cancer and the 2:16-OH ratio, with mixed results.[81-86] Possible explanations for these disparate findings include small sample sizes, retrospective study designs, and the use of prevalent breast cancer cases. Metabolite levels in women with breast cancer may not reflect the hormonal milieu during the etiologically relevant period. Moreover, the use of prevalent cases may mask any association, because estrogen metabolism may be altered by treatment.[87] Notably, the only two prospective studies to date,[83,84] have found a decreased risk associated with a high urinary 2:16-OH ratio; however, the results were not statistically significant in either study. Moreover, in one study,[84] the association was limited to premenopausal women only.

In summary, although there is evidence to suggest an association between estrogen metabolism and risk of breast cancer, supporting data from large, population-based studies is lacking.

EXOGENOUS HORMONES: ORAL CONTRACEPTIVES AND POSTMENOPAUSAL HORMONE THERAPY

Exposure to exogenous estrogen has been related to the risk of breast cancer. In the general population, oral contraceptive (OC) use is weakly associated with such risk. In 1996, the Collaborative Group on Hormonal Factors in Breast Cancer analyzed the worldwide epidemiologic evidence on the relation between risk of breast cancer and use of hormonal contraceptives.[88] This large meta-analysis combined individual data on 53,297 women with breast cancer and 100,239 women without breast cancer from 54 epidemiologic studies conducted in 25 countries. Results showed that women who used OCs had a slight but significant increased risk of breast cancer, compared with nonusers (RR 1.24; 95% CI 1.15–1.33). Reassuringly, the risk diminished steadily after cessation of use, with no increase in risk 10 years after cessation of OC use, irrespective of family history of breast cancer, reproductive history, geographic area of residence, ethnic background, differences in study designs, dose and type of hormone, and duration of use.

More recent population-based studies of the risk of breast cancer in former and current users of OCs do not suggest that these drugs increase risk.[89,90] In women 35 to 64 years of age participating in a population-based, case-control study (The National Institute of Child Health and Human Development Women's Contraceptive and Reproductive Experiences Study [CARE]), current or former OC use was not associated with a significantly increased risk of breast cancer.[90]

A retrospective cohort study evaluated the effect of OCs in women with a familial predisposition to breast cancer.[91] A total of 394 sisters and daughters of the probands, 3002 granddaughters and nieces, and 2754 women who married into the families were studied.

After accounting for age and birth cohort, any OC use was significantly associated with increased risk of breast cancer in first-degree relatives only (RR 3.3; 95% CI 1.6–6.7). The elevated risk in women with a first-degree family history of breast cancer was most evident for OC use during or prior to 1975, when formulations were likely to contain higher dosages of estrogen and progestins.

In 1997, the Collaborative Group on Hormonal Factors in Breast Cancer[92] brought together and reanalyzed about 90% of the worldwide epidemiologic evidence on the relation between risk of breast cancer and use of postmenopausal HT. In current users of HT, or those who ceased use 1 to 4 years previously, the risk of having breast cancer diagnosed increased by 2.3% for each year of use; the RR was 1.35 for women who had used HT for 5 years or longer. A more recent meta-analysis also found an increased risk of breast cancer associated with the use of HT.[93]

The results of the Women's Health Initiative (WHI), however, showed that this increased risk may occur only in users of combined estrogen and progestin regimens[94] and not in women using unopposed estrogen.[95] The WHI conducted two separate randomized, controlled primary prevention trials of HT use in postmenopausal women 50 to 79 years of age. One was a trial of conjugated equine estrogens, 0.625 mg daily, plus medroxyprogesterone acetate, 2.5 mg daily, in a single tablet (n = 8506) versus placebo (n = 8102) in women with an intact uterus. The other was a trial of conjugated equine estrogens, 0.625 mg daily (n = 5310) versus placebo (n = 5429) in women with a hysterectomy. Women randomized to take the combination of estrogen and progestin had a 24% increase in risk of invasive breast cancer compared with those randomized to placebo (hazard ratio 1.24; 95% CI 1.01–1.54).[94] However, in the unopposed estrogen trial, women randomized to active treatment had a similar risk of invasive breast cancer as women randomized to placebo.[95] The duration of follow-up in WHI may not have been long enough to observe an association between breast cancer and unopposed estrogen use. Recently, the Nurse's Health Study, an observational study of women's health, reported that the risk of breast cancer increased with the duration of unopposed estrogen use. The multivariate RRs and 95% CIs for breast cancer with current HT use for less than 5 years, 5 to 9.9 years, 10 to 14.9 years, 15 to 19.9 years, and 20 years or more were, respectively, 0.96 (0.75–1.22), 0.90 (0.73–1.12), 1.06 (0.87–1.30), 1.18 (0.95–1.48), and 1.42 (1.13–1.77; P for trend < 0.001).[96] The relationship was more notable in estrogen receptor–positive and progesterone receptor–positive tumors, and it became statistically significant after 15 years of use (RR 1.48).

PREECLAMPSIA

Preeclampsia, a common complication of pregnancy, may be a particularly sensitive marker for endogenous hormonal factors associated with the development of breast cancer. In a review of the connection between preeclampsia and the risk of breast cancer, the data suggest that both a personal and maternal history of preeclampsia are inversely and independently associated with subsequent risk of breast cancer.[97] Preeclampsia may be a novel marker of endogenous hormonal factors that are related to breast cancer development, including reduced levels of estrogens and insulin-like growth factor I (IGF-I), as well as elevated levels of progesterone, androgens, and IGF-I binding protein. These factors may act both individually and synergistically to decrease the risk of breast cancer.

INDUCED ABORTION

It has been hypothesized that an interrupted pregnancy might increase a woman's risk of breast cancer because of proliferation of breast cells without the later protective effect of differentiation. In a cohort of 1.5 million women (28.5 million person-years) and after adjustment for known risk factors, induced abortion as determined by a national Danish registry was not associated with an increased risk of breast cancer. No increases in risk were found in subgroups defined according to age at abortion, parity, time since abortion, or age at diagnosis of breast cancer.[98] The RR of breast cancer increased with increasing gestational age of the fetus at the time of the most recent induced abortion: less than 7 weeks, 0.81 (95% CI 0.58–1.13); greater than 12 weeks, 1.38 (1–1.9; reference category, 9 to 10 weeks). Induced abortions appear to have no overall effect on the risk of breast cancer.

MAMMOGRAPHIC BREAST DENSITY

Mammographic breast density is determined by the relative proportions of fat and structural tissues in the breast as viewed on a mammogram. Both qualitative and quantitative methods of measuring breast density exist, although quantitative methods are typically used in contemporary studies. Breast density is most often measured as the percentage of the breast composed of dense tissue.

Numerous studies have investigated associations between breast density and breast cancer since Wolfe hypothesized such a relationship more than 30 years ago. A recent meta-analysis of such studies[99] showed a high degree of consistency. The combined RR from incidence studies of the general population using qualitative Wolfe patterns was 1.76 (95% CI 1.41–2.19) for P1 versus N1, 3.05 (95% CI 2.54–3.66) for P2 versus N1, and 3.98 (95% CI 2.53–6.27) for DY versus N1. Combined RR estimates of studies using the Breast Imaging Reporting and Data System (BIRADS) qualitative classification with fatty breast as the referent group were 2.04 for scattered density, 2.81 for heterogeneously dense, and 4.08 for extremely dense.

Similar combined estimates of RRs using quantitative percent density assessments were also reported. Compared with having less than 5% breast density, incidence studies had combined RRs of 1.79 (95% CI 1.48–2.16) for 5% to 24% density, 2.11 (95% CI 1.70–2.63) for 25% to 49% density, 2.92 (95% CI 2.49–3.42) for 50%

to 74% density, and 4.64 (95% CI 3.64–5.91) for density of 75% or more. The combined RR estimates for prevalence studies were similar but slightly lower: 1.39 (95% CI 1.10–1.76) for 5% to 24% density, 2.22 (95% CI 1.75–2.81) for 25% to 49% density, 2.93 (95% CI 2.27–3.79) for 50% to 74% density, and 3.67 (95% CI 2.72–4.96) for 75% density or more versus less than 5% density.[99]

Presence of masking bias would result in underestimated RRs reported by prevalence studies, in which cancers were detected at the time of screening, and overestimated RRs reported by incidence studies; this is consistent with the results of the previously mentioned meta-analysis. The review and meta-analysis also reported that breast density remains associated with the risk of breast cancer regardless of age, menopausal status, or race.[99] Mammographic breast density may be a stronger risk factor for postmenopausal breast cancer than for premenopausal breast cancer, however.[100,101]

Mitchell and colleagues reported that higher-percent breast density remains a strong risk factor for breast cancer in women with known *BRCA1/BRCA2* mutations.[102] The odds of breast cancer in mutation carriers with density greater than or equal to 50% were twice that of mutation carriers with less than 50% density (OR 2.29).[102]

Few studies have reported how changes in breast density relate to changes in the risk of breast cancer.[103] One study reported that women who consistently had high-risk Wolfe patterns (P2 or DY) had more than twice the risk of breast cancer (RR 2.2; 95% CI 1.2–3.9) compared with women who consistently had low-risk Wolfe patterns (N1 or P1). Those women whose patterns on the first mammogram were either P2 or DY but then had a low-risk pattern on a subsequent mammogram had similar risk to women with consistently low-risk Wolfe patterns (RR 1.2; 95% CI 0.5–2.8).[104] Although the ability of breast density to change in response to known risk factors for breast cancer, such as use of postmenopausal HT, has been established, it is unclear what these changes in breast density mean in terms of altering breast cancer risk.[105]

Mammographic Breast Density and Breast Cancer Risk Factors

In general, risk factors for breast cancer increase mammographic breast density. For example, nulliparity and later age at first birth have been associated with increased density.[106] On the other hand, breast density has been shown to decrease with increasing age,[106,107] although increased age is a risk factor for breast cancer. This apparent contradiction has been explained by noting that breast density may be related to the rate of change in breast cancer incidence rather than the incidence of breast cancer itself.[101]

Age may not be related to breast density in women older than 70 years of age.[108] A study of 239 participants from the Study of Osteoporotic Fractures (SOF) reported that only BMI, parity, surgical menopause, and current smoking status were significantly associated with mammographic breast density in multivariable analyses. The mean age of these women at the time of consent for obtaining the most recent mammogram was 78.6 years,

thus indicating that the factors associated with breast density in older women may differ from premenopausal and younger postmenopausal women.[108] Genetic factors explain 60% to 75% of the variability in percent breast density.[109] Specific genes responsible for differences in breast density have yet to be conclusively identified, however. Despite the relationships between breast cancer risk factors and breast density, presence of other breast cancer risk factors does not fully account for the association between increased breast density and risk of breast cancer.[101] Mammographic breast density is indeed an independent risk factor for breast cancer.

Exogenous Hormones and Mammographic Density

Studies have repeatedly shown that increased breast density is related to postmenopausal hormone replacement therapy (HRT).[110–112] The percent of women whose breast density changes after initiating HRT varies by type of HRT used, with increased density occurring more often in estrogen-plus-progestin regimens than with estrogen-alone regimens.[110,111] In the WHI, investigators reported that 75% of women on active treatment experienced an increase in breast density after 1 year. The mean change in percent density from baseline to year 1 was 6% (95% CI 4.6–7.5) in the treatment group compared with −0.9% (95% CI −1.5 to −0.2) in the placebo group.[112] Short-term cessation of HRT use prior to mammography results in a decrease in breast density[113] or less frequent increase in density compared with women who continue to take HRT,[111] and even months after cessation of therapy there appears to be residual effects of HRT on breast density.[114]

Data on the effect of OC use on breast density are limited, probably because the majority of women for whom screening mammography is recommended (age ≥40) are postmenopausal and would not be currently using oral contraceptives. One study has reported, however, that use of OCs prior to first birth was not related to breast density later in life.[115]

Dietary Fat and Mammographic Breast Density

The few studies that have assessed the role of dietary fat on mammographic density have revealed that diet may influence percent breast density. A 2-year intervention with a low-fat, high-carbohydrate diet reduced breast density by 6.1% in the experimental group compared with 2.1% in the control group (P = 0.02).[116] Positive associations between total fat intake and high mammographic density have been observed.[117,118] However, decreased density and null findings have also been associated with total fat intake.[119–121] As with total fat, positive and null relationships have been found between total polyunsaturated fat intake and breast density.[117–121] Two studies assessed the effects of total meat intake and breast density. A nonsignificant, positive association (OR 1.59; 95% CI 0.83, 3.04) was observed in one study; however, no relationship was found between total meat intake and breast density in the other.[121,122]

PHYSICAL ACTIVITY

Interest in physical activity as a means for reducing the risk of breast cancer is growing, although evidence for an association between physical activity and breast cancer is not entirely consistent. A review of such studies showed that the strength of association between physical activity and breast cancer ranges from 0.3 to 1.6.[123] Thirty-two of 44 studies reviewed observed a reduction in the risk of breast cancer in women who were most physically active, and the risk reduction averaged between 30% and 40%. An inverse dose-response relationship between increasing activity levels and decreased risk of breast cancer was found in 20 of 23 studies that examined this trend. Only two studies observed an opposite trend such that breast cancer risk increased with increasing physical activity levels; the remaining studies found no association at all.

ALCOHOL CONSUMPTION

Although the association of alcohol consumption with increased risk of breast cancer has been a consistent finding in the majority of epidemiologic studies during the past two decades, questions remain regarding the interactions between alcohol and other risk factors and the biologic mechanisms involved. A meta-analysis of epidemiologic studies carried out through 1999 examined the dose-response relation and assessed whether effect estimates differed according to various study characteristics.[124] Overall, there was an increase in the RR of breast cancer with alcohol consumption, but the magnitude of the effect was small; in comparison with nondrinkers, women consuming an average of 12 grams per day of alcohol (approximately one typical drink) had an RR of 1.10. Estimates of RR were 7% greater in hospital-based case control studies than in cohort studies or community-based case control studies, 3% greater in studies published before 1990 than in later studies, and 5% greater in studies conducted outside of the United States than inside the country. The findings of five U.S. cohort studies published since 1990 yielded an increased risk of 6% for consumers of 12 grams per day of alcohol compared with nondrinkers. Cohort studies with less than 10 years of follow-up yielded estimates 11% higher than studies with longer follow-up periods. No meaningful differences are seen by either menopausal status or type of beverage consumed.

Alcohol-related risk of breast cancer may be associated with endogenous hormone levels.[125] Recent results from 44,187 postmenopausal women participating in the Nurses' Health Study are consistent with the hypothesis that the use of alcohol increases the risk of breast cancer through a hormonal mechanism. Risk of breast cancer was about 30% higher in women who currently used postmenopausal hormones for 5 or more years and did not drink alcohol (RR 1.32; 95% CI 1.05–1.66). Those who never used postmenopausal hormones but consumed 1.5 to 2 drinks or more of alcohol daily had a nonsignificantly increased risk of 28%. Current users of postmenopausal hormones for 5 or more years who consumed 20 or more grams of alcohol daily had an RR for breast cancer nearly twice that of nondrinking nonusers of postmenopausal hormones (RR 1.99; 95% CI 1.42–2.79). Women who are making decisions about alcohol and postmenopausal hormone use may want to consider the added risks associated with breast cancer.[126]

SMOKING

The role of active and passive smoking in breast cancer remains controversial, largely because of the fact that breast cancer is hormone-dependent and cigarette smoking appears to have antiestrogenic effects in women.[127,128] Most reports demonstrated no association between smoking and risk of breast cancer; however, many studies included passive smokers within the referent category, possibly diluting any true effect that active or passive smoking exposure might have on risk of breast cancer.[129] In a review of 11 studies, five found significantly increased ORs of at least 1.5 for passive smokers versus unexposed, and six reported significantly increased risk of breast cancer for active smokers versus nonsmoking women, suggesting a similar strength of association between active or passive smoking and risk of breast cancer. Some of the inconsistency in the relationship of breast cancer to cigarette smoking may also result from the influence of age at diagnosis and menopausal status on the response of breast cells to exposure to cigarette smoke.[128]

The risk of breast cancer is significantly higher (70%) in parous women who initiated smoking within 5 years postmenarche and in nulliparous women who smoked 20 cigarettes per day or more (sevenfold increase in risk) and for 20 cumulative pack-years or more (OR 7.48; 95% CI 1.59–35.2).[130] On the contrary, postmenopausal women who began smoking after their first full-term pregnancy and whose BMI increased from 18 years of age had half the risk of breast cancer. Cigarette smoke appears to exert a dual action on the breast, with different effects in premenopausal and postmenopausal women, thus reinforcing the importance of smoking prevention. Furthermore, the timing of exposure in relation to windows of susceptibility is extremely important in the design of studies to investigate relationships between exposure to cigarette smoke and risk of breast cancer.

BREAST IMPLANTS

There is no convincing evidence of a causal association between breast implants and breast cancer. Scientific studies have consistently determined that when women with breast implants are compared to women without implants, the women with implants are not at increased risk for breast cancer incidence or recurrence, are not diagnosed with later-stage breast malignancies, and do not have a decreased length of survival.[131]

IONIZING RADIATION

There is a well-established relationship between exposure to ionizing radiation and the risk of breast cancer.[132,133] Increased risk of breast cancer has been consistently observed in association with a variety of exposures, such as the Hiroshima or Nagasaki atomic explosions, fluoroscopy for tuberculosis, and radiation treatments for medical conditions (e.g., Hodgkin's disease). Although risk is inversely associated with age at radiation exposure, exposures past the menopausal age seem to carry a low risk. Although an estimate of the risk of breast cancer associated with medical radiology puts the figure at less than 1% of the total,[134] certain populations, such as women who are heterozygous for ataxia-telangiectasia, may be at increased risk from usual sources of radiation exposure.[135]

Women with a history of benign breast disease or a family history of breast cancer appear to have greater risk of breast cancer following relatively low ionizing radiation exposure compared with other women.[136] Risk of breast cancer is elevated in women exposed to medical radiation prior to 20 years of age versus women who are not unexposed, and this increased risk is observed only in women with a history of benign breast disease. Overall, risk is not associated with exposure to medical radiation after 20 years of age, although in women with a positive family history of breast or ovarian cancer, exposed women have an increased risk. The elevated risks are attributable to exposures and radiation doses that are no longer common, hampering study generalizability to younger cohorts. In theory, patients with breast cancer who are treated with lumpectomy and radiation therapy may be at increased risk for second breast or other malignancies compared with those treated with mastectomy. Outcome studies after a median follow-up of 15 years show no difference, however, in the risk of second malignancies.[137]

REFERENCES

1. American Cancer Society: Cancer Facts & Figures 2008. Atlanta, American Cancer Society, 2008.
2. American Cancer Society: Breast Cancer Facts & Figures 2005–2006. Atlanta, American Cancer Society, 2005.
3. Surveillance, Epidemiology, and End Results (SEER) Program (www.seer.cancer.gov): SEER*Stat Database: Incidence–SEER 9 Regs Public Use, Nov 2005 Sub (1973–2003), National Cancer Institute, Division of Cancer Control and Population Sciences, Surveillance Research Program, Cancer Statistics Branch, released April 2006, based on the November 2005 submission.
4. Surveillance, Epidemiology, and End Results (SEER) Program (www.seer.cancer.gov): SEER*Stat Database: Mortality–All COD, Public Use With State, Total U.S. for Expanded Races/Hispanics (1990–2003), National Cancer Institute, Division of Cancer Control and Population Sciences, Surveillance Research Program, Cancer Statistics Branch, released April 2006. Underlying mortality data provided by National Center for Health Statistics (www.cdc.gov/nchs).
5. Moorman PG, Jones BA, Millikan RC, et al: Race, anthropometric factors, and stage at diagnosis of breast cancer. Am J Epidemiol 153:284–291, 2001.
6. Jatoi I, Becher H, Leake CR: Widening disparity in survival between white and African-American patients with breast carcinoma treated in the U.S. Department of Defense Healthcare system. Cancer 98:894–899, 2003.
7. Yood MU, Johnson CC, Blount A, et al: Race and differences in breast cancer survival in a managed care population. J Natl Cancer Inst 91:1487–1491, 1999.
8. Nanda R, Schumm LP, Cummings S, et al: Genetic testing in an ethnically diverse cohort of high-risk women: A comparative analysis of BRCA1 and BRCA2 mutations in American families of European and African ancestry. JAMA 294:1925–1933, 2005.
9. Pal T, Permuth-Wey J, Holtje T, et al: BRCA1 and BRCA2 mutations in a study of African American breast cancer patients. Cancer Epidemiol Biomarkers Prev 13:1794–1799, 2004.
10. Olopade OI, Fackenthal JD, Dunston G, et al: Breast cancer genetics in African Americans. Cancer 97:236–245, 2003.
11. Health, United States, 2004, with Chartbook on Trends in the Health of Americans: Hyattsville, MD, National Center for Health Statistics, 2004.
12. Hall IJ, Newman B, Millikan RC, et al: Body size and breast cancer risk in black women and white women: The Carolina Breast Cancer Study. Am J Epidemiol 151:754–764, 2000.
13. Zhu K, Caulfield J, Hunter S, et al: Body mass index and breast cancer risk in African American women. Ann Epidemiol 15:123–128, 2005.
14. Anderson WF, Chatterjee N, Ershler WB, et al: Estrogen receptor breast cancer phenotypes in the Surveillance, Epidemiology, and End Results database. Breast Cancer Res Treat 76:27–36, 2002.
15. Chlebowski RT, Chen Z, Anderson GL, et al: Ethnicity and breast cancer: factors influencing differences in incidence and outcome. J Natl Cancer Inst 97:439–448, 2005.
16. Cunningham JE, Butler WM: Racial disparities in female breast cancer in South Carolina: clinical evidence for a biological basis. Breast Cancer Res Treat 88:161–176, 2004.
17. Henson DE, Chu KC, Levine PH: Histologic grade, stage, and survival in breast carcinoma: Comparison of African American and Caucasian women. Cancer 98:908–917, 2003.
18. Schairer C, Mink PJ, Carroll L, et al: Probabilities of death from breast cancer and other causes among female breast cancer patients. J Natl Cancer Inst 96:1311–1321, 2004.
19. Tammemagi CM, Nerenz D, Neslund-Dudas C, et al: Comorbidity and survival disparities among black and white patients with breast cancer. JAMA 294:1765–1772, 2005.
20. Ziegler RG, Hoover RN, Pike MC, et al: Migration patterns and breast cancer risk in Asian-American women. J Natl Cancer Inst 85:1819–1827, 1993.
21. Deapen D, Liu L, Perkins C, et al: Rapidly rising breast cancer incidence rates among Asian-American women. Int J Cancer 99: 747–750, 2002.
22. Santen RJ, Mansel R: Benign breast disorders. N Engl J Med 353:275–285, 2005.
23. Fitzgibbons PL, Henson DE, Hutter RV: Benign breast changes and the risk for subsequent breast cancer: an update of the 1985 consensus statement. Cancer Committee of the College of American Pathologists. Arch Pathol Lab Med 122:1053–1055, 1998.
24. Colditz GA, Rosner B: Cumulative risk of breast cancer to age 70 years according to risk factor status: Data from the Nurses' Health Study. Am J Epidemiol 152:950–964, 2000.
25. Marshall LM, Hunter DJ, Connolly JL, et al: Risk of breast cancer associated with atypical hyperplasia of lobular and ductal types. Cancer Epidemiol Biomarkers Prev 6:297–301, 1997.
26. Loman N, Johannsson O, Kristoffersson U, et al: Family history of breast and ovarian cancers and BRCA1 and BRCA2 mutations in a population-based series of early-onset breast cancer. J Natl Cancer Inst 93:1215–1223, 2001.
27. Familial breast cancer: collaborative reanalysis of individual data from 52 epidemiological studies including 58,209 women with breast cancer and 101,986 women without the disease. Lancet 358:1389–1399, 2001.
28. Hulka BS, Moorman PG: Breast cancer: Hormones and other risk factors. Maturitas 38:103–113, 2001.
29. National Cancer Institute: Genetics of Breast and Ovarian Cancer (PDQ®), Health Professional Version. Available at http://www.cancer.gov/cancertopics/pdq/genetics/breast-and-ovarian/health professional/allpages. Accessed September 18, 2005.
30. Kelsey JL, Gammon MD, John EM: Reproductive factors and breast cancer. Epidemiol Rev 15:36–47, 1993.
31. Newcomb PA, Storer BE, Longnecker MP, et al: Lactation and a reduced risk of premenopausal breast cancer. N Engl J Med 330: 81–87, 1994.
32. Clavel-Chapelon F, Gerber M: Reproductive factors and breast cancer risk. Do they differ according to age at diagnosis? Breast Cancer Res Treat 72:107–115, 2002.
33. Cui Y, Whiteman MK, Langenberg P, et al: Can obesity explain the racial difference in stage of breast cancer at diagnosis between black and white women? J Womens Health Gend Based Med 11: 527–536, 2002.

34. Jones BA, Kasi SV, Curnen MG, et al: Severe obesity as an explanatory factor for the black/white difference in stage at diagnosis of breast cancer. Am J Epidemiol 146:394–404, 1997.

35. den Tonkelaar I, Seidell JC, Collette HJ, et al: A prospective study on obesity and subcutaneous fat patterning in relation to breast cancer in post-menopausal women participating in the DOM project. Br J Cancer 69:352–357, 1994.

36. van den Brandt PA, Spiegelman D, Yaun SS, et al: Pooled analysis of prospective cohort studies on height, weight, and breast cancer risk. Am J Epidemiol 152:514–527, 2000.

37. Trentham-Dietz A, Newcomb PA, Egan KM, et al: Weight change and risk of postmenopausal breast cancer. Cancer Causes Control 11:533–542, 2000.

38. Key TJ, Appleby PN, Reeves GK, et al: Body mass index, serum sex hormones, and breast cancer risk in postmenopausal women. J Natl Cancer Inst 95:1218–1226, 2003.

39. Carpenter CL, Ross RK, Paganini-Hill A, et al: Effect of family history, obesity and exercise on breast cancer risk among postmenopausal women. Int J Cancer 106:96–102, 2003.

40. La Vecchia C, Negri E, Franceschi S, et al: Body mass index and post-menopausal breast cancer: An age-specific analysis. Br J Cancer 75:441–444, 1997.

41. Lahmann PH, Lissner L, Gullberg B, et al: A prospective study of adiposity and postmenopausal breast cancer risk: The Malmo Diet and Cancer Study. Int J Cancer 103:246–252, 2003.

42. Li CI, Malone KE, Daling JR: Interactions between body mass index and hormone therapy and postmenopausal breast cancer risk. Cancer Causes Control 17:695–703, 2006.

43. Morimoto LM, White E, Chen Z, et al: Obesity, body size, and risk of postmenopausal breast cancer: The Women's Health Initiative. Cancer Causes Control 13:741–751, 2002.

44. Huang Z, Willett WC, Colditz GA, et al: Waist circumference, waist:hip ratio, and risk of breast cancer in the Nurses' Health Study. Am J Epidemiol 150:1316–1324, 1999.

45. Connolly BS, Barnett C, Vogt KN, et al: A meta-analysis of published literature on waist-to-hip ratio and risk of breast cancer. Nutr Cancer 44:127–138, 2002.

46. Verla-Tebit E, Chang-Claude J: Anthropometric factors and the risk of premenopausal breast cancer in Germany. Eur J Cancer Prev 14:419–426, 2005.

47. Harvie M, Howell A, Vierkant RA, et al: Association of gain and loss of weight before and after menopause with risk of postmenopausal breast cancer in the Iowa women's health study. Cancer Epidemiol Biomarkers Prev 14:656–661, 2005.

48. Parker ED, Folsom AR: Intentional weight loss and incidence of obesity-related cancers: The Iowa Women's Health Study. Int J Obes Relat Metab Disord 27:1447–1452, 2003.

49. Chu SY, Lee NC, Wingo PA, et al: The relationship between body mass and breast cancer among women enrolled in the Cancer and Steroid Hormone Study. J Clin Epidemiol 44:1197–1206, 1991.

50. Tehard B, Clavel-Chapelon F. Several anthropometric measurements and breast cancer risk: results of the E3N cohort study. Int J Obes 30:156–163, 2006.

51. Swanson CA, Coates RJ, Schoenberg JB, et al: Body size and breast cancer risk among women under age 45 years. Am J Epidemiol 143:698–706, 1996.

52. Yoo K, Tajima K, Park S, et al: Postmenopausal obesity as a breast cancer risk factor according to estrogen and progesterone receptor status. Cancer Lett 167:57–63, 2001.

53. Freni SC, Eberhardt MS, Turturro A, et al: Anthropometric measures and metabolic rate in association with risk of breast cancer. Cancer Causes Control 7:358–365, 1996.

54. Huang Z, Hankinson SE, Colditz GA, et al: Dual effects of weight and weight gain on breast cancer risk. JAMA 278:1407–1411, 1997.

55. Wenten M, Gilliland FD, Baumgartner K, et al: Associations of weight, weight change, and body mass with breast cancer risk in Hispanic and non-Hispanic white women. Ann Epidemiol 12:435–434, 2002.

56. Williams G, Anderson E, Howell A, et al: Oral contraceptive (OCP) use increases proliferation and decreases oestrogen receptor content of epithelial cells in the normal human breast. Int J Cancer 48:206–210, 1991.

57. Clavel-Chapelon F: Differential effects of reproductive factors on the risk of pre- and postmenopausal breast cancer. Results from a large cohort of French women. Br J Cancer 86:723–727, 2002.

58. Titus-Ernstoff L, Longnecker MP, Newcomb PA, et al: Menstrual factors in relation to breast cancer risk. Cancer Epidemiol Biomarkers Prev 7:783–789, 1998.

59. Lilienfeld AM: The relationship of cancer of the female breast to artificial menopause and marital status. Cancer 9:927–934, 1956.

60. Zmuda JM, Cauley JA, Ljung BM, et al: Bone mass and breast cancer risk in older women: Differences by stage at diagnosis. J Natl Cancer Inst 93:930–936, 2001.

61. Kaaks R, Rinaldi S, Key TJ, et al: Postmenopausal serum androgens, oestrogens and breast cancer risk: The European prospective investigation into cancer and nutrition. Endocr Relat Cancer 12: 1071–1082, 2005.

62. Key T, Appleby P, Barnes I, et al: Endogenous sex hormones and breast cancer in postmenopausal women: Reanalysis of nine prospective studies. J Natl Cancer Inst 94:606–616, 2002.

63. Carr BR, Bradshaw KD: Disorders of the ovary and female reproductive tract. In Braunwald E, Fauci AS, Kasper DL, et al (eds): Harrison's principles of internal medicine, 15th ed. New York, McGraw-Hill, 2001, pp 2154–2168.

64. Eliassen AH, Missmer SA, Tworoger SS, et al: Endogenous steroid hormone concentrations and risk of breast cancer among premenopausal women. J Natl Cancer Inst 98:1406–1415, 2006.

65. Kabuto M, Akiba S, Stevens RG, et al: A prospective study of estradiol and breast cancer in Japanese women. Cancer Epidemiol Biomarkers Prev 9:575–579, 2000.

66. Kaaks R, Berrino F, Key T, et al: Serum sex steroids in premenopausal women and breast cancer risk within the European Prospective Investigation into Cancer and Nutrition (EPIC). J Natl Cancer Inst 97:755–765, 2005.

67. Key TJ: Serum oestradiol and breast cancer risk. Endocr Relat Cancer 6:175–180, 1999.

68. Yu H, Shu X-O, Shi R, et al: Plasma sex steroid hormones and breast cancer risk in Chinese women. Int J Cancer 105:92–97, 2003.

69. Cummings SR, Duong T, Kenyon E, et al: Serum estradiol level and risk of breast cancer during treatment with raloxifene. JAMA 287:216–220, 2002.

70. Fisher B, Costantino JP, Wickerham DL, et al: Tamoxifen for prevention of breast cancer: Report of the National Surgical Adjuvant Breast and Bowel Project P-1 Study. J Natl Cancer Inst 90:1371–1388, 1998.

71. Lippman ME, Krueger KA, Eckert S, et al: Indicators of lifetime estrogen exposure: effect on breast cancer incidence and interaction with raloxifene therapy in the multiple outcomes of raloxifene evaluation study participants. J Clin Oncol 19:3111–3116, 2001.

72. Wu AH, Pike MC, Stram DO: Meta-analysis: Dietary fat intake, serum estrogen levels, and the risk of breast cancer. J Natl Cancer Inst 91:529–534, 1999.

73. Berrino F, Bellati C, Secreto G, et al: Reducing bioavailable sex hormones through a comprehensive change in diet: the diet and androgens (DIANA) randomized trial. Cancer Epidemiol Biomarkers Prev 10:25–33, 2001.

74. Holmes MD, Spiegelman D, Willett WC, et al: Dietary fat intake and endogenous sex steroid hormone levels in postmenopausal women. J Clin Oncol 18:3668–3676, 2000.

75. Bruning PF, Bonfrer JM: Free fatty acid concentrations correlated with the available fraction of estradiol in human plasma. Cancer Res 46:2606–2609, 1986.

76. Reed MJ, Cheng RW, Beranek PA, et al: The regulation of the biologically available fractions of oestradiol and testosterone in plasma. J Steroid Biochem 24:317–320, 1986.

77. Bradlow HL, Hershcopf R, Martucci C, et al: 16 Alpha-hydroxylation of estradiol: A possible risk marker for breast cancer. Ann N Y Acad Sci 464:138–151, 1986.

78. Bradlow HL, Telang NT, Sepkovic DW, et al: 2-hydroxyestrone: The "good" estrogen. J Endocrinol 150(suppl):S259–S265, 1996.

79. Fishman J, Martucci C. Biological properties of 16 alpha-hydroxyestrone: Implications in estrogen physiology and pathophysiology. J Clin Endocrinol Metab 51:611–615, 1980.

80. Schneider J, Huh MM, Bradlow HL, et al: Antiestrogen action of 2-hydroxyestrone on MCF-7 human breast cancer cells. J Biol Chem 259:4840–4845, 1984.

81. Adlercreutz H, Fotsis T, Hockerstedt K, et al: Diet and urinary estrogen profile in premenopausal omnivorous and vegetarian women and in premenopausal women with breast cancer. J Steroid Biochem 34:527–530, 1989.

82. Kabat GC, Chang CJ, Sparano JA, et al: Urinary estrogen metabolites and breast cancer: A case-control study. Cancer Epidemiol Biomarkers Prev 6:505–509, 1997.

83. Meilahn EN, De Stavola B, Allen DS, et al: Do urinary oestrogen metabolites predict breast cancer? Guernsey III cohort follow-up. Br J Cancer 78:1250–1255, 1998.

84. Muti P, Bradlow HL, Micheli A, et al: Estrogen metabolism and risk of breast cancer: A prospective study of the 2:16alpha-hydroxyestrone ratio in premenopausal and postmenopausal women. Epidemiology 11:635–640, 2000.

85. Schneider J, Kinne D, Fracchia A, et al: Abnormal oxidative metabolism of estradiol in women with breast cancer. Proc Natl Acad Sci USA 79:3047–3051, 1982.

86. Ursin G, London S, Stanczyk FZ, et al: Urinary 2-hydroxyestrone/16 alpha-hydroxyestrone ratio and risk of breast cancer in postmenopausal women. J Natl Cancer Inst 91:1067–1072, 1999.

87. Osborne MP, Telang NT, Kaur S, et al: Influence of chemopreventive agents on estradiol metabolism and mammary preneoplasia in the C3H mouse. Steroids 55:114–119, 1990.

88. Collaborative Group on Hormonal Factors in Breast Cancer: Breast cancer and hormonal contraceptives: collaborative reanalysis of individual data on 53,297 women with breast cancer and 100,239 women without breast cancer from 54 epidemiological studies. Lancet 347:1713–1727, 1996.

89. Hankinson SE, Colditz GA, Manson JE, et al: A prospective study of oral contraceptive use and risk of breast cancer. Cancer Causes Control 8:65–72, 1997.

90. Marchbanks PA, McDonald JA, Wilson HG, et al: Oral contraceptives and the risk of breast cancer. N Engl J Med 346:2025–2032, 2002.

91. Grabrick DM, Hartmann LC, Cerhan JR, et al: Risk of breast cancer with oral contraceptive use in women with a family history of breast cancer. JAMA 284:1791–1798, 2000.

92. Collaborative Group on Hormonal Factors in Breast Cancer: Breast cancer and hormone replacement therapy: Collaborative reanalysis of data from 51 epidemiological studies of 52,705 women with breast cancer and 108,411 women without breast cancer. Lancet 350:1047–1059, 1997.

93. Beral V: Breast cancer and hormone-replacement therapy in the Million Women Study. Lancet 362:419–427, 2003.

94. Chlebowski RT, Hendrix SL, Langer RD, et al: Influence of estrogen plus progestin on breast cancer and mammography in healthy postmenopausal women: the Women's Health Initiative Randomized Trial. JAMA 289:3243–3253, 2003.

95. Stefanick ML, Anderson GL, Margolis KL, et al: Effects of conjugated equine estrogens on breast cancer and mammography screening in postmenopausal women with hysterectomy. JAMA 295:1647–1657, 2006.

96. Chen WY, Manson JE, Hankinson SE, et al: Unopposed estrogen therapy and the risk of invasive breast cancer. Arch Intern Med 166:1027–1032, 2006.

97. Innes KE, Byers TE: Preeclampsia and breast cancer risk. Epidemiology 10:722–732, 1999.

98. Melbye M, Wohlfahrt J, Olsen JH, et al: Induced abortion and the risk of breast cancer. N Engl J Med 336:81–85, 1997.

99. McCormack VA, dos Santos Silva I: Breast density and parenchymal patterns as markers of breast cancer risk: A meta-analysis. Cancer Epidemiol Biomarkers Prev 15:1159–1169, 2006.

100. Byrne C, Schairer C, Wolfe J, et al: Mammographic features and breast cancer risk: Effects with time, age, and menopause status. J Natl Cancer Inst 87:1622–1629, 1995.

101. Boyd NF, Lockwood GA, Byng JW, et al: Mammographic densities and breast cancer risk. Cancer Epidemiol Biomarkers Prev 7:1133–1144, 1998.

102. Mitchell G, Antoniou AC, Warren R, et al: Mammographic density and breast cancer risk in BRCA1 and BRCA2 mutation carriers. Cancer Res 66:1866–1872, 2006.

103. Vachon CM, Pankratz VS, Scott CG, et al: Longitudinal trends in mammographic percent density and breast cancer risk. Cancer Epidemiol Biomarkers Prev 16:921–928, 2007.

104. Salminen TM, Saarenmaa IE, Heikkila MM, et al: Risk of breast cancer and changes in mammographic parenchymal patterns over time. Acta Oncol 37:547–551, 1998.

105. Chlebowski RT, McTiernan A: Biological significance of interventions that change breast density. J Natl Cancer Inst 95:4–5, 2003.

106. Bergkvist L, Tabar L, Bergstrom R, et al: Epidemiologic determinants of the mammographic parenchymal pattern. A population-based study within a mammographic screening program. Am J Epidemiol 126:1075–1081, 1987.

107. Hart BL, Steinbock RT, Mettler FA Jr, et al: Age and race related changes in mammographic parenchymal patterns. Cancer 63:2537–2539, 1989.

108. Modugno F, Ngo DL, Allen GO, et al: Breast cancer risk factors and mammographic breast density in women over age 70. Breast Cancer Res Treat 97:157–166, 2006.

109. Boyd NF, Dite GS, Stone J, et al: Heritability of mammographic density, a risk factor for breast cancer. N Engl J Med 347:886–894, 2002.

110. Greendale GA, Reboussin BA, Slone S, et al: Postmenopausal hormone therapy and change in mammographic density. J Natl Cancer Inst 95:30–37, 2003.

111. Colacurci N, Fornaro F, De Franciscis P, et al: Effects of a short-term suspension of hormone replacement therapy on mammographic density. Fertil Steril 76:451–455, 2001.

112. McTiernan A, Martin CF, Peck JD, et al: Estrogen-plus-progestin use and mammographic density in postmenopausal women: Women's health initiative randomized trial. J Natl Cancer Inst 97:1366–1376, 2005.

113. Harvey JA, Pinkerton JV, Herman CR: Short-term cessation of hormone replacement therapy and improvement of mammographic specificity. J Natl Cancer Inst 89:1623–1625, 1997.

114. Crandall C, Palla S, Reboussin BA, et al: Positive association between mammographic breast density and bone mineral density in the Postmenopausal Estrogen/Progestin Interventions Study. Breast Cancer Res 7:R922–R928, 2005.

115. Jeffreys M, Warren R, Gunnell D, et al: Life course breast cancer risk factors and adult breast density. Cancer Causes Control 15:947–955, 2004.

116. Boyd NF, Greenberg C, Lockwood G, et al: Effects at two years of a low-fat, high-carbohydrate diet on radiologic features of the breast: Results from a randomized trial. Can Diet Breast Cancer Prev Study Group. J Natl Cancer Inst 89:488–496, 1997.

117. Knight JA, Martin LJ, Greenberg CV, et al: Macronutrient intake and change in mammographic density at menopause: results from a randomized trial. Cancer Epidemiol Biomarkers Prev 8:123–128, 1999.

118. Nagata C, Matsubara T, Fujita H, et al: Associations of mammographic density with dietary factors in Japanese women. Cancer Epidemiol Biomarkers Prev 14:2877–2880, 2005.

119. Masala G, Ambrogetti D, Assedi M, et al: Dietary and lifestyle determinants of mammographic breast density. A longitudinal study in a Mediterranean population. Int J Cancer 118: 1782–1789, 2006.

120. Vachon CM, Kuni CC, Anderson K, et al: Association of mammographically defined percent breast density with epidemiologic risk factors for breast cancer. Cancer Causes Control 11:653–662, 2000.

121. Thomson CA, Arendell LA, Bruhn RL, et al: Pilot study of dietary influences on mammographic density in pre- and postmenopausal Hispanic and non-Hispanic white women. Menopause 14:243–250, 2007.

122. Sala E, Warren R, McCann J, et al: High-risk mammographic parenchymal patterns, hormone replacement therapy and other risk factors: a case-control study. Int J Epidemiol 29:629–636, 2000.

123. Friedenreich CM, Orenstein MR: Physical activity and cancer prevention: Etiologic evidence and biological mechanisms. J Nutr 132:3456S–3464S, 2002.

124. Ellison RC, Zhang Y, McLennan CE, et al: Exploring the relation of alcohol consumption to risk of breast cancer. Am J Epidemiol 154:740–747, 2001.

125. Singletary KW, Gapstur SM: Alcohol and breast cancer: Review of epidemiologic and experimental evidence and potential mechanisms. JAMA 286:2143–2151, 2001.

126. Summaries for patients: Alcohol, postmenopausal hormone therapy, and breast cancer. Ann Intern Med 137:1–43, 2002.

127. Egan KM, Stampfer MJ, Hunter D, et al: Active and passive smoking in breast cancer: Prospective results from the Nurses' Health Study. Epidemiology 13:138–145, 2002.

128. Russo IH: Cigarette smoking and risk of breast cancer in women. Lancet 360:1033–1034, 2002.

129. Morabia A: Smoking (active and passive) and breast cancer: Epidemiologic evidence up to June 2001. Environ Mol Mutagen 39:89–95, 2002.

130. Band PR, Le ND, Fang R, et al: Carcinogenic and endocrine disrupting effects of cigarette smoke and risk of breast cancer. Lancet 360:1044–1049, 2002.

131. Hoshaw SJ, Klein PJ, Clark BD, et al: Breast implants and cancer: Causation, delayed detection, and survival. Plast Reconstr Surg 107:1393–1407, 2001.

132. Boice JD Jr: Radiation and breast carcinogenesis. Med Pediatr Oncol 36:508–513, 2001.

133. Tokunaga M, Land CE, Yamamoto T, et al: Incidence of female breast cancer among atomic bomb survivors, Hiroshima and Nagasaki, 1950–1980. Radiat Res 112:243–272, 1987.

134. Evans JS, Wennberg JE, McNeil BJ: The influence of diagnostic radiography on the incidence of breast cancer and leukemia. N Engl J Med 315:810–815, 1986.

135. Swift M, Morrell D, Massey RB, et al: Incidence of cancer in 161 families affected by ataxia-telangiectasia. N Engl J Med 325:1831–1836, 1991.

136. Hill DA, Preston-Martin S, Ross RK, et al: Medical radiation, family history of cancer, and benign breast disease in relation to breast cancer risk in young women, USA. Cancer Causes Control 13:711–718, 2002.

137. Obedian E, Fischer DB, Haffty BG: Second malignancies after treatment of early-stage breast cancer: lumpectomy and radiation therapy versus mastectomy. J Clin Oncol 18:2406–2412, 2000.

chapter 20

Primary Prevention of Breast Cancer

MEHRET BIRRU | KRISTEN SANFILIPPO |
VICTOR G. VOGEL

Identifying Women at Risk

Chemoprevention can be defined as the use of natural or synthetic chemical agents to reverse, suppress, or prevent carcinogenic progression to invasive cancer.[1-5] Epidemiologic data suggesting that breast cancer is preventable through drug intervention include time trends in cancer incidence and mortality, geographic variations and the effects of migration, identification of specific causative factors, and the observation that most human cancers do not show simple patterns of genetic inheritance.

Chemoprevention may be recommended for certain women who are at increased risk of breast cancer. Indeed, the need for effective breast cancer preventive strategies is apparent based solely on the number of women who are at increased risk for the disease. More than 30 million women in the United States are older than 50 years of age, and at least 2 million of these women have first-degree relatives with breast cancer. At least 6 million postmenopausal women have undergone biopsy for benign breast disease, and one in four of these women have proliferative changes. As many as 10 million older women are obese, and one in six women 40 years of age or older is nulliparous.[6] A substantial proportion of breast cancer occurs in women with these characteristics, and strategies to reduce this risk may have a significant effect on the burden of breast cancer in the United States.

The clinician's role in identifying candidates for chemoprophylaxis should include a detailed assessment of familial breast cancer, the opportunity for genetic testing when appropriate, comprehensive quantitative risk assessment, and a specific management prescription.[7] Clinicians should also address the risks and benefits of screening, prophylactic surgery when indicated, and risk reduction using approved chemopreventive agents.

Familial breast cancer—often in a mother, aunt, and/or sister—is a leading reason why women seek counseling from their physicians about their own risks of developing breast cancer. Well-characterized breast cancer susceptibility genes, including *BRCA1* and *BRCA2*, account for approximately 25% of breast cancers.[8] The cumulative lifetime risk of developing breast cancer can approach 50% for some carriers of *BRCA* mutations, as estimated by the number of relatives with positive breast diagnoses prior to 50 years of age. If there is a suspicion that one of the susceptibility genes may be involved in the etiology of the breast cancers in a woman's family, further risk assessment is recommended.[9] A strategy to guide consideration of risk-reducing chemoprevention interventions in these women is discussed later in this chapter.

Clinicians should strive to ensure that the patient understands her objective risk and its implications for making a decision about chemoprevention. In addition to genetic susceptibility, hormonally linked adult reproductive and anthropometric risk factors have been well established in the etiology of pre- and postmenopausal breast cancers[10-11] and early life exposures have been evaluated only more recently.[12]

THE GAIL MODEL AND THE BREAST CANCER RISK ASSESSMENT TOOL

The Gail model[13] estimates the probability that a woman who engages in annual mammographic screening will develop invasive or in situ ductal or lobular cancer over a particular age interval. It was derived using 4496 matched pairs of subjects from the Breast Cancer Detection and Demonstration Project, a mammography screening project carried out between 1973 and 1980 that involved more than 280,000 women. The risk factors were adjusted simultaneously for the presence of the other risk factors, and only six factors were shown to be significant predictors of the lifetime risk of breast cancer:

1. Current age
2. Age at menarche
3. Number of breast biopsies
4. Age at first live birth (or nulliparity)
5. Family history of breast cancer in first-degree relatives
6. Race

The average American woman's Gail score is 0.3%, which represents her estimated risk of developing invasive breast cancer over the next 5 years; the lifetime risk for the average American woman is 10.1%. A previous diagnosis of atypical lobular or ductal hyperplasia nearly doubles the estimated risk.

Costantino and coworkers[14] used data from 5969 white women in the placebo arm of the Breast Cancer Prevention Trial (BCPT) who were screened annually to explore the accuracy of the Gail model. With an average follow-up period of 48.4 months, they compared the observed number of breast cancers with the predicted numbers from the model. The ratio of total expected to observed numbers of cancers was 1.03 (range, 0.88–1.21), indicating high predictive accuracy. The Gail model is optimal for breast cancer risk estimation in high-risk women who do not present with the genetic susceptibility genes.

Because the clinical trials used to develop the Gail model recruited predominately Caucasian women, the relevance of the race/ethnicity component of the model has been debated. In 1999, Costantino and colleagues[15] further modified the Gail model to estimate the absolute risk of developing invasive breast cancer only in women 35 years and older. The tool was not designed for women with prior diagnoses of breast cancer, lobular carcinoma in situ (LCIS), or ductal carcinoma in situ (DCIS).

The most recent iteration of the Breast Cancer Risk Assessment tool (www.cancer.gov/bcrisktool) may now have enhanced validity for estimating risk in African-American women. In 2007, the Women's Contraceptive and Reproductive Experiences (CARE) study enrolled African-American women with invasive breast cancer and controls; relative and attributable risks based on most questions of the Breast Cancer Risk Assessment tool were calculated for this group.[16] The Breast Cancer Risk Assessment model has been updated using data from the CARE study in addition to the National Cancer Institute (NCI)'s Surveillance, Epidemiology, and End Results (SEER) program for more accurate risk assessment for African-American women. In the absence of clinical trials that have enrolled sufficient numbers of American Indian, Alaskan Native, Pacific Islander, and Asian women, the Breast Cancer Risk Assessment model may be somewhat inaccurate. Despite the limitations of the race and ethnicity components of the Gail model/Breast Cancer Risk Assessment tool, it represents one of the easiest, least expensive, and enduring ways to assess objectively those women who are at greatest risk of developing breast cancer.

MAMMOGRAPHIC DENSITY

Increased mammographic density is associated with greater risk of breast cancer than any other breast cancer risk factor except genetic predisposition. Dense breasts are radiographically opaque but appear light via mammography, because of extensive stromal and glandular tissues. The extent of hormonally active and proliferative breast tissue is positively associated with increased breast cancer risk. Women with dense tissue in at least 75% of their breasts have a risk of breast cancer four to six times as high as women with low or normal breast densities.

The associations between mammographic density and both DCIS and invasive breast cancer are similar in magnitude.[17]

Breast density appears to have a strong genetic basis: monozygotic twins 40 to 70 years of age show a correlation with mammographic density approximately twice as strong as that between dizygotic twins; genetic factors explain 60% to 75% of the variation in mammographic density. An additional 20% to 30% of the age-adjusted variation in the percentage of dense tissue is attributed to menopausal status, body mass index, and parity.[18-22] The increased risk of breast cancer associated with dense breasts persists for at least 8 years after initial screening and is higher in younger women.

Mammographic density is also associated with an increased risk of estrogen receptor (ER)– and progesterone receptor–positive tumors, which suggests a hormonal etiology for mammographic density. Indeed, endogenous sex hormone levels are strongly and independently related to the risk of breast cancer in postmenopausal women.[23] Mammographic density may reflect high levels of circulating sex hormones or sensitivity to hormones but has a stronger predictive association with breast cancer than serum hormone levels alone. No enhanced risk assessment model has yet been developed to combine mammographic density testing and/or endogenous hormone levels with the Gail model/Breast Cancer Risk Assessment tool.[24]

Ultimately, not all of the variation in the Gail model assessments is explained by mammographic density.[25] One strategy may be to include mammographic density assessment and endogenous hormone assays for women who have an intermediate risk of breast cancer according to the Gail model, although reliable clinical measurements of these hormones are not readily available. These additional data may inform the clinician as to whether chemoprevention will be beneficial to the patient.

CLINICAL RISK COUNSELING

The major steps in risk assessment of breast cancer include (1) assessment of genetic susceptibility via genetic counseling and (2) quantitative risk assessment via the Gail model/Breast Cancer Risk Assessment tool and/or mammographic density analysis. These steps are outlined in Figure 20-1. Women at lower risk of breast cancer qualify for routine surveillance, including annual mammography for women older than 40 years of age as well as annual clinical breast examinations and self-breast examinations starting at 20 years of age. High-risk women who have a 5-year risk of breast cancer of 1.67% according to the Gail model/Breast Cancer Risk Assessment tool may qualify for chemoprevention in addition to routine surveillance. Those options will be discussed in the following sections.

Chemoprevention

There are three areas unique to the field of chemoprevention that must be considered in all stages of the clinical evaluation of a new chemopreventive agent.[25]

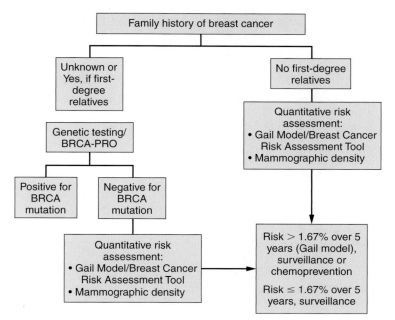

Figure 20-1 Algorithm for clinical management of breast cancer risk.

First, the characteristics of the target population must be clearly defined. For breast cancer chemoprevention, the target is a group of healthy women who may have had a previous diagnosis of breast cancer or who may be known to have a condition that predisposes them to the development of breast cancer. Second, the frequency and severity of side effects of the chemopreventive agent should be acceptable to the individual and ethically justifiable in the target population. Third, the duration of use of the chemopreventive agent must be defined. For most preventable malignancies, this requires a sustained period of drug administration that may be lifelong.

Epidemiologic studies indicate that estrogen-mediated events are integral to the development of breast cancer[26-28] and support the hypothesis that intact ovarian function is required to develop breast cancer. Oophorectomy or radiation-induced ovarian ablation can reduce the incidence of breast cancer by up to 75%.[29] These observations suggest that estrogen antagonists may be instrumental in the primary prevention of breast cancer.

TAMOXIFEN

Hormones, especially estrogens, have been linked to breast cancer,[30,31] with their role being attributed to their ability to stimulate cell proliferation. This cellular proliferation leads to the accumulation of random genetic errors that result in neoplastic transformation.[28] According to this concept, chemoprevention of breast cancer is targeted to reduce the rate of cell proliferation through administration of hormonal modulators. Tamoxifen, a triphenylethylene compound, was synthesized in 1966 as a potential fertility agent. Demethylation to the active metabolite, N-desmethyl tamoxifen, is the principal metabolic pathway in humans. Maximum serum concentration of N-desmethyl tamoxifen is observed within 12 to 24 hours after dosing; its serum half-life is approximately 12 days.[32-35] Tamoxifen suppresses the appearance of chemically induced breast tumors in laboratory animals. In rats, ovariectomy or the injection of antiestrogens after carcinogen administration results in the appearance of very few mammary tumors. In the mature reproductive-age animal, tamoxifen acts as an estrogen antagonist, inducing atrophy of lobular structures. In postmenopausal women, tamoxifen treatment results in upregulation of the proportion of ductal cells that express ER.[36] Several mechanisms have been proposed regarding tamoxifen's ability to prevent or suppress breast carcinogenesis, and these are listed in Table 20-1.

RALOXIFENE

Raloxifene hydrochloride, like tamoxifen, is a selective estrogen receptor modulator (SERM) that has antiestrogenic effects on breast and endometrial tissue and estrogenic effects on bone, lipid metabolism, and blood clotting.[37] It is a benzothiophene with characteristics similar to but distinct from the triphenylethylene SERMs such as tamoxifen. It inhibits the growth of ER-dependent, dimethylbenzanthracene-induced mammary tumors and reduces the occurrence of N-nitrosomethyl urea-induced mammary tumors in rats. In preclinical studies, raloxifene inhibited binding of estradiol to the ER and inhibited estradiol-dependent proliferation of MCF-7 breast cancer cells. Consistent with these observations, in vivo studies demonstrated antitumor activity in carcinogen-induced tumors in rodents of a magnitude similar to that observed previously with tamoxifen.

In vitro, raloxifene binds to both the alpha and beta subtypes of the ER (α and β, respectively).[38] Compared with 17β-estradiol, raloxifene has a relative binding affinity of 46% at the human ERα and 26% at the rat ERβ. In functional transactivation studies, raloxifene antagonizes 17β-estradiol-induced estrogen response element–mediated activity via ERα and ERβ. In contrast, raloxifene acts as an agonist at ERα and ERβ in an estrogen response

TABLE 20-1

Possible Mechanisms of Inhibition of Cell Proliferation by Tamoxifen

1. Modulating the production of transforming growth factors (TGF-α and TGF-β) that regulate breast cancer cell proliferation, including proliferation of estrogen receptor–negative cell lines[a]

2. Binding to cytoplasmic antiestrogenic binding sites, increasing intracellular drug levels[b]

3. Increasing sex hormone–binding globulin levels, which may decrease the availability of free estrogen for diffusion into tumor cells[c]

4. Increasing levels of natural killer cells[d]

5. Decreasing circulating insulin-like growth factor-I levels, which may modify the hormonal regulation of breast cancer cell kinetics[e]

[a]From Noguchi S, Motomura K, Inaji H, et al: Down regulation of transforming growth factor-α by tamoxifen in human breast cancer. Cancer 72:131–136, 1993; Butta A, MacLennan K, Flanders KC, et al: Induction of transforming growth factor β in human breast cancer in vivo following tamoxifen treatment. Cancer Res 52:4261–4264, 1992; Grainger DJ, Metcaffe JC: Tamoxifen: Teaching an old drug new tricks? Nat Med 2:381–385, 1996; and Dickens T-A, Colletta AA: The pharmacological manipulation of members of the transforming growth factor beta family in the chemoprevention of breast cancer. Bioessays 15:71–74, 1993.
[b]From Murphy LC, Sutherland RL: Antitumor activity of clomiphene analogs in vitro: Relationship to affinity for the estrogen receptor and another high affinity antiestrogen-binding site. J Clin Endocrinol Metab 57:373–379, 1983.
[c]From Jordan VC, Fritz NF, Tormey DC: Long term adjuvant therapy with tamoxifen: Effects on sex hormone binding globulin and antithrombin III. Cancer Res 47:4517–4519, 1987.
[d]From Berry J, Green BJ, Matheson DS: Modulation of natural killer cell activity by tamoxifen in stage I postmenopausal breast cancer. Eur J Cancer Clin Oncol 23:517–520, 1987.
[e]From Pollak MN, Huymh HT, Lefebre SP: Tamoxifen reduces serum insulin-like growth factor I (IGF-I). Breast Cancer Res Treat 22:91, 1992; Friedl A, Jordan VC, Pollack M: Suppression of serum insulin-like growth factor-1 levels in breast cancer patients during adjuvant tamoxifen therapy. Eur J Cancer 29A:1368, 1993; Lien EA, Johannessen DC, Aakvaag A, Lonning PE: Influence of tamoxifen, aminoglutethimide and goserelin on human plasma IGF-I levels in breast cancer patients. J Steroid Biochem Molec Biol 41:541, 1992; and Lonning PE, Hall K, Aakvaag A, Lien EA: Influence of tamoxifen on plasma levels of insulin-like growth factor β and insulin-like growth factor binding protein I in breast cancer patients. Cancer Res 52:4719, 1992.

element transactivation system. The conformation of ER when occupied by 17β-estradiol is different from its conformation when occupied by raloxifene.[39] SERMs interact either with membrane-bound ER as part of the cell surface receptor signal transduction phosphorylation cascade or with the nuclear ER. The shape of the SERM determines optimal antiestrogenic folding of the ER complex.[40]

For both raloxifene and tamoxifen, minor differences in SERM-ligand interaction with specific amino acids produce different intrinsic estrogen actions. The tamoxifen-ER complex is more estrogen-like in vitro, reflecting more estrogen-like action in the uterus. In contrast, the raloxifene-ER complex is much less estrogen-like and has fewer estrogen-like properties in the uterus.

Chemoprevention Risk Reduction Trials

Four prospective studies evaluating tamoxifen for reducing the risk of invasive breast cancer have been published: the National Surgical Adjuvant Breast and Bowel Project (NSABP) Breast Cancer Prevention Trial (BCPT, P-1),[41,42] the Royal Marsden Hospital (RMH) Tamoxifen Chemoprevention Trial,[43,44] the Italian Tamoxifen Prevention Study,[45-47] and the International Breast Intervention Study I (IBIS I).[48,49] A summary of the results of these trials is shown in Table 20-2. We review the findings from each of these studies,

BREAST CANCER PREVENTION TRIAL

The BCPT, a randomized, placebo-controlled, double-blind clinical trial, was initiated in June 1992 by collaboration of the NCI and the NSABP to evaluate whether tamoxifen reduced risk of invasive breast cancer in women at increased risk. To date, it represents the largest, prospective, controlled trial of tamoxifen's risks and benefits in a high-risk population.

The primary aim of the trial was to evaluate the effectiveness of 20 mg/day of tamoxifen orally for 5 years in preventing the occurrence of invasive breast cancer in women at high risk. Secondary aims of the trial were to assess osteoporotic fractures and cardiovascular disease in women taking tamoxifen compared with those in the control group.

Between June 1992 and September 1997, 13,388 women deemed at high risk for developing breast cancer were enrolled in the trial. Women were chosen if they were determined to be at high risk for developing breast cancer within the next 5 years if they met the following criteria: were 60 years of age or older, were between 35 and 59 years of age with a 5-year predicted risk of breast cancer of at least 1.66% as indicated by the Gail model, or had a history of LCIS. These women were then randomized to receive either 20 mg/day of tamoxifen (n = 6681) or placebo (n = 6707) for a period of 5 years.

In March, 1998, the trial was terminated early when an interim analysis showed that statistical significance had occurred in a number of end points. This decrease was evident only in ER-positive breast cancers, with no significant change seen in ER-negative tumors. The median follow-up time at the end point was 48 months, at which time a 49% ($P < 0.00001$) decreased risk of invasive breast cancer in the total study population was documented, with the greatest benefit seen in women 60 years of age and older. Overall, a total of 264 invasive cases were documented out of a total of 13,175 women with measurable end points at the time of the interim analysis. Of the 264 cases, 175 cases occurred in the placebo group, compared with 89 cases in the tamoxifen group (risk ratio [RR] = 0.51; 95% confidence interval [CI]: 0.39–0.66; $P < 0.00001$). The cumulative events are depicted in Figure 20-2. The annual event rate for invasive breast cancer was 3.4 per 1000 in the tamoxifen group and 6.8 per 1000 in the placebo group. There were

TABLE 20-2

Summary of Breast Cancer Risk Reduction in Randomized Trials of Tamoxifen for Women at Increased Risk for Breast Cancer

	Breast Cancer Prevention Trial (BCPT)	Royal Marsden Hospital Chemoprevention Trial	Italian Tamoxifen Prevention Study	International Breast Intervention Study I (IBIS I)
Subject characteristics	High breast cancer risk (age ≥60 years or a combination of risk factors using the Gail model); 39% age <50 years	Family history of breast cancer age <50 years or 2 or more affected first-degree relatives	Women with hysterectomy (48% bilateral oophorectomy); median age: 51 years	Women 35–70 years of age who were at increased risk for breast cancer
Number randomized	13,175	2494	5408	7152
Daily treatment	Tamoxifen 20 mg	Tamoxifen 20 mg	Tamoxifen 20 mg	Tamoxifen 20 mg
Proportion who took estrogen	<10%	26%	14%	50%
Median follow-up, years	7	13	9.1	8
Cases of invasive breast cancer	Placebo: 250 Tamoxifen: 145	Placebo: 82 Tamoxifen: 104	Placebo: 68 Tamoxifen: 53	Placebo: 168 Tamoxifen: 124
Breast cancer rates per 1000 woman–years and relative risk of cancer (95% CI)	Invasive Placebo: 6.8 Tamoxifen: 3.4 RR: 0.57 (0.46–0.70) Noninvasive Placebo: 2.7 Tamoxifen: 1.4 RR: 0.63 (0.45–0.89)	All cases Placebo: 5 Tamoxifen: 4.7 RR: 0.78 (0.58–1.04)	All cases Placebo: 2.3 Tamoxifen: 2.1 RR: 0.84 (0.60–1.17)	Invasive Placebo: 5.7 Tamoxifen: 4.2 RR: 0.74 Noninvasive Placebo: 1.1 Tamoxifen: 0.3 RR: 0.31
Number and relative risk of estrogen receptor–positive breast cancer	Placebo: 130 Tamoxifen: 41 RR: 0.31 (0.22–0.45)	Not available	Placebo: 10 Tamoxifen: 8	Placebo: 60 Tamoxifen: 43 RR: 0.71

CI, confidence interval; RR, relative risk.

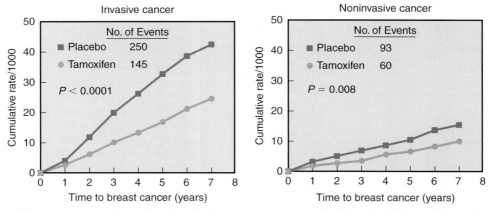

Figure 20-2 Cumulative rates of invasive and noninvasive breast cancer events after 7 years of follow-up in the National Surgical Adjuvant Breast and Bowel Project Breast Cancer Prevention Trial. (From Fisher B, Costantino JP, Wickerham DL, et al: Tamoxifen for the prevention of breast cancer: Current status of the National Surgical Adjuvant Breast and Bowel Project P-1 Study. J Natl Cancer Inst 97:1652–1662, 2005.)

104 cases of noninvasive breast cancer; 69 of these occurred in the placebo group and 35 in the tamoxifen group. Thus, there was a 50% reduction in rate of noninvasive breast cancer in women taking tamoxifen. The annual event rate for noninvasive breast cancer was 1.35 per 1000 in the tamoxifen group and 2.68 per 1000 in the placebo group. The relative risks of invasive breast cancer reduction were 0.56 (95% CI = 0.37–0.85) for women less than 50 years of age; 0.49 (95% CI = 0.29–0.81) for women 50 to 59 years of age; and 0.45 (95% CI = 0.27–0.74) for women 60 years of age and older.

Women with a previous history of breast disease (either LCIS or atypical hyperplasia) were also found to have a decreased risk with tamoxifen, with relative risks being 0.44 (95% CI = 0.16–1.06) in women with a prior history of LCIS and 0.14 (95% CI = 0.03–0.47) in women with a prior history of atypical lobular or ductal hyperplasia, an 86% reduction in risk.

Other Outcomes in the Breast Cancer Prevention Trial

Secondary outcomes in the BCPT included osteoporotic fractures and cardiovascular events. Tamoxifen is known to have estrogen agonist-like effects on both mineral density and serum cholesterol levels in postmenopausal women.[50,51] During the BCPT, 955 women experienced skeletal fractures. Women in the tamoxifen group had a 19% reduction in hip, spine, and distal radius fractures

(111 vs. 137 events in the tamoxifen and placebo groups, respectively). Thirty-four of the women enrolled in the trial experienced a hip fracture; when the tamoxifen versus the placebo group were compared, there was a 45% reduction. However, because of the small number of events that occurred, this reduction failed to reach statistical significance. In the incidence of cardiovascular events (namely, stroke and transient ischemic attack), no statistically significant difference was noted between the tamoxifen and placebo group. This was likely a result of the short interval time of follow-up of only 4 years and the fact that only 30% of women in the trial were 60 years of age or older.

Other Unfavorable Outcomes in the Breast Cancer Prevention Trial

Adverse outcomes related to tamoxifen in the BCPT are summarized in Table 20-3 and include pulmonary embolism (PE), deep vein thrombosis (DVT), endometrial carcinoma, cataracts, and vasomotor symptoms. These outcomes were significantly higher in women older than 50 years of age when compared with their younger counterparts. Women on tamoxifen were found to have a statistically significant higher incidence of PE than those on placebo. Although incidences of DVT, stroke, and transient ischemic attack in these women were not statistically significant, incidence in women on tamoxifen was higher, and thus the concern lies for development of these events in women on tamoxifen.

TABLE 20-3

Events and Incidence Rates of Invasive and in Situ Endometrial Cancer in the Placebo and Tamoxifen Groups by Age at Study Entry*

Type of Cancer	No. of Events		Rate per 1000 Women		Difference[†]	RR[‡]	95% CI
	Placebo	Tamoxifen	Placebo	Tamoxifen			
Invasive	17	53	0.68	2.24	−1.56	3.28	1.87–6.03
≤49 y at entry	9	12	0.82	1.16	−0.34	1.42	0.55–3.81
>50 y at entry	8	41	0.58	3.08	−2.50	5.33	2.47–13.17
In situ cancer	3	1	0.12	0.04	0.08	0.35	0.01–4.36
Stroke	50	71	1.23	1.75	−0.52	1.42	0.97–2.08
≤49	8	9	0.50	0.57	−0.07	1.13	0.39–3.36
≤50	42	62	1.70	2.50	−0.80	1.47	0.97–2.22
Transient ischemic attack	34	31	0.84	0.76	0.08	0.91	0.54–1.52
≤49	7	4	0.44	0.25	0.19	0.57	0.12–2.25
≥50	27	27	1.10	1.09	0.01	0.99	0.56–1.76
Pulmonary embolism	13	28	0.32	0.69	−0.37	2.15	1.08–4.51
≤49	2	4	0.13	0.25	−0.12	2.01	0.29–22.19
≥50	11	24	0.44	0.96	−0.52	2.16	1.02–4.89
Deep venous thrombosis	34	49	0.84	1.21	−0.37	1.44	0.91–2.30
≤49	12	16	0.76	1.01	−0.25	1.34	0.59–3.10
≥50	22	33	0.89	1.33	−0.44	1.49	0.84–2.68

RR, risk ratio; CI, confidence interval.
*Women at risk were those with an intact uterus.
[†]Rate in the placebo group minus rate in the tamoxifen group.
[‡]Risk ratio for women in the tamoxifen group relative to women in the placebo group.
Data from Fisher B, Costantino JP, Wickerham DL, et al: Tamoxifen for prevention of breast cancer: Report of the National Surgical Adjuvant Breast and Bowel Project P-1 Study. J Natl Cancer Inst 1998;90:1371–1388.

Women in the tamoxifen arm of the trial were found to have a 2.5 times greater risk of developing invasive endometrial carcinoma than women in the placebo arm, with an annual incidence of 2.3 per 1000 in the tamoxifen arm and 0.9 per 1000 in the placebo arm. This increased risk was greater in postmenopausal women. All cases of endometrial carcinoma that occurred in the BCPT (n = 36) were International Federation of Gynecology and Obstetrics (FIGO) stages 0 or I and thus had excellent clinical prognoses with treatment. A marginal increase of 14% in the development of cataracts was seen in women who were free of cataracts at initiation of the trial. The number of cataract surgeries was also increased in women taking tamoxifen. Vasomotor symptoms, mainly hot flashes, were reported by 46% of women on tamoxifen and only 29% of women in the placebo arm, whereas an increase in vaginal discharge was reported in 29% of women taking tamoxifen and 13% of women taking placebo.

Very few clinically significant differences in quality-of-life outcomes were seen when comparing the tamoxifen and placebo groups,[52] and tamoxifen was not associated with an increased risk of developing depressive symptoms in the BCPT.[53]

After 7 years of follow-up in BCPT,[42] the cumulative rate of invasive breast cancer was reduced from 42.5 per 1000 in the placebo group to 24.8 per 1000 in the tamoxifen group (RR = 0.57; 95% CI = 0.46–0.70) and the cumulative rate of noninvasive breast cancer was reduced from 15.8 per 1000 in the placebo group to 10.2 per 1000 in the tamoxifen group (RR = 0.63; 95% CI = 0.45–0.89). Tamoxifen continued to reduce the occurrence of ER-positive tumors by 69%, but no difference was seen in the occurrence of ER-negative tumors.

Risks of PE were approximately 11% lower than in the original report, and risks of endometrial cancer were about 29% higher, but these differences were not statistically significant. The net benefit achieved with tamoxifen varied according to age, race, and level of breast cancer risk. Despite the potential bias caused by the unblinding of the P-1 trial and subsequent crossover between the treatment groups, the magnitudes of all beneficial and undesirable treatment effects of tamoxifen were similar to those initially reported, with notable reductions in breast cancer and increased risks of thromboembolic events and endometrial cancer. The incidence of all osteoporotic fractures was reduced by 19% in women taking tamoxifen compared with those in the placebo group (111 events vs. 137 events, respectively). There was a 45% reduction in fractures of the hip that missed reaching statistical significance because of the small number of events reported.

In summary, the BCPT found that tamoxifen greatly reduced the incidence of ER-positive invasive and noninvasive breast cancers when compared with placebo over the 48-month follow-up time.

ROYAL MARSDEN HOSPITAL TAMOXIFEN CHEMOPREVENTION TRIAL

The RMH Tamoxifen Chemoprevention Trial was a randomized, placebo-controlled clinical trial initiated in 1986 to assess the effects of tamoxifen in preventing breast cancer in healthy women at increased risk for developing breast cancer based on family history.[43,44] The RMH Tamoxifen Chemoprevention Trial served as a preliminary pilot trial for the IBIS I trial described later.[48,49] The primary aim of the RMH trial was to evaluate the effectiveness of oral tamoxifen in preventing the occurrence of invasive breast cancer in women at high risk based on family history.

Between October 1986 and April 1996, 2494 women were enrolled in the trial and randomized to either receive tamoxifen 20 mg/day or placebo for up to 8 years. Eligible women were 30 to 70 years of age with one of the following: at least one first-degree relative diagnosed with breast cancer at younger than 50 years of age, one first-degree relative with bilateral breast cancer, or one first-degree relative with breast cancer of any age plus an additional affected first- or second-degree relative. Women in the trial were permitted to use hormone replacement therapy (HRT) during the trial, of which concomitant use occurred during 13% of the tamoxifen therapy time.

Interim analysis at median follow-up of 70 months revealed no significant difference in the incidence of breast cancer between the tamoxifen and placebo groups in 2471 women. A total of 70 cases of breast cancer occurred, including both invasive and noninvasive, with 34 cases in the tamoxifen group and 36 cases in the placebo group (RR = 1.06; 95% CI = 0.7–1.7) at the time of interim analysis. No interaction was noted between the concomitant use of HRT and incidence of breast cancer.

Early analysis of this trial was controversial for several reasons[54]: (1) there was poor compliance in both arms of the study, with 877 patients prematurely discontinuing therapy; (2) the trial permitted concomitant use of HRT and tamoxifen with an overlap occurring during 13% of tamoxifen therapy, which may have inhibited the antiestrogenic effect of tamoxifen on breast tissue; and (3) the small sample size limited the statistical power of the trial to detect a difference between the study's treatment arms. Long-term analysis of the trial confirmed the effectiveness of tamoxifen in reducing the risk of invasive breast cancer.[44]

ITALIAN TAMOXIFEN PREVENTION TRIAL

The Italian Tamoxifen Prevention Trial was a randomized, placebo-controlled, double-blind clinical trial initiated in October 1992 at the European Institute of Oncology, the F. Addarii Cancer Institute in Bologna, Italy, and the Cancer Institute of Naples, Italy, to evaluate the effectiveness of tamoxifen in preventing breast cancer.[45] The primary aim of this trial was to evaluate the effectiveness of 20 mg/day of tamoxifen orally for 5 years in preventing the occurrence of breast cancer versus placebo in healthy women, with the primary end points being reduction in the incidence and mortality from breast cancer.

Between October 1992, and July 1997, 5408 women were randomized into either the tamoxifen 20 mg/day or the placebo group. Women were eligible for the trial if they were between 35 and 70 years of age and had undergone hysterectomy for benign disease, because of the associated risk of endometrial cancer in patients taking tamoxifen. Women in the trial were not required to undergo standard breast cancer risk assessment. Thus, some of the participants in the trial were at decreased risk for developing breast cancer at randomization because they had had previous oophorectomy (48.3%) prior to menopause. Concomitant use of HRT was also permitted.

Accrual to the trial was ended prematurely because of a 26.3% dropout rate for women already randomized secondary to side effects, decreased interest, and fear. There were 5378 women with complete data for analysis of the trial. At an extended median follow-up of 81.2 months, there was no significant benefit for women at average or slightly reduced risk of breast cancer in taking tamoxifen.[46] A total of 79 cases of breast cancer were identified, with 34 cases in the tamoxifen arm and 45 cases in the placebo arm (RR = 0.76; 95% CI = 0.47–1.60). Thus, the difference was not statistically significant, yet it correlates with that found in other chemoprevention trials with tamoxifen. Subanalysis of the incidence of breast cancer in users of HRT revealed a significant benefit from concomitant use of tamoxifen. Within the subgroup of HRT users, 17 cases of breast cancer occurred in 791 HRT users receiving placebo (2.58%) compared with 7 cases in 793 HRT users receiving tamoxifen (0.92%).

In an additional subgroup analysis,[47] Italian investigators identified a group of women at increased risk for ER-positive breast cancer. This group included women taller than 160 cm (the median height of the group), with at least one functioning ovary, who had menarche no older than 13 years, and who had no full-term pregnancy before 24 years of age. This group of 702 women (13% of the trial population) was classified as high risk. The remaining group of 4693 women (87%) was classified as low risk. In the high-risk group, the risk of breast cancer was increased threefold over that of the low-risk group. Tamoxifen reduced the incidence of breast cancer in the high-risk group (n = 3 vs. n = 15 in the placebo group; P = 0.003), but it had no effect in the low-risk group. After 11 years of follow-up, 136 women developed breast cancer (RR = 0.84; 95% CI = 0.60–1.17).[47] In the group defined as "high risk" with at least one functioning ovary, there was a 77% reduction in the incidence of breast cancer (hazard ratio [HR] = 0.24; 95% CI = 0.10–0.59). This trial demonstrated that appropriate selection of women at high risk for developing hormone receptor–positive breast cancer led to benefit from tamoxifen intervention. The update after 11 years of follow-up also confirmed the finding that tamoxifen in addition to estrogen replacement therapy is protective against breast cancer development, although this approach is not used in North America and is called into question by the IBIS I results.

Overall, the Italian Tamoxifen Prevention Study found that tamoxifen did not greatly reduce the risk of breast cancer in healthy women at normal or slightly decreased risk of breast cancer. The results of this trial have been criticized, however, like those of the RMH chemoprevention trial, because the study was not powered to detect a statistically significant difference between tamoxifen and placebo. The updated data support the original conclusion that tamoxifen provides some benefit in the prevention of breast cancer, but the difference was not significant in women at normal or slightly reduced risk of the disease.

INTERNATIONAL BREAST CANCER INTERVENTION STUDY I

The IBIS I trial, a randomized, placebo-controlled study, with design and outcomes similar to that of BCPT, was initiated in 1992 to evaluate whether tamoxifen reduced the risk of invasive breast cancer in women at increased risk.[48] The primary aim of the trial was to evaluate the effectiveness of 20 mg/day of tamoxifen orally (for 5 years) in preventing the occurrence of both invasive and in situ breast cancer in women deemed at high risk compared to placebo.

Between April 1992 and March 2001, more than 7000 women 35 to 70 years of age evaluated as high risk for development of breast cancer (invasive or in situ) were enrolled into the trial and randomized to either the tamoxifen (n = 3578) or placebo group (n = 3566) for five years. Selection criteria for the trial's high-risk patients required that women 45 to 70 years of age have at least a twofold relative risk, women 40 to 44 years of age at least a fourfold relative risk, and women 35 to 39 years of age at least a tenfold relative risk of developing breast cancer.[55] Risk factors involved in determining the relative risk of breast cancer development included family history, history of LCIS, history of atypical hyperplasia, benign breast biopsies, and nulliparity. Of the women enrolled in the trial, 60% had two or more first-degree relatives with a history of breast cancer, 60% had an estimated 5% to 10% 10-year risk of developing breast cancer, one-third had prior hysterectomies, and a few of the women had a history of LCIS or atypical hyperplasia. Unlike the BCPT, women in this trial were permitted use of HRT, with approximately 40% of women using HRT at some time during the trial. Based on the published model, women in this trial were at moderately increased risk of development of breast cancer.

At interim analysis with a median follow-up of 50 months, 170 cases of breast cancers had been diagnosed, with 69 cases in the tamoxifen arm and 101 cases in the placebo arm (RR = 32%; 95% CI = 8–50, P = 0.013). This risk reduction result was virtually identical to that found in the BCPT in women who did not have atypical hyperplasia. As with the BCPT, that risk reduction was seen only with ER-positive tumors and not with ER-negative tumors. Of women in the trial who concomitantly used HRT with tamoxifen, there were 29 cases of breast cancer in the tamoxifen arm and 38 cases in the placebo arm (odds ratio [OR] = 0.76; 95% CI = 0.47–1.23). Although there was no significant reduction in the incidence of breast cancer in women concomitantly using HRT and tamoxifen, a risk reduction was seen in women who had a history of HRT use and were assigned tamoxifen in the trial. Women who had used HRT before their enrollment in the trial experienced a 57% risk reduction in their risk of breast cancer, with only 9 cases of breast cancer occurring in those on tamoxifen compared with 21 cases of breast cancer in previous HRT users in the placebo arm (OR = 0.43; 95% CI = 0.20–0.91).

Additional analysis with a median follow-up of 96 months after randomization in IBIS I revealed a total of 337 cases of breast cancer that had been diagnosed, 142 breast cancers were diagnosed in the 3579 women in the tamoxifen group and 195 in the 3575 women in the placebo group (4.97 vs. 6.82/1000 woman-years, respectively [RR = 0.73; 95% CI = 0.58–0.91; P = 0.004]).[49] The risk-reducing effect of tamoxifen was fairly constant for the entire follow-up period, and no lessening of benefit was observed for up to 10 years after randomization. The data from the IBIS I trial by subcategories are summarized in Figure 20-3.

Again in this later analysis, there was a statistically insignificant interaction between HRT use and treatment with tamoxifen in women in IBIS I, as was seen in the evaluation at 50 months of follow-up. In women who never used HRT or who used it only before the trial, there was a statistically significant reduction in ER-positive breast cancers in the tamoxifen group compared with the placebo group (for all breast cancers, 76 vs. 126 cases, RR = 0.62, 95% CI = 0.46–0.83; for ER-positive cancers, 37 vs. 77 cases, RR = 0.49, 95% CI = 0.32–0.74). For women who used HRT during any point of the trial, no clear benefit of tamoxifen was seen in reducing the risk of breast cancer, either overall (66 vs. 69 cases, RR = 0.92, 95% CI = 0–1.31) or for ER-positive tumors (40 vs. 43 cases, RR = 0.89,

95% CI = 0.57–1.41). Results were similar regardless of the HRT preparations used (i.e., either estrogen only or combined estrogen and progestin). HRT use was not associated with the development of ER-negative breast cancers, either during the active treatment period or during subsequent follow-up. The risk reduction observed may be smaller that that seen in the BCPT both because patients enrolled onto IBIS I were allowed to take HRT during the trial and because few women in IBIS I had atypical hyperplasia, whereas a large reduction in incidence of invasive breast cancer was seen in BCPT.

As in the BCPT trial, adverse outcomes in the tamoxifen arm in the IBIS I included an increase in thromboembolic events, a marginal increase in risk of endometrial cancer, and an overall increase in risk of death from all causes. The overall risk of clotting events was increased in tamoxifen users, with a 2.5-fold increase in risk of venous thromboembolism. As with the BCPT, this risk was seen predominately in women older than 50 years of age and in those women with a recent history of surgery. Although the risk was not significant, there was a marginal increase in risk of endometrial cancer in women taking tamoxifen, especially in women 50 years of age or older. As observed in the BCPT, all cases of endometrial cancer diagnosed were FIGO stages 0 or I.

Overall the IBIS I trial found that tamoxifen reduced the incidence of ER-positive breast cancers in women at

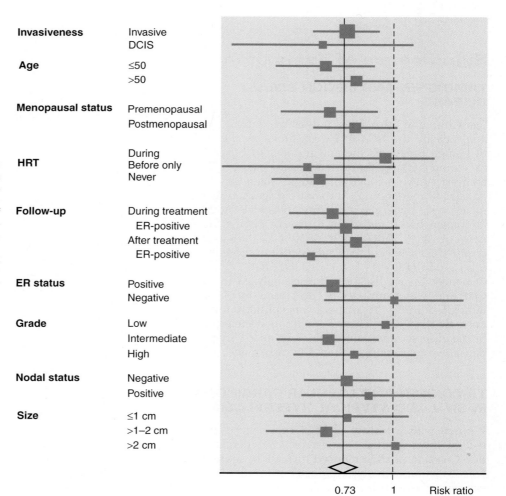

Figure 20-3 Point estimates and 95% confidence intervals for various subgroup outcomes within the International Breast Cancer Intervention Study I trial. Numbers on the left of the vertical dashed line show reduction in the event rate with tamoxifen compared with placebo. The vertical solid line indicates the overall risk ratio of 0.73 for all subsets combined in the entire trial. DCIS, ductal carcinoma in situ; ER, estrogen receptor. (From Cuzick J, Forbes JF, Sestak I, et al: Long-term results of tamoxifen prophylaxis for breast cancer: 96-month follow-up of the randomized IBIS-I trial. J Natl Cancer Inst 99:272–282, 2007.)

increased risk, while increasing the risk of venous thromboembolism 2.5-fold and marginally increasing the risk of endometrial cancer in women older than 50 years of age, when compared with those in the placebo group.

SUMMARY OF THE TAMOXIFEN CHEMOPREVENTION TRIALS

In 2003, a summary of the four trials using tamoxifen for breast cancer risk reduction was published by Cuzick and colleagues,[56] and the trials were compared in Table 20-2. Data from all four trials combined concluded that tamoxifen decreased breast cancer incidence by 38% (RR = 0.62; 95% CI = 28–46; $P < 0.0001$). The risk reduction for development of ER-positive breast cancers was 48% (RR = 0.52; 95% CI = 0.36–0.58; $P < 0.0001$). No significant risk reduction was seen in the incidence of ER-negative breast cancers. Venous thromboembolic events were found to be increased in women using tamoxifen in all trials (RR = 1.9; 95% CI = 1.4–2.6; $P < 0.0001$), with reduction in this risk seen with concomitant use of low-dose aspirin. Rates of endometrial cancer were also found to be increased in all trials in women using tamoxifen (RR = 2.4; 95% CI = 1.5–4; $P < 0.0005$), with a reduction in this risk seen by excluding women at increased risk for endometrial cancer and higher risks in women of 50 years of age. Overall, there was no effect on mortality from all causes; however, these trials were not powered or designed to analyze all-cause mortality events.

Significance of Tamoxifen

TAMOXIFEN AND BENIGN BREAST DISEASE

Tan-Chiu and associates published data on evidence analyzed by the NSABP investigators on the incidence of benign breast disease and number of breast biopsies in women taking tamoxifen versus placebo.[57] In this analysis, they included histologic diagnoses of ductal ectasia, fibroadenoma, fibrocystic disease, fibrosis, adenosis, cyst, hyperplasia, or metaplasia. Women taking tamoxifen had a reduction in risk of benign breast disease of 28% (RR = 0.72; 95% CI = 0.65–0.79) and required 29% fewer breast biopsies than those in the placebo group (RR = 0.71; 95% CI = 0.66–0.77). Incidence of benign breast disease was also analyzed in the IBIS I trial and was found to be decreased by 31% in the tamoxifen group; breast pain was similarly found to be decreased by 32%. These benefits in decreasing benign breast disease were predominately noted in premenopausal women younger than 50 years of age.

TAMOXIFEN AND LOBULAR CARCINOMA IN SITU AND ATYPICAL HYPERPLASIA

Women with a history of LCIS experienced an annual risk of invasive breast cancer of 1.3% per year in the BCPT, and tamoxifen reduced this risk by approximately 55%. Women with atypical ductal or lobular hyperplasia experience an increased risk of subsequent invasive breast cancer, and tamoxifen reduced this risk by 86% in BCPT. Women with either LCIS or atypical hyperplasia should, therefore, be considered candidates for primary reduction of breast cancer risk with tamoxifen if there are no absolute contraindications to its use.

POPULATION-BASED BENEFITS OF TAMOXIFEN

Based on data from 2000, Freedman and coworkers published data estimating that 9 million of the 65 million women 35 to 79 years of age in the United States with no history of breast cancer were eligible for tamoxifen chemoprevention based on inclusion criteria from the BCPT.[6] Of these 9 million women, approximately 2.4 million would have derived a net benefit from taking tamoxifen based on their 5-year risk of developing breast cancer. An estimated 58,000 cases of invasive breast cancer would develop over the ensuing 5 years in that population. Based on the 49% risk reduction associated with tamoxifen in the BCPT, if all 2.4 million women had taken tamoxifen, 24,492 cases of breast cancer may have been prevented.

ASSESSING RISKS AND BENEFITS OF TAMOXIFEN FOR CHEMOPREVENTION

Despite its favorable potential for risk reduction of breast cancer, however, chemoprevention with tamoxifen is not yet routine management among physicians. This is likely because of the perception by both patients and physicians that side effects associated with tamoxifen use are potentially serious and include PE, DVT, stroke, uterine malignancy, and cataracts. With these risks in mind, Gail and colleagues[15] published data summarizing a workshop sponsored by the NCI to aid physicians in identifying women in whom the benefits of tamoxifen outweigh the risks based on data from the BCPT.

Recommendations from the NCI workshop began with calculating the 5-year risk of breast cancer in women based on the Gail model. Women with a calculated risk of 1.66% or greater should be considered as high-risk individuals and should be deemed potential candidates for SERM therapy. In response to findings from the BCPT, the U.S. Food and Drug Administration (FDA) approved the use of tamoxifen to reduce the incidence of breast cancer in women older than 35 years of age whose 5-year risk of breast cancer is 1.66% or greater as determined by the Gail model. The risks and benefits of using tamoxifen depend on age and race, as well as on a woman's specific risk factors for breast cancer. In particular, the absolute risks of endometrial cancer, stroke, PE, and DVT associated with tamoxifen use increase with age, as does the protective effect of tamoxifen on fractures.

Once women are classified in terms of their risk of breast cancer, high-risk women should be assessed further to determine their individual specific risk-benefit profile. A woman's risk can change over time, and it is important to revisit risk assessment at multiple stages of a woman's life. The workshop found that, by using a series of risk-benefit models, tamoxifen has positive net benefit in women younger than 50 years of age with elevated risk of both invasive and in situ breast cancer. Women older than 70 years of age have adverse events associated with tamoxifen use regardless of race or ethnicity.[58]

Not included in the preceding models are other factors that may increase a woman's calculated risk of breast cancer over a specified 5-year period. For example, each woman's calculated 5-year risk should be adjusted to account for both invasive and in situ cancers that will occur.[15] Risk of in situ cancer is also reduced by tamoxifen therapy. In the BCPT, in the women in the placebo group undergoing annual screening, the relative incidence of in situ cancer was 0.53 times the invasive cancer rate in women 49 years of age and younger, and it was 0.31 times the invasive cancer rate in women 50 years of age and older.

The workshop produced several tables useful in assessing a "high-risk" woman's risk-benefit profile narrowed by age and race that may be helpful in determining which patients would benefit most from tamoxifen chemoprevention (Table 20-4). Adverse events related to stroke and thromboembolism were seen more often in women 60 years of age and older. In women 50 to 59 years of age with a uterus (increasing the risk of endometrial cancer), there is evidence for net benefit with tamoxifen if the overall 5-year risk of breast cancer is 6% or greater and only moderate benefit for those with a projected 5-year risk of 4% to 5.9%. The published quantitative analyses can assist both health care providers and women in weighing the risks and benefits of tamoxifen for reducing breast cancer risk.

In 2002, the American Society of Clinical Oncology (ASCO) Technology Assessment Working Group, evaluating data based on all of the tamoxifen chemoprevention trials, recommended that 20 mg/day of tamoxifen for 5 years could be offered to decrease risk of breast cancer in women with a 5-year risk of 1.66% or more. The greatest benefit with the least risk would be seen in younger premenopausal women who are less likely to develop thromboembolism or uterine cancer, women who have had a hysterectomy, and women at higher risk of breast cancer such as those with a history of atypical hyperplasia or LCIS.[59]

In July 2002, the U.S. Preventive Services Task Force (USPSTF) listed use of tamoxifen for breast cancer prevention in women with increased risk as a grade "B" recommendation, suggesting fair evidence that treatment with tamoxifen significantly decreased the risk of ER-positive invasive breast cancer in women at high risk of breast cancer based on 5-year risk assessment.[60] Evidence was increased for use in women with increasing risk of breast cancer. These recommendations were made for women who were at low risk for development of adverse events with no specific recommendations given for postmenopausal women.

All three organizations (i.e., FDA, ASCO, USPSTF) recommended assessing the risk-benefit profile of women and informing them of the risks associated with tamoxifen as part of an informed-decision making process. The USPSTF did not recommend tamoxifen in women at low or average risk of breast cancer because the risks outweigh the benefits. The greatest net benefit for tamoxifen use was associated with both age and the presence of factors that increase the risk of toxicity.

INDICATIONS AND CONTRAINDICATIONS OF TAMOXIFEN

Indications for chemoprevention with tamoxifen therapy are summarized in Table 20-5. These include history of

TABLE 20-4

Numbers of Favorable and Adverse Events, Incidence Rates per 1000 Women-Years, and Relative Risks in the Breast Cancer Prevention Trial

Type of Event	No. of Events		Average Annual Incidence Rate per 1000		Relative Risk	95% CI
	Placebo	Tamoxifen	Placebo	Tamoxifen		
Life-Threatening Events						
1. Invasive breast cancer	175	89	6.76	3.43	0.51	0.39–0.66
2. Hip fracture	22	12	0.84	0.46	0.55	0.25–1.15
3. Endometrial cancer						
All women	15	36	0.91	2.30	2.53	1.35–4.97
Women age ≥50 yr at entry	7	27	0.76	3.05	4.01	1.70–10.90
4. Stroke	24	38	0.92	1.45	1.59	0.93–2.77
5. Pulmonary embolism	6	18	0.23	0.69	3.01	1.15–9.27
Severe Events						
6. In situ breast cancer	69	35	2.68	1.35	0.50	0.33–0.77
7. Deep vein thrombosis	22	35	0.84	1.34	1.60	0.91–2.86
Other Events						
8. Colles' fracture	23	14	0.88	0.54	0.61	0.29–1.23
9. Spine fracture	31	23	1.18	0.88	0.74	0.41–1.32
10. Cataracts	507	574	21.72	24.82	1.14	1.01–1.29

CI, confidence interval.
From Gail MH, Costantino JP, Bryant J, et al: Weighing the risks and benefits of tamoxifen treatment for preventing breast cancer. J Natl Cancer Inst 91:1829–1846, 1999.

TABLE 20-5

Women in Whom Selective Estrogen Receptor Modulators Should Be Considered for Reducing the Incidence of Invasive Breast Cancer

Women with a history of one of the following:
- Lobular carcinoma in situ (LCIS)
- Ductal carcinoma in situ (DCIS)
- Atypical ductal or lobular hyperplasia

Premenopausal women with mutations in either the *BRCA1* or *BRCA2* genes

Premenopausal women at least 35 years of age with 5-year probability of breast cancer of 1.66%

Women aged 60 years with Gail model 5-year probability of breast cancer of 5%

DCIS or LCIS, history of atypical ductal or lobular hyperplasia, history of *BRCA1* or *BRCA2* mutation, or a 5-year predicted risk of invasive breast cancer of 1.66% or more. Tamoxifen is also indicated as adjuvant therapy in ER-positive breast cancer to prevent contralateral breast cancer.

Absolute contraindications for tamoxifen use include a history of DVT or PE as well as concurrent warfarin therapy. Relative contraindications include history of transient ischemic attack or stroke, poorly controlled diabetes, hypertension, or atrial fibrillation, immobility, mitral valve disease, and ischemic heart disease. Postmenopausal women are at increased risk for adverse events; thus, alternate therapy with an agent such as raloxifene should be considered. Women taking oral contraceptives, estrogen, progesterone, or androgens should discontinue these prior to initiation of tamoxifen therapy. Women should be advised against becoming pregnant while on tamoxifen, because the drug has a class D pregnancy recommendation and has been associated with birth defects in rats.

The optimal duration of risk-reducing therapy is unknown, but adjuvant therapy studies with tamoxifen indicate that therapy of less than 5 years is not as effective in reducing the incidence of second contralateral invasive breast cancer as therapy for at least 5 years. Whether using tamoxifen for longer than 5 years is more effective in preventing the recurrence of breast cancer than using it for only 5 years is the subject of ongoing clinical trials; however, no trials are currently being conducted or planned to examine the ideal duration of therapy in the risk-reduction setting. The optimal age at which to start therapy is unknown. Acceptance of tamoxifen may be poor in eligible subjects who elect prophylactic surgery instead of a chemopreventive risk-reduction strategy. Toxicity is a concern in postmenopausal women.

EFFECT OF TAMOXIFEN IN CARRIERS OF PREDISPOSING GENETIC MUTATIONS

Consideration of familial history of breast cancer is an integral component to assessing a patient's lifetime risk of breast cancer. Specific genetic mutations markedly increase the likelihood of breast cancer incidence over the lifespan. Well-characterized breast cancer susceptibility genes, including *BRCA1* and *BRCA2*, account for approximately 25% of breast cancers.[8] *BRCA1* acts, in part, as a tumor suppressor gene. Reduction in *BRCA1* expression in vitro results in the accelerated growth of breast and ovarian cell lines, although overexpression of *BRCA1* results in inhibited growth.[61] *BRCA1* also serves as a substrate for certain cyclin-dependent kinases, and estradiol induces *BRCA1* through an increase in DNA synthesis, which suggests that *BRCA1* may serve as a negative modulator of estradiol-induced growth.[62,63]

The cumulative lifetime risk of developing breast cancer can exceed 50% for some carriers of *BRCA* mutations, as estimated by the number of relatives with breast cancer diagnosed prior to 50 years of age. To assess whether a women without a breast cancer diagnosis may carry *BRCA1* or *BRCA2* genetic variants, a detailed family history of breast and ovarian cancers must first be assessed, with particular emphasis given to the number of family members who were diagnosed with either cancer prior to 50 years of age.

High-risk family histories raise the suspicion that one of the *BRCA* susceptibility genes may be involved in the etiology of the breast cancers; further risk assessment is recommended for these patients. BRCAPRO, a statistical software package, assesses an individual's probability of carrying a *BRCA1* or *BRCA2* mutation with 85% sensitivity.[9] Patients may test positively, negatively, or indeterminately for the *BRCA* mutations.

Like *BRCA1*, *BRCA2* expression in the breast is induced during puberty and pregnancy as well as after treatment with estradiol and progesterone. In multiple fetal and adult tissues, the temporal expression of *BRCA2* mRNA is indistinguishable from that of *BRCA1*,[61,64] and it seems that both *BRCA1* and *BRCA2* expression may be regulated through similar pathways. Expression of both genes is differentially regulated by hormones during the development of specific target tissues, but the upregulation of mRNA expression in the breast by ovarian steroid hormones is greater for *BRCA1* than for *BRCA2*.

Although carriers of *BRCA1* mutations are more likely to develop ER-negative tumors,[65,66] prophylactic oophorectomy reduces the risk of breast cancer by approximately 30% in women who carry mutations in either the *BRCA1* or *BRCA2* gene.[67] More importantly, Narod and colleagues[68,69] compared 209 women with bilateral breast cancer and *BRCA1* or *BRCA2* mutations (bilateral disease cases) with 384 women with unilateral disease and *BRCA1* or *BRCA2* mutations (controls) in a matched case-control study. The multivariate OR for contralateral breast cancer associated with tamoxifen use was 0.50 (95% CI = 0.28–0.89). Tamoxifen protected against contralateral breast cancer for carriers of *BRCA1* mutations (OR = 0.38; 95% CI = 0.19–0.74) and for those with *BRCA2* mutations (OR = 0.63; 95% CI = 0.20–1.50). The greater apparent benefit of tamoxifen in carriers of *BRCA1* mutations as compared with carriers of *BRCA2* mutations is paradoxical given the greater prevalence of ER-positive breast cancer reported in carriers of *BRCA2* mutations. This observation needs to be validated in additional studies.

Narod and colleagues[68] also observed similar results in their study of carriers of *BRCA* mutations with contralateral breast cancer. Compared with mutation carriers who used no chemoprevention, tamoxifen protected against contralateral breast cancer for *BRCA1* mutation carriers (OR = 0.38; 95% CI = 0.19–0.74). Women who used tamoxifen for 2 to 4 years had a 75% lowered risk of contralateral breast cancer. The effectiveness of tamoxifen in preventing contralateral, second breast cancers is related to the high concordance of the ER status of the first and second cancers.[70] Other data suggest a 50% reduction in the risk of contralateral, second primary breast tumors in carriers of *BRCA1* mutations who take tamoxifen after a first breast cancer and a 58% reduction of second cancers in *BRCA2* mutation carriers.[71] These results imply that, in mutation carriers who develop breast cancer, secondary breast cancers can be prevented using tamoxifen; similar risk reductions are thus likely to be seen for primary breast cancers. However, it remains unclear whether tamoxifen has the greatest efficacy in *BRCA1* or *BRCA2* carriers.

The only prospective evaluation of the effect of tamoxifen in carriers of predisposing mutations was carried out in the BCPT.[72] To evaluate the effect of tamoxifen on the incidence of breast cancer in women with inherited *BRCA1* or *BRCA2* mutations, genomic analysis of *BRCA1* and *BRCA2* was performed in 288 women who developed breast cancer after entry into the trial. Of the 288 cases of breast cancers, 19 (6.6%) inherited disease-predisposing *BRCA1* or *BRCA2* mutations. Of eight patients with *BRCA1* mutations, five received tamoxifen and three received placebo (RR = 1.67; 95% CI = 0.32–10.70). Of 11 patients with *BRCA2* mutations, three received tamoxifen and eight received placebo (RR = 0.38; 95% CI = 0.06–1.56).

In the BCPT, therefore, tamoxifen reduced the incidence of breast cancer in healthy *BRCA2* carriers by 62%, similar to the reduction in incidence of ER-positive breast cancer in all women in the trial. In contrast, tamoxifen use did not reduce breast cancer incidence in healthy women with inherited *BRCA1* mutations. These results must be interpreted with caution, however, because of the small number of women with mutations of either *BRCA1* or *BRCA2* who were identified in the trial. Larger prospective studies of women with predisposing mutations are required to provide conclusive evidence of either protection or lack of effect by tamoxifen in women with these mutations.

Using a simulated cohort of 30-year-old women who tested positive for either *BRCA1* or *BRCA2* mutations, Grann and coworkers[73] estimated that a 30-year-old woman with a mutation of either gene could prolong survival by undergoing a bilateral oophorectomy and/ or bilateral mastectomy, compared with surveillance alone. In their simulation model, chemoprevention with tamoxifen increased survival time by 1.6 years (95% CI = 1–2.1) and yielded more quality-adjusted life-years than did prophylactic surgery, even when treatment was delayed until 40 or 50 years of age. All of these procedures were cost-effective or cost-saving procedures when compared with surveillance alone.

Others have calculated that, compared with surveillance alone, 30-year-old patients with early-stage breast cancer with *BRCA1* or *BRCA2* mutations gain 0.4 to 1.3 years of life expectancy from tamoxifen therapy, 0.2 to 1.8 years from prophylactic oophorectomy and 0.6 to 2.1 years from prophylactic mastectomy. The magnitude of these gains is least for women with low-penetrance mutations and greatest for those with high-penetrance mutations.[74]

CLINICAL MONITORING OF WOMEN TAKING TAMOXIFEN

Endometrial hyperplasia and cancer were more frequent in women taking tamoxifen than in women taking placebo in the BCPT, but there was no evidence of elevated risk from tamoxifen use in women younger than 50 years of age (RR = 1.21; 95% CI = 0.41–3.60). The utility of endometrial cancer screening with either endometrial biopsy or transvaginal ultrasound in asymptomatic tamoxifen-treated women is limited and is not recommended outside the setting of a clinical trial. Rather, women receiving tamoxifen should have annual cervical cytology and pelvic examinations. Any abnormal bleeding should be evaluated with appropriate diagnostic testing, and women should be counseled about the risk of benign and malignant conditions associated with tamoxifen.

Routine screening with hematologic or chemical blood tests is not indicated because no hematologic or hepatic toxicities attributable to tamoxifen were demonstrated in the BCPT or in clinical trials using tamoxifen as adjuvant therapy. Because of the modest increase in risk of cataracts (RR = 1.14) and cataract surgery in women using tamoxifen compared with women taking placebo, women taking tamoxifen should be questioned about symptoms of cataracts during follow-up and should discuss with their health care provider the value of periodic eye examinations.

TAMOXIFEN METABOLITES

Tamoxifen can be considered a classic "prodrug," requiring metabolic activation to elicit pharmacologic activity. The cytochrome P450 (CYP) enzyme 2D6 is the rate-limiting step catalyzing the conversion of tamoxifen into metabolites with significantly greater affinity for the ER and greater ability to inhibit cell proliferation. Both genetic and pharmacologic factors that alter CYP2D6 enzyme activity directly affect the concentrations of the active tamoxifen metabolites and the outcomes of patients receiving adjuvant tamoxifen.[75]

Tamoxifen is hydroxylated by CYP2D6 to the potent metabolites 4-hydroxytamoxifen (4OH-tam) and 4-hydroxy-*N*-desmethyl tamoxifen (4OHNDtam), which are both conjugated by sulphotransferase (SULT)1A1. Clinical studies indicate that CYP2D6 and SULT1A1 genotypes are predictors for treatment response to tamoxifen. The levels of 4OHtam, 4OHNDtam, and *N*-desmethyl tamoxifen are associated with CYP2D6 predicted enzymatic activity ($P < 0.05$). The SULT1A1 genotype or copy number does not influence the levels of tamoxifen and its metabolites. However, the ratios of *N*-desmethyl tamoxifen/tamoxifen and *N*-dedimethyl tamoxifen/*N*-desmethyl tamoxifen are related to SULT1A1 genotype. CYP2D6 and SULT1A1 genotypes may partly explain the wide interindividual variations in the serum levels of tamoxifen and its metabolites. Use of therapeutic drug monitoring has not been included in studies linking CYP2D6 and SULT1A1 genotypes to clinical outcome.[76]

N-desmethyl tamoxifen (NDM), resulting from the CYP3A4/5-mediated catalysis of tamoxifen, is quantitatively the major primary metabolite of tamoxifen and accounts for approximately 92% of primary tamoxifen oxidation. NDM is predominantly biotransformed to α-hydroxy N-desmethyl-, N-didesmethyl-, and 4-hydroxy-N-desmethyl-tamoxifen (endoxifen). Recent clinical studies have demonstrated that common CYP2D6 genetic variation (leading to low or absent CYP2D6 activity), or the inhibition of CYP2D6 enzyme activity significantly lowers the plasma concentrations of endoxifen. Patients homozygous for a CYP2D6 null allele have significantly lower endoxifen concentrations than patients with one or two CYP2D6 functional alleles.

The CYP2D6 phenotypes associated with different alleles include poor, intermediate, extensive, and ultra-rapid metabolizers. Carriers of any two of approximately 20 known null alleles are phenotypic poor metabolizers, representing 7% to 10% of the European and North American Caucasian population. One of the most important functionally altered null variants, in others, includes CYP2D6*4 (15%–21% in Caucasians). Individuals at the high end of the activity spectrum (ultra-rapid metabolizers) carry gene duplications and multiduplications of functional alleles, which lead to higher CYP2D6 expression and enzyme activity, with relatively low frequency observed in Caucasians and Asians.[77]

For premenopausal breast cancer, there are no published data regarding CYP2D6 genotype and treatment outcomes. In the setting of chemoprevention, a small case-control study from the Italian chemoprevention group demonstrated a higher likelihood that tamoxifen-treated women homozygous for the *4 allele would develop breast cancer compared with those who did not carry a *4 allele.[78] These data are considered preliminary, and further research is needed in premenopausal women before using CYP2D6 genotype to exclude patients from tamoxifen.

Clinical Data with Raloxifene

During the past decade, a number of clinical trials have been conducted to assess the benefit of raloxifene on osteoporosis and fracture. After the publication of the results of the BCPT, these osteoporosis trials reported data related to the incidence of invasive breast cancer in women taking raloxifene compared with those taking placebo. They are summarized in Table 20-6 along with two prospective trials designed to assess the effect of raloxifene on the risk of breast cancer. A trial in women who were at increased risk of coronary heart disease (CHD) also reported breast cancer end points.[79] The design of each of these trials will be described separately, and the breast cancer outcomes will be reviewed. The toxicities associated with raloxifene in each of the trials will also be reviewed. Finally, the data from the Study of Tamoxifen and Raloxifene will be reviewed in great detail because they comprise the majority of the prospective data related specifically to the reduction of risk of breast cancer.

MULTIPLE OUTCOMES OF RALOXIFENE EVALUATION TRIAL

The Multiple Outcomes of Raloxifene Evaluation (MORE) trial, a multicenter, randomized, double-blind trial, was initiated in 1994 at 180 clinical centers in 25 countries, mainly in the United States and Europe. Its purpose was to evaluate whether postmenopausal women with osteoporosis using raloxifene for a period of 3 years would have a reduced risk of fracture.[80,81] A secondary end point of this trial was incidence of invasive breast cancer in women using raloxifene versus placebo.

The primary aim of this trial was to evaluate reduced risk of fracture in postmenopausal women taking raloxifene versus placebo for a period of 3 years, already at high risk for developing fractures secondary to osteoporosis. Secondary outcomes included the incidence of breast cancer between women in the raloxifene groups versus women in the placebo group.

From 1994 to 1998, 7705 postmenopausal women were enrolled in the trial. Women were chosen for the trial if they were postmenopausal, younger than 81 years of age, and had radiographic evidence of osteoporosis along with at least one osteoporotic fracture. Women were excluded from the trial if they had taken estrogens within 6 months prior to randomization, and they were not allowed the use of HRT while taking raloxifene. These women were randomized to receive either raloxifene 120 mg/day, raloxifene 60 mg/day, or placebo for a period of 3 years.

Analysis at a median follow-up of 40 months revealed that raloxifene significantly reduced the risk of invasive breast cancer in postmenopausal women with osteoporosis by 76%. This reduction was in large part a result of the 90% decrease in risk of ER-positive breast cancer (RR = 0.10; 95% CI = 0.04–0.24), with no risk reduction seen with ER-negative breast cancer (RR = 0.88; 95% CI = 0.26–3). In all, 40 cases of invasive breast cancer were documented, with 13 cases total occurring in the 5129 women in the raloxifene arms of the trial and 27 cases in the 2576 women in the placebo arm of the trial (RR = 0.24; 95% CI = 0.13–0.44; $P < 0.001$). Women in the study had also been divided into prespecified subgroups, allowing a more detailed analysis of who had the greatest benefit from raloxifene. The subgroups were divided by age (<65 and ≥65 years of age), age at menopause (<49 and ≥49 years of age), body mass index (<25 and ≥25 kg/m²), family history of breast cancer, serum estradiol level (5–10 vs. <5; >10 vs. < 10 pmol/L), prior estrogen therapy use, bone mass at time of randomization, and lastly 5-year predicted risk of breast cancer as assessed by the Gail model. Women with the highest risk reduction of development of breast cancer were those with a positive family history in first-degree relatives.

Overall, raloxifene decreased the risk of vertebral fractures in postmenopausal women with osteoporosis. Raloxifene was also found to decrease serum levels of low-density lipoprotein cholesterol. Unlike tamoxifen, raloxifene was not found to increase the risk of endometrial cancer (RR = 0.80; 95% CI = 0.2–2.7). Similar to tamoxifen, raloxifene was found to increase the risk of

TABLE 20-6

Prospective, Randomized, Placebo-Controlled Clinical Studies of Raloxifene with Invasive Breast Cancer as an End Point

Study	MORE[80,81]	CORE[82]	RUTH[79]	STAR[83]
Study population	Older postmenopausal women with at least one osteoporotic fracture	Continuation of the MORE study	Older postmenopausal women with a history of CHD or risk factors for CHD	Postmenopausal women who were at increased risk of breast cancer
No. of subjects	7705	5213	10,101	19,747
Primary outcome	Fractures	Fractures	CHD events and invasive breast cancer	Invasive breast cancer
Secondary outcomes	Breast cancer	Breast cancer	Death from coronary or cardiovascular causes and noncoronary cardiovascular causes; death from any cause	Fracture, CHD events
Major toxicities reported	Thromboembolic events, uterine malignancy	Thromboembolic events, uterine malignancy	Thromboembolic events, uterine malignancy	Thromboembolic events, uterine malignancy, other cancers, total deaths
Formal quality-of-life study	No	No	No	Yes
Event rate in raloxifene group (per 1000 woman–years)	0.9	1.4	1.5	4.4
No. of breast cancers in comparison group	27	58	533	163
Event rate in comparison group (per 1000 woman–years)	3.6	4.2	2.7	4.3
Risk reduction (hazard rate or risk ratio) and 95% confidence interval	0.24 (0.13–0.44)	0.34 (0.22–5.50)	0.56 (0.38–0.83)	Not applicable (no placebo group)

CHD, coronary heart disease; CORE, Continuing Outcomes Relevant to Evista; MORE, Multiple Outcomes of Raloxifene Evaluation; RUTH, Raloxifene Use for the Heart; STAR, Study of Tamoxifen and Raloxifene.
From Vogel VG: Raloxifene: A second-generation selective estrogen receptor modulator for reducing the risk of invasive breast cancer in postmenopausal women. Women's Health 3:139–153, 2007.

thromboembolic events almost threefold (RR = 3.1; 95% CI = 1.5–6.2). It was also found to increase the incidence of vasomotor symptoms, including hot flashes, leg cramps, and peripheral edema.

CONTINUING OUTCOMES RELEVANT TO EVISTA TRIAL

The Continuing Outcomes Relevant to Evista (CORE) was an extension to examine the effect of an additional 4 years of raloxifene therapy on the reduction of the incidence of breast cancer in participants of the MORE trial.[82] A total of 5213 participants in the MORE trial agreed to participate in the CORE trial. Of the participants, 3510 women who had been assigned to either the 120 mg/day or 60 mg/day raloxifene arm were assigned to receive 60 mg/day of raloxifene for 4 years; 1703 women in the placebo arm of the MORE trial remained in the placebo arm of the CORE trial. During the additional 4 years, there was a total of 61 cases of breast cancer in the 5213 participants: 31 in the

raloxifene arm and 30 in the placebo arm (11–12.3). Of these cases, 52 were classified as invasive. Of the invasive cases of breast cancer, 24 were in the raloxifene arm, and 28 in the placebo arm; thus, women in the raloxifene arm had a 59% reduction in occurrence when compared with placebo (2.1 vs. 5.2 cases/1000 woman-years; HR = 0.41; 95% CI = 0.24–0.71). Of the invasive cases, 46 were ER positive. The largest benefit (66%) was seen in ER-positive tumors in women taking raloxifene compared with placebo (1.3 vs. 3.9 cases/1000 woman-years; HR = 0.34; 95% CI = 0.18–0.66). As with tamoxifen chemoprevention trials, there was no reduction in the risk of developing ER-negative breast cancer.

As with its predecessor, there was an increased incidence in the number of thromboembolic events in participants taking raloxifene (2.9 events/1000 woman-years) compared with those taking placebo (1.3 events/1000 woman-years; RR = 3.11; 95% CI = 0.92–10.44). Overall, during the 4 years of the CORE trial, 9 cases of PE occurred in the raloxifene group compared with no cases in the placebo group (P = 0.066).

COMBINED RESULTS OF MULTIPLE OUTCOMES OF RALOXIFENE EVALUATION AND CONTINUING OUTCOMES RELEVANT TO EVISTA TRIALS

Data available from the CORE trial is a continuation of the MORE trial, and it summarizes a total of 8 years of therapy with either placebo or raloxifene. Of the 7705 participants in the MORE and CORE trials, there were 121 cases of breast cancer, 98 of which were invasive. Of these 98 cases, 40 cases occurred in women taking raloxifene, compared with 65 cases in women taking placebo, for an overall risk reduction of 66% (1.4 vs. 4.2/1000 woman-years; HR = 0.34; 85% CI = 0.22–0.50). Consistent with findings in the MORE trial, reductions were seen only with ER-positive tumors (76% reduction) and no reduction in risk was seen in ER-negative tumors. Over the 8-year period of the MORE and CORE trials, regardless of invasiveness, the overall incidence of breast cancer was reduced in the raloxifene arm by 58% compared with placebo (HR = 0.42; 95% CI = 0.29–0.60; $P = 0.001$).

Cardiovascular outcomes were also measured in participants in the MORE and CORE trials. Throughout the duration of the 8-year analyses, overall there was no increased incidence of serious adverse cardiovascular events in the raloxifene arm (5.5%) compared with the placebo (4.7%) arm (HR = 1.1; 95% CI = 0.86–1.56). There was also no statistically significant difference in either coronary (HR = 1.22; 95% CI = 0.82–1.83) or cerebrovascular events (HR = 1.19; 95% CI = 0.78–1.84) in the two groups. Thus, raloxifene offers neither a risk nor a benefit with regard to cardiovascular events in postmenopausal women at low risk of having an event. A subgroup analysis of women in the MORE trial also revealed that raloxifene has no effect on lipids and lipoproteins.

Consistent with the results of the individual trials, the combined data from the MORE and CORE trials revealed an increase in the incidence of thromboembolic events in participants taking raloxifene over an 8-year period. The overall incidence was 2.2 versus 1.3 events/1000 woman-years in the raloxifene versus the placebo group, respectively. Incidence of PE was 17 cases in the raloxifene group (0.62%) with one death compared with only two cases in the placebo group (0.16%) with no deaths.

RALOXIFENE USE FOR THE HEART TRIAL

The Raloxifene Use for the Heart (RUTH) trial was assembled after the observation that raloxifene was found to decrease serum levels of lipoprotein cholesterol, homocysteine, and fibrinogen in correlation with observational studies showing that treatment with estrogen decreased risk of CHD in postmenopausal women. It was also designed to assess the clinical effect of raloxifene on reduction of coronary events in postmenopausal women.[79]

During enrollment, 10,101 postmenopausal women (mean age, 67.5 years) with a history of CHD or with documented multiple risk factors for CHD were randomized to either receive raloxifene 60 mg/day or placebo and were followed for a median of 5.7 years. The primary outcomes of the trial were (1) coronary events (including, but not limited to, death from coronary causes, myocardial infarction, or hospitalization from acute coronary syndrome) and (2) occurrence of invasive breast cancer in postmenopausal women. A secondary outcome in the trial was incidence in vertebral fractures.

Raloxifene was found to reduce the risk of breast cancer in the population study of women (older, postmenopausal women, at lower risk for breast cancer) by 44% (RR = 0.56; 95% CI = 0.38–0.83). As with previous trials, this reduction was seen with ER-positive tumors, with no effect on ER-negative tumors. In the 5044 women randomized to the raloxifene group, there were 1.5 events per 1000 woman-years compared with 2.7 events per 1000 woman-years in the placebo group.

Other outcomes in the RUTH trial included risk of fracture and cardiovascular events. The risk of vertebral fracture was significantly decreased in women taking raloxifene by 35% (RR = 0.65; 95% CI = 0.47–0.89). Despite previous documented reduction in lipoproteins, homocysteine, and fibrinogen, there was no decrease in risk of cardiovascular events in women on raloxifene compared with placebo in the RUTH trial. Within the raloxifene group, there were 553 cardiovascular events in the 5044 women on raloxifene, compared with 533 cases of 5057 women on placebo (RR = 0.95; 95% CI = 0.84–1.07). Thus, in the outcomes measured, there was no significant difference in the incidence of death from coronary events, nonfatal myocardial infarction, or hospitalization for acute coronary syndrome in women taking raloxifene. These findings were true for both women with a previous history of CHD and for those with multiple documented risk factors for the development of CHD.

Of the adverse outcomes, four were more common in the placebo group, including acute coronary syndrome, anxiety, constipation, and osteoporosis. In the raloxifene group, there were seven symptoms (or adverse events) with higher frequency, including arthritis, cholelithiasis, dyspepsia, hot flushes, intermittent claudication, muscle spasms, and peripheral edema. Importantly, there was no difference in the incidence of endometrial cancer between the two groups, unlike studies of similar design that used tamoxifen as the SERM.

Data from the RUTH trial were used to assess the net risk-benefit ratio of raloxifene use in older, postmenopausal women at lower risk for development of breast cancer (not in women at high risk for development of breast cancer). Although the incidence of breast cancer and vertebral fractures was decreased in this population, the incidence of venous thromboembolic events and fatal stroke was increased.

Like tamoxifen, raloxifene increased the risk of venous thromboembolic disease threefold (RR = 3.1; 95% CI = 1.5–6.2), but unlike tamoxifen, it did not increase the risk of endometrial cancer (RR = 0.8; 95% CI = 0.2–2.7). However, this finding was based on only 10 total cases of invasive endometrial cancer (six in women taking either 60 or 120 mg of raloxifene and four in those taking placebo) and requires additional years of observation. Endometrial cancer was a rare event, occurring at a rate of only two to three cases per 1000 person-years, and these results are based on only 25,000 total person-years of observation. Raloxifene at either 60 or 120 mg/day was also associated with statistically significant increases in the incidence of influenza-like symptoms, hot flashes, leg cramps, and endometrial cavity fluid.

Study of Tamoxifen and Raloxifene Trial

The findings of the BCPT and IBIS I, coupled with the observations from the MORE trial, led the NSABP to design and launch the Study of Tamoxifen and Raloxifene (STAR) trial. Eligible women were at least 35 years of age and postmenopausal, and they must have had either LCIS or a 5-year risk of invasive breast cancer of at least 1.67% as determined by the Gail model. Subjects were randomly assigned to receive either tamoxifen 20 mg/day or raloxifene 60 mg/day in a double-blind, double-dummy design. No group of women in the trial received placebo alone.[83]

The primary aim of the trial was to evaluate the statistical equivalence of 20 mg/day of tamoxifen orally for over 5 years versus 60 mg/day of raloxifene in decreasing the incidence of breast cancer. Secondary aims were to assess the incidence of noninvasive breast cancer, endometrial cancer, skeletal fractures, and venous thromboembolic events in women on chemoprevention therapy. During 5 years of enrollment, 19,747 postmenopausal women (mean age, 58.5 years) with an increased risk of breast cancer were randomly assigned either to receive tamoxifen 20 mg/day or raloxifene 60 mg/day for a period of at least 5 years. Women were evaluated as having an increased risk of breast cancer by using criteria from the Gail model with a mean risk in those randomized of 4%.

The trial was powered to report data when 327 cases of invasive breast cancer had occurred. After a median follow-up of 3.2 years, 331 cases of invasive breast cancer had been reported. Overall, there were 163 cases of invasive breast cancer in women in the tamoxifen arm (4.3 cases/1000 woman-years) compared with 168 cases in the raloxifene arm (4.41 cases/1000 woman-years; RR = 1.02; 95% CI = 0.82–1.28). After a total of 6 years of follow-up, incidence was 25.1 cases/1000 woman-years in the tamoxifen arm and 24.8/1000 woman-years in the raloxifene arm ($P = 0.83$). When subpopulations in the study groups were compared based on categories of age, history of LCIS, history of atypical hyperplasia, 5-year predicted risk of breast cancer, and the number of family members with a history of breast cancer, there was no difference in the incidence of invasive breast cancer between the treatment groups. There was also no difference in tumor size, nodal status, or ER level between compatible subgroups in the two treatment groups. In the tamoxifen arm of the trial, there were fewer incidences of both LCIS and DCIS over a 6-year follow-up. There was a total of 57 cases of noninvasive breast cancer in the tamoxifen arm compared with 80 cases in women on raloxifene (1.51 vs. 2.11 cases/1000 woman-years, respectively; RR = 1.40; 95% CI = 0.98–2).

Incidences of endometrial cancer, cardiovascular events, venous thromboembolic events, osteoporotic fractures, and cataracts were also analyzed in the trial. There were more cases of uterine cancer in the tamoxifen group compared with the raloxifene group: 36 vs. 23, respectively (RR = 0.62; 95% CI = 0.35–1.08). There was no significant difference in the number of cerebrovascular events between the two arms (53 vs. 51 strokes). The number of thromboembolic events, including PE and DVT, was also higher in the tamoxifen group (RR = 0.70; 95% CI = 0.54–0.91). The rate of venous thromboembolism was 2.6 cases per 1000 woman-years in the raloxifene group and 3.7 cases per 1000 woman-years in the tamoxifen group. The incidence of PE was 54 versus 35 (RR = 0.64; 95% CI = 0.41–1), and the incidence of DVT was 87 versus 65 in the tamoxifen and raloxifene groups, respectively (RR = 0.74; 95% CI = 0.53–1.03). Osteoporotic fractures were comparable in the two groups. Women on raloxifene also experienced fewer incidences of cataracts (RR = 0.79; 95% CI = 0.68–0.92) and surgery for cataracts (RR = 0.82; 95% CI = 0.68–0.99) at 6 years follow-up.

Adverse effects experienced by patients in the STAR trial were reported by participants using a 36-item symptom checklist.[84] Questionnaires were given to participants before treatment, every 6 months for 5 years, and then again at 6 years. Of the almost 20,000 enrolled in the trial, a subgroup of 1983 were selected to fill out the questionnaires in a quality-of-life analysis. Both physical and mental components were evaluated, with scores worsening modestly over increasing treatment duration, but with no significant difference seen between the two treatment groups. Sexual dysfunction was slightly more prominent in the raloxifene arm.

In summary, raloxifene proved as effective as tamoxifen in reducing the incidence of invasive breast cancer in younger, postmenopausal women at increased risk, with a reduced incidence of both endometrial cancers and thromboembolic events. However, raloxifene is less effective in reducing the incidence of in situ carcinoma when compared with tamoxifen. Considerations for choosing raloxifene over tamoxifen in postmenopausal women who are at increased risk for breast cancer are summarized in Table 20-7.

Future Strategies: Aromatase Inhibitors

Tamoxifen is not the ideal drug to reduce the incidence of primary invasive breast cancer for a number of reasons, and it has neither the safety nor the efficacy desired to be the optimal agent. Raloxifene is an acceptable alternative for many postmenopausal women, but it is not ideal, either. Because of this, several agents are being evaluated as possibly being more suitable alternatives to tamoxifen for reducing the risk of breast cancer in high-risk women.

In postmenopausal women, the main source of estrogen is the peripheral conversion of androstenedione, produced by the adrenal glands, to estrone and estradiol in breast, muscle, and fat tissue. This conversion requires the aromatase enzyme.[85,86] In postmenopausal women, estrogen is synthesized in these peripheral tissues and

TABLE 20-7

Clinical Management Considerations for Selective Estrogen Receptor Modulators in Breast Cancer Risk Reduction

Positive Considerations	Negative Considerations and Cautions
Premenopausal women older than 35 years of age with Gail model risks of breast cancer greater than 1.67% in 5 years or lobular carcinoma in situ should be offered tamoxifen for the reduction of breast cancer risk.	No study has evaluated the *optimal age* at which to begin tamoxifen to reduce breast cancer risk; premenopausal women at increased risk derive the greatest net benefit because of the absence of increased risks of either thromboembolic events or uterine cancer in this group.
IBIS I study data suggest that the *benefit* from tamoxifen chemoprevention *extends beyond treatment* into the post-treatment period.	There are no primary prevention studies to evaluate the *optimum duration* of tamoxifen therapy for reducing the risk of breast cancer. Ongoing clinical trials will determine whether using tamoxifen for more than 5 years would be beneficial. No trials are being conducted or are planned to examine the ideal duration of therapy in the risk-reduction setting.
When used for reducing the risk of breast cancer, *tamoxifen* should be given in a dose of *20 mg once daily;* alternate doses and schedules have not been evaluated for either safety or efficacy.	In *Europe,* tamoxifen is not recommended as a preventive agent, except possibly in very high-risk women wishing to avoid or delay prophylactic mastectomy.
Chemoprevention with a SERM may be particularly beneficial to women with *atypical hyperplasia*, a 5-year Gail model risk of more than 5%, lobular carcinoma in situ, or two or more first-degree relatives with breast cancer.	*Clotting increases with age,* and both stroke and pulmonary embolism are potentially life-threatening consequences of tamoxifen therapy. Care must be given to risks versus benefits in older postmenopausal women who are considering tamoxifen for risk reduction.
Raloxifene 60 mg orally daily for 5 years offers an acceptable alternative to tamoxifen for the reduction of breast cancer risk in high-risk postmenopausal women, and it is associated with lower associated risks of both benign and malignant uterine events as well as significantly less thromboembolic toxicity.	*Pregnant women* or women who may become pregnant should also *avoid tamoxifen.*
Raloxifene use should be restricted to *postmenopausal* women.	*Early ambulation* following surgery, *discontinuation of tamoxifen* in the *perioperative* setting, and the use of concomitant low-dose aspirin may be helpful (but as yet unproven) methods of thromboembolism prevention.
Women currently taking **estrogen, progesterone, androgens, or birth control pills** *should discontinue these for 30 to 90 days before initiating SERM therapy.*	*Absolute contraindications* to tamoxifen use for risk reduction include a history of deep venous thrombosis or pulmonary embolism; a history of stroke or transient ischemic attack; and a history of uncontrolled diabetes, hypertension, or atrial fibrillation.

IBIS I, International Breast Intervention Study I; SERM, selective estrogen receptor modulator.

circulates at a relatively low and constant level. The selective aromatase inhibitors (AIs) markedly suppress the concentration of estrogen in plasma via inhibition or inactivation of aromatase. The use of AIs is restricted to postmenopausal women, however, because in premenopausal women, high levels of androstenedione compete with AIs at the enzyme complex such that estrogen synthesis is not completely blocked. Moreover, the initial decrease in estrogen levels causes a reflex increase in gonadotropin levels, provoking ovarian hyperstimulation, thereby increasing aromatase in the ovary and consequently overcoming the initial blockade. Unlike tamoxifen, AIs lack partial estrogen agonist activity and are, therefore, not associated with an increased risk of the development of endometrial cancer.

Anastrozole and letrozole are reversible, nonsteroidal inhibitors of the aromatase enzyme, whereas exemestane is an irreversible steroidal inhibitor. AIs have significant antitumor activity in postmenopausal patients with breast cancer, and a number of randomized trials have evaluated the adjuvant use of aromatase inhibitors in postmenopausal women. The Arimidex, Tamoxifen Alone, or in Combination (ATAC) trial is the largest and most mature AI adjuvant therapy trial; it compared 5 years of anastrozole with 5 years of tamoxifen as initial adjuvant therapy.[87-89] The ATAC trial enrolled 9366 postmenopausal women with early breast cancer. The incidence of contralateral breast cancer was reduced by 58% with anastrozole (RR = 0.42; 95% CI = 0.22-0.79; $P = 0.007$) when compared with tamoxifen. The updated data at 47 and 100 months continued to show that anastrozole was superior to tamoxifen in reducing the incidence of new ER-positive breast cancer, but the results were not as dramatic as the initial report (OR = 0.60; 95% CI = 0.42-0.85; $P = 0.004$).[88,89]

Similar results were reported in the reduction of the risk of contralateral, second breast primary tumors by letrozole when it was used following five years of tamoxifen in the extended adjuvant therapy of early, postmenopausal breast cancer. The National Cancer Institute of Canada (NCIC) Clinical Trials Group MA-17 Trial compared letrozole with placebo after 5 years of tamoxifen. It demonstrated a 46% relative reduction of new primary contralateral breast cancers in women treated with letrozole.[90] When the trial was unblinded, patients who received placebo were offered letrozole.

Efficacy outcomes of women who chose letrozole were compared with those who did not use HRs and P values calculated from Cox models that adjusted for imbalances between the groups. There were 1579 women in the letrozole group (median time from tamoxifen, 2.8 years) and 804 in the placebo group. Patients in the letrozole group were younger; had a better performance status; and were more likely to have had node-positive disease, axillary dissection, and adjuvant chemotherapy than those in the placebo group. At a median follow-up of 5.3 years, disease-free survival (DFS; adjusted HR = 0.37; 95% CI = 0.23–0.61; $P < 0.0001$) and distant DFS (HR = 0.39; 95% CI = 0.2–0.74; $P = 0.004$) were superior in the letrozole group. Relevant to the question of chemoprevention and risk reduction of breast cancer, incidence of new, contralateral, second breast primary tumors was reduced by 79% in women taking letrozole (HR = 0.21; 95% CI = 0.06–0.71; $P = 12$).

AIs are yet to be approved by the FDA for the chemoprevention of breast cancer, but data from the adjuvant setting have provided the rationale for study of their potential use as chemopreventive agents. Ongoing randomized, placebo-controlled trials investigating the use of third-generation AIs in the chemoprevention of breast cancer in postmenopausal women include the NCIC Clinical Trials Group MAP3 Exemestane in Preventing Cancer in Postmenopausal Women at Increased Risk of Developing Breast Cancer (ExCel) Trial and the IBIS II (International Breast Cancer Intervention Study II) trial.[85] The North American MAP3 study randomizes patients to exemestane or placebo in patients who refuse treatment with a SERM, and the international IBIS II trial compares anastrozole for 5 years versus placebo for chemoprevention in patients at increased risk. Until they are completed, it is not appropriate to use AIs to reduce the risk of breast cancer in postmenopausal women. For the reasons we have shown, AIs do not yet have an approved role in preventing breast cancer in premenopausal women.

REFERENCES

1. Wattenberg LW: Chemoprevention of cancer. Cancer Res 45:1–8, 1985.
2. Lippman SM, Benner SE, Hong WK: Cancer chemoprevention. J Clin Oncol 12:851–873, 1994.
3. O'Shaughnessy JA: Chemoprevention of breast cancer. JAMA 275:1349–1353, 1996.
4. Sporn MB, Suh N: Chemoprevention of cancer. Carcinogenesis 21:525–530, 2000.
5. Sporn MB, Suh N: Chemoprevention: An essential approach to controlling cancer. Nature Rev Cancer 2:537–543, 2002.
6. Freedman AN, Graubard BI, Rao SR, et al: Estimates of the number of U.S. women who could benefit from tamoxifen for breast cancer chemoprevention. J Natl Cancer Inst 95:526–532, 2003.
7. Vogel VG: Chemoprevention: Reducing breast cancer risk. In Vogel VG (ed): Management of patients at high risk for breast cancer. Malden, MA, Blackwell Science, 2001.
8. Antoniou AC, Easton DF: Models of genetic susceptibility to breast cancer. Oncogene 25:5898–5905, 2006.
9. Berry DA, Iversen ES Jr, Gudbjartsson DF, et al: BRCAPRO validation, sensitivity of genetic testing of BRCA1/BRCA2, and prevalence of other breast cancer susceptibility genes. J Clin Oncol 2701–2712, 2002.
10. Bernstein L: Epidemiology of endocrine-related risk factors for breast cancer. J Mammary Gland Biol Neoplasia 7:3–15, 2002.
11. Kelsey JL, Gammon MD, John EM: Reproductive factors and breast cancer. Epidemiol Rev 15:36–47, 1993.
12. Velie EM, Nechuta S, Osuch JR: Lifetime reproductive and anthropometric risk factors for breast cancer in postmenopausal women. Breast Dis 24:17–35, 2005–2006.
13. Gail MH, Brinton LA, Byar DP, et al: Projecting individualized probabilities of developing breast cancer for white females who are being examined annually. J Natl Cancer Inst 81:1879–1886, 1989.
14. Costantino JP, Gail MH, Pee D, et al: Validation studies for models projecting the risk of invasive and total breast cancer incidence. J Natl Cancer Inst 91:1541–1548, 1999.
15. Gail MH, Costantino JP, Bryant J, et al: Weighing the risks and benefits of tamoxifen treatment for preventing breast cancer. J Natl Cancer Inst 91:1829–1846, 1999.
16. Gail MH, Anderson WF, Garcia-Closas M, et al: Absolute risk models for subtypes of breast cancer. J Natl Cancer Inst 99:1657–1659, 2007.
17. Gill JK, Maskarinec G, Pagano I, Kolonel LN: The association of mammographic density with ductal carcinoma in situ of the breast: The Multiethnic Cohort. Breast Cancer Res 8:R30, 2006.
18. Tice JA, Cummings SR, Ziv E, et al: Mammographic breast density and the Gail model for breast cancer risk prediction in a screening population. Breast Cancer Res Treat 94:115–122, 2005.
19. Boyd NF, Martin LJ, Yaffe MJ, et al: Mammographic density: A hormonally responsive risk factor for breast cancer. J Brit Menopause Soc 12:186–193, 2006.
20. Chen J, Pee D, Ayyagari R, et al: Projecting absolute invasive breast cancer risk in white women with a model that includes mammographic density. J Natl Cancer Inst 98:1215–1226, 2006.
21. Boyd NF, Guo H, Martin LJ, et al: Mammographic density and the risk and detection of breast cancer. N Engl J Med 356:227–236, 2007.
22. Kerlikowske K, Ichikawa L, Miglioretti DL, et al: Longitudinal measurement of clinical mammographic breast density to improve estimation of breast cancer risk. J Natl Cancer Inst 99:386–395, 2007.
23. Tamimi RM, Byrne C, Colditz GA, et al: Endogenous hormone levels, mammographic density, and subsequent risk of breast cancer in postmenopausal women. J Natl Cancer Inst 99:1178–1187, 2007.
24. Chlebowski RT, Anderson GL, Lane DS, et al: Predicting risk of breast cancer in postmenopausal women by hormone receptor status. J Natl Cancer Inst 99:1695–1705, 2007.
25. Palomares MR, Machia JRB, Lehman CD, et al: Mammographic density correlation with Gail model breast cancer risk estimates and component risk factors. Cancer Epidemiol Biomarkers Prev 15: 1324–1330, 2006.
26. Kelsey JL, Berkowitz GS: Breast cancer epidemiology. Cancer Res 48:5615–5623, 1988.
27. Kelsey JL: A review of the epidemiology of human breast cancer. Epidemiol Rev 1:74–109, 1979.
28. Petrakis NL, Ernster VL, King MC: Breast. In Schottenfeld D, Fraumeni JF Jr (eds): Cancer epidemiology and prevention. Philadelphia, WB Saunders, 1982.
29. Henderson BE, Ross RK, Pike MC, Casagrande JT: Endogenous hormones as a major factor in human cancer. Cancer Res 42: 3232–3239, 1982.
30. Russo J, Russo IH: Toward a physiological approach to breast cancer prevention. Cancer Epidemiol Biomarkers Prev 3:354–364, 1994.
31. Henderson BE, Ross RK, Pike MC: Hormonal chemoprevention of cancer in women. Science 259:633–638, 1993.
32. Jordan VC: Effect of tamoxifen (ICI 46,474) on initiation and growth of DMBA-induced rat mammary carcinomata. Eur J Cancer 12:419–424, 1976.
33. Jordan VC: Antiestrogenic and antitumor properties of tamoxifen in laboratory animals. Cancer Treat Rep 60:1409–1419, 1976.
34. Jordan VC, Murphy CS: Endocrine pharmacology of antiestrogens as antitumor agents. Endocr Rev 11:578–610, 1990.
35. Jordan VC: Chemosuppression of breast cancer with long-term tamoxifen therapy. Prev Med 20:3–14, 1991.
36. Walker KJ, Price-Thomas JM, Candlish W, Nicholson RI: Influence of the antiestrogen on normal breast tissue. Br J Cancer 64:764–768, 1991.
37. Vogel VG: Raloxifene: a second-generation selective estrogen receptor modulator for reducing the risk of invasive breast cancer in postmenopausal women. Women's Health 3:139–153, 2007.

38. Clemett D, Spencer CM. Raloxifene: A review of its use in postmenopausal osteoporosis. Drugs 60:379–411, 2000.

39. Loose-Mitchell DS, Stancel GM: Estrogens and progestins. In Hardman JG, Linbird LE (eds): The pharmacological basis of therapeutics. McGraw-Hill, New York, 2001, p 615.

40. Jordan VC: The science of selective estrogen receptor modulators: Concept to clinical practice. Clin Cancer Res 12:5010–5013, 2006.

41. Fisher B, Costantino JP, Wickerham DL, et al: Tamoxifen for prevention of breast cancer: Report of the National Surgical Adjuvant Breast and Bowel Project P-1 Study. J Natl Cancer Inst 90:1371–1388, 1998.

42. Fisher B, Costantino JP, Wickerham DL, et al: Tamoxifen for the prevention of breast cancer: Current status of the National Surgical Adjuvant Breast and Bowel Project P-1 Study. J Natl Cancer Inst 97:1652–1662, 2005.

43. Powles TJ: The Royal Marsden Hospital (RMH) trial: Key points and remaining questions. Ann NY Acad Sci 949:109–112, 2001.

44. Powles TJ: Twenty-year follow-up of the Royal Marsden randomized, double-blinded Tamoxifen Breast Cancer Prevention Trial. J Natl Cancer Inst 99:283–290, 2007.

45. Veronesi U, Sacchini V, Rotmensz N, Boyle P, and Italian Tamoxifen Study Group: Tamoxifen for breast cancer among hysterectomised women. Lancet 359:1122–1124, 2002.

46. Veronesi U, Mariani L, Decensi A, et al: Fifteen-year results of a randomized phase III trial of fenretinide to prevent second breast cancer. Ann Oncol 17:1065–1071, 2006.

47. Veronesi U, Maisonneuve P, Rotmensz N, et al: Tamoxifen for the prevention of breast cancer: late results of the Italian randomized tamoxifen prevention trial among women with hysterectomy. J Natl Cancer Inst 99:727–737, 2007.

48. IBIS Investigators: First results from the International Breast Cancer Intervention Study (IBIS-I): a randomised prevention trial. Lancet 360:817–824, 2002.

49. Cuzick J, Forbes JF, Sestak I, et al: Long-term results of tamoxifen prophylaxis for breast cancer: 96-month follow-up of the randomized IBIS-I trial. J Natl Cancer Inst 99:272–282, 2007.

50. Love RR, Mazess RB, Barden HS, et al: Effects of tamoxifen on bone mineral density in postmenopausal women with breast cancer. N Engl J Med 326:852–856, 1992.

51. Love RR, Wiebe DA, Newcomb PA, et al: Effects of tamoxifen on cardiovascular risk factors in postmenopausal women. Ann Intern Med 115:860–864, 1991.

52. Day R, Ganz PA, Costantino JP, et al: Health-related quality of life and tamoxifen in breast cancer prevention: A report from the National Surgical Adjuvant Breast and Bowel Project P-1 Study. J Clin Oncol 17:2659–2669, 1999.

53. Day R, Ganz PA, Costantino JP: Tamoxifen and depression: More evidence from the National Surgical Adjuvant Breast and Bowel Project's Breast Cancer Prevention (P-1) randomized study. J Natl Cancer Inst 93:1615–1623, 2001.

54. Costantino JP, Vogel VG: Results and implications of the Royal Marsden and other tamoxifen chemoprevention trials: An alternative view. Clin Breast Cancer 2:41–46, 2001.

55. Tyrer J, Duffy SW, Cuzick J: A breast cancer prediction model incorporating familial and personal risk factors. Stat Med 23:1111–1130, 2004.

56. Cuzick J, Powles T, Veronesi U, et al: Overview of the main outcomes in breast-cancer prevention trials. Lancet 361:296–300, 2003.

57. Tan-Chiu E, Wang J, Costantino JP, et al: Effects of tamoxifen on benign breast disease in women at high risk for breast cancer. J Natl Cancer Inst 95:302–307, 2003.

58. McCaskill-Stevens W, Wilson J, et al: Contralateral breast cancer and thromboembolic events in African American women treated with tamoxifen. J Natl Cancer Inst 96:1762–1769, 2004.

59. Chlebowski RT, Col N, Winer EP, et al: American Society of Clinical Oncology technology assessment of pharmacologic interventions for breast cancer risk reduction including tamoxifen, raloxifene, and aromatase inhibition. J Clin Oncol 20:3328–3343, 2002.

60. Kinsinger LS, Harris R, Woolf SH, et al: Chemoprevention of breast cancer: a summary of the evidence for the U.S. Preventive Services Task Force. Ann Intern Med 137:59–69, 2002.

61. Rajan JV, Marquis ST, Gardner HP, Chodosh LA: Developmental expression of BRCA2 co-localizes with BRCA1 and is associated with proliferation and differentiation in multiple tissues. Dev Biol 184:385–401, 1997.

62. Marks JR, Huper G, Vaughn JP, et al: BRCA1 expression is not directly responsive to estrogen. Oncogene 14:115–121, 1997.

63. Fan S, Wang J, Yuan R, et al: BRCA1 inhibition of estrogen receptor signaling in transfected cells. Science 284:1354–1356, 1999.

64. Marquis ST, Rajan JV, Wynshaw-Boris A, et al: The developmental pattern of BRCA1 expression implies a role in differentiation of the breast and other tissues. Nat Genet 11:17–26, 1995.

65. Karp SE, Tonin PN, Bégin LR, et al: Influence of BRCA1 mutations on nuclear grade and estrogen receptor status of breast carcinoma in Ashkenazi Jewish women. Cancer 80:435–441, 1997.

66. Loman N, Johannsson O, Bendahl PO, et al: Steroid receptors in hereditary breast carcinomas associated with BRCA1 or BRCA2 mutations or unknown susceptibility genes. Cancer 83:310–319, 1998.

67. Rebbeck TR, Levin AM, Eisen A, et al: Breast cancer risk after bilateral prophylactic oophorectomy in BRCA1 mutation carriers. J Natl Cancer Inst 91:1475–1479, 1999.

68. Narod SA, Brunet JS, Ghadirian P, et al: Tamoxifen and risk of contralateral breast cancer in BRCA1 and BRCA2 mutation carriers: A case-control study—Hereditary Breast Cancer Clinical Study Group. Lancet 356:1876–1881, 2000.

69. Narod SA: Modifiers of risk of hereditary breast cancer. Oncogene 25:5832–5836, 2006.

70. Weitzel JN, Robson M, Pasini B, et al: A comparison of bilateral breast cancers in BRCA carriers. Cancer Epidemiol Biomarkers Prev 14:1534–1538, 2005.

71. Gronwald J, Tung N, Foulkes WD, et al: Hereditary Breast Cancer Clinical Study Group. Tamoxifen and contralateral breast cancer in BRCA1 and BRCA2 carriers: An update. Int J Cancer 118: 2281–2284, 2006.

72. King M-C, Wieand S, Hale K, et al: Tamoxifen and breast cancer incidence among women with inherited mutations in BRCA1 and BRCA2. National Surgical Adjuvant Breast and Bowel Project (NSABP-P1) Breast Cancer Prevention Trial. JAMA 286:2251–2256, 2001.

73. Grann VR, Jacobson JS, Whang W, et al: Prevention with tamoxifen or other hormones versus prophylactic surgery in BRCA1/2-positive women: A decision analysis. Cancer J Sci Am 6:13–20, 2000.

74. Schrag D, Kuntz KM, Garber JE, Weeks JC: Life expectancy gains from cancer prevention strategies for women with breast cancer and BRCA1 or BRCA2 mutations. JAMA 283:617–624, 2000.

75. Goetz MP, Kamal A, Ames MM: Tamoxifen pharmacogenomics: The role of CYP2D6 as a predictor of drug response. Clin Pharmacol Ther 83:160–166, 2008.

76. Gjerde J, Hauglid M, Breilid H, et al: Effects of CYP2D6 and SULT1A1 genotypes including SULT1A1 gene copy number on tamoxifen metabolism. Ann Oncol 19:56–61, 2008.

77. Ingelman-Sundberg, M: Genetic polymorphisms of cytochrome P450 2D6 (CYP2D6): Clinical consequences, evolutionary aspects and functional diversity. Pharmacogenomics J 5:6–13, 2005.

78. Bonanni B, Macis D, Maisonneuve P, et al: Polymorphism in the CYP2D6 tamoxifen-metabolizing gene influences clinical effect but not hot flashes: Data from the Italian Tamoxifen Trial. J Clin Oncol 24:3708–3709, 2006.

79. Barrett-Connor E, Mosca L, Collins P, et al: Raloxifene Use for The Heart (RUTH) Trial Investigators. Effects of raloxifene on cardiovascular events and breast cancer in postmenopausal women. N Engl J Med 355:125–137, 2006.

80. Cummings SR, Eckert S, Krueger KA, et al: The effect of raloxifene on risk of breast cancer in postmenopausal women: Results from the MORE randomized trial. JAMA 281:2189–2197, 1999.

81. Cauley JA, Norton L, Lippman ME, et al: Continued breast cancer risk reduction in postmenopausal women treated with raloxifene: 4-year results from the MORE trial. Breast Cancer Res Treat 65:125–134, 2001.

82. Martino S, Cauley JA, Barrett-Connor E, et al: Continuing outcomes relevant to Evista: Breast cancer incidence in postmenopausal osteoporotic women in a randomized trial of raloxifene. J Natl Cancer Inst 96:1751–1761, 2004.

83. Vogel VG, Costantino JP, Wickerham DL, et al: Effects of tamoxifen vs. raloxifene on the risk of developing invasive breast cancer and other disease outcomes: The NSABP Study of Tamoxifen and Raloxifene (STAR) P-2 Trial. JAMA 295:2727–2741, 2006.

84. Land SR, Wickerham DL, Costantino JP, et al: Patient-reported symptoms and quality of life during treatment with tamoxifen or raloxifene for breast cancer prevention: The NSABP Study of Tamoxifen and Raloxifene (STAR) P-2 Trial. JAMA 295: 2742–2751, 2006.

85. Goss PE, Strasser-Weippl K: Aromatase inhibitors for chemoprevention. Best Practice Res Clin Endocrinol Metabol 18:113–130, 2004.

86. Geller BA, Vogel VG: Chemoprevention of breast cancer in postmenopausal women. Breast Dis 24:79–92, 2005–2006.

87. Baum M, Buzdar A, Cuzik M, et al: Anastrozole alone or in combination with tamoxifen versus alone for adjuvant treatment of postmenopausal women with early stage breast cancer: results of the ATAC (Arimidex, tamoxifen alone or in combination) trial efficacy and safety update analyses. Cancer 98:1802–1810, 2003.

88. Howell A, Cuzick J, Baum M, et al: Results of the ATAC (Arimidex, Tamoxifen, Alone or in Combination) trial after completion of 5 years' adjuvant treatment for breast cancer, Lancet 365:60–62, 2005.

89. The Arimidex, Tamoxifen, Alone or in Combination (ATAC) Trialists' Group: Effect of anastrozole and tamoxifen as adjuvant treatment for early-stage breast cancer: 100-month analysis of the ATAC trial. Lancet Oncol 9:45–53, 2008.

90. Goss PE, Ingle JN, Martino S, et al: A randomized trial of letrozole in postmenopausal women after five years of tamoxifen therapy for early-stage breast cancer. N Engl J Med 349:1793–1802, 2003.

Breast Cancer Genetics: Syndromes, Genes, Pathology, Counseling, Testing, and Treatment

HENRY T. LYNCH | JOSEPH N. MARCUS | JANE LYNCH | CARRIE L. SNYDER | WENDY S. RUBINSTEIN

Approximately 1,444,920 new cases of cancer occurred in the United States in 2007 (males 766,860, females 678,060), 180,510 involving the breast.[1] Using a conservative estimate that 5% to 10% of the total breast cancer burden is hereditary, then in 2007, 9025 to 18,050 new cases of breast cancer fit a hereditary etiology. Most published estimates of the prevalence of BRCA1 mutations have used techniques with less than ideal sensitivities,[2] and up to 15% of BRCA1 and BRCA2 mutations may be undetectable by DNA sequencing[3]; thus, the contribution of these genes to hereditary cancer is known somewhat imprecisely. Additional "breast cancer genes" continue to be reported.[4,5] As the knowledge gap narrows for genetic and environmental etiologies and these interactions are clarified, cancer control can be better targeted to a smaller fraction of the population at highest risk.[6,7]

The etiology of breast cancer remains enigmatic. Madigan and colleagues[8] calculated incidence rates, relative risks (RRs), and population-attributable risks for breast cancer risk factors. They have extended these results to the U. S. population using data from the National Health and Nutrition Examination Survey (NHANES I) and Epidemiologic Follow-up Study (NHEFS). Their findings disclosed that estimates of population-attributable risks suggest that later age at first birth and nulliparity accounted for 29.5% of U. S. breast cancer cases (95% confidence interval [CI] = 5.6–53.3), higher income 18.9% (95% CI = 4.3–42.1), and family history of breast cancer 9.1% (95% CI = 3–15.2). Taken together, these well-established risk factors accounted for approximately 47% (95% CI = 17–77) of breast cancer cases in the NHEFS cohort and about 4% (95% CI = 2–80) in the U.S. population. The authors concluded that the RRs in the majority of these risk factors were modest. However, their prevalence as a group was high, thereby suggesting that a large proportion of breast cancer cases in the United States can be explained by well-established risk factors.

The prevalence and type of breast cancer susceptibility genes fall into three classes: (1) high-penetrance alleles (e.g., BRCA1, BRCA2, TP53), (2) rare moderate-penetrance alleles (e.g., CHEK2, ATM), and (3) common low-penetrance alleles (e.g., FGFR2, TOX).[9] BRCA1, BRCA2, and other rare, high-risk susceptibility genes account for approximately 20% of familial risk.

Few systematic studies have defined these breast cancer risk factors in concert with primary genetic susceptibility to this disease. Narod and colleagues[10] studied the reproductive histories of 333 North American women who were found by haplotype analysis to carry BRCA1 mutations. An increased risk of breast cancer was associated with menarche below the age of 12 years (RR = 1.57), parity of less than 3 (RR = 2.04), and year of birth after 1930 (RR = 2.72). The risk of ovarian cancer (OC), however, increased with increasing parity and earlier age at last childbirth. Will BRCA1 germline mutation carriers who have had a late menarche, early age of onset of a full-term pregnancy, and a late menopause, likely be protected from developing breast cancer or OC? Would such patients experience a later age of cancer onset? Is tamoxifen an effective chemoprevention agent for women with germline mutations? In some instances, the effect of hormonal[11] and other[12] risk factors may actually be opposite of those seen for sporadic breast cancer. For example, BRCA1 and BRCA2 carriers who have children have an increased risk of breast cancer compared with nulliparous carriers.[11] These are the types of research questions that genetic epidemiologists should pursue and that may be answerable given the present ability to identify BRCA1 mutation carriers.

The authors' purpose in this chapter is to provide a comprehensive study of hereditary breast cancer (HBC), with particular attention given to its molecular genetic basis (when known), natural history, pathology, phenotypic and genotypic heterogeneity, as well as implications for its control through risk assessment, genetic counseling, and genetic testing.

Genetic Predisposition to Breast Cancer

HEREDITARY BREAST CANCER: A HISTORY

Research during the past several decades has taught us more about the genetic etiology of breast cancer than perhaps all of the knowledge that had been accrued on the subject since Paul Broca, the famed French surgeon, first described his wife's pedigree in 1865 (Fig. 21-1).[13] Her family showed four generations of breast cancer and occurrences of cancer of the gastrointestinal tract, making this the first report of the tumor heterogeneity of HBC.

The importance of genetic and clinical heterogeneity in HBC received very little attention until a century later, when Lynch and coworkers[14] described 34 families with two or more first-degree relatives affected with

breast cancer in association with a variety of other cancers, including the first description of the now well-known hereditary breast/ovarian cancer (HBOC) syndrome. Thus, up to that time, risk of breast cancer was computed primarily on the patient's position within the pedigree, often when there were multiple first- and second-degree relatives affected with breast cancer and/or OC. Therefore, these publications, more than three decades ago, constituted the first reports of what is now known as the HBOC syndrome.[14,15] These studies also contributed to the identification of the profound heterogeneity in HBC (Fig. 21-2).

Understanding of the genetic etiology of breast cancer advanced dramatically in 1990 when Hall and associates[16] identified linkage for early site-specific breast cancer on chromosome 17q. Shortly thereafter, Narod and coworkers[17] showed linkage to this same locus in concert with OC in the HBOC syndrome (Fig. 21-3). The gene, now known as *BRCA1*, has been cloned.[18] Subsequently, a second breast cancer gene, *BRCA2*, was identified and shown to be linked to chromosome 13q.[19,20] These important events are discussed in greater detail throughout this chapter.

The gates were then opened for a new era for genetic counseling, all of which rapidly evolved thanks to the cloning of *BRCA1* and *BRCA2*. Prior to *BRCA* mutation discovery, we had to rely solely on an individual's family history; now we can determine lifetime risks for breast cancer and

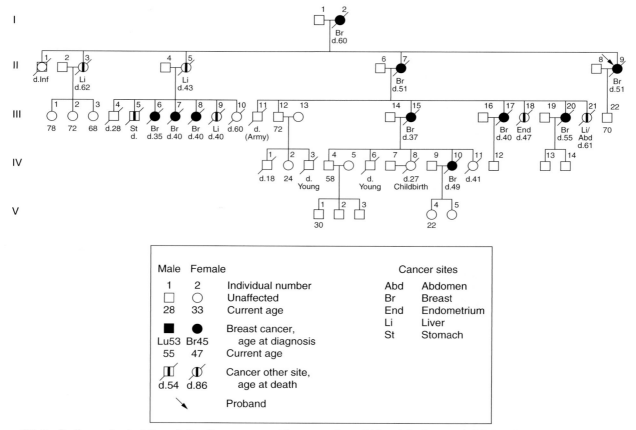

Figure 21-1 Pedigree chart of Broca's family constructed from a review of his original paper published in 1866. (Lynch HT, Krush AJ, Lemon HM, et al: Tumor variation in families with breast cancer. JAMA 222:1631–1635, 1972. Copyright 1972, American Medical Association. All rights reserved.)

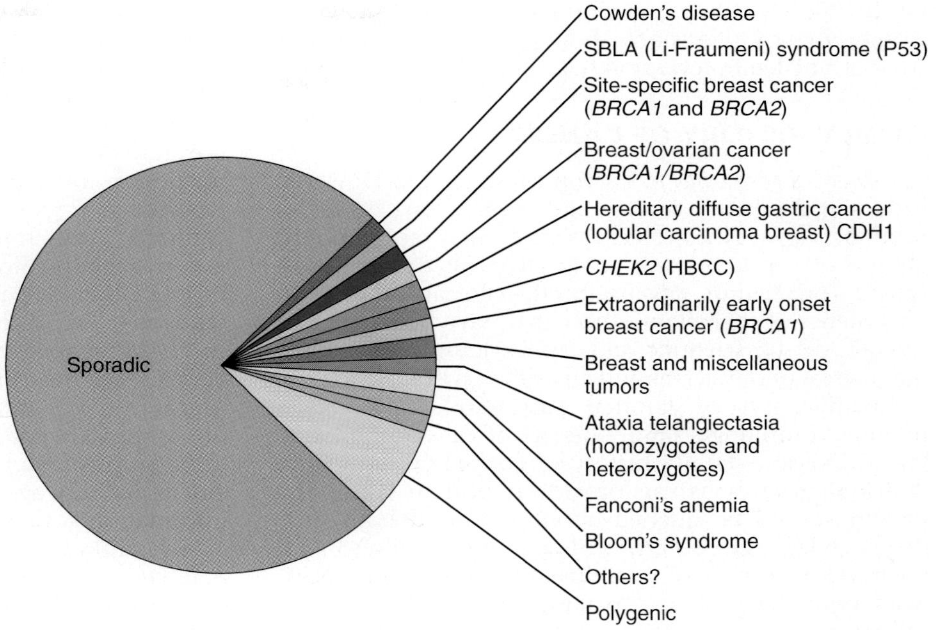
Sporadic
Cowden's disease
SBLA (Li-Fraumeni) syndrome (P53)
Site-specific breast cancer (*BRCA1* and *BRCA2*)
Breast/ovarian cancer (*BRCA1/BRCA2*)
Hereditary diffuse gastric cancer (lobular carcinoma breast) CDH1
CHEK2 (HBCC)
Extraordinarily early onset breast cancer (*BRCA1*)
Breast and miscellaneous tumors
Ataxia telangiectasia (homozygotes and heterozygotes)
Fanconi's anemia
Bloom's syndrome
Others?
Polygenic

Figure 21-2 Schematic depicting heterogeneity in breast cancer. (Adapted from Lynch HT, Fitzgibbons RJ Jr, Lynch JF: Heterogeneity and natural history of hereditary breast cancer. Surg Clin North Am 70:753–774, 1990. Reprinted with permission.)

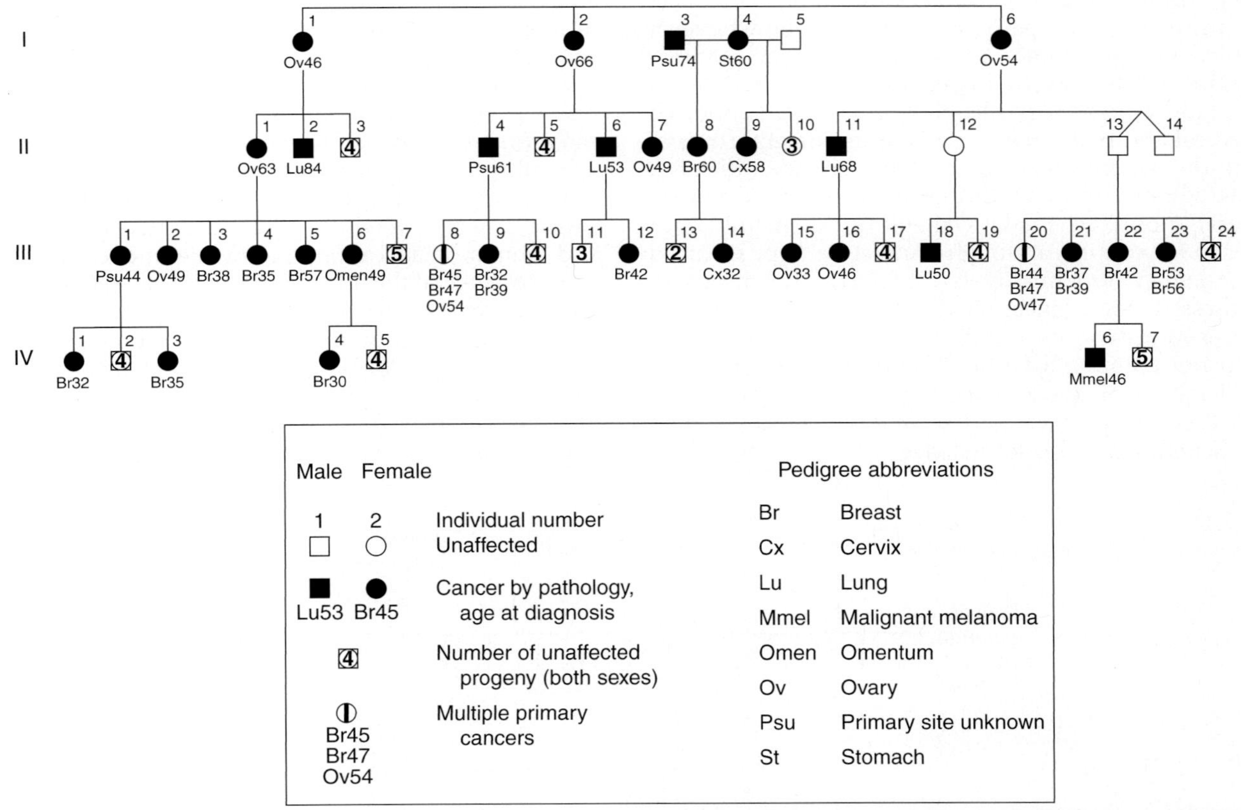
I
Ov46
Ov66
Psu74
St60
Ov54
II
Ov63 Lu84
Psu61
Lu53 Ov49 Br60 Cx58
Lu68
III
Psu44 Ov49 Br38 Br35 Br57 Omen49
Br45 Br47 Ov54
Br32 Br39
Br42
Cx32
Ov33 Ov46
Lu50
Br44 Br47 Ov47
Br37 Br39
Br42
Br53 Br56
IV
Br32
Br35
Br30
Mmel46
Male Female
1 2 Individual number
Unaffected
Lu53 Br45 Cancer by pathology, age at diagnosis
Number of unaffected progeny (both sexes)
Br45 Br47 Ov54 Multiple primary cancers
Pedigree abbreviations
Br Breast
Cx Cervix
Lu Lung
Mmel Malignant melanoma
Omen Omentum
Ov Ovary
Psu Primary site unknown
St Stomach

Figure 21-3 The pedigree of one of the families involved in the linkage studies that demonstrated that the 17q12-q23 locus for **early-onset breast cancer was also associated with hereditary ovarian cancer.** (Reprinted from Lenior GM, Lynch HT, Watson P, et al: Familial breast-ovarian cancer locus on chromosome 17q12-q23, Lancet 388:82–83, 1991. Copyright 1991, with permission from Elsevier.)

OC by *BRCA1/BCRA2* mutation testing. This then enables women to make decisions about screening, prophylactic surgery, or chemoprevention (e.g., tamoxifen).

FAMILY HISTORY OF CANCER

The study of genealogy has become fashionable. However, gathering the family history and investigating causes of death or serious illnesses such as cancer may raise concerns about how one's heritage could affect his or her risk of cancer. The scientific advances in the clinical and molecular genetics of hereditary cancer that have been reported recently in the scientific and lay literature have piqued the interest of physicians as well as the general public.

Identification of familial susceptibility to cancer requires compiling a family history of cancer of all anatomical sites. A family history of congenital anomalies and benign growths can provide important clues. The patient should be queried about cancer in both first-degree relatives (parents, siblings, and children) and second-degree relatives (grandparents, aunts, and uncles) from both maternal and paternal lineages (Fig. 21-4). Information on older relatives is more genetically significant because most cancers are of adult onset, making the phenotypic expression more likely than in younger relatives (children, cousins, nephews, and nieces of probands). The compilation should include age of cancer onset, primary source, pathology confirmation whenever possible, and occurrence of multiple primary cancers (including bilaterality of paired organs). This detailed cancer family history, particularly when it is supported by medical and pathology records, is an integral component of the patient's medical work-up. The identification of a hereditary cancer syndrome with its cancer control potential should be made available to all members of the extended family, although it must be kept in mind that patient confidentiality is a concern that needs to be addressed when cancer family history is being shared. However, our experience indicates that clinicians generally do not compile a family history of cancer in sufficient detail to diagnose a hereditary cancer syndrome, and if they do, primary and secondary at-risk relatives rarely benefit from this knowledge.

Lynch and colleagues[21] interviewed 200 consecutive cancer patients who were undergoing treatment in an oncology clinic. They noted numerous examples of familial cancer clusters, as well as several hereditary cancer syndromes. However, in the overwhelming majority of cases, the family history of cancer, as reported in patients' initial medical records, had either been entirely omitted or reported as negative, despite substantial evidence to the contrary. Furthermore, even when the family history was strongly positive, the information was not used to benefit either the patient or his or her close relatives. Subsequently, David and Steiner-Grossman[22] conducted a survey of 76 acute care, nonpsychiatric hospitals in New York City to determine the notation of family history of cancer in the medical charts. Only four of the 64 reporting hospitals reported any notation of cancer family history. Surprisingly, the American College of Surgeons and accrediting agencies of hospitals did not require this information at that time (1991).

A careful assessment of cancer of all anatomic sites is mandatory in compiling a cancer family history, since diagnosis of a hereditary cancer syndrome may often be established through recognition of the pattern of multiple primary cancers in the family. This, of course, is most evident in the HBOC syndrome. Other examples include colorectal cancer and carcinoma of the endometrium and ovary among other cancer types in the Lynch syndrome; in the Li-Fraumeni (SBLA) syndrome, sarcomas, breast, brain, lung, leukemia, lymphoma, and adrenal cortical carcinoma; in multiple endocrine neoplasia 1 (MEN1),as well as MEN2a and 2b; in medullary thyroid carcinoma and pheochromocytoma; in the familial atypical multiple mole melanoma (FAMMM) syndrome, melanoma, and pancreatic cancer; in the hereditary diffuse gastric cancer (HDGC) syndrome, diffuse gastric cancer, and lobular breast cancer; and many other conditions.

Knowledge of the integral tumors in the differing hereditary cancer syndromes provides important diagnostic clues through the natural history of their cancer complement. Therein, screening and management may differ strikingly based on the differences in the tumor; age of onset (frequently earlier than their sporadic counterparts); pathology; accelerated carcinogenesis, which has

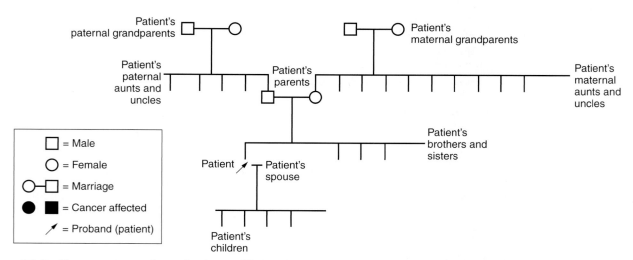

Figure 21-4 Diagram representing a simple, modified nuclear pedigree for clinical use. (From Lynch HT, et al: Surv Dig Dis 2:244–260, 1984. Reproduced by permission.)

an impact on the frequency of screening; and bilaterality in paired organs, which can provide the need for prophylactic surgery as in the contralateral breast in the case of ipsilateral breast cancer with *BRCA1* or *BRCA2* mutation. The location of the cancer may also be important, as in the case of colorectal cancer and its proximal proclivity in the Lynch syndrome. All of this information must be transmitted to the patient in the genetic counseling sessions.

Unfortunately, family history is still notoriously neglected by physicians as well as their patients. However, genetic counselors have been contributing immensely to rectifying this problem and are making a difference. It is important to realize that genetic counseling must be considered to be mandatory prior to DNA testing and when DNA results are disclosed. However, this dictum has not been routinely followed by commercial testing laboratories; some may send a blood collection kit to the physician or directly to the patient and thus do not demand genetic counseling prior to the DNA collection.

DEFINITIONS OF SPORADIC, FAMILIAL, AND HEREDITARY BREAST CANCER

Sporadic Breast Cancer

Sporadic breast cancer is breast cancer with no other family history of breast carcinoma through two generations including siblings, offspring, parents, and both maternal and paternal aunts, uncles, and grandparents.

Familial Breast Cancer

Familial breast cancer is breast cancer with a family history of one or more first- or second-degree relatives with breast cancer that does not fit the HBC definition given later. It is important to note that a patient with one or more first-degree relatives with breast cancer in this familial breast cancer category has a substantial excess lifetime risk of breast cancer when compared with patients in the general population who do not have affected first-degree relatives. A collaborative reanalysis of data from 52 epidemiologic studies provides the largest data source for risk estimation in familial breast cancer.[23] This study found that risk ratios for breast cancer increased with increasing numbers of affected first-degree relatives (1.80, 2.93, and 3.90, respectively, for one, two, and three first-degree relatives) compared with women who had no affected relative.

As yet, genetic and environmental causes of familial (as opposed to hereditary) cancer are incompletely described. Therefore, genetic testing is not feasible in the setting of familial breast cancer. A case has been made for *CHEK2* gene testing in familial breast cancer, but the impact on clinical management remains unclear. The vast majority of moderate penetrance genes are yet to be discovered. Some cases that demonstrate a familial pattern are found on germline testing to have *BRCA1* or *BRCA2* mutations, and it is difficult to know exactly where to set the threshold for genetic testing. However, quantitative risk assessment of breast cancer is extremely useful for the familial category of at-risk women[24] and guides medical decision making about chemoprevention, high-risk surveillance using breast magnetic resonance imaging (MRI),[25] and prophylactic mastectomy.

Hereditary Breast Cancer

Hereditary breast cancer is characterized by a significantly earlier age of onset of breast cancer (average, 45 years of age, beginning in the early 20s with high risk extending throughout life), an excess of bilateral breast cancer, a greater frequency of multiple primary cancer such as cancer of the breast and ovary in the HBOC syndrome, and an autosomal dominant inheritance pattern for cancer susceptibility.[26,27] Surveillance and management strategies for HBC must be in accord with these clinical features and address the risk to relatives; therefore, they clearly differ from that required for sporadic cases.[26,27] Figure 21-5 shows the pedigree of a site-specific HBC family. Figures 21-6 and 21-7 are pedigrees for two families with classical HBOC syndrome.

SCREENING AND MANAGEMENT MELDED TO GENETIC AND NATURAL HISTORY

The natural history of hereditary breast cancer mandates that high-risk patients (i.e., germline mutation carriers and first-degree relatives of women affected with breast cancer and/or OC) receive special attention with regard to the screening and management practices. Physicians must keep in mind that these high-risk women often present with a heightened sense of fear of developing breast cancer and/or OC, which has likely been amplified through living with this fear for years and having seen loved ones become affected by, and sometimes succumb to, these cancers.

Genetic counseling is mandatory, particularly when matters of germline mutation testing are considered. Such counseling should be initiated prior to DNA collection and provided again, in person, at the time of disclosure of results. All matters concerning psychological issues, costs, potential insurance and/or employment discrimination, and confidentiality must be discussed with the patient.[28-32] Available options such as prophylactic bilateral mastectomy[33] and prophylactic bilateral oophorectomy,[34] chemoprevention such as tamoxifen,[35] as well as the limitations of these preventive strategies, need to be discussed in detail (Table 21-1).[36-38] Prophylactic contralateral mastectomy in the case of ipsilateral breast cancer or prophylactic bilateral mastectomy may be discussed as an option for women with excessive fear of breast cancer and/or who may be noncompliant with screening because of fear of finding a tumor or because fibrocystic disease has increased the difficulty of examination.[33,37]

High-risk surveillance using annual breast MRI coupled with mammography starting at 20 to 25 years of age, with biannual clinical breast examination and monthly self-breast examination, is crucial in women who do not choose prophylactic mastectomy. Breast MRI and mammography are complementary techniques and although MRI is more sensitive, some breast tumors are detected solely by mammography. Although there is some concern about the potential carcinogenic effects of radiation from screening mammograms in young high-risk women,[39,40] the importance of early detection must be stressed in medical decision making. We also discuss ovarian screening procedures and their limitations, with the option for prophylactic oophorectomy

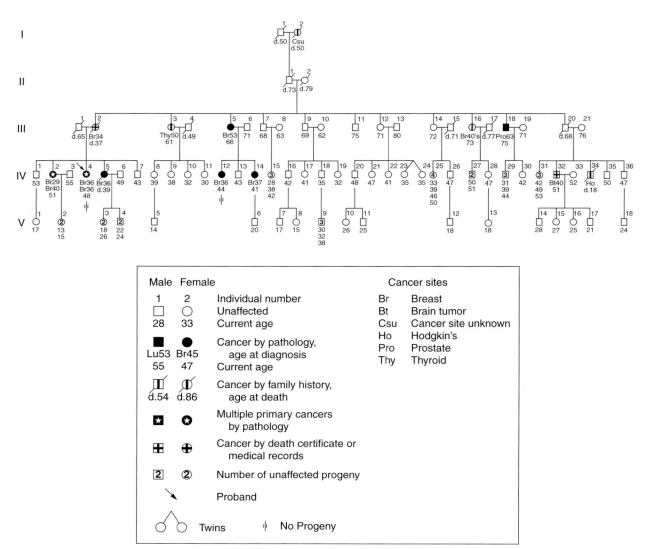

Figure 21-5 A classical hereditary breast cancer family with eight cases (III-2, III-5, III-16, IV-2, IV-4, IV-5, IV-12, and IV-14) of breast cancer over two generations. Note the classical sign of bilateral breast cancer primaries in two cases (IV-2 and IV-4).

once the family has been completed.[41] The severe limitations of current OC screening and typical presentation of OC at advanced stage essentially mandate risk-reducing salpingo-oophorectomy after the completion of childbearing and merit priority attention to new technologies for early diagnosis of OC.[42–44]

Hereditary Breast and Ovarian Cancer Syndrome and *BRCA1* and *BRCA2* Mutations

HBC, inclusive of HBOC, is genotypically and phenotypically heterogeneous (see Fig. 21-2). It is estimated that approximately 45% of hereditary early-onset site-specific breast cancer and about 80% of HBOC kindreds show linkage to *BRCA1*. The majority of the remaining families are attributable to *BRCA2*. The predominant cancer types in the HBOC syndrome are breast and ovary. The lifetime risk of breast cancer in *BRCA1* and *BRCA2* mutation carriers is estimated to be as high as 85%.[45] The lifetime risk of OC is estimated to be 40% to 60% for *BRCA1* carriers[46] and 15% for *BRCA2* carriers.[45,47] *BRCA2* is more highly associated with male breast cancer than *BRCA1*. In one study, results showed that, among male patients with breast cancer, about one third of *BRCA*-positive cases involved *BRCA1* and two thirds involved *BRCA2*.[48] The risk of a second female breast cancer in a putative gene carrier already affected with breast cancer was estimated to be 65% by 70 years of age (95% CI, 47–77).[45] When allowing for the fact that such women only have one breast at risk, the corresponding penetrance estimate was 87% by 70 years of age [CI = 72–95]. The corresponding estimate for OC was 44% by 70 years of age [CI = 28–56].

Lower penetrance estimates have been found in studies where ascertainment is population- or clinic-based. A recent meta-analysis indicates a risk of breast cancer of

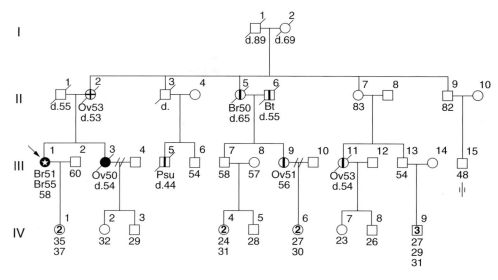

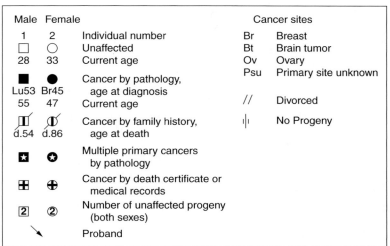

Figure 21-6 A classical hereditary breast/ovarian cancer pedigree showing two breast cancer cases (II-5 and III-1) and four ovarian cancer cases (II-2, III-3, III-9, and III-11). Note the decreased penetrance in II-7, who remains unaffected with breast or ovarian cancer even though she is an obligate gene carrier with a daughter who developed ovarian cancer at 53 years of age.

57% (95% CI = 47–66) for *BRCA1* and 49% (95% CI = 40–57) for *BRCA2* mutation carriers. Risks of OC were 40% (95% CI = 35–46) for *BRCA1* and 18% (95% CI = 13–23) for *BRCA2* mutation carriers.[49] Because all of these risks are high, we do not think that differences between these and previous risk estimates have a significant bearing on clinical management. Figure 21-8 shows the pedigree of a family in which a *BRCA1* mutation segregates primarily with OC.

BRCA1

Easton and colleagues computed RRs for breast cancer and OC in *BRCA1* carriers and compared them with general population risks for England and Wales for 1978 to 1982. The RR for breast cancer based on the contralateral breast cancer data declined significantly with age, from over 200-fold below 40 years of age to 15-fold in the 60- to 69-year-old age group ($P < 0.0001$). The RR for OC, based on the second cancer data, also declined significantly ($P < 0.001$), but it was not as dramatic as that for breast cancer.[45]

Ford and Easton[46] suggest that the majority of multiple-case families that segregate both breast cancer and OC in a dominant manner, consistent with the HBOC syndrome, manifest mutations in the *BRCA1* gene. These researchers combined penetrance estimates for *BRCA1* with results from two population-based genetic epidemiologic investigations to estimate the gene frequency of *BRCA1*. Using the assumption that the excess risk of OC in first-degree relatives of patients with breast cancer, and conversely that the breast cancer excess in relatives of patients with OC are both entirely accounted for by *BRCA1*, they estimate that the *BRCA1* gene frequency is 0.0006 (95% CI = 0.0002–0.001) and that the proportion of breast cancer cases in the general population caused by *BRCA1* is 5.3% below 40 years of age, 2.2% between 40 and 49 year of age, and 1.1% between 50 and 70 years of age. The corresponding estimates for OC are 5.7%, 4.6%, and 2.1%, respectively. These investigators concluded that the occurrence of cancer in the majority of families with breast cancer with less than four cases and no OC is likely to be due either to chance or to more common genes of lower penetrance.

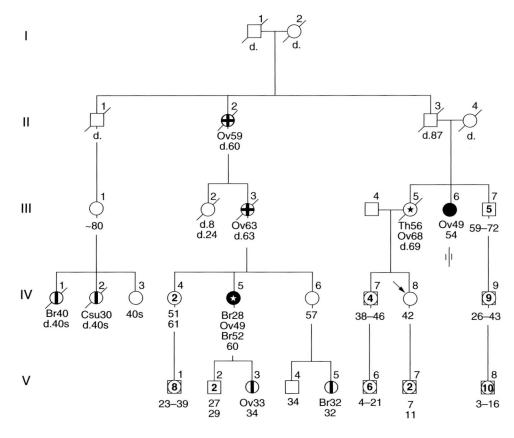

Figure 21-7 A classical hereditary breast/ovarian cancer pedigree demonstrating four generations of ovarian cancer cases (II-2, III-3, IV-5, and V-3). Also, note the very early onset of breast cancer in IV-5 and V-5. Individual II-3 is shown as an obligate gene carrier with two daughters (III-5 and III-6) who are affected by ovarian cancer.

Ford and coworkers[50] examined cancers of other anatomic sites in individuals affected with breast cancer or OC and their first-degree relatives in *BRCA1*-linked families. They observed 87 cancers (other than breast or ovarian) in individuals with breast cancer or OC and their first-degree relatives compared with 69.3 expected based on national incidence rates. Significant excesses were observed for colon cancer (estimated RR to gene carriers, 4.11 [95% CI = 2.36–7.15] and prostate cancer, 3.33 [95% CI = 1.78–6.20]).

Molecular Biology and Mutations in BRCA1

BRCA1 is a large gene that contains 22 coding exons and produces a protein of 1863 amino acids. *BRCA2* has 26 coding exons and produces a protein of 3418 amino acids. One thousand six hundred forty-three distinct mutations, polymorphisms and variants have been reported in *BRCA1*, of which 890 have been reported only once. For *BRCA2*, 1856 distinct mutations, polymorphisms and variants have been reported, and

TABLE 21-1

Surveillance and Management for Hereditary Breast Cancer

I. Education about genetics, natural history, surveillance, and management—initiate midteens; genetic counseling can take place at 18 years of age; when indicated, *BRCA1/BRCA2* mutation testing can take place at that age.

II. Instruction in breast self-examination—initiate at 18 years of age.

III. Clinical breast examination—begin at 20 years of age and repeat semiannually.

IV. Mammography—begin at 25 years of age and carry out every 6–12 months after that.

V. Ovarian cancer screening (transvaginal ovarian ultrasound, Doppler color blood flow imagery, CA-125, annual pelvic examinations)—begin at 30 years of age and carry out annually thereafter.

VI. Option for contralateral prophylactic mastectomy in patient with ipsilateral breast cancer, and bilateral prophylactic mastectomy and prophylactic oophorectomy—consider when family completed.

VII. Emphasis on clinical and self-breast examination in male carriers

VIII. Consideration of tamoxifen or selective estrogen receptor modulator

IX. Consideration of annual bilateral breast MRI under research protocol

X. Surveillance and chemoprevention for at-risk relatives; surgical prevention is guided by result of gene testing.

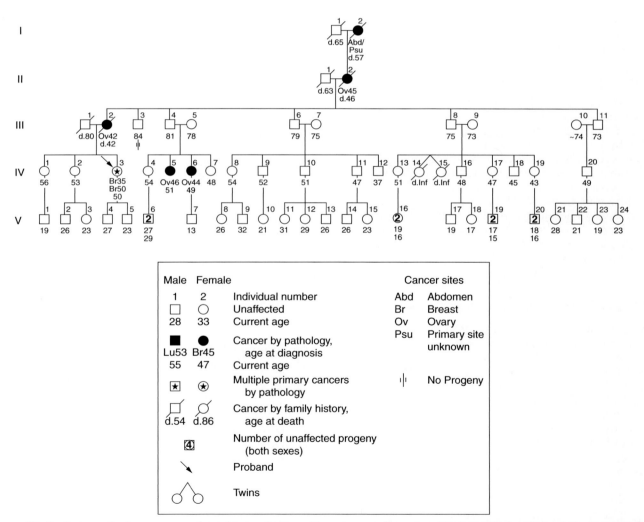

Figure 21-8 Noteworthy is an excess of ovarian carcinoma with early age of onset and its transmission through three generations (II-2, III-2, IV-5, IV-6), and possibly a fourth generation (I-2), namely, the putative progenitor who died of abdominal cancer, site unknown. We speculate that it was possibly ovarian carcinoma. It is noteworthy that individual IV-3, with bilateral breast cancer with first onset at 35 years of age, is to date the only family member who has had breast cancer. This family has the *BRCA1* mutation. A potential confounder is the predominance of males in the direct lineage in the third generation, one of whom (III-4) is a progenitor, namely the father of two individuals affected by ovarian cancer (IV-5, IV-6).

about 975 are as yet unique to one family (Breast Cancer Information Core web site: http://www.nhgri.nih.gov/Intramural_research/Lab_transfer/Bic/index.html; accessed 2 March 2008). The occurrence of numerous unique mutations is of clinical importance: When genetic testing is first performed in a given family, complete analysis of both genes is generally required (unless the individual's ancestry can guide initial analysis to founder mutations). Most mutations that have been identified in *BRCA1* are frame shifts, nonsense mutations, or splice mutations.[48,51,52] These mutations presumably lead to premature truncation of the BRCA1 protein. General methods used to scan for mutations, including DNA sequencing, fail to identify large duplications, deletions, and rearrangements, which may account for approximately 10% of mutations.[53] Enhancement of testing to ascertain these types of mutations using multiplex ligation-dependent probe amplification (MLPA) is now available and adds about one to three percentage points to overall sensitivity in high-risk families. The higher rate of MLPA-detected mutations in families with a high calculated risk of a *BRCA1* and/or *BRCA2* mutation demonstrates the importance of using enhanced mutation detection methods in very high-risk families.[49]

Phenotypic Variation in BRCA1

Based on linkage analysis, Easton and coworkers[45] predicted the existence of two variants of families with *BRCA1*: (1) those showing a high penetrance of OC (84% by 70 years of age) and (2) those showing a low penetrance of OC (32% by 70 years of age).

Gayther and associates[54] studied 60 families with a history of breast or ovarian carcinoma, or both, for *BRCA1* germline mutations. They found 22 different mutations detected in 32 families (53%). A significant correlation was observed between the location of the mutation in the gene and the ratio of breast to OC incidence within each family. They suggested that mutations in the 3′ third of the gene are associated with a lower proportion of OC.

PTEN and Breast Cancers with BRCA1 Mutation

Saal and colleagues[55] note that *Pten* contributes to the formation of basal-like mammary tumors in mice. In humans, loss of PTEN expression is significantly associated with the basal-like breast cancer subtype of breast cancer with poor prognosis. Importantly, *BRCA1* is a cancer-susceptibility gene involved in double-stranded DNA break repair, which leads to breast cancers that are nearly always of the basal-like breast cancer type.

Basal-like breast cancer comprises 10% to 20% of all breast cancer and is one of the subtypes with the worst prognosis. These types of breast cancer are highly proliferative, poorly differentiated, and genomically unstable. They are positive for estrogen receptor (ER), progesterone receptor (PR), and Her2/*neu*; these are initiated by a *BRCA1* mutation.

PTEN is a tumor suppressor that inhibits downstream signaling. The model developed by Saal and colleagues implies that basal-like breast cancers may be strongly associated with aberrant *PTEN-PI3K* pathway signaling.

Importantly, therapy targeted to this pathway may be an effective way to treat and possibly even prevent some sporadic and hereditary basal-like breast cancers.

The double-stranded DNA break repair pathway in breast cancer may make it possible for other grossly rearranged tumors to contribute to tumor suppression—observations that are analogous to those in Lynch syndrome, where lack of mismatch repair leads to microsatellite instability. This in turn leads to mutation of *TGFBR2* and other genes that drive tumor progression.

BRCA2

A second susceptibility gene, *BRCA2*, was mapped to chromosome 13 in 1994[19] and was subsequently identified.[20] The majority of *BRCA*-associated cases of male breast cancer appear to be associated with *BRCA2*.[48] *BRCA2* confers a high risk of breast cancer and a lower risk of OC ($\approx$15%). Pancreatic cancer, prostate cancer, and malignant melanoma also have been described as integral cancers in *BRCA2*.

Figure 21-9 shows a *BRCA2* family with three males affected with breast cancer; two of these males also developed prostate cancer. Note that in this family the proband's father (see Fig. 21-9, III-1), paternal grandfather (II-2), and paternal great-uncle (II-3) each developed breast cancer, at 53, 57, and 60 years of age, respectively. Furthermore, the father and grandfather also developed prostate cancer at 64 and 79 years of age, respectively. A *BRCA2* mutation has been identified in this family. Wooster and colleagues[20] report on the identification of *BRCA2* mutation in five different families with breast cancer. Each of these mutations was found to disrupt the open reading frame of the transcriptional unit.

In the course of the mutational screen of candidate coding sequences from the *BRCA2* region, the first detected sequence variant that was predicted to this rough translation of an encoded protein was observed in a Creighton University breast cancer–prone family. This family is strongly linked to *BRCA2*, with a multipoint log of the odds score of 3.01 using D13S260 and D13S267. Wooster and coworkers[20] reported a six–base pair deletion in this family, resulting in a premature termination codon. This mutation has been detected in two other cases of early-onset breast cancer in this family.

Modifiers of Breast Cancer Risk in BRCA2 Mutation Carriers

Risk of breast cancer in mutation carriers is modified by variable genetic or environmental factors that cluster in families. *BRCA1* and *BRCA2* interact with *RAD51*, which has a single nucleotide polymorphism (SNP) that has been suggested as a possible modifier of risk of breast cancer in *BRCA1* and *BRCA2* mutation carriers.[56] Findings disclosed a statistically significant increased risk in *BRCA2* mutation carriers through 135G → C. This may modify risk of breast cancer in *BRCA2* mutation carriers by altering expression of *RAD51*, which is the first gene to be reliably identified as a modifier of risk in *BRCA* mutation carriers.[56]

Stacey and coworkers[57] investigated a missense BARD1 variant, Cys557Ser, which has been reported to be at increased frequency in breast cancer–prone families. They investigated this variant in a population-based cohort of

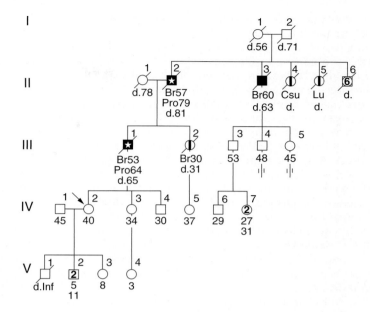

Figure 21-9 Pedigree showing a *BRCA2* family with three males affected with breast cancer; two of these males also developed prostate cancer.

1090 Icelandic patients with invasive breast cancer and 703 controls. According to their report, their findings "...suggest that BARD1 Cys557Ser is an ancient variant that confers risk of single and multiple primary breast cancers, and this risk extends to carriers of the *BRCA2* 999del5 mutation."

ESTIMATED *BRCA1* AND *BRCA2* MUTATION PROBABILITIES: CLINICAL IMPLICATIONS

Berry and colleagues[3] compared results for mutations involving *BRCA1* and *BRCA2* with estimated probabilities of harboring these mutations to assess sensitivity of genetic testing as well as the relevance of other susceptibility genes in familial breast cancer and OC. They used BRCAPRO,[58,59] a computer program that implements a statistical model enabling the calculation of an individual's probability of harboring a *BRCA1* or *BRCA2* mutation, neither of these, or even both, based on the individual's cancer status in concert with the history of

breast cancer and OC in that individual's first- and second-degree relatives. Data were collected and analyzed from six high-risk genetic counseling clinics and focused on individuals from families containing at least one member who was tested for *BRCA1* and *BRCA2* mutations. Findings disclosed that BRCAPRO:

> ...is an accurate counseling tool for determining the probability of carrying mutations of *BRCA1* and *BRCA2*. Genetic testing for *BRCA1* and *BRCA2* is highly sensitive, missing an estimated 15% of mutations. In the population studied, breast cancer susceptibility genes other than *BRCA1* and *BRCA2* either do not exist, are rare, or are associated with low disease penetrance.[3]

The accuracy of BRCAPRO compares well when tested against other risk assessment models.[24,60]

From a very practical standpoint, BRCAPRO is widely used in the clinical setting to assist in advising individuals whether they are sufficient candidates to undergo genetic testing. Of note, experienced genetic counselors perform as accurately as BRCAPRO in predicting *BRCA1* and/or *BRCA2* risk; individual counselors may outperform the model.[61]

BRCAPRO may underestimate *BRCA1* and *BRCA2* pretest probability in families whose structures include few female relatives (or ones who have died young from noncancer-related causes). In this situation, corrective factors can be applied to modify BRCAPRO in cases of early-onset breast cancer with limited family structure (e.g., fewer than two first- or second-degree relatives surviving beyond 45 years of age in either lineage).[62]

BRCAPRO uses a carrier frequency based on whites and adjusts for carrier frequency in individuals of Ashkenazi Jewish ancestry but not other ethnic groups. To assess the accuracy of BRCAPRO in minorities, the area under the receiver operating characteristic curves was measured in African-American[63] and Hispanic[64] patients. Test performance was found to be similar to that of whites, indicating that BRCAPRO performs equally in African-American and Hispanic populations.

BRCAPRO and other assessment models have important research potential, particularly as a guide to determine who to test and to judge the utility of such testing as well as a substitute for testing.[24] Thus, a researcher

> ...who contemplates genetic testing for subjects involved in a clinical trial or subjects in a research database can use BRCAPRO to determine the expected number of mutations in each subset of study participants. This allows for judging whether the scientific question can be addressed with sufficient statistical power.[3]

BRCAPRO also allows for selecting the most informative subset of individuals for testing in a setting where funds for genetic testing are limited. Additional models to gauge pretest probabilities have also emerged.[65]

BRCA1 and *BRCA2* testing for breast cancer and OC clearly has important cancer control implications. However, this testing is expensive and may be beyond the financial reach of many patients. Antoniou and colleagues[65] note that there are several algorithms that predict the likelihood of a patient harboring a *BRCA1* or *BRCA2* mutation, some of which are currently used in clinical practice to focus on such inordinately high-risk individuals. These authors studied the performance of the carrier prediction algorithms BOADICEA, BRCAPRO, IBIS, the Manchester scoring system, and the Myriad tables, for the study of 1934 families evaluated in cancer genetic clinics in the United Kingdom in which an index patient had been screened for *BRCA1* and/or *BRCA2* mutations. These models were evaluated for calibration, discrimination, and accuracy of their predictions. Findings disclosed that of the five algorithms, only BOADICEA

> ...predicted the overall observed number of mutations detected accurately (i.e., was well calibrated). BOADICEA also provided the best discrimination, being significantly better ($P < 0.05$) than all models except BRCAPRO (area under the receiver operating characteristic curve statistics: BOADICEA = 0.77, BRCAPRO = 0.76, IBIS = 0.74, Manchester = 0.75, Myriad = 0.72). All models underpredicted the number of *BRCA1* and *BRCA2* mutations in the low estimated risk category.

These investigators concluded that these carrier prediction algorithms for *BRCA1* and *BRCA2* mutations were sufficiently sensitive so that their widespread use could not only improve equity of access but also contribute to cost-effectiveness of mutation testing.

BRCA1 AND *BRCA2* IN ASHKENAZI JEWS

Struewing and coworkers[66] studied the frequency of the 185delAG frameshift mutation in *BRCA1* in 858 Ashkenazi Jewish individuals who had sought genetic testing for conditions that were unrelated to cancer. They observed the 185delAG mutation in 0.9% of Ashkenazi DNA samples (95% CI = 0.4–1.8). They concluded that approximately 1 in 100 women of Ashkenazi descent may be at increased risk for developing breast or ovarian carcinoma, or both.[66] Subsequent studies have confirmed the increased prevalence of the 185delAG *BRCA1* mutation in the Ashkenazi Jewish population. Roa and coworkers[67] performed a large-scale population study for the 185delAG mutation in 3000 Ashkenazi Jewish blood samples collected for relatively common diseases among this population and found a carrier frequency of 1.09%.[67] Offit and colleagues evaluated the frequency of the 185delAG mutation in Ashkenazi Jewish women with early-onset breast cancer seen at medical oncology and genetic counseling clinics in New York. They found that 20% of 80 women with breast cancer diagnosed before 42 years of age carried this mutation. They concluded that screening for the 185delAG mutation in the Ashkenazi Jewish population may serve as a useful tool in the genetic counseling of these families.[68] In addition, Modan and coworkers identified an increased prevalence of the 185delAG mutation in OC cases in Israel compared to healthy controls.[69]

As a result of the specificity of 185delAG, it appears to be the result of a founder effect in the Ashkenazi Jewish population. Therefore, Struewing and coworkers[66] reasoned that inherited breast cancer possibly represents a higher proportion of breast cancer in this population than in others. Specifically, a higher proportion of breast cancer is attributable to *BRCA1* and/or *BRCA2* in Ashkenazi Jewish women; for example, 21% to 30% of Ashkenazi Jewish women diagnosed with breast cancer when younger than 40 years of age have founder mutations compared with 6.1% of non-Jewish women diagnosed under age 50.[24]

Family history of breast cancer conveys a higher RR in Jewish versus non-Jewish women, an effect that is magnified for early-onset breast cancer.[24] Helmrich and colleagues[70] evaluated risk factors for breast cancer in a hospital-based case-control study of 1185 women with breast cancer (90% United States, 4% Canada, 6% Israel). Jewish ethnicity was associated with an RR of 2.8 compared to Catholics (95% CI = 2.3–3.4) and was "not confounded materially" by parity, age at first birth, or years of education. The increased prevalence of the Ashkenazi Jewish founder mutations might partially explain the possibly increased risk of breast cancer in Jewish women.[66] Although clear data are not available regarding the incidence of breast cancer in Jewish women, unless *BRCA1* and *BRCA2* penetrance rates are lower in Ashkenazi Jews (a concept refuted by the study of King and colleagues[71]), the incidence of breast cancer in Jewish women is likely elevated.

The *BRCA2* mutation 6174delT has been identified as characteristic in Ashkenazi Jewish women, and appears to have an approximately 1.5% prevalence rate in this population.[67,72] Therefore, the 185delAG *BRCA1* and 6174delT *BRCA2* mutations appear to constitute the two most frequent mutation alleles predisposing to HBC in Ashkenazi Jewish women. The *BRCA2* 6174delT mutation is less penetrant than the *BRCA1* 185delAG mutation. It has been found less frequently in Ashkenazi Jewish women with breast cancer than the 185delAG mutation.[72] Phenotypic variation in *BRCA2* has also been identified. Gayther and colleagues studied the distribution of *BRCA2* mutations in 25 families with multiple cases of breast cancer or OC, or both, and found mutations in families with a high proportion of OC to cluster in exon 11.[73] Mutations in the ovarian cancer cluster region (OCCR) appear to convey as high a risk of OC as do mutations in *BRCA1*. Furthermore, colorectal, stomach, pancreatic, and prostate cancer occurred in excess in first-degree relatives of carriers of OCCR mutations compared with mutations in other regions of *BRCA2*.[74]

Although these studies focused on Ashkenazi Jewish women, it is vital to keep in mind that Ashkenazi Jewish males can also carry these mutations. Of note, male *BRCA1* or *BRCA2* carriers face high relative risks of prostate cancer, and *BRCA2* carriers appear to develop more aggressive prostate cancer.[75]

Frank and coworkers[48] investigated 10,000 consecutive gene sequence analyses for the identification of mutations anywhere in the *BRCA1* and *BRCA2* genes and correlated these results with personal and family history of cancer, ancestry, invasive versus noninvasive breast neoplasia, and sex. They identified mutations in 1720 (17.2%) of the 10,000 individuals tested, including 968 (20%) of 4843 women with breast cancer and 281 (34%) of 824 women with OC; prevalence was correlated with specific features of the individuals' personal and family histories.

...Mutations were as prevalent in high-risk women of African (25 [19%] of 133) and other non-Ashkenazi ancestries as those of European ancestry (712 [16%] of 4379) and were significantly less prevalent in women diagnosed before 50 years of age with ductal carcinoma in situ than with invasive breast cancer (13% v 24%, $P = 0.0007$)....Twenty-one (28%) of 76 men with breast cancer carried mutations, of which more than one third occurred in *BRCA1*.

These authors concluded that certain features of personal and family history can be used effectively for assessment in a clinical setting of the likelihood of identifying a mutation in *BRCA1* or *BRCA2*.

PROBABILISTIC IMPLICATIONS OF HEREDITARY CANCER

When evaluating families with hereditary cancer, it is important to realize that genetic information is probabilistic. Not all carriers of *BRCA1* and *BRCA2* germline

mutations develop cancer (penetrance of the genes is about 85% to 90%), and conversely, some noncarriers do not remain cancer-free because these cancers are relatively common in the general population. In addition, there is always uncertainty in a mutation carrier about whether and when cancer will occur. The unaffected proband of the family depicted in Figure 21-10, an HBC family, sought *BRCA* testing because her mother (also unaffected with cancer) and the proband's maternal aunt (affected with breast cancer in her 30s) refused to undergo genetic testing. The family history and the proband's desire to be tested led to *BRCA* testing in the proband, even though the probability of her carrying a *BRCA* mutation was low. A *BRCA2* mutation was found. Given the fact that these cancers are common, affected individuals within a pedigree cannot invariably be assumed to be gene carriers because they may in fact represent a sporadic (phenocopy) case. This consideration has importance for genetic counseling, selection of individuals for genetic testing, and ultimate medical management of the offspring of such sporadic cases.

VARIABLE AGE OF ONSET IN HEREDITARY BREAST CANCER

Extremely early age of onset of breast cancer appears to be another example of heterogeneity in HBC (Fig. 21-11). In this category, we see breast cancer clustering in the 20s and early 30s in certain families. In contrast, we see clustering of late age of onset in selected families (discussed subsequently).

The authors studied the relationship between age of onset of breast cancer in 328 breast cancer probands (consecutively ascertained patients from Creighton's oncology clinic) and breast cancer incidence and age of onset in their female relatives.[76] A family history of early-onset breast cancer was associated with a higher risk of early onset breast cancer. A family history of early-onset breast cancer occurred more frequently in young (<40 years of age) breast cancer probands than among older ones (>40 years of age; odds ratio [OR] = 23; $P < 0.001$). This relationship was particularly evident when the analysis was restricted to HBC (OR = 3.3; $P < 0.001$). The authors also observed a positive family history of breast cancer (at any age) more frequently in young breast cancer probands than in older breast cancer probands (OR = 2.9; $P < 0.001$). These observations have important pragmatic implications for surveillance. Specifically, the authors recommend that intense surveillance for breast cancer be initiated earlier for women who have close relatives with early-onset breast cancer.[76] Such women are important candidates for detailed pedigree studies.

From the genetic and epidemiologic standpoint, there are two questions to address. Is earlier age at breast cancer onset more likely to predict genetic susceptibility than later age at onset? Are some families characterized by early-onset breast cancer, whereas others show familial aggregation of later age at onset? The case-control study by Claus and coworkers[77] (4730 histologically confirmed cases of breast cancer in women 20 to 54 years of age and 4688 controls) showed that a major factor influencing breast cancer risk in first-degree relatives

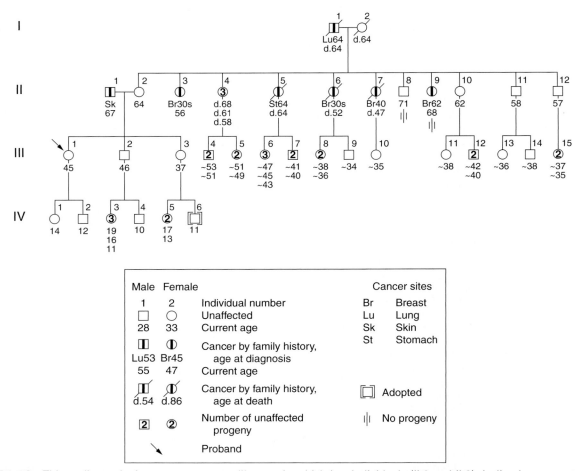

Figure 21-10 This pedigree depicts an uncommon dilemma in which key individuals (II-2 and II-3) declined an opportunity to be tested for *BRCA* mutations. We note early-onset breast cancer (II-3 in the 30s, II-6 at 30 years of age, and II-7 at 40 years of age). Because the proband's mother (II-2) refused testing, we tested the proband (III-1), who did show a *BRCA2* mutation. Before consenting to testing, the proband understood from genetic counseling that her risk for carrying a mutation would be approximately 25%, because her mother was not affected by breast cancer. Despite this relatively low probability, we proceeded with testing because of the strong family history of breast cancer and the proband's strong desire to be tested.

of cases was the age at which the woman was affected with breast cancer.

Mettlin and colleagues[78] suggest that some families are characterized by early-onset breast cancer, whereas others show familial aggregations of later age at onset of breast cancer. They hypothesized that breast cancers in younger and older women were distinct epidemiologic entities. Of interest is the finding that the occurrence of breast cancer in an immediate family member at an older age may increase risk specifically for the disease to occur in a person at older ages; conversely, it may be that only when diagnosis of breast cancer occurs in a close relative at a young age that it poses a risk in younger women.

GENETIC FACTORS IN PROGNOSIS AND SURVIVAL

BRCA1 Mutation and Young Age Predict Rapid Breast Cancer Growth

Tumor volume doubling time was assessed in 100 breast cancer cases through MRI and/or mammography. Forty-three were women with *BRCA1* mutation, 16 with

BRCA2 mutation, and 41 were at high risk in absence of an identified mutation through MRI and/or mammography. Growth rate slowed continuously with increased age ($P = 0.004$) but was twice as fast in *BRCA1* ($P = 0.003$) or *BRCA2* ($P = 0.03$) carriers as in other high-risk patients of the same age.[79] Pathologic tumor size decreased with increasing age ($P = 0.001$). Specifically, median size was 15 mm for patients younger than 40 years of age compared with 9 mm in older patients ($P = 0.003$); tumors were largest in young women with *BRCA1* mutations. It was concluded that young age and *BRCA1* mutation carrier status both contribute to increased speed of tumor growth. A patient's age and risk group should therefore be taken into account in screening protocols.[79] For this reason, we have recommended annual mammography because of this alleged accelerated carcinogenesis. Because of the early age of onset in *BRCA1* and *BRCA2*, we initiate screening at 20 to 25 years of age. Breast MRI as an adjunct to mammography is recommended in these young and high-risk patients by the American Cancer Society.[25] Recently, we and others have recommended alternating MRI with mammography every 6 months.

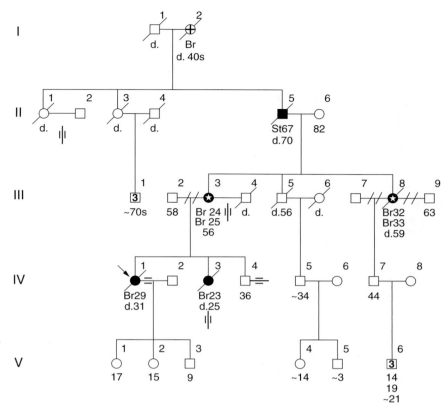

Figure 21-11 Pedigree of a hereditary breast cancer family showing extraordinarily early age of cancer onset. (Lynch HT, Conway T, Watson P, et al: Extremely early onset hereditary breast cancer: Surveillance/ management implications. Neb Med J 73:97–100, 1988. Reprinted with permission.)

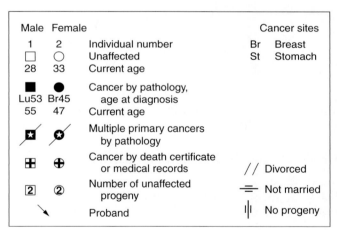

"Watchful waiting" can be dangerous as evidenced in patient III-8 (Fig. 21-12) who had a lump in her breast and knew about her family history consistent with HBOC. Unfortunately, her physician elected to "watch it," and the lesion grew significantly over a period of only 3 months. Biopsy at that time confirmed stage III invasive carcinoma with positive lymph nodes. Also, her health insurance carrier delayed coverage for cancer treatment. Final diagnosis was stage III invasive breast cancer, ER-negative, PR-negative, HER2-negative ("triple negative").

Although most HBC literature has shown early age at onset as an important predictor of risk of breast cancer in the patient's primary relatives, systematic investigation of familial clustering of late age at onset of breast cancer has been virtually ignored. However, we have identified a number of putative HBC kindreds characterized by late-onset breast cancer (H.T. Lynch, unpublished data, 2009). Perhaps the lack of attention to late-onset breast cancer occurs because it is more difficult to determine the genetic significance of a familial aggregation of patients with onset of breast cancer in the seventh, eighth, or ninth decades of life. For example, many high-risk relatives may have died from comorbidities or other competing causes. It is also much more difficult to secure documentation of cancer in the parents, aunts, uncles,

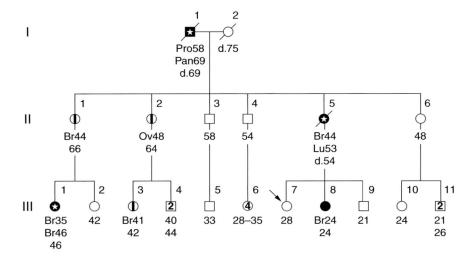

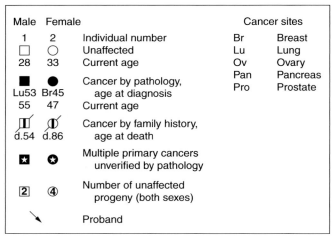

Figure 21-12 The proband (III-7) is a 28-year-old woman whose sister (III-8) had very early onset (24 years of age) breast cancer. Their mother (II-5) had breast cancer at 44 years of age with a second primary of the lung. There is other evidence of breast (II-1, III-1, and III-3) and ovarian (II-2) cancer in the family. In this case, the proband had her blood drawn once we knew a mutation was present in the family, and the *BRCA1* mutation was identified (in individual III-3). This is of importance because the proband's sister (III-8) had a lump in her breast and the family history was known to the provider. However, it was elected to follow the lump with the admonition that, should it increase in size, a biopsy would be performed. The lump, unfortunately, progressed, and mastectomy showed this to be stage III, "triple-negative" breast cancer with axillary lymph node positivity. Further confounding this problem was the fact that the insurer delayed consideration for funding treatment for several months in spite of the fact that it was known that she had "triple-negative" cancer.

and grandparents of these older-onset patients, many of whom may be deceased.

Survival in BRCA1 and BRCA2 Mutation Carriers

Clinical outcome of breast cancer in women with a *BRCA1* or *BRCA2* mutation has been inconclusive. In a Finnish study of 359 patients with familial breast cancer (32 from *BRCA1*-positive families, 43 from *BRCA2*-positive families, and 284 from *BRCA1* or *BRCA2*-negative breast cancer families), there was no difference in cumulative survival rates as compared with sporadic breast cancer (adjusted for age, stage, and year of diagnosis).[80] However, a study of paraffin tumor blocks from 118 Ashkenazi Jewish patients with breast cancer and negative axillary lymph nodes found that *BRCA1* mutation carrier status was a significant prognostic factor of death (risk ratio = 5.8, 95% CI = 1.5–22, $P = 0.009$).[81] Furthermore, a French study of 183 women with breast cancer and a family history of breast cancer and/or OC found a worse prognosis for *BRCA1* carriers in terms of overall survival and metastasis-free interval.[82]

Rennert and colleagues[83] compiled data on all incident cases of invasive breast cancer from January 1, 1987, to December 31, 1988, which had been recorded in the Israel National Cancer Registry. Pathology samples were obtained from 1794 of 2514 subjects (71%) for founder mutation testing, and medical records were reviewed in 1545 of the cases (86%). DNA was extracted from the tumor specimens and analyzed for the three Ashkenazi founder mutations in *BRCA1* and *BRCA2*. Findings disclosed that a *BRCA1* or *BRCA2* mutation had been identified in 10% of women who were of Ashkenazi Jewish ancestry. The adjusted hazard ratios for death attributable to breast cancer "...were not significantly different among mutation carriers and noncarriers (hazard ratio among *BRCA1* carriers, 0.76; 95% confidence interval [CI], 0.45 to 1.30; $P = 0.31$; hazard ratio among *BRCA2* carriers, 1.31; 95% CI, 0.80 to 2.15; $P = 0.28$)." Treatment with chemotherapy among *BRCA1* carriers showed a nonsignificant hazard ratio for death. It was concluded that breast cancer–specific rates of death were similar for carriers of a BRCA founder mutation and noncarriers, among Israeli women. Due caution is advised for any generalization of these data beyond carriers of an Ashkenazi BRCA founder mutation.

The present evidence, described subsequently, presents a paradox. *BRCA1* HBC has poor prognostic markers (aneuploidy, high-grade, high cell-proliferation rates) but better disease-free survival rates in some studies, whereas *BRCA2* HBC has neutral markers but poorer survival behavior, albeit controversial. This paradox is as yet unexplained and requires more investigation.

PATHOBIOLOGY OF *BRCA1*, *BRCA2*, AND NON-*BRCA1* OR *BRCA2* HEREDITARY BREAST CANCER

Even before the discovery and isolation of the major breast cancer genes *BRCA1* and *BRCA2*, there were clues that the pathology of HBC differed from that of its sporadic counterpart.[84,85] Earlier work showed (1) more medullary carcinoma (Fig. 21-13)—a proliferative, high-grade special type with good prognosis—in familial and HBC settings[86-89]; (2) a higher mitotic grade (Fig. 21-14) in the no special type (NST, or ductal) invasive carcinoma in HBC[84,87]; (3) a statistically insignificant association of invasive lobular[90-92] or tubular[93,94] carcinomas in familial settings; and (4) conflicting positive[95,96] and negative[90] associations of lobular carcinoma in situ (LCIS) with family history. Only one of these, a positive association, was statistically significant.[84,95] In the sections that follow, we review the histopathology and biomarkers in *BRCA1*, *BRCA2*, and non-*BRCA1* and *BRCA2* HBC, considering invasive and in situ disease in turn. To highlight trends in original published data, it was sometimes necessary to compute or recompute *P*-values for significances of differences, using Yates-corrected chi-square or Fisher's exact tests. These we designate as *P**, in distinction to original published values, *P*.

BRCA1 Hereditary Breast Cancer Phenotype

At Creighton University, the authors have been investigating the clinical and pathologic features of HBC with one of the largest and most long-standing pathology resources. By 1994, sufficient linkage information on *BRCA1* had become available to assign the high mitotic grade of the NST carcinomas in the cohort[87] to the *BRCA1*-related HBC subset.[84,97-100] This result has been confirmed in all subsequent studies of *BRCA1* HBCs

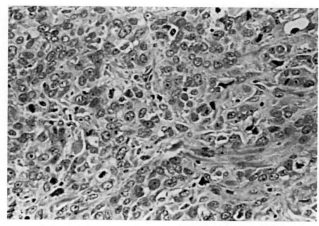

Figure 21-14 "No special type" (ductal) carcinoma with a high mitotic grade. Increased tumor cell proliferative rates are characteristic of *BRCA1* hereditary breast cancer. (×375.)

(Table 21-2).[101-105] The early claim that the high mitotic grade segregates with mutations in the two terminus regions of the gene[106] has not been confirmed by other groups,[104,107,108] including ours. In addition to mitotic grade, tubular and nuclear, and overall grades also are increased in *BRCA1* HBC (Table 21-3; and see Table 21-2). In the Breast Cancer Linkage Consortium[101] database, for example, 66% of *BRCA1* HBCs are high overall grade, compared with 36% for age-matched controls with sporadic breast cancer (*P** < 0.00001).

The excess of medullary and atypical medullary carcinomas, which had long been observed in the Creighton HBC cases,[88] was assigned by the authors to the *BRCA1* subset shortly after the gene was isolated.[97,99,100] This result was confirmed by the Breast Cancer Linkage Consortium[101] and other groups (see Table 21-2).[105,109-112] Like HBC, medullary carcinoma is more common in early-onset breast cancer,[84] but the excess of medullary and atypical medullary carcinoma in *BRCA1* HBC as compared with sporadic breast cancer is independent of this age covariate.[97,101,105,112] In one study of 139 *BRCA1* HBCs, the excess of medullary carcinoma is striking—35.3% versus 3.4% in age-matched control non-*BRCA1* breast cancers (*P* < 10^{-12}).[105] Compared with 101 sporadic breast cancers[99] or with *BRCA2* HBC (see Table 21-3), *BRCA1* HBC shows significantly more of a superfamily of types that we term "medullary group" carcinomas (medullary, atypical medullary, and NST with medullary features). These have in common a heavy infiltration of lymphocytes and plasma cells in the tumor stroma and often pushing borders, which are prominent features of *BRCA1* HBCs.[101,103,113,114]

We have also found a deficit in low-grade special type carcinomas that we call "tubular-lobular group," or TLG, carcinomas, comprised of lobular, tubulolobular, tubular, and invasive cribriform types (Fig. 21-15; and see Tables 21-2 and 21-3). These special types were considered together (see Marcus and colleagues[100] and references therein) because they share certain histologic features (including the hybrid type, tubulolobular), secretory properties, epidemiologic risk factors, an association with family history in earlier reports, and

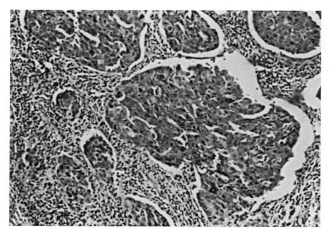

Figure 21-13 Medullary breast carcinoma in a 24-year-old woman who, 1 year later, developed a "no special type" carcinoma in the contralateral breast. Note the expansive islands of large tumor cells with intervening stroma filled with lymphocytes. Medullary and atypical medullary carcinomas are common in *BRCA1* hereditary breast cancer. (×125.)

TABLE 21-2

Pathobiologic Characteristics of *BRCA1* and *BRCA2* Compared with Nonhereditary Breast Cancers: Literature Summary*

Characteristic	BRCA1	BRCA2	non-BRCA1/ BRCA2	References
Histologic Type				
Medullary and atypical medullary	↑	↔?	↔	97,99–101,105,109–113
Lobular and variants	↓	↑?	↔	BRCA1: 97 BRCA2: 105,109,111–113
Tubular-lobular group	↓	↑?	?	97,99,105[†]
Primary DCIS	↓	?	?	105,113,163,164,166
Any DCIS	↓	↔	↔?	97,100,101,113,144,166,167
Any lobular carinoma in situ	↓	↔?	↔	99,101
Histologic Grade				
Total	↑	↔?	↓	79,97,99–102,104,105,107,109,111–113,118,153,154,167
Tubular	↑	↑	↔	97,99,101–103,113,144
Nuclear	↑	↔?	↓	BRCA1: 102 BRCA1 and BRCA2: 101,113
Mitotic	↑	↔?	↓	97,99–104,113
DNA Cytometry				
Diploidy	↓	↔	?	97,99,100,107[†]
Nondiploid S-phase fraction	↑	↔	?	97,99,100,107[†]
Protein Markers				
Estrogen receptor	↓	↔	↔	82,104,105,107,111,112,117–119, 144,148–150,153, 154,167
Progesterone receptor	↓	↔	↔ ↑ ?	82,104,105,107,112,117,144,149,150,153,154,167
p53	↑	↔	↔ ↓	104,111,116–120,144,153,154
HER2/*neu*	↓	↔	↔ ↓	107,111,117,118,144,153
Gene Expression				
Basal-like	↑	↓ #	↔	124–126,136,153,154
Luminal-like	↓	↑ #	↑	136,144,154

DCIS, ductal carcinoma in situ.
*Symbols in columns 2 to 4 indicate increased (↑), decreased (↓), or similar (↔) incidence of a characteristic as compared with nonhereditary breast cancer. "?" indicates nonunanimity in the literature and evidence for possible syndrome heterogeneity. "#" indicates a tentative result.
[†]See also data in Table 21-3.

in the case of lobular carcinoma, a virtual lack of somatic alteration at the 17q *BRCA1* site and more microsatellite instability, in contrast to ductal carcinomas. The deficit in TLG carcinomas in *BRCA1* HBC has been confirmed by other groups.[105,112] In the investigation of Brekelmans and coworkers,[112] only 3.6% of 165 *BRCA1* HBCs were lobular type, compared with 10.4% of 759 age-matched non-HBC control cases (*P** = 0.001).

As further evidence for a proliferative phenotype, we found that a high DNA S-phase fraction originally observed in the whole HBC cohort[115] was confined to the *BRCA1* subset.[84,97,99] Jóhannsson and colleagues[107] have confirmed this observation (see Table 21-2). The Creighton data also showed that *BRCA1* HBC is more prevalently aneuploid than non-HBC (see Table 21-3) and that the average aneuploid DNA index (DI) is less compared with non-HBC (age-adjusted OR = 4.89 for DI < 1.7, *P* = 0.0078).[97] The tumor suppressor protein p53 is more frequently increased in *BRCA1* breast cancers compared with sporadic breast cancers,[104,116–118]

BRCA2 HBC,[119] and non-*BRCA1* and *BRCA2* breast cancers.[111] This had been observed earlier in the Creighton breast-ovary HBC family cases,[120] most of which were later identified as *BRCA1* HBC. Overexpression of p53, almost always the result of a mutation in the *TP53* gene, has been observed in general in highly proliferating breast carcinomas.[121] The *TP53* mutations in *BRCA1* and *BRCA2* breast cancers are unusual in that most of them are not in usual "hotspots," and they are distributed in a region of the protein on the opposite side of its DNA-binding surface.[122]

Based on patterns of gene expression measured by DNA microarrays, breast cancers[123,124] can be subdivided into five basic expression profiles: basal-like, HER/2-overexpressing, luminal A, luminal B, and normal breast tissue-like.[125] Most *BRCA1* HBCs fall into the basal-like group, alluded to earlier, so-called because its phenotype parallels that of the myoepithelial, or "basal," stem cell of the non-neoplastic breast duct, rather than the luminal-like phenotypes (see

TABLE 21-3

BRCA1 vs. BRCA2 Hereditary Breast Cancer: The Creighton University Series*

	BRCA1	BRCA2	P†
Number of families with pathology assessment	29	10	
Number of invasive carcinomas in females	108‡	37‡	
Clinical Features			
Age of onset (mean ± SD) (yr)	42.9±12.6	49.1±12.3	0.011
Bilateral cases	34 (31.5%)	8 (21.6%)	0.30
Male cases (excluded)	2	2	
Tumor size (mean ± SD) (cm)	2.1±1.3	1.8±1.2	0.25
Lymph node-positive cases	30 (31.9%)	12 (50%)	0.15
Pathologic Types and Features			
Medullary group (medullary, atypical medullary, ductal with medullary features)	43 (40.6%)	4 (12.5%)	0.003
Tubular-lobular group (lobular, tubulolobular, tubular, cribiform special types and variants)	14 (13.2%)	15 (46.9%)	0.0001
Any DCIS	31 (28.7%)	20 (54%)	0.009
Any LCIS	2 (1.9%)	5 (13.5%)	0.012
Any lobular neoplasia (LCIS–positive atypical lobular hyperplasia)	3 (2.5%)	11 (29.7%)	<0.0001
Mononuclear cell infiltration absent	3 (9.4%)	9 (27.5%)	0.019
Pathologic Grades			
Mitotic grade 3	43 (53.1%)	6 (25%)	0.020
Nuclear grade 3	45 (55.1%)	2 (8.3%)	<0.0005
Tubular grade 3	72 (88.9%)	19 (79.2%)	0.30
Final grade 3	39 (56.5%)	4 (21.1%)	0.009
DNA Cytometry			
Diploid	10 (14.9%)	10 (50%)	0.002
Nondiploid	57 (85.1%)	10 (50%)	
S-phase fraction, diploids (mean ± SD, %)	2.78 ± 1.73 $n = 10$	3.53 ± 1.73 $n = 10$	0.48
S-phase fraction, nondiploids (mean ± SD, %)	15.77 ± 6.82 $n = 56$	7.36 ± 4.87 $n = 10$	<0.0005

DCIS, ductal carcinoma in situ; LCIS, lobular carcinoma in situ.
*Data presented at Department of Defense Era of Hope Breast Cancer Research Program Meeting, Atlanta, Georgia, June 8–11, 2000. Supported by U.S. Army grant award DAMD17-97-1-7112.
†Fisher's exact test for 2 × 2 tables or 2-tailed Student t-test for means and standard errors of the means (SDs).
‡The numbers of cases simultaneously reviewed by the project pathologists (J.N. Marcus and D.L. Page). The denominators implicit from the percent figures that follow are sometimes less than these totals if not every tumor was available for assessment of a given feature.

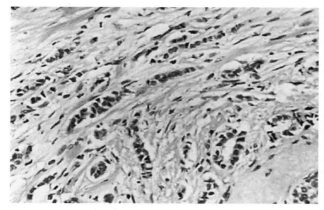

Figure 21-15 Invasive tubulolobular (TLG) breast carcinoma. Note that the cancer cells form single "Indian files" such as lobular carcinoma and tubules such as tubular carcinoma. This histologic type is a member of the so-called TLG group that includes lobular, tubular, and cribiform carcinoma. TLG carcinomas are decreased in BRCA1 hereditary breast cancers (HBCs) and possibly increased in BRCA2 HBCs. (×400.)

Table 21-2).[124,125] Basal-like breast cancers are characterized by the expression of basal cytokeratins 5/6 and 14[126] and P-cadherin, among other markers.[114] Most studies find BRCA1 HBCs to be negative for ER, PR, and HER2/neu oncogene amplification and overexpression.[105,107,117,119] This so-called "triple negative" phenotype (see Table 21-2) is characteristic of BRCA1 HBCs and of the basal phenotype.[114,127] Moreover, medullary carcinomas[128] and carcinomas with medullary features,[129] which are such integral components of BRCA1 HBC pathology (see Tables 21-2 and 21-3), display the basal-like phenotype.

All of the evidence thus indicates a remarkable proliferative phenotype in BRCA1 breast cancers, and high proliferation rates are a characteristic of the OCs in the Creighton families with breast-ovary (and mostly BRCA1) HBC as well.[130] The distinctive pathobiology of BRCA1 HBC can be understood in context with a model of tumor genetic evolution. In the model,[131,132] intermediate and transformed cells suffer small losses or gains of chromosomal material while remaining near diploid in DNA content (DI $\cong$ 1). At some point the chromosome complement endoreduplicates to near-tetraploidy (DI $\cong$ 2), with continuing and more severe segmental or complete chromosomal loss, which progressively lessens the DI. In this scenario, hyperdiploid breast cancers with $1.3 \leq DI \leq 1.7$, higher S-phase fractions, [TP53] mutations, and increased chromosomal gains and losses are among the most "evolved."[133–136] The BRCA1 phenotype—aneuploidy, lower aneuploid DI,[97,99,100] high proliferation, and p53 overexpression (see Tables 21-2 and 21-3)—fits the profile of a genetically evolved tumor. To evolve genetically, the target cell must proliferate. In the model, the BRCA1 mutation would put the intermediate target cell[137,138] on a fast track of increased or unregulated proliferation, beginning near the time of menarche. At transformation, the intrinsic high proliferation rate is locked in to the tumor as a fossil phenotype of the intermediate cell.[139] The BRCA1 protein fulfills the role required in this model. When mutated, its well-established antiproliferative function[140–142] is lost, which sends the target cells into unregulated proliferation.

Liu and colleagues[127] have established that in addition to its role as a check on cell proliferation, functioning BRCA1 protein is also required for the differentiation of the ER-negative progenitor basal stem cell into ER-positive luminal cells. In mutation carriers, the authors observed whole breast lobules that have lost heterozygosity for BRCA1 and manifest no ER expression, whereas adjacent lobules without loss of heterozygosity do. These same defective lobules display only basal phenotype markers, indicating loss of maturation. Interestingly, the two types of lobules appear histologically indistinguishable. In effect, Liu and coworkers have directly observed the putative BRCA1 tumor progenitor cell, which bears the same ER-negative basal phenotype as the breast cancers that arise from it.

BRCA2 Hereditary Breast Cancer Phenotype

The BRCA2 HBC phenotype is less well determined than that of BRCA1 HBC because there are fewer cases and probably greater intrinsic heterogeneity, leading to less concordance in the literature. Most studies agree that the age of onset is significantly greater than in BRCA1 HBC (see Table 21-3) but still considerably less than in non-HBC. All studies agree that there is a lesser propensity for the NST (ductal) carcinomas to form tubules (see Table 21-3), as in BRCA1 HBC. The pathologists in the blinded Creighton studies[97,99,100] have made special efforts to not underdiagnose the TLG carcinomas. They find that TLG group carcinoma is a powerful discriminator between BRCA1 and BRCA2 HBC, scarce in the former but prevalent in the latter (see Table 21-3). Consistent with this result, Armes and colleagues[109] also find increased lobular carcinoma in BRCA2 HBC, but other groups do not,[101,111,112,143,144] for reasons that may relate to differing diagnostic thresholds or to intrinsic differences in the data sets.

The Breast Cancer Linkage Consortium[101] claims a higher grade for BRCA2 HBC than for age-matched non-HBC controls, but this result is questionable. Higher nuclear, mitotic, and total grades are not seen in the large Creighton data set displayed in Table 21-3, and higher total grades are not seen in most other studies.[79,104,109,111,112,118,125] The problem is that the Consortium BRCA2 pathology data set is dominated by the Icelandic founder 999del5 mutation, which comprises nearly half (49%) of its cases. The pathology associated with this mutation, reported in a separate publication by non-Consortium pathologists,[143] is remarkable for very high grades that do not appear typical of the non-999del5 BRCA2 cases in other data sets. Because the Consortium cases are so heavily weighted with this specific mutation, its overall results may be skewed toward higher grade. Thus, despite its large size, the Consortium data base may not be representative of BRCA2 HBC at large. In a similar vein, Bane and colleagues[144] report higher nuclear, mitotic, and total grades in BRCA2 HBC compared with age-matched SBC controls, but in their large series, the Ashkenazi 6174delT mutation comprises 30.4% of their BRCA2 cases.[145] There are no definitive data on potential pathology grade differences between BRCA2 breast cancers with this specific mutation and those without it, but the fact that all five 6174delT BRCA2 cases in one early study were high grade[146] raises concern that the data set presented by Bane and colleagues[144] could also be skewed toward higher grades. Certainly BRCA2 HBC is known to be heterogeneous. In addition to the high grade associated with 999del5, the positions of mutations on the gene modulate the relative frequencies of ovarian, pancreatic, and male breast cancer in the syndrome.[147]

The DNA cytometric characteristics of BRCA2 HBC differ from those of BRCA1 HBC (see Table 21-3); there is lesser aneuploidy and a lower mean aneuploid S-phase fraction, which is more in line with the characteristics of non-HBC (see Table 21-3). ER, PR, p53, and HER2/neu proteins also appear to be generally expressed at levels comparable to those in non-HBC (see Table 21-2),[104,107,111,112,116–118,120,144,148–150] although two studies[112,144] find more cases positive for ER. A recent report[119] suggests that cyclin D1 cell cycle protein is expressed in most BRCA2 HBCs (11/15 = 73%), compared with 12/21 (57%) in non-BRCA1 and 2 HBCs ($P = 0.029$) and near absence in BRCA1 HBCs (1/20 = 5%, $P* = 0.00003$). However, a larger study[144] finds no difference in cyclin D1 expression between BRCA2 HBC and non-BRCA1 or BRCA2 HBC.

Sorlie and colleagues[125] note that the two BRCA2 cases in the data set of van't Veer and colleagues[124] are luminal A in phenotype. Of 16 BRCA2 cases, Melchor and coworkers[136] report 2 luminal A, 6 luminal B, 5 unclassified, and only 3 basal-like phenotypes. Compared to age-matched noncarriers, Bane and colleagues[144] find a slight increase in luminal phenotype and a slight decrease in basal-like phenotype in BRCA2 HBCs, using cytokeratin 5 as a basal-like marker, and ER-positive cytokeratins 8/18 as a luminal phenotype markers. These results are treated as preliminary ("#") in Table 21-2 because as yet there are no other such comparative studies.

Non-BRCA1 and BRCA2 Hereditary Breast Cancer Phenotypes

Estimates of the prevalence of HBC due to mutations in genes other than *BRCA1* or *BRCA2* range from 16% in the Breast Cancer Linkage Consortium database[151] to as high as 84%.[9] Such wide variance surely relates to differences in population selection criteria and stringency of the definition of family risk. Using the relatively stringent definition of HBC given earlier in this chapter, and accepting estimates of the prevalences of *BRCA1* and *BRCA2* mutations in breast cancer cases as 2.4% and 2.3% in a recent population-based study,[152] we believe that the fraction of non-*BRCA1* and *BRCA2* HBC cases is closer to 50%. Keeping in mind the heterogeneity in definitional criteria, non-*BRCA1* and *BRCA2* HBCs have been investigated as an agglomerated, "generic" group in comparison with age-matched controls with sporadic breast cancer. These studies find no difference in the incidences of either medullary/atypical medullary or lobular and lobular variant special type carcinomas,[111–113] lower histologic grade,[111–113,153,154] particularly the nuclear (OR = 0.26, P = 0.0002) and mitotic (OR = 0.33, P = 0.003) grades,[113] and either the same[153] or statistically insignificantly increased[112] ER and PR expression (see Table 21-2). Reinforcing the finding of lower grades, Ki-67 proliferation index is less.[153] Expression of *p53* is decreased in two studies,[153,154] and is the same as in the controls in another.[111] HER-2 as assayed by gene amplification is less than in age-matched controls with sporadic breast cancer,[153] but variously decreased[153] or the same[154] as measured by protein overexpression. Unlike *BRCA1* HBC and like *BRCA2* HBC, non-*BRCA1* or *BRCA2* HBC has no increase in the "basal-like" phenotype as defined by P-cadherin[153] or basal cytokeratin 5/14 expression[126] (see Table 21-2). Rather, Honrado and colleagues[154] find that the gene expression profile distributes into all five of the breast cancer subtypes, in proportions similar to those in sporadic breast cancer, leading them to conclude that "familial non-*BRCA1/2* tumors are heterogeneous" and suggest "a polygenic model for explaining the majority of BRCAX families," rather than a single undiscovered major HBC predisposition gene.

A small subset of non-*BRCA1* and *BRCA2* HBCs results from mutations in other known genes, leading to a predisposition to lobular carcinoma in two examples. Germline mutations in the CDH1 (E-cadherin) gene confer a 40% to 70% lifetime risk of hereditary diffuse gastric carcinoma, and a 39% to 52% lifetime risk of invasive lobular breast carcinoma in female carriers.[155–158] CDH1 codes for the E-cadherin cell adhesion protein, which is lost in sporadic lobular carcinoma of the breast through somatic mutation. Likewise, the specific truncating mutation 1157T in the CHEK2 gene—but interestingly, not other mutations in that gene—results in a six-fold relative risk for developing invasive lobular carcinoma.[159] In contrast, breast cancers occurring in ATM gene variant heterozygotes, who have an increased RR of breast cancer, show no obvious histopathologic differences with sporadic breast cancers in a solitary study limited by its small size (21 heterozygotes with 25 breast cancers).[160] In the case of Li-Fraumeni (SBLA) cancer syndrome, involving germline mutations in *TP53*, the first gene to be associated with hereditary risk of breast cancer, the histopathologic characteristics of the breast cancers have not been elucidated.

Less in Situ Carcinoma in BRCA1 Hereditary Breast Cancer than in BRCA2 Hereditary Breast Cancer, Non-BRCA1 and BRCA2 Hereditary Breast Cancer, and Nonhereditary Breast Cancer

Some studies have reported fewer cases of in situ carcinoma in "BRCA" carriers,[48,161,162] combining *BRCA1* and *BRCA2* HBC into one group as though they were the same syndrome. This "apples-oranges" approach is problematic at best and misleading at worst. When carefully separated into *BRCA1* and *BRCA2* carrier status, striking differences emerge in the incidence of in situ carcinoma.

Soon after the *BRCA1* and *BRCA2* genes were discovered, the incidence of primary ductal carcinoma in situ (DCIS) was independently reported to be significantly less in *BRCA1* mutation carriers than in noncarriers followed at Creighton University[163] and in France.[164] At the same time, large studies at Creighton University and by Breast Cancer Linkage Consortium in Europe reported significant deficits of any primary or accompanying DCIS or LCIS in *BRCA1* HBC in comparison with *BRCA2* HBC and non-HBC (see Tables 21-2 and 21-3).[97,100,101] These findings have held up in more recent studies by other groups. Of 369 unselected cases of primary DCIS cases in Connecticut, 3 *BRCA1* and 9 *BRCA2* mutations were found (0.8% and 2.4%, respectively).[165] The authors did not analyze the difference, but when compared with the numbers of cases with *BRCA1* and *BRCA2* mutations in the Myriad Genetics data set in 2002 (689 and 440, respectively),[48] we compute that the trend in this study for less DCIS in *BRCA1* carriers than in *BRCA2* carriers reaches formal statistical significance ($P*$ = 0.025). Lubinski and coworkers[105] find marginally less primary DCIS in Polish *BRCA1* carriers than in noncarriers, 4/139 (2.9%) versus 11/147 (7.5%; P = 0.07). In a study at the Nottingham Breast Institute by Hamilton and colleagues,[166] there were no (0%) primary DCIS diagnoses in 20 *BRCA1* carriers, compared with 4 (36%) in 11 *BRCA2* carriers ($P*$ = 0.010). The invasive carcinomas had a DCIS component in 2 (10%) *BRCA1* carriers, compared with 3 (27%) *BRCA2* carriers ($P*$ = 0.32) and 24 (44%) of 54 age-matched sporadic controls ($P*$ = 0.006). When scored for the presence of any DCIS there were only the 2 (10%) occurrences in *BRCA1* carriers compared with 7 (64%) in the *BRCA2* carriers ($P*$ = 0.003). Similarly, in French women 46 years of age or less, Bonadona and colleagues[167] find significantly less accompanying DCIS in the breast cancers of *BRCA1* mutation carriers (4/10 = 40%) than in noncarriers (137/169 = 81%; $P*$ = 0.0072).

The study by Hamilton and colleagues[166] is of special interest because it correlates the pathology to mammography findings. Microcalcifications were the predominant mammographic feature in 8 of the 11 (73%) *BRCA2* breast cancers, but in only 2 of 18 (12%) *BRCA1* breast cancers, again a striking difference (*P* = 0.0007). The radiology and pathology findings in *BRCA2* breast cancers are thus quite concordant, because microcalcification is a prominent feature of DCIS. At the same time, only 4 of 11 (36%) *BRCA2* breast cancers mammographically presented predominantly as a mass, compared to 13 of 18 (73%) *BRCA1* breast cancers, but the difference in these small samples was not statistically significant (*P** = 0.12). In another pathology-radiology study,[168] which used clinical breast examination, mammography, ultrasound, and MRI to screen *BRCA* gene mutation carriers, all of the DCIS cases were detected in *BRCA2* gene carriers, and comprised the majority (6/11) of the *BRCA2* breast cancers. None of the 11 breast cancers detected in *BRCA1* carriers were DCIS (*P** = 0.012). The authors write: "Mammography appears to be a valuable adjunct to MRI for *BRCA2* carriers because of the high incidence of DCIS in this subgroup."[168]

Most studies report that the incidence of DCIS (and LCIS) accompanying the invasive breast cancers in *BRCA2* mutation carriers is about the same as in non-HBC (see Table 21-2).[101,144,166] However, the incidence of primary DCIS in *BRCA2* mutation carriers, in formal comparison with sporadic breast cancer age-matched controls, is currently unknown (see Table 21-2), even if two of the studies[166,168] previously cited anecdotally suggest that it may be quite common. In Poland, the missense *BRCA2* mutation variant C5972T predisposes to DCIS accompanied by microinvasive carcinoma.[169] In the Creighton *BRCA2* HBC data set, there is prevalent lobular neoplasia, defined as LCIS or atypical lobular hyperplasia (Fig. 21-16).[100] In one *BRCA2* HBC family, 10 of 13 invasive breast carcinomas were accompanied by lobular neoplasia. Of interest, TLG carcinomas have a high prevalence of lobular neoplasia (see Marcus and colleagues[100] and references therein). As seen in Tables 21-2 and 21-3, lobular and TLG carcinomas and lobular neoplasia appear to coordinately discriminate the *BRCA1* and *BRCA2* HBC subsets.

Little has been reported about in-situ carcinoma in non-*BRCA1* or *BRCA2* HBC. Lakhani and coworkers[113]

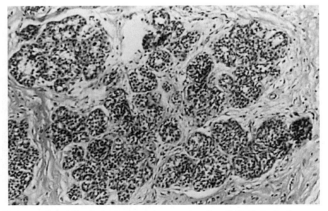

Figure 21-16 Lobular carcinoma in situ (LCIS). Lobular neoplasia (LCIS and atypical lobular hyperplasia) is prevalent in affected members of this *BRCA2* family. (×200.)

have found a nonsignificant trend for less primary or accompanying DCIS (OR = 0.69, *P* = 0.10), and no difference in primary or accompanying LCIS, as compared to SBC controls. The incidence of primary DCIS compared to SBC controls is unknown (see Table 21-2).

CLINICAL IMPLICATIONS OF *BRCA1* AND *BRCA2* HEREDITARY BREAST CANCER PATHOPHENOTYPES

The decreased ER and PR expression suggests that *BRCA1* breast cancer generally will not respond as well to therapy with hormone receptor modulators such as tamoxifen when compared with its *BRCA2* counterpart. However, we and others have cautioned[170,171] that this supposition should not preclude consideration of such therapy in chemoprevention trials, for there is no evidence that the pretransformed target intermediate cell lacks receptors. Indeed, as noted elsewhere in this chapter, tamoxifen appears to significantly reduce the risk of bilateral breast cancer in *BRCA1* carriers and may well do so in *BRCA2* carriers as well.[35]

The prognosis of *BRCA1* HBC has been a matter of ongoing debate. The issue is important because it weighs in the decisions on prophylactic therapies. Most studies find no significant differences in survival in comparison with non-HBC,[99,112,150,167,170,172–174] but better[175] and worse[82,167,176,177] outcomes have also been reported. Methodologic differences may account in part for the variability in results.[178] Why the prognosis of *BRCA1*-related HBC, with its adverse pathology markers, would be no worse than non-HBC is a conundrum that is deepened by the observation that in the Creighton families, *BRCA1*-related HBC cases fare better than non-*BRCA1*–related HBC cases, which have neutral pathology indicators.[99,170] But there are clues that *BRCA1* HBC is not an ordinary high-grade breast cancer. As we have seen, it does not overexpress HER-2/*neu*, a marker of poor prognosis,[107,117] and a high proportion are medullary carcinomas,[97,99–101,105,109–112] which in pure forms are prognostically favorable, despite their otherwise prognostically adverse high mitotic and nuclear grades[179] and basal-like phenotype.[125,128,129] Basal-like breast cancers have markedly poor disease-free and overall survivals.[125] However, medullary carcinoma is a subtype of the basal-like breast cancer that expresses genes related to immune reaction and apoptosis.[180] These features may then ameliorate the bad prognostic characteristics of the basal-like phenotype and account for why the prognosis of *BRCA1* HBC is not as bad as it could be. Another ameliorating prognostic factor might be the genetic instability in *BRCA1* HBC—manifested by the prevalent aneuploidy, low aneuploid DI, and increased p53 expression described previously—which could confer increased genomic fragility and possibly increased susceptibility to chemotherapy and radiation therapy. These observations and questions point to directions for future investigation.

Less is known about the prognosis of *BRCA2* and non-*BRCA1* and *BRCA2* HBC. The best available evidence from several studies is that survivals probably do not differ significantly among *BRCA1*, *BRCA2*, non-BRCA1 and BRCA2 HBC, and non-HBC groups when adjusted for other variables such as stage.[112,167,181]

Recurrence at the biopsy site is a frequent complication of inadequately excised DCIS. The lesser prevalence of DCIS in BRCA1 HBC in comparison with non-BRCA1 HBC and sporadic breast cancer could reasonably prompt more serious consideration of conservation therapy in BRCA1 mutation carriers than in these other groups.[164]

The pathobiologic features of BRCA1 and BRCA2 HBC summarized in Tables 21-2 and 21-3 offer some clues as to whether a patient in a family untested for the genes may lie in one or another syndrome, and various authors have offered algorithms to increase the accuracy of syndrome prediction.[117,182–184] However, these should not be regarded as sufficiently sensitive and specific to serve as a substitute for syndrome identification by direct genetic testing for germline mutations. Molecular genetic approaches to the classification of breast cancer are progressing,[123,125] and these hold great promise for the diagnosis of HBC syndromes.

RADIATION SENSITIVITY IN *BRCA1* AND *BRCA2* MUTATION CARRIERS[185–197]

The BRCA1 and BRCA2 genes function in several important cellular pathways, including (1) mediating the cellular response to DNA damage, (2) as a cell cycle checkpoint protein, and (3) in the regulation of transcription.[37,191] Of clinical[197] concern is the substantial evidence that BRCA1 and BRCA2 are key components of the repair pathway for double stranded DNA breaks, a form of damage induced by ionizing radiation. The main scenarios in which to consider the potential clinical impact of impaired DNA repair function are (1) low-dose exposure to ionizing radiation from screening mammography, particularly in young, high-risk women, and (2) the effect of radiotherapy in BRCA carriers with breast cancer who opt for breast-conserving therapy (BCT) (lumpectomy plus radiation) instead of mastectomy.

There is considerable biologic plausibility to support the concern that radiation from screening and diagnostic procedures may pose additional risks to BRCA1 and BRCA2 mutation carriers. BRCA1 associates in nuclear dots with Rad51, which mediates the repair of double-stranded DNA breaks.[193] The RAD51 gene has a single nucleotide polymorphism that increases the risk of breast but not OC in carriers of BRCA2 mutations.[198] BRCA1 is phosphorylated by the ATM (ataxia telangiectasia–mutated) protein kinase in response to DNA damage induced by gamma radiation. Epidemiologic evidence has suggested that ATM heterozygotes, who comprise about 1% of the population, may be at increased risk of breast cancer,[195] a theory supported by some but not all molecular studies.[187] Furthermore, Brca2-deficient mouse embryos are acutely sensitive to ionizing radiation.[194] In surviving Brca2-deficient mice with partial gene function, repair of double-stranded DNA is impaired.[189] The extreme sensitivity of human BRCA2-deficient cancer cells to agents that cause double-stranded DNA breaks[185] may ultimately serve as a specific molecular target for genotype-based therapy in mutation carriers.[186] Radiation sensitization may also be a viable strategy.[188]

It is difficult to predict the clinical impact of basic research findings. On the one hand, radiation exposure could induce mutations that accumulate because of limited repair function, inducing a higher rate of cancer. On the other hand, radiation-induced damage could induce programmed cell death (apoptosis), limiting the potential for invasive cancer to develop. Although basic research helps frame the relevant clinical questions, medical decision making must be based on clinical studies on BRCA carriers.

There are no prospective controlled trials assessing the possible adverse effects of radiation from mammography screening in BRCA carriers. However, a retrospective cohort study of 1601 female BRCA1 or BRCA2 mutation carriers found an increased risk of breast cancer (hazard ratio [HR] = 1.54, $P = 0.007$) for women with any reported exposure to chest x-rays. This risk was particularly pronounced in women exposed only before 20 years of age (HR = 4.64, $P < 0.001$).[39] In a case-control study of 1600 BRCA1 or BRCA2 mutation carriers and an equal number of matched controls, no association was found between screening mammography and risk of breast cancer, although a subgroup analysis showed a slight increase in risk of breast cancer before 40 years of age for women who initiated screening between 31 and 40 years of age (multivariate OR 1.56 [95% CI = 1.07–2.27], $P = 0.02$).[40] Although breast MRI surveillance is an appealing surveillance technique in that there are no associated risks from radiation, as of yet there is insufficient evidence to replace screening mammography with breast MRI.[199] The hypothetical sequelae[190] must be balanced against the need for surveillance in high-risk individuals and the emerging evidence that mammographic screening is valuable.[38] Nevertheless, alternating mammography with MRI at 6-month intervals is a reasonable consideration.

BCT and the potential consequences of radiation have been explored by Pierce and colleagues[192] and Turner and associates.[196] Pierce and colleagues[192] compared rates of radiation-associated complications, in-breast tumor recurrence, and distant relapse in 71 women with BRCA1 or BRCA2 mutations treated with BCT using radiation therapy with rates observed in 213 matched controls with sporadic breast cancer. Comparable rates of tumor control and 5-year survival rates were observed among the sporadic and germline cases, providing reassurance regarding the safety of administering radiation therapy to germline BRCA1 or BRCA2 mutation carriers. BRCA1 and BRCA2 carriers do not appear to be susceptible to acute or late radiation toxicities. In a study of 55 BRCA carriers at four centers, with median follow-up of 6.75 years for carriers and 7.75 years for controls, no increase in radiation toxicity was observed, including late effects such as rib fractures, lung fibrosis, tissue necrosis, or pericarditis.[200]

Turner and associates[196] examined the rate of ipsilateral breast tumor recurrence (IBTR) in BRCA mutation carriers by estimating the frequency of BRCA1 and BRCA2 mutations in breast cancer patients with IBTR treated with

BCT. Among 52 patients with IBTR, 8 (15%) had deleterious *BRCA1 and BRCA2* mutations, compared with 6.6% of matched control patients without IBTR (*P* = 0.03). The median time to IBTR for mutation carriers was prolonged (7.8 years) compared with noncarriers (4.7 years; *P* = 0.03). Considering the long time to recurrence, as well as histologic and clinical criteria, IBTRs in mutation carriers were interpreted as representing new primary breast cancers. These data suggest that radiation therapy is effective in treating primary breast cancers and highlight the risk of second primaries in *BRCA* mutation carriers, which may be best addressed at the time of initial diagnosis, if not before. However, the possible role of radiation in inducing second primary breast cancers is raised by the high rate of late IBTRs observed in the study. If so, the radiation therapist and medical oncologist must then become concerned about recommendations for lumpectomy followed by radiation therapy. It is clear that molecular genetic discoveries in HBC and their clinical implications have barely begun to be translated to patient care.

BREAST CANCER IN *BRCA* MALES

Tai and associates[201] note that men who harbor mutations in the *BRCA2* gene have an increased risk of breast carcinoma when compared to men in the general population. They have found that men with a *BRCA1* gene mutation may also show a higher risk of developing carcinoma of the breast; however, this risk is lower than that for *BRCA2* mutation carrier males.

They confirm data for 1939 families in which 97 males with breast cancer were evaluated. When considering all ages, cumulative risks of male breast cancer were increased in both *BRCA1* and *BRCA2* mutation carriers when compared to noncarriers. Specifically, the RR for breast cancer was highest for men in their 30s and 40s, which decreased with increasing age. The relative and cumulative risks were higher for those males with *BRCA2* mutations than for their counterparts with *BRCA1* mutations.

> The estimated cumulative risk of breast carcinoma for male *BRCA1* mutation carriers at age 70 years was 1.2% (95% confidence interval [CI] = 0.22% to 2.8%) and for *BRCA2* mutation carriers, 6.8% (95% CI = 3.2% to 12%).[201]

PROSTATE CANCER IN *BRCA* MALES

Rosen and colleagues[202] have described the possible etiologic relationship between *BRCA1* and prostate cancer. In their review, they found that a positive family history of prostate cancer confers an approximate two- to three-fold greater risk of prostate cancer to first-degree relatives of affected men as opposed to men without a family history.[203–205] Rosen and colleagues[202] suggested that only a minority (<10%) of patients with prostate cancer are clearly familial in origin.[206] Their review[202] disclosed that certain epidemiologic studies documented a statistically significant linkage between prostate cancers and other tumor types such as carcinoma of the breast, ovary, and uterus.[204,207–210] In one

such study[207] involving 143 families with three or more cases of OC, males showed a 4.5-fold increase in the RR of prostate cancer while females had a 2.5-fold increased risk of breast cancer and a 5-fold higher risk of uterine cancer.[208]

In the case of *BRCA1* and *BRCA2* mutations, investigators have shown an association between these mutations and prostate cancer in male probands and in these settings the prostate cancers occurred at a younger age than in their sporadic counterparts. In the case of Ashkenazi Jews, a population-based study involving two *BRCA1* founder mutations (185delAG and 5382insC) showed an increased lifetime risk of prostate cancer.[211] Carriers of these mutations harbored risk estimates of 20% occurrence of prostate cancer by 70 years of age and 35% by 80 years of age when compared with 5% and 10%, respectively, for noncarriers. An increased proportion of *BRCA1* and *BRCA2* mutation carriers had a family history of prostate cancer in first-degree relatives (14%) compared with noncarriers (8%; *P* < 0.01).

Rosen and colleagues[202] suggest that genetic linkage studies support "...the existence of a prostate tumor suppressor gene located on chromosome 17q at or near the *BRCA1* locus (D17S855-D17S856)." Other studies[212–214] support these findings. Allelic loss at this location was observed in about 25% to 50% of localized prostate cancer cases in these studies. Furthermore, fragments of normal chromosomal region 17q that include the *BRCA1* gene inhibited tumorigenicity of a human prostate cancer cell line.[215] A further analysis of sporadic localized prostate cancers suggests the existence of a second prostate tumor suppressor gene on chromosome 17q distal to *BRCA1*.[216]

Prostate cancer was the most common cancer type following carcinoma of the breast in seven Icelandic families who were characterized by HBOC.[217] Two of the families showed linkage to *BRCA1*, wherein 44% of the males harboring the putative breast cancer gene alleles had a history of prostate cancer.

Heterogeneity: Multiple Breast Cancer Syndromes

GENOME-WIDE HIGH-DENSITY SINGLE NUCLEOTIDE POLYMORPHISM LINKAGE ANALYSIS OF NON-*BRCA1* AND *BRCA2* BREAST CANCER FAMILIES

Gonzalesz-Neira and associates[218] estimate that approximately 30% of cases of HBC involve *BRCA1* or *BCRA2* mutations. Search for an additional high-risk breast cancer predisposition gene(s), to date, has been unsuccessful. However, these authors[218] used SNP markers for whole-genome screening of 19 non-*BRCA1* or *BRCA2* breast cancer families using 4720 genome-wide SNPs with technology from Illumina, Inc. (San Diego, California). They identified five regions on chromosomes 2, 4, 7, 11, and 14, as candidates to contain breast cancer susceptibility genes. These results clearly indicate the power increase that SNPs can supply in linkage studies.

LOW-PENETRANCE BREAST CANCER SUSCEPTIBILITY MUTATIONS

Meijers-Heijboer and coworkers[4] more recently described a low-penetrant breast cancer susceptibility locus, namely CHEK, which encodes a cell-cycle checkpoint kinase that is implicated in the DNA repair process involving BRCA1 and p53. CHEK2*1100delC is a truncating variant that abrogates the kinase activity. It occurs in 1.1% of healthy individuals and in 5.1% of individuals with breast cancer. This finding is based on the study of 718 families that do not carry mutations in BRCA1 or BRCA2 ($P = 0.00000003$). Interestingly, 15.5% of individuals with breast cancer from families with male breast cancer and no mutations in BRCA1 or BRCA2 harbor CHEK2 ($P = 0.00015$).

It is estimated that the CHEK2*1100delC variant results in an approximate two-fold increase of breast cancer risk in females and an approximate ten-fold increase of risk in males. The variant confers no increased cancer risk in carriers of BRCA1 or BRCA2 mutations.

Weischer and colleagues[219] investigated CHEK2* 1100delC heterozygosity with respect to its increased risk of breast cancer through meta-analysis of 26,000 patient cases and 26,000 controls to determine whether the evidence was sufficient to recommend genotyping for this mutation. Their findings disclosed aggregated odds ratios of

> ...2.7 (95% CI, 2.1 to 3.4) for unselected breast cancer, 2.6 (95% CI, 1.3 to 5.5) for early-onset breast cancer, and 4.8 (95% CI, 3.3 to 7.2) for familial breast cancer. For familial breast cancer, this corresponds to a cumulative risk of breast cancer at age 70 years in CHEK2*1100delC heterozygotes of 37% (95% CI, 25% to 56%)....

CHEK2-related breast cancer risks were compared with risks derived from the meta-analysis of Chen and associates[49] of 57% for BRCA1 mutation carriers and 49% for BRCA2 mutation carriers.

These authors concluded that CHEK2*1100delC is an important breast cancer predisposing gene that they note increases the risk three- to fivefold, which is almost as high as that for BRCA1 and BRCA2 heterozygotes. The authors opined that these findings support genotyping for CHEK2*1100delC and that CHEK2 testing should be considered together with BRCA1 and BRCA2 mutation screening in women who have a family history of breast cancer.

However, an editorial on the subject by Offit and Garber[220] takes a contrary position with respect to available data; they do not believe that there is compelling evidence to justify routine clinical testing for CHEK2*1100delC in order to guide the management of breast cancer–prone families. They point out that although Weischer and colleagues sought to limit their study to population-based ascertainment, their upper band of the risk estimate derives from familial studies. The meta-analysis by Chen and associates includes several population-based studies, so a direct comparison of penetrance estimates may not be reasonable. Furthermore, the issues of phenocopies (individuals in a family who appear to have hereditary cancer but do not carry the familial mutation), variable penetrance, and

multiple susceptibility genes can make the meaning of true positive and true negative tests unclear. Accordingly, it is not yet clear whether an individual who tests negative for a familial CHEK2 mutation faces average cancer risks and should follow routine management guidelines.

An additional class of common low-penetrance susceptibility alleles is beginning to emerge, based on large-scale association studies of candidate genes and genome-wide tag SNP searches.[9] Thus far only seven susceptibility loci have been reported and convincingly confirmed. The reported SNPs may be causal but might instead be in linkage disequilibrium with the causal variant. Not all loci map to regions with known protein-coding genes, leaving open the possibility of susceptibility based on cryptic genetic elements. The magnitude of increased RRs conferred by these susceptibility alleles is very low compared to moderate and high-risk genes and ranges from 1.07 to 1.26. However, the population prevalence is high, ranging from 28% to 87%. Only about 4% of familial risk is attributable to known susceptibility alleles of this kind.

The elucidation of breast cancer susceptibility genes has the potential to improve on current risk prediction methods for individuals as well as populations. Currently identified risk factors can stratify just 62% of individuals into high-risk and low-risk halves of the population. In contrast, a population-based study of breast cancer found that if all susceptibility genes could be identified, then we could efficiently discriminate between low- and high-risk groups, and the half of the population at highest risk would account for 88% of all affected individuals.[7]

SPECIFIC SYNDROMES

Li-Fraumeni Syndrome

Lynch and colleagues[221] described an extended kindred that showed a broad spectrum of cancer: namely, sarcoma, breast cancer and brain tumors, lung and laryngeal cancer, leukemia, lymphoma, and adrenal cortical carcinoma (Li-Fraumeni [SBLA] syndrome). A limited description of the elements of this syndrome previously had been recognized in four nuclear kindreds by Li and Fraumeni,[222] who subsequently published a prospective observation of these families that covered a 12-year time frame (1969 through 1981).[223,224] Of interest[224] was the fact that in 31 surviving family members, 16 additional cancers developed (the expected number was 0.5). Five of these were carcinomas of the breast, four were soft tissue sarcomas, and seven were cancers of other anatomic sites. Eight of the patients had multiple primary cancers. Four cancers occurred at sites of prior radiotherapy (three soft tissue sarcomas and one mesothelioma).

The SBLA syndrome is pertinent to this chapter because of the occurrence of breast cancer (particularly with remarkably early age at onset), as well as recent reports of germ cell tumors of the ovary. The SBLA syndrome is caused by the p53 germline mutation, which, like many cancer-prone genes, gives rise to a spectrum of cancers as a result of its carcinogenic pleiotropic effects.[225,226]

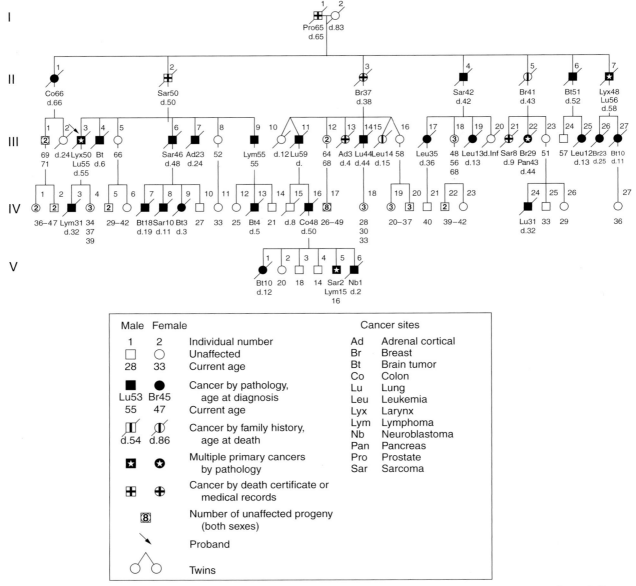

Figure 21-17 An updated pedigree of a Li-Fraumeni (SBLA) syndrome kindred showing cancer occurrences through five generations. (Lynch HT, Mulcahy GM, Harris RE, et al: Genetic and pathologic findings in a kindred with hereditary sarcoma, breast cancer, brain tumors, leukemia, lung, laryngeal, and adrenal cortical carcinoma. Cancer 41:2055–2064, 1978. Copyright 1978 American Cancer Society. Reprinted by permission of Wiley Liss Inc., a subsidiary of John Wiley & Sons, Inc.)

The authors have continued to follow the SBLA syndrome kindred that they first described in 1978 (Fig. 21-17).[221] They republished the pedigree in 1985, when children in the fifth generation began to develop cancer. The father (see Fig. 21-17, IV-16) of these affected children did not have cancer when that study was first published. He was considered to be an obligate gene carrier. Since then, however, he developed colorectal cancer and died from this disease. A further update of this family has been noteworthy for a marked excess of brain tumors.[226]

SBLA is obviously an exceedingly complex syndrome and requires investigation of cancer of all anatomical sites with a vigorous effort to histopathologically verify cancer. Problems in pedigree analysis in the SBLA syndrome are compounded by the fact that in addition to reduced penetrance of the deleterious gene, two age-specific modes of cancer expression are encountered, one in childhood and the second in adult life. Figure 21-18 shows a classical SBLA family with the *p53* pathogenic mutation.

Cowden Disease

Brownstein and associates[227] described in detail a cancer-associated genodermatosis known as Cowden disease. This hereditary disorder, also known as multiple hamartoma syndrome, is inherited as an autosomal dominant trait and is characterized by distinctive mucocutaneous lesions and cancer of the breast, thyroid, and female genitourinary tract.

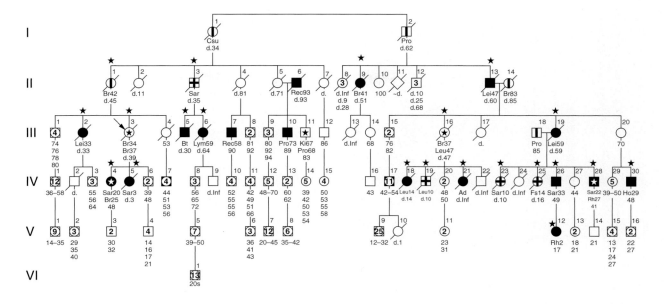

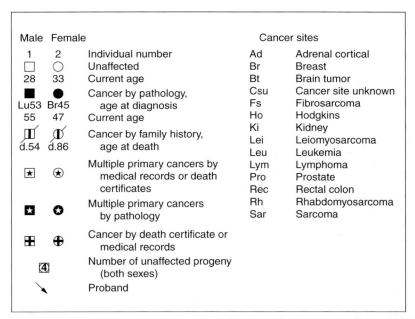

Figure 21-18 Classical Li-Fraumeni (SBLA) syndrome pedigree which harbors the *p53* mutation. The stars show the intense cancer association, which is classical for this syndrome. Noteworthy are the increased numbers of sarcomas in generation IV, coupled with the strikingly early breast cancer onset (proband at 34 years of age, with a second primary at 39). Also noteworthy is the proband's daughter (IV-4) with sarcoma at 20 years of age and breast cancer at age 25, and a second daughter of the proband (IV-5) with sarcoma at 3 years of age.

Germline mutations in the *PTEN* gene[228,229] are associated with Cowden disease as well as Bannayan-Riley-Ruvalcaba syndrome. Because the major malignancies in Cowden disease, namely breast and thyroid cancer, can be detected in early stages by surveillance, recognition of the syndrome is critical. The International Cowden Syndrome Consortium operational criteria for diagnosis are useful for weighting the pleiotropic manifestations according to major and minor criteria to make a formal diagnosis.[230,231]

The cutaneous manifestations of Cowden disease involve multiple trichilemmomas, the presence of which appears to be pathognomonic. These multiple cutaneous lesions are often located on the face (Fig. 21-19) and on the dorsal and ventral aspects of the hands, feet, and forearms. These are hyperkeratotic, slightly brownish lesions, but they show the histologic pattern of benign keratoses. The stratum corneum is thick, compact, and largely orthokeratotic. The granular layer is prominent; the malpighian layer is papillomatous, acanthotic, and well differentiated but shows no distinguishing features. Additional skin features include multiple facial papules, acral and palmoplantar keratoses, multiple skin tags, and subcutaneous lipomas. Cobblestone-like gingival and buccal mucosa papules, as well as papillomatous tongue are hallmarks. Merkel cell carcinoma (primary neuroendocrine carcinoma of the skin) is a distinguishing feature.

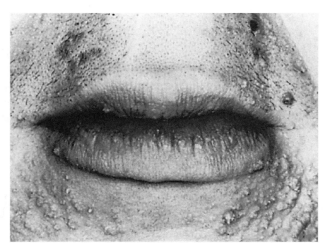

Figure 21-19 Multiple trichilemmomas in a patient with Cowden's disease, which is frequently associated with breast cancer. (From Brownstein MH: Breast cancer in Cowden's syndrome. In Lynch HT [ed]: Genetics and breast cancer. New York, Van Nostrand Reinhold, 1981. Reprinted by permission.)

In their review of the literature, Williard and coworkers[232] noted that 30% of women with Cowden disease manifested infiltrating ductal carcinoma of the breast, and a third of these individuals had bilateral primary breast carcinomas. The median age at breast cancer onset was 41 years of age, with a range of 20 to 62 years, leading some authors to recommend prophylactic mastectomy.[233] Williard and colleagues[232] suggest that those patients showing clinical manifestations of this disorder should be considered as candidates for prophylactic bilateral total mastectomy. They suggest that this procedure be considered by the third decade of life.

Our recommendation is that, should the patient decline surgical prophylaxis, she should consider monthly breast self-examination, physician examination every 3 to 6 months, and bilateral mammograms every 6 to 12 months, which could alternate with MRI, with appropriate biopsy of suspicious lesions.

In addition to the susceptibility to breast cancer, women may show virginal hypertrophy of the breasts. Breast hamartomas, as well as an array of benign breast findings, may occur, including ductal hyperplasia, intraductal papillomatosis, adenosis, lobular atrophy, fibroadenomas, fibrocystic change, densely fibrotic hyalinized breast nodules, and nipple and areolar malformations.[234] The risk of fibrocystic breast disease may be as high as 67%. Males and females who have the cutaneous lesions may also manifest thyroid goiter, thyroid adenoma, and hyper- or hypothyroidism, as well as carcinoma of the thyroid, mainly of the follicular type. Thyroid disease is seen in 5% to 75% of individuals, and there is a 3% to 10% chance of epithelial thyroid carcinoma. Multiple, early-onset uterine leiomyomas are characteristic, and brain tumors (meningiomas, glioblastoma multiforme) also occur. Hamartomatous polyps are relatively common and have been observed throughout the gastrointestinal tract, including the esophagus. Adenocarcinoma of the colon has been reported in patients with Cowden disease, but the risk is yet to be clearly defined.

Dysmorphic features are part of the Cowden phenotype and are especially useful for diagnosis.[230] The pleiotropic effects of the *PTEN* gene in development are highlighted by the numerous affected organ systems: neurologic (Lhermitte-Duclos disease, mild to moderate mental retardation in 12%, cerebellar gangliocytoma manifesting as seizure and tremor); head and neck (progressive macrocephaly, "birdlike" facies, high-arched palate, scrotal tongue); skeletal (pectus excavatum, scoliosis, kyphosis); genitourinary (hydrocele, varicocele, vaginal and vulvar cysts, ovarian cysts and leiomyomas); and the endocrine, gastrointestinal, oncologic, and dermatologic features noted previously.

Although Cowden syndrome is said to be rare, underdiagnosis is likely because of general lack of awareness of the syndrome, as well as its variable expressivity and its sometimes subtle manifestations.[235] In addition, there may be lack of a family history. De novo mutations may occur. Regardless of whether there is a family history, the risk of transmission by affected individuals is 50%; therefore, institution of cancer surveillance is crucial in at-risk relatives.

Ataxia-Telangiectasia

A mutated gene that is responsible for the rare childhood neurologic disorder ataxia-telangiectasia (AT) has been identified on chromosome 11q.[236,237] AT is characterized by progressive cerebellar and neuromotor deterioration, telangiectasia of the conjunctivae and facial skin, cellular and humoral immune deficiencies, growth retardation, clinical and cellular hypersensitivity to ionizing radiation, and cancer.[238] The disease follows an autosomal recessive pattern of inheritance, with homozygous affected individuals having a cancer risk 61 to 184 times greater than the general population.[239] Obligate heterozygous carriers of the gene have been found to have three- to four-fold the population risk for cancer.[240,241] Female carriers of the mutated AT gene (*ATM*) are at five times the population risk for developing breast cancers.[241]

In younger patients with AT, there is an increased frequency of lymphoreticular neoplasms or leukemia. However, an association with epithelial cancers is rare in young AT patients. In contrast, older patients with AT show an excess of epithelial neoplasms, but interestingly, lymphoreticular cancer and leukemia rarely occur in the older patients. At least two young patients with AT who developed dysgerminomas have been reported.[242,243]

It is estimated that as many as 1% of the general population carry the *ATM* gene,[244] which may predispose to as many as 9% to 18% of all breast cancers.[241] It is of interest that the *ATM* gene seems also to convey susceptibility to cancers of the lung, pancreas, gallbladder, and stomach, but in obligate heterozygous carriers of the gene, colorectal cancers were observed less frequently than expected.[240] This autosomal recessive disease and the somatic effects of the heterozygous carrier state of *ATM* are exceedingly important models for future study, and they present a dilemma to the physician for clinical management. Homozygotic individuals are excessively sensitive to the necrotizing effects of radiation therapy, and in vitro their cells show several repair and growth defects following radiation exposure. Heterozygotic carriers of *ATM*, however, are susceptible to early-onset breast cancers and therefore might benefit from screening mammography, yet it is speculated that they may be particularly susceptible to malignant transformation induced by this radiation exposure.[245] DNA screening for mutations is clinically feasible, although test sensitivity is imperfect. It is possible to identify those individuals who are at increased genetic risk for neoplasms associated with this specific genetic defect; however, clear screening guidelines have not been developed.

Lobular Breast Cancer in the Hereditary Diffuse Gastric Cancer Syndrome

Hereditary diffuse gastric cancer (HDGC) is an autosomal dominantly inherited disorder caused by mutations of the E-cadherin gene (*CDH1*, epithelial cadherin, OMIM#19209). These mutations have been identified in approximately 40% to 50% of well-defined HDGC families from low-incident populations.[157,246,247] There is also an excess of lobular carcinoma of the breast in women from those HDGC families with CDH1 mutations.[155,248,249] These mutations are associated with a 70% life-time risk for diffuse gastric cancer and a 40% risk for lobular breast cancer in females.

Diagnostic Considerations and Implications

ENDOCRINE SIGNALING

The substantial interindividual variability in the occurrence of breast cancer in *BRCA1* and *BRCA2* mutation carriers has been partially attributed to endocrine signaling, which may modify the *BRCA1* and *BRCA2*–associated age-specific breast cancer penetrance.[250] This hypothesis was supported by the finding that women showed a significantly higher breast cancer risk

> ...if they carried alleles with at least 28 or 29 polyglutamine repeats at *AIB1*, compared with women who carried alleles with fewer polyglutamine repeats [odds ratio (OR), 1.59; 95% confidence interval (CI), 1.03–2.47 and OR, 2.85; 95% CI, 1.64–4.96, respectively]...Women were at significantly increased risk if they were nulliparous or had a late age at first live birth and had *AIB1* alleles no shorter than 28 or 29 or more *AIB1* polyglutamine repeats (OR, 4.62; 95% CI, 2.02–10.56 and OR, 6.97; 95% CI, 1.71–28.43, respectively) than women with none of these risk factors.

Clearly, endocrine signaling, as evidenced through *AIB1* genotype and reproductive history, may show a powerful effect on *BRCA1* and *BRCA2*-associated breast cancer risk.[250]

POLYMORPHIC ANDROGEN-RECEPTOR CAG REPEAT

As in the case of breast cancer risk modification in *BRCA1* and *BRCA2* mutation carriers by *AIB1* genotype and reproductive history, endocrine signaling in concert with the CAG repeat-length polymorphism found in exon 1 of the androgen-receptor (*AR*) gene (*AR-CAG*) may also modify the *BRCA1*-associated age-specific breast cancer risk. For example, Rebbeck and colleagues[251] found that all of the women who harbored at least one *AR-CAG* allele with at least 29 repeats had breast cancer. Results from this study were in support of the hypothesis that age at breast cancer diagnosis, "...is earlier among *BRCA1* mutation carriers who carry very long *AR-CAG* repeats. ...[indicating that] pathways involving androgen signaling may affect the risk of *BRCA1*-associated breast cancer."

DUCTAL LAVAGE

Fabian and associates[252] studied ductal epithelial cells from 480 high-risk women wherein they used random, four-quadrant periareolar fine-needle aspiration for cytologic analysis. The women were then prospectively followed for a median of 45 months. Importantly, 15% of the women showing both atypical cytology and an elevated 10-year Gail risk manifested carcinoma of the breast within the first 3 years of follow-up. In comparison, only 4% of women who were at an elevated 10-year Gail risk but who lacked atypical cytology manifested breast cancer within that same time period.

Given the safety of ductal lavage (DL) and its ability to provide additional information regarding risk of breast cancer in women who are already at an elevated risk for this disease and who do not have a history of biopsy-proven atypical hyperplasia, the finding of cytologic atypia in DL

> ...provides risk assessment information that is independent of her Gail risk. This information can assist the woman and her physician in weighing the risks and benefits of hormone replacement therapy, antiestrogen therapy, and, in very high-risk women, prophylactic mastectomies.[253]

Thus, DL provides additional information regarding breast cancer risk to these women as well as their physicians so that women can become more informed about physicians' advice, given the DL findings. Thus, they can participate in a more informed manner with decision logic relevant to hormone replacement therapy and anti-estrogen risk-reduction therapy.[253]

Dooley and colleagues[254] described a new procedure for collecting ductal cells with a microcatheter and compared this with nipple aspiration with respect to safety, tolerability, and the ability to detect abnormal breast epithelial cells. They found that DL detected abnormal intraductal breast cells 3.2 times more often than nipple aspiration (79 vs. 25 breasts; McNemar's tests, $P < 0.001$). There was no report of any serious procedure-related adverse events. They concluded that large numbers of ductal cells can be collected by DL, identifying atypical cellular changes in this safe and well-tolerated procedure; they conclude that this is a more sensitive method for detecting cellular atypia when compared to nipple aspiration.

These methods of DL merit meticulous examination in a clinical trial setting, preferably involving women who are harbingers of *BRCA1* and *BRCA2* germline mutations in order to test its efficacy. However, at this time, DL should not be considered a substitute for mammography, breast self-examination, or clinical breast examination.

EXPRESSION PROFILING OF BREAST CANCER

Novel scientific terms have been adopted into popular parlance, such as "DNA fingerprinting" and "genetic profiling." This new "technospeak" attempts to explain the mystery of our biologic selves as being attributable to the result of our unique, individual genetic programs. When the interaction with the outside world is added to the equation, we have the classic nature versus nurture theory (or more accurately, nature "plus" nurture). Our genetic blueprint, or DNA code, is essentially the same in each of our cells, yet our cells are visibly and functionally different. Lung, nerve, heart, and breast cells all have different functions and different morphologies reflecting that functionality. A particular set of genes from the master blueprint is activated/deactivated in specialized cells, which defines those cells. Although we can distinguish colonic epithelium from cerebral cortex with hematoxylin and eosin staining and microscopy, another approach would be to isolate the messenger RNA from each specimen, create a DNA copy (cDNA) of the RNA to work with (because RNA is highly degradable) and review the pattern of each sample. The set of genes turned on and off in each specimen would provide a colon or brain fingerprint, and we could tell the specimens apart.

Although pathologic specimens from different tissues are readily distinguished with the use of a microscope, histopathologic techniques have approached a limit in terms of discerning the finer steps of malignant progression from benign tissue to atypia to preinvasive lesions to invasive malignancies and metastases. A finer "microscope" is needed, and comes in the form of discerning molecular techniques. The fingerprinting process described previously is termed "genetic expression profiling" and is technically feasible using "microarrays" that can analyze the expression of hundreds to thousands of genes on a small slide, or chip. Among the many applications of this technology is the potential to assess individual cancers for their genetic fingerprint. Genes of interest in oncogenic pathways are selected for analysis, printed onto slides, and then hybridized with the test sample (e.g., RNAs from different breast cancer specimens). Gene expression levels for each tumor are compared with a control or median level of expression among samples and color-coded (red = high, green = low). Samples are then compared using clustering algorithms, which assign a hierarchy of similarity (i.e., identify the closest neighbors).

The traditional approach in biology has been to evaluate one or a few genes at a time and elucidate relevant pathways; microarray technology supplements this approach by discovering "molecular portraits" of tumors. This new approach has begun to lead to a subclassification of tumors that cannot otherwise be distinguished using histopathologic techniques. First effectively applied to the subclassification of lymphomas, tumor profiling has defined breast cancer portraits as well.[255] Correlations between clinical outcomes and tumor profiles are beginning to emerge.[256,257] The divergence of breast cancer evolutionary pathways according to ER status is confirmed by tumor profiling and does not strictly correlate with estrogen responsiveness.[258] The clinical need to distinguish between primary and secondary breast tumors is also amenable to molecular profiling analysis; distantly located metachronous ipsilateral breast tumors may be shown to be genetically related,[259] and lymph node metastases can be confirmed to have arisen from the primary tumor.[255]

Hedenfalk and colleagues[123] distinguished *BRCA1*, *BRCA2*, and sporadic breast cancers using gene expression profiling. Review of 176 differentially expressed genes revealed a common theme in *BRCA1* mutated samples, involving the coordinated transcriptional activation of two major cellular processes, DNA repair and apoptosis.[123] A *BRCA1* signature was also discerned in a study that used gene expression profiling to identify "poor prognosis" signatures in breast tumors from young women with node-negative disease.[257] Using an optimal set of 100 *BRCA1* reporter genes, the investigators were able to distinguish *BRCA1* from sporadic ER-negative breast cancers with an accuracy of 95%. "Misclassified" sporadic tumors in these studies had decreased *BRCA1* expression and promoter hypermethylation, reflecting a common biology between germline and somatically inactivated tumors and showing the centrality of *BRCA1* in determining the molecular phenotype. All of the *BRCA1* tumors fell within the basal subgroup, indicative of a distinctive biology associated with a poor prognosis.[125] Gene expression profiling studies demonstrate that a highly penetrant susceptibility gene can markedly influence the molecular phenotype, histology, and prognosis of the resulting breast tumor. Moreover, the molecular phenotype can be examined to gain insight into the specific cellular pathways that have been disrupted.

The delineation of molecular targets has led to a few success stories in targeted therapeutics, namely trastuzumab (Herceptin) for Her2/*neu*-positive breast cancers and STK571 for gastric intestinal stromal tumors. Initial work in breast tumor profiling demonstrates significant potential to identify new diagnostic and prognostic markers and therapeutic targets. For example, doxorubicin resistance correlates with a particular gene expression profile, which could theoretically be used for chemotherapy selection and to develop strategies to undermine resistance.[260] Expression profiling of disseminated breast tumor cells in peripheral blood may be a viable approach to early cancer detection.[259] In the case of *BRCA1* and *BRCA2*, profiling based on a hereditary phenotype may provide a strategy for targeted therapies such as PARP1 inhibitors.

Treatment Interventions

HORMONAL EFFECTS ON RISK

Tubal Ligation and Risk of Ovarian Cancer in BRCA1 or BRCA2 Mutation Carriers

Narod and colleagues,[261] in a matched case-control study, assessed women with a pathogenic mutation in BRCA1 or BRCA2, in order to determine the potential reduction in the risk of OC through tubal ligation. Cases were 232 women with a history of invasive OC and controls were 232 women without OC who had both ovaries intact. Cases and controls were matched for year of birth and mutation (BRCA1 or BRCA2) status. The odds ratio for OC occurrence was estimated for tubal ligation with adjustment for parity, breast cancer history, oral contraceptive use, and ethnic background.

Findings disclosed that in an unadjusted analysis among BRCA1 carriers

> ...significantly fewer cases than controls had ever had tubal ligation (30 of 173 [18%] vs. 60 of 173 [35%], odds ratio 0.37 [95% CI 0.21-0.63]; $P = 0.0003$). After adjustment for oral contraceptive use, parity, history of breast cancer, and ethnic group, the odds ratio was 0.39 ($P = 0.002$). Combination of tubal ligation and past use of an oral contraceptive was associated with an odds ratio of 0.28 (0.15-0.52). No protective effect of tubal ligation was seen among carriers of the BRCA2 mutation.[261]

It was therefore concluded that tubal ligation may be a feasible option for the reduction of OC in women with BRCA1 mutations who have completed their childbearing. However, we consider it mandatory that genetic counselors emphasize the fact that these statistical findings need to be confirmed in additional studies, that the magnitude of protection is much less for tubal ligation than prophylactic oophorectomy, and that due caution must be exercised when considering tubal ligation as a preventive measure for reduction of risk of OC in BRCA1 carriers.

Tamoxifen and Risk of Contralateral Breast Cancer in BRCA1 and BRCA2 Mutation Carriers

Tamoxifen has been shown to protect against contralateral breast cancer in women with a prior history of ER-positive breast cancer, and to be protective for women without a prior history of breast cancer who are at increased risk. To evaluate the effect of tamoxifen on contralateral breast cancer in BRCA1 and BRCA2 mutation carriers, Narod and colleagues[35] compared 209 women with bilateral breast cancer and a BRCA1 or BRCA2 mutation with 384 women with unilateral breast cancer and BRCA1 or BRCA2 mutation (controls) in a matched case-control study. Findings disclosed that

> ...the multivariate odds ratio for contralateral breast cancer associated with tamoxifen use was 0.50 (95% CI, 0.28-0.89). Tamoxifen protected against contralateral breast cancer for carriers of BRCA1 mutations (odds ratio 0.38, 95% CI 0.19-0.74) and those with BRCA2

mutations (0.63, 0.20-1.50). In women who used tamoxifen for 2-4 years, the risk of contralateral breast cancer was reduced by 75%. A reduction in risk of contralateral breast cancer was also seen with oophorectomy (0.42, 0.22-0.83) and with chemotherapy (0.40, 0.26-0.60).[35]

It was therefore concluded that there was a reduction of contralateral breast cancer in women harboring BRCA1 or BRCA2 mutations, and herein the protective effect of tamoxifen appeared to be independent of that of oophorectomy.

Oral Contraceptives and Risk of Hereditary Ovarian Cancer

Oral contraceptives have been shown to protect against OC in the general population. Narod and colleagues[262] showed that oral contraceptive use may provide a reduction in the risk of OC in women harboring BRCA1 or BRCA2 germline mutations.

Marchbanks and colleagues[263] studied oral contraceptive use in 4575 breast cancer–affected women and 4683 controls who were 35 to 64 years of age. Conditional logistical regression for calculating ORs revealed the RR of 1 (95% CI = 0.8-1.3) for women currently using oral contraceptives and 0.9 (95% CI = 0.8-1) for those who had previously used oral contraceptives. Interestingly, there was no increase in women who had longer periods of use or who had higher doses of estrogen. There were no differences between white and black women.

In support of the results obtained by Narod and associates,[262] those obtained by Marchbanks and colleagues[263] showed that neither use of oral contraceptives nor the initiation of use of oral contraceptives at a young age was associated with an increased risk of breast cancer in women with a family history of breast cancer.

PROPHYLACTIC BILATERAL MASTECTOMY AND OOPHORECTOMY IN HEREDITARY BREAST AND OVARIAN CANCER

History

Prophylactic mastectomy and prophylactic oophorectomy among patients at inordinately high risk for HBOC were initially discussed in the early 1970s.[14,15,264-268] Prophylactic contralateral mastectomy in high-risk women with ipsilateral breast cancer was considered a logical option, given the enormous risk of bilaterality in hereditary cases.[269] This was predicated by the concern that women at inordinately high risk of familial breast cancer and OC required special cancer control measures. Prophylactic mastectomy, for example, was suggested as an option for members of breast cancer–prone families wherein the risk to first-degree relatives of the proband, "...approach 50%, consistent with an autosomal dominant factor...."[267] In turn, a relative who developed a crippling cancer phobia resulting from her awareness of this disease in her family may express a strong desire to have what she correctly considers her extremely highly cancer-prone breast tissue excised.

Patients who were candidates for the option of prophylactic mastectomy included those who failed to comply with screening recommendations, often because of their fear of "finding" breast cancer.[265] Also included were women at high risk for HBC who manifested severe fibrocystic breast disease that made it difficult for them and their physicians to determine which palpable masses were significant.[267] In those "early days" prior to BRCA testing, counseling and consultation with a medical geneticist was recommended when weighing genetic risk factors relevant to considerations of prophylactic surgery.[265,268]

Prophylactic mastectomy has long been a controversial issue, raising such questions as, "Will it work?" "Will patients accept it?" "Will physicians recommend it?" "Will insurance companies cover the cost?" "Will it effectively reduce breast cancer's and OC's morbidity and mortality?" "Is it considered to be such a radical medical and surgical concern that patients who harbor BRCA1 or BRCA2 germline mutations with a lifetime risk for breast cancer of 70% to 85%, and/or some of their physicians, may remain reluctant to advocate it?"

Recent Surgical Prophylaxis Studies

Hartmann and colleagues[270] initially used "high-risk" criteria such as the number of breast cancer–affected first- and second-degree relatives for consideration of prophylactic mastectomy. They found that prophylactic mastectomy was effective in these high-risk women in that there was a 90% reduction in the risk of breast cancer, with a significant reduction in mortality.

Seven breast cancers occurred in their study after subcutaneous bilateral mastectomy; there were none after total mastectomy.[270] Subsequently,[33] they used genetic testing to distinguish the BRCA1 or BRCA2 mutation carriers in this cohort and proved that prophylactic mastectomy works in these BRCA1 or BRCA2 mutation carriers.[33] For example, breast cancer did not develop in any of the women with a confirmed BRCA1 or BRCA2 mutation after a median follow-up of 16 years.[33] Therefore, prophylactic mastectomy appears to reduce the long-term risk of breast cancer in those women with a BRCA1 or BRCA2 mutation.

A prospective study by Meijers-Heijboer and colleagues[271] also showed significant benefit of prophylactic mastectomy among BRCA1 and BRCA2 mutation carriers. These investigators studied 139 women with a BRCA1 or BRCA2 mutation who were part of a prospective study of the effectiveness of prophylactic mastectomy in a breast-cancer surveillance program at the Rotterdam Family Cancer Clinic in The Netherlands. Seventy-six of these women eventually underwent prophylactic mastectomy, and 63 declined prophylactic mastectomy in preference to regular surveillance. The Cox proportional-hazards method evaluated the incidence of breast cancer as a time-dependent covariate for the effect of mastectomy on the incidence of breast cancer. Findings disclosed an absence of breast cancer in those undergoing prophylactic mastectomy during a follow-up of 2.9 ($\pm$1.4) years; in comparison, eight breast cancers developed in those women who elected regular surveillance after a mean follow-up of 3 ($\pm$1.5) years ($P = 0.003$, hazard ratio, 0; 95% CI, 0–0.36). The authors concluded that, "...in women with a BRCA1 or BRCA2 mutation, prophylactic bilateral total mastectomy reduces the incidence of breast cancer at three years of follow-up." It was of particular interest that of the eight cancers identified in the screening group, four were identified between screening sessions, consonant with so-called interval cancers, and herein "...the interval from screening to diagnosis was two to five months." Cancers in the remaining four patients were detected during a screening session. Thus, it is possible that some were "missed lesions" versus accelerated breast carcinogenesis.

A significantly greater number of women in the prophylactic mastectomy group, as opposed to those in the surveillance group, had undergone a premenopausal oophorectomy (44 vs. 24 [58% vs. 38%], $P = 0.03$). Thus, there was a likely protective effect from prophylactic oophorectomy, consistent with the findings of Rebbeck and colleagues,[34] discussed subsequently.

Given the assumption that within 10 years breast cancer will develop in approximately 25% of the high-risk women undergoing regular surveillance, these authors[271] estimated that 10% to 20% of high-risk women who choose surveillance instead of prophylactic mastectomy will die of breast cancer within 20 years, and 35% to 50% of women under surveillance who develop primary breast cancer will die of distant metastases within 10 to 15 years.[150,272]

Meijers-Heijboer and colleagues[271] suggest that the use of high-resolution imaging as well as more frequent screening might be effective in early breast cancer detection in women with a BRCA1 or BRCA2 mutation. Specifically, in their study, MRI was performed in six women at the time of breast cancer diagnosis and it detected all six cancers. In contrast, mammography was diagnostic in only two of the eight women with breast cancer.

Contralateral Prophylactic Mastectomy

Metcalfe and associates[273] evaluated the rate of prophylactic contralateral mastectomy in an international cohort of women with HBOC. This dealt with BRCA1 or BRCA2 mutation positive women who had manifested unilateral breast cancer and were followed prospectively for a minimum of 1.5 years, following which, information was obtained on prophylactic surgery, tamoxifen use, as well as the occurrence of contralateral breast cancer. The study comprised 927 women, of whom 253 (27.3%) underwent a contralateral prophylactic mastectomy following the diagnosis of breast cancer. This international study involved 43 centers in 8 countries (Austria, Canada, France, Israel, Italy, Norway, Poland, and the United States). Once a BRCA1 or BRCA2 mutation was found in a proband or in her relative, DNA testing was offered to additional at-risk women in her family. Eligibility of the women was obtained for study when her status as a mutation carrier was established. Unaffected and affected women with breast cancer were part of the study. Large differences in uptake of contralateral prophylactic mastectomy by country, ranging from 0% in Norway to 49.3% in the United States, were identified. In addition,

...Among women from North America, those who had a prophylactic contralateral mastectomy were significantly younger at breast cancer diagnosis (mean age, 39 years) than were those without preventive surgery (mean age, 43 years). Women who initially underwent breast-conserving surgery were less likely to undergo contralateral prophylactic mastectomy than were women who underwent a mastectomy (12% vs. 40%, $P < 10^{-4}$). Women who had elected for a prophylactic bilateral oophorectomy were more likely to have had their contralateral breast removed than those with intact ovaries (33% vs. 18%, $P < 10^{-4}$).[273]

These authors concluded that patients' age, type of initial cancer surgery, as well as prophylactic oophorectomy, were all predictive of prophylactic contralateral mastectomy in breast cancer–affected women with a BRCA mutation. Acceptance of contralateral prophylactic mastectomy appeared to be significantly higher in North America than in Europe. Tuttle and colleagues[274] have shown that contralateral prophylactic mastectomy increased by 150% from 1998 to 2003 in the United States.

Bilateral Prophylactic Oophorectomy in BRCA1 Mutation Carriers

Recent studies[41,275] have provided prospective findings about the risk-reducing effects on both breast cancer and OC in patients who were harbingers of BRCA1 and BRCA2 and who underwent prophylactic salpingo-oophorectomy.

Rebbeck and colleagues[34] studied a cohort of women with BRCA1 mutations who underwent bilateral prophylactic oophorectomy (BPO) in order to test the hypothesis that decreases in ovarian hormone exposure following BPO may alter risk of breast cancer in BRCA1 mutation carriers. This study showed a statistically significant reduction in risk of breast cancer following BPO, which was greater in women who were followed 5 to 10 years, or for at least 10 years, after surgery. BPO also provided a potential for reduction of risk of OC. Hormone replacement therapy did not negate this reduction in risk of breast cancer following BPO. The researchers concluded that BPO "...is associated with a reduced breast cancer risk in women who carry a BRCA1 mutation. The likely mechanism is reduction of ovarian hormone exposure...."[34]

Rebbeck and colleagues,[41] in a prospective study, evaluated a total of 551 women with BRCA1 or BRCA2 germline mutations identified from registries, 259 of whom had undergone BPO and 292 who were matched controls who had not undergone the procedure. They then investigated these women for the occurrence of carcinoma of the breast and ovary. Among a subgroup of 241 women who lacked a history of carcinoma of the breast and of prophylactic mastectomy, the incidence of breast cancer was determined in 99 women who had undergone bilateral prophylactic oophorectomy and in 142 matched controls. Postoperative

follow-up with both groups was at least 8 years. Findings disclosed that

...Six women who underwent prophylactic oophorectomy (2.3%) received a diagnosis of stage I ovarian cancer at the time of the procedure; two women (0.8%) received a diagnosis of papillary serous peritoneal carcinoma, 3.8 and 8.6 years after bilateral prophylactic oophorectomy. Among the controls, 58 women (19.9%) received a diagnosis of ovarian cancer, after a mean follow-up of 8.8 years. With the exclusion of the six women whose cancer was diagnosed at surgery, prophylactic oophorectomy significantly reduced the risk of coelomic epithelial cancer (hazard ratio 0.04, 95% CI 0.01–0.16). Of 99 women who underwent bilateral prophylactic oophorectomy and who were studied to determine the risk of breast cancer, breast cancer developed in 21 (21.2%), as compared with 60 (42.3%) in the control group (hazard ratio, 0.47, 95% CI 0.29–0.77).

In conclusion, BPO reduced the risk of OC and breast cancer in those women who were harbingers of BRCA1 or BRCA2 germline mutations.

Kauff and colleagues[275] compared the effect of risk-reducing salpingo-oophorectomy to that of surveillance for OC on the incidence of carcinoma of the breast cancer and OC in harbingers of BRCA mutations. They studied 170 women 35 years of age or older who had declined bilateral oophorectomy in preference to other surveillance for OC. Kaplan-Meier analysis and a Cox proportional-hazards model were used in order to compare the time to cancer in both groups. Herein, it was found that, "...The time to breast cancer or BRCA-related gynecologic cancer was longer in the salpingo-oophorectomy group, with a hazard ratio for subsequent breast cancer or BRCA-related gynecologic cancer of 0.25 (95% CI, 0.08–0.72)."

A more recent study by Kauff and colleagues[276] notes that risk-reducing salpingo-oophorectomy (RRSO) now provides an option for the reduction of both breast and ovarian cancer for women with BRCA1 and BRCA2 mutations. These authors studied 1079 women 30 years of age and older who had their ovaries retained in situ in concert with a deleterious BRCA1 or BRCA2 mutation and who were enrolled into prospective follow-up studies at one of 11 centers in the United States. Women self-selected RRSO or observation and underwent a questionnaire and medical record review. Analysis of the effect of RRSO on time to diagnosis of breast cancer or BRCA-associated gynecologic cancer were analyzed by a Cox proportional-hazards model. A 3-year follow-up was performed, during which time RRSO was associated with

...an 85% reduction in BRCA1-associated gynecologic cancer risk (hazard ratio [HR] = 0.15; 95% CI 0.04–0.56) and a 72% reduction in BRCA2-associated breast cancer risk (HR = 0.28; 95% CI 0.08–0.92). While protection against BRCA1-associated breast cancer (HR = 0.61; 95% CI 0.30–1.22) and BRCA2-associated gynecologic cancer (HR = 0; 95% CI not estimable) was suggested, neither effect reached statistical significance.[276]

The authors concluded that the protection conferred by RRSO against breast and gynecologic cancers may differ between carriers of BRCA1 and BRCA2 mutations. They also noted that studies evaluating the efficacy of risk-reduction strategies in *BRCA* mutation carriers should stratify by the specific gene mutated.

BRCA1 and BRCA2 Concerns about Prophylactic Surgery

We have identified the *BRCA1* and *BRCA2* germline mutation status of 1855 individuals from 174 families with HBOC (H.T. Lynch, unpublished data, 2009). To date, we have counseled 819 women from 127 of these families. Pertinent insights about their interest in surgical prophylaxis have emerged. For example, prior to receiving their DNA results, 609 of these women were asked if they would consider the option of prophylactic mastectomy. Two hundred seventy-seven of 609 (45%) said they would consider prophylactic mastectomy if they were positive for the mutation. Conversely, 17 out of 530 (3%) said they would still consider prophylactic mastectomy even if negative for the mutation, reflecting, in part, their concern about the 1:8 lifetime risk of breast cancer in the general population and personal experiences with breast cancer suggesting that it cannot be survived. It may also reflect a lack of belief that a negative mutation finding would remove them from the greater lifetime breast cancer risk of HBOC, given that they may have been labeled high-risk for years and/or that so many of their relatives may have been affected with breast cancer. If positive for the mutation, 350 (64%) of the 549 who answered the question said that they would consider BPO and, if *BRCA*-negative, 45 (9%) of 494 would still consider BPO. Following disclosure, our follow-up survey found that 59 of 226 (26%) mutation-positive women had undergone prophylactic mastectomy and that 87 of 201 (43%) had a BPO.

Genetic counseling is mandatory when working with patients from high-risk families.[265] But will it make a difference? With the discovery of mutations in the *BRCA1* and *BRCA2* genes that predispose to breast cancer, we have been able to counsel these women with greater precision not only about their cancer risk but also about screening and management options, including chemoprevention and prophylactic surgery.

Attitudes about Prophylactic Surgery

Meiser and colleagues[277] showed that cancer worry as opposed to objective risk estimates strongly influences consideration of prophylactic oophorectomy. Lerman and associates[278] suggested that many women will likely postpone prophylactic surgery until they obtain results of their mutation status testing. Decisions about surgical prophylaxis are conditioned strongly by assessing the positive and negative issues surrounding the outcome of surgery. It does appear that the majority of women decide on their preferences about prophylactic surgery at an early stage and that the desire to avoid later regret is a motivating factor.[279]

Hallowell and colleagues[280] studied a cohort of women who had at least two first- or second-degree relatives with carcinoma of the ovary or breast, for the assessment of attitudes that influence decisions about prophylactic oophorectomy. Knowledge about *BRCA1* or *BRCA2* mutation status, prior to prophylactic surgery, was an important consideration. These findings were in accord with studies showing that many women undergo *BRCA1* and *BRCA2* testing in order to facilitate their decisions relevant to prophylactic surgery.[281,282] Hallowell and colleagues[280] also noted less anxiety among women who did not have close relatives with cancer, and none of the women in the screening group would, at the time of the study, absolutely exclude the possibility of prophylactic surgery at some future date.

Racial and Sociocultural Variation in Breast Cancer Rates

The international variation in breast cancer incidence, particularly with respect to ethnic, racial, and socioethnic populations such as Ashkenazi Jews, must be considered when interpreting the etiologic role of hereditary factors in these disorders. For example, Deapen and colleagues[283] have shown marked fluctuation in breast cancer incidence rates over relatively short time spans in various racial groups, particularly Asian-American women. These authors note that, overall, breast cancer incidence rates remained stable in the Los Angeles, California, area during the late 1980s and early 1990s. However, data from the most recent 5-year period suggest that the breast cancer incidence may be increasing for Asian-American and non-Hispanic white women older than 50 years of age.

These changes occurred in the face of little change in breast cancer incidence in black and Hispanic women. Attention was given to sorting breast cancer rate differences in specific subsets of the Asian population. For example, Filipinas, who historically had higher rates of breast cancer than their other Asian-American counterparts, were shown to not have as rapid a rate of increase as Japanese women; nevertheless, they remain relatively high. Women of Japanese and Filipino ancestry had breast cancer rates that were twice that of Chinese and Korean women. Asian women, who commonly have low breast cancer rates in their native countries, typically experience increasing breast cancer incidence after immigrating to the United States. How much of this variation in breast cancer rates is attributable to host factors, environmental-culture exposures, and/or their interaction? Do *BRCA1* or *BRCA2* mutations behave differently with respect to such parameters as age of onset, bilaterality, virulence, and association with carcinomas of the ovary and other anatomic sites in these racial and ethnic population subtypes?

Psychological Aspects of Familial Breast Cancer

QUALITY OF LIFE AND HEALTH BEHAVIOR

As our knowledge of breast cancer risk factors has increased, so has attention to the impact of risk assessment on women's quality of life. In one of the first empirical studies to examine this systematically, Kash and colleagues[284] showed that over one fourth of women with a family history of breast cancer exhibited psychological distress that warranted counseling. Significant distress was also reported in a subsequent population-based study of first-degree relatives of breast cancer patients.[285] In this study, 53% of women reported intrusive thoughts about breast cancer, 33% reported impairments in daily functioning resulting from breast cancer worries, and 20% reported sleep disturbance. Psychological distress in high-risk women parallels that of women diagnosed with invasive breast cancer,[286] and it is increased significantly compared with women who do not have a family history of this disease.[287] Younger high-risk women, those 35 years of age and younger, appear to be at greatest risk for cancer-related distress.[288,289]

In addition to its effects on quality of life, breast cancer–related distress can also influence health behavior in high-risk women. One adaptive aspect of distress is that it may motivate women to seek counseling about their breast cancer risk and options for prevention and surveillance. In a study of predictors of participation in a breast cancer health promotion trial, high-risk women who were more distressed about their risk were significantly more likely to participate than those with low levels of distress.[290] However, although distress may increase motivation for counseling, it may interfere with comprehension of the information provided during the counseling session. In the same study, Lerman and colleagues[291] found that women who had high levels of breast cancer–related distress before the risk counseling session were significantly less likely to improve in terms of their comprehension of personal risk. Moreover, anxieties and fears about breast cancer can lead some high-risk women to avoid breast cancer detection practices. Psychological distress has been associated with decreased adherence to guidelines for clinical breast examination, breast self-examination, and mammography.[284,285]

INTEREST IN GENETIC TESTING FOR BREAST CANCER SUSCEPTIBILITY

In anticipation of the widespread availability of genetic testing for breast cancer susceptibility, several studies have examined interest in testing and anticipated reactions to positive and negative test results. Overall, interest in genetic testing for inherited breast cancer risk has been reported to be very high. In a sample of women with a family history of OC, 75% said they would definitely want to be tested for mutations in the BRCA1 gene and 20% said they probably would want to be tested.[290] Interest in testing was significantly greater among women who perceived themselves to be at higher risk for cancer and those who were more worried about their risk. Similar levels of interest have been observed among women in the general population,[292] women with a family history of breast cancer,[291] and female members of families with HBOC.[66,76] However, with the possible exception of the study by Lynch and colleagues,[76] these studies used hypothetical scenarios to assess interest in testing and actual test results were not available.

It is, therefore, possible that the actual demand for genetic testing for breast cancer susceptibility is not as great as that suggested by these preliminary studies. For example, before the initiation of predictive testing for Huntington's disease (HD), more than two thirds of persons at risk expressed interest in testing.[133] Since predictive testing for HD has become available, fewer than 15% of those who initially expressed interest have come forward.[293,294] However, one critical difference between HD and breast cancer is that breast cancer can be treated and has the potential to be cured if it is found early. This potential for early detection and treatment of breast cancer and the high levels of anxiety about this disease have generated great demand for genetic testing now that it is commercially available.

For those persons who ultimately do decide to receive genetic testing for breast cancer susceptibility, there may be a significant burden associated with the knowledge that one is a carrier of a cancer-predisposing mutation. In the hypothetical studies described earlier, a substantial proportion of women indicated that they would become very depressed and anxious if they received positive results.[291,292] Interestingly, many women also anticipated adverse effects of negative results, including "survivor guilt" (i.e., that other family members had inherited the mutation but they had not) and continued worry.

An earlier descriptive report by Lynch and colleagues did not contain evidence for serious adverse emotional effects of disclosure of BRCA1 mutation status in families with HBOC. However, the need for controlled trials of the impact of testing was acknowledged.[76]

INSURANCE ISSUES

Hudson and colleagues[295] discuss the Genetic Information Nondiscrimination Act (GINA) of 2008, which has been officially signed by the President. It is important to note that GINA addresses only employment and health insurance, excluding life insurance, disability insurance, or long-term-care insurance. Importantly, it prohibits health insurers from using an individual's genetic information for determining eligibility or premiums; in addition, an insurer is prohibited from requesting or requiring that a person undergo a genetic test.

GINA is timely, given the fact that genomic information has grown exponentially, wherein it has revolutionized "...nearly all areas of biomedical research and, many believe, promising an eventual transformation of health care...." This law, along with the Health Insurance Portability and Accountability Act (HIPAA) should assuage the fears and anxieties of patients contemplating DNA mutation testing or those who have already been tested and may remain concerned about being discriminated against by health insurers or employers.

INSURANCE ADJUDICATION FAVORING PROPHYLACTIC OOPHORECTOMY IN HEREDITARY BREAST OR OVARIAN CANCER

Many patients contemplating prophylactic surgery are concerned about whether their insurance will cover the costs for these procedures. The authors provide a case

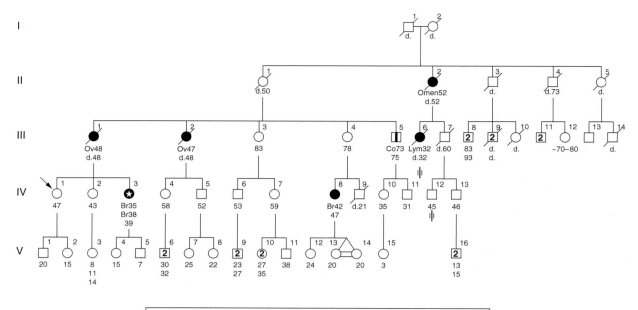

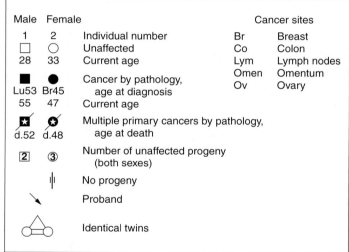

Figure 21-20   Pedigree of a family showing linkage to *BRCA1* and clinical findings consistent with the hereditary breast/ovarian cancer syndrome. The proband initially was denied insurance coverage for prophylactic oophorectomy. (Lynch HT, Severin MJ, Mooney MJ, Lynch JF: Insurance adjudication favoring prophylactic surgery in hereditary breast-ovarian cancer syndrome. Gynecol Oncol 57:23–26, 1995. Reproduced by permission.)

report that we hope will become a legal precedent in support of insurance coverage for indicated prophylactic surgery.[296]

The proband was from a classic HBOC family in which the *BRCA1* gene was subsequently identified. She met the authors' criteria for prophylactic oophorectomy based on her estimated cancer risk status in an HBOC syndrome pedigree (Fig. 21-20).[296] Payment for this procedure was initially denied by the insurer, and the decision was later upheld in a summary judgment issued by the Nebraska District Court, which ruled in favor of the insurance company against the patient. On appeal, the Nebraska Supreme Court concluded that the patient did in fact suffer from a bodily disorder or disease.[297] The Nebraska Supreme Court's decision hinged on descriptions of the term "disease" that were used in several prior court decisions based, in part, on definitions of disease found in standard general and professional dictionaries. The Nebraska Supreme Court applied wording from court decisions concerning related cases, using these definitions to expand the criteria for identifying human conditions in which genetic aberrations result in the impairment of function or damage to tissue.[298–300]

The Decision-Making Process and Genetic Testing

ETHICAL, LEGAL, AND SOCIAL CONSIDERATIONS AND GENETIC TESTING

Burke and colleagues[301] discuss the ethical, legal, and social implications (ELSI) of genetic tests as part of the genetic counseling process, as well as the manner in which certain genetic testing decisions should be determined by personal values. These issues (genetic testing vs. no testing) strike an important balance relevant to their potential benefits for ultimate treatment versus potential harms of "genetic labeling," which must be carefully weighed. Pertinent to hereditary breast cancer, there may exist uncertainty

...concerning both clinical validity and effectiveness of treatment, as in the case of *BRCA1/BRCA2* mutation testing, the value of testing may vary according to different testing contexts. This approach to test categorization allows a rapid determination of the predominant ELSI concerns with different kinds of genetic tests and identifies the data most urgently needed for test evaluation.[301]

We must strive to include the patient as a responsible decision-making participant in this genetic testing decision process, which in fact is the art of medical judgment during the course of the genetic counseling process.

WHO SHOULD BE TESTED?

Lynch and colleagues[302] discussed strategies for genetic testing in hereditary colorectal cancer syndromes and have used this as a model for all forms of hereditary cancer syndromes. It was found to be crucial that the patient receive genetic counseling, once he or she is thoroughly familiar with the Health Insurance Portability and Accountability Act (HIPAA)[303] consenting process. Needed prior to testing is a pedigree of the individual's family that is highly consistent with an HBOC syndrome. It would be helpful if the known germline mutation predisposing to cancer is present in the family. Patients at acceptable high cancer risk status, and therefore informative, should be the one(s) offered testing initially; this will help should there be a distinguishing syndrome stigmata (phenotype) such as multiple trichilemmomas in Cowden syndrome. Risks and benefits must be understood and conveyed through genetic counseling, and consent should be given. A full explanation of surveillance and management strategies should be provided. A major question is the issue of how one determines high cancer-risk status and what one should look for. The answer centers around the ideal setting; that is, one where a mentioned cancer-causing mutation is known to be segregating in the family and the patient is in the direct line of descent—through an affected parent, sibling, or progeny. Reliance, therefore, is placed on the family history and the presence of the mutation.

Ideally, one should inform first- and second-degree relatives of their risk status and the potential for DNA testing. Patients, particularly those who attended a Family Information Service and are sufficiently informed about the presence of the syndrome in their family and its association with the germline mutation, should then encourage their relatives to take responsibility for informing as many people at high risk as possible. Whenever possible, distribution of educational brochures will prove to be helpful. Finally, one should consider a Family Information Service.[304] This service may be highly cost effective in that it poses an efficient way of educating and counseling all available family members from a geographic catchment area during a single session. It makes the best use of a physician's time and effort and has a group therapy potential, which usually makes patients welcome it.

SUMMARY

Considerations for DNA Testing

- Pedigree consistent with HBOC syndrome or other HBC syndrome
- Known germline mutation predisposing to cancer
- Patients at acceptable high cancer-risk status
- Presence of cancer syndrome stigmata (phenotype), such as multiple trichilemmomas in Cowden's syndrome
- Genetic counseling, with understanding of risks and benefits
- Consent
- Results, with a full explanation of the surveillance/management recommendations.

Determining "High Cancer-Risk Status"

- Look for cancer-causing mutation known to be segregating in family
- Look for a patient in direct line of descent (affected parent, sibling, progeny)
- Rely on family history

At-Risk Relatives of Highly Informed Patient(s)

- Ideally, inform first- and/or second-degree relatives, particularly those in clinical catchment area
- Encourage patients to take the responsibility for informing at-risk relatives
- When possible, distribute educational brochures
- Consider Family Information Service

Future of Research in Genetics in Hereditary Cancer

SUMMARY AND FUTURE QUESTIONS

Eisen and Weber[305] conclude that in considering the imperfect surveillance tools for early detection of cancer, especially OC, coupled with the difficult surgical choices for women with *BRCA1* and *BRCA2* mutations, it appears that prophylactic mastectomy is clearly

...the right choice for some women. For the remainder, oophorectomy and tamoxifen in conjunction with intensive screening that includes MRI is a viable alternative. More important, ongoing and novel prospective studies to define the role of prophylactic surgery, new chemopreventive agents, and optimal screening strategies must be supported, and women at very high risk should be encouraged to participate.

Grann and colleagues[306] found that women who were positive for *BRCA1* or *BRCA2* mutations

> ...may derive greater survival and quality adjusted survival benefits than previously reported from chemoprevention, prophylactic surgery, or a combination. Observational studies and clinical trials are needed to verify the results of this analysis of the long-term benefits of preventive strategies among *BRCA1/BRCA2*-positive women.

We believe that third-party carriers should defray the expenses of not only surveillance but, moreover, prophylactic mastectomy and prophylactic salpingo-oophorectomy in women at inordinately high risk for carcinoma of the breast, inclusive of those who are harbingers of *BRCA1* or *BRCA2* germline mutations.

What will be the public health impact of the recent studies showing benefits of prophylactic surgery for mutation carriers, given the enormous magnitude of breast cancer in the general population, particularly in women indigenous to western highly industrialized nations? How will women determine if they are at high risk?[37] Will physicians take family histories that are sufficiently detailed to enable them to make hereditary cancer risk determinations? Are there enough genetic counselors who are sufficiently knowledgeable about cancer genetics and the pros and cons of prophylactic mastectomy and BPO, particularly the potential physical and psychologic sequelae, to adequately and responsibly advise their patients? Indeed, should offering such options be the responsibility of the nonmedically trained genetic counselor? Are the skills of these counselors being sufficiently used? Will insurers defray the cost of genetic counseling, genetic testing, and prophylactic surgery? Will there be insurance discrimination? Will women accept the loss of sexual stimulation following prophylactic mastectomy, particularly with sacrifice of the nipple–areola complex, and/or the change in their body image due to disfigurement? Will women accept the cardiovascular, osteoporotic, and physiologic/sexual risks of BPO? What will be the spouse response? Only time will tell!

FUTURE PROJECTIONS

We predict that as molecular genetic discoveries advance in the throes of this molecular genetic revolution, they will continue to improve our understanding of the diagnostic and pathogenic pathways of breast cancer, contribute to the development of molecular-based designer drugs, provide new insights about prophylactic surgery, and contribute to improved cancer control in hereditary forms of breast cancer. New imaging studies in their developmental stage will aid in earlier diagnosis, thereby maximizing the potential for curative radiation and chemotherapy.

The authors have attempted to review what they consider to be the most salient clinical and research aspects of HBC genetics. However, the reader will realize immediately that progress has been so rapid in this field that by the day this work is sent to the printer, new concepts and developments in all facets of HBC research will probably have taken place. Therefore, the best use of material in this chapter is to provide background, much of which will become historical, thereby compelling the reader to search the current literature.

Finally, society will have to find ways for DNA testing costs to be contained and, whenever possible, covered by third-party payers. Legislation may become necessary to prohibit employers or insurance companies from discrimination because an individual happens to have been found to harbor a deleterious cancer-prone gene. Clearly, the task will be an enormous one, but it must be initiated at this time because progress in the field of molecular genetics and cancer epidemiology is moving ahead at an almost logarithmic pace. The professional and lay literature is keeping abreast of these advances, and as a consequence, patient demand for genetic services, including DNA testing, has increased at almost exponential proportions.

Acknowledgments

We greatly appreciate funding support for the several research projects on hereditary breast and ovarian cancer, which provided us material for inclusion in this chapter. This includes revenue from Nebraska cigarette taxes awarded to Creighton University by the Nebraska Department of Health and Human Services. The contents of this chapter are solely the responsibility of the authors and do not necessarily represent the official views of the State of Nebraska or the Nebraska Department of Health and Human Services. Funding support was also provided through the following NIH/NCI Grants: #1U01 CA 86389; 1 U01 CZ 77165; and 1 RO1 CA 838555-01. Dr. Henry Lynch's work is partially funded through the Charles F. and Mary C. Heider Chair in Cancer Research, which he holds at Creighton University.

We gratefully acknowledge the painstaking effort provided by Trudy Shaw, MA, throughout the updating of this chapter. We also extend our gratitude to the literally thousands of high cancer-risk patients who have allowed us to study them and their families in order to learn about breast cancer genetics, so that this knowledge could be used in the writing of this chapter. These studies have allowed us to grasp some degree of understanding of this exceedingly complex subject.

REFERENCES

1. Jemal A, Siegel R, Ward E, et al: Cancer statistics, 2007. CA Cancer J Clin 57:43–66, 2007.
2. Eng C, Brody LC, Wagner TMU, et al: Interpreting epidemiological research: Blinded comparison of methods used to estimate the prevalence of inherited mutations in *BRCA1*. J Med Genet 38:824–833, 2001.
3. Berry DA, Iversen ES Jr, Gudbjartsson DF, et al: BRCAPRO validation, sensitivity of genetic testing of *BRCA1/BRCA2* and prevalence of other breast cancer susceptibility genes. J Clin Oncol 20:2701–2712, 2002.
4. Meijers-Heijboer H, van den Ouweland A, Klijn J, et al: Low-penetrance susceptibility to breast cancer due to *CHEK2*1100delC* in noncarriers of *BRCA1* and *BRCA2* mutations. Nat Genet 31:55–59, 2002.
5. Howlett NG, Taniguchi T, Olson S, et al: Biallelic inactivation of *BRCA2* in Fanconi anemia. Science 297:606–609, 2002.

6. Pharoah PDP, Antoniou AC, Easton DF, Ponder BAJ: Polygenes, risk prediction, and targeted prevention of breast cancer. N Engl J Med 358:2796–2803, 2008.

7. Pharoah PD, Antoniou A, Bobrow M, et al: Polygenic susceptibility to breast cancer and implications for prevention. Nat Genet 31:33–36, 2002.

8. Madigan MP, Ziegler RG, Benichou J, et al: Proportion of breast cancer cases in the United States explained by well-established risk factors. J Natl Cancer Inst 87:1681–1685, 1995.

9. Stratton MR, Rahman N: The emerging landscape of breast cancer susceptibility. Nat Genet 40:17–22, 2008.

10. Narod SA, Goldgar D, Cannon-Albright L, et al: Risk modifiers in carriers of BRCA1 mutations. Int J Cancer (Pred Oncol) 64:394–398, 1995.

11. Jernstrom H, Lerman C, Ghadirian P, et al: Pregnancy and risk of early breast cancer in carriers of BRCA1 and BRCA2. Lancet 354:1846–1850, 1999.

12. Brunet J-S, Ghadirian P, Rebbeck TR, et al: Effect of smoking on breast cancer in carriers of mutant BRCA1 or BRCA2 genes. J Natl Cancer Inst 90:761–766, 1998.

13. Broca PP: Traité des tumeurs. Paris, Asselin, 1866.

14. Lynch HT, Krush AJ, Lemon HM, et al: Tumor variation in families with breast cancer. JAMA 222:1631–1635, 1972.

15. Lynch HT, Krush AJ: Carcinoma of the breast and ovary in three families. Surg Gynecol Obstet 133:644–648, 1971.

16. Hall JM, Lee MK, Newman B, et al: Linkage of early-onset breast cancer to chromosome 17q21. Science 250:1684–1689, 1990.

17. Narod SA, Feunteun J, Lynch HT, et al: Familial breast-ovarian cancer locus on chromosome 17q12-q23. Lancet 388:82–83, 1991.

18. Miki Y, Swensen J, Shattuck-Eidens D, et al: A strong candidate for the breast and ovarian cancer susceptibility gene BRCA1. Science 266:66–71, 1994.

19. Wooster R, Neuhausen SL, Mangion J, et al: Localization of a breast cancer susceptibility gene, BRCA2, to chromosome 13q12-13. Science 265:2088–2090, 1994.

20. Wooster R, Bignell G, Lancaster J, et al: Identification of the breast cancer susceptibility gene BRCA2. Nature 378:789–792, 1995.

21. Lynch HT, Follett KL, Lynch PM, et al: Family history in an oncology clinic: Implications for cancer genetics. JAMA 242:1268–1272, 1979.

22. David KL, Steiner-Grossman P: The potential use of tumor registry data in the recognition and prevention of hereditary and familial cancer. NY State J Med 91:150–152, 1991.

23. Collaborative Group on Hormonal Factors in Breast Cancer: Familial breast cancer: Collaborative reanalysis of individual data from 52 epidemiological studies including 58,209 women with breast cancer and 101,986 women without the disease. Lancet 358:1389–1399, 2001.

24. Rubinstein WS, O'Neill SM: Quantitative risk assessment. Advanced therapy of breast disease. New York, BC Decker, 2004.

25. Saslow D, Boetes C, Burke W, et al: American Cancer Society guidelines for breast screening with MRI as an adjunct to mammography. CA Cancer J Clin 57:75–89, 2007.

26. Lynch HT, Lynch J, Conway T, et al: Hereditary breast cancer and family cancer syndromes. World J Surg 18:21–31, 1994.

27. Lynch HT, Watson P, Conway TA, et al: DNA screening for breast/ovarian cancer susceptibility based on linked markers: A family study. Arch Intern Med 153:1979–1987, 1993.

28. Kauff ND, Scheuer L, Robson ME, et al: Insurance reimbursement for risk-reducing mastectomy and oophorectomy in women with BRCA1 or BRCA2 mutations. Genet Med 3:422–425, 2001.

29. Lynch HT, Lemon SJ, Durham C, et al: A descriptive study of BRCA1 testing and reactions to disclosure of test results. Cancer 79:2219–2228, 1997.

30. Peters J: Familial cancer risk–Part I: Impact on today's oncology practice. J Oncol Manage 3:18–30, 1994.

31. Peters J: Familial cancer risk–Part II. Breast cancer risk counseling and genetic susceptiblity testing. J Oncol Manage 3:14–22, 1994.

32. Peterson EA, Milliron KJ, Lewis KE, et al: Health insurance and discrimination concerns and BRCA1/2 testing in a clinic population. Cancer Epidemiol Biomarkers Prev 11:79–87, 2002.

33. Hartmann LC, Sellers TA, Schaid DJ, et al: Efficacy of bilateral prophylactic mastectomy in BRCA1 and BRCA2 gene mutation carriers. J Natl Cancer Inst 93:1633–1637, 2001.

34. Rebbeck TR, Levin AM, Eisen A, et al: Breast cancer risk after bilateral prophylactic oophorectomy in BRCA1 mutation carriers. J Natl Cancer Inst 91:1475–1479, 1999.

35. Narod SA, Brunet J-S, Ghadirian P, et al: Tamoxifen and risk of contralateral breast cancer in BRCA1 and BRCA2 mutation carriers: A case-control study. Lancet 356:1876–1881, 2000.

36. Eisen A, Rebbeck TR, Wood WC, Weber BL: Prophylactic surgery in women with a hereditary predisposition to breast and ovarian cancer. J Clin Oncol 18:1980–1995, 2000.

37. Lynch HT, Lynch JF, Rubinstein WS: Prophylactic mastectomy: Obstacles and benefits. J Natl Cancer Inst 93:1586–1587, 2001.

38. Scheuer L, Kauff N, Robson M, et al: Outcome of preventive surgery and screening for breast and ovarian cancer in BRCA mutation carriers. J Clin Oncol 20:1260–1268, 2002.

39. Andrieu N, Easton DF, Chang-Claude J, et al: Effect of chest x-rays on the risk of breast cancer among BRCA1/2 mutation carriers in the BRCA1/2 Carrier Cohort Study: A report from the EMBRACE, GENEPSO, GEO-HEBON, and IBCCS Collaborators' Group. J Clin Oncol 24:3361–3366, 2006.

40. Narod SA, Lubinski J, Ghadirian P, et al: Screening mammography and risk of breast cancer in BRCA1 and BRCA2 mutation carriers: A case-control study. Lancet Oncol 7:402–406, 2006.

41. Rebbeck TR, Lynch HT, Neuhausen SL, et al: Prophylactic oophorectomy in carriers of BRCA1 or BRCA2 mutations. N Engl J Med 346:1616–1622, 2002.

42. Dyck HG, Hamilton TC, Godwin AK, et al: Autonomy of the epithelial phenotype in human ovarian surface epithelium: Changes with neoplastic progression and with a family history of ovarian cancer. Int J Cancer (Pred Oncol) 69:429–436, 1996.

43. Hensley ML, Castiel M, Robson ME: Screening for ovarian cancer: What we know, what we need to know. Oncology 14:1601–1607, 2001.

44. Petricoin EF, III, Ardekani AM, Hitt BA, et al: Use of proteomic patterns in serum to identify ovarian cancer. Lancet 359:572–577, 2002.

45. Easton DF, Ford D, Bishop DT, and the The Breast Cancer Linkage Consortium: Breast and ovarian cancer incidence in BRCA1 mutation carriers. Am J Hum Genet 56:265–271, 1995.

46. Ford D, Easton DF: The genetics of breast and ovarian cancer. Br J Cancer 72:805–812, 1995.

47. Easton DF, Bishop DT, Ford D, et al: Genetic linkage analysis in familial breast and ovarian cancer: results from 214 families. Am J Hum Genet 52:678–701, 1993.

48. Frank TS, Deffenbaugh AM, Reid JE, et al: Clinical characteristics of individuals with germline mutations in BRCA1 and BRCA2: Analysis of 10,000 individuals. J Clin Oncol 20:1480–1490, 2002.

49. Chen S, Parmigiani G: Meta-analysis of BRCA1 and BRCA2 penetrance. J Clin Oncol 25:1329–1333, 2007.

50. Ford D, Easton DF, Bishop DT, et al: Risks of cancer in BRCA1-mutation carriers. Lancet 343:692–695, 1994.

51. Serova O, Montagna M, Torchard D, et al: A high incidence of BRCA1 mutations in 20 breast-ovarian cancer families. Am J Hum Genet 58:42–51, 1996.

52. Shattuck-Eidens D, McClure M, Simard J, et al: A collaborative survey of 80 mutations in the BRCA1 breast and ovarian cancer susceptibility gene: Implications for presymptomatic testing and screening. JAMA 273:535–541, 1995.

53. Bressac-de-Paillerets B, Di Rocco ZC, Gad S, et al: Comparative analysis of methods for detecting BRCA1 rearrangements in breast-ovarian cancer families. Am J Hum Genet 69(suppl 4):248, 2001 [Abstract 377].

54. Gayther SA, Warren W, Mazoyer S, et al: Germline mutations of the BRCA1 gene in breast and ovarian cancer families provide evidence for a genotype-phenotype correlation. Nat Genet 11:428–433, 1995.

55. Saal LH, Gruvberger-Saal SK, Persson C, et al: Recurrent gross mutations of the PTEN tumor suppressor gene in breast cancers with deficient DSB repair. Nat Genet 40:102–107, 2008.

56. Antoniou AC, Sinilnikova OM, Simard J, et al: RAD51 135G → C modifies breast cancer risk among BRCA2 mutation carriers: Results from a combined analysis of 19 studies. Am J Hum Genet 81:1186–1200, 2007.

57. Stacey SN, Sulem P, Johannsson OT, et al: The BARD1 Cys557Ser variant and breast cancer risk in Iceland. PLoS Med 3:e217, 2006.

58. Parmigiani G, Berry DA, Aguilar O: Determining carrier probabilities for breast cancer-susceptibility genes *BRCA1* and *BRCA2*. Am J Hum Genet 62:145–158, 1998.
59. Parmigiani G, Berry DA, Iversen E, et al: Modeling risk of breast cancer and decisions about genetic testing. In Gatsonis C, Kass RE, Carlin B, et al (eds): Case studies in Bayesian statistics IV. New York, Springer, 1999, pp 173–268.
60. Parmigiani G, Chen S, Iversen ES Jr, et al: Validity of models for predicting *BRCA1* and *BRCA2* mutations. Ann Intern Med 147:441–450, 2007.
61. Euhus DM, Smith KC, Robinson L, et al: Pretest prediction of *BRCA1* or *BRCA2* mutation by risk counselors and the computer model BRCAPRO. J Natl Cancer Inst 94:844–851, 2002.
62. Weitzel JN, Lagos VI, Cullinane CA, et al: Limited family structure and BRCA gene mutation status in single cases of breast cancer. JAMA 297:2587–2595, 2007.
63. Nanda R, Schumm LP, Cummings S, et al: Genetic testing in an ethnically diverse cohort of high-risk women: A comparative analysis of *BRCA1* and *BRCA2* mutations in American families of European and African ancestry. JAMA 294:1925–1933, 2005.
64. Vogel KJ, Atchley DP, Erlichman J, et al: *BRCA1* and *BRCA2* genetic testing in Hispanic patients: Mutation prevalence and evaluation of the BRCAPRO risk assessment model. J Clin Oncol 25:4635–4641, 2007.
65. Antoniou AC, Hardy R, Walker L, et al: Predicting the likelihood of carrying a *BRCA1* or *BRCA2* mutation: Validation of BOADICEA, BRCAPRO, IBIS, Myriad and the Manchester scoring system using data from UK genetics clinics. J Med Genet 45:425–431, 2008.
66. Struewing JP, Brody LC, Erdos MR, et al: Detection of eight *BRCA1* mutations in 10 breast/ovarian cancer families, including 1 family with male breast cancer. Am J Hum Genet 57:1–7, 1995.
67. Roa BB, Boyd AA, Volcik K, Richards CS: Ashkenazi Jewish population frequencies for common mutations in *BRCA1* and *BRCA2*. Nat Genet 14:185–187, 1996.
68. Offit K, Gilewski T, McGuire P, et al: Germline *BRCA1* 185delAG mutations in Jewish women with breast cancer. Lancet 347:1642–1645, 1996.
69. Modan B, Gak E, Sade-Bruchim RB, et al: High frequency of *BRCA1* 185delAG mutation in ovarian cancer in Israel. JAMA 276:1823–1825, 1996.
70. Helmrich SP, Shapiro S, Rosenberg L, et al: Risk factors for breast cancer. Am J Epidemiol 117:35–45, 1983.
71. King MC, Marks JH, Mandell JB, and the New York Breast Cancer Study Group: Breast and ovarian cancer risks due to inherited mutations in *BRCA1* and *BRCA2*. Science 302:643–646, 2003.
72. Oddoux C, Struewing JP, Clayton CM, et al: The carrier frequency of the *BRCA2* 6174delT mutation among Ashkenazi Jewish individuals is approximately 1%. Nat Genet 14:188–190, 1996.
73. Gayther SA, Mangion J, Russell P, et al: Variation of risks of breast and ovarian cancer associated with different germline mutations of the *BRCA2* gene. Nat Genet 15:103–105, 1997.
74. Risch HA, McLaughlin JR, Cole DEC, et al: Prevalence and penetrance of germline *BRCA1* and *BRCA2* mutations in a population series of 649 women with ovarian cancer. Am J Hum Genet 68:700–710, 2001.
75. Mitra A, Fisher C, Foster CS, et al: Prostate cancer in male *BRCA1* and *BRCA2* mutation carriers has a more aggressive phenotype. Br J Cancer 98:502–507, 2008.
76. Lynch HT, Watson P, Conway T, et al: Breast cancer family history as a risk factor for early onset breast cancer. Breast Cancer Res Treat 11:263–267, 1988.
77. Claus EB, Risch N, Thompson WD: Age of onset as an indicator of familial risk of breast cancer. Am J Epidemiol 131:961–972, 1990.
78. Mettlin C, Croghan I, Natarajan N, Lane W: The association of age and familial risk in a case-control study of breast cancer. Am J Epidemiol 131:973–983, 1990.
79. Tilanus-Linthorst MMA, Obdeijn I-M, Hop WCJ, et al: *BRCA1* mutation and young age predict fast breast cancer growth in the Dutch, United Kingdom, and Canadian Magnetic Resonance Imaging Screening Trials. Clin Cancer Res 13:7357–7362, 2007.
80. Eerola H, Vahteristo P, Sarantaus L, et al: Survival of breast cancer patients in *BRCA1*, *BRCA2*, and non-*BRCA1/2* breast cancer families: A relative survival analysis from Finland. Int J Cancer 93:368–372, 2001.
81. Foulkes WD, Chappuis PO, Wong N, et al: Primary node negative breast cancer in *BRCA1* mutation carriers has a poor outcome. Ann Oncol 11:307–313, 2000.
82. Stoppa-Lyonnet D, Ansquer Y, Dreyfus H, et al: Familial invasive breast cancers: Worse outcome related to *BRCA1* mutations. J Clin Oncol 18:4053–4059, 2000.
83. Rennert G, Bisland-Naggan S, Barnett-Griness O, et al: Clinical outcomes of breast cancer in carriers of *BRCA1* and *BRCA2* mutations. N Engl J Med 357:115–123, 2007.
84. Marcus J, Watson P, Linder-Stephenson L, et al: The pathobiology of *BRCA1*-linked and -unlinked hereditary breast cancer (HBC). Modern Pathol 7:18A,1994 [Abstract].
85. Lynch HT, Marcus JN, Watson P, Lynch J: Familial breast cancer, cancer family syndromes, and predisposition to breast neoplasms. In Bland K, Copeland EM (eds): The breast. Philadelphia, WB Saunders, 1991, pp 262–291.
86. Claus EB, Risch N, Thompson WD, et al: Relationship between breast histopathology and family history of breast cancer. Am J Epidemiol 131:961–972, 1990.
87. Marcus J, Page D, Watson P, et al: High mitotic grade in hereditary breast cancer. Lab Investig 56:61A, 1988 [Abstract].
88. Mulcahy GM, Platt R: Pathologic aspects of familial carcinoma of the breast. In Lynch HT (ed): Genetics and breast cancer. New York, Van Nostrand Reinhold, 1981, pp 65–97.
89. Rosen PP, Lesser ML, Senie MA, Kinne DW: Epidemiology of breast carcinoma III: Relationship of family history to tumor type. Cancer 50:171–179, 1982.
90. Erdreich LS, Asal NR, Hoge AF: Morphologic types of breast cancer: Age, bilaterality, and family history. South Med J 73:28–32, 1980.
91. LiVolsi VA, Kelsey JL, Fischer DB, et al: Effect of age at first child-birth on risk of developing specific histologic subtype of breast cancer. Cancer 49:1937–1940, 1982.
92. Stalsberg H, Thomas DB, Noonan EA: The WHO collaborative study of neoplasia and steroid contraceptives. Histologic types of breast carcinoma in relation to international variation and breast cancer risk factors. Cancer 44:399–409, 1989.
93. Lagios MD, Rose MR, Margolin FR: Tubular carcinoma of the breast: Association with multicentricity, bilaterality, and family history of mammary carcinoma. Am J Clin Pathol 73:25–30, 1980.
94. Mosimann S, Torhorst JKH, Weber W, Muller H: Histopathological aspects of familial breast cancer. In Weber W, Laffer UT, Durig M (eds): Hereditary cancer and preventive surgery. Karger, Basel, 1990, pp 1–7.
95. Claus EB, Risch N, Thompson WD, Carter D: Relationship between breast histopathology and family history of breast cancer. Cancer 71:147–153, 1993.
96. Glebov OK, McKenzie KE, White CA, Sukumar S: Frequent p53 gene mutations and novel alleles in familial breast cancer. Cancer Res 54:3703–3709, 1994.
97. Marcus JN, Page DL, Watson P, et al: *BRCA1* and *BRCA2* hereditary breast carcinoma phenotypes. Cancer 80(suppl):543–556, 1997.
98. Marcus JN, Watson P, Page DL, Lynch HT: The pathology and heredity of breast cancer in younger women. J Natl Cancer Inst Monogr 16:23–34, 1994.
99. Marcus JN, Watson P, Page DL, et al: Hereditary breast cancer: Pathobiology, prognosis, and *BRCA1* and *BRCA2* gene linkage. Cancer 77:697–709, 1996.
100. Marcus JN, Watson P, Page DL, et al: *BRCA2* hereditary breast cancer pathophenotype. Breast Cancer Res Treat 44:275–277, 1997.
101. Breast Cancer Linkage Consortium: Pathology of familial breast cancer: differences between breast cancers in carriers of *BRCA1* or *BRCA2* mutations and sporadic cases. Lancet 349:1505–1510, 1997.
102. Eisinger F, Stoppa-Lyonnet D, Longy M, et al: Germ line mutation at *BRCA1* affects the histoprognostic grade in hereditary breast cancer. Cancer Res 56:471–474, 1996.
103. Lakhani SR, Jacquemier J, Sloane JP, et al: Multifactorial analysis of differences between sporadic breast cancers and cancers involving *BRCA1* and *BRCA2* mutations. J Natl Cancer Inst 90:1138–1145, 1998.

104. Lynch BJ, Holden JA, Buys SS, et al: Pathobiologic characteristics of hereditary breast cancer. Hum Pathol 29:1140–1144, 1998.

105. Lubinski J, Gorski B, Huzarski T, et al: BRCA1-positive breast cancers in young women from Poland. Cancer Res Treat 99:71–76, 2006.

106. Sobol H, Stoppa-Lyonnet D, Bressac-de-Paillerets B, et al: Truncation at conserved terminal regions of BRCA1 protein is associated with highly proliferating hereditary breast cancers. Cancer Res 56:3216–3219, 1996.

107. Jóhannsson OT, Idvall I, Anderson C, et al: Tumour biological features of BRCA1-induced breast and ovarian cancer. Eur J Cancer 33:362–371, 1997.

108. Rahman N, Stratton MR: The genetics of breast cancer susceptibility. Annu Rev Genet 32:95–121, 1998.

109. Armes JE, Egan AJM, Southey MC, et al: The histologic phenotypes of breast carcinoma occurring before age 40 years in women with and without BRCA1 or BRCA2 germline mutations: A population-based study. Cancer 83:2335–2345, 1998.

110. Eisinger F, Jacquemier J, Charpin C, et al: Mutations at BRCA1: The medullary breast carcinoma revisited. Cancer Res 58: 1588–1592, 1998.

111. Eerola H, Heikkilä P, Tamminen A, et al: Histopathological features of breast tumors in BRCA1, BRCA2 and mutation-negative breast cancer families. Breast Cancer Res 7:R93–R100, 2005.

112. Brekelmans CTM, Tilanus-Linthorst MMA, Seynaeve C, et al: Tumour characteristics, survival and prognostic factors of hereditary breast cancer from BRCA2-, BRCA1- and non-BRCA1/2 families as compared to sporadic breast cancer cases. Eur J Cancer 43:867–876, 2007.

113. Lakhani SR, Gusterson BA, Jacquemier J, et al: The pathology of familial breast cancer: Histologic features of cancers in families not attributable to mutations in BRCA1 or BRCA2. Clin Cancer Res 6:782–789, 2000.

114. Honrado E, Osorio A, Palacios J, Benitez J: Pathology and gene expression of hereditary breast tumors associated with BRCA1, BRCA2 and CHEK2 gene mutations. Oncogene 25:5837–5845, 2006.

115. Marcus J, Linder-Stephenson L, Conway T, et al: High S phase fraction in hereditary breast carcinoma. Cytometry. 14(suppl 6): 34, 1993.

116. Armes JE, Trute L, White D, et al: Distinct molecular pathogeneses of early-onset breast cancers in BRCA1 and BRCA2 mutation carriers: A population-based study. Cancer Res 59:2011–2017, 1999.

117. Lakhani SR, van de Vijver MJ, Jacquermier J, et al: The pathology of familial breast cancer: Predictive value of immunohistochemical markers estrogen receptor, progesterone receptor, HER-2, and p53 in patients with mutations in BRCA1 and BRCA2. J Clin Oncol 20:2310–2318, 2002.

118. Noguchi S, Kasugai T, Miki Y, et al: Clinicopathologic analysis of BRCA1- or BRCA2-associated hereditary breast carcinoma in Japanese women, Cancer 85:2200–2205, 1999.

119. Colombo M, Giarola M, Mariani L, et al: Cyclin D1 expression analysis in familial breast cancers may discriminate BRCAX from BRCA2-linked cases. Mod Pathol 21:1262–1270, 2008.

120. Thor AD, Moore DH, II, Edgerton SM, et al: Accumulation of p53 tumor suppressor gene protein: An independent marker of prognosis in breast cancers. J Natl Cancer Inst 84:845–855, 1992.

121. Meyer JS, He W: High proliferative rates demonstrated by bromodeoxyuridine labeling index in breast carcinomas with p53 overexpression. J Surg Oncol 156:146–152, 1994.

122. Greenblatt M, Chappuis P, Bond J, et al: TP53 Mutations in breast cancer associated with BRCA1 and BRCA2 germline mutations: Distinctive spectrum and structural distribution. Cancer Res 61:4092–4097, 2001.

123. Hedenfalk I, Duggan D, Chen Y, et al: Gene expression profiles in hereditary breast cancer. N Engl J Med 344:539–548, 2001.

124. van't Veer LJ, Dai H, van de Vijver M, et al: Gene expression profiling predicts clinical outcome of breast cancer. J Clin Pathol 59:611–617, 2002.

125. Sørlie T, Tibshirani R, Parker J, et al: Repeated observation of breast tumor subtypes in independent gene expression data sets. Proc Natl Acad Sci USA 100:8418–8423, 2003.

126. Laasko M, Loman N, Borg Å, Isola J: Cytokeratin 5/14-positive breast cancer: True basal phenotype confined to BRCA1 tumors. Mod Pathol 18:1321–1328, 2005.

127. Liu S, Ginestier C, Charafe-Jauffret E, et al: BRCA1 regulates human mammary stem/progenitor cell fate. Proc Natl Acad Sci USA 105:1680–1685, 2008.

128. Jacquemier J, Padovani L, Rabayrol L, et al: Typical medullary breast carcinomas have a basal/myoepithelial phenotype. J Pathol 207:260–268, 2005.

129. Rodriguez-Pinilla SM, Rodriguez-Gil Y, Moreno-Bueno G, et al: Sporadic invasive breast carcinomas with medullary features display a basal-like phenotype: An immunohistochemical and gene amplification study. Am J Surg Pathol 31:501–508, 2007.

130. Bewtra C, Watson P, Conway T, et al: Hereditary ovarian cancer: A clinicopathological study. Int J Gynecol Pathol 11:180–187, 1992.

131. Hartwell LH, Kastan MB: Cell cycle control and cancer. Science 266:1821–1928, 1994.

132. Shackney SE, Smith CA, Miller BW, et al: Model for the genetic evolution of solid tumors. Cancer Res 49:3344–3354, 1989.

133. Cornelisse CJ, Kuipers-Dijkhoorn N, van Vliet M, et al: Fractional allelic imbalance in human breast cancer increases with tetraploidization and chromosome loss. Int J Cancer 50:544–548, 1992.

134. Dutrillaux B, Gerbault-Seureau M, Remvikos Y, et al: Breast cancer genetic evolution: I. Data from cytogenetics and DNA content. Breast Cancer Res Treat 19:245–255, 1991.

135. Remvikos Y, Gerbault-Seureau M, Magdelénat H, et al: Proliferative activity of breast cancers increases in the course of genetic evolution as defined by cytogenetic analysis. Breast Cancer Res Treat 23:43–49, 1992.

136. Melchor L, Honrado E, Garcia MJ, et al: Distinct genomic aberration patterns are found in familial breast cancer associated with different immunohistochemical subtypes. Oncogene 27: 3165–3175, 2008.

137. Meyer JS: Cellular proliferation in normal human breast ducts, fibroadenomas, and other ductal hyperplasias measured by nuclear labeling with tritiated thymidine: Effects of menstrual phase, age, and oral contraceptive hormones. Human Pathol 8:67–81, 1977.

138. Russo J, Calaf G, Roi L, Russo IH: Influence of age and gland topography on cell kinetics of normal human breast tissue. J Natl Cancer Inst 78:413–418, 1987.

139. Olsson H, Ranstam J, Baldetorp B, et al: Proliferation and DNA ploidy in malignant breast tumors in relation to early oral contraceptive use and early abortions. Cancer 67:1285–1290, 1991.

140. Holt JT, Thompson ME, Szabo CI, et al: Growth retardation and tumour inhibition by BRCA1. Nat Genet 12:298–302, 1996.

141. Jarvis EM, Kirk JA, Clarke CL: Loss of nuclear BRCA1 expression in breast cancers is associated with a highly proliferative tumor phenotype. Cancer Genet Cytogenet 101:109–115, 1998.

142. Thompson ME, Jensen RA, Obermiler PS, et al: Decreased expression of BRCA1 accelerates growth and is often present during sporadic breast cancer progression, Nat Genet 9:444–450, 1995.

143. Agnarsson BA, Jonasson JG, Björnsdottir IB, et al: Inherited BRCA2 mutation associated with high grade breast cancer. Breast Cancer Res Treat 47:121–127, 1998.

144. Bane AL, Beck JC, Bleiweiss I, et al: BRCA2 mutation-associated breast cancers exhibit a distinguishing phenotype based on morphology and molecular profiles from tissue microarrays. Am J Surg Pathol 31:121–128, 2007.

145. John EM, Hopper JL, Beck JC: The Breast Cancer Family Registry: An infrastructure for cooperative multinational, interdisciplinary and translational studies of the genetic epidemiology of breast cancer. Breast Cancer Res 6:R375–R389, 2004.

146. Robson M, Rajan P, Rosen PP, et al: BRCA-associated breast cancer: Absence of a characteristic immunophenotype? Cancer Res 58:1839–1842, 1998.

147. Lubinski J, Phelan CM, Ghadirian P, et al: Cancer variation associated with the position of the mutation in the BRCA2 gene. Fam Cancer 3:1–10, 2004.

148. Karp SE, Tonin PN, Begin LR, et al: Influence of BRCA1 mutations on nuclear grade and estrogen receptor status of breast carcinoma in Ashkenazi Jewish women. Cancer 80:435–441, 1997.

149. Loman N, Johannsson O, Bendahl P-O, et al: Steroid receptors in hereditary breast carcinomas associated with *BRCA1* or *BRCA2* mutations or unknown susceptibility genes. Cancer 83:310–319, 1998.

150. Verhoog LC, Brekelmans CTM, Seynaeve C, et al: Survival and tumour characteristics of breast-cancer patients with germline mutations of *BRCA1*. Lancet 351:316–321, 1998.

151. Ford D, Easton DF, Stratton M, et al: Genetic heterogeneity and penetrance analysis of the *BRCA1* and *BRCA2* genes in breast cancer families. Am J Hum Genet 62:676–689, 1998.

152. Malone KE, Daling JR, Doody DR, et al: Prevalence and predictors of *BRCA1* and *BRCA2* mutations in a population-based study of breast cancer in white and black American women ages 35 to 64 years. Cancer Res 66:8297–8308, 2006.

153. Palacios J, Honrado E, Osorio A, et al: Immunohistochemical characteristics defined by tissue microarray of hereditary breast cancer not attributable to *BRCA1* or *BRCA2* mutations: Differences from breast carcinomas arising in *BRCA1* and *BRCA2* mutation carriers. Clin Cancer Res 9:3606–3614, 2003.

154. Honrado E, Osorio A, Milne RL, et al: Immunohistochemical classification of non-*BRCA1/2* tumors identifies different groups that demonstrate the heterogeneity of *BRCAX* families. Modern Pathol 20:1298–1306, 2007.

155. Keller G, Vogelsang H, Becker I, et al: Diffuse type gastric and lobular breast carcinoma in a familial gastric cancer patient with an E-cadherin germline mutation. Am J Pathol 155:337–342, 1999.

156. Pharoah PDP, Guilford P, Caldas C, and the International Gastric Cancer Linkage Consortium: Incidence of gastric cancer and breast cancer in *CDH1* (E-cadherin) mutation carriers from hereditary diffuse gastric cancer families. Gastroenterology 121:1348–1353, 2001.

157. Kaurah P, MacMillan A, Boyd N, et al: Founder and recurrent *CDH1* mutations in families with hereditary diffuse gastric cancer. JAMA 297:2360–2372, 2007.

158. Lynch HT, Kaurah P, Wirtzfeld D, et al: Hereditary diffuse gastric cancer: Diagnosis, genetic counseling, and prophylactic total gastrectomy. Cancer 112:2655–2663, 2008.

159. Huzarski T, Cybulski C, Domagala W, et al: Pathology of breast cancer in women with constitutional *CHEK2* mutations. Breast Cancer Res Treat 90:187–189, 2005.

160. Balleine RL, Murali R, Bilious AM, et al: Histopathologic features of breast cancer in carriers of *ATM* gene variants. Histopathology 49:523–532, 2006.

161. Kauff ND, Brogi E, Scheuer L, et al: Epithelial lesions in prophylactic mastectomy specimens from women with *BRCA* mutations. Cancer 97:1601–1608, 2003.

162. Smith KL, Adank M, Kauff N, et al: *BRCA* mutations in women with ductal carcinoma in situ. Clin Cancer Res 13:4306–4310, 2007.

163. Sun CC, Lenoir G, Lynch H, Narod SA: In-situ breast cancer and *BRCA1*. Lancet 348:408, 1996.

164. Jacquemier J, Eisinger F, Guinebretiere J-M, et al: Intraductal component and *BRCA1*-associated breast cancer. Lancet 350:1098, 1996.

165. Claus EB, Petruzella S, Matloff E, Carter D: Prevalence of *BRCA1* and *BRCA1* mutations in women diagnosed with ductal carcinoma in situ. JAMA 293:964–969, 2005.

166. Hamilton LJ, Evans AJ, Wilson AR, et al: Breast imaging findings in women with *BRCA1*- and *BRCA1*-associated breast carcinoma. Clin Radiol 59:895–902, 2004.

167. Bonadona V, Dussart-Moser S, Voirin N, et al: Prognosis of early-onset breast cancer based on *BRCA1/2* mutation status in a French population-based cohort and review. Breast Cancer Res Treat 101:233–245, 2007.

168. Warner E, Plewes DB, Hill KA, et al: Surveillance of *BRCA1* and *BRCA2* mutation carriers with magnetic resonance imaging, ultrasound, mammography, and clinical breast examination. JAMA 292:1317–1325, 2004.

169. Górski B, Narod SA, Lubinski J: A common missense variant in *BRCA2* predisposes to early onset breast cancer. Breast Cancer Res 7:1023–1027, 2005.

170. Watson P, Marcus JN, Lynch HT: Prognosis of *BRCA1* hereditary breast cancer. Lancet 351:304–305, 1998.

171. Foulkes WD, Goffin J, Brunet JS, et al: Tamoxifen may be an effective adjuvant treatment for *BRCA1*-related breast cancer irrespective of estrogen receptor status. J Natl Cancer Inst 94:1504–1506, 2002.

172. Gaffney DK, Brohet RM, Holden JA, et al: Response to radiation therapy and prognosis in breast cancer patients with *BRCA1* and *BRCA2* mutations, Radiother Oncol 47:129–136, 1998.

173. Hamann U, Sinn H-P: Survival and tumor characteristics of German hereditary breast cancer patients. Breast Cancer Res Treat 59:185–192, 2000.

174. Jóhannsson OT, Ranstam J, Borg Å, Olsson H: Survival of *BRCA1* breast and ovarian cancer patients: A population-based study from southern Sweden. J Clin Oncol 16:397–404, 1998.

175. Porter DE, Cohen BB, Wallace MR, et al: Breast cancer incidence, penetrance and survival in probable carriers of *BRCA1* gene mutation in families linked to *BRCA1* on chromosome 17q12-21. Br J Surg 81:1512–1515, 1994.

176. Foulkes WD, Wong N, Brunet J-S, et al: Germ-line *BRCA1* mutation is an adverse prognostic factor in Ashkenazi Jewish women with breast cancer. Clin Cancer Res 3:2465–2469, 1997.

177. Møller P, Borg A, Evans DG, et al: Survival in prospectively ascertained familial breast cancer: Analysis of a series stratified by tumour characteristics, *BRCA* mutations and oophorectomy. Int J Cancer 101:555–559, 2002.

178. Phillips K-A, Andrulis IL, Goodwin PJ: Breast carcinomas arising in carriers of mutations in *BRCA1* or *BRCA2*: Are they prognostically different? J Clin Oncol 17:3653–3663, 1999.

179. Ridolfi RL, Rosen PP, Port A, et al: Medullary carcinoma of the breast: A clinicopathologic study with 10 year follow-up. Cancer 40:1365–1385, 1977.

180. Bertucci F, Finetti P, Cervera N, et al: Gene expression profiling shows medullary breast cancer is a subgroup of basal breast cancers. Cancer Res 66:4633–4636, 2006.

181. Verhoog LC, Berns EM, Brekelmans CT, et al: Prognostic significance of germline *BRCA2* mutations in hereditary breast cancer patients. J Clin Oncol 18:119s–124s, 2000.

182. James PA, Doherty R, Harris M, et al: Optimal selection of individuals for *BRCA* mutation testing: A comparison of available methods. J Clin Oncol 24:707–715, 2006.

183. Farshid G, Balleine RL, Cummings M, Waring P: Morphology of breast cancer as means of triage of patients for *BRCA1* genetic testing. Am J Surg Pathol 30:1357–1366, 2006.

184. van der Groep P, Bouter A, van der Zanden R, et al: Distinction between hereditary and sporadic breast cancer on the basis of clinicopathological data. J Clin Pathol 59:611–617, 2006.

185. Abbott DW, Freeman ML, Holt JT: Double-strand break repair deficiency and radiation sensitivity in *BRCA2* mutant cancer cells. J Natl Cancer Inst 90:978–985, 1998.

186. Biggs PJ, Bradley A: A step toward genotype-based therapeutic regimens for breast cancer in patients with *BRCA2* mutations? J Natl Cancer Inst 90:951–953, 1998.

187. Broeks A, Urbanus JH, Floore AN, et al: *ATM*-heterozygous germline mutations contribute to breast cancer susceptibility. Hum Genet 66:494–500, 2000.

188. Coleman CN: Molecular biology in radiation oncology. Radiation oncology perspective of *BRCA1* and *BRCA2*. Acta Oncologica 38(suppl):55–59, 1999.

189. Connor F, Bertwistle D, Mee PJ, et al: Tumorigenesis and a DNA repair defect in mice with a truncating *BRCA2* mutation. Nat Genet 17:423–430, 1997.

190. Friedenson B: Is mammography indicated for women with defective BRCA genes? Implications of recent scientific advances for the diagnosis, treatment, and prevention of hereditary breast cancer. Medscape General Medicine. 2:2000; Medscape Portals, Inc. Available at: http://www.medscape.com/viewarticle/408048. Accessed 4 September 2008.

191. Harkin DP: Uncovering functionally relevant signaling pathways using microarray-based expression profiling. Oncologist 5:501–507, 2000.

192. Pierce LJ, Strawderman M, Narod SA, et al: Effect of radiotherapy after breast-conserving treatment in women with breast cancer and germline *BRCA1/2* mutations. J Clin Oncol 18:3360–3369, 2000.

193. Scully R, Chen J, Plug A, et al: Association of *BRCA1* with Rad51 in mitotic and meiotic cells. Cell 88:265–275, 1997.

194. Sharan SK, Morimatsu M, Albrecht U, et al: Embryonic lethality and radiation hypersensitivity mediated by Rad51 in mice lacking *BRCA2*. Nature 386:804–810, 1997.

195. Swift M, Morrell D, Massey RB, Chase CL: Incidence of cancer in 161 families affected by ataxia-telangiectasia. N Engl J Med 325:1831–1836, 1991.

196. Turner B, Harrold E, Matloff E, et al: *BRCA1/BRCA2* germline mutations in locally recurrent breast cancer patients after lumpectomy and radiation therapy: implications for breast-conserving management in patients with *BRCA1/BRCA2* mutations. J Clin Oncol 17:3017–3024, 1999.

197. Venkitaraman AR: Breast cancer genes and DNA repair. Science 286:1100–1102, 1999.

198. Levy-Lahad E, Lahad A, Eisenberg S, et al: A single nucleotide polymorphism in the RAD51 gene modifies cancer risk in *BRCA2* but not *BRCA1* carriers. Proc Natl Acad Sci USA 98:3232–3236, 2001.

199. Bradbury A, Olopade OI: The case for individualized screening recommendations for breast cancer. J Clin Oncol 24:3328–3330, 2006.

200. Shanley S, McReynolds K, Ardern-Jones A, et al: Late toxicity is not increased in *BRCA1/BRCA2* mutation carriers undergoing breast radiotherapy in the United Kingdom. Clin Cancer Res 12:7025–7032, 2006.

201. Tai YC, Domchek S, Parmigiani G, Chen S: Breast cancer risk among male *BRCA1* and *BRCA2* mutation carriers. J Natl Cancer Inst 99:1811–1814, 2007.

202. Rosen EM, Fan S, Goldberg ID: *BRCA1* and prostate cancer. Cancer Invest 19:396–412, 2001.

203. Carter BS, Beaty TH, Steinberg GD et al: Mendelian inheritance of familial prostate cancer. Proc Natl Acad Sci USA 89:3367–3371, 1992.

204. Thiessen EU: Concerning a familial association between breast cancer and both prostatic and uterine malignancies. Cancer 34:1102–1107, 1974.

205. Whittemore AS, Wu AH, Kolonel LN, et al: Family history and prostate cancer risk in black, white, and Asian men in the United States and Canada. Am J Epidemiol 141:732–740, 1995.

206. Bishop DT, Kiemeney LA: Family studies and the evidence for genetic susceptibility to prostate cancer. Semin Cancer Biol 8:45–51, 1997.

207. Anderson DE, Badzioch MD: Familial breast cancer risks: Effects of prostate and other cancers. Cancer 72:114–119, 2001.

208. Jishi MF, Itnyre JH, Oakley-Girvan IA, et al: Risks of cancer among members of families in the Gilda Radner Familial Ovarian Cancer Registry. Cancer 76:1416–1421, 1995.

209. Sellers TA, Potter JD, Rich SS, et al: Familial clustering of breast and prostate cancers and risk of postmenopausal breast cancer. J Natl Cancer Inst 86:1860–1865, 1994.

210. Tulinius H, Egilsson V, Olafsdottir GH, et al: Risk of prostate, ovarian, and endometrial cancer among relatives of women with breast cancer. Br Med J 305:855, 1992.

211. Struewing JP, Hartge P, Wacholder S, et al: The risk of cancer associated with specific mutations of *BRCA1* and *BRCA2* among Ashkenazi Jews. N Engl J Med 336:1401–1408, 1997.

212. Brothman AR, Steele MR, Williams BJ, et al: Loss of chromosome 17 loci in prostate cancer detected by polymerase chain reaction quantitation of allelic markers. Genes Chromosomes Cancer 13:278–284, 1995.

213. Gao X, Zacharek A, Grignon DJ, et al: Localization of potential tumor suppressor loci to a <2 Mb region on chromosome 17q in human prostate cancer. Oncogene 11:1241–1247, 1995.

214. Gao X, Zacharek A, Salkowski A, et al: Loss of heterozygosity of the *BRCA1* and other loci on chromosome 17q in human prostate cancer. Cancer Res 55:1002–1005, 1995.

215. Murakami YS, Brothman AR, Leach RJ, et al: Suppression of malignant phenotype in a human prostate cancer cell line by fragments of normal chromosome region 17q. Cancer Res 55:3389–3394, 1995.

216. Williams BJ, Jones E, Zhu XL, et al: Evidence for a tumor suppressor gene distal to *BRCA1* in prostate cancer, J Urol 155:720–725, 1996.

217. Arason A, Barkardóttir RB, Egilsson V: Linkage analysis of chromosome 17q markers and breast-ovarian cancer in Icelandic families, and possible relationship to prostatic cancer. Am J Hum Genet 52:711–717, 1993.

218. Gonzalez-Neira A, Rosa-Rosa JM, Osorio A, et al: Genomewide high-density SNP linkage analysis of non-*BRCA1/2* breast cancer families identifies various candidate regions and has greater power than microsatellite studies. BMC Genomics 8:299, 2007.

219. Weischer M, Bojesen SE, Ellervik C, et al: *CHEK2**1100delC genotyping for clinical assessment of breast cancer risk: meta-analyses of 26,000 patient cases and 27,000 controls. J Clin Oncol 26:542–548, 2008.

220. Offit K, Garber JE: Time to check *CHEK2* in families with breast cancer? J Clin Oncol 26:519–520, 2008.

221. Lynch HT, Mulcahy GM, Harris RE, et al: Genetic and pathologic findings in a kindred with hereditary sarcoma, breast cancer, brain tumors, leukemia, lung, laryngeal, and adrenal cortical carcinoma. Cancer 41:2055–2064, 1978.

222. Li FP, Fraumeni JF: Soft-tissue sarcomas, breast cancer, and other neoplasms: A familial syndrome? Ann Intern Med 71:747–752, 1969.

223. Li FP, Fraumeni JF: Familial breast cancer, soft-tissue sarcomas, and other neoplasms. Ann Intern Med 83:833–834, 1975.

224. Li FP, Fraumeni JF: Prospective study of a family cancer syndrome. JAMA 247:2692–2694, 1982.

225. Malkin D, Li FP, Stron LC, et al: Germ line *p53* mutations in a familial syndrome of breast cancer, sarcomas and other neoplasms. Science 250:1233–1238, 1990.

226. Lynch HT, McComb RD, Osborn NK, et al: Predominance of brain tumors in an extended Li-Fraumeni (SBLA) kindred, including a case of Sturge-Weber syndrome. Cancer 88:433–439, 2000.

227. Brownstein MH, Wolf M, Bikowski JB: Cowden's disease: A cutaneous marker of breast cancer. Cancer 41:2393–2398, 1978.

228. Liaw D, Marsh DJ, Li J, et al: Germline mutations of the PTEN gene in Cowden disease, an inherited breast and thyroid cancer syndrome. Nat Genet 16:64–67, 1997.

229. Nelen MR, van Stavernen WC, Peeters EA, et al: Germline mutations in the *PTEN/MMAC1* gene in patients with Cowden disease. Hum Mol Genet 6:1383–1387, 1997.

230. Eng C: Cowden syndrome. J Genet Counsel 6:181–192, 1997.

231. Marsh DJ, Dahia PLM, Caron S, et al: Germline *PTEN* mutations in Cowden syndrome-like families. J Med Genet 35:881–885, 1998.

232. Williard W, Borgen P, Bol R, et al: Cowden's disease: A case report with analyses at the molecular level. Cancer 69:2969–2974, 1992.

233. Walton BJ, Morain WB, Baughman RD, et al: A further indication for prophylactic mastectomy. Surgery 99:82–86, 1986.

234. Schrager CA, Schneider D, Gruener AC, et al: Clinical and pathological features of breast disease in Cowden's syndrome: An underrecognized syndrome with an increased risk of breast cancer. Hum Pathol 29:47–53, 1998.

235. Lynch ED, Ostermeyer EA, Lee MK, et al: Inherited mutations in PTEN that are associated with breast cancer, Cowden disease, and juvenile polyposis. Am J Hum Genet 61:1254–1260, 1997.

236. Gatti RA, Berkel I, Boder E, et al: Localization of an ataxia-telangiectasia gene to chromosome 11q22-23. Nature 366:577–580, 1988.

237. Savitsky K, Bar-Shira A, Gilad S, et al: A single ataxia telangiectasia gene with a product similar to PI-3 kinase. Science 268:1749–1753, 1995.

238. Swift M: Genetic aspects of ataxia-telangiectasia. Immunodefic Rev 2:67–81, 1990.

239. Morrell D, Cromartic E, Swift M: Mortality and cancer incidence in 263 patients with ataxia- telangiectasia. J Natl Cancer Inst 77:89–92, 1986.

240. Morrell D, Chase CL, Swift M: Cancers in 44 families with ataxia-telangiectasia. Cancer Genet Cytogenet 50:119–123, 1990.

241. Swift M, Chase CL, Morrell D: Cancer predisposition of ataxia-telangiectasia heterozygotes. Cancer Genet Cytogenet 46:21–27, 1990.

242. Buyse M, Hartman CT, Wilson MG: Gonadoblastoma and dysgerminoma with ataxia-telangiectasia. Birth Defects 12:165–169, 1976.

243. Narita T, Takagi K: Ataxia-telangiectasia with dysgerminomas of the right ovary, papillary carcinoma of the thyroid and adenocarcinoma of the pancreas. Cancer 54:1113–1116, 1984.

244. Swift M, Morrell D, Cromartie E, et al: The incidence and gene frequency of ataxia-telangiectasia in the United States. Am J Hum Genet 39:573–583, 1986.

245. Lavin MF, Khanna KK, Beamish H, et al: Defect in radiation signal transduction in ataxia-telangiectasia. Int J Radiat Biol 66(suppl 6):S151–S156, 1994.

246. Lynch HT, Grady W, Suriano G, Huntsman D: Gastric cancer: New genetic developments, J Surg Oncol 90:114–133, 2005.
247. Suriano G, Oliveira C, Ferreira P, et al: Identification of *CDH1* germline missense mutations associated with functional inactivation of the E-cadherin protein in young gastric cancer probands. Hum Mol Genet 12:575–582, 2003.
248. Suriano G, Yew S, Ferreira P, et al: Characterization of a recurrent germ line mutation of the E-cadherin gene: Implications for genetic testing and clinical management. Clin Cancer Res 11: 5401–5409, 2005.
249. Oliveira C, Seruca R, Caldas C: Genetic screening for hereditary diffuse gastric cancer. Expert Rev Mol Diagn 3:201–215, 2003.
250. Rebbeck TR, Wang Y, Kantoff PW, et al: Modification of *BRCA1*- and *BRCA2*-associated breast cancer risk by *AIB1* genotype and reproductive history, Cancer Res 61:5420–5424, 2001.
251. Rebbeck TR, Kantoff PA, Krithivas K, et al: Modification of *BRCA1*-associated breast cancer penetrance by androgen receptor CAG repeat length variants. Am J Hum Genet 64:1371–1377, 1999.
252. Fabian CJ, Kimler BF, Zalles CM, et al: Short-term breast cancer prediction by random periareolar fine-needle aspiration cytology and the Gail risk model. J Natl Cancer Inst 92:1217–1227, 2000.
253. O'Shaughnessy JA, Ljung B-M, Dooley WC, et al: Ductal lavage and the clinical management of women at high risk for breast carcinoma: A commentary. Cancer 94:292–298, 2002.
254. Dooley WC, Ljung B-M, Veronesi U, et al: Ductal lavage for detection of cellular atypia in women at high risk for breast cancer. J Natl Cancer Inst 93:1624–1632, 2001.
255. Perou CM, Sorlie T, Eisen MB, et al: Molecular portraits of human breast tumours. Nature 406:747–752, 2000.
256. Sørlie T, Perou CM, Tibshirani R, et al: Gene expression patterns of breast carcinomas distinguish tumor subclasses with clinical implications. Proc Natl Acad Sci USA 98:10869–10874, 2001.
257. van 't Veer LJ, Dai H, van de Vijver MJ, et al: Gene expression profiling predicts clinical outcome of breast cancer. Nature 415:530–536, 2002.
258. Gruvberger S, Ringner M, Chen Y, et al: Estrogen receptor status in breast cancer is associated with remarkably distinct gene expression patterns. Cancer Res 61:5979–5984, 2001.
259. Martin KJ, Graner E, Li Y, et al: High sensitivity array analysis of gene expression for the early detection of disseminated breast tumor cells in peripheral blood. Proc Natl Acad Sci USA 98: 2646–2651, 2001.
260. Kudoh K, Ramanna M, Ravatn R, et al: Monitoring the expression profiles of doxorubicin-induced and doxorubicin-resistant cancer cells by cDNA microarray. Cancer Res 60:4161–4166, 2000.
261. Narod SA, Sun P, Ghadirian P, et al: Tubal ligation and risk of ovarian cancer in carriers of *BRCA1* or *BRCA2* mutations: A case-control study. Lancet 357:1467–1470, 2001.
262. Narod SA, Risch H, Moslehi R, et al: Oral contraceptives and the risk of hereditary ovarian cancer, N Engl J Med 339:424–428, 1998.
263. Marchbanks PA, McDonald JA, Wilson HG, et al: Oral contraceptives and the risk of breast cancer. N Engl J Med 346:2025–2032, 2002.
264. Lynch HT: Hereditary factors in carcinoma. In Lynch HT (ed): Recent results in cancer research, vol 12. New York, Springer-Verlag, 1967.
265. Lynch HT: Dynamic genetics counseling for clinicians. Springfield, IL, CC Thomas, 1969.
266. Lynch HT, Guirgis HA, Brodkey F, et al: Early age of onset in familial breast cancer: Genetic and cancer control implications. Arch Surg 111:126–131, 1976.
267. Lynch HT, Krush AJ: Genetic predictability in breast cancer risk: Surgical implications. Arch Surg 103:84–88, 1971.
268. Lynch HT, Lynch PM, Albano WA, et al: Hereditary cancer: Ascertainment and management. CA Cancer J Clin 29:216–232, 1979.
269. Harris RE, Lynch HT, Guirgis HA: Familial breast cancer: Risk to the contralateral breast. J Natl Cancer Inst 60:955–960, 1978.
270. Hartmann LC, Schaid DJ, Woods JE, et al: Efficacy of bilateral prophylactic mastectomy in women with a family history of breast cancer. N Engl J Med 340:77–84, 1999.
271. Meijers-Heijboer H, van Geel B, van Putten WLJ, et al: Breast cancer after prophylactic bilateral mastectomy in women with a *BRCA1* or *BRCA2* mutation. N Engl J Med 345:159–164, 2001.
272. Verhoog LC, Brekelmans CTM, Seynaeve C, et al: Survival in hereditary breast cancer associated with germline mutations of *BRCA2*. J Clin Oncol 17:3396–3402, 1999.
273. Metcalfe KA, Lubinski J, Ghadirian P, et al: Predictors of contralateral prophylactic mastectomy in women with a *BRCA1* or *BRCA2* mutation: The Hereditary Breast Cancer Clinical Study Group. J Clin Oncol 26:1093–1097, 2008.
274. Tuttle TM, Habermann EB, Grund EH, et al: Increasing use of contralateral prophylactic mastectomy for breast cancer patients: A trend toward more aggressive surgical treatment. J Clin Oncol 25:5203–5209, 2007.
275. Kauff ND, Satagopan JM, Robson ME, et al: Risk-reducing salpingo-oophorectomy in women with a *BRCA1* or *BRCA2* mutation. N Engl J Med 346:1609–1615, 2002.
276. Kauff ND, Domchek SM, Friebel TM, et al: Risk-reducing salpingo-oophorectomy for the prevention of *BRCA1*- and *BRCA2*-associated breast and gynecologic cancer: a multicenter, prospective study. J Clin Oncol 26:1331–1337, 2008.
277. Meiser B, Butow P, Barratt A, et al: Attitudes toward prophylactic oophorectomy and screening utilization in women at increased risk of developing hereditary breast/ovarian cancer. Gynecol Oncol 75:122–129, 1999.
278. Lerman C, Hughes C, Croyle RT, et al: Prophylactic surgery decisions and surveillance practices one year following *BRCA1/2* testing. Prev Med 31:75–80, 2000.
279. van Dijk S, van Roosmalen MS, Otten W, Stalmeier PFM: Decision making regarding prophylactic mastectomy: Stability of preferences and the impact of anticipated feelings of regret. J Clin Oncol 26:2358–2363, 2008.
280. Hallowell N, Jacobs I, Richards M, et al: Surveillance or surgery? A description of the factors that influence high risk premenopausal women's decisions about prophylactic oophorectomy. J Med Genet 38:683–691, 2001.
281. Droegemueller W: Screening for ovarian cancer: Hopeful and wishful thinking. Am J Obstet Gynecol 170:1095–1098, 1994.
282. National Institutes of Health Consensus Development Conference Statement: Ovarian cancer: Screening, treatment, and follow-up. Gynecol Oncol 55:S4–S14, 1994.
283. Deapen D, Liu L, Perkins C, et al: Rapidly rising breast cancer incidence rates among Asian-American women. Int J Cancer 99:747–750, 2002.
284. Kash KM, Holland JC, Halper MS, Miller DG: Psychological distress and surveillance behaviors of women with a family history of breast cancer. J Natl Cancer Inst 84:24–30, 1992.
285. Lerman C, Daly M, Sands C, et al: Mammography adherence and psychological distress among women at risk for breast cancer. J Natl Cancer Inst 85:1074–1080, 1993.
286. Lerman C, Schwartz M: Adherence and psychological adjustment among women at high risk for breast cancer. Breast Cancer Res Treat 28:145–155, 1993.
287. Valdimarsdottir HB, Bovbjerg DH, Kash KM, et al: Psychological distress in women with a familial risk of breast cancer. Psycho-Oncology 4:133–141, 1995.
288. Lerman C, Kash K, Stefanek M: Younger women at increased risk for breast cancer: Perceived risk, psychological well-being, and surveillance behavior. J Natl Cancer Inst Monogr 16:171–176, 1994.
289. Schwartz M, Lerman C, Daly M, et al: Utilization of ovarian cancer screening by women at increased risk. Cancer Epidemiol Biomarkers Prev 4:269–273, 1995.
290. Lerman C, Rimer BK, Daly M, et al: Recruiting high risk women into a breast cancer health promotion trial. Cancer Epidemiol Biomarkers Prev 3:271–276, 1994.
291. Lerman C, Lustbader E, Rimer B, et al: Effects of individualized breast cancer risk counseling: A randomized trial. J Natl Cancer Inst 87:286–292, 1995.
292. Chaliki H, Loader S, Levenkron JC, et al: Women's receptivity to testing for a genetic susceptibility to breast cancer. Am J Public Health 85:1133–1135, 1995.
293. Bloch M, Fahy M, Fox S, Hayden MR: Predictive testing for Huntington disease II. Demographic characteristics, life-style patterns, attitudes, and psychosocial assessments of the first fifty-one test candidates. Am J Med Genet 32:217–224, 1989.

294. Craufurd D, Dodge A, Kerzin-Storrar L, Harris R: Uptake of pre-symptomatic predictive testing for Huntington's disease. Lancet 2:603–605, 1989.

295. Hudson KL, Holohan MK, Collins FS: Keeping pace with the times—the Genetic Information Nondiscrimination Act of 2008. N Engl J Med 358:2661–2663, 2008.

296. Lynch HT, Severin MJ, Mooney MJ, Lynch JF: Insurance adjudication favoring prophylactic surgery in hereditary breast-ovarian cancer syndrome. Gynecol Oncol 57:23–26, 1995.

297. Katskee A: Katskee v. Blue Cross/Blue Shield of Nebraska, Nebraska Supreme Court No. S-92-1002, 1994.

298. Beggs v. Pacific Mutual Life Insurance Company, 171 Ga.App. 204, 218 S.E.2d 836, 1984.

299. Cheney v. Bell National Life, 315 Md. 761, 556 A.2d 1135, 1989.

300. Silverstein v. Metropolitan Life Insurance Company, 171 N.E. 914, 1930.

301. Burke W, Pinsky LE, Press NA: Categorizing genetic tests to identify their ethical, legal, and social implications. Am J Med Genet (Semin Med Genet) 106:233–240, 2001.

302. Lynch HT, Boland CR, Rodriguez-Bigas MA, et al: Who should be sent for genetic testing in hereditary colorectal cancer syndromes? J Clin Oncol 25:3534–3542, 2007.

303. U.S. Department of Health and Human Services: HIPAA—General information, 2005. Available at: http://www.cms.hhs.gov/HIPAAGenInfo/. Accessed 29 January 2007.

304. Lynch HT: Family Information Service and hereditary cancer. Cancer 91:625–628, 2001.

305. Eisen A, Weber BL: Prophylactic mastectomy for women with *BRCA1* and *BRCA2* mutations—facts and controversy. N Engl J Med 345:207–208, 2001.

306. Grann VR, Jacobson JS, Thomason D, et al: Effect of prevention strategies on survival and quality-adjusted survival of women with *BRCA1/2* mutations: An updated decision analysis. J Clin Oncol 20:2520–2529, 2002.

chapter 22

Patterns of Recurrence in Breast Cancer

DAVID P. WINCHESTER | DAVID J. WINCHESTER |
MAHMOUD EL-TAMER

Recurrent breast cancer may present as local, regional, or systemic disease, isolated or in combination. Recurrences are related to the type or characteristics of the tumor. These factors include the stage of the tumor at presentation, for example, tumor size, axillary nodal status, and presence or absence of metastatic disease. Multiple histologic and biologic parameters play a role.

Another predictor of recurrence is the type of treatment rendered: surgery, radiation, chemotherapy, or a combination thereof. The type and extent of surgical treatment has an impact on locoregional recurrence (positive margins, the omission of axillary node surgery, and the number of nodes dissected). The addition of radiation therapy has clearly shown to lead to better local control of the disease. In addition to improved local control, there have been reports of increased survival with radiation therapy in high-risk women undergoing mastectomy.[1,2] Adjuvant chemotherapy has proved its efficacy in improving survival by decreasing both systemic and local recurrence.

Future trends for patterns of breast cancer recurrence likely will change with improved surgical, radiation, and targeted systemic therapies.

The site of local recurrence is related to the initial surgical procedure. After mastectomy, the most common local recurrences present as a cutaneous or subcutaneous mass palpated on physical examination. More advanced local recurrences include nodules involving skin, pectoral muscle, and occasionally, deeper chest wall structures. The most ominous postmastectomy local recurrence presents with widespread skin infiltration with or without inflammatory changes.

After breast-conserving surgery, a true local recurrence is defined as regrowth of tumor at the lumpectomy site in the same quadrant of the breast. An in-breast tumor recurrence definition is broadened to include tumor recurrence anywhere in the ipsilateral breast.

A regional recurrence is defined as recurrence of disease in the ipsilateral axillary nodal basin, internal mammary nodal chain, or supraclavicular nodal basin. A previous edition of the American Joint Committee on Cancer Staging Manual[3] categorized supraclavicular nodal metastasis as distant metastatic disease. The most recent edition of the staging manual[4] classifies supraclavicular nodal involvement at initial presentation as N_{3c} rather than M_1. This change occurred because improved survival rates were observed with more aggressive management of supraclavicular disease rather than palliation therapy. Following the same logic, supraclavicular nodal recurrence most likely was present as occult disease at initial diagnosis.

Systemic recurrence refers to evidence of metastatic breast cancer at sites other than local or regional, such as bone, liver, or pleura.

Importance of Minimizing Local Recurrence

All breast cancer patients should be afforded optimal local and regional therapy. Local recurrence should be regarded as a significantly adverse event; all available means should be used to minimize this risk. Even in highly curable ductal carcinoma in situ (DCIS), the 10-year disease-specific survival decreases from nearly 100% to 92% with local recurrence.[5,6] The overall survival rates for patients with early-stage breast cancers undergoing breast-conserving therapy (BCT) who subsequently develop a local recurrence is 81% at 5 years[7] and 39% at 10 years.[8] The 5-year overall survival rate for patients experiencing local recurrence following mastectomy is 42%.[9] In a retrospective analysis of 1043 patients with consecutive stage I and II breast cancers who underwent BCT at MD Anderson Cancer Center, Meric and colleagues found in a multivariate analysis that ipsilateral breast tumor recurrence was an independent predictor of systemic recurrence and disease-specific survival.[10]

An excellent review of local therapy and survival in breast cancer by Punglia and associates[11] challenges the theory of predetermined systemic disease. The authors cite evidence that mammographic screening reduces breast cancer mortality. Evidence is cited from randomized clinical trials demonstrating a link between local control and overall survival in breast cancer.

The Early Breast Cancer Trialist's Collaborative Group (EBCTCG) meta-analysis from 78 randomized clinical trials evaluating the extent of surgery and the use of radiation therapy, which analyzes data from 42,000 patients treated in trials before 1995, has provided important information linking local therapy with survival.[12] This study has demonstrated a highly statistically significant improvement in both breast cancer survival and overall survival at 15 years with improvement of local control observed 10 years earlier. With studies reporting at least a 10% reduction in the 5-year risk of local recurrence, breast cancer mortality was reduced by 1.6% at 5 years, 3.7% at 10 years, and 4.9% at 15 years. For the studies in the meta-analysis evaluating radiation therapy, the addition of radiation therapy significantly improved the 15-year absolute overall survival after breast conservation surgery by 5.3% ($P = 0.005$) and after mastectomy in node-positive patients by 4.4% ($P = 0.001$). Punglia and associates[11] probed a possible biologic explanation for the association between local control and survival. In citing the EBCTCG meta-analysis, for every four local recurrences that were prevented at 5 years, there was approximately one less death from breast cancer at 15 years. It is suggested that in about 25% of local recurrences, the cancer cells in the recurrent tumor have developed metastatic capability.

Local Recurrence Patterns and Risk Factors

Prospectively and retrospectively identified risk factors for local recurrence must be considered in the context of both the histology of the primary tumor and treatment.

Several prospective randomized controlled trials have reported similar rates of distant disease-free and overall survival, as well as local control following both treatments (Table 22-1).

Local Recurrence following Breast Conservation Therapy

DUCTAL CARCINOMA IN SITU

BCT is defined as complete excision of DCIS, verified by pathologic clear margins and, in most cases, radiation therapy. Paradoxically, DCIS, a less aggressive tumor than infiltrating carcinomas, has a higher local recurrence rate than its invasive counterpart. This is believed to be a result of the fact that it is often occult, with disease distribution in discontinuous ducts. About 90% of DCIS is diagnosed with mammography, but recent data suggest that mammography underestimates the histopathologic extent of the disease. Using magnetic resonance imaging (MRI), Berg and colleagues found that mammography missed 17 of 38 cases of DCIS.[13]

Following BCT for DCIS, patients should be on a surveillance program that includes breast imaging and clinical breast examination. In a review of the literature, Huston and Simmons[14] reported that local recurrences were detected by mammography alone 42% to 75% of the time, by physical examination alone in 10% to 33% of cases and by a combination of the two in 12% to 25% of the time. In up to 5% of cases, MRI was useful.

A variety of risk factors have been reported for local recurrence following BCT for patients with DCIS. They are broadly categorized as associated with the patient, tumor, and treatment. Table 22-2 summarizes these risk

TABLE 22-1

Incidence of Locoregional Recurrence after Mastectomy and Breast Conservation Therapy in Prospective Randomized Trials

Trial	Stage	n	Follow-Up (years)	LLR (%)	
				BCT	Mastectomy
Milan[a]	I	701	20	8.8	2.3
IGR[b]	I	179	10	7	10
NSABP B-06[c]	I–II	1219	20	12.8	14.7
NCI[d]	I–II	237	10	18	10
EORTC 10801[e]	I–II	874	8	13	9
DBCG[f]	I–III	904	6	3	4

BCT, breast conservation therapy; DBCG, Danish Breast Cancer Group; EORTC, European Organization for Research and Treatment of Cancer; IGR, Institute Gustave Roussy; LRR, locoregional recurrence; NCI, National Cancer Institute; NSABP, National Surgical Adjuvant Breast and Bowel Project.

[a]From Veronesi U, Cascinelli N, Mariani L, et al: Twenty-year follow-up of a randomized study comparing breast conserving surgery with radical mastectomy for early breast cancer. N Engl J Med 347:1227–1232, 2002.

[b]From Sarrazin D, Lê MG, Arriagada R, et al: Ten-year results of a randomized trial comparing a conservative treatment to mastectomy in early breast cancer. Radiother Oncol 14:177–184, 1989.

[c]From Fisher B, Anderson S, Bryant J, et al: Twenty-year follow-up of a randomized trial comparing total mastectomy, lumpectomy, and lumpectomy plus irradiation for the treatment of invasive breast cancer. N Engl J Med 347:1233–1241, 2002.

[d]From Jacobson JA, Danforth DN, Cowan KH, et al: Ten-year results of a comparison of conservation with mastectomy in the treatment of stage I and II breast cancer. N Engl J Med 332:907–911,1995.

[e]From van Dongen JA, Bartelink H, Fentiman IS, et al: Randomized clinical trial to assess the value of breast-conserving therapy in stage I and II breast cancer. EORTC 10801 trial. J Natl Cancer Inst Monogr 11:15–18, 1992.

[f]From Blichert-Toft M, Rose C, Anderson JA, et al: Danish randomized trial comparing breast conservation therapy with mastectomy: Six years of life table analysis. J Natl Cancer Inst Monogr 11:19–25,1992.

TABLE 22-2

Ductal Carcinoma in Situ Risk Factors for Local Recurrence following Breast Conservation Treatment

Tumor Factors	Treatment Factors	Patient Factors
Size[a]	Radiation therapy[b]	Young age[c]
Grade[a,c]	Doubtful margins[c]	Symptomatic detection[c]
HER2/neu[d]	Positive margins[e]	
p53[d]	Margin size[a]	
	Tamoxifen[f]	

[a]From Silverstein M.[18]

[b]From Fisher B, Dignam J, Wolmark N, et al[15]; EORTC Breast Cancer Cooperative Group, EORTC Radiotherapy Group, Bijker N, Meijnen P, Peterse JL, et al[16]; and de Roos MA, de Bock GH, de Vries J, et al: p53 overexpression is a predictor of local recurrence after treatment for both in situ and invasive ductal carcinoma of the breast. J Surg Res 140:109–114, 2007.

[c]From EORTC Breast Cancer Cooperative Group, EORTC Radiotherapy Group, Bijker N, Meijnen P, Peterse JL, et al.[16]

[d]From de Roos MA, de Bock GH, de Vries J, et al: p53 overexpression is a predictor of local recurrence after treatment for both in situ and invasive ductal carcinoma of the breast. J Surg Res 140:109–114, 2007; and Kepple J, Henry-Tillman RS, Klimberg VS, et al: The receptor expression pattern in ductal carcinoma in situ predicts recurrence. Am J Surg 192:68–71, 2006.

[e]From Punglia R, Morrow M, Winer EP, Harris JR.[11]

[f]From Fisher B, Dignam J, Wolmark N, et al.[19]

factors. In all three prospective randomized trials evaluating the benefit of adding radiation therapy to breast-conserving surgery, there was a statistically significant reduction in the risk of local recurrence.[15–17] However, with a careful selection of tumor and treatment factors, local recurrence rates are low for excision alone.[18] Tamoxifen has been shown to reduce the risk of local recurrence in one randomized trial[19] but was not found effective in a subsequent trial.[17]

INVASIVE CARCINOMA

After BCT, local recurrence most commonly is detected on routine mammography or as a palpable clinical finding proximate to the initial site of disease and within the same quadrant as the primary tumor. However, any ipsilateral breast recurrence arising in a different quadrant is usually considered a new breast cancer. Comparing the histology and tumor markers between the different sites of disease may provide a distinction between a recurrence and a new primary tumor. In reviewing the experience of the Joint Center for Radiation Therapy, Recht and coworkers[20] classified recurrences following BCT as true recurrences (TRs), marginal miss (MM), or new primaries. TRs occur in the original tumor bed, whereas MM is a recurrence in the same quadrant of the original primary tumor. New primaries are recurrences that occur several centimeters from the boosted volume. Occasionally, recurrences after BCT may present as a widespread skin involvement, within other quadrants, or as carcinoma en cuirasse. TRs, MM, new primaries, and skin recurrences occurred

in 50%, 22.4%, 18%, and 10% of patients, respectively. Gage and associates[21] updated the same series 10 years later. They found the annual incidence rate of local recurrence following BCT to be relatively constant during the first 10 years. TR/MM was the most common type of ipsilateral breast cancer recurrence and was highest during years 2 through 7. The risk of a recurrence elsewhere in the breast increased with longer follow-up and was highest during years 8 through 10. The study notes that any decrease in ipsilateral breast tumor recurrence (IBTR) is not a result of patterns of local recurrence but rather improvements in mammographic and pathologic evaluation, patient selection, and increased use of reexcision.

The incidence of IBTR in the literature has been variable and clearly depends on many factors, including the size of the primary tumor, adequacy of resection, status of margins, addition of radiation therapy, boost dose, and tumor, as well as patient characteristics. In the 15-year update of the findings of the National Surgical Adjuvant Breast and Bowel Project (NSABP) Protocol B-06, Fisher and colleagues assessed 31 pathologic and 6 clinical features in 1039 patients with breast cancer to determine their value in predicting IBTR and survival rates.[22] In addition to nodal status and nuclear grade, factors that were correlated with a greater risk of breast cancer recurrence that have not yet been mentioned were race (African-American descent), histologic tumor type, and detection of tumoral blood vessel extension.

In an extensive review of the literature, Clemons and associates[23] approximated the incidence of locoregional recurrence (LRR) 10 years after BCT and radiation therapy as being 12% (interquartile range [IQR], 7%–15%). The incidence of IBTR is approximately 1.5% to 2% per year for the first 7 to 8 years. At 10 to 15 years of follow-up, IBTR stabilizes at an incidence of 10% to 20%.[24,25] Approximately 10% (IQR, 6.5%–22%) of patients with IBTR after BCT and radiation therapy present with prior or synchronous systemic disease.[23] With systemic and radiotherapy, the incidence of IBTR has decreased. With these treatment modalities, the NSABP reported a 6% local recurrence rate with more than 10 years of follow-up in B-06.[26]

The impact of radiation therapy on local recurrence patterns for BCT was studied carefully in the NSABP B-06 trial. At 12 years of follow-up, the incidence of IBTR was 10% with radiation compared with 35% without radiation. Other studies report a similar reduction in IBTR with radiotherapy.[27–31]

As in DCIS, patient, tumor, and treatment factors influence the development of local recurrence following BCT for invasive breast cancer. These are summarized in Table 22-3.

Local Recurrence following Mastectomy

DUCTAL CARCINOMA IN SITU

There is a significant local recurrence rate in patients with DCIS treated with breast conservation, but this is an unusual event when total mastectomy is performed.

TABLE 22-3

Invasive Breast Cancer Risk Factors for Local Recurrence following Breast Conservation Treatment

Tumor Factors	Treatment Factors	Patient Factors
Size[a]	Close margin[b,c]	Young age[a,b,d,e]
Nodal status[a,b,f]	Positive margin[b,c]	African-American race[f]
Grade[f]	Radiation therapy[g]	
Type[b,f]	Systemic therapy[b]	
Vascular invasion[b,d]		
Estrogen receptor– negative[a]		
Progesterone receptor–negative[a]		
HER2/neu[h]		
p53[h]		

[a]From Wapnir IL, Anderson SJ, Mamounas EP, et al: Prognosis after ipsilateral breast tumor recurrence and locoregional recurrences in five national surgical adjuvant breast and bowel project node-positive adjuvant breast cancer trials. J Clin Oncol 24:2028–2037, 2006.
[b]From Clark M, Collins R, Darby S, et al.[11]
[c]From Horst KC, Smitt MC, Goffinet DR, Carlson RW: Predictors of local recurrence after breast-conservation therapy. Clin Breast Cancer 5:425–438, 2005.
[d]From Bollet MA, Sigal-Zafrani B, Mazeau V, et al: Age remains the first prognostic factor for loco-regional breast cancer recurrence in young (<40 years) women treated with breast conserving surgery first. Radiother Oncol 82:272–280, 2007.
[e]From Kim JH, Tavossoli F, Haffty BG.[33]
[f]From Fisher ER, Anderson S, Tan-Chiu E, et al.[22]
[g]From Liljegren G, Holmberg L, Adami HO, et al; Veronesi U, Luini A, Del Vecchio M, et al; Clark RM, Whelan T, Levine M, et al; Forrest AP, Stewart HJ, Everington D, et al; and Renton SC, Gazet JC, Ford HT, et al.[27–31]
[h]From de Roos MA, de Bock GH, de Vries J, et al: p53 overexpression is a predictor of local recurrence after treatment for both in situ and invasive ductal carcinoma of the breast. J Surg Res 140:109–114, 2007.

It is estimated that the local recurrence rate in this setting is 1% to 3%.[32] Kim and associates[33] reported 10 cases of chest wall relapse following mastectomy for DCIS. All chest wall relapses were treated with radiation therapy, with or without adjuvant systemic therapy. Of the 10 cases, nine patients remain alive without evidence of disease. Young patient age, multiquadrant disease, and the presence of residual normal breast tissue were common features in the cases of chest wall relapse. Similarly, in a review of the Emory University experience, Carlson and colleagues identified 7 (3.3%) of 223 consecutive patients with DCIS who developed a local recurrence following skin-sparing mastectomy with immediate reconstruction.[34] This finding confirms the low rate of local recurrence following mastectomy and also supports the role of skin-sparing mastectomy in patients with DCIS.

Other authors reporting chest wall recurrence cite failure to completely remove breast tissue with DCIS, the presence of occult invasive carcinoma at the time of mastectomy, de novo DCIS or invasive cancer arising in residual breast tissue, and tumor seeding at the time of surgery.[35–37]

INVASIVE CARCINOMA

Wong and Harris[38] summarized risk factors for local recurrence after mastectomy to include an increasing number of positive axillary lymph nodes, lack of systemic therapy, positive margin of resection, close margin of resection, tumor size, young age, and lymphovascular invasion. In analyzing these data, Punglia and associates ranked the consistency of association of these factors with local recurrence in the same descending order.[11]

Buchanan and coworkers reported a prospective database of 1057 patients undergoing mastectomy for invasive cancer at the Memorial-Sloan Kettering Cancer Center from 1995 to 1999.[39] Median follow-up was 6 years. Overall, LRR developed in 93 of 1057 (8.8%) patients. Thirty-four of these 93 patients had synchronous metastatic disease, and 31 patients developed metachronous metastases. Twenty-eight of 93 had isolated recurrence; 24 experienced chest wall recurrence, 2 at the axillary nodal basin, and 2 at more than one additional local site. The authors point out that this latter group of patients should receive aggressive multimodality therapy because many were rendered disease free (22 of 28), although there have not been any randomized prospective clinical trials to define optimal therapy. Treatment may include systemic treatment, hormonal therapy, and radiation therapy, depending on the extent of recurrence, functional status, receptor assays, and prior therapy. Multivariant analysis revealed that age younger than 35 years, lymphovascular invasion, and multi-centricity were major predictors for isolated LRR.

Carreño and colleagues analyzed the clinicopathologic, biologic, and prognostic characteristics of 1087 women undergoing mastectomy for breast cancer.[40] Ninety-eight of these patients developed local recurrence as the first manifestation of tumor progression. The patients with local recurrence showed a significantly higher percentage of larger primary tumors, node-positive status and higher grade than patients without evidence of local recurrence. Tumor size, histologic grade, estrogen receptor (ER) and progesterone (PR) status, and a shorter disease-free interval (<12 months) were significantly associated with overall survival in patients who had mastectomies who later developed isolated local recurrence. There was significant concordance between primary tumors and local recurrences regarding the expression of ER, PR, and p53.

Vaughan and associates from Washington University School of Medicine described the patterns of local breast cancer recurrence after skin-sparing mastectomy and immediate breast reconstruction.[41] In skin-sparing mastectomies with immediate reconstruction from 1998 to 2006, there were 11 patients with a local recurrence (5.3%). Nine developed in the quadrant of the corresponding primary tumor. There were no significant differences between patients who recurred and those who did not with respect to tumor size/stage, margin status, ER/PR/HER2/neu status, lymph node metastasis, or radiation therapy. A predictive factor for local recurrence was grade III tumors.

Regional Recurrences

Regional recurrences are considered recurrences in the regional nodal basins and are divided into axillary, supraclavicular, infraclavicular, and internal mammary nodal basins. The delineation between level III axillary nodes, Rotter's nodes, and infraclavicular nodes is not clear, and perhaps all are lumped together under the broad subheading of infraclavicular nodes.

With 5 years of follow-up, most LRRs following mastectomy occur within the chest wall skin or scar.[23] Approximately 72% of the regional recurrences arise within the supraclavicular fossa, infraclavicular fossa, and internal mammary chain,[23] presumably from surgically inaccessible tumor deposits left following the initial operation. A smaller percentage[23] may be found in incompletely dissected axillae, representing true regional recurrences. Multiple recurrences occur in 16% of patients,[23] suggesting that some regional recurrences may be related to metastasis from a local recurrence.

Axillary lymph node dissection (ALND) has traditionally been performed as part of the treatment of invasive breast cancer. Large patient series are required to compile data about the risk factors of axillary recurrence because it is an uncommon event following ALND, with an incidence of 0.25% to 3%.[23,42-47] The incidence of axillary recurrence is directly related to the extent of initial axillary dissection or the number of lymph nodes removed. With complete node dissection, Haagensen[44] noticed two axillary recurrences in 794 patients. The Danish Breast Cancer Group reviewed 3128 patients and found a direct relationship between the number of negative lymph nodes sampled and the incidence of axillary recurrence. Over 5 years, the risk of axillary recurrence varied from 19% when no node dissection was performed, 10% when fewer than three nodes were removed, 5% following removal of fewer than five nodes, to 3% when more than five negative axillary nodes were dissected.[48] Later, the same group recommended the removal of a minimum of 10 axillary nodes to achieve optimal regional control of the disease.[49]

Similar findings were noticed in the NSABP B-04 trial, where patients had been randomized into three arms: radical mastectomy, total mastectomy with axillary radiation, and total mastectomy alone for clinically node negative disease. Axillary recurrence in the total mastectomy arm was directly related to the number of axillary nodes removed. The incidence of axillary recurrence was 21% when no axillary nodes were dissected, 12% when six or fewer nodes were dissected, and 0.3% when more than 10 nodes were excised.[46] In this prospective randomized study, 40% of patients in the radical mastectomy arm had histologically positive axillary nodes. It is assumed that a similar number in the total mastectomy arm would have histologically positive nodes. Only 17.8% of the 365 patients in the total mastectomy arm who had no axillary treatment underwent a delayed axillary node dissection for isolated axillary recurrences. The median time for axillary recurrence from mastectomy was 14.7 months (range, 3 to 112.6). Most recurrences (78.5%) occurred within 24 months of mastectomy.[41,47]

In the literature review by Clemons and coworkers,[23] the authors estimate the incidence of supraclavicular nodal recurrence after 5 years to be 2% following mastectomy. With an average of 36 months of follow-up in the initial report of NSABP B-04, 0.8% of women with clinically negative axillae treated with radical mastectomy developed a supraclavicular recurrence. For the same group of women who were clinically node positive, the supraclavicular recurrence rate was 3.6% at 3 years.[45] The incidence of internal mammary node recurrence is extremely low. None were identified in B-04.[45] With 25 years of follow-up for all 1665 clinically node-negative and node-positive women in NSABP B-04, the overall risk of regional recurrence (including supraclavicular, infraclavicular, axillary, and internal mammary) was 6%. This is remarkably low, considering that this was a patient population that did not receive adjuvant therapy and presented with palpation-detected tumors, averaging between 3.1 and 3.8 cm.[45]

Cranenbroek and associates[50] studied 6000 patients from a population-based registry in the Netherlands. The authors defined internal mammary lymph node recurrence as breast cancer recurrence in an internal mammary lymph node without a distant metastasis before the recurrence and confirmed by cytology and/or computed tomography (CT). The time interval between diagnosis of the primary tumor and the recurrence vary between 5 and 102 months. Only six patients were observed to have internal mammary lymph node recurrence. One patient showed no symptoms and the other five had parasternal swelling. Treatment resulted in complete remission in four patients, but in five of six patients, distant metastasis occurred in 0 to 37 months. This study suggests that isolated internal mammary lymph node recurrence may be a forerunner of metastatic disease.

With the shift in axillary management and the widespread application of sentinel node biopsy that includes more intensive analysis of relevant nodes and more accurate staging and more consistent utilization of adjuvant therapy, axillary recurrence rates have diminished greatly compared with historical controls. Sentinel node biopsy has a false-negative rate of 5% to 10%. In the NSABP B-04 trial, only 50% of patients with untreated axillae and presumed residual axillary disease presented with isolated axillary recurrences. If we extrapolate from this finding, an axillary recurrence of about 2.5% after sentinel node biopsy can be anticipated. However, adjuvant systemic therapy has become commonplace, and irradiation to the breast with BCT, which may include part of the axilla, may contribute to the reduction of the incidence of axillary recurrences to perhaps less than 1%. Guiliano and colleagues[51] reported a 0% recurrence after 4 years of follow-up. Several additional studies confirm a very low rate of axillary recurrence following sentinel lymphadenectomy.

Jeruss and associates[52] prospectively followed 864 patients with sentinel lymph node biopsies for a median follow-up of 27.4 months. The median number of sentinel nodes harvested was two, and 633 (73%) patients had negative sentinel nodes. Thirty (4.7%) of those sentinel node–negative patients underwent completion axillary dissections, whereas 592 (94%) patients were followed with observation. A total of 231 (27%) had positive sentinel nodes; 158 (68%) of these patients underwent completion axillary dissection, and 73 (32%) were managed with observation alone. No patient in the observed sentinel node–positive group had an axillary recurrence. The authors concluded that on the basis of a median follow-up of 27.4 months, axillary recurrence after sentinel node biopsy is extraordinarily rare regardless of nodal involvement. This indicates that this technique provides an accurate measure of axillary disease and may afford regional control for patients with node-positive disease.

Systemic Recurrences

Systemic recurrences in patients with breast cancer can occur in any organ of the body but primarily occur in the bone, the liver, and the lungs. Metastasis is the invasion of cancer into distant healthy tissue. Scientists have known for more than 100 years that metastasis is not a random phenomenon. Cancer cells preferentially grow in organs that promote and provide an adequate environment—the "soil and seed theory." More recently, the "homing theory" postulates that different organs have the ability to attract or arrest cancer cells through specific chemotactic factors.[53] Currently, studies have focused on the role of chemokines in cancer metastasis. Chemokines are a large family of proteins crucial to the function and circulation of leukocytes. Muller and associates[54] found increased levels of two chemokine receptor genes in human breast cancer cells. In addition, extracts of organs consistently targeted by breast cancer metastasis (lungs, liver, bone marrow, and lymph nodes) were found to have chemotactic ability for breast cancer cells that could be neutralized by antibodies against one of the chemokines.

Patterns of systemic recurrence are derived from different types of studies. Historically, studies have relied on data collected from autopsy series performed on patients who have been diagnosed as having breast cancer (Table 22-4). The most common cause of death in these series is assumed to be breast cancer. Such data do not reflect the site of first recurrence or the time or interval to such events. However, autopsy data are an accurate assessment of the final pattern of metastasis at death. Lee[55] reviewed the American experience between 1943 and 1977 and concluded that the pattern of metastasis did not change over the 35-year span. The reported median incidence in the six most common sites were as follows: lung, 71% (57%–77%); bone, 71% (49%–74%); lymph nodes, 67% (50%–67%); liver, 62% (50%–71%); pleura, 50% (36%–65%); and adrenal glands, 41% (30%–54%). Similar observations were documented in Europe.[56,57]

The pattern of recurrence in breast cancer is perhaps better derived from longitudinal observational studies documenting the first site of recurrence (Table 22-5). In many of these studies, multiple sites of first recurrences were included as separate first sites; hence the total percentage may have exceeded 100%. The most common site of recurrence was systemic, with bone being the most common organ, followed by LRR, the lung, and the liver. Such data are limited by many factors, including their retrospective nature. Furthermore, the first site of recurrence is dependent on the type and intensity of screening during follow-up. Extensive screening may entail a frequent detailed history and physical examination only or may include blood testing (alkaline phosphatase, liver function tests, and tumor markers), bone scans, liver scan or ultrasound, chest films or CT, CT scans of the abdomen and pelvis, as well as CT scans or MRI of the brain. It has been documented that such extensive screening may detect metastasis before the development of any symptoms.

The incidence of recurrences and perhaps the pattern may vary with the stage of disease and administration of adjuvant chemotherapy. Breast cancer is increasingly being diagnosed at an earlier stage, and the indication

---

TABLE 22-4

Site of Metastasis of Breast Cancer: Autopsy Series

Author	Year	n	Lung (%)	Pleura (%)	Liver (%)	Bone (%)	Skin/Soft Tissue (%)	CNS (%)	GI (%)
Walther[a]	1948	186	62	—	35	73	19	—	—
Trauth[b]	1978	116	71	46	59	59	21	—	—
Cifuentes and Pickren[c]	1979	676	67	50	62	71	—	44	16
Lee[d]	1983	2147	71	50	62	71	—	—	—
Hagemeister[e]	1980	166	75*		71	67	30	38	—
Haagensen[f]	1986	100	69	51	65	71	30	22	18

CNS, central nervous system; GI, gastrointestinal.
*75% respiratory organs (including lung, pleura, and trachea).
[a]From Walther H.[56]
[b]From Trauth H.[57]
[c]From Cifuentes N, Pickren JW: Metastases from carcinoma of the mammary gland: An autopsy study. J Surg Oncol 11:193, 1979.
[d]From Lee T-Y.[55]
[e]From Hagemeister FB, Buzdar AU, Luna MA, Blumenschien GR: Causes of death in breast cancer: A clinicopathologic study. Cancer 46:142–167, 1980.
[f]From Haagensen C: Diseases of the breast. Philadelphia, WB Saunders, 1986.

TABLE 22-5

Site of First Recurrence in Retrospective Studies Presented as Percentages

Author	Year	n	Locoregional (%)*	Bone (%)	Lung and Pleura (%)	Liver (%)	Soft Tissue (%)	Brain (%)
Hatschek[a]	1989	81	36	30	22	11	—	—
Tomin and Donegan[b]	1987	248	32	28	16	5	—	—
Kambyl[c]	1988	401	65	31	29	15	—	2
Rutgers, van Slooten and Kluck[d]	1989	194	23	62	26	22	—	—
Stierer and Rosen[e]	1989	133	30	29.3	21	5.25	5.5	2.25
Zwaveling[f]	1987	128	11	43	18	15	—	—
Hannisdal[g]	1993	126	29	43.7	24	10	—	5.5
Mirza[h]	2001	261	47.9	26.4	20.3	13.4	—	3

*Locoregional recurrences without systemic disease were excluded.
[a]From Hatschek T, Carstensen J, Fagerberg G, et al: Influence of S-phase fraction on metastatic pattern and post-recurrence survival in a randomized mammography screening trial. Breast Cancer Res Treat 14:321, 1989.
[b]From Tomin R, Donegan WL: Screening for recurrent breast cancer—its effectiveness and prognostic value. J Clin Oncol 5:62,1987.
[c]From Kamby C, Vejborg I, Kristensen B, et al: Metastatic pattern in recurrent breast cancer. Cancer 62:2226, 1988.
[d]From Rutgers E, van Slooten EA, Kluck H: Follow-up after treatment of primary breast cancer. Br J Surg 76:187, 1989.
[e]From Steirer M, Rosen HR: Influence of early diagnosis on prognosis of recurrent breast cancer. Cancer 64:1128, 1989.
[f]From Zwaveling A, Albers GH, Felthius W, Hermans J: An evaluation of routine follow up for detection of breast cancer recurrences. J Surg Oncol 34:194,1987.
[g]From Hannisdal E, Gundersen S, Kvaløy S, et al: Follow-up of breast cancer patients stage I–II: A baseline strategy. Eur J Cancer 29:992, 1993.
[h]From Mirza N, Valstos G, Meric F, et al: Predictors of systemic recurrence and impact of local failure among early stage breast cancer patients treated with breast conserving therapy. Abstracts of 24th Annual San Antonio Breast Cancer Symposium, San Antonio, December 2001.

for adjuvant chemotherapy has changed. Furthermore, histologic tumor type has been shown to affect the pattern of recurrence. In a study comparing the metastatic patterns of invasive lobular carcinoma to invasive ductal carcinoma of the breast, Borst and Ingold[58] retrospectively examined 2605 cases of invasive lobular and ductal carcinoma. Their findings, as well as those of others, have demonstrated that invasive lobular carcinoma has a higher incidence of metastasis to the gastrointestinal system, gynecologic organs, peritoneum and retroperitoneum, adrenal glands, and bone marrow, whereas invasive ductal carcinoma has been found to have a higher incidence of metastasis to the lungs and pleura. In both histologic types the incidence of metastasis to the axillary lymph nodes, liver, central nervous system, and soft tissue has been shown to be similar.[59–61]

Patients with triple-negative tumors (ER-negative, PR-negative and HER2/neu-negative) have an increased likelihood of distant recurrence. When compared with other breast cancers, patients with triple-negative tumors more frequently presented with visceral metastasis and with a shorter time interval from diagnosis. This observation did not hold for bony metastasis. Interestingly, patients with triple-negative breast cancer did not develop any visceral metastasis after 8 years of follow-up.[62]

A more reliable representation of the first site of metastasis can be seen in the prospective clinical trials shown in Table 22-6. Similarly, these studies have shown the bone to be the most common first site of recurrence in up to 35% of the patients with metastasis, followed by LRR, the lungs, and the liver. Two studies investigating the value of intensive follow-up are valuable in describing the pattern of recurrences. In a study

by the Interdisciplinary Group for Cancer Care Evaluation (GIVIO) investigators, a total of 1320 women diagnosed as having stage I to III breast cancer, with the exclusion of T_4N_2, were followed up either intensively or regularly, and the difference in outcome was examined based on the type of survival. The intensive follow-up group had a chest film every 6 months and a bone scan and liver sonogram yearly. LRRs and distant metastases were reviewed, whereas new primaries, contralateral disease, and deaths from other causes were ignored. A total of 322 such events occurred in both groups, with a distribution detailed in Table 22-6. At a median follow-up of 71 months, no difference was apparent in overall survival between the two groups. Bone was the most common site of first recurrence, consisting of 32.6% of the total events, followed by LRR, the lungs, and the pleura, as well as the liver.[58]

In a study by Roselli Del Turco[63] and colleagues, 1243 women with stage I to III (no exclusion) breast cancer who had undergone BCT were studied to assess whether the early detection of intrathoracic and bone metastases was effective in reducing mortality in patients with breast cancer. All patients were given a physical examination and underwent mammography, but patients in the intensive follow-up group received a chest x-ray study and a bone scan every 6 months. After 5 years, 393 patients had developed a similar pattern of metastasis as those in the GIVIO study (see Table 22-6). Relapse-free survival was significantly better for the clinical follow-up group ($P = 0.01$), probably attributable to lead-time bias because the overall survival over 5 years was the same for both groups (18.6% vs. 19.5%).[64]

TABLE 22-6

Pattern of Recurrences in Prospective Series

Author	Year	Follow-up Year	Stage	Locoregional (%)	Bone (%)	Lung/ Pleura (%)	Liver (%)	Multiple (%)	Other (%)
Veronesi[a]	1981	5	I–II	27	50	38	15	Listed separately	8
NSABP B-04[b]	1985	10	I–II	23.9	22.3	16.9	—	22.9	14
GIVIO[c]	1994	5	I–III	21.1	32.6	7.8	13.9	9.6	14.3
Roselli Del Turco, Palli, and Cariddi[d]	1994	5	I–III	26.5	34.8	11.7	—	16	10.9

[a]From Veronesi U, Saccozzi R, Del Vecchio M, et al: Comparing radical mastectomy with quadrantectomy, axillary dissection, and radiotherapy in patients with small cancer of the breast. N Engl J Med 305:6, 1981.
[b]From Fisher B, Redmond C, Fisher ER, et al.[47]
[c]From the GIVIO Investigators.[64]
[d]From Roselli Del Turco M, Palli D, Cariddi A.[63]

Time of Recurrence

Although there is no cutoff period beyond which patients are assumed cured from breast cancer, most systemic recurrences occur within the first 10 years. Most studies have noted a peak in LRRs and distant recurrences during the first to fifth years after diagnosis and initiation of treatment. There has been a uniform observation that most recurrences plateau after the first decade, although they continue to occur at a much smaller rate. Demicheli and colleagues[65] from the Milan Cancer Institute reviewed the incidence of recurrence at a given time in 1173 patients with breast cancer who had undergone mastectomy by using the cause-specific hazard function. The results produced a graph with two peaks, demonstrating a hazard function for first failure at approximately 18 months after surgery, followed by another peak at approximately 60 months, and tapering off with a plateau-like tail extending up to 15 years. A similar pattern for local recurrence and distant metastases was observed in all tumors, but the size of the tumor was shown to be a determinant in the time frame of local or distant recurrence. The risk of early local and distant recurrences was lower for T_1 tumors than for larger tumors, whereas the risk of late recurrence was similar for all tumors regardless of size. Demonstrating an increased risk of local and distant recurrence, node-positive patients showed peaks four to five times higher than node-negative patients. The division of node-positive patients into those with one to three positive nodes and those with more than three positive nodes did not substantially affect the general time frame of tumor recurrence, although the height of the peaks was double for those with more than three positive nodes. Data regarding recurrences in premenopausal and postmenopausal patients resulted in hazard functions that were virtually superimposable, showing no difference in the rates of local or distant recurrence on the basis of menopausal status. The time frame for distant metastasis was reported to be similar for 2233 patients with breast cancer who underwent BCT.[65]

In a follow-up article, Demicheli and coworkers[66] compared the risk of recurrence over time for the 877 patients who were given 6 or 12 cycles of adjuvant cyclophosphamide/methotrexate/fluorouracil (CMF) therapy with 575 who received no adjuvant treatment. The recurrence risk for this group of patients was estimated based on the event-specific hazard rate to ascertain the time of first failure and distant metastases, and following Efron, hazard rates were fitted with logistic regression models. Again a double-peaked pattern was observed for both treated patients and controls, with the first hazard peak occurring at approximately 18 to 24 months after surgery (defined as early metastases), a second minor peak occurring at the fifth to sixth year, and a tapered, plateau-like tail extending over 10 years after surgery (late metastases). Compared with the previous trial, the recurrence risk of CMF-treated patients was lower than the corresponding risk of patients who had undergone only surgery—an expected result. However, the difference between recurrence risks was highly evident only for early recurrences and disappeared after approximately 2 years.[66]

Models of tumor growth play a key role in understanding breast cancer as a systemic disease. Demicheli[67] disagrees with the exponential Gompertzian model (i.e., the explanation of uncontrolled tumor growth as a result of tumor seeding). He rejects this theory because of the inadequacy of the model in explaining clinical findings concerning the long-lasting recurrence risk, as well as the time distribution of the first treatment failure and mortality for patients undergoing mastectomy. According to Demicheli, the theory of tumor dormancy provides a more reasonable description of the natural history of breast cancer, assuming that for some patients during the preclinical phase, micrometastases present in the breast do not grow for a given time interval that is dependent on tumor and/or host characteristics. Using the tumor dormancy model facilitates the treatment of patients with recurrent disease. If the recurrence is related to the growth of micrometastases that were latent during adjuvant chemotherapy, the patient can be considered previously untreated and full-treatment options are available. This model explains the response of patients who had a recurrence more than 1 year after the end of adjuvant CMF to the same chemotherapy, an observation consistent with the hypothesis that the metastases were dormant and had not yet been treated.[67]

The pattern of recurrence of breast cancer provides a valuable insight into the behavior of the disease and may direct future research in the prevention of such occurrences. Based on the concept previously described, the "soil and seed theory" as it relates to breast cancer metastasis to the bone. The role of bisphosphonates in breast cancer bone metastasis was explored in a prospective randomized study.[68] This study had shown that bisphosphonates significantly decreased the incidence of bony metastasis compared with placebo, although only during the 2-year medication period. This significant advantage was lost after the medication was stopped (patients were followed up for the total 5-year study period). A better understanding of the tumor dormancy concept and tumor-host interaction may change the therapeutic strategies and result in different treatment modalities other than cytotoxic chemotherapeutic agents.

REFERENCES

1. Overgaard M, et al: Postoperative radiotherapy in high-risk premenopausal women with breast cancer who receive adjuvant chemotherapy. Danish Breast Cancer Cooperative Group 82b Trial. N Engl J Med 337:949, 1997.
2. Ragaz J, et al: Adjuvant radiotherapy and chemotherapy in node-positive premenopausal women with breast cancer. N Engl J Med 337:956, 1997.
3. Beahrs OH, Myers MH (eds): Manual for the staging of cancer, 2nd ed. Philadelphia, JB Lippincott, 1983.
4. Greene FL, Page DL, Fleming ID, et al (eds): AJCC Cancer Staging Manual, 6th ed. New York, Springer-Verlag, 2002.
5. Ernster VL, Barclay J, Kerlikowske K, et al: Mortality among women with ductal carcinoma in situ of the breast in the population-based Surveillance, Epidemiology and End Results program. Arch Intern Med 160:953, 2000.
6. Solin LJ, Fourquet A, Vicini FA, et al: Salvage treatment for local recurrence after breast conserving surgery and radiation as initial treatment for mammographically detected ductal carcinoma in situ of the breast. Cancer 91:1090, 2001.
7. Voogd AC, Van Oost FJ, Rutgers EJT, et al, for the Dutch Study Group on Local Recurrence after Breast Conservation (BORST Group). Long-term prognosis of patients with local recurrence after conservative surgery and radiotherapy for early breast cancer. Eur J Cancer 41:2637, 2005.
8. Galper S, Blood E, Gelman R, et al: Prognosis after local recurrence after conservative surgery and radiation for early-stage breast cancer. Int J Radiat Oncol Biol Phys 61:348, 2005.
9. Willner J, Kiricuta IC, Kölbi O: Locoregional recurrence of breast cancer following mastectomy: always a fatal event? Results of univariate and multivariate analysis. Int J Radiat Oncol Biol Phys 37:853–863, 1997.
10. Meric F, Mirza NQ, Vlastos G, et al: Positive surgical margins and ipsilateral breast tumor recurrence predict disease-specific survival after breast-conserving therapy [see comment]. Cancer 97:926–933, 2003.
11. Punglia R, Morrow M, Winer EP, Harris JR: Local therapy and survival in breast cancer. N Engl J Med 356:2399–2405, 2007.
12. Clarke M, Collins R, Darby S, et al: Effects of radiotherapy and of differences in the extent of surgery for early breast cancer on local recurrence and 15-year survival: An overview of the randomized trials. Lancet 366:2087–2106, 2005.
13. Berg WA, Gutierrez L, NessAiver MS, et al: Diagnostic accuracy of mammography, clinical examination, US, and MR imaging in preoperative assessment of breast cancer. Radiology 23:830–849, 2004.
14. Huston TL, Simmons RM: Locally recurrent breast cancer after conservation therapy. Am J Surg 189:229–235, 2005.
15. Fisher B, Dignam J, Wolmark N, et al: Lumpectomy and radiation therapy for the treatment of intraductal breast cancer: Findings from National Surgical Adjuvant Breast and Bowel Project B-17. J Clin Oncol 16:441–452, 1998.
16. EORTC Breast Cancer Cooperative Group, EORTC Radiotherapy Group, Bijker N, Meijnen P, Peterse JL, et al: Breast-conserving treatment with or without radiotherapy in ductal carcinoma-in-situ: Ten-year results of European Organisation for Research and Treatment of Cancer randomized phase III trial 10853—a study by the EORTC Breast Cancer Cooperative Group and EORTC Radiotherapy Group [see comment]. J Clin Oncol 24:3381–3387, 2006.
17. Houghton J, George WD, Cuzick J, et al: UK Coordinating Committee on Cancer Research. Ductal Carcinoma in situ Working Party. DCIS trialists in the UK, Australia, and New Zealand. Radiotherapy and tamoxifen in women with completely excised ductal carcinoma in situ of the breast in the UK, Australia, and New Zealand: randomised controlled trial [see comment]. Lancet 362:95–102, 2003.
18. Silverstein M: Van Nuys Prognostic Index for DCIS. In Silverstein M (ed): Ductal carcinoma in situ of the breast. Baltimore, Williams & Wilkins, 1977.
19. Fisher B, Dignam J, Wolmark N, et al: Tamoxifen in treatment of intraductal breast cancer: National Surgical Adjuvant Breast and Bowel Project B-24 randomised controlled trial [see comment]. Lancet 353:1993–2000, 1999.
20. Recht A, et al: Time-course of local recurrence following conservative surgery and radiotherapy for early stage breast cancer. Int J Radiat Oncol Biol Phys 15:255, 1988.
21. Gage I, et al: Long-term outcome following breast-conserving surgery and radiation therapy. Int J Radiat Oncol Biol Phys 33:245, 1995.
22. Fisher ER, et al: Fifteen-year prognostic discriminants for invasive breast carcinoma: National Surgical Adjuvant Breast and Bowel Project Protocol-06. Cancer 91:1679, 2001.
23. Clemons M, et al: Locoregionally recurrent breast cancer: Incidence, risk factors and survival. Cancer Treat Rev 27:67, 2001.
24. Hafty BG, et al: Ipsilateral breast tumor recurrence as a predictor of distant disease: Implication for systemic therapy at the time of local relapse. J Clin Oncol 14:52, 1996.
25. Fourquet A, et al: Prognostic factors of breast recurrences in the conservative management of early breast cancer: a 25-year follow-up. Int J Radiat Oncol Biol Phys 17:719, 1989.
26. NSABP progress report 2001. Pittsburgh, PA, National Surgical Adjuvant Breast and Bowel Project:84, 94, 140; May 2002.
27. Liljegren G, et al: Sector resection with or without postoperative radiation therapy for stage I breast cancer: five years results of a randomized trial. Uppsala-Orebro breast cancer study group. J Natl Cancer Inst 86:717, 1994.
28. Veronesi U, et al: Radiotherapy after breast preserving surgery in women with localized cancer of the breast. N Engl J Med 328:1587, 1993.
29. Clark RM, et al: Randomized clinical trial of irradiation following lumpectomy and axillary dissection of node-negative breast cancer: An update. Ontario Clinical Oncology Group. J Natl Cancer Inst 88:1659, 1996.
30. Forrest AP, et al: Randomized controlled trial of conservative therapy for breast cancer: 6-year analysis of the Scottish trial. Scottish Cancer Trial Breast Group. Lancet 348:708, 1996.
31. Renton SC, et al: The importance of resection margin in conservative surgery for breast cancer. Eur J Surg Oncol 22:17, 1996.
32. Silverstein MJ, Barth A, Poller DN, et al: Ten-year results comparing mastectomy to excision and radiation therapy for ductal carcinoma in situ of the breast. Eur J Cancer 31A:1425–1427, 1995.
33. Kim JH, Tavassoli F, Haffty BG: Chest wall relapse after mastectomy for ductal carcinoma in situ: A report of 10 cases with a review of the literature. Cancer J 12:92–101, 2006.
34. Carlson GW, Page A, Johnson E, et al: Local recurrence of ductal carcinoma in situ after skin-sparing mastectomy. J Am Coll of Surg 204:1074–1080, 2007.
35. Deutsch M: Ductal carcinoma in situ recurrent on the chest wall after mastectomy. Clin Oncol (R Coll Radiol) 11:61–62, 1999.
36. Salas AP, Helvie MA, Wilkins EG, et al: Is mammography useful in screening for local recurrences in patients with TRAM flap breast

reconstruction after mastectomy for multifocal DCIS? Ann Surg Oncol 5:456–463, 1998.

37. Price P, Sinnett HD, Gusterson B, et al: Duct carcinoma in situ: Predictors of local recurrence and progression in patients treated by surgery alone. Br J Cancer 61:869–872, 1990.
38. Wong JS, Harris JR: Postmastectomy radiation therapy. In Harris JR, Lippman ME, Morrow M, Osborne CK (eds): Diseases of the breast, 3rd ed. Philadelphia, Lippincott Williams & Wilkins, 2004, pp 785–799.
39. Buchanan CL, Dorn PL, Fey J, et al: Locoregional recurrence after mastectomy: Incidence and outcomes. J Am Coll Surg 469–474, 2006.
40. Carreño G, del Casar JM, Cort MD, et al: Local recurrence after mastectomy for breast cancer: Analysis of clinicopathological, biological and prognostic characteristics. Breast Cancer Res Treat 102:61–73, 2007.
41. Vaughan A, Dietz JR, Aft R, et al: Patterns of local breast cancer recurrence after skin-sparing mastectomy and immediate breast reconstruction. Am J Surg 194:438–44, 2007.
42. Newman LA, et al: Presentation, management and outcome of axillary recurrence from breast cancer. Am J Surg 180:252, 2000.
43. de Boer R, et al: Detection, treatment and outcome of axillary recurrence after axillary clearance for invasive breast cancer. Br J Surg 88:118, 2001.
44. Haagensen CD: The surgical treatment of mammary carcinoma. In Diseases of the breast, 2nd ed. Philadelphia, WB Saunders, 1971.
45. Fisher B, Montague E, Redmond C, et al: Comparison of radical mastectomy with alternative treatments for primary breast cancer. A first report of results from a prospective randomized clinical trial. Cancer 39(6 suppl):2827–2839, 1977.
46. Fisher B, et al: The accuracy of clinical nodal staging and of limited axillary dissection as a determinant of histologic nodal status in carcinoma of the breast. Surg Gynecol Obstet 152:765, 1981.
47. Fisher B, Redmond C, Fisher ER, et al: Ten-year results of a randomized clinical trial comparing radical mastectomy and total mastectomy with or without radiation. N Engl J Med 312:674, 1985.
48. Graversen H, et al: Breast cancer: Risk of axillary recurrence in node negative patients following partial dissection of the axilla. Eur J Surg Oncol 14:407, 1988.
49. Axelsson CK, et al: Axillary dissection of level I and II lymph nodes is important in breast cancer classification. The Danish Breast Cancer Cooperative Group (DBCG). Eur J Cancer 28A: 1415, 1992.
50. Cranenbroek S, van der Sangen MJC, Kuijt GP, Voogd AC: Diagnosis, treatment and prognosis of internal mammary lymph node recurrence in breast cancer patients. Breast Cancer Res Treat 89:271–275, 2005.
51. Giuliano AE, et al: Prospective observational study of sentinel lymphadenectomy without further axillary dissection in patients with sentinel node-negative breast cancer. J Clin Oncol 18:2553, 2000.
52. Jeruss JS, Winchester DJ, Sener SF, et al: Axillary recurrence after sentinel node biopsy. Ann Surg Oncol 12:34–40, 2005.
53. Murphy PM: Chemokines and the molecular basis of cancer metastasis. N Engl J Med 345:833, 2001.
54. Muller A, et al: Involvement of chemokine receptors in breast cancer metastasis. Nature 410:50, 2001.
55. Lee Y-T: Breast carcinoma: Pattern of metastases at autopsy. J Surg Oncol 23:175, 1983.
56. Walther H (ed): Kerbsmetastasen. Basel, Schwabe, 1948.
57. Trauth H: Zur pathologie der hamatogenen metastasierung des mammakarzinoms. In Pathologieder Brustedruse. Berlin, Springer, 1978.
58. Borst MJ, Ingold JA: Metastatic patterns of invasive lobular versus invasive ductal carcinoma of the breast. Surgery 114:637, 1993.
59. Lamovec J, Bracko M: Metastatic pattern of infiltrating lobular carcinoma of the breast: An autopsy study. J Surg Oncol 48:28, 1991.
60. Harris M, et al: A comparison of the metastatic pattern of infiltrating lobular carcinoma and infiltrating duct carcinoma of the breast. Br J Cancer 50:23, 1984.
61. Weiss MC, et al: Outcome of conservative therapy for invasive breast cancer by histologic subtype. Int J Radiat Oncol Biol Phys 23:941, 1992.
62. Dent R, Trudeau M, Sun P, Narod S: San Antonio Breast Conference, 2007. Abstract 1053.
63. Roselli Del Turco M, Palli D, Cariddi A: Intensive diagnostic follow-up after treatment of primary breast cancer: A randomized trial. JAMA 271:1593, 1994.
64. The GIVIO Investigators: Impact of follow-up and testing on survival and health related quality of life in breast cancer patients: A multicenter randomized controlled trial. JAMA 271:1587, 1994.
65. Demicheli R, et al: Time distribution of the recurrence risk for breast cancer patients undergoing mastectomy: Further support about the concept of tumor dormancy. Breast Cancer Res Treat 41:177, 1996.
66. Demicheli R, et al: Comparative analysis of breast cancer recurrence risk for patients receiving or not receiving adjuvant cyclophosphamide, methotrexate, fluorouracil (CMF). Data supporting the occurrence of "cures." Breast Cancer Res Treat 53:209, 1999.
67. Demicheli R: Tumour dormancy: Findings and hypotheses from clinical research on breast cancer. Semin Cancer Biol 11:297, 2001.
68. Powles TJ, et al: A randomized placebo controlled trial to evaluate the effect of the bisphosphonate, clodronate, on the incidence of metastases and mortality in patients with primary operable breast cancer. Breast Cancer Res Treat 69:209, 2001.

SECTION VI

Staging of Breast Cancer

chapter 23

Assessment and Designation of Breast Cancer Stage

ALFREDO A. SANTILLAN | JOHN V. KILUK |
CHARLES E. COX

Staging: Past, Present, and Future

Staging plays an integral role in the management of breast cancer. Classifying patients by stage places them in prognostic groupings based on the best current available evidence gained from observation studies or clinical trials. The role of the surgical oncologist both past and present has been to acquire with precision the pathologic tissues required to accurately diagnose, measure size, and determine nodal staging of patients' tumors. Current and future roles include the harvesting of tissues to achieve the previously stated goals as well as to biochemically, molecularly, and genetically catalog primary tumors antecedent to treatment regimens. The major disciplines of surgery, medical oncology, and radiation oncology use current breast cancer staging classifications for determining the extent of disease, predicting overall survival, and providing guidance for therapy. This process requires objective analysis of pertinent, well-organized, uniformly reproducible clinical and pathologic data. Furthermore, epidemiologists and public health researchers rely on uniform breast cancer staging methods to evaluate trends in breast cancer incidence, screening programs, treatment outcomes, and risk factors worldwide. Finally, staging also plays an integral part in advances in breast cancer research and in the application of basic science to clinical science (translational research).

In the past, the cancer staging system was quite simplistic. Neoplasms were staged on the basis of clinical evaluation alone as operable or inoperable and classified as local, regional, or metastatic. However, there were limitations of the clinical staging in accurately predicting the outcome in patients, and therefore the importance of deriving a more sophisticated staging system has been realized. Its predictive power is largely based on simple physical measurements such as size of the tumor or extent of anatomic spread of the disease to regional lymph nodes and distant organ sites at the time of diagnosis. These measurements are static and permit only limited evaluation of an ever-changing, heterogenous neoplasm that often has been in existence for years before the initiation of the staging process. Furthermore, advancements in breast cancer research and the development of new therapies have led to more treatment options (e.g., systemic chemotherapy, hormonal and other novel biologic therapies). In addition, the impact of treatment on long-term prognosis is not incorporated. Even today, the classification schemas for staging patients are limited by the inability to accurately assess the biologic behavior of tumors and only minimal levels of molecular data are available.

Breast cancers, in general, are considered relatively indolent tumors with a long natural history. However, breast cancer in different patients progresses at different rates, despite similarities in the clinical parameters at the time of diagnosis. The growth rate may range from a few to as many as 25 years, making it difficult to predict the biologic behavior of each tumor. The rate of tumor progression depends on a number of factors, such as size and lymph node status, histologic type, DNA ploidy, and others that have not yet been identified.

Future staging systems will likely include new technologies and in-depth molecular, genetic, and pathologic analysis of the tissue specimens. The introduction of the sentinel lymph node (SLN) technique has allowed more accurate staging with much less morbidity to the patient compared with a complete axillary node dissection. With improvements in the sensitivity of detection methods, including histopathologic assays and molecular techniques, microscopic and submicroscopic tumor metastases can be detected. The recent expansion of genetic knowledge associated with the Human Genome Project has provided a large number of molecular tools that may prove valuable in the evaluation of tumor progression and overall survival. Molecular staging using reverse transcriptase–polymerase chain reaction (RT-PCR), microarray analysis, and proteomics to identify unique gene and protein expression profiles may allow the detection of occult cancer before it becomes clinically evident and may provide more accurate information to help determine prognosis and survival with minimal morbidity to the patient. Finally, more accurate molecular staging may allow ablative rather than extirpative procedures and molecular-directed systemic therapies to be used. The increasing use of molecular staging and assessment of tumor response could potentially affect future staging systems by including biologic markers to pretreatment clinical stage and post-treatment pathologic staging.

Central to any staging system are identifiable objective tumor and host characteristics that are prognostic of tumor progression. A number of clinical and pathologic factors have been identified that may predict the long-term outcome in patients with breast cancer. Generally accepted prognostic factors include age, tumor size, lymph node status, histologic tumor and grade, mitotic rate, hormone receptor, and human epidermal growth factor receptor 2 (HER2/neu). A number of other biologic factors have also been studied and provide information regarding the potential for aggressive behavior of tumors (Table 23-1).

Clinical and pathologic staging systems are both useful in providing prognostic information. Clinical parameters historically have been used to predict survival because of the simplicity in obtaining the data. The clinical system may serve to guide initial therapy based on all available preoperative data that include history, physical and laboratory examinations, and biopsy material. However, tumors are now detected at very early stages, before they become clinically evident; as a result, histopathologic staging based on the primary tumor and local/regional lymph nodes has proved to be more accurate in predicting survival. The pathologic system, because of its ability to precisely define the histology and the extent of disease, is more accurate for grouping of patients with similar prognoses and for planning subsequent therapies.

Clinical, Pathologic, and Biologic Markers and Factors in Determining Prognosis

Prognostic factors are important for forecasting outcomes in individual patients and can be used to help refine treatment choices. A prognostic factor is capable of providing information on clinical outcome at the time of diagnosis, independent of therapy. Such markers are usually indicators of growth, invasion, and metastatic potential. Nodal status is the most important parameter used to define risk category in early breast cancer and is considered a "pure" prognostic factor; that is, nodal status does not affect response to systemic therapy. On the other hand, a predictive factor is capable of providing information on the likelihood of response to a given therapeutic modality. Such markers are either within the target of the treatment, or serve as modulators related to expression and/or function of the target. Estrogen receptor status is a predictive factor because it indicates the likelihood of response to endocrine therapy, but its role as an independent prognostic factor is controversial. In contrast, expression of the HER2/neu oncogenes may not only be an important prognostic factor in at least some subsets of patients with breast cancer; it may also provide some indication of the likelihood of response to certain chemotherapeutic agents. Therefore, the HER2/neu oncogene has a dual role as prognostic and predictive factor.

Traditionally the dogma has been that prognostic factors help physicians determine which patients with breast cancer need adjuvant therapy, whereas predictive factors indicate which adjuvant therapy is most appropriate. The most important benefit of prognostic classification may be to help physicians identify patients in whom adjuvant therapy could be avoided, thus preventing treatment-related side effects. In theory, the identification, validation, and application of suitable predictive and prognostic factors helps ensure that only those patients likely to benefit will receive a given treatment.

CLINICAL FACTORS

Clinical staging is based on a thorough physical examination of the breast tissue, skin overlying the breasts, and the regional lymph nodes (axillary, infraclavicular, supraclavicular, cervical) and various imaging modalities. On physical examination, important characteristics to note are the tumor size, whether there is extension into the chest wall, involvement of the overlying skin (e.g., erythema, induration, or edema) and the regional lymph nodes. Mobility of the involved regional lymph nodes is important to note as a prognosticating indicator, with fixed nodes with extracapsular extension having a worse prognosis.

TABLE 23-1	
Prognostic Factors in Breast Cancer	
Clinical Histopathologic Factors	**Biologic Factors**
Age	Angiogenesis (VEGF)
Tumor size	Proliferation (MIBI/Ki67/mitotic index)
Tumor location	Growth factor receptor (EGFR/HER2/neu)
Tumor histology	Cell cycle regulators (p53/c-myc/cyclins)
Tumor grade	Proteases (uPA/PAI-1/cathepsin D)
Hormone receptor status	Bone marrow micrometastasis
Vascular invasion	Circulating tumor cells
Lymph node status	Molecular subtype
Distant metastasis	Multiparameter gene expression analysis (MammaPrint/Oncotype DX)

Modified from Bundred NJ: Prognostic and predictive factors in breast cancer. Cancer Treat Rev 27:137–142, 2001.

Imaging modalities such as mammograms, ultrasound, and computed tomography (CT) scans are available and useful as an adjuvant to the physical examination. Newer imaging modalities that are currently under intense clinical investigation as a diagnostic screening tool include digital mammography, contrast enhanced magnetic resonance imaging (MRI), and positron emission tomography (PET). In particular, digital mammography and MRI could play an important role in screening patients with dense breasts, young age, and hereditary breast cancer. MRI may also be considered in the evaluation of the extent of disease in the affected breast (including the detection of chest wall invasion), the detection of cancer in the contralateral breast, the evaluation of occult cancer, and the detection of response to preoperative neoadjuvant therapy. The role of PET in the initial staging evaluation of breast cancer is uncertain, because it does not add significant information over the other imaging modalities for locoregional disease, either the primary site or axillary nodal status. Positron emission mammography (PEM) is currently under investigation for the evaluation of the breast itself.

PRIMARY TUMOR CHARACTERISTICS

Tumor Size

Tumor size is one of the most important prognostic markers of invasive breast cancer. It is defined as the maximal size of the invasive component of the primary tumor on pathologic examination. Clinical evaluation of tumor size has been included in many staging systems as an independent predictor of survival.[1-3] The potential for metastasis increases in a linear relationship with the size of the primary tumor (Fig. 23-1).[1] Metastasis does not occur in 50% of the cases until the primary tumor reaches a size of 3.6 cm in diameter. Furthermore, there is a distinct relationship between increasing tumor size and the probability of axillary nodal metastasis.[4] These investigators demonstrated that tumors must reach 3.1 to 4 cm in diameter to generate axillary metastasis in 50% of patients (Table 23-2). Fisher[5] has likewise shown that tumor size correlates with disease-free survival at 10 years, even when controlled for nodal metastases (Fig. 23-2). Tumor size is particularly useful as a prognostic tool in patients with no involvement of regional lymph nodes. Tumor size alone may alter adjuvant treatment options. Patients with small tumors (<1 cm) who have lymph node–negative disease have an excellent overall prognosis. A recent study from the Surveillance, Epidemiology, and End Results (SEER) Program demonstrated that the 10-year breast cancer–specific mortality in this group of patients is only 4%, whereas their overall mortality is 24%.[6] Thus, patients with small tumors with lymph node–negative disease have a fivefold higher risk of dying from causes other than breast cancer. It is also true, however, that patients with small tumors can have metastasis to the axillary lymph nodes, and conversely, more than one third of patients with tumors greater than 6 cm in palpable diameter have negative lymph nodes, thus demonstrating the limited predictiveness of tumor size alone.[7]

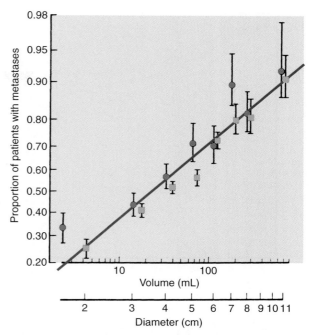

Figure 23-1 A linear relationship exists between tumor size (volume or diameter) and potential for metastases. (From Koscielny S, Tubiana M, Lê MG, et al: Breast cancer: Relationship between the size of the primary tumour and the probability of metastatic dissemination. Br J Cancer 49:709, 1984.)

Tumor Location

Tumor site is generally not included as a prognostic factor to identify patients at higher risk of relapse. However, tumor location has a significant prognostic utility, especially for axillary lymph node–negative patients. Although the risk of metastasis to the axillary lymph nodes is greater for lateral versus medial breast cancers, one study by Fisher and colleagues[8] showed that patients with medial tumors fare more poorly than those with lateral tumors because of a greater risk of local recurrence. Another study demonstrated that the prognosis is quite similar between groups of patients with tumors in the medial or lateral half of the breast.[9] More recently, other investigators from single institutions and data obtained from SEER have found that medial and central locations of tumor are associated with a 29% to 46%

TABLE 23-2

Relationship between Tumor Size and Axillary Metastases

Tumor Diameter (cm)	No. of Patients	Axillary Node–Positive (%)
0.1–0.5	147	28.6
0.6–1	960	24.7
1.1–2	4044	34.1
2.1–3	3546	42.1
3.1–4	1917	50.1
4.1–5	1135	56.5
>5	1232	64.5

Modified from Nemoto T, Vana J, Bedwani RN, et al.[4]

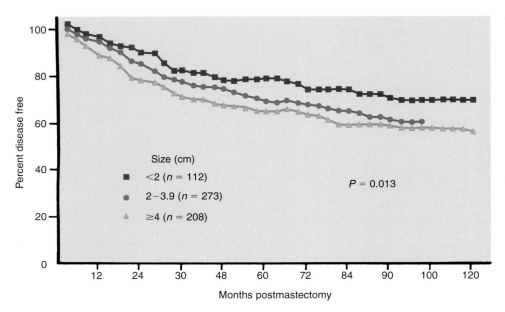

Figure 23-2 Primary tumor size correlates with disease-free survival in patients undergoing curative surgery. (From Fisher ER: Prognostic and therapeutic significance of pathological features of breast cancer. NCI Monogr 1:29, 1986.)

increase risk of developing systemic relapse and 20% to 46% increase risk of breast cancer–related death compared with the lateral location.[10–12] A study from the International Breast Cancer Study Group trials that included more than 8000 patients confirmed these results but also demonstrated that the risk of relapse for patients with medial tumors was largest for the lymph node–negative patients and for patients with tumors larger than 2 cm (Fig. 23-3).[13] Furthermore,

a recent study demonstrated that lower inner quadrant tumors have the highest risk of mortality compared with other locations in women with early lymph node–negative breast cancer.[14] A proposed mechanism for the increased risk of metastases and death from breast cancer from medial tumors is occult involvement of internal mammary nodes (IMNs) that are not systematically treated with either surgery or radiation therapy. In fact, there is growing evidence that the lower inner quadrant drains more often to the IMNs than the other quadrants.[15,16]

Tumor Histology

The great majority of breast carcinomas are adenocarcinomas that derive from the mammary glandular epithelial cells, most commonly cells from terminal ductal lobular units. Approximately two thirds of invasive breast cancers are classified as invasive ductal carcinoma or not otherwise specified (NOS). The other third invasive breast cancers are classified as special types of breast cancer and show distinctive growth patterns, cytologic features, clinical presentation, and behavior.[17] Next to inflammatory carcinoma, which is the most aggressive form of primary breast cancer with a 5-year survival rate of approximately 50%,[18] invasive ductal carcinoma and micropapillary carcinoma carries a poor prognosis. Tubular, cribriform, mucinous, papillary, and adenoid cystic subtypes have a more favorable prognosis than invasive cancers; in contrast, medullary, secretory, metaplastic, and invasive lobular (classic type) have an intermediate prognosis.[17,19–21]

Tumor Grade

Histologic grading is a strong predictor of overall and disease-free survival in patients with invasive breast cancer. Nuclear grading is the cytologic assessment of tumor cells and it is applied to all invasive and in situ carcinoma of the breast. The World Health Organization (WHO) endorses a histologic grading system based on

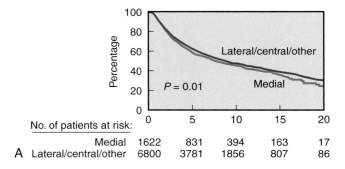

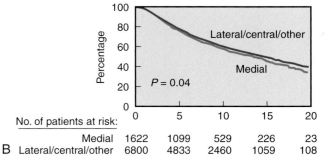

Figure 23-3 **(A)** Disease-free survival and **(B)** overall survival according to predominant site of primary tumor. (From Colleoni M, Zahrieh D, Gelber RD, et al: Site of primary tumor has a prognostic role in operable breast cancer: The international breast cancer study group experience. J Clin Oncol 23:1390, 2005.)

criteria established by Bloom and Richardson and Elston and Ellis.[22,23] This grading system incorporates cytoplasmic and nuclear characteristics such as size, shape, and hyperchromatism along with number of mitotic features and tubules. Other systems of grading based on nuclear characteristics alone have also been developed.[24] Hutter[20] has reviewed this topic and reports that overall survivorship is related to differentiation of tumor cells. Survival at 20 years was estimated to be 41% for grade I (well differentiated), 29% for grade II (moderately differentiated), and 21% for grade III (poorly differentiated). Fisher and colleagues[25] examined histologic grade in relationship to 5-year treatment failures and found that there is a significant correlation between these two factors in patients with absent nodal metastases or with four or more positive lymph nodes. The importance of predictive and prognostic value of poor nuclear grade is also revealed with a significant better outcome for patients treated with L-phenylalanine mustard regimens whose tumors exhibited high or poor histologic grade compared with patients in whom the grade was good.[26] Furthermore, poor nuclear grade is a significant predictor of pathologic complete response (26%) compared with good nuclear grade (14%) in the setting of neoadjuvant chemotherapy.[27,28]

Histopathologic Features of Tumor

Fisher and associates[29] examined the relationship of pathologic and clinical characteristics to 5-year survival in 1000 patients treated with radical mastectomy. Although they found that pathologic nodal status was the most dominant influence on treatment failure rates and corresponding survival, they also identified a number of other important predictors of short-term (<24 months) treatment failure. Characteristics such as noncircumscription, perineural invasion, absence of sinus histiocytosis, presence of glycogen, and skin involvement correlated with poor long-term survival. Tumor necrosis was also associated with a poor clinical outcome. However, independent prognostic significance of this histologic feature is not established in the literature. Furthermore, quantification of necrosis has not been standardized.

Other histologic characteristics have also been found to bear prognostic information. These include blood vessel invasion, lymphatic extension, elastosis, glycogen staining, and the presence or absence of numerous host inflammatory responses. Evaluation of vascular/lymphatic invasion is particularly important in small lesions without nodal involvement because it can identify patients with high risk of recurrence. These and other histologic characteristics often can be identified in many patients. Unfortunately, histologic criteria can rarely be used to modify the management of a patient by stratification into different substages; when these characteristics are present, the prognosis is usually guarded.

Estrogen and Progesterone Receptors

Both estrogen receptors (ERs) and progesterone receptors (PRs) are essential prognostic indicators in patients with breast cancer, and more importantly, they are highly predictive of benefit from endocrine therapy in both the adjuvant and metastatic settings. Knight and colleagues[30] and Osborne and McGuire[31] have shown that ER status affects survival, independent of axillary nodal status. Similarly, another study has demonstrated longer survivorship for PR-positive patients than for PR-negative patients.[32] ER and PR positivity generally correlates with a better prognosis and a better response to chemotherapy, with or without the concomitant use of tamoxifen. Reports of the beneficial use of chemotherapy and/or tamoxifen have suggested that receptor status may be important in patients with known systemic disease, as well as in patients without axillary metastasis. In the neoadjuvant setting, several studies have confirmed that ER-negative tumors are more likely to decrease in size and response to chemotherapy.[28,33,34] However, although ER-negative tumors are more likely to achieve pathologic complete response with neoadjuvant chemotherapy, affected patients have less favorable 5-year overall and progression-free survival rates when compared with those with ER-positive disease. One proposed explanation for this finding was the beneficial impact of postoperative hormonal therapy available to patients with ER-positive tumors, which could supersede the significance of achieving pathologic complete response in this setting.[34]

Tumor Growth Rate and Proliferation

Anatomic methods for staging breast cancer have withstood the test of time and remain the gold standard; however, these methods often provide only a static or instantaneous view of what is actually occurring at the molecular and cellular level. Attempts at measuring dynamic characteristics (clinical and pathologic) have also been predictive of tumor progression. Clinical measurements of flux of tumor volume over time and pathologic determinations of cell kinetics have both been useful. Charlson and Feinstein[35] developed a clinical index of growth rate based on the first clinical manifestation of disease and then on subsequent unfavorable transition events. Their methods were used in conjunction with the anatomic tumor, node, metastasis (TNM) system to better predict which subgroups of patients would have predictably good 10-year survival rates despite poor anatomic status. Conversely, patients with rapidly progressing lesions could be identified despite favorable anatomic staging.

Most of breast cancer prognostic factors are directly or indirectly related to proliferation, and increased proliferation correlates strongly with poor prognosis, irrespective of the methodology used to assess proliferation. Measurements of tumor doubling time, although not clinically practical, have been shown to correlate with prognosis. Multiple studies have demonstrated a wide range of doubling times, not only between patients but also within the same patient over time.[36-38] This heterogeneity is typical of breast cancer. Serial mammography has also been used for this purpose and has shown that shorter doubling times correlate with diminished survival.[39] Recently, evaluation of tumor cell kinetics through growth fraction estimates has been used for the assessment of proliferation rate and its relation to prognosis.[40] The growth fraction can be assessed by immunohistochemistry (IHC) of proliferation-associated antigens, such as Ki-67, cyclin A, cyclin D, cyclin E, p27, p21, thymidine kinase (TK), topoisomerase IIα, proliferating cell nuclear antigen (PCNA), geminin, or minichromosome maintenance (McM) proteins. Of these, Ki-67 has extensively been studied alone or with MIB1, which is an antibody that reacts against Ki-67. There is a good correlation between Ki-67 and MIB1 staining,[41] and a pronounced decrease in the Ki-67/MIB-1 labelling index is associated with a good response to preoperative treatment with chemotherapy or tamoxifen.[42-44]

Flow cytometry has recently been used to estimate cellular kinetics and to detect the presence of aneuploidy. Flow cytometry permits rapid, single-cell analysis of DNA content per cell, enabling the determination of the fraction of cells within the S phase and the ploidy levels within a tumor cell proliferation. However, despite extensive literature on flow cytometry, the results obtained by this method are still not widely used in everyday practice, because there is high intratumor heterogeneity of the S-phase fraction and multiple methodologies to determine S-phase fraction by flow cytometry.[45,46] In general, a high S-phase fraction is associated with a higher risk of metastatic recurrence in lymph node–negative patients. Furthermore, it has been suggested that flow cytometry also influences the response to chemotherapy in neoadjuvant, adjuvant, and metastatic settings.[47-56]

Other methods used to assess the growth fraction are the incorporation techniques with tritium-labeled thymidine (3H-TdR) and bromodeoxyuridine (BrdU), which theoretically provide the gold standard of cellular proliferation.[57,58] These methods are more sensitive than standard histologic tests that enumerate the relative number of mitoses and have demonstrated some promise in their ability to identify aggressive, rapidly growing tumors. With tritiated thymidine, tumor cells are sampled from the specimen and then incubated with 3H-TdR, which is taken up by cells in the DNA synthetic or S phase. Measuring 3H-TdR uptake then permits the estimation of the percentage of cells in the S phase (thymidine labeling index). Many studies have shown that a high thymidine labeling index is associated with poor prognosis in lymph node–positive and –negative patients with breast cancer,[59-61] and patients with a high index benefit from adjuvant chemotherapy.[62] However, incorporation techniques can be tedious and time consuming, and they are impractical for routine use; this hampers their worldwide application, despite the very good prognostic value of the thymidine labeling index. This index does, however, correlate with histologic characteristics such as tumor grade and may be important in the staging of lymph node–negative patients.[63]

One the most powerful, practical, and well-reproduced indicators of proliferation and prognosis is the mitotic activity index (MAI).[64-66] As mentioned previously, MAI is part of the histologic grade system and represents by far the most important contributor to the prognostic value of histologic grade. The proliferation factor MAI is one of the strongest prognostic factors in patients younger than 71 years of age with lymph node–negative invasive

breast cancer, without adjuvant systemic treatment and with long-term follow-up.[67] Moreover, patients with rapidly proliferating tumors significantly benefit from adjuvant systemic therapy, in contrast to those with low proliferation.[68] Recently, Baak and colleagues[67] demonstrated that among women with small, low-grade, lymph node–negative invasive breast cancer who usually do not receive systemic therapy, MAI ($\geq 10/1.6$ mm^2) was able to identify accurately those patients at high risk of distant metastatic disease or death. The 10-year overall survival rates for MAI less than 10 versus 10 or higher in women with tumor diameter less than 1 cm were 94% and 67%, respectively (Fig. 23-4). The authors concluded that these high-risk patients identified by MAI should be considered for adjuvant systemic therapy.

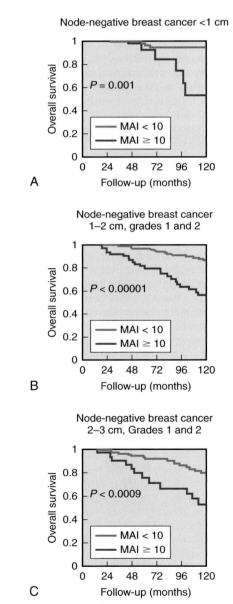

Figure 23-4 Overall survival associated with mitotic activity index (MAI) in patients with tumors less than 1 cm diameter (all grades) **(A)**, 1 to 2 cm (grades 1+2) **(B)**, and 2 to 3 cm (grades 1+2) **(C)**. (From Baak JP, van Diest PJ, Janssen EA, et al: Proliferation accurately identifies the high-risk patients among small, low-grade, lymph node-negative invasive breast cancers. Ann Oncol 19:649–654, 2008.)

BIOLOGIC MARKERS

With the development of monoclonal antibody technology, antibodies specific for breast cancer have been developed. These antibodies can be used to detect microscopic disease not easily seen on routine histopathology by using immunoperoxidase technology and radioimmunoassay. They may be useful in accurately staging the anatomic extent of axillary disease and distant disease such as tumor infiltration of bone marrow.[69] The presence of isolated tumor cells in the bone marrow of women with early-stage breast cancer may be an independent marker of disease recurrence and shortened survival.[70] However, controversy exists regarding the independent influence of occult metastatic cells on prognosis. Recently, Braun and colleagues[71] performed a pooled analysis involving more than 4700 patients from several prospective studies and revealed that bone marrow micrometastases did predict an independent poor outcome (Fig. 23-5). The presence of bone marrow micrometastases was found in 30% of patients with stage I, II, or III disease. Compared with women without bone marrow micrometastases, patients with bone marrow micrometastases had larger tumors, tumor with a higher histologic grade, more frequent lymph node metastases, and more hormone receptor–negative tumors. Furthermore, in a subgroup analysis of low-risk patients with tumors less than 2 cm and without lymph node metastases who did not receive chemotherapy, the difference in distant disease-free survival between those patients who had micrometastases versus those who did not was very small (Fig. 23-6). These data suggest that the presence of bone marrow micrometastases may often reflect other prognostic factors already discerned from the primary tumor characteristics and lymph node status. Finally, bone marrow micrometastases add little prognostic information in low-risk patients; therefore, routine assay of bone marrow for disseminated tumor cells should not be widely adopted as a routine staging procedure.[46] The American College of Surgeons Oncology Group (ACOSOG) Z10 study should help answer some questions regarding the significance of bone marrow micrometastases.

Other novel methods that measure circulating tumor cells (CTCs) in the peripheral blood have been

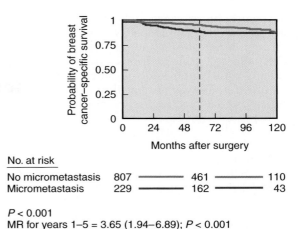

No. at risk

No micrometastasis	807	461	110
Micrometastasis	229	162	43

$P < 0.001$
MR for years 1–5 = 3.65 (1.94–6.89); $P < 0.001$
MR for years 6–10 = 0.42 (0.12–1.48); $P = 0.16$

Figure 23-6 Breast cancer–specific survival in low-risk patients with no adjuvant systemic therapy, according to the presence or absence of bone marrow micrometastasis. (From Braun S, Vogl FD, Naume B, et al: A pooled analysis of bone marrow micrometastasis in breast cancer. N Engl J Med 353:793, 2005. Copyright © 2005 Massachusetts Medical Society. All rights reserved.)

developed.[72–74] In particular, the CellSearch assay (Veridex, Warren, New Jersey) is based on the enumeration of epithelial cells, which are separated from the blood by antibody-coated magnetic beds and identified with the use of fluorescently labeled antibodies against cytokeratin and with fluorescent nuclear stain and fluorescent cytokeratin antibodies. Several studies have confirmed that the presence of CTCs is associated with a poor outcome in patients with metastatic disease.[75–77] Cristofanilli and associates[78] measured CTCs prior to systemic treatment in patients with metastatic disease and found that levels of CTCs equal to or higher than 5 per mL of whole blood were the most significant predictors of progression-free and overall survival. Furthermore, these CTCs levels after the first course of hormone therapy or chemotherapy predicted no treatment response.

Tumor markers, such as CA 15–3, CA27–29, and carcinoembryonic antigen (CEA), are not very sensitive and specific for breast cancer and are not recommended for screening, diagnosis, and staging.[46] Cathepsin D, a lysosomal proteolytic enzyme with a critical role in protein catabolism and tissue remodeling,[79] has been used as a marker of invasion and poor prognosis in breast cancer.[80,81] However, the magnitude in predicting outcome is relatively small and routine clinical use of this marker is also not recommended.[46] Other novel biologic markers recently found to be associated with prognosis are the urokinase plasminogen activator (uPA) and the plasminogen activator inhibitor (PAI-1), which are part of the plasminogen activating system. This system has been shown experimentally to be associated with invasion, angiogenesis, and metastasis.[82] Several studies have suggested that overexpression of uPA and/or PAI-1 are strongly associated with poor prognosis in lymph node–negative cancer, and when these two factors are combined they are associated with twofold to eightfold higher risk of recurrence and death.[83,84] Currently, uPA and/or PAI-1 measured by enzyme-linked immunosorbent assay (ELISA) has been recommended for the determination of prognosis in patients with newly diagnosed, lymph

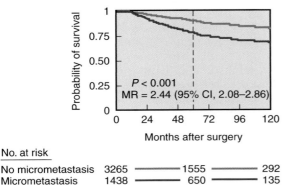

No. at risk

No micrometastasis	3265	1555	292
Micrometastasis	1438	650	135

Figure 23-5 Breast cancer–specific survival according to the presence or absence of bone marrow micrometastasis. (From Braun S, Vogl FD, Naume B, et al: A pooled analysis of bone marrow micrometastasis in breast cancer. N Engl J Med 353:793, 2005. Copyright © 2005 Massachusetts Medical Society. All rights reserved.)

node–negative breast cancer.[46] Furthermore, Janicke and coworkers[85] found in a prospective randomized trial that low or high levels of uPA and/or PAI-1 can help stratify patients who will benefit from adjuvant chemotherapy in patients with lymph node–negative breast cancer. In their study, for all women treated without systemic chemotherapy, the 3-year recurrence rate was significantly lower for those with low expression of uPA and PAI-1 (6.7% vs. 14.7%). Patients whose tumors showed elevated uPA and/or PAI-1 levels were randomly assigned to adjuvant chemotherapy. The hazard rate for recurrence in the group for patients treated with adjuvant chemotherapy was 0.56 of that for patients who were not treated. The independent prognostic value of high levels of uPA and/or PAI-1 was confirmed in a pooled analysis involving 8377 breast cancer patients by the European Organization of Research and Treatment of Cancer-Receptor and Biomarker Group (EORT-RBG).[86] In both lymph node–positive and lymph node–negative patients, higher levels of uPA and/or PAI-1 were independently associated with poor relapse-free and overall survival (Fig. 23-7).

Oncogenes may be related to the complex phenomenon of human breast cancer initiation and progression through the process of gene amplification, mutation, chromosomal breakage, or insertion of retroviral promoters near oncogenes.[87] With current technology, both their number and their expressed gene products may be measured. Amplification or overexpression of HER2/neu has recently been found to portend a poor prognosis, correlating with other factors associated with poor prognosis such as tumor grade, size, nodal status, and hormone receptor status.[88] This oncogene, however, has independent prognostic significance only in patients with lymph node–positive breast cancer.[89-91] The prognostic value of HER2/neu in lymph node–negative patients is more controversial. It has been suggested that HER2/neu may be useful for identifying subsets of lymph node–negative patients within otherwise low-risk groups who might have a poorer prognosis.[92] Other oncogenes or tumor suppressor genes, such as myc[93] and p53,[94,95] are also under current study and have been associated with poor prognosis. In particular, a meta-analysis that looked to the association of p53 mutations and clinical outcomes showed that p53 conferred an independent relative risk of 1.7 (95% confidence interval 1.2–2.3) for both disease-free and overall survival in node-negative patients.[96] However, in contrast to HER2/neu, there is no consensus that p53 testing should be performed routinely in clinical practice.[46]

Although studies of individual oncogenes and tumor suppressor genes may prove fruitful in identifying poor patient prognosis, simultaneous analysis of expression of multiple genes in individual tumors is a new approach to breast cancer classification and has shown promise in providing greater accuracy in predicting outcomes and in aiding selection of therapies for individual patients. Using RNA expression array technology, initially four and then after further refinement, five breast cancer molecular subtypes were identified and validated in both clinically and ethnically diverse patient populations.[97-100] These five subtypes include basal-like, HER2/neu-overexpressing, luminal A, luminal B, and

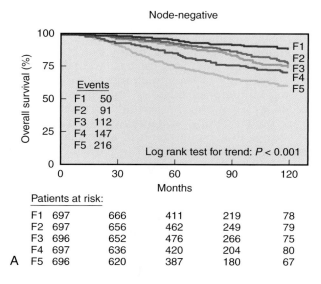

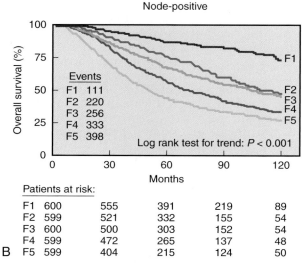

Figure 23-7 Overall survival as a function of categorized prognostic scores of urokinase-type plasminogen activator (uPA) and its inhibitor (PAI-1) in lymph node-negative **(A)** and lymph node-positive **(B)** breast cancer patients. Prognostic scores were divided in five groups (F1 to F5) with the use of their 20th, 40th, 60th, and 80th percentiles. (From Look MP, van Putten WL, Duffy MJ, et al: Pooled analysis of prognostic impact of urokinase-type plasminogen activator and its inhibitor PAI-1 in 8377 breast cancer patients. J Natl Cancer Inst 94:116, 2002.)

normal breastlike (Fig. 23-8). These subtypes have been compared to clinical outcomes; luminal-type cancers tend to have the most favorable long-term survival, whereas the basal-like and HER2/neu-overexpressing are most sensitive to chemotherapy but have the worst prognosis overall (Fig. 23-9).[98,101,102]

The true prognostic or predictive value of the molecular classes is unknown because there is a strong correlation between molecular class and conventional histopathologic prognostic factors. For example, Pusztai and colleagues[103] found that all luminal-type cancers were ER-positive and 63% of these were also low or intermediate histologic grade. This contrasted with their finding that 95% of basal-like cancers were ER-negative and 91% were high histologic grade. Furthermore, the

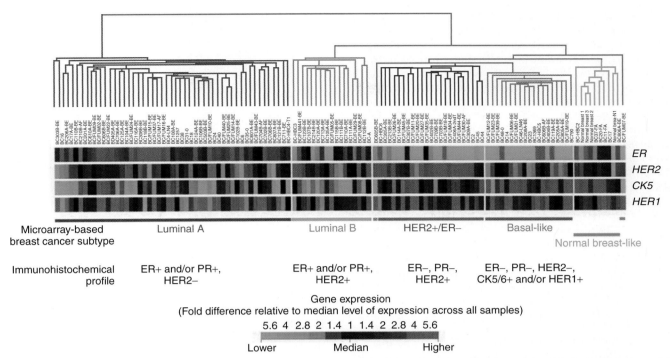

Figure 23-8 Microarray-based breast cancer subtypes and their immunohistochemical profile. (From Carey LA, Perou CM, Livasy CA, et al: Race, breast cancer subtypes, and survival in the Carolina Breast Cancer Study. JAMA 295:2492, 2006.)

majority of basal-like cancers are characterized by the absence of ER receptor, PR receptor, and *HER2/neu* expression, and they are also associated with *p53* gene mutations and a high proliferation rate.[104] Because of these characteristics, basal-like cancer is usually referred to as "triple-negative" breast cancer in daily practice.

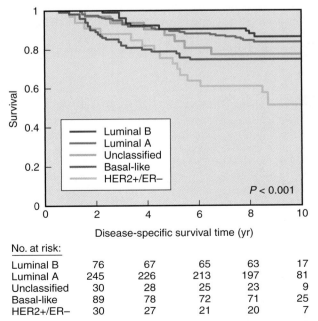

Figure 23-9 Survival of patients with breast cancer according to molecular subtype. (From Carey LA, Perou CM, Livasy CA, et al: Race, breast cancer subtypes, and survival in the Carolina Breast Cancer Study. JAMA 295:2492, 2006.)

However, although the terms tend to be used interchangeably, they are not completely synonymous, because a small proportion of basal-like cancers do express hormone receptors or *HER2/neu*. Several studies have confirmed that triple-negative breast cancers are characterized by an aggressive clinical history, an earlier age of onset, and *BRCA1*-related breast cancer.[105,106] Recently, Bauer and colleagues[106] found that the relative survival for women with triple-negative breast cancer was poorer than for women with other types of breast cancer, with 77% of women surviving 5 years after diagnosis, compared with 93%. Finally, several studies have confirmed that African-American women and Hispanic women were found to have a higher incidence of triple-negative phenotype.[101,106] These recent results may explain biologic disparities in long-term survival of breast cancer associated with race.

Molecular profiling has also been used to stratify patients with early breast cancer into prognostic groups, and information gained by these methods may outperform standard clinical and pathologic prognostic features. Several multiparameter assays that do not overlap have been developed and include the Rotterdam signature,[107] the Breast Cancer Gene Expression Ratio,[108] MammaPrint,[109] and Oncotype DX,[110] but only the last two are currently commercially available. For instance, MammaPrint (Agendia BV, Amsterdam, the Netherlands), is a 70-gene signature (largely consisting of genes regulating proliferation, invasion, metastasis, stromal integrity, and angiogenesis) used to stratify patients into a prognostic group using DNA microarrays in fresh frozen tissue.[109] This was designed by comparing gene expression in lymph node–negative patients, younger than 53 years of age with T₁ or

T_2 breast cancers who developed metastases within 5 years of diagnosis, compared with a matched group that did not develop metastasis. At 10 years, van de Vijver and colleagues[111] demonstrated that both overall survival (95% vs. 55%), and distant metastasis-free survival (85% vs. 51%) were significantly greater in those classified as having a good prognosis according to their gene expression profile alone (Table 23-3). The estimated hazard ratio for distant metastases by signature was 5.1 ($P < 0.001$) and remained significant when adjusted for lymph node status. This signature has since been validated with an independent data set and is currently being utilized in the Microarray In Node Negative Disease May Avoid Chemotherapy (MINDACT) trial, which is accruing patients.[112,113]

On the other hand, Oncotype DX (Genomic Health Inc, Redwood City, California) is a 21-gene real-time RT-PCR assay on formalin-fixed, paraffin-embedded tissue—with 15 cancer-related genes and six reference genes—that is currently being studied to help predict the chance of recurrence in patients with lymph node–negative, ER-positive breast cancer. The assay calculates a recurrence score, which stratifies patients into low, intermediate, and high risk of recurrence.[114,115] Paik and colleagues evaluated this assay among women treated with tamoxifen in the National Surgical Adjuvant Breast and Bowel Project (NSABP) B-14 trial. Kaplan-Meir estimates of 10-year disease recurrence rate in the three groups were 6.8%, 14.3%, and 30.5% (Fig. 23-10), respectively, and there was also a significant relationship between recurrence score and overall survival.[115] Currently this assay is being studied in a clinical trial (Trial Assigning IndividuaLized Options for Treatment [TAILORx]), evaluating the role of chemotherapy in lymph node–negative patients. Patients deemed to be high risk are given chemotherapy and hormone therapy, patients in the intermediate group are randomized to hormonal therapy alone or combination chemotherapy plus hormonal therapy, and patients in the low-risk group are treated with hormone therapy alone.[113]

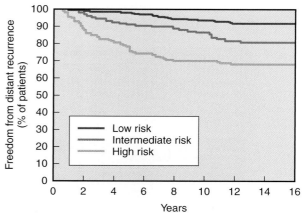

No. at risk:								
Low risk	338	328	313	298	276	258	231	170	38
Intermediate risk	149	139	128	116	104	96	80	66	16
High risk	181	154	137	119	105	91	83	63	13

Figure 23-10 Likelihood of distant recurrence according to recurrence score categories of a 21-gene prognostic signature (Oncotype DX). (From Paik S, Shak S, Tang G, et al: A multigene assay to predict recurrence of tamoxifen-treated, node-negative breast cancer. N Engl J Med 351;2817, 2004. Copyright © 2004 Massachusetts Medical Society. All rights reserved.)

In addition to gene expression–based molecular profiling, other technologies are emerging that may ultimately assist in creating prognostic signatures in breast cancer. These include comparative genomic hybridization, CpG island profiling for patterns of DNA promoter methylation silencing, single-cell whole genome sequencing for mutation detection, and phosphoprotein analysis via mass spectrometry to profile the entire phosphotyrosine proteome (proteomics). For instance, Jacquemier and associates[116] used IHC on tissue microarrays to profile the expression of 26 selected proteins from 552 patients with early breast cancer. Supervised cluster analysis identified a set of 21 proteins whose combined expression significantly correlated with metastasis-free

TABLE 23-3

Survival and Probability That Patients Would Remain Free of Distant Metastasis According to a 70-Gene Prognostic Signature (MammaPrint)

Group	No. of Patients	Free of Distant Metastases (%)		Overall Survival (%)	
		5 Years	10 Years	5 Years	10 Years
All patients					
Good prognosis signature	115	95	85	97	95
Poor prognosis signature	180	61	51	74	55
Lymph node–negative disease					
Good prognosis signature	60	93	87	97	97
Poor prognosis signature	91	56	44	72	50
Lymph node–positive disease					
Good prognosis signature	55	95	83	98	92
Poor prognosis signature	89	66	57	77	60

Modified from van de Vijver MJ, He YD, van't Veer LJ, et al.[111] Copyright © 2002 Massachusetts Medical Society. All rights reserved.

survival. Among the 552 patients, the 5-year metastasis-free survival was 90% for patients classified in the "good prognosis class" and 61% for those classified in the "poor prognosis class." In multivariate analysis, the 21-protein set was the strongest independent predictor of clinical outcome. Despite these results, the emerging field of proteomics is complex and none of the proteomic profiling techniques has been validated sufficiently to be used for patient care.

LYMPH NODE STATUS

In the late nineteenth century, Halsted[117] described how breast cancer spreads systematically from the primary breast tissue to the ipsilateral axilla and is finally disseminated into the systemic circulation. The presence of axillary nodal metastasis was considered a poorer prognostic factor compared with improvement in survival with a more radical operation. However, this theory has been challenged over the years when it became evident that more extensive mastectomies proved to have survival benefit equal to that of less extensive, breast-conserving operations.[118,119] Furthermore, up to 30% of patients with lymph node–negative disease eventually develop recurrent metastatic disease.[120] However, once the diagnosis of breast cancer has been established, the lymph node status remains the most powerful predictor for long-term survival.[121] Over the years, lymph node staging has been refined to include the number of lymph nodes, and more recently, the amount of tumor burden within these nodes. Not only does the lymph node status give prognostic information, it is important in making therapeutic decisions.

The clinical assessment of regional lymph nodes must include ipsilateral axillary nodes and interpectoral (Rotter's) nodes. Other regional nodes include the internal mammary nodes in the intercostal spaces along the sternum and supraclavicular nodes. For a lymph node to be considered supraclavicular, it must be located in a triangle bound by the clavicle at the base, the internal jugular vein medially, and omohyoid muscle and tendon laterally and superiorly. Physical examination, however, is notoriously inaccurate in preoperative assessment of the presence of lymph node metastasis. In fact, microscopic evidence of tumor can be demonstrated in one third of patients in the absence of palpable axillary lymph nodes. Clinical examination has a false-positive rate for detection of axillary metastases ranging from 25% to 31%. False-negative rates range from 27% to 33%.[122,123]

Axillary Nodal Disease

Results of a national survey by the American College of Surgeons (ACS) involving 20,547 women with breast cancer clearly demonstrated a strong linear association between the number of histologically involved axillary nodes and 5-year survival (Fig. 23-11).[4] Furthermore, in a 10-year clinical trial, Fisher, Fisher, and Redmond,[124] reporting for the NSABP, found that patients with negative axillary lymph nodes had 5- and 10-year survival rates

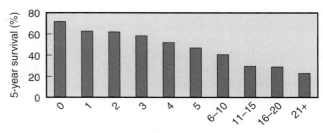

Figure 23-11 Survival of breast cancer according to number of histologically involved axillary lymph nodes. (From Nemoto T, Vana J, Bedwani RN, et al: Management and survival of female breast cancer: Results of a national survey by the American College of Surgeons. Cancer 45:2917, 1980.)

of 78% and 65%, respectively. Similarly, the number of positive nodes correlated with the 5- and 10-year treatment failures. No positive nodes was associated with a 20% treatment failure rate at 10 years, whereas more than four positive nodes was associated with a 71% treatment failure rate. Diab and associates[125] have shown that the presence of more than 10 positive lymph nodes is associated with an increased risk in locoregional and distant failure rates. Not only is axillary lymph node metastasis a time-dependent variable, but it also seems to be a marker for a more aggressive tumor phenotype. Jatoi and associates[126] have shown that patients with four or more involved lymph nodes at the time of initial diagnosis have a significantly worse outcome after their first recurrence (Fig. 23-12).

The location of the positive axillary lymph nodes is important. Involvement of apical axillary (level 3) or infraclavicular lymph nodes carries a grim prognosis.[127] Another issue is the level of axillary lymph nodes that must be removed to obtain accurate prognostic information. Certainly, complete dissection of all three levels of

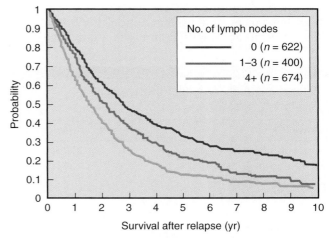

Figure 23-12 Survival after first relapse by number of positive axillary lymph nodes. (From Jatoi I, Hilsenbeck SG, Clark GM, Osborne CK: Significance of axillary lymph node metastasis in primary breast cancer. J Clin Oncol 17:2334, 1999.)

lymph nodes (Patey dissection) not only provides the maximum amount of prognostic information but also clears the axilla of gross disease and obviates the need for axillary irradiation. In fact, total axillary clearance has been supported by some authors as the only acceptable method of assessing axillary nodal status.[128] Several studies, however, have addressed this topic and have concluded that, in certain cases, a level 1 dissection can be predictive of the actual involvement of the remaining nodal basin. Boova and colleagues[129] examined the contents of 200 consecutive mastectomy and total axillary dissection specimens. The average number of lymph nodes recovered from each level was 14 at level 1, 11 at level 2, and 8 at level 3. Of the patients, 40% had axillary metastases, with half of these involving only level 1 (Table 23-4). Interestingly, seven patients (3.5% of all patients and 8.7% of those with lymph node metastases) had positive nodes at level 2 and/or 3 without positive nodes at level 1 (skip metastasis). These authors concluded that level 1 dissections can be accurate predictors of the status of the entire axillary lymph node basin, assuming that an adequate number of lymph nodes has been sampled. Fisher and coworkers[123] have also suggested that dissection of level 1 and 2 is more than adequate in most cases to accurately predict prognosis. Their report found that qualitative disease (positive vs. negative) in the axilla could be determined equally well by studying 3 to 5 or 27 or more lymph nodes; however, to quantitatively determine the true axillary involvement, sampling of more than 10 lymph nodes is required. The current standard of care for a complete axillary lymph node dissection includes both level 1 and level 2 lymph nodes with procurement of at least 10 lymph nodes. Sentinel lymph node (SLN) technique is also changing the current standard of nodal staging in breast cancer patients.

Sentinel Lymph Node Mapping

The recent introduction of SLN mapping technology has challenged the classic approach to breast cancer staging that involves routine axillary lymph node dissection. The SLN concept supports the notion that breast cancer cells spread in an orderly fashion via a direct lymphatic communication from the primary tumor to the SLN. Therefore, the SLN is the most likely to be the first site of metastasis within the lymph node basin. Currently, SLN mapping for breast cancer has become the primary means for accurately assessing nodal metastasis. On average, one to three SLNs may be found within an axillary basin. A number of large, single, and multi-institutional trials have now demonstrated the accurate predictability of the SLN technique in staging the axilla in breast cancer patients by using various injection techniques with technetium sulfur colloid, isosulfan blue, or a combination of both agents.[130-133] The optimal technique for most is a combination of blue dye and technetium sulfur colloid. A SLN identification rate of more than 95% is the rule, with accuracy rates exceeding 95% and a false-negative rate of approximately 2%. A well-trained multidisciplinary team must be systematically assembled to ensure the success of the procedure. Long-term follow-up is needed to define the true false-negative rate—that is, to identify axillary recurrences in patients with breast cancer with negative SLNs and no complete axillary dissections. Initial studies suggest that this risk is less than 1% (0.2%–0.3%).[134,135]

In addition, the accuracy of the SLN mapping technique is enhanced by the ability to improve on the histologic examination of the lymph node when 1 to 3 lymph nodes, as opposed to 15 to 20 lymph nodes in a complete node dissection are submitted for a more detailed examination. Routine histologic examination with serial step sectioning and hematoxylin and eosin (H&E) staining is performed to identify tumor deposits within the lymph node. Furthermore, IHC, with cytokeratin assays, shows an increased rate of detection of occult micrometastatic disease, further improving the accuracy of the technique.[136] Cote and colleagues[137] have shown the importance of IHC and serial sectioning for accurate evaluation of sentinel lymph nodes. Occult nodal metastases were detected in 7% of patients with H&E sections and in 20% with IHC. Other investigators have also shown the increase in detection of rate of occult micrometastatic disease in patients who were determined to be lymph node–negative based on routine histologic methods.[138,139] In a study by Schreiber and associates,[140] up to 9.4% of the patients were upstaged with the addition of IHC and serial sectioning. However, to date, the clinical significance of identifying micrometastatic and submicrometastatic disease as a prognostic variable is controversial. A recent population-based analysis by Chen and coworkers[141] evaluated a total of 209,720 patients with invasive breast cancer without distant metastases and no more than three axillary nodes using the SEER registries. Overall, patients with micrometastases no larger than 2 mm had a significant worse 5-year survival (86%) than patients without nodal metastases (90%) and better than patients with macrometastases in no more than three nodes (82%; Fig. 23-13). Our institution has noted that 16% of patients with micrometastasis (>0.2 mm and <2 mm) and 9% of patients with isolated tumor cells or small-cell clusters not greater than 0.2 mm by IHC on SLN biopsy will have additional positive nonsentinel lymph nodes if an axillary lymph node dissection is performed.[142] Prospective trials are

TABLE 23-4

Patterns of Axillary Nodal Involvement: Levels 1, 2, and 3

Nodal Status	No. of Patients (%)
All levels negative	120 (60)
Level 1 positive	39 (19.5)
Levels 1 and 2 positive	19 (9.5)
Levels 1, 2, and 3 positive	11 (5.5)
Levels 1 and 3 positive	4 (2)
Level 2 positive*	5 (2.5)
Level 3 positive*	1 (0.5)
Levels 2 and 3 positive*	1 (0.5)

*Skip metastasis group.
Modified from Boova RS, Roseann B, Rosato F.[129]

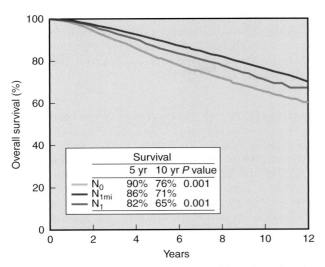

Figure 23-13 Prognostic significance of lymph node micrometastases in breast cancer. (From Chen SL, Hoehne FM, Giuliano AE: The prognostic significance of micrometastases in breast cancer: A SEER population-based analysis. Ann Surg Oncol 14;3378, 2007.)

currently underway to define the clinical significance of micrometastatic disease within SLN. In the meantime, it is apparent that the diagnosis of micrometastasis may provide additional prognostic information.

Internal Mammary Nodal Disease

The status of the IMNs has been a point of controversy since the time of Halsted in the 1890s. Prospective randomized trials have failed to demonstrate a benefit in survival for women who had complete IMN dissections (extended radical mastectomy) while incurring significant operative morbidity. However, other studies have shown a prognostic significance of metastasis to the IMNs.[143–146] Veronesi and associates[147] reported 10-year overall survival rates according to IMN disease and/or axillary lymph node disease among patients who had extended radical mastectomy (Fig. 23-14). The study clearly demonstrated a marked difference in overall survival between patients without any nodal disease (80%) and patients with only IMN disease and only

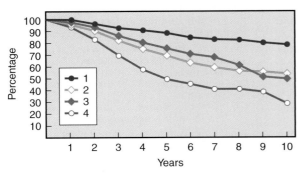

Figure 23-14 Ten-year overall survival in patients without lymph node metastases (1), with axillary lymph node metastases only (2), with internal mammary node metastases (3), and with both groups involved (4). (From Veronesi U, Cascinelli N, Greco M, et al: Prognosis of breast cancer patients after mastectomy and dissection of internal mammary nodes. Ann Surg 202:702, 1985.)

axillary lymph node disease, with an overall survival of 53% and 55%, respectively. Furthermore, the presence of both IMN disease and axillary lymph node disease was associated with the worst outcome with an overall survival of 30%. Positive IMNs can be found in up to 10% of cases when axillary nodes are negative and in as many as 26% of cases when the primary tumor location is medial.[148] The emergence of the lymphatic mapping technique may lead to the ability to sample IMNs with improved morbidity to provide additional staging information that may have an impact on radiation planning.

Supraclavicular Nodal Disease

Historically, supraclavicular lymph nodes involved with tumor indicated advanced disease and were associated with a poor prognosis. Positive supraclavicular lymph nodes were considered to have survival rates similar to those with distant spread rather than of regional nodal disease.[149,150] More recent studies suggest that the outcomes of patients with these tumors are comparable to the outcomes of those with locally advanced disease rather than those with distant metastatic disease.[151]

Currently, routine scalene lymph node biopsies are not indicated. In the prechemotherapy era, scalene lymph node biopsy was performed to determine operability of breast cancer patients with advanced local disease but without evidence of distant metastases. It was noted by Papaioannou and Urban,[152] however, that when scalene lymph nodes were pathologically positive, despite the use of radical mastectomy with adjuvant radiotherapy, no patients were disease free after 1 year, and more than 50% were dead within 3 years. These data once again suggested that metastases to lymph node beds other than regional (axillary, clavicular, and internal mammary) suggest the presence of distant systemic disease.

Intramammary Nodal Disease

Intramammary lymph nodes (intraMLNs) have received little attention as potential prognostic indicators for patients with breast carcinoma and are largely overlooked by radiologists, pathologists, and surgeons. Recently, interest for intraMLNs as a marker of disease severity has increased with the introduction of SLN biopsy and lymphatic mapping, because detection of intraMLNs is likely to occur more frequently by preoperative lymphoscintigraphy and intraoperative gamma probe scanning of the breast. By definition, intraMLNs are surrounded by breast parenchyma, a feature that distinguishes them from low axillary lymph nodes. Histopathologic studies of breast specimens containing intraMLNs have revealed that these lymph nodes may be present in any quadrant of the breast and can yield a variety of pathologic findings, including metastatic carcinoma in the ipsilateral breast.

The prevalence of intraMLNs has been reported to range between 1% and 28%.[153,154] Egan and McSweeney[153] were the first to address the prognostic significance of intraMLN in breast cancer. They found that in stage I disease, positive intraMLNs were associated with a poor prognosis (10-year survival rate, 79%); however, intraMLNs were not found to be associated with poorer prognosis in stage II disease. Because of this, patients with breast carcinoma accompanied by intraMLN metastases are traditionally considered to have stage II disease, even in the absence of axillary lymph node involvement. Recently, Shen and colleagues[155] evaluated 130 patients with intraMLNs. IntraMLN metastases were found in 28% of all cases, and isolated intraMLN metastases were documented in 5% of all cases. The presence of intraMLN metastases was associated with poorer 5-year overall survival compared with non-intraMLN involvement (64% vs. 88%). Furthermore, intraMLN was found to be a significant independent predictor of survival in patients with axillary lymph node involvement as well as among those without axillary involvement. Similar results have reported that intraMLN metastases is a marker of disease severity and that the presence of metastatic disease in an intraMLN is associated with a high rate of axillary nodal involvement.[156]

Pathologic Assessment of Lymph Nodes

Molecular staging using techniques such as RT-PCR is allowing the detection of one tumor cell in the background of a million. Adoption of these technologies has raised the likelihood of finding micrometastases. Furthermore, accurate molecular analysis of all or part of the SLN offers the potential to reduce false-negative findings significantly and overcome limitations that occur with standard methods of intraoperative SLN analysis. Currently, intraoperative SLN analysis methods such as imprint cytology (touch preparation) and frozen section suffer from poor and variable sensitivity and a lack of standardization.[157,158] When compared with final pathology results, the reported sensitivity of frozen section SLN analysis varies from 58% to 87%.[159] Imprint cytology has similar limitations in sensitivity.[160] Recently, Backus and colleagues[161] were able to identify an optimal two-gene expression marker set (mammaglobin, cytokeratin 19) for detection of clinically actionable metastasis in breast SLNs using microarray methods. Furthermore, they developed a rapid RT-PCR assay (GeneSearch Breast Lymph Node [BLN] Assay; Veridex, Warren, New Jersey) using these two markers; it generates a result in less than 30 minutes. The authors assessed the utility of RT-PCR assay in SLNs of 254 breast cancer patients, reporting a sensitivity of 90% and specificity of 94%. Blumencranz and associates[162] recently validated this RT-PCR assay in a prospective study at 11 clinical sites. The assay detected 98% of metastases larger than 2 mm and 88% of metastases larger than 0.2 mm. Micrometastases were less frequently detected (57%), and assay positive results in nodes found to be negative by histology were rare (4%). The authors concluded that the use of the BLN assay overcomes conventional histologic sampling errors, and can reduce the need for second surgeries to complete the axillary dissection on SLN-positive patients. Similar results have been reported by other authors who used this commercially available assay, and prospective trials are underway to further

characterize its utility in daily practice.[163] Other indices that portend an unfavorable prognosis for breast cancer relate to the presence of gross rather than microscopic disease in the lymph nodes and/or the presence of extranodal disease.[164,165]

Evolution of Staging Systems

Early staging systems for breast cancer were based on the feasibility of operative intervention. Most tumors were classified as either operable or inoperable; however, this grouping did not offer any significant prognostic information. In 1905, the German physician Steinthal[166] recommended three different classifications for patients with breast cancer: (1) tumors not larger than "a plum" and clinically not associated with skin or axillary lymph node involvement; (2) large tumors adherent to the skin with palpable enlarged axillary lymph nodes; and (3) large tumors diffusely involving the breast with skin, deep muscle, and supraclavicular lymph node involvement. This classification was based on clinical factors that were perceived as important in predicting prognosis. Early on, it was clear that surgeons had identified some of the most ominous prognostic indicators for breast cancer. It is also interesting to note the inclusion of primary tumor size in this primitive staging scheme. An unpopular but insightful system was proposed by Lee and Stubenbord[167] in 1928. Their system included an index of the rate of tumor growth. This method was the first to attempt assessment of the biology of individual tumors and their potential for progression.

In 1940, the four-stage Manchester classification was introduced (Table 23-5).[168] It permitted staging based solely on clinical criteria, including the extent of local involvement by the primary tumor, the presence and

TABLE 23-5

Manchester System

Stage I	The tumor is confined to the breast. Involvement of the skin may be present, provided the area is small in relation to the size of the breast
Stage II	The tumor is confined to the breast and associated lymph nodes are present in the axilla
Stage III	The tumor extends beyond the breast as demonstrated by the following: a. Skin invasion or fixation of a large area in relation to the size of the breast or skin ulceration b. Tumor fixation to the underlying muscle or fascia; mobile axillary nodes
Stage IV	The tumor extends beyond the breast as shown by the following: a. Fixation or matting of the axillary nodes b. Fixation of tumor to chest wall c. Deposits in supraclavicular nodes or in the opposite breast d. Satellite nodules or distant metastases

Modified from Patterson R: The treatment of malignant disease by radium and x-rays. London, Edward Arnold, 1948.

TABLE 23-6

Portmann Classification

Stage I

–	Skin–not involved
+	Tumor–localized to breast, mobile
–	Metastases–none

Stage II

–	Skin–not involved
+	Tumor–localized to breast, mobile
+	Metastases–few axillary lymph nodes involved in microscopic evaluation; no other metastases

Stage III

–	Skin–edematous; brawny red induration and inflammation not obviously caused by infection; extensive ulceration; multiple secondary nodules
++	Tumor–diffusely infiltrating breast; fixation of tumor or breast to chest wall; edema of breast; secondary tumors
++	Metastases–many axillary lymph nodes involved or fixed; no clinical or roentgenologic evidence of distant metastases

Stage IV

+/–	Skin–involved or not involved
+/++	Tumor–localized or diffuse
+++	Metastases–axillary and supraclavicular lymph nodes extensively involved; clinical or roentgenologic evidence of more distant metastases

Modified from Portmann, UV: Clinical and pathological criteria as a basis for classifying cases of primary breast cancer. Cleve Clin Q 10:41–47, 1943.

mobility of palpable enlarged axillary lymph nodes, and the presence of distant metastases. Neither pathologic information nor tumor size was included in this system. In 1943, Portmann[169] described a staging system that incorporated clinical, pathologic, and roentgenographic characteristics of breast cancers and evaluated each lesion based on three categories: skin involvement, the location and mobility of the primary tumor, and the extent of local and distant metastases (Table 23-6). Haagensen and Stout[170] evaluated 568 patients with breast cancer who were treated with radical mastectomy. In 1943, they published the following criteria of inoperability, which were based on the clinical characteristics of patients who were clearly incurable by aggressive surgery alone:

- Extensive edema of the skin overlying the breast or edema of the arm
- Satellite nodules of the breast or parasternal tumor nodules
- Inflammatory carcinoma
- Supraclavicular or distant metastases
- Two or more of the five "grave signs" of locally advanced cancer:
  1. Breast skin edema
  2. Breast skin ulceration
  3. Tumor fixation to chest wall
  4. Axillary lymph node fixation to skin or deep tissues
  5. Enlarged axillary lymph nodes larger than 2.5 cm in diameter

Haagensen and Stout also advocated the use of biopsy material in the determination of inoperability. Their proposed "triple biopsy" included sampling the primary tumor, apical axillary nodes, and IMNs as part of the pretreatment evaluation. This represented the first attempt at including pathologic data in the staging process.

Although largely derived from Haagensen and Stout's criteria of inoperability, the Columbia Clinical Classification (CCC) ignored the use of tumor size and any biopsy material or other pathologic data. It has, however, been successfully used to separate different groups of patients with distinctly different survival rates.[171] Staging was determined on the basis of physical examination and other roentgenographic information in an attempt to simplify and streamline the staging process. Four stages were defined (Table 23-7). Stages A and B were both used to describe operable cancers, but stage B referred to palpably enlarged, unfixed axillary lymph nodes (presumed to represent regional metastases). Based on the five "grave signs" listed previously, stage C defined a group of patients with cancers that were locally advanced. In stage D, the tumors were considered inoperable as defined by the "criteria of inoperability." Patients with stage A and B disease were treated with radical mastectomy, whereas those with stage C and D disease underwent radiation therapy.

TABLE 23-7

Columbia Clinical Classification

Stage A	No skin involvement or fixation of the tumor to the chest wall. Axillary nodes are not palpable.
Stage B	No skin involvement or fixation of the tumor to the chest wall. Clinically palpable nodes, but <2.5 cm in transverse diameter and not fixed to overlying skin or deeper structures of the axilla
Stage C	Any one of the five grave signs of advanced breast carcinoma: 1. Limited edema of the skin involving less than one third of the skin over the breast 2. Skin ulceration 3. Fixation of the tumor to the chest wall 4. Massive involvement of axillary lymph nodes measuring >2.5 cm in transverse diameter 5. Fixation of the axillary nodes to overlying skin or deeper structures of the axilla
Stage D	Any patient with signs of advanced breast carcinoma: 1. A combination of any two or more of the five grave signs listed under stage C 2. Extensive edema of the skin (involving more than one third of the skin over the breast) 3. Satellite skin nodules 4. The inflammatory type of carcinoma 5. Clinically involved supraclavicular lymph nodes 6. Internal mammary metastases as evidenced by a parasternal tumor 7. Edema of the arm 8. Distant metastases

Modified from Haagensen CD, et al.[171]

Despite initial acceptance, the CCC has since been replaced by the current TNM system, which incorporates both clinical and pathologic features. This system was adopted for many reasons, including its initial simplicity, clinical applicability, and universal utility. Moreover, it is clear that in the past two decades, because of the widespread use of screening mammography and public education, breast cancers are being detected earlier, with smaller delays in diagnosis. This has necessarily shifted the contemporary population of patients being studied to earlier stages at diagnosis. In turn, the need for elaborate classification schemes based on generally advanced clinical criteria has become obsolete. At present, patients need to be stratified into groups based on more subtle, less advanced characteristics of disease progression. This is necessary not only because many women now have small or nonpalpable tumors but also because not all small tumors have the same biologic behavior (e.g., growth, metastases).

The TNM system, developed by Pierre Denoix[172] in the 1940s in France, represented an attempt to classify cancer based on the major morphologic attributes of malignant tumors thought to influence prognosis: size of the primary tumor (T), presence and extent of regional lymph node involvement (N), and presence of distant metastases (M). In 1958, the International Union Against Cancer (UICC) described the first recommendations for the staging of breast cancer based on the TNM system.[173] Simultaneously, the American Joint Committee on Cancer (AJCC) published a breast cancer staging system based on the TNM in their first cancer staging manual in 1977.[174] Since then, the proposals of the AJCC have undergone somewhat parallel and confluent evolutionary changes to those of the UICC, meaning that in 1987, for the first time, a truly universal staging system was developed and differences between them were eliminated. The current UICC and AJCC staging systems for breast cancer are now identical. This alliance now permits collaboration in multi-institutional trials on an international level.

The TNM system was originally conceived to be a simple system that would classify patients into various groups, each with a different survival rate and prognosis. There were binary choices for each evaluable patient and tumor characteristic. For instance, T_0 represented the absence of tumor; T_1 represented the presence of tumor. Similarly, N_0/M_0 and N_1/M_1 represented the absence or presence of regional or distant metastatic disease. Any patient could be rapidly classified into one of eight possible groups that could then be stratified into any number of stages based on observed survival frequencies. Such a classification system would have been simple, logical, and easy to commit to memory for future use. Although the TNM system was originally simple in design, modifications were necessary to improve prognostic power and stage definition. A large number of clinical and pathologic prognostic indicators have been identified since the inception of the TNM system (see section on clinical and pathologic correlates with prognosis). The TNM system, to date, is the only system that has successfully incorporated many of these factors. For this reason, despite the observation that this method of staging for breast cancer is the most complicated, it is also highly practical and adaptable. It provides more prognostic information and better stratifies patients for the purpose of guiding therapy than do other systems that are based largely on clinical criteria alone.

The more precise the clinician is able to define specific groups of patients who should undergo equivalent therapeutic regimens, the greater the probability that medical scientists should be able to reduce the number of patients with aggressive disease who are undertreated and those with limited disease who are overtreated. As more and more prognostic indices are identified and successful therapeutic modalities discovered, more subcategories will be required; for this reason, binary choices have become quaternary (N_0, N_1, N_2, N_3) or greater (T_0, Tis, T_1, T_2, T_3, T_4). Further delineation within each subcategory has also been added.

Current Staging System

Currently, the most popular staging system is the TNM system, based on the AJCC, sponsored by the American Cancer Society (ACS) and the American College of Surgeons (ACS). The updated sixth edition represents the culmination of many years of evolution of the AJCC and ACS and was modified extensively in 2002.[175] Despite these unified efforts, however, the current system will certainly undergo future changes. The best staging system will be flexible and continue to evolve with new prognostic data.

The current staging system requires microscopic confirmation and histologic typing of the tumor before attempting any stage classification. Any patient with documented breast cancer may then be staged by clinical (clinical or preoperative, designated by a "c" prefix) or pathologic criteria (pathologic or postoperative, designated by a "p" prefix). The clinical-diagnostic staging process requires a complete physical examination, with determination of the extent of ipsilateral and contralateral neoplastic involvement of skin, breast tissue, regional and distant lymph nodes, and underlying muscles. The microscopic diagnosis of breast cancer must be confirmed by examination of breast tissue. Routine laboratory examinations, chest x-ray films, and bilateral mammograms are also recommended. The pathologic classification involves all the data used in clinical staging; however, this more definitive staging system can be implemented only after the resection of the primary tumor and regional lymph nodes. It requires that no gross tumor be present at margins of resection and that at least the level 1 axillary lymph nodes be resected and histologically examined. Should tumor be present at the margins on gross examination of the resected specimen, the code TX is applied, indicating that the pathologic stage cannot yet be determined. The current TNM staging system based on the sixth edition of the AJCC staging manual is summarized in the following sections.

SPECIFIC STAGES

T Stage (Tumor Size)

Clinical tumor stage is the size of the tumor (reported in centimeters) based on the physical examination and various imaging modalities (e.g., mammogram, ultrasound, CT scans, MRI scans; Table 23-8). The pathologic T stage is based on the tumor size on the final pathologic specimen measuring only the invasive component. For multiple synchronous ipsilateral primary carcinomas, the largest tumor is used for the T classification and the physician should document that there are multiple primaries with their corresponding sizes and characteristics. Bilateral synchronous breast cancers are staged separately as separate primaries.

Tis includes ductal carcinoma in situ, lobular carcinoma in situ, or Paget's disease of the nipple with no invasive tumor. Paget's disease of the nipple with an associated invasive tumor is classified based on the invasive component. Although there is controversy regarding lobular carcinoma in situ, whether this is merely a marker for increased risk of developing breast cancer or a precursor of invasive lobular carcinoma, lobular carcinoma in situ is reported as a malignancy. T_1 is designated for tumors that are 2 cm or smaller and subclassified as T_{1mic}, T_{1a}, T_{1b}, and T_{1c}. Microinvasive breast cancer is defined as a focus of tumor less than or equal to 0.1 cm in greatest dimension. When

TABLE 23-8

AJCC Primary Tumor (T) Classification for Breast Cancer

T_x	Primary tumor cannot be assessed
T_0	No evidence of primary tumor
Tis	Carcinoma in situ
Tis (DCIS)	DCIS
Tis (LCIS)	LCIS
Tis (Paget)	Paget disease of the nipple with no tumor
T_1	Tumor ≤2 cm in greatest dimension
T_{1mic}	Microinvasion ≤0.1 cm in greatest dimension
T_{1a}	Tumor >0.1 cm but ≤0.5 cm in greatest dimension
T_{1b}	Tumor >0.5 cm but ≤1 cm in greatest dimension
T_{1c}	Tumor >1 cm but ≤2 cm in greatest dimension
T_2	Tumor > 2 cm but ≤5 cm in greatest dimension
T_3	Tumor > 5 cm in greatest dimension
T_4	Tumor of any size with direct extension to chest wall or skin, only as described below
T_{4a}	Extension to chest wall, not including pectoralis muscle
T_{4b}	Edema (including peau d'orange or ulceration of the skin of the breast or satellite skin nodules confined to the same breast)
T_{4c}	Both T_{4a} and T_{4b}
T_{4d}	Inflammatory carcinoma

DCIS, ductal carcinoma in situ; LCIS, lobular carcinoma in situ.
Modified from Greene FL, et al.[175]

TABLE 23-9

AJCC Clinical Regional Lymph Nodes (N) Classification for Breast Cancer

N_x	Regional lymph nodes cannot be assessed (e.g., previously removed)
N_0	No regional lymph node metastases
N_1	Metastasis in movable ipsilateral axillary lymph node(s)
N_2	Metastases in ipsilateral axillary lymph nodes fixed or matted, or in clinically apparent* ipsilateral internal mammary nodes in the absence of clinically evident axillary lymph node metastases
N_{2a}	Metastasis in ipsilateral axillary lymph nodes fixed to one another (matted) or to other structures
N_{2b}	Metastasis only in clinically apparent ipsilateral internal mammary nodes and in the absence of clinically evident axillary lymph node metastases
N_3	Metastasis in ipsilateral infraclavicular lymph node(s), or in clinically apparent ipsilateral internal mammary lymph node(s) and in the presence of clinically evident axillary lymph node metastases; or metastasis in ipsilateral supraclavicular lymph node(s) with or without axillary or internal mammary lymph node involvement
N_{3a}	Metastasis in ipsilateral infraclavicular lymph node(s) and axillary lymph node(s)
N_{3b}	Metastasis in ipsilateral internal mammary node(s) and axillary lymph node(s)
N_{3c}	Metastasis in ipsilateral supraclavicular lymph node(s)

*Clinically apparent is defined as detected by imaging studies (excluding lymphoscintigraphy) or by clinical examination.
Modified from Greene FL, et al.[175]

there are multiple foci of microinvasion, the T designation is based on the largest of the foci and not the additive sum of these. T_2 tumors are between 2 and 5 cm, and T_3 tumors larger than 5 cm. Tumors with direct invasion into the chest wall or skin are designated as T_4 tumors, with subclassification based on edema, extension to chest wall, skin ulceration, peau d'orange, or inflammation.

N Stage

Clinical nodal staging is based on physical examination or imaging studies, including CT scans and ultrasound but excluding lymphoscintigraphy (Table 23-9). If the regional lymph nodes cannot be assessed clinically (previously removed or not removed for pathologic examination), they are designated N_X. If no regional nodes are involved with tumor, it is designated as N_0. Categorization of clinical regional lymph node involvement is based on whether the lymph nodes are mobile (N_1) or fixed (N_{2a}) and evidence of involvement of the ipsilateral IMNs (N_{2b}) and ipsilateral infraclavicular lymph nodes (N_{3a}). Metastasis to ipsilateral supraclavicular lymph node disease was considered to have prognosis similar to that for patients with distant disease; however, the overall survival is better and was changed to stage N_{3c} in the revised 2002 AJCC staging system.

SLN biopsy techniques have dramatically changed the pathologic staging of patients with breast cancer. Patients are now being diagnosed with earlier tumor stages with the detection of microscopic and submicroscopic metastatic tumor deposits. This is reflected and incorporated into the revised 2002 AJCC pathologic staging system for the first time. This revised system also incorporates the assessment of microscopic disease based on IHC and molecular techniques (RT-PCR).

Pathologic staging of the lymph nodes is based on biopsies taken from SLN or complete axillary lymph node dissections (Table 23-10). If the regional nodes cannot be assessed pathologically (previously removed or not removed for pathologic examination), they are designated pN_X. If no regional lymph nodes are involved with tumor, it is designated as pN_0. Further subclassification of pN_0 allows the distinction between the identification of microscopic cells based on IHC or molecular techniques (RT-PCR). Isolated tumor cells are defined as single tumor cells or small clusters not greater than 0.2 mm, usually detected with IHC or molecular methods but that may be verified on H&E stains. Isolated tumor cells usually show no

evidence of metastatic activity. Pathologic node positivity is based on the number of lymph nodes involved (pN). pN_1 is divided into four categories, including pN_{1mic} (>0.2 mm, <2 mm), pN_1 (1 to 3 positive nodes, microscopic IMNs positive as determined with SLN dissection), pN_2 (4 to 9 positive nodes, positive IMNs with at least one tumor deposit >2 mm), and pN_3 (>10, or positive infraclavicular lymph nodes, or both internal mammary and axillary nodes positive, or ipsilateral supraclavicular lymph nodes). In the previous AJCC 1997 staging system, the designation of fixed, matted nodes were separate categories. In the revised AJCC 2002 staging system, there is not a distinction for fixed or matted lymph nodes.

One of the major changes in the revised staging system was to subclassify internal mammary nodal metastasis. This subclassification is, for the most part, dependent on SLN biopsies because small metastatic tumor burden within the IMNs is difficult to detect clinically, and routine IMN dissection is not performed. IMN microscopic disease without evidence of axillary disease is designated as pN_{1b}, and IMN microscopic disease with the presence of 1 to 3 ipsilateral axillary disease is designated pN_{1c}.

TABLE 23–10

AJCC Pathologic Regional Lymph Nodes (pN) Classification for Breast Cancer

pN_x	Regional lymph nodes cannot be assessed (e.g., previously removed or not removed for pathologic study)
pN_0	No regional lymph node metastasis histologically; no additional examination for isolated tumor cells*
$pN_{0(i-)}$	No regional lymph node metastasis histologically; negative immunohistochemical staining
$pN_{0(i+)}$	Isolated tumor cells identified histologically; negative immunohistochemical staining
$pN_{0(mol-)}$	No regional lymph node metastasis histologically; negative molecular findings (RT-PCR)
$pN_{0(mol+)}$	No regional lymph node metastasis histologically; positive molecular findings (RT-PCR)
pN_1	Metastasis is one to three axillary lymph nodes and/or in internal mammary nodes with microscopic disease detected by sentinel lymph node dissection but no clinically apparent
pN_{1mi}	Micrometastases (>0.2 mm, none > 2 mm)
pN_{1a}	Metastasis in one to three axillary lymph nodes
pN_{1b}	Metastasis in internal mammary nodes with microscopic disease detected by sentinel lymph node dissection but not clinically apparent
pN_{1c}	Metastasis in one to three axillary lymph nodes[†] and in internal mammary lymph nodes with microscopic disease detected by sentinel lymph node dissection but not clinically apparent
pN_2	Metastasis in four to nine axillary lymph nodes or in clinically apparent internal mammary lymph nodes in the absence of axillary lymph node metastasis
pN_{2a}	Metastasis in four to nine axillary lymph nodes (at least one tumor deposit >2 mm)
pN_{2b}	Metastasis in clinically apparent internal mammary lymph nodes in the absence of axillary lymph node metastasis
pN_3	Metastasis in 10 or more axillary lymph nodes, or in infraclavicular lymph nodes, or in clinically apparent ipsilateral internal mammary lymph nodes in the presence of one or more positive axillary lymph nodes; or in more than three axillary lymph nodes with clinically negative microscopic metastasis in internal mammary lymph nodes; or in ipsilateral supraclavicular lymph nodes
pN_{3a}	Metastasis in 10 or more axillary nodes (at least one deposit > 2 mm) or metastasis to the infraclavicular lymph nodes
pN_{3b}	Metastasis in clinically apparent ipsilateral internal mammary lymph nodes in the presence of one or more positive axillary lymph nodes; or in more than three axillary lymph nodes and in internal mammary lymph nodes with microscopic disease detected by sentinel lymph node dissection but not clinically apparent
pN_{3c}	Metastasis in ipsilateral supraclavicular lymph nodes

RT-PCR, reverse transcriptase polymerase chain reaction.

*Isolated tumor cells are defined as single tumor cells or small cell clusters ≤0.2 mm, usually detected only by immunohistochemical or molecular methods but which may be verified on hematoxylin and eosin stains.

[†]If associated with more than three positive axillary lymph nodes, the internal mammary nodes are classified as pN3b to reflect increased tumor burden.

Modified from Greene FL, et al.[175]

TABLE 23-11	
AJCC Distant Metastasis (M) Classification for Breast Cancer	
M_x	Distant metastasis cannot be assessed
M_0	No distant metastasis
M_1	Distant metastasis

Modified from Greene FL, et al.[175]

M Stage

Distant metastatic disease is designated as M_1 disease (Table 23-11). Ipsilateral supraclavicular lymph node disease is no longer considered distant metastatic disease but rather locally advanced disease (N_3). Evidence of metastatic disease may be based on clinical history and physical examination, with or without the assistance of various imaging modalities and biochemical markers.

STAGE GROUPINGS

There are five stage groupings (0, I, II, III, and IV) in the new TNM staging system, with stage II being subdivided into A and B and stage III into A, B, and C (Table 23-12). Stage 0 (Tis N_0 M_0) refers to preinvasive cancers (carcinoma in situ) that have not penetrated the basement

TABLE 23-12	
AJCC Stage Grouping and Histopathologic Grading System Classification for Breast Cancer	
Stage Grouping	
Stage 0	Tis N_0 M_0
Stage I	T_1* N_0 M_0
Stage IIA	T_0 N_1 M_0
	T_1* N_1 M_0
	T_2 N_0 M_0
Stage IIB	T_2 N_1 M_0
	T_3 N_0 M_0
Stage IIIA	T_0 N_2 M_0
	T_1* N_2 M_0
	T_2 N_2 M_0
	T_3 N_1 M_0
	T_3 N_2 M_0
Stage IIIB	T_4 N_0 M_0
	T_4 N_1 M_0
	T_4 N_2 M_0
Stage IIIC	Any T N_3 M_0
Stage IV	Any T Any N M_1
Histologic Grade	
G_x	Grade cannot be assessed
G_1	Low combined histologic grade (favorable)
G_2	Intermediate combined histologic grade (moderate favorable)
G_3	High combined histologic grade (unfavorable)

*T_1 includes T_{1mtc}.
Modified from Greene Fl, et al.[175]

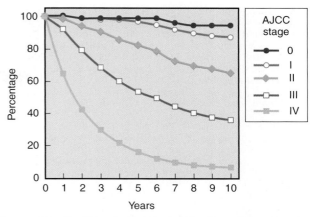

Figure 23-15 The relative survival for breast cancer patients according to the American Joint Committee on Cancer (AJCC) stage group. (From Bland KI, Menck HR, Scott-Conner CE, et al: The National Cancer Data Base 10-year survey of breast carcinoma treatment at hospitals in the United States. Cancer 86:1262, 1998.)

membrane of the duct or lobule. There are no regional or distant metastases associated with this stage at initial diagnosis and treatment. Stage 0 tumors have an excellent prognosis of nearly 100% cure. Stage I (T_{1mic} N_0 M_0) refers to tumors that are micrometastatic; these patients also have an excellent prognosis. Stage I cancers are localized to the breast and are small (T_1 N_0 M_0). Stage IIA (T_0 N_1 M_0, T_1 N_1 M_0, T_{1mic} N_1 M_0, T_2 N_0 M_0) and stage IIB (T_2 N_1 M_0, T_3 N_0 M_0) are reserved for cases with regional lymph node metastases and carry a worse prognosis. Stage IIIA (T_0 N_2 M_0, T_1 N_2 M_0, T_2 N_2 M_0, T_3 N_1 M_0, T_3 N_2 M_0), stage IIIB (T_4 N_0 M_0, T_4 N_1 M_0, T_4 N_2 M_0), and stage IIIC (any T N_3 M_0) refer to larger tumors that are locally advanced and thus have a worse prognosis. Stage IV (any T any N M_1) refers to distant systemic spread of disease with a significantly poor survival (Fig. 23-15).

HISTOPATHOLOGIC GRADE

The AJCC-recommended histologic grading system is based on the Nottingham combined histologic grade (see Table 23-12).[23] The grade "G" of the tumor is designated based on the morphologic features of the primary tumor (tubule formation, nuclear pleomorphism, and mitotic count) by assigning a value of 1 to 3 (1, favorable; 3, unfavorable). The scores are added together for each feature. Grade 1 tumors have a combined score of 3 to 5 points; grade 2, 6 to 7 points; and grade 3, 8 to 9 points.

REFERENCES

1. Koscielny S, Tubiana M, Lê MG, et al: Breast cancer: Relationship between the size of the primary tumour and the probability of metastatic dissemination. Br J Cancer 49:709–715, 1984.
2. Carter CL, Allen C, Henson DE: Relation of tumor size, lymph node status, and survival in 24,740 breast cancer cases. Cancer 63:181–187, 1989.
3. McGuire WL, Clark GM: Prognostic factors and treatment decisions in axillary-node-negative breast cancer. N Engl J Med 326:1756–1761, 1992.
4. Nemoto T, Vana J, Bedwani RN, et al: Management and survival of female breast cancer: Results of a national survey by the American College of Surgeons. Cancer 45:2917–2924, 1980.

5. Fisher ER: Prognostic and therapeutic significance of pathological features of breast cancer. NCI Monogr 1:29–34, 1986.
6. Hanrahan EO, Gonzalez-Angulo AM, Giordano SH, et al: Overall survival and cause-specific mortality of patients with stage $T_{1a,b}$ N_0M_0 breast carcinoma. J Clin Oncol 25:4952–4960, 2007.
7. Fisher B, Slack NH, Bross ID: Cancer of the breast: size of neoplasm and prognosis. Cancer 24:1071–1080, 1969.
8. Fisher B, Slack NH, Ausman RK, Bross ID: Location of breast carcinoma and prognosis. Surg Gynecol Obstet 129:705–716, 1969.
9. Nemoto T, Natarajan N, Bedwani R, et al: Breast cancer in the medial half. Results of 1978 National Survey of the American College of Surgeons. Cancer 51:1333–1338, 1983.
10. Zucali R, Mariani L, Marubini E, et al: Early breast cancer: Evaluation of the prognostic role of the site of the primary tumor. J Clin Oncol 16:1363–1366, 1998.
11. Lohrisch C, Jackson J, Jones A, et al: Relationship between tumor location and relapse in 6,781 women with early invasive breast cancer. J Clin Oncol 18:2828–2835, 2000.
12. Gaffney DK, Tsodikov A, Wiggins CL: Diminished survival in patients with inner versus outer quadrant breast cancers. J Clin Oncol 21:467–472, 2003.
13. Colleoni M, Zahrieh D, Gelber RD, et al: Site of primary tumor has a prognostic role in operable breast cancer: The international breast cancer study group experience. J Clin Oncol 23:1390–1400, 2005.
14. Sarp S, Fioretta G, Verkooijen HM, et al: Tumor location of the lower-inner quadrant is associated with an impaired survival for women with early-stage breast cancer. Ann Surg Oncol 14:1031–1039, 2007.
15. Shahar KH, Buchholz TA, Delpassand E, et al: Lower and central tumor location correlates with lymphoscintigraphy drainage to the internal mammary lymph nodes in breast carcinoma. Cancer 103:1323–1329, 2005.
16. Estourgie SH, Nieweg OE, Olmos RA, et al: Lymphatic drainage patterns from the breast. Ann Surg 239:232–237, 2004.
17. Page DL: Special types of invasive breast cancer, with clinical implications. Am J Surg Pathol 27:832–835, 2003.
18. Gonzalez-Angulo AM, Hennessy BT, Broglio K, et al: Trends for inflammatory breast cancer: Is survival improving? Oncologist 12:904–912, 2007.
19. Di Saverio S, Gutierrez J, Avisar E: A retrospective review with long term follow up of 11,400 cases of pure mucinous breast carcinoma. Breast Cancer Res Treat 111:541–547, 2008.
20. Hutter RV: The influence of pathologic factors on breast cancer management. Cancer 46(suppl):961–976, 1980.
21. Hoge AF, Asal N, Owen W, Anderson P: Histologic and staging classification of breast cancer: Implications for therapy. South Med J 75:1329–1334, 1987.
22. Bloom HJ, Richardson WW: Histological grading and prognosis in breast cancer: A study of 1409 cases of which 359 have been followed for 15 years. Br J Cancer 11:359–377, 1957.
23. Elston CW, Ellis IO: Pathological prognostic factors in breast cancer. I. The value of histological grade in breast cancer: Experience from a large study with long-term follow-up. Histopathology 19:403–410, 1991.
24. Black MM, Speer FD: Nuclear structure in cancer tissues. Surg Gynecol Obstet 105:97–102, 1957.
25. Fisher ER, Swamidoss S, Lee CH, et al: Detection and significance of occult axillary node metastases in patients with invasive breast cancer. Cancer 42:2025–2031, 1978.
26. Fisher ER, Redmond C, Fisher B: Pathologic findings from the National Surgical Adjuvant Breast Project. VIII. Relationship of chemotherapeutic responsiveness to tumor differentiation. Cancer 51:181–191, 1983.
27. Fisher ER, Costantino JP, Leon ME, et al: Pathobiology of small invasive breast cancers without metastases (T1a/b, N0, M0): National Surgical Adjuvant Breast and Bowel Project (NSABP) protocol B-21. Cancer 110:1929–1936, 2007.
28. Fisher ER, Wang J, Bryant J, et al: Pathobiology of preoperative chemotherapy: Findings from the National Surgical Adjuvant Breast and Bowel (NSABP) protocol B-18. Cancer 95:681–695, 2002.
29. Fisher ER, Gregorio RM, Fisher B, et al: The pathology of invasive breast cancer. A syllabus derived from findings of the National Surgical Adjuvant Breast Project (protocol no. 4). Cancer 36:1–85, 1975.
30. Knight WA, Livingston RB, Gregory EJ, McGuire WL: Estrogen receptor as an independent prognostic factor for early recurrence in breast cancer. Cancer Res 37:4669–4671, 1977.
31. Osborne CK, McGuire WL: Current use of steroid hormone receptor assays in the treatment of breast cancer. Surg Clin North Am 58:777–788, 1978.
32. Pichon MF, Pallud C, Brunet M, Milgrom E: Relationship of presence of progesterone receptors to prognosis in early breast cancer. Cancer Res 40:3357–3360, 1980.
33. Jeruss JS, Mittendorf EA, Tucker SL, et al: Combined use of clinical and pathologic staging variables to define outcomes for breast cancer patients treated with neoadjuvant therapy. J Clin Oncol 26:246–252, 2008.
34. Guarneri V, Broglio K, Kau SW, et al: Prognostic value of pathologic complete response after primary chemotherapy in relation to hormone receptor status and other factors. J Clin Oncol 24:1037–1044, 2006.
35. Charlson ME, Feinstein AR: A new clinical index of growth rate in the staging of breast cancer. Am J Med 69:527–536, 1980.
36. Gershon-Cohen J, Berger SM, Klickstein HS: Roentgenography of breast cancer moderating concept of "biologic predeterminism." Cancer 16:961–964, 1963.
37. Lee YT: The lognormal distribution of growth rates of soft tissue metastases of breast cancer. J Surg Oncol 4:81–88, 1972.
38. Philippe E, Le Gal Y: Growth of seventy-eight recurrent mammary cancers. Quantitative study. Cancer 21:461–467, 1968.
39. Heuser LS, Spratt JS, Kuhns JG, et al: The association of pathologic and mammographic characteristics of primary human breast cancers with "slow" and "fast" growth rates and with axillary lymph node metastases. Cancer 53:96–98, 1984.
40. van Diest PJ, Brugal G, Baak JP: Proliferation markers in tumours: Interpretation and clinical value. J Clin Pathol 51:716–724, 1998.
41. Clahsen PC, van de Velde CJ, Duval C, et al: The utility of mitotic index, oestrogen receptor and Ki-67 measurements in the creation of novel prognostic indices for node-negative breast cancer. Eur J Surg Oncol 25:356–363, 1999.
42. Billgren AM, Rutqvist LE, Tani E, et al: Proliferating fraction during neoadjuvant chemotherapy of primary breast cancer in relation to objective local response and relapse-free survival. Acta Oncol 38:597–601, 1999.
43. Chang J, Powles TJ, Allred DC, et al: Prediction of clinical outcome from primary tamoxifen by expression of biologic markers in breast cancer patients. Clin Cancer Res 6:616–621, 2000.
44. Nole F, Minchella I, Colleoni M, et al: Primary chemotherapy in operable breast cancer with favorable prognostic factors: A pilot study evaluating the efficacy of a regimen with a low subjective toxic burden containing vinorelbine, 5-fluorouracil and folinic acid (FLN). Ann Oncol 10:993–996, 1999.
45. Bergers E, van Diest PJ, Baak JP: Tumour heterogeneity of DNA cell cycle variables in breast cancer measured by flow cytometry. J Clin Pathol 49:931–937, 1996.
46. Harris L, Fritsche H, Mennel R, et al: American Society of Clinical Oncology 2007 update of recommendations for the use of tumor markers in breast cancer. J Clin Oncol 25:5287–5312, 2007.
47. Ewers SB, Langstrom E, Baldetorp B, Killander D: Flow-cytometric DNA analysis in primary breast carcinomas and clinicopathological correlations. Cytometry 5:408–419, 1984.
48. Hedley DW, Friedlander ML, Taylor IW: Application of DNA flow cytometry to paraffin-embedded archival material for the study of aneuploidy and its clinical significance. Cytometry 6:327–333, 1985.
49. Moran RE, Black MM, Alpert L, Straus MJ: Correlation of cell-cycle kinetics, hormone receptors, histopathology, and nodal status in human breast cancer. Cancer 54:1586–1590, 1984.
50. Camplejohn RS, Ash CM, Gillett CE, et al: The prognostic significance of DNA flow cytometry in breast cancer: Results from 881 patients treated in a single centre. Br J Cancer 71:140–145, 1995.
51. Bryant J, Fisher B, Gunduz N, et al: S-phase fraction combined with other patient and tumor characteristics for the prognosis of node-negative, estrogen-receptor-positive breast cancer. Breast Cancer Res Treat 51:239–253, 1998.
52. Moureau-Zabotto L, Bouchet C, Cesari D, et al: Combined flow cytometry determination of S-phase fraction and DNA ploidy is an independent prognostic factor in node-negative invasive breast

carcinoma: analysis of a series of 271 patients with stage I and II breast cancer. Breast Cancer Res Treat 91:61–71, 2005.

53. Chevillard S, Lebeau J, Pouillart P, et al: Biological and clinical significance of concurrent p53 gene alterations, MDR1 gene expression, and S-phase fraction analyses in breast cancer patients treated with primary chemotherapy or radiotherapy. Clin Cancer Res 3(pt 1):2471–2478, 1997.

54. Stal O, Skoog L, Rutqvist LE, et al: S-phase fraction and survival benefit from adjuvant chemotherapy or radiotherapy of breast cancer. Br J Cancer 70:1258–1262, 1994.

55. Silvestrini R, Luisi A, Zambetti M, et al: Cell proliferation and outcome following doxorubicin plus CMF regimens in node-positive breast cancer. Int J Cancer 87:405–411, 2008.

56. Pinto AE, Andre S, Pereira T, Nobrega S, Soares J: Prognostic comparative study of S-phase fraction and Ki-67 index in breast carcinoma. J Clin Pathol 54:543–549, 2001.

57. van Diest PJ, van der Wall E, Baak JP: Prognostic value of proliferation in invasive breast cancer: A review. J Clin Pathol 57:675–681, 2004.

58. Colozza M, Azambuja E, Cardoso F, et al: Proliferative markers as prognostic and predictive tools in early breast cancer: Where are we now? Ann Oncol 16:1723–1739, 2005.

59. Silvestrini R, Daidone MG, Luisi A, et al: Cell proliferation in 3,800 node-negative breast cancers: consistency over time of biological and clinical information provided by 3H-thymidine labelling index. Int J Cancer 74:122–127, 1997.

60. Nio Y, Tamura K, Kan N, et al: In vitro DNA synthesis in freshly separated human breast cancer cells assessed by tritiated thymidine incorporation assay: Relationship to the long-term outcome of patients. Br J Surg 86:1463–1469, 1999.

61. Tubiana M, Pejovic MH, Chavaudra N, et al: The long-term prognostic significance of the thymidine labelling index in breast cancer. Int J Cancer 33:441–445, 1984.

62. Paradiso A, Schittulli F, Cellamare G, et al: Randomized clinical trial of adjuvant fluorouracil, epirubicin, and cyclophosphamide chemotherapy for patients with fast-proliferating, node-negative breast cancer. J Clin Oncol 19:3929–3937, 2001.

63. Schwartz GF, Feig SA, Patchefsky AS: Significance and staging of nonpalpable carcinomas of the breast. Surg Gynecol Obstet 166:6–10, 1988.

64. Meyer JS, Alvarez C, Milikowski C, et al: Breast carcinoma malignancy grading by Bloom-Richardson system vs proliferation index: reproducibility of grade and advantages of proliferation index. Mod Pathol 18:1067–1078, 2005.

65. Baak JP, van Diest PJ, Voorhorst FJ, et al: Prospective multicenter validation of the independent prognostic value of the mitotic activity index in lymph node-negative breast cancer patients younger than 55 years. J Clin Oncol 23:5993–6001, 2005.

66. Baak JP, van Diest PJ, Voorhorst FJ, et al: The prognostic value of proliferation in lymph-node-negative breast cancer patients is age dependent. Eur J Cancer 43:527–535, 2007.

67. Baak JP, van Diest PJ, Janssen EA, et al: Proliferation accurately identifies the high-risk patients among small, low-grade, lymph node-negative invasive breast cancers. Ann Oncol 19:649–654, 2008.

68. Andre F, Khalil A, Slimane K, et al: Mitotic index and benefit of adjuvant anthracycline-based chemotherapy in patients with early breast cancer. J Clin Oncol 23:2996–3000, 2005.

69. Redding WH, Coombes RC, Monaghan P, et al: Detection of micrometastases in patients with primary breast cancer. Lancet 2:1271–1274, 1983.

70. Braun S, Pantel K, Muller P, et al: Cytokeratin-positive cells in the bone marrow and survival of patients with stage I, II, or III breast cancer. N Engl J Med 342:525–533, 2000.

71. Braun S, Vogl FD, Naume B, et al: A pooled analysis of bone marrow micrometastasis in breast cancer. N Engl J Med 353:793–802, 2005.

72. Demel U, Tilz GP, Foeldes-Papp Z, et al: Detection of tumour cells in the peripheral blood of patients with breast cancer. Development of a new sensitive and specific immunomolecular assay. J Exp Clin Cancer Res 23:465–468, 2004.

73. Schroder CP, Ruiters MH, de Jong S, et al: Detection of micrometastatic breast cancer by means of real time quantitative RT-PCR and immunostaining in perioperative blood samples and sentinel nodes. Int J Cancer 106:611–618, 2003.

74. Taback B, Chan AD, Kuo CT, et al: Detection of occult metastatic breast cancer cells in blood by a multimolecular marker assay: Correlation with clinical stage of disease. Cancer Res 61:8845–8850, 2001.

75. Weigelt B, Bosma AJ, Hart AA, et al: Marker genes for circulating tumour cells predict survival in metastasized breast cancer patients. Br J Cancer 88:1091–1094, 2003.

76. Cristofanilli M, Hayes DF, Budd GT, et al: Circulating tumor cells: A novel prognostic factor for newly diagnosed metastatic breast cancer. J Clin Oncol 3:1420–1430, 2005.

77. Hayes DF, Cristofanilli M, Budd GT, et al: Circulating tumor cells at each follow-up time point during therapy of metastatic breast cancer patients predict progression-free and overall survival. Clin Cancer Res 12(pt 1):4218–422, 2006.

78. Cristofanilli M, Budd GT, Ellis MJ, et al: Circulating tumor cells, disease progression, and survival in metastatic breast cancer. N Engl J Med 351:781–791, 2004.

79. Westley BR, May FE: Cathepsin D and breast cancer. Eur J Cancer 32A:15–24, 1996.

80. Foekens JA, Look MP, Bolt-de Vries J, et al: Cathepsin-D in primary breast cancer: Prognostic evaluation involving 2810 patients. Br J Cancer 79:300–307, 1999.

81. Billgren AM, Tani E, Liedberg A, et al: Prognostic significance of tumor cell proliferation analyzed in fine needle aspirates from primary breast cancer. Breast Cancer Res Treat 71:161–170, 2002.

82. Stephens RW, Brunner N, Janicke F, Schmitt M: The urokinase plasminogen activator system as a target for prognostic studies in breast cancer. Breast Cancer Res Treat 52:99–111, 1998.

83. Duffy MJ: Urokinase plasminogen activator and its inhibitor, PAI-1, as prognostic markers in breast cancer: From pilot to level 1 evidence studies. Clin Chem 48:1194–1197, 2002.

84. Harbeck N, Schmitt M, Kates RE, et al: Clinical utility of urokinase-type plasminogen activator and plasminogen activator inhibitor-1 determination in primary breast cancer tissue for individualized therapy concepts. Clin Breast Cancer 3:196–200, 2002.

85. Janicke F, Prechtl A, Thomssen C, et al: Randomized adjuvant chemotherapy trial in high-risk, lymph node-negative breast cancer patients identified by urokinase-type plasminogen activator and plasminogen activator inhibitor type 1. J Natl Cancer Inst 93:913–920, 2001.

86. Look MP, van Putten WL, Duffy MJ, et al: Pooled analysis of prognostic impact of urokinase-type plasminogen activator and its inhibitor PAI-1 in 8377 breast cancer patients. J Natl Cancer Inst 94:116–128, 2002.

87. Cline MJ, Battifora H, Yokota J: Proto-oncogene abnormalities in human breast cancer: Correlations with anatomic features and clinical course of disease. J Clin Oncol 5:999–1006, 1987.

88. Taucher S, Rudas M, Mader RM, et al: Do we need HER-2/neu testing for all patients with primary breast carcinoma? Cancer 98:2547–2553, 2003.

89. Kroger N, Milde-Langosch K, Riethdorf S, et al: Prognostic and predictive effects of immunohistochemical factors in high-risk primary breast cancer patients. Clin Cancer Res 12:159–168, 2006.

90. Slamon DJ, Clark GM, Wong SG, et al: Human breast cancer: Correlation of relapse and survival with amplification of the HER-2/neu oncogene. Science 235:177–182, 1987.

91. Gusterson BA, Gelber RD, Goldhirsch A, et al: Prognostic importance of c-erbB-2 expression in breast cancer. International (Ludwig) Breast Cancer Study Group. J Clin Oncol 10:1049–1056, 1992.

92. Volpi A, Nanni O, De Paola F, et al: HER-2 expression and cell proliferation: Prognostic markers in patients with node-negative breast cancer. J Clin Oncol 21:2708–2712, 2003.

93. Varley JM, Swallow JE, Brammar WJ, et al: Alterations to either c-erbB-2(neu) or c-myc proto-oncogenes in breast carcinomas correlate with poor short-term prognosis. Oncogene 1:423–430, 1987.

94. Thor AD, Moore DH, II, Edgerton SM, et al: Accumulation of p53 tumor suppressor gene protein: An independent marker of prognosis in breast cancers. J Natl Cancer Inst 84:845–855, 1992.

95. Olivier M, Langerod A, Carrieri P, et al: The clinical value of somatic TP53 gene mutations in 1,794 patients with breast cancer. Clin Cancer Res 12:1157–1167, 2006.

96. Pharoah PD, Day NE, Caldas C: Somatic mutations in the p53 gene and prognosis in breast cancer: A meta-analysis. Br J Cancer 80:1968–1973, 1999.

97. Perou CM, Sorlie T, Eisen MB, et al: Molecular portraits of human breast tumours. Nature 406:747–752, 2000.

98. Sorlie T, Perou CM, Tibshirani R, et al: Gene expression patterns of breast carcinomas distinguish tumor subclasses with clinical implications. Proc Natl Acad Sci USA 98:10869–10874, 2001.

99. Sorlie T, Tibshirani R, Parker J, et al: Repeated observation of breast tumor subtypes in independent gene expression data sets. Proc Natl Acad Sci USA 100:8418–8423, 2003.

100. Perreard L, Fan C, Quackenbush JF, et al: Classification and risk stratification of invasive breast carcinomas using a real-time quantitative RT-PCR assay. Breast Cancer Res 8:1–11, 2006.

101. Carey LA, Perou CM, Livasy CA, et al: Race, breast cancer subtypes, and survival in the Carolina Breast Cancer Study. JAMA 295:2492–2502, 2006.

102. Rouzier R, Perou CM, Symmans WF, et al: Breast cancer molecular subtypes respond differently to preoperative chemotherapy. Clin Cancer Res 11:5678–5685, 2005.

103. Pusztai L, Ayers M, Stec J, et al: Gene expression profiles obtained from fine-needle aspirations of breast cancer reliably identify routine prognostic markers and reveal large-scale molecular differences between estrogen-negative and estrogen-positive tumors. Clin Cancer Res 9:2406–2415, 2003.

104. Cleator S, Heller W, Coombes RC: Triple-negative breast cancer: Therapeutic options. Lancet Oncol 8:235–244, 2007.

105. Foulkes WD, Stefansson IM, Chappuis PO, et al: Germline BRCA1 mutations and a basal epithelial phenotype in breast cancer. J Natl Cancer Inst 95:1482–1485, 2003.

106. Bauer KR, Brown M, Cress RD, et al: Descriptive analysis of estrogen receptor (ER)-negative, progesterone receptor (PR)-negative, and HER2-negative invasive breast cancer, the so-called triple-negative phenotype: A population-based study from the California Cancer Registry. Cancer 109:1721–1728, 2007.

107. Wang Y, Klijn JG, Zhang Y, et al: Gene-expression profiles to predict distant metastasis of lymph-node-negative primary breast cancer. Lancet 365:671–679, 2005.

108. Goetz MP, Suman VJ, Ingle JN, et al: A two-gene expression ratio of homeobox 13 and interleukin-17B receptor for prediction of recurrence and survival in women receiving adjuvant tamoxifen. Clin Cancer Res 12(pt 1):2080–2087, 2006.

109. van't Veer LJ, Dai H, van de Vijver MJ, et al: Gene expression profiling predicts clinical outcome of breast cancer. Nature 415:530–5, 2002.

110. Cronin M, Pho M, Dutta D, et al: Measurement of gene expression in archival paraffin-embedded tissues: Development and performance of a 92-gene reverse transcriptase-polymerase chain reaction assay. Am J Pathol 164:35–42, 2004.

111. van de Vijver MJ, He YD, van't Veer LJ, et al: A gene-expression signature as a predictor of survival in breast cancer. N Engl J Med 347:1999–2009, 2002.

112. Buyse M, Loi S, van't Veer L, et al: Validation and clinical utility of a 70-gene prognostic signature for women with node-negative breast cancer. J Natl Cancer Inst 98:1183–1192, 2006.

113. Morris SR, Carey LA: Gene expression profiling in breast cancer. Curr Opin Oncol 19:547–551, 2007.

114. Paik S, Tang G, Shak S, et al: Gene expression and benefit of chemotherapy in women with node-negative, estrogen receptor-positive breast cancer. J Clin Oncol 24:3726–3734, 2006.

115. Paik S, Shak S, Tang G, et al: A multigene assay to predict recurrence of tamoxifen-treated, node-negative breast cancer. N Engl J Med 351:2817–2826, 2004.

116. Jacquemier J, Ginestier C, Rougemont J, et al: Protein expression profiling identifies subclasses of breast cancer and predicts prognosis. Cancer Res 65:767–779, 2005.

117. Halsted W: The results of operations for the cure of cancer of the breast performed at the Johns Hopkins Hospital from June, 1889 to January, 1894. Johns Hopkins Hosp Bull 4:297–321, 1895.

118. Fisher B, Redmond C, Fisher ER, et al: Ten-year results of a randomized clinical trial comparing radical mastectomy and total mastectomy with or without radiation. N Engl J Med 312:674–681, 1985.

119. Cancer Research Campaign Working Party: Cancer research campaign (King's/Cambridge) trial for early breast cancer. A detailed update at the tenth year. Lancet 2:55–60, 1980.

120. Bonadonna G: Evolving concepts in the systemic adjuvant treatment of breast cancer. Cancer Res 52:2127–2137, 1992.

121. Fisher B, Slack NH: Number of lymph nodes examined and the prognosis of breast carcinoma. Surg Gynecol Obstet 131:79–88, 1970.

122. Wallace IW, Champion HR: Axillary nodes in breast cancer. Lancet 1:217–218, 1972.

123. Fisher B, Wolmark N, Bauer M, et al: The accuracy of clinical nodal staging and of limited axillary dissection as a determinant of histologic nodal status in carcinoma of the breast. Surg Gynecol Obstet 152:765–772, 1981.

124. Fisher B, Fisher ER, Redmond C: Ten-year results from the National Surgical Adjuvant Breast and Bowel Project (NSABP) clinical trial evaluating the use of L-phenylalanine mustard (L-PAM) in the management of primary breast cancer. J Clin Oncol 4:929–941, 1986.

125. Diab SG, Hilsenbeck SG, de Moor C, et al: Radiation therapy and survival in breast cancer patients with 10 or more positive axillary lymph nodes treated with mastectomy. J Clin Oncol 16:1655–1660, 1998.

126. Jatoi I, Hilsenbeck SG, Clark GM, Osborne CK: Significance of axillary lymph node metastasis in primary breast cancer. J Clin Oncol 17:2334–2340, 1999.

127. Adair F, Berg J, Joubert L, Robbins GF: Long-term followup of breast cancer patients: The 30-year report. Cancer 33:1145–1150, 1974.

128. Davies GC, Millis RR, Hayward JL: Assessment of axillary lymph node status. Ann Surg 192:148–151, 1980.

129. Boova RS, Bonanni R, Rosato FE: Patterns of axillary nodal involvement in breast cancer. Predictability of level one dissection. Ann Surg 196:642–664, 1982.

130. Veronesi U, Paganelli G, Galimberti V, et al: Sentinel-node biopsy to avoid axillary dissection in breast cancer with clinically negative lymph-nodes. Lancet 349:1864–1867, 1997.

131. Albertini JJ, Lyman GH, Cox C, et al: Lymphatic mapping and sentinel node biopsy in the patient with breast cancer. JAMA 276:1818–1822, 1996.

132. Giuliano AE, Jones RC, Brennan M, Statman R: Sentinel lymphadenectomy in breast cancer. J Clin Oncol 15:2345–2350, 1997.

133. Cox CE, Pendas S, Cox JM, et al: Guidelines for sentinel node biopsy and lymphatic mapping of patients with breast cancer. Ann Surg 227:645–651, 1998.

134. Jeruss JS, Winchester DJ, Sener SF, et al: Axillary recurrence after sentinel node biopsy. Ann Surg Oncol 12:34–40, 2005.

135. Naik AM, Fey J, Gemignani M, et al: The risk of axillary relapse after sentinel lymph node biopsy for breast cancer is comparable with that of axillary lymph node dissection: A follow-up study of 4008 procedures. Ann Surg 240:462–468, discussion 468–471, 2004.

136. Giuliano AE, Haigh PI, Brennan MB, et al: Prospective observational study of sentinel lymphadenectomy without further axillary dissection in patients with sentinel node-negative breast cancer. J Clin Oncol 18:2553–2559, 2000.

137. Cote RJ, Peterson HF, Chaiwun B, et al: Role of immunohistochemical detection of lymph-node metastases in management of breast cancer. International Breast Cancer Study Group. Lancet 354:896–900, 1999.

138. Cox CE, Bass SS, McCann CR, et al: Lymphatic mapping and sentinel lymph node biopsy in patients with breast cancer. Annu Rev Med 51:525–542, 2000.

139. Turner RR, Ollila DW, Krasne DL, Giuliano AE: Histopathologic validation of the sentinel lymph node hypothesis for breast carcinoma. Ann Surg 226:271–276, discussion 276–278, 1997.

140. Schreiber RH, Pendas S, Ku NN, et al: Microstaging of breast cancer patients using cytokeratin staining of the sentinel lymph node. Ann Surg Oncol 6:95–101, 1999.

141. Chen SL, Hoehne FM, Giuliano AE: The prognostic significance of micrometastases in breast cancer: A SEER population-based analysis. Ann Surg Oncol 14:3378–3384, 2007.

142. Cox CE, Kiluk JV, Riker AI, et al: Significance of sentinel lymph node micrometastases in human breast cancer. J Am Coll Surg 206:261–268, 2008.

143. Veronesi U, Cascinelli N, Bufalino R, et al: Risk of internal mammary lymph node metastases and its relevance on prognosis of breast cancer patients. Ann Surg 198:681–684, 1983.

144. Cody HS III, Urban JA: Internal mammary node status: A major prognosticator in axillary node-negative breast cancer. Ann Surg Oncol 2:32–37, 1995.

145. Sugg SL, Ferguson DJ, Posner MC, Heimann R: Should internal mammary nodes be sampled in the sentinel lymph node era? Ann Surg Oncol 7:188–192, 2000.

146. Veronesi U, Marubini E, Mariani L, et al: The dissection of internal mammary nodes does not improve the survival of breast

cancer patients. 30-year results of a randomised trial. Eur J Cancer 35:1320–1325, 1999.

147. Veronesi U, Cascinelli N, Greco M, et al: Prognosis of breast cancer patients after mastectomy and dissection of internal mammary nodes. Ann Surg 202:702–707, 1985.

148. Morrow M, Foster RS Jr: Staging of breast cancer: A new rationale for internal mammary node biopsy. Arch Surg 116:748–751, 1981.

149. Kiricuta IC, Willner J, Kolbl O, Bohndorf W: The prognostic significance of the supraclavicular lymph node metastases in breast cancer patients. Int J Radiat Oncol Biol Phys 28:387–393, 1994.

150. Debois JM: The significance of a supraclavicular node metastasis in patients with breast cancer. A literature review. Strahlenther Onkol 173:1–12, 1997.

151. Brito RA, Valero V, Buzdar AU, et al: Long-term results of combined-modality therapy for locally advanced breast cancer with ipsilateral supraclavicular metastases: The University of Texas MD Anderson Cancer Center experience. J Clin Oncol 19:628–633, 2001.

152. Papaioannou AN, Urban JA: Scalene node biopsy in locally advanced primary breast cancer of questionable operability. Cancer 17:1006–1011, 1964.

153. Egan RL, McSweeney MB: Intramammary lymph nodes. Cancer 51:1838–1842, 1983.

154. Jadusingh IH: Intramammary lymph nodes. J Clin Pathol 45:1023–1026, 1992.

155. Shen J, Hunt KK, Mirza NQ, et al: Intramammary lymph node metastases are an independent predictor of poor outcome in patients with breast carcinoma. Cancer 101:1330–1337, 2004.

156. Guth AA, Mercado C, Roses DF, et al: Intramammary lymph nodes and breast cancer: A marker for disease severity, or just another lymph node? Am J Surg 192:502–50, 2006.

157. Weiser MR, Montgomery LL, Susnik B, et al: Is routine intraoperative frozen-section examination of sentinel lymph nodes in breast cancer worthwhile? Ann Surg Oncol 7:651–655, 2000.

158. Van Diest PJ, Torrenga H, Borgstein PJ, et al: Reliability of intraoperative frozen section and imprint cytological investigation of sentinel lymph nodes in breast cancer. Histopathology 35:14–18, 1999.

159. Creager AJ, Geisinger KR: Intraoperative evaluation of sentinel lymph nodes for breast carcinoma: Current methodologies. Adv Anat Pathol 9:233–243, 2002.

160. Creager AJ, Geisinger KR, Shiver SA, et al: Intraoperative evaluation of sentinel lymph nodes for metastatic breast carcinoma by imprint cytology. Mod Pathol 15:1140–1147, 2002.

161. Backus J, Laughlin T, Wang Y, et al: Identification and characterization of optimal gene expression markers for detection of breast cancer metastasis. J Mol Diagn 7:327–336, 2005.

162. Blumencranz P, Whitworth PW, Deck K, et al: Scientific Impact Recognition Award. Sentinel node staging for breast cancer: Intraoperative molecular pathology overcomes conventional histologic sampling errors. Am J Surg 194:426–432, 2007.

163. Viale G, Dell'orto P, Biasi MO, et al: Comparative evaluation of an extensive histopathologic examination and a real-time reverse-transcription-polymerase chain reaction assay for mammaglobin and cytokeratin 19 on axillary sentinel lymph nodes of breast carcinoma patients. Ann Surg 247:136–142, 2008.

164. Pierce LJ, Oberman HA, Strawderman MH, Lichter AS: Microscopic extracapsular extension in the axilla: Is this an indication for axillary radiotherapy? Int J Radiat Oncol Biol Phys 33:253–259, 1995.

165. Mambo NC, Gallager HS: Carcinoma of the breast: The prognostic significance of extranodal extension of axillary disease. Cancer 39:2280–2285, 1977.

166. Steinthal C: Dauerheilung des brustkerbses. Beitr Z Kin Chir 47:226, 1905.

167. Lee B, Stubenbord J: Clinical index of malignancy for carcinoma of the breast. Surg Gynecol Obstet 47:812, 1928.

168. Paterson R: Treatment of malignant diseases by radium and x-rays. London, Edward Arnold, 1948.

169. Portman U: Clinical and pathological criteria as a basis for classifying cases of primary cancer of the breast. Cleve Clin Q 10:41, 1943.

170. Haagensen C, Stout A: Carcinoma of the breast: II. Criteria of operability. Ann Surg 118:859–870, 1943.

171. Haagensen CD, Cooley E, Kennedy CS, et al: Treatment of early mammary carcinoma: A Cooperative International Study. Ann Surg 157:157–179, 1963.

172. Denoix P: De l'importance d'une nomeclature uniflee dans Petude du cancer. Rev Med Franc. 28:130–132, 1947.

173. International Union Against Cancer: Clinical Stage Classification and Presentation Results, Malignant Tumors of the Breast and Larynx. Paris, International Union Against Cancer, 1958.

174. Beahrs O, Carr D, Rubin P: Manual for staging of cancer. Philadelphia, JB Lippincott, 1977.

175. Greene F, Page D, Fleming I, et al: AJCC cancer staging manual, 6th ed. New York, Springer, 2002.

SECTION VII

Prognostic Factors for Breast Cancer

chapter 24

Clinically Established Prognostic Factors in Breast Cancer

TONCRED M. STYBLO | WILLIAM C. WOOD

Nomenclature

Prognostic factors have grown in importance as the options for the treatment of breast cancer have increased. By definition, prognostic factors (Table 24-1) are quantifiable data about the tumor or host that provide information about the expected outcome of a population of patients with similar defining characteristics in the absence of systemic therapy. Several facts that follow from this definition are often overlooked in clinical medicine. The first is that the prognostic value, which may be clearly defined for a population, bears only limited application to any individual within that population. Patients should not be terrorized by membership in a high-risk population, and they should not be made to feel invincible by membership in a favorable risk group. The second fact is that with the broad application of systemic therapy, less and less information will become available about prognostic factors in the absence of such therapy. The best example of a prognostic factor is lymph node status, the degree to which the axillary lymph nodes have been colonized by metastatic breast cancer.[1-5]

Some parameters of a tumor that were measured and originally described as prognostic factors are now considered primarily predictive factors (see Table 24-1). The best example of a predictive factor is estrogen receptor (ER) status. It is of great clinical importance as a predictor of response to hormonal therapy. Certain tumor parameters, such as hormone receptor status, are both prognostic factors and predictive factors and may be considered separately for their contributions to each of these areas.

In the past, prognostic indicators were valued both for their ability to offer a glimpse of risk—desired by both the patient and the physician—and in a related way, the importance of systemic adjuvant therapy. Prognostic factors can be used to define a population of patients at so little risk of progression or recurrence of breast cancer that systemic therapy may be avoided.[6,7] This is recognized as increasingly important now that the series of overviews from the Early Breast Cancer Trialists' Collaborative Group have demonstrated that the relative value of adjuvant therapy applies to all women with breast cancer.[8-11] Only those with truly minimal risk can be dismissed from consideration because the absolute benefit is so small. On the other hand, studies of the adverse effects of adjuvant therapy that were initially focused on dose-limiting toxicities are beginning to quantify other toxicities, such as neurocognitive dysfunction associated with cytotoxic chemotherapy.[12-14] With the recognition that an improvement in survival accruing to 2% to 3% of certain subgroups may be achieved at a cost of toxicity accruing to 20% or more of the patients, the need for more precise prognostic factors has grown. Can we divide the most favorable groups of women into those at greater and lesser risk in the future? And of at least as great importance, can we identify predictive factors that will allow us to determine—independent of risk—whether the contemplated therapy will be effective against her tumor?

Clinically established prognostic factors are those that meet the following criteria:
- Are reproducibly associated with a better or worse prognosis at a level of clinical utility
- Provide independent information not available by more easily measured parameters (this requires multivariate analysis with other established factors)
- Are reproducible in multiple clinics or laboratories
- Have demonstrated prognostic value in prospective trials

The literature of prognostic and predictive factors is replete with retrospective analysis of data sets. Although these are useful in generating hypotheses, any of multiple parameters may relate to outcome by play of chance in a given data set. If the data set is large, the statistical significance value of such chance associations may appear great. It is only when evaluated prospectively, at

TABLE 24-1

Prognostic and Predictive Factors for Breast Cancer

Standard Prognostic Factors

Lymph node status

Tumor size

Histologic grade

Age

Predictive Factors

Estrogen and/or progesterone receptor status

HER2 overexpression

---

best, or in multiple other data sets retrospectively, that prognostic value may be validated. Of such prognostic values, some may be associated with other values, such as nodal status or tumor size. Unless significant additional prognostic information is added, as evaluated with multivariate statistical methods, they lack clinical utility.

The two best-established prognostic factors form the basis of clinical and pathologic staging (Table 24-2).

Both nodal status and tumor size represent a summation of biologic effects in both the host and tumor that relate to the rate of tumor progression and the time from the initiation of the tumor or the development of its blood supply. Thus, a very indolent cancer biologically, long undetected, may present at an identical stage to an extremely biologically aggressive tumor present for a lesser time. Other prognostic factors, such as markers of proliferation, may distinguish between these two scenarios in a specific individual.

The most powerful adjuvant therapy demonstrated to date—tamoxifen in a premenopausal receptor-positive individual or third-generation aromatase inhibitor in a postmenopausal individual—achieved only a 50% reduction in annual risk of recurrence.[10,15] Although the ability to identify individuals who lack ERs or progesterone receptors (PRs) and who will consequently not benefit at all from tamoxifen therapy is a great triumph, greater still will be the ability to define predictive factors that will identify the responders from the nonresponders in the receptor-positive population. This is even more true in the case of cytotoxic chemotherapy.[6,16] Dose-dense

---

TABLE 24-2

TNM Classification of Breast Cancer

Classification	Definition
Primary Tumor (T)	
T_X	Primary tumor cannot be assessed
T_0	No evidence of primary tumor
Tis	Carcinoma in situ
Tis (DCIS)	Ductal carcinoma in situ
Tis (LCIS)	Lobular carcinoma in situ
Tis (Paget)	Paget disease of the nipple with no tumor (Paget disease associated with a tumor is classified according to the size of the tumor.)
T_1	Tumor ≤ 2 cm in greatest dimension
T_1mic	Microinvasion ≤ 0.1 cm in greatest dimension
T_{1a}	Tumor >0.1 cm but ≤ 0.5 cm in greatest dimension
T_{1b}	Tumor >0.5 cm but ≤ 1 cm in greatest dimension
T_{1c}	Tumor >1 cm but ≤ 2 cm in greatest dimension
T_2	Tumor >2 cm but ≤ 5 cm in greatest dimension
T_3	Tumor >5 cm in greatest dimension
T_4	Tumor of any size with direct extension to chest wall or skin, only as described below
T_{4a}	Extension to chest wall, not including pectoralis muscle
T_{4b}	Edema (including peau d'orange) or ulceration of the skin of the breast, or satellite skin nodules confined to the same breast
T_{4c}	Both T_{4a} and T_{4b}
T_{4d}	Inflammatory carcinoma
Regional Lymph Nodes (N)	
N_X	Regional lymph nodes cannot be assessed (eg, previously removed)
N_0	No regional lymph node metastasis
N_1	Metastasis in movable ipsilateral axillary lymph node(s)
N_2	Metastases in ipsilateral axillary lymph nodes fixed or matted, or in clinically apparent* ipsilateral internal mammary nodes in the absence of clinically evident axillary lymph node metastasis
N_{2a}	Metastasis in ipsilateral axillary lymph nodes fixed to one another (matted) or to other structures
N_{2b}	Metastasis only in clinically apparent* ipsilateral internal mammary nodes and in the absence of clinically evident axillary axillary lymph node metastasis

TABLE 24-2—Cont.

TNM Classification of Breast Cancer

Classification	Definition
N_3	Metastasis in ipsilateral infraclavicular lymph node(s), or in clinically apparent* ipsilateral internal mammary lymph node(s) and in the presence of clinically evident axillary lymph node metastasis; or metastasis in ipsilateral supraclavicular lymph node(s) with or without axillary or internal mammary lymph node involvement
N_{3a}	Metastasis in ipsilateral infraclavicular lymph node(s) and axillary lymph node(s)
N_{3b}	Metastasis in ipsilateral internal mammary lymph node(s) and axillary lymph node(s)
N_{3c}	Metastasis in ipsilateral supraclavicular lymph node(s)
Regional Lymph Nodes (pN)[†]	
pN_X	Regional lymph nodes cannot be assessed (eg, previously removed or not removed for pathologic study)
pN_0	No regional lymph node metastasis histologically, no additional examination for isolated tumor cells[‡]
$pN_0(i-)$	No regional lymph node metastasis histologically, negative immunohistochemical staining
$pN_0(i+)$	Isolated tumor cells identified histologically or by positive immunohistochemical staining, no cluster >0.2 mm[§]
$pN_0(mol-)$	No regional lymph node metastasis histologically, negative molecular findings (RT-PCR)
$pN_0(mol+)$	No regional lymph node metastasis histologically, positive molecular findings (RT-PCR)
pN_1	Metastasis in one to three axillary lymph nodes, and/or internal mammary nodes with microscopic disease detected by sentinel lymph node dissection but not clinically apparent*
pN_{1mi}	Micrometastasis (>0.2 mm, non >2mm)
pN_{1a}	Metastasis in one to three axillary lymph nodes
pN_{1b}	Metastasis in internal mammary nodes with microscopic disease detected by sentinel lymph node dissection but not clinically apparent*
pN_{1c}	Metastasis in one to three axillary lymph nodes[‖] and in internal mammary lymph nodes with microscopic disease detected by sentinel lymph node dissection but not clinically apparent*
pN_2	Metastasis in four to nine axillary lymph nodes, or in clinically apparent* internal mammary lymph nodes in the absence of axillary lymph node metastasis

RT-PCR, reverse transcriptase–polymerase chain reaction.
*Clinically apparent is defined as detected by imaging studies (excluding lymphoscintigraphy) or by clinical examination.
[†]Classification is based on axillary lymph node dissection with or without sentinel lymph node dissection.
[‡]Classification based solely on sentinel lymph node dissection without subsequent axillary lymph node dissection is designated (sn) for "sentinel node," such as $pN_0(i+)(sn)$.
[§]Isolated tumor cells are defined as single tumor cells or small cell clusters 0.2 mm, usually detected only by immunohistochemical or molecular methods but they may be verified on hematoxylin and eosin stains. Isolated tumor cells do not usually show evidence of metastatic activity (e.g., proliferation or stromal reaction). Definition of (i+) was adapted in 2003 to be consistent with the updated International Union Against Cancer (UICC) classification.[20]
[‖]If associated with more than three positive axillary lymph nodes, the internal mammary nodes are classified as pN_{3b} to reflect increased tumor burden.
Adapted from Greene FL, Page DL, Fleming ID, et al: AJCC cancer staging manual, 6th ed. New York, Springer, 2002.

therapy is associated with greater population benefit than less intensive chemotherapy in clinical adjuvant trials. Certain data suggest that this benefit accrues from a subpopulation of individuals who require this greater dose density and that many other individuals would do as well with less aggressive chemotherapy.[6,16] Predictive factors that will reproducibly define these subpopulations are the subject of active investigation.

Prognostic Factors

AXILLARY LYMPH NODES

The degree of involvement of axillary lymph nodes by metastatic tumor cells is the dominant prognostic factor for later systemic disease.[2] Oncologists believe that virtually all women with axillary lymph node involvement should receive adjuvant systemic therapy.[17-19] Other prognostic factors and combinations of such factors have repeatedly been shown to be of equal or greater value in a given retrospective database, but when such factors or combination of factors have been tested prospectively, axillary lymph node status has been shown to be more predictive. This is understandable because any parameters of the primary tumor are surrogates for the likelihood of metastatic involvement. The potential for metastatic spread also depends on interaction with host resistance. Axillary lymph node status reflects actual end-results data on the interaction between tumor aggressiveness and host defense mechanisms. Therefore, it is not surprising that it provides the most important prognostic measure available in clinical decision making.

Clinical staging of axillary lymph nodes is notoriously inaccurate: The difference is 33% in clinical evaluation of axillary nodes, even by experienced clinicians. Cutler and Connelly[20] found that among patients who have clinically negative nodes, 38% had evidence of nodal metastases on pathologic examination and in those who had clinically suspicious nodes, the nodes were pathologically negative 38% of the time. Fisher and colleagues reported that the false-positive and false-negative clinical evaluation rates for axillary nodes were 24% and 39%, respectively, and the overall error in clinical staging was 32%.[21,22] Smart, Myers, and Gloeckler[23] reported that 35% of clinically negative lymph nodes had metastases detected on pathologic examination, and 87% of those considered clinically positive contained metastases. Because the clinical staging of axillary nodes is so inaccurate and accurate staging is so important, histopathologic axillary lymph node staging is necessary to stage patients accurately and assign population risks for considering adjuvant therapy. To avoid the consequences of axillary dissection for those with negative axillae, a variety of radiologic and nuclear medicine techniques for diagnosis have been attempted. They have all proved less than accurate in predicting the presence or absence of small axillary nodal metastases, even though some of the techniques (e.g., positron emission tomography) may surpass clinical examination in accuracy. The use of sentinel lymph node biopsy to limit axillary dissection in those with nodal metastases has revolutionized axillary lymph node staging.

The adoption of sentinel lymph node biopsy has, however, introduced other areas of controversy in prognostic factor research. The first issue concerns the additional value of the number of involved lymph nodes in planning adjuvant systemic therapy. If a patient has a clinically positive node, the risk of systemic failure is roughly 70% at 10 years.[24] Independent of the question of control of axillary disease is the question of additional prognostic information related to the number of involved lymph nodes. Clinical trials are under way to better define this question.

The identification of a limited number of sentinel lymph nodes invited a focused pathologic examination of these nodes. This has included multiple histologic sections (versus one or two),[25] the use of immunohistochemistry (IHC) with cytokeratin stains to identify tiny foci of breast cancer cells that escape notice on hematoxylin and eosin (H&E) staining,[26,27] and the use of polymerase chain reaction (PCR) to search for "breast cancer RNA" in these lymph nodes. Complicating this question is the pervasive use of core needle biopsy for diagnosis with the introduction of tumor cell clumps into local lymphatics. This has been demonstrated to lead to in transit cell clumps in the subcapsular spaces of axillary lymph nodes. Although this is clearly different than an established metastasis in an axillary lymph node, it may also reflect tumor volume, lack of tumor cellular adhesion, or other factors that may be of prognostic influence.

Micrometastases to axillary lymph nodes, defined as metastases less than 2 mm in diameter, have been found in some studies to have the same prognostic significance as negative nodes.[3,28,29] Other authors have suggested a worse prognosis.[30–32] However, any difference in outcome between the populations is not dramatic and calls into question whether this is additional prognostic information that should influence individual therapeutic decision making. Cells seen in lymph nodes with IHC but not with H&E are similarly of uncertain significance. The present consensus is that axillary micrometastases identified only with IHC should be noted but that the patient be staged as "node negative." Any such clinical consensus is fragile.

Because virtually all women with axillary lymph nodes involved by breast cancer metastases will be offered adjuvant systemic therapy, it is in advising node-negative patients concerning adjuvant therapy decisions that all the other prognostic and predictive factors are considered.

TUMOR SIZE

Tumor size is probably the most important single, secondary prognostic factor for risk of recurrence and consequent benefit from systemic therapy in axillary node–negative breast cancer. Tumor size also affects axillary node involvement. Axillary nodes were involved in 15% of patients with tumors smaller than 1.1 cm in diameter and in 60% of those with tumors 5.5 cm in diameter or larger. Small tumors associated with positive nodes had a better prognosis than large tumors with positive nodes. Survival decreased with increasing tumor size in all node categories (Fig. 24-1).[33] There is a clear relationship between the size of the primary tumor and recurrence and survival rates. Tumor size 1 cm or smaller was associated with a very favorable prognosis in studies by Rosen and colleagues[29] and Carter, Allen, and Henson.[34] Subsequent studies have reinforced the importance of a prognostic break at 1 cm for node-negative tumors with 98% to 99% distant disease-free outcomes.[7,35] Node-negative patients with tumors 1 cm or smaller should receive adjuvant systemic therapy only on investigative protocols. Patients with tumors larger than 2 cm benefit significantly from adjuvant therapy, and those with tumors measuring 1 to 2 cm should be evaluated for risks and benefits based on careful examination of other prognostic factors.

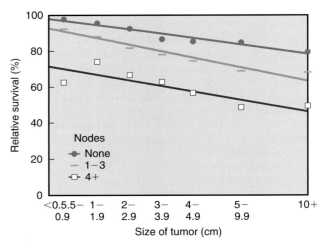

Figure 24-1 Invasive female breast cancer. Five-year relative survival rates by tumor size and number of positive regional lymph nodes, excluding cases with further extension or distant metastasis. (Surveillance, Epidemiology, and End Results [SEER] data, 1977 to 1982.)

HISTOLOGIC GRADING SYSTEM

Histopathologic analysis is based on individual characteristics such as nuclear grade, gland formation (e.g., tumor grading), or the clustering of various cytologic and histologic features into special types of breast carcinoma. Several histologic grading systems have been described and have prognostic value in the evaluation of breast carcinoma. Two commonly used grading systems were those of Scarff, Blume, Richardson, and Fisher and coworkers.[36] Both evaluated architectural arrangement of cells or tubule formation, degree of nuclear differentiation, and mitotic rate, although each system used distinct and differently weighted histologic criteria. These grading systems have been shown to be poorly reproducible and to have marked interobserver variation. Today the Nottingham combined histologic grade is recommended.[37] Nuclear grading is also subjective, but there is more concordance on grade I of III and grade III of III.

Regardless of the grading system used, grade I or its equivalent identifies a small subset of axillary node–negative patients at very low risk of recurrence and death from breast cancer. Grade I cancers up to 2 cm in diameter have a systemic failure rate of only 2% at 5 years.[38]

In addition to nuclear grade, another important indicator of favorable prognosis is histologic tumor type. A number of classifications are aimed at grouping breast cancer according to the histologic growth pattern and structural characteristics.[39–41] Breast cancers generally arise from the two major functional units of the breast: lobules and ducts. Invasive ductal and invasive lobular histologies behave similarly, and the differentiation has no particular prognostic significance. They are further classified as noninvasive or cancers in situ if the malignant cells fail to traverse the basement membrane and as infiltrating or invasive if the malignant cells do invade the basement membrane.

Certain histologic types of breast cancer, even though they are invasive, have a more favorable prognosis. About 20% to 30% of all breast cancers are classified as special, and their frequency has increased as a result of mammographic detection of smaller carcinomas.[42] The histologic features that define special types of carcinomas are present homogeneously throughout more than 90% of the lesion; however, when these features are present throughout only 75% to 90% of the carcinoma, the prognosis may be only slightly better. The three special types of invasive breast cancer are tubular, mucinous (or colloid), and medullary.

Tubular carcinoma has an excellent prognosis.[43,44] It accounts for some 3% to 5% of all breast cancers but may be the most prevalent of the special breast cancers. It is associated with a favorable prognosis when it occurs in its pure form and meets the histologic criteria. Invasive cribriform carcinoma is very similar, both histologically and biologically, to tubular carcinoma.

Colloid carcinoma is a glandular papillary or glandular cystic tumor that demonstrates a high degree of maturity and prominent mucin surrounding the cellular aggregates. It has also been called mucinous or gelatinous carcinoma. A favorable prognosis is associated with colloid carcinoma only when it occurs in the pure form. It accounts for 2% to 4% of all invasive breast cancers and usually affects older women. Women who have pure mucinous carcinomas have a 10-year survival rate of about 90%. It is more often seen in the mixed form and, in that context, does not have the favorable prognosis.[22,45–49] Generally, special-type carcinomas are low grade. An exception is medullary carcinoma.

Medullary carcinoma is a parenchyma-rich tumor with little stroma that shows a marked lymphoid infiltrate. These tumors have a favorable prognosis despite a high degree of cellular pleomorphism and a high mitotic rate. Generally, the tumors are well circumscribed and may be large, but size does not seem to affect prognosis adversely.[50,51] Medullary carcinomas account for 5% to 7% of all breast cancers. Bloom, Richardson, and Field,[52] in a 20-year follow-up, reported a 74% survival rate for patients with medullary carcinoma, as compared with 14% for those who had other types. Typical medullary breast carcinoma is a favorable histologic type of breast carcinoma with very good prognosis for pathologically node-negative patients.[53]

Pure infiltrating papillary carcinoma is rare: It accounts for only 0.3% to 1.5% of all breast cancers. Intraductal papillary growth is a common component of breast cancer of many other histologic types, and like colloid carcinoma, unless the papillary carcinoma is present in the pure form, it is not associated with a more favorable prognosis.[54]

Adverse histologic features such as lymphatic vessel or blood vessel invasion may be noted at the time of diagnosis. These findings are strongly related to the presence of lymph node metastases and are consequently of moderate prognostic significance. Despite their association with increased risk, they are not of independent significance sufficient for them to influence clinical decision making regarding such things as systemic therapy.

AGE AND RACE

Age at diagnosis has proved to be an important prognostic factor. Younger age is a major risk factor for bad outcome in breast cancer. A multivariate analysis of more than 4000 women younger than 50 years of age demonstrated that the hazard ratio set at 1 for women 40 to 44 years of age and 45 to 49 years of age, was 1.8 for those younger than 30 years of age, 1.7 for those 30 to 34, and 1.5 for those 35 to 39. These differences were highly statistically significant.[55] There have been numerous reviews of population studies examining race as an independent prognostic marker in breast cancer. Using Surveillance, Epidemiology, and End Results (SEER) data, Eley and colleagues noted a higher mortality for African Americans, but this was not statistically significant when other variables were controlled.[56] Simon and Severson did not identify race as an independent predictor of survival in their study.[57] Joslyn and West also used SEER data to examine race and breast cancer survival. Race was an independent predictor of survival in this study and others.[58–60] This epidemiologic observation that race is associated with mortality almost certainly reflect differences in the molecular biology of breast cancer in these populations.[61]

Predictive Factors

STEROID RECEPTORS

The measurement of ERs and PRs has become standard practice in the evaluation of patients with primary breast cancer. The measurement can be performed accurately on paraffin-embedded sections of formaldehyde-fixed breast tissue by using immunohistochemical assays, and results correlate well with those of the biochemical (Dextran-coated charcoal) assays. Results from paraffin-embedded sections agree very closely with those from frozen sections, so frozen tissue is not needed for optimal results.[62]

Although there is a modest prognostic effect of receptor status, it disappears by 5 years. Much data on the prognostic significance of hormone receptor assays is confounded by the predictive value of receptor positivity. Data from both the National Surgical Adjuvant Breast Project (NSABP) and the National Cancer Institute (NCI) Breast Intergroup have been confirmed by the Early Breast Cancer Trialists' Collaborative Overview of all randomized trials.[10] These all show that the benefits of tamoxifen, the most potent therapy in preventing systemic failure of breast cancer, are confined to patients with receptor-positive tumors. Thus, the treatment benefit prediction confounds the prognostic value except when it is measured in patients who have not received systemic therapy.

DNA AND S PHASE

Proliferative rate can be determined by studying the percentage of cells in the DNA synthetic phase (S phase) of the cell cycle. It does not require fresh tissue but can be performed on frozen or formalin-fixed paraffin-embedded material. Cell proliferation can also be assessed with an immunohistochemical assay that detects and quantifies cellular proteins unique to proliferating cells in either single cells or tissue sections. Proliferation-dependent antigens have been identified, including Ki-67 and proliferating cell nuclear antigen (PCNA).[63] Recent reports demonstrate that an increased percentage of S phase predicts early recurrence or poor survival for breast cancer patients who are either axillary node negative or axillary node positive. This is the only factor, other than size and grade that has been shown in multivariate analysis to add prognostic information in multiple population studies. It is unclear whether measures of proliferation are superior to the less expensive measure of histologic grade assessed at the time of diagnosis.

EPIDERMAL GROWTH FACTOR RECEPTOR FAMILY

Over the past decade, many growth factors and their receptors have been found to be expressed in primary breast cancers.[64] Some of these are estrogen regulated, some are prognostically important, and the role of many remains unknown.[65] Epidermal growth factor receptors are upregulated in approximately 25% to 40% of breast cancers, usually ER-negative cases.[66] The upregulation occurs at a transcriptional level. Overexpression of epidermal growth factor receptor is associated with poor prognosis and hormone resistance[55,67] in lymph node–positive and lymph node–negative cases. Another member of the family, ERB2, or HER2, is overexpressed in 20% to 30% of cases, usually as a result of gene amplification.[68] It usually results in overexpression of the encoded transmembrane protein p185. This is associated with poorer prognosis for lymph node–positive cases, and coexpression with epidermal growth factor receptors contributes to a particularly poor outcome.[69] The value of HER2 overexpression is a predictive factor for response to the anti-erbB2 drug trastuzumab (Herceptin) and to the small-molecule inhibitor of the tyrosine kinase domains of HER1 and HER2 lapatinib (Tykerb).[70] It is best assayed with fluorescence in situ hybridization (FISH), although immunohistochemical stains can be used to select candidates for FISH analysis. IHC negative or 1+ tissue is extremely unlikely to overexpress HER2 when studied with FISH. Results may vary among studies depending on the type of assay used and the target of the antibody in IHC assays. Controversy reigns over the role of HER2 overexpression as a predictive factor for tamoxifen resistance, sensitivity to certain cytotoxic agents, or dose density of chemotherapy. In the past, it has been suggested that pregnancy-associated breast cancer has a poor prognosis. When pregnant patients are matched stage for stage with control subjects, survival seems equivalent, although pregnant patients have more advanced-stage disease.[69,71]

Summary

How can all of these various prognostic factors be used to make rational treatment decisions? The first step in the process is to determine recurrence probability for the subpopulation of patients with a similar profile of established prognostic factors. Oncologists agree that axillary nodal metastases mark a population of breast cancer patients who should receive adjuvant systemic therapy. Within this group of patients the number of involved axillary lymph nodes remains the most powerful predictor of prognosis, overwhelming the results of the other factors.

In the absence of nodal metastases, tumor size and grade or proliferative index, together with the possibility of special histologies, allow patients to be sorted into groups of extremely low risk or increasing risk. The following have a very low risk of distant metastatic disease and, hence, the most favorable prognosis:
- In situ breast carcinoma: <1% at 10 yr
- T_{1a} or T_{1b} N_0 M_0 invasive breast carcinoma: <2% at 10 yr
- T_1 N_0 M_0 histologic grade I invasive breast carcinoma: ~2% at 5 yr

Some oncologists have suggested that adjuvant systemic therapy is appropriate for all patients with invasive breast cancer, regardless of prognostic factors. With evidence of neurocognitive deficits detectable in roughly 20% of women receiving cytotoxic chemotherapy, it is difficult to propose its use outside of a prospective clinical trial in the subpopulation with only a 2% risk of failure in the next decade who can expect a benefit of 1% or less. For any not in this group with a most favorable prognosis, adjuvant systemic therapy should be considered.

If prognostic factors can identify the populations at risk, predictive factors can identify therapies that will not be effective for certain subgroups. Hormone receptor–negative tumors will not respond to tamoxifen, and tumors that do not overexpress HER2 will not respond to trastuzumab. Decades of basic and clinical research have identified breast cancer as a heterogeneous disease with ever evolving prognostic and predictive indicators. Targeted therapies have been developed for subclasses of breast cancer, such as hormonal therapies (Tamoxifen, AI) and biologic therapies (trastuzumab and lapatinib). These targeted therapies have initiated a molecular revolution in an effort to explain them. Gene expression profiling seems to confirm that the biologic heterogeneity of breast cancer has implications for treatment. One such predictor is the intrinsic-subtype classifier, which uses gene-expression profiles to distinguish among breast cancers on the basis of either their cell type of origin—the luminal cell (which is ER-positive) or the basal cell (which lacks expression of ER, the progesterone receptor, and HER2)—or whether the tumor is HER2-positive.[72]

The prognostic value of several multiple gene expression patterns or signatures using cDNA arrays has been reported. The Amsterdam group identified a 70-gene signature as an independent predicting factor for the risk of early distant metastasis.[73] Another multiple-gene approach has been developed in the United States using multiple reverse-transcriptase polymerase chain reaction (RT-PCR) assays to quantify expression of several genes in formalin-fixed paraffin embedded tissue. The 21-gene signature was analyzed as a prognostic factor and a predictive factor. The results suggest that the high recurrence score group is also predictive of response to chemotherapy (with little or no benefit of chemotherapy in the low and intermediate groups). When the recurrence score was added to age and tumor size in a multivariate Cox model, the recurrence score remains the only independent prognostic factor with a hazard ratio of 3.21 (95% CI = 2.23–4.61, $P < 0.001$).[15] DNA microarrays have made a significant contribution to classifying tumor samples into groups that can predict clinical behavior. In the 21-gene assay, neither size nor patient ages were independent prognostic factors.[72]

Can the traditional anatomic prognostic indicators be supplanted by biologic ones? At present, is not clear that the quantification of the level of expression of dozens or hundreds of genes provides more information about the potential of a cancer for metastasis, virulence,[74] and response to therapy for an individual patient than does an optimal analysis of the standard and readily available histopathologic prognostic factors. These diagnostic advances have led to the Microarray in Node-Negative Disease May Avoid Chemotherapy (MINDACT) and the Trial Assigning Individualized Options for Treatment (Rx; TAILORx) studies. These trials will use the 70-gene profile and the recurrence score, respectively, to determine prospectively which patients with ER-positive, node-negative breast cancer benefit from adjuvant chemotherapy and which patients have a risk of recurrence sufficiently low that chemotherapy is unlikely to change their outcome. The results of these trials will probably alter the standard practice eliminating the need for adjuvant chemotherapy for ER-positive breast cancer.

REFERENCES

1. Hayes DF, Isaacs C, Stearns V: Prognostic factors in breast cancer: Current and new predictors of metastasis. J Mammary Gland Biol Neoplasia 6:375–392, 2001.
2. Henderson IC, Patek AJ: The relationship between prognostic and predictive factors in the management of breast cancer. Breast Cancer Res Treat 52:261–288, 1998.
3. Clayton F, Hopkins CL: Pathologic correlates of prognosis in lymph node-positive breast carcinomas. Cancer 71:1780–1790, 1993.
4. Isaacs C, Stearns V, Hayes DF: New prognostic factors for breast cancer recurrence. Semin Oncol 28:53–67, 2001.
5. Beenken SW, Urist MM, Zhang Y, et al: Nodal status, but not tumor size, predicts local/regional recurrence after standardized surgery for breast cancer. Ann Surg 237:732–739, 2003.
6. Wood WC, Budman DR, Korzun AH, et al: Dose and dose intensity of adjuvant chemotherapy for stage II, node-positive breast carcinoma. N Engl J Med 330:1253–1259, 1994.
7. Arnesson LG, Smeds S, Fagerberg G: Recurrence-free survival in patients with small breast cancers. Eur J Surg 160:271–276, 1994.
8. Early Breast Cancer Trialists' Collaborative Group: Effects of adjuvant tamoxifen and of cytotoxic therapy on mortality in early breast cancer: An overview of 61 randomized trials among 28,896 women. N Engl J Med 319:1681–1692, 1988.
9. Early Breast Cancer Trialists' Collaborative Group: Systemic treatment of early breast cancer by hormonal, cytotoxic, or immune therapy: 133 randomised trials involving 31,000 recurrences and 24,000 deaths among 75,000 women. Lancet 339:71–85, 1992.
10. Early Breast Cancer Trialists' Collaborative Group: Tamoxifen for early breast cancer: An overview of the randomized trials. Lancet 351:1451–1467, 1998.
11. Early Breast Cancer Trialists' Collaborative Group: Polychemotherapy for early breast cancer: An overview of the randomized trials. Lancet 352:930–942, 1998.
12. van Dam FS, Schagen SB, Muller MJ, et al: Impairment of cognitive function in women receiving adjuvant treatment for high-risk breast cancer: High-dose versus standard-dose chemotherapy. J Natl Cancer Inst 90:210–219, 1998.
13. Brezden CB, Phillips KA, Abdolell M, et al: Cognitive function in breast cancer patients receiving adjuvant chemotherapy. J Clin Oncol 18:2695–2701, 2000.
14. Paganini-Hill A, Clark LJ: Preliminary assessment of cognitive function in breast cancer patients treated with tamoxifen. Breast Cancer Res Treat 64:165–181, 2000.
15. Paik S, Shak S, Tang G, et al: A multigene assay to predict recurrence of tamoxifen-treated, node-negative breast cancer. N Engl J Med 351:2817–2826, 2004.
16. Muss HB, Thor AD, Berry DA, et al: c-erbB-2 expression and response to adjuvant therapy in women with node-positive early breast cancer [published erratum appears in 331:211, 1994]. N Engl J Med 330:1260–1266, 1994.
17. Consensus Statement: Treatment of early-stage breast cancer. J Natl Cancer Inst Monogr 11:1–5, 1992.
18. Goldhirsch A, Glick JH, Gelber RD, et al: Meeting highlights: International Consensus Panel on the treatment of primary breast cancer. J Clin Oncol 19:3817–3827, 2001.
19. NIH Consensus Development Conference Statement: Adjuvant chemotherapy for breast cancer, September 9–11, 1985. CA Cancer J Clin 36, 1986.
20. Cutler SJ, Connelly RE: Mammary cancer trends. Cancer 23:767–771, 1969.
21. Fisher ER, Gregorio R, Fisher B: Prognostic significance of histopathology. London, Heinemann, 1976.
22. Fisher ER, Gregorio R, Redmond C, et al: Pathologic findings from the national surgical adjuvant breast project (protocol no. 4). II. The significance of regional node histology other than sinus histiocytosis in invasive mammary cancer. Am J Clin Pathol 65:21–30, 1987.

23. Smart CR, Myers MH, Gloeckler LA: Implications from SEER data on breast cancer management. Cancer 41:787–789, 1978.
24. Elledge RM, McGuire WL: Prognostic factors and therapeutic decisions in axillary node-negative breast cancer. Annu Rev Med 44:210, 1993.
25. Colpaert C, Vermeulen P, Jeuris W, et al: Early distant relapse in "node-negative" breast cancer patients is not predicted by occult axillary lymph node metastases, but by the features of the primary tumour. J Pathol 193:442–449, 2001.
26. Carcoforo P, Bergosi L, Basaglia E, et al: Prognostic and therapeutic impact of sentinel node micrometastasis in patients with invasive breast cancer. Tumori 88:S4–S5, 2002.
27. Tjan-Heijnen VC, Buit B, de Widt-Evert LM, et al: Micro-metastases in axillary lymph nodes: An increasing classification and treatment dilemma in breast cancer due to the introduction of the sentinel lymph node procedure. Breast Cancer Res Treat 70:81–88, 2001.
28. Huvos AG, Hutter RV, Berg JW: Significance of axillary macrometastases and micrometastases in mammary cancer. Ann Surg 173:44–46, 1971.
29. Rosen PP, Saigo PE, Braun DW Jr, et al: Occult axillary lymph node metastases from breast cancers with intramammary lymphatic tumor emboli. Am J Surg Pathol 6:639–641, 1982.
30. International (Ludwig) Breast Cancer Study Group: Prognostic importance of occult axillary lymph node micrometastases from breast cancers. Lancet 335:1565–1568, 1990.
31. Sedmak DD, Meineke TA, Knechtges DS, Anderson J: Prognostic significance of cytokeratin-positive breast cancer metastases. Mod Pathol 2: 516–520, 1989.
32. Trojani M, de Mascarel I, Bonichon F, et al: Micrometastases to axillary lymph nodes from carcinoma of breast: Detection by immunohistochemistry and prognostic significance. Br J Cancer 50:303–306, 1987.
33. Ries LA, Henson DE, Harras A: Survival from breast cancer according to tumor size and nodal status. Surg Oncol Clin North Am 3, 1994.
34. Carter CL, Allen C, Henson DE: Relation of tumor size, lymph node status, and survival in 24,740 breast cancer cases. The Surveillance, Epidemiology, End Result (SEER) Program of the National Cancer Institute. Cancer 63:181–187, 1989.
35. Wood WC, Anderson M, Lyles RH, et al: Can we select which patients with small breast cancers should receive adjuvant chemotherapy? Ann Surg 235:859–862, 2002.
36. Fisher B, Redmond C, Fisher ER, Caplan R: Relative worth of estrogen or progesterone receptor and pathologic characteristics of differentiation as indicators of prognosis in node-negative breast cancer patients: Findings from National Surgical Adjuvant Breast and Bowel Project Protocol B-06. J Clin Oncol 6:1076–1078, 1988.
37. Fitzgibbons PL, Page DL, Weaver D, et al: Prognostic factors in breast cancer. Arch Pathol Lab Med 124:966–978, 2000.
38. Lundin J, Lundin M, Holli K, et al: Omission of histologic grading from clinical decision making may result in overuse of adjuvant therapies in breast cancer: Results from a nationwide study. J Clin Oncol 19:28–36, 2001.
39. Fisher ER, Gregorio RM, Fisher B: The pathology of invasive breast cancer: A syllabus derived from the findings of the National Surgical Adjuvant Breast Project (Protocol No 4). Cancer 36:1–85, 1975.
40. Leis HP: Prognosis and recurrence of breast cancer. In Diagnosis and treatment of breast lesions. Flushing, NY, Medical Examination, 1970.
41. Robbins GF, Leis HP Jr, Hutter RVP: A rational approach to end-result of women with breast carcinoma. J Breast 3, 1977.
42. Simpson JF, Page DL: Prognostic value of histopathology in the breast. Semin Oncol 19:254–262, 1992.
43. Carstens PH, Huvos AG, Foote FW Jr, Ashikari R: Tubular carcinoma of the breast: A clinicopathologic study of 35 cases. Am J Clin Pathol 58:231–238, 1972.
44. Taylor HB, Norris HJ: Well-differentiated carcinoma of the breast. Cancer 25:687–692, 1970.
45. Geshickter CF: Gelatinous mammary cancer. Ann Surg 1938; 108:321.
46. Haagensen C: Diseases of the breast. Philadelphia, WB Saunders, 1971.
47. Hutter RVP: The influence of pathologic factors on breast cancer. Cancer 1980;46:961.
48. Melamed MR, Robbins GF, Foote FW Jr: Prognostic significance of gelatinous mammary carcinoma. Cancer 14:699–704, 1961.
49. Nemoto T, Vana J, Bedwani RN, et al: Management of survival of female breast cancer: Results of a national survey by the American College of Surgeons. Cancer 45:2917–2924,1980.
50. Moore OS, Foote FW Jr: The relatively favorable prognosis of medullary carcinoma of the breast. Cancer 2:635–642, 1949.
51. Ridolfi RL, Rosen PP, Port A, et al: Medullary carcinoma of the breast: A clinicopathologic study with a ten-year follow-up. Cancer 40:1365–1385, 1977.
52. Bloom HJ, Richardson WW, Field JR: Host resistance and survival in carcinoma of the breast: Study of 104 cases of medullary carcinoma in a series of 1411 cases of breast cancer followed for twenty years. Br Med J 3:181–188, 1970.
53. Reinfuss M, Stelmach A, Mitus J, et al: Typical medullary carcinoma of the breast: A clinical and pathological analysis of 52 cases. J Surg Oncol 60:89–94, 1995.
54. McDivitt RW, Stewart FW, Berg JW: Tumors of the breast. In Firminger HI (ed): Atlas of tumor pathology. Washington, DC: Armed Forces Institute of Pathology, 1968.
55. Bernstein V, Trong P, Speers C, et al: How young is too young? The impact of age on premenopausal breast cancer prognosis. Breast Cancer Res Treat 76:A137, 2002.
56. Eley JW, Hill HA, Chen VW, et al: Racial differences in survival from breast cancer. Results of the National Cancer Institute Black/White Cancer Survival Study. JAMA 272:947–954, 1994.
57. Simon MS, Severson RK: Racial differences in survival of female breast cancer in the Detroit metropolitan area. Cancer 77:308–414, 1996.
58. Joslyn SA, West MM: Racial differences in breast carcinoma survival. Cancer 88:114–123, 2000.
59. Coates RJ, Clark WS, Eley JW, et al: Race, nutritional status, and survival from breast cancer. J Natl Cancer Inst 82:1684–1692, 1990.
60. Heimann R, Ferguson D, Powers C, et al: Race and clinical outcome in breast cancer in a series with long-term follow-up evaluation. J Clin Oncol 15:2329–2337, 1997.
61. Porter PL, Lund MJ, Lin MG, et al: Racial differences in the expression of cell cycle-regulatory proteins in breast carcinoma. Cancer 100:2533–2542, 2004.
62. Miller RT, Hapke MR, Greene GL: Immunocytochemical assay for estrogen receptor with monoclonal antibody in routinely processed formaldehyde-fixed breast tissue: Comparison with frozen section assay with monoclonal antibody. Cancer 71:3541–3546, 1993.
63. Oza AM, Tannock IF: Clinical relevance of breast cancer biology. Hematol Oncol Clin North Am 8:1–14, 1994.
64. Lupu R: Growth control of normal and malignant breast epithelium. In Lippman ME (ed): The therapeutic implications of the molecular biology of breast cancer. Rome: John Libbey, 1991.
65. Plowman GD, Culouscou JM, Whitney GS, et al: Ligand-specific activation of HER4. Proc Natl Acad Sci USA 90:1746–1750, 1993.
66. Harris AL, Nicholson S, Sainsbury R, et al: Epidermal growth factor receptor and other oncogenes as prognostic markers. J Natl Cancer Inst Monogr 11:181–187, 1992.
67. Anderson BO, Senie RT, Vetto JT, et al: Improved survival in young women with breast cancer. Ann Surg Oncol 2:407–415, 1995.
68. Nicholson S, Sainsbury JR, Halcrow P, et al: Expression of epidermal growth factor receptors associated with lack of response to endocrine therapy in recurrent breast cancer. Lancet i:182–185, 1989.
69. Wright C, Angus B, Nicholson S, et al: Expression of c-erbB-2 oncoprotein: A prognostic indicator in breast cancer. Cancer Res 49:2087–2090, 1989.
70. Geyer CE, Forster J, Lindquist D, et al: Lapatinib plus capecitabine for HER2-positive advanced breast cancer. N Engl J Med 355:2733–2743, 2006.
71. Petrek JA: Breast cancer during pregnancy. Cancer 74 (suppl):518–527, 1994.
72. Perou CM, Sorlie T, Eisen MB, et al: Molecular portraits of human breast tumours. Nature 406:747–752, 2000.
73. van 't Veer LJ, Dai H, van de Vijver MJ, et al: Gene expression profiling predicts clinical outcome of breast cancer. Nature 415:530–536, 2002.
74. Heimann R, Hellman S: Clinical progression of breast cancer malignant behavior: What to expect and when to expect it. J Clin Oncol 18:591–599, 2000.

chapter 25

Investigational Molecular Prognostic Factors for Breast Carcinoma

HEATHER SHAH | **LISLE NABELL**

Prognostic and Predictive Factors

The identification of accurate prognostic factors that can reliably aid in assessing risk of recurrence or specific therapies remains a critical area of investigation in breast carcinoma. This search is spurred onward by two major concerns. First, we have a desire to better discern those patients who will not benefit significantly from chemotherapy; our inability to separate prognostic groups in the past has led to a pattern of overtreatment of large numbers of women in order to affect the recurrence risk of a small proportion of patients. Second, there is a need to better tailor individual therapy on the basis of gene expression. There is increasing recognition of the remarkable amount of heterogeneity in breast cancers at a molecular level, referred to as a "molecular portrait" by Perou and colleagues in their seminal paper in 2000.[1] This genetic diversity is responsible for the natural history of breast cancer and likely for differences in the responses of individual tumors to selected chemotherapeutic regimens. With improved understanding of the processes that initiate and promote tumorigenesis, we will be able to begin to truly individualize treatment regimens.

Drawing a distinction between prognostic factors and predictive factors remains relevant with regard to distinguishing models that define risk of recurrence, as opposed to calculating a response to specific interventions.[2] Prognostic factors are those measurable clinical or biologic features of a cancer that provide information about potential patient outcomes prior to initiation of any therapy. These features undoubtedly reflect inherent tumor biology relating to growth, invasion, and metastases. The major prognostic factors associated with breast cancer include the number of involved lymph nodes, tumor size, histologic grade, and hormone receptor status.[3] For example, the presence of cancer in a locoregional nodal basin is a commonly used and robust prognostic factor, one that is associated with an increased risk of recurrence.[4] In contrast, predictive factors provide information about likelihood of response to a particular therapy. The use of the estrogen receptor (ER), for example, is important clinically as a predictor of the likelihood of response to hormonal therapy. Frequently, factors may be both prognostic and predictive, blurring the distinction between these two entities. One example of this is the use of HER2, which has significant predictive value for gauging responsiveness to drugs such as trastuzumab or lapatinib, but also carries prognostic value in many studies.[5]

However, our current models of prognostic and predictive factors are quite limited. A large number of tumors recur, despite being found at an early stage, and the ability to better characterize tumors has spurred on research for other more robust prognostic and predictive markers. The critical objectives of ongoing research are to develop improved prognostic markers, which are sensitive and specific in their ability to identify individuals who do not require adjuvant treatment, as well as to develop robust predictive markers that will aid in identifying optimal treatment regimens. These two goals were named as the top research priorities in a multinational focus group charged with identifying the top ten research goals (http://www.toptenresearch.org/).

Development of Biomarkers

Despite substantial efforts, the number of reliable and informative prognostic markers has changed little over the last decade. The lack of substantive improvement has been attributed to a variety of problems, including poorly designed and analyzed clinical studies, varied approaches to scoring markers of interest, inadequate sample sizes, and technological challenges that preclude widespread usage.[6-8] In large part, the failure to move the field forward has been hampered by a significant lack of cohesion in the development of biomarkers that can be rigorously ascertained and validated externally. One of the first stumbling blocks has been the ability to define a prognostic marker by widely available and standardized methodologies. There is considerable interest about the prognostic and predictive capabilities of the marker HER2; however, the use of both gene amplification with fluorescent in situ hybridization (FISH) and immunohistochemistry (IHC) to describe the presence of amplification in laboratories without substantial experience has created difficulties with regard to inconsistent results.[9] Development of a standardized approach for measurement of HER2 expression has been addressed by the American Society of Clinical Oncology (ASCO) and College of American Pathologists (CAP) Committee on HER2 interpretation.[10] This move to formalize expectations for laboratories to develop high-quality testing of a biomarker, however, is relatively rare. Other putative markers remain of uncertain value, despite promising early studies, given difficulties with small studies or technological processing. For example, incorporation of cathepsin-D, urokinase plasminogen activator (uPA), and plasminogen activator inhibitor (PAI-1), has remained difficult outside of clinical trials because of technically demanding methodology.[11-13] Despite evidence of usefulness in assessing recurrence of breast cancer, inherent difficulties in measurement and standardization are examples of the limitations imposed by technology.[12,14] Another active area of investigation has centered around markers of increased proliferation, which have generally been correlated with a worse prognosis in newly diagnosed breast cancers.[15] However, with significant technical variation in determination of S phase, the lack of standard methodologies again has limited the standard incorporation of S phase in a routine fashion.[14] Other markers of proliferation, such as Ki-67, have multiple small studies that support its potential usefulness, but technological differences among these studies, including lack of consistent scoring methodologies, limit inclusion of Ki-67.[14-16] Thus, as new molecular markers are evaluated for their promise to improve prediction of recurrence, it will be increasingly critical that investigators apply stringent guidelines with regard to reporting and standardizing end points and results to render new markers and studies relevant.

In addressing these problems, the National Cancer Institute–European Organization for Research and Treatment of Cancer (NCI-EORTC) International Meeting on Cancer Diagnostics task force developed reporting guidelines for prognostic markers designed to build a common lexicon that would promote improved quality of new marker assessment.[7] These guidelines recommend including a descriptive overview of the study design, statistical analysis methods, and demographic information, and they endorse univariate analyses to examine the relationship of the marker of interest and clinical outcome. The use of a hazard ratio to estimate the effect of a given marker along with confidence intervals is strongly recommended.[7] This move to develop standard guidelines for prognostic markers complements general

guidelines developed by the NCI Office of Biorepositories and Biospecimens Research (http://biospecimens.cancer.gov/) for specimen acquisition and processing. A similar effort extends to the use of standardized terminology and end points for clinical trials in breast carcinoma.[17,18] It is hoped that this more structured approach will improve the usefulness of new trials exploring putative biomarkers.

Assessing prognosis of an established breast cancer has historically relied on specific clinical characteristics of the cancer, which may or may not be reflective of the inherent tumor biology. Size of the tumor, lymph node involvement, and the presence or absence of ERs and progesterone receptors (PRs) have been used to develop a calculated risk of recurrence and have influenced decisions regarding adjuvant therapy.[3] However, staging criteria and limited use of some prognostic markers by IHC have proven inadequate to separate out groups of patients on the basis of prognosis, as reflected by the percentage of stage I, node-negative patients who experience recurrent disease following appropriate care to the breast.[19] Use of biochemical and molecular makers to aid in more consistent and accurate prognostication of risk of recurrence has, however, remained elusive. Table 25-1 summarizes evidence-based conclusions

TABLE 25-1

Evidence-Based Consensus on Prognostic Factors in Breast Cancer

Prognostic Marker	CAP	ASCO	AJCC
Tumor size	↑	—	↑
Histologic grade	↑	—	↑
Estrogen receptor	↓	↑	—
HER/neu	→	→	→
Cathepsin-D	↓	—	—
Immunohistochemically based markers of proliferation*	→	—	↑
DNA ploidy	↓	—	↓
p53	→	↓	—
Urokinase plasminogen activator	—	↑	—
Bone Marrow Micrometastases	—	—	—
Multiparameter gene expression†	—	↑	↓

↑, Usefulness as prognostic factor supported by multiple studies; →, mixed results; ↓, present data do not support usefulness as a prognostic factor; —, data not available.
*Proliferation markers include Ki67, cyclin D, cyclin E, p27, p21, thymidine kinase, and topoisomerase II.
†Multiparameter gene expression assays include the Oncotype DX assay, the MammaPrint assay, the Rotterdam Signature, and the Breast Cancer Gene Expression Ratio; currently only the Oncotype DX assay was recommended by the panel for assessment of recurrence in patients treated with tamoxifen.
Data from Fitzgibbons PL, Page DL, Weaver D, et al: Prognostic factors in breast cancer. College of American Pathologists consensus statement. Arch Pathol Lab Med 124:966–978, 2000; Harris H, Fritsche H, Mennel R, et al: American Society of Clinical Oncology 2007 update of recommendations for the use of tumor markers in breast cancer. J Clin Oncol 25:5287–5312, 2007; and Singletary SE, Allred C, Ashley P, et al: Staging system for breast cancer: Revisions for the 6th edition of the AJCC cancer staging manual. Surg Clin North Am 83:803–819, 2003.

regarding several widely studied prognostic factors from the CAP Consensus Report,[4] the clinical practice guidelines from ASCO,[14] and the American Joint Committee on Cancer (AJCC) Staging Manual, sixth edition.[3]

Despite the proliferation of putative biomarkers, we have failed thus far to develop a novel biomarker that predicts outcome. However, technological advances now allow for assessment of a number of genes at one time, rather than in isolation. It is our increasing ability to deconstruct the molecular "fingerprint" of a cancer that gives us insight into the biologic behavior of breast cancer, and this has led to an explosion of new putative "molecular markers" that are currently being subjected to scrutiny in the setting of clinical trials. Relevant to this discussion is the description of a clinically relevant prognostic factor as one that (1) can be reproducibly measured; (2) is reproducibly associated with a good or poor outcome, at a level clinically significant to the patient; and (3) provides independent information that cannot be obtained more easily by measuring some other factor.[2,3,18]

Breast Cancer Tumorigenesis

Cancers are thought to arise from a series of sequential mutations that occur as a result of inherited genetic predisposition, genetic instability, or environmental effects. A common approach to studying the genetic basis of tumorigenesis involves comparing genetic changes in neoplastic breast lesions with the genetic characteristics of normal tissue. The development of immunohistochemical and molecular techniques for the identification of specific genes and gene products in archived tissue samples has made a broad patient base available to study the genetic basis of breast cancer. With the understanding that some genes have multiple roles in tumorigenesis, such studies have looked at specific genes implicated in the early stages of tumor development, including oncogenes, tumor suppressor genes, growth factor receptor genes, genes associated with the regulation of the cell cycle, and genes involved in apoptosis, as well as the presence of putative breast stem cells. In addition, researchers are attempting to identify specific genes that mark a cell's progression from early, nonaggressive cancer to aggressive metastatic disease. This process includes an increase in invasiveness, the ability to migrate and evade the immune system, and the development of angiogenesis. Biomarkers are surrogates for the underlying genetic changes that occur, leading to cancer development or resistance to therapy. Two main approaches exist in the development of predictive markers as illustrated in Figure 25-1. The first approach is the "bottom-up" approach in which a targeted pathway is deconstructed and examined in detail. A prognostic signature is built on the basis of mechanistic pathways and is then tested in preclinical and clinical models. In contrast, the "top-down" approach uses clinical outcomes to produce predictive signatures that may then implicate altered pathways of transformation.[20]

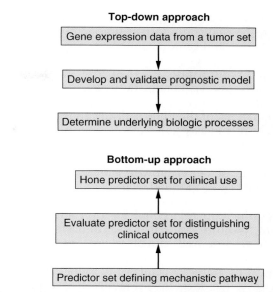

Figure 25-1 Two main approaches to the development of predictive markers. (Adapted from Liu ET: Mechanism-derived gene expression signatures and predictive biomarkers in clinical oncology. Proc Natl Acad Sci USA 102:3531–3532, 2005. Copyright 2005 National Academy of Sciences, USA.)

Investigational Molecular Markers

BREAST STEM CELLS

There is increasing evidence that within a tumor only small subsets of cells are actually capable of continued self-renewal and that these cells originate from the stem cell compartment.[21-23] Although investigators have viewed the general concept of tumor growth as an unregulated, continual process, they have suggested that the majority of cells that comprise a tumor do not actually have the capacity for unlimited self-renewal. Rather, they propose that this ability for self-renewal may rest with a subpopulation of cells that can be defined by an invasive gene signature.[21,23] These cells are thought to account for a minority of the tumor bulk, and this may explain the difficulty in characterizing these cells unless a population is enriched for their presence. Work by Al-Hajj[21] and others has helped define this putative stem cell phenotype phenotypically as CD44$^+$/CD24$^{-/lo}$, findings subsequently confirmed by other researchers.[24] These cells can be further characterized as lacking differentiated epithelial cell lineage markers, resembling stem cells, and having a significantly increased capacity to form tumors in an in vitro model when compared with the majority of tumor cells.[21,25] The shared ability to carry out self-renewal between stem cells and cancer has suggested that the cellular machinery, which drives self-renewal by stem cells, may be co-opted by cancer cells.

Although a number of pathways have been implicated, tumor suppressor genes such as phosphatase and tensin homolog deleted on chromosome 10 (PTEN), as well as tumor protein p53 (TP53), are thought to play a critical role in governing stem cell growth. PTEN is reported to be frequently lost in cancer through mutation or deletion, and germline mutations appear to occur commonly in hereditary cancer syndrome.[26] A dual protein/lipid phosphatase, PTEN opposes the action of phosphatidylinositol 3-kinase (PI3K) and Akt to reduce signaling through this critical growth-promoting pathway.[27] Alterations of the PI3K pathway appear common in a variety of cancers, and PI3K is often identified as having activating mutations. Many components of this system have been described as integral in the process of the promotion of cancer growth, with recent activating mutations described in the PI3K gene linked specifically to the appearance of breast cancer.[27] Other signaling pathways, which appear central in governing stem cell growth, include the epidermal growth factor receptor (EGFR), platelet-derived growth factor (PDGF), Wnt/β-catenin, and Notch. The Wnt pathway, in particular, has emerged as a crucial regulator of stem cell growth and renewal.[22] Members of this family of glycoproteins inhibit phosphorylation of β-catenin, which is involved in cell-cell adhesion and integral in activation of several signal-transduction pathways, which result in proliferation and invasion.[28] These pathways control self-renewal, and in conjunction with increased drug efflux transporter systems present in stem cells, have been implicated as critical pathways in driving cancer progression.[22,29] Pathologists have identified features of a migratory phenotype by tumor cells, which occurs at the periphery of cancers, as reflecting invasive potential. The phenotypic changes which appear to result in this "epithelial-mesenchymal transition," termed EMT, appear to be driven by transforming growth factor-β (TGF-β) and activation of tyrosine kinase pathways, with repression of E-cadherin.[30] EMT has been implicated as a process whereby early stem cells gain invasive properties, thought to account for the findings of putative stem cells at sites distant from the primary tumor.[29] For a comprehensive review of stem cell research, refer to the excellent review by Mimeault and associates.[29]

There is preliminary evidence to suggest that cancer stem cells may be particularly resistant to cytotoxic agents and to radiotherapy. Perhaps this may occur because of infrequent cycling or the presence of multidrug efflux transporters, including P-glycoprotein encoded by the MDR1 (ABCB1) gene, the multidrug resistance-associated protein 1 (MRP1), and breast cancer resistance protein-1 gene products, which are frequently overexpressed in cancer cells.[31,32] It has been hypothesized that the presence of these highly resistant stem cells may account for our current failure to eradicate established tumors with common cytotoxic agents.[22,32] In this theory, there is a disconnect from the gratifying shrinkage that occurs from most cancers following chemotherapy administration in that a reduction in size of the cancer is not accompanied by a reduction in the size of the stem cell population. This failure to reduce the number of tumor stem cells may occur because of slow inherent growth rates and intrinsic resistance to most conventional therapies, resulting from the embryonic nature of the stem cell, which potentially explains the common regrowth of cancers and/or late recurrences. Thus, to effectively eradicate a tumor, therapy

would need to be directed at the bulk of differentiated cells as well as the more primitive stem cells.[32,33]

Liu and collaborators have shown that tumors that could be characterized by having a high proportion of tumorigenic cells, defined by the CD44$^+$/CD24$^{-/lo}$ phenotype, were associated with a higher likelihood of recurrence. These findings were replicated in breast cancer, lung cancer, prostate carcinoma, and medulloblastoma.[23] Additional studies have suggested that these cells are particularly resistant to chemotherapy, hormonal therapy and also to radiation.[34-37] Li and coworkers[33] recently performed an elegant clinical trial evaluating the response of putative breast stem cells to more targeted therapies. Building on the hypothesis that conventional chemotherapy may cause cytoreduction in tumor bulk only, without affecting stem cells, they designed a trial using targeted therapy first, followed by chemotherapy. Based on observations that the EGFR/HER2 pathway is particularly important in promoting growth of stem cells, they used a small molecule inhibitor of the epidermal growth factor tyrosine kinase receptor, lapatinib, as a 6-week treatment prior to chemotherapy with trastuzumab in HER2-amplified, locally advanced breast cancers. The authors found that the HER2-positive tumors treated with lapatinib demonstrated a slight decrease in CD44$^+$/CD24$^{-/lo}$ cells and a decrease in the number of cells capable of self-renewal.[33] This stands in stark contrast to the group of patients treated only with chemotherapy who demonstrated increased numbers of self-renewal cells. There is thus increasing evidence that agents used to block the earliest signaling pathways in self-renewal may ultimately prove to be more effective in reducing cancer recurrence. The ability to identify these cells accurately and target them effectively may prove to be important steps forward in improving cancer treatment.

BONE MARROW MICROMETASTASES AND CIRCULATING TUMOR CELLS

Circulating tumor cells (CTCs) are cells detected in the blood that possess the genetic and protein characteristics of breast cancer. These cells can be isolated from the more common leukocytes by the use of an antibody-coated immunomagnetic bead or by sorting on the basis of surface antigen expression.[38] The importance of CTCs has been the subject of some debate in the literature, as a result of the observation that not all CTCs are capable of forming tumors; this phenomenon is potentially explained by tumor heterogeneity.[1] Gene expression profiling using the reverse-transcriptase polymerase chain reaction (RT-PCR) process overcomes the technical limitations of IHC and can be performed on peripheral blood to aid in identification of the CTCs. Although some studies have used this process to provide early information regarding response to therapies,[39] assays for CTCs could potentially be more important if they are able to provide additional prognostic information in early-stage breast cancer. Several studies have tackled the use of this potential marker in early-stage breast cancer and linked CTCs to disease-free survival.[40,41] Using IHC or RT-PCR methodology, most studies have correlated the presence of CTCs after surgery with adverse outcomes. However, many of the earlier studies were underpowered and used differing techniques to denote a tumor cell. Preliminary studies assessing the prognostic value of circulating cytokeratin-19 positive cells seem promising,[40–42] but developing a consistent methodology and defining markers that correlates with prognosis in early-stage breast cancer has proved daunting. Much like molecular profiling of breast cancers, discussed later in this chapter, most studies demonstrate improved correlation with prognosis when several genes are assayed as opposed to one marker in isolation.

Similar to the process of detection of CTCs, the detection of microscopic disease in the bone marrow is of considerable interest with regard to refining our current staging processes. Although a meta-analysis recently reported the presence of IHC-detected tumor cells in bone marrow in patients with operable breast cancer correlated with early relapse,[43] other studies have not found a consistent association.[44] Conventional assessment by routine stains, IHC and RT-PCR have been used to evaluate the presence of micrometastases in the bone marrow. The specificity of these assays however, has been unclear and importantly there appears to be considerable false-positive rates depending the on detection assay.[44] Nevertheless, most studies show that detection of disseminated tumor cells in the bone marrow of patients with breast cancer is an independent risk factor for the subsequent development of metastatic disease.[43]

Stromal Gene Expression

Evidence over the past several years has suggested that the tumoral stroma do not play a passive role in cancer progression. In fact, there is increasing evidence that interactions between tumor cells and stromal cells are intimately linked to the processes of tumorigenesis, invasion, and metastasis.[45–47] A number of diverse growth factors, chemokines, metalloproteinases, vascular endothelial growth factor (VEGF), stromal cell–derived factor-1 (SDG-1) and uPA appear to participate in autocrine or paracrine signaling, which influences tumor cell behavior.[46,47] In support of these interactions, Allinen and associates have described transcriptional profiles of cells both comprising and surrounding in situ breast cancer, invasive breast cancer, and adjacent normal breast tissue through use of a sequential isolation technique.[48] They have found that transcriptional changes occur during all cell types during the process of cancer progression, although only the epithelial cancer cells contain genomic alterations.[48] Similar work by Patocs used microdissection to examine the epithelial and stromal components of primary breast cancers.[47] These investigators found, contrary to prior studies, that the stromal cells harbored TP53 mutations that differed from the genetic changes in the epithelial cells and that moreover, the presence of TP53 mutations in the stromal cells was associated with an increase in lymph node metastases.[47]

Using a set of 26 genes important in signaling tissue hypoxia, angiogenic response, and chemokine signaling,

Finak and colleagues[49] constructed a stroma predictor that significantly predicted for poor outcome independent of traditional prognostic factors such as ER and HER2/neu status. These findings suggest that increasingly, investigators will be mining genetic and epigenetic changes to generate prognostic models. Moreover, targeted therapies, which are directed at the stroma, are likely to become molecular targets for therapy. One example of this is the use of the anti-VEGF monoclonal antibody bevacizumab, which appears to disrupt the vascular microenvironment of brainstem cells and the process of angiogenesis.[50]

Markers of Proliferation

Markers of proliferation have commonly reflected the tumor grade and have been exhaustively studied in breast cancer as potential prognostic markers. As noted by Harris in a review of tumor markers, the category of proliferation markers has included Ki-67, thymidine kinase, topoisomerase II, cyclin D, cyclin E, and p21, among others.[14] The proliferation antigen Ki-67, has long been used as a measure of cell cycle proliferation, and high levels of expression have generally been correlated with an increased risk of recurrence, as noted in a recent meta-analysis.[51] However, varied scoring patterns and cutoff points for immunoreactivity have hampered widespread usage of this marker. Of interest, Ki-67 is included as one of the core 16 genes in the Oncotype DX assay, suggesting that when applied in a standardized fashion, this marker aids in assessing prognosis.

A large body of literature has detailed the importance of the cyclin-dependent kinases (cdks) as critical in the regulation of cell cycle progression, summarized in an elegant review by Shapiro.[52] Cyclin D–dependent kinases 4 and 6 and cyclin E-cdk2 are of particular interest as potential markers given their role in promoting cell cycle progression. Although several studies have documented elevated levels of cyclin D with breast cancer prognosis, particularly in tumors that are resistant to tamoxifen, there are conflicting studies in the literature, and difficulty in quantifying the impact of cyclin D has limited its prognostic importance.[14]

HER2/neu

The HER2 gene, a member of the EGFR family, is amplified in approximately 20% of breast cancers, where it is associated with an adverse outcome.[5] Although testing for HER2 is performed now routinely for decisions regarding adjuvant therapy with trastuzumab, there is increasing evidence that HER2 positivity may be associated with resistance to some forms of endocrine therapy and non–anthracycline-containing chemotherapy regimens.[53–55] Initial reports of improved response to neoadjuvant letrozole as compared with tamoxifen suggested that HER2 status might dictate the type of hormonal therapy chosen.[53] However, follow-up studies have not confirmed these earlier reports, and at this time, HER2 status cannot be used as a predictor of endocrine manipulation.[56,57] If HER2 is not predictive of response to hormonal manipulation, can it be used to select chemotherapy regimens? A large number of publications have suggested that HER2-positive tumors benefit from treatment with anthracycline-containing regimens.[58-60] Anthracyclines are known to inhibit the topoisomerase II alpha enzyme (TOP2A), which results in double-stranded DNA breaks and initiation of apoptosis.[61] Although there is no clear interaction of anthracyclines with HER2, it has been postulated that HER2 may serve as a marker because of the proximity of TOP2A to HER2 on chromosome 17q.[59] Many of the early reports of the potential association of HER2 status and anthracycline effect were, however, hampered by being small, underpowered studies. A recent comprehensive review of 10 trials by Pritchard and coworkers[60] suggests that HER2 status remains predictive of a response to anthracycline-containing regimens but fails to find sufficient evidence to warrant the use of TOP2A to predict response to anthracyclines.

Molecular Profiling

In the last several years, high-throughput molecular profiling, with the ability to analyze hundreds of genes of interest simultaneously, has rapidly changed the process of subdividing breast cancer into clinically distinct groups on the basis of gene expression patterns. These technological improvements, coupled with effective analytical tools, have changed our ability to assess genes that may by implicated in tumorigenesis or biologic behavior of a given tumor. Investigators are now using molecular profiling to generate a genetic blueprint of a given tumor, based on specific gene activity. These assessments have allowed further subdivision of breast cancers into relevant subclasses that appear to carry significant prognostic associations.[1,24,62] Using a cDNA expression microarray, Perou and colleagues[1] subclassified breast cancer into four distinct molecular subtypes on the basis of gene expression patterns, which segregated broadly on the basis of ER and HER2 expression. These subtypes were first identified using 65 surgical specimens, with external validation performed by application of the subtypes to independent data sets from three different patient populations. Based on gene expression profiles, the tumors were separated into a luminal epithelial/ER-positive group, a basal epithelial-like group negative for ER expression, a HER2-positive group, and a group exhibiting a "normal-like" expression signature.[1] Further extension of this work has demonstrated that there were two subgroups within the luminal group, each with a distinct profile, termed luminal A and luminal B.[63]

The molecular subtypes are clinically important in that these subgroups have different responses to treatment and different clinical courses; they have been linked to some ethnic groups and genetic changes. Further work has suggested that the luminal A, HER2, and basal type tumors are the most homogenous and reproducible. Prognostically, the luminal A type tumors have a better overall survival and are generally sensitive to endocrine

therapy, with the highest expression of ER.[63] Aggressiveness varies between the different subtypes; basal-like and HER2/neu–positive tumors tend to have higher nuclear and histologic grade and mitotic indices, with greater sensitivity to chemotherapy when compared with luminal tumors. A higher rate of recurrences with HER2 and basal subtypes is noted in most studies.[63,64] HER2-amplified tumors can be treated with targeted therapy such as trastuzumab, but they have also been found to have better response to chemotherapy than HER2-negative tumors.[65] Although the presence of amplified HER2 denotes this group, it is the absence of expression that has characterized the basal group. The basal-like tumors typically lack surface expression of ER and PR as well as HER2 expression, and thus they have been termed "triple-negative" tumors. In addition, germline *BRCA1* mutations are much more common in basal-like tumors, as is overexpression of EGFR and c-Kit.[66,67] Racial differences with regard to subtypes of breast cancer have been noted as well, suggesting further genetic predisposition to this subtype of tumor in some groups. In a population-based study of 196 African-American and 300 non–African-American women, premenopausal African-American women had an incidence of 39% basal-like tumor subtype, whereas postmenopausal women of all ethnicities and premenopausal non–African-American women had an incidence of only 15% of these basal-like tumors.[64]

One of the features of molecular subclassification of breast tumors has been the ability to use differing cytokeratin expression between these classes, which to some degree, mimics the molecular distinctions. In normal tissue, luminal epithelial cells stain with cytokeratins 8 and 18, whereas basal epithelial cells stain with cytokeratins 5 and 17.[63] This ability to distinguish basal from luminal tumors on the basis of cytokeratin expression has been observed by other researchers.[68-70] Thus, existing and commonly used IHC panels can be used to differentiate between the molecular subclasses, although without the precision of molecular profiling.

Gene Expression Signatures: Top Down

Although investigators have focused on gene expression signatures from defined groups, van't Veer and associates initially reported on the use of a 231-gene expression profile in node-negative breast cancers, which strongly predicted disease-free survival at 5 years.[62,71] Using the development of distant metastases as a dividing line with a supervised method of classification led to the identification of a core set of 70 genes derived from the original set that correlated with clinical outcome. These genes were comprised largely of genes associated with proliferation, invasion, and metastasis, and they commonly are known now as the "Amsterdam signature." Internal validation of this profile showed accurate prediction of outcome with regard to the development of metastasis in 83% of patients[62] and was later externally validated using young patients with tumors less than 5 cm in diameter; approximately half of these patients were node-negative. Using a multivariate analysis, the Amsterdam gene expression signature predicted risk of distant metastasis better than age, lymph node status, tumor dimensions, grade, invasiveness, ER expression, mastectomy, or treatment.[71] A second retrospective validation[72] evaluated 302 early-stage (T_1 to T_2) tumors in lymph node–negative women younger than 60 years of age who received no adjuvant therapy. These patients had follow-up data over 10 years, and the same 70-gene set was superior in predicting time to distant metastases and overall survival as compared to the clinical variables used in Adjuvant! Online.[72] Tissue handling was of paramount importance, given that specimens had to be snap-frozen within one hour following surgery and depended heavily on the purity of the specimen submitted.[62] The prognostic capability of this test is undergoing further evaluation in identifying patients who may not benefit from adjuvant therapy. Evaluation of this assay, known now as MammaPrint, is ongoing through the Microarray in Node-Negative Disease May Avoid Chemotherapy (MINDACT) study.

Another gene expression test requiring freshly processed tissue, referred to as the "Rotterdam signature," was reported in 2006 by Wang and coworkers.[73] This 76-gene signature evaluated patients with ER-positive and ER-negative disease, in hopes of distinguishing patients who would benefit from adjuvant chemotherapy regardless of hormonal status. The Rotterdam signature was created using 115 node-negative breast tumors from patients of all ages and then applied to 171 node-negative patients. Using a gene panel that demonstrated little overlap with the 70-gene assay or Oncotype DX, this molecular profile in node-negative patients was subsequently validated in a multicenter study[74]; there it was prognostically significant in both pre- and postmenopausal women with tumors measuring 1 to 2 cm with statistically significant hazard ratios between the good and poor signatures.

A different approach taken by Paik and colleagues studied a 21-gene panel by using RNA extracted from formalin-fixed, paraffin-embedded breast cancers and subsequently quantified by RT-PCR.[75,76] This group of 16 cancer-related genes and 5 reference controls was selected from a larger group of candidate genes derived from a clinical trial in node-negative, ER-positive cancers. Because of the ability to use formalin-fixed, paraffin-embedded tumor tissue, which is widely available, this methodology has generated significant interest given its ease of use. Based on the level of expression of the genes, a recurrence risk score is generated from a mathematical algorithm, assigning a recurrence risk as low, intermediate, or high.[75] The most influential pathways assessed in this calculation are proliferation and ER, followed by the HER2/neu pathway. Using a multivariate Cox analysis, the recurrence risk was found to be an independent predictor of recurrence, irrespective of the patient's age or tumor size in an external validation study from patients enrolled on National Surgical Adjuvant Breast and Bowel Project (NSABP) trial B-14.[75] Patients were stratified into risk categories based on recurrence score, which was strongly predictive of distant recurrence with 10-year rates of 6.8% in the low-risk group as compared to 30.5% in the high-risk group.[75] There has been some controversy, however, with regard to the predictive values of this test. A recent single-center study that evaluated Oncotype DX in 149 untreated patients failed to find a clear association with risk for distant metastases within 10 years, although tumor grade did not correlate, either.[77] Given the heavy weight toward the proliferative, ER, and HER2 pathways, the most likely benefit of this assay is in determining the sensitivity to hormonal therapy as compared to chemotherapy. Currently, a large trial conducted by the Breast Cancer Intergroup is underway to assess the ability of this assay, Oncotype DX, to discriminate further groups of patients who may not benefit from the use of adjuvant chemotherapy in the Trial Assigning Individualized Options for Treatment (TailorRx).

Prognostic Gene Signatures: Bottom Up

Chang and associates[24] took a distinctly different approach as they sought to construct a gene expression signature that reflected a mechanistic pathway. These authors built on prior research into tissue injury that had identified a "wound response" signature in response to changes that occurred with wound healing. Using a set of core serum response genes identified as being induced or repressed in activated fibroblasts, researchers developed a surrogate marker for a wound environment.[24,78] These expression cassettes included genes that appear integral in wound healing such as motility and angiogenesis—pathways that likely play a pivotal role in cancer progression, invasiveness, and metastasis. A quantitative wound response signature was generated based on how closely a given tumor reflected the activated signaling profile.[24] This signature was statistically accurate in identifying a low-risk and high-risk population of breast cancer and proved to be superior to established clinical models of assessing risk.[74] Defining the biologic underpinnings of cellular growth may aid improved understanding of the coordinated events that occur in carcinogenesis and has the capacity to transcend tumor types.[24,78] Interestingly, the authors note that the cassette of genes invoked in the wound response pathway demonstrated little overlap with the 70-gene prognostic signature. However, when compared with the 70-gene profile, both forms of molecular profiling segregated largely the same group of patients into good and poor risk groups.

This use of gene expression profiling using a biologically defined gene set has been applied as well to circulating putative tumor cells, which can be identified phenotypically as $CD44^+/CD24^{-/lo}$. Liu and others[23] used the differential gene expression patterns of these tumorigenic cells to create a 186-gene signature termed the "invasiveness" gene signature (IGS). The genes that comprised the IGS were distinct from previous gene signatures in breast cancer and importantly were genes that were differentially expressed between tumorigenic breast cells and breast epithelial cells. When applied to patients with early breast cancer in the Netherlands Cancer Institute database and the Erasmus Medical Center database, the IGS correlated with significantly reduced metastasis-free and overall survival.[23] These associations remained significant even when patients were stratified for tumor size, patient age, ER status, tumor differentiation, or lymph node status.[23] Focusing on the detection of breast stem cells, researchers also found an 11-gene signature that was able to pinpoint stem cells that possessed self-renewal capability. This gene signature identified the oncogenic pathway of BMI1: an oncogene involved in the proliferation of stem cells as being of prime importance. Application of this gene signature to tumor samples revealed that expression of this stem cell profile portended a poor prognosis with higher risk of metastatic disease and poor response to therapy.[79]

Similar studies defining other pathways that may reflect mechanisms of cancer progression have been performed. A recent example is a study exploring genetic changes that occur with increased proliferation. This study was undertaken in an attempt to improve the ability to assess grade in ER-positive subtypes of breast cancer.[80,81] In these studies, investigators evaluated tumors of different histologic grade for differential gene expression patterns. Using tumor specimens from more than 600 patients, histologic tumor grade was reviewed centrally as a comparator to microarray analysis. An initial set of ER-positive samples underwent microarray analysis with a resulting gene expression grade index (GGI) derived from the results. Application of the GGI to different patient samples confirmed a strong association between genomic grade and relapse-free survival.[80] The authors then applied the GGI to the different molecular subtypes of breast cancer as defined earlier by Perou and coworkers, to assess the basal-like and HER2 tumor types had high GGI scores, whereas the normal-like tumor types had low ones. They found, however, diverse genomic grading in the ER-positive luminal subtype tumors. Using this information, they applied the GGI to a large group of ER-positive samples and defined two subtypes of ER-positive tumors based on genomic grade. The subtype with the high GGI scores had worse survival rates in both treated and untreated patients. Further analysis revealed significant correlation of the GGI to the recurrence score of Oncotype DX.[81] The GGI assay is now licensed for further commercial development. Other studies have used pathways involved in cellular response to hypoxia or in response to p53 mutations to generate gene signatures that have, at least in early studies, suggested a correlation with outcome.[82,83] These ongoing studies illustrate the potential for improved understanding of the complex pathways leading to breast carcinomas. How the differing profiles compare with each other and with more established clinical prognostic factors has been the subject of intense research.

Concordance

When evaluating the prospective gene signatures as a whole, there appears to be a high degree of concordance between them, despite a low level of overlap in the genes used in each of the previously discussed signatures. Despite the lack of common priority genes, the major biologic pathways emphasized in most of these panels continue to be proliferation, ER, and HER2. One study has evaluated five gene expression profiles for comparative predictive value;[84] these profiles included the 70-gene profile, wound response, recurrence score, the two-gene ratio (discussed later), and intrinsic subtypes. This study found excellent agreement in classification between the recurrence score and 70-gene profile models. As well, this study noted that tumors classified as basal-like or luminal B subtypes had poor outcomes as determined by the 70-gene, wound response, and recurrence score prognostic profiles.[85] Of interest, the smallest gene set, which used only two genes in the profile, failed to significantly distinguish different outcomes compared with the other four models. These observations suggest that examining small sets of gene markers in isolation may not be as helpful as microarray profiling, in which there is an ability to examine large gene sets. Moreover, different approaches to building prognostic models may complement each other, with numerous genes within important pathways able to correlate with clinical outcome.[23,73,85]

There is considerable interest in furthering gene profiling and using genetic signatures to provide improved estimates of breast cancer recurrence. These approaches to fingerprinting individual cancers offer the promise of improved prognostication on the basis of gene expression. One central area that will affect further profiling studies is the platform used for analysis. The method of tissue processing and preservation is quite different between the two most fully developed assays (Oncotype DX and MammaPrint) and both offer different advantages and disadvantages: The Mamma-Print test is a prognostic test and includes a wider number of assayed genes. However, it requires freshly prepared mRNA extracts that have inherent problems with tissue heterogeneity. The Oncotype DX test has been validated as a stand-alone prognostic and predictive test with greater ease of handling tissue given that formalin-fixed, paraffin-embedded tissue can be used for RT-PCR with excellent sensitivity. Here again, however, results depend heavily on the presence of tumor tissue weighed against benign tissue.[86] Similar to ongoing work to standardize biomarkers, efforts are underway to develop a consistent methodology for microarray technology and analysis.[87] Whether platforms examining a plethora of gene activity or ones that detail specific cellular processes will prove to more successful is unclear at this time. However, both approaches appear to predict with some degree of accuracy which patients with early-stage breast cancer are more likely to develop recurrence of their cancer. Ongoing studies suggest the ability to begin to more accurately predict the likelihood to respond to neoadjuvant chemotherapy or specific regimes.[75,88] The follow-up of this approach is the promise of individualized approach to risk assessment and ultimately management of the choices of adjuvant therapy.

Predictive Gene Signatures

ESTROGEN

Although quantitative ER/PR expression is currently the best predictor of clinical response to tamoxifen,[89] a significant number of hormonal receptor–positive tumors do not respond to tamoxifen or develop early resistance to this drug.[90,91] The underlying mechanisms of tamoxifen resistance are poorly understood, but the use of DNA microarray technology offers some promise of identifying tumors that may be resistant to endocrine manipulation and similarly, predict response to specific chemotherapeutic regimens. Several investigators have published gene signatures reputed to more accurately predict response to tamoxifen. One such signature, developed by Jansen and colleagues,[88] was derived from 81 genes that were differentially expressed in tamoxifen-responsive and tamoxifen-resistant tumors in the setting of metastatic disease. This set was honed down to create a 44-gene signature including genes involved in estrogen action, apoptosis, immune response, and extracellular matrix formation. This signature was validated on an independent set of 66 tumors and was found to have 80% accuracy for prediction of resistance to tamoxifen therapy. This signature was more predictive of response to tamoxifen than traditional factors such as menopausal status, ER/PR status, disease-free interval, and first dominant site of relapse.[88]

Another test currently marketed for assessment of response to tamoxifen, is the so-called "two-gene" expression ratio based on the relative mRNA expression of two genes—the homeobox gene-B13 (*HOXB13*) and the interleukin-17B receptor gene (*IL17BR*).[92] Using a group of patients who were ER-positive, lymph node–negative, researchers evaluated differing gene expression between those patients who developed distant metastasis and those who remained disease-free. This test uses formalin-fixed, paraffin-embedded tissue as the source for the RT-PCR assay. Reflecting again the proliferative pathway, the *HOXB13* gene is expressed almost exclusively in breast tumors, whereas the *IL17BR* gene is typically absent in invasive tumors.[93,94] This test has demonstrated prognostic significance with regard to tumor aggressiveness and failure of tamoxifen.[95,96] However, there has been some question as to external validation of this model by other investigators, who found a poor correlation between this two-gene test and outcome.[97] Moreover, concordance between these profiles is not uniform. In comparing the available molecular signatures, the two-gene ratio, Oncotype DX, and the gene set described by Jansen and colleagues, investigators demonstrated a significant association using multivariate analysis only for the 21-gene and the Jansen gene set when applied to a single data set of first-line treatment for relapsed disease.[98] Several potential problems are evident with the number of new studies seeking to define prognostic assays that are illustrated by these different results. These problems include heterogeneous populations of patients from which data sets are derived, small studies, and lack of independent validation studies.[99]

A similar trial used clusters of correlated genes to develop an outcome-based predictor of response to tamoxifen based on earlier studies.[80,81] These investigators used more than 250 cases to develop a predictor set with 181 genes made up of 13 clusters. Here again, proliferation and cell cycle genes played a major role, comprising more than 50% of the gene clusters, with at least one gene set proving to be predictive of response to tamoxifen.[81] Other trials have suggested gene expression signatures for responsiveness to tamoxifen using gene sets involved with estrogen action, apoptosis, immune response, and extracellular matrix formation.[88]

CHEMOTHERAPY

Analogous to the situation with tamoxifen, not all patients manifest a response to the use of chemotherapy. Application of DNA microarray analysis to this area has led to hope that targeting chemotherapeutic agents to particular tumors lies in the not-so-distant future. Several investigators have developed potential predictive gene sets based on observed responses to chemotherapy in the setting of neoadjuvant chemotherapy, where responses can be ascertained. Several gene signatures have been reported as predictive of a pathologic complete response in response to multiagent regimens.[100,101] Other investigators have targeted specific responses to anthracyclines[102] and taxanes.[103-105] Because the taxanes have a very well defined mechanism of action in paralyzing the microtubule assembly, specific mechanisms of resistance have been proposed as prognostic with regard to response. These include overexpression of P-glycoprotein, β-tubulin mutations, and shift in β-III-tubulin isoforms.[106] Low expression of the microtubule-associated protein tau has been suggested as a marker that could identify patients with increased sensitivity to paclitaxel based on responses to neoadjuvant chemotherapy.[107] As these gene sets become validated, it is likely that they will prove to be informative as to pathways mediating resistance. However, to date they have not been widely used because of problems with relatively low sensitivity and a paucity of information regarding benefits of alternative therapies.[103,108]

Use of gene profiling has also been reported to aid in decisions regarding chemotherapy in lymph node–positive patients.[109] Using the candidate genes of Oncotype DX as well as an additional panel of genes related by biologic functions including ER, proliferation, HER2, and macrophage clustering, researchers demonstrated an ability to separate out prognostic groups, even in a node-positive group of patients.[109] A similar approach has been used to predict responses to neoadjuvant chemotherapy, suggesting that again, combinations of genes are more powerful predictors of response than single genes.[110] Conversely, pathways of signal transduction that are currently well understood may serve as vehicles for predictive assays that reflect the activation status of one or more pathways. For example, delineating pathways that are involved with angiogenesis, adhesion, and invasion frequently implicate Src, a member of the nonreceptor protein tyrosine kinase family, Ras, β-catenin, and Myc.[111] This mechanistic approach has been used to identify genes that would predict for resistance to various chemotherapeutic agents.[104] At least one study has attempted to use activated profiles to develop relapse risk scores and help refine prognosis on early stage breast carcinomas.[85]

Pharmacogenomics

Pharmacogenomics, a term coined by Weinshilboum,[112] relates the relationship of a patient's genetic makeup and response to a given drug. This has become an increasingly pertinent topic, given that a wide variety of drugs are metabolized by a group of liver enzymes known as the cytochrome P450 or CYP enzymes. Referable to tamoxifen, the CYP2D6 enzyme metabolizes tamoxifen to endoxifen, an active metabolite. It is now recognized that there is a subset of women with low levels of CYP2D6, who fail to activate tamoxifen, and thus do not benefit from its protective effects. The importance of this with regard to clinical practice in some settings is well known (e.g., the potential for resistance to drugs such as warfarin [Coumadin]).[113] In the case of ER-positive breast cancer, some investigators have reported substantial variability of tamoxifen and its active metabolites at the standard dose of 20 mg/day.[114] These authors noted that the active metabolite, endoxifen was produced through the activity of the cytochrome P450 enzyme CYP2D6 somewhat variably.[114] Single-nucleotide polymorphisms are relatively common in this gene, and the effect of genotype on endoxifen levels was examined, with the finding of significantly reduced levels with low-activity polymorphisms.[115,116] Goetz and associates examined a specific polymorphism (*4 genotype) that accounts for the majority of the low metabolization seen in Caucasian women and found a reduced disease-free survival and time to recurrence in women homozygous for the 4 genotype (*4/*4).[117] These findings appeared to correlate with absence of symptoms of estrogen deprivation such as hot flashes.[117] Although others have reported similar findings,[118] conflicting studies have been published, with at least one other study failing to find an adverse outcome in women homozygous or heterozygous for the CYP2D6*4 genotype treated with tamoxifen.[119] Additional studies to detail the potential impact of genotype-based predictions of response or resistance to specific chemotherapeutic agents are ongoing.[120]

Summary

Development of a cancer is a complex process involving the accumulation of independent mutations that ultimately lead to unregulated cell signaling pathways, resulting in uncontrolled cell growth. Our understanding of the biology of breast cancer has been dramatically improved by the technology of DNA microarray. It has become increasingly clear that breast cancers are extremely heterogeneous in their composition. Clustering tumors based on pathway signatures aids in defining prognosis in patient subsets. Linking pathway deregulation with sensitivity to therapeutic drugs that target components of the pathways provides an opportunity to make use of these oncogenic pathway signatures to guide the use of targeted therapeutics.

Integration of genetic profiling into clinic trial design will allow prospective correlative studies to be performed and molecular stratification of patients for treatment arms. It is increasingly important that future trials adopt a standardized approach to technology use to allow comparison within and across data sets. Substantial differences in prognosis are discernible with molecular profiling, but the data sets have thus far consisted of very heterogeneous patients, small sample size, and lack of external validation, and these are the same problems that have hampered development of biomarker development.

Currently, strong claims cannot be made regarding superiority of genomic profiling over standard histologic or clinical parameters. Nevertheless, many of these gene expression profiles appear to augment existing classification schemes. An important potential of microarray-based tests is that multiple predictions, including prognosis and sensitivity, to various treatment modalities may be generated from relatively small clinical trials. Too often, however, studies may enhance our understanding of breast cancer biology but fail to shed light on the oncogenic pathways that drive tumor growth and development. To provide a truly personalized treatment recommendation, it is important to understand the risk of relapse and the probability of benefit from endocrine therapy and chemotherapy separately. It is likely that the next improvements will come from development of functional hypotheses incorporated into genomic analyses of patients undergoing therapy for breast carcinoma.

REFERENCES

1. Perou CM, et al: Molecular portraits of human breast tumours. Nature 406:747–752, 2000.
2. Henderson IC, Patek AJ: The relationship between prognostic and predictive factors in the management of breast cancer. Breast Cancer Res Treat 52:261, 1998.
3. Singletary SE, Allred C, Ashley P, et al: Staging system for breast cancer: Revisions for the 6th edition of the AJCC cancer staging manual. Surg Clin North Am 83:803–819, 2003.
4. Fitzgibbons PL, Page DL, Weaver D, et al: Prognostic factors in breast cancer. College of American Pathologists consensus statement. Arch Pathol Lab Med 124:966–978, 2000.
5. Slamon DJ, Clark GM, Wong SG, et al: Amplification of a novel v-erbB-related gene in a human mammary carcinoma. Science 235:177–182, 1987.
6. Bartlett JMS: Translational research and the development of novel biomarkers in breast cancer. Advan Breast Cancer 3;76–85, 2006.
7. McShane LM, Altman DG, Sauerberi W, et al: Reporting recommendations for tumor marker prognostic studies, J Clin Oncol 23;9067–9072, 2005.
8. Hammond MEH, Taube SE: Issues and barriers to development of clinically useful tumor markers: A development pathway proposal. Semin Oncol 29:213–221, 2002.
9. Perez EA, Romond EH, Suman VJ, et al: Updated results of the combined analysis of NCCTG N9831 and NSABP B-31 adjuvant chemotherapy with/without trastuzumab in patients with HER2-postive breast cancer. J Clin Oncol 25, 2007 [Abstract 512].
10. Wolff AC, Hammond ME, Schwartz JN, et al: American Society of Clinical Oncology/College of American Pathologists guideline recommendations for human epidermal growth factor receptor 2 testing in breast cancer. J Clin Oncol 25:118–145, 2007.
11. Billgren AM, Tani E, Liedberg A, et al: Prognostic significance of tumor cell proliferation analyzed in fine needle aspirates from primary breast cancer. Breast Cancer Res Treat 71:161–170, 2002.
12. Look MP, van Putten WL, Duffy MJ, et al: Pooled analysis of prognostic impact of urokinase-type plasminogen activator and its inhibitor PAI-1 in 8377 breast cancer patients. J Natl Cancer Inst 94:116–128, 2002.
13. Schmitt M, Sturmheit AS, Welk A, et al: Procedures for the quantitative protein determination of urokinase and its inhibitor, PAI-1, in human breast cancer tissue extracts by ELISA. Methods Mol Med 120:245–265, 2006.
14. Harris H, Fritsche H, Mennel R, et al: American Society of Clinical Oncology 2007 update of recommendations for the use of tumor markers in breast cancer. J Clin Oncol 25:5287–5312, 2007.

15. Colozza M, Azambuja E, Cardoso F, et al: Proliferative markers as prognostic and predictive tools in early breast cancer: Where are we now? Ann Oncol 16:1723–1739, 2005.
16. Viale G, Regan MM, Mastropasqua MG, et al: Predictive value of tumor Ki-67 expression in two randomized trials of adjuvant chemoendocrine therapy for node-negative breast cancer. J Natl Cancer Inst 100:207–212, 2008.
17. Hudis CA, Barlow WE, Costantino, JP, et al: Proposal for standardized definitions for efficacy end points in adjuvant breast cancer trials: The STEEP system. J Clin Oncol 25:2127–2132, 2007.
18. Ransohoff DF: How to improve reliability and efficiency of research about molecular markers: Roles of phases, guidelines, and study design. J Clin Epidemiol 60:1205–1219, 2004.
19. Fisher B, Jeong JH, Bryant J, et al: Treatment of lymph-node-negative, oestrogen-receptor-positive breast cancer: Long-term findings from National Surgical Adjuvant Breast and Bowel Project randomized clinical trials. Lancet 364:858–868, 2004.
20. Liu ET: Mechanism-derived gene expression signatures and predictive biomarkers in clinical oncology. Proc Natl Acad Sci USA 102:3531–3532, 2005.
21. Al-Hajj M, Wicha MS, Benito-Hernandez A, et al: Prospective identification of tumorigenic breast cancer cells. Proc Natl Acad Sci USA 100:3983–3988, 2003. [Erratum, 100:6890]
22. Reya T, Morrison SJ, Clarke MF Weissman IL: Stem cells, cancer, and cancer stem cells. Nature 414:105–111, 2001.
23. Liu R, Wang X, Chen GY, Dalerba P, et al: The prognostic role of a gene signature from tumorigenic breast-cancer cells. New Engl J Med 356:217–226, 2007.
24. Chang HY, Nuyten DSA, Sneddon JB, et al: Robustness, scalability, and integration of a wound-response gene expression signature in predicting breast cancer survival. Proc Natl Acad Sci USA 102:3738–3743, 2005.
25. Ponti D, Costa A, Zaffaroni N, et al: Isolation and in vitro propagation of tumorigenic breast cancer cells with stem/cell progenitors. Cancer Res 65:5506–5511, 2005.
26. Sansal I, Sellers WR: The biology and clinical relevance of the PTEN tumor suppressor pathway. J Clin Oncol 22:2954–2963, 2004.
27. Dillon RL, White DE, Muller WJ: The phosphatidy inositol 3-kinase signaling network: Implications for human breast cancer. Oncogene 26:1338–1345, 2007.
28. Seldin DC, Landesman-Bollag E, et al: CK2 as a positive regulator of Wnt signaling and tumourigenesis. Mol Cell Biochem 274:63–67, 2005.
29. Mimeault M, Hauke R, Mehta PP, Gatra SK: Recent advances in cancer stem progenitor cell research: Therapeutic implications for overcoming resistance to the most aggressive cancers. J Cell Mol Med 11:981–1011, 2007.
30. Thiery JP: Epithelial-mesenchymal transitions in development and pathologies. Curr Opin Cell Biol 15:740–746, 2003.
31. Wicha MS: Cancer stem cell heterogeneity in hereditary breast cancer. Breast Cancer Res 10:105, 2008.
32. Wicha MS, Liu S, Dontu G: Cancer stem cells: An old idea—a paradigm shift. Cancer Res 66:1883–1890, 2006.
33. Li X, Lewis MT, Huang J, et al: Intrinsic resistance of tumorigenic breast cancer cells to chemotherapy. J Natl Cancer Inst 100:672–679, 2008.
34. Woodward WA, Chen MS, Behbod F, Rosen JM: On mammary stem cells. J Cell Sci 118:3585–3594, 2005.
35. Lindvall C, Evans NC, Zylstra CR, et al: The Wnt signaling receptor Lrp5 is required for mammary ductal stem cell activity and Wnt1-induced tumorigenesis. J Biol Chem 281:35081–35087, 2006.
36. Liu S, Dontu G, Mantle ID, et al: Hedgehog signaling and Bmi-1 regulate self-renewal of normal and malignant human mammary stem cells. Cancer Res 66:6063–6071, 2006.
37. Woodward, WA, Chen MS, et al: Wnt/b-catenin mediates radiation resistance of mouse mammary progenitor cells. Proc Natl Acad Sci USA 104:618–623, 2007.
38. Dawood S, Cristofanilli M: Integrating circulating tumor cell assay into the management of breast cancer. Curr Treat Options Oncol 8:89–95, 2007.
39. Pachmann K, Camara O, Kavallaris A, et al: Quantification of the response of circulating epithelial cells to neoadjuvant treatment for breast cancer: A new tool for therapy monitoring. Breast Cancer Res 7:975–979, 2005.
40. Bidard FC, Vincent-Salomon A, Gomme S, et al: Disseminated tumor cells of breast cancer patients: A strong prognostic factor for distant and local relapse. Clin Cancer Res 14:3306–3311, 2008.
41. Xenidis N, Perraki M, Kafousi M, et al: Predictive and prognostic value of peripheral blood cytokeratin-19 mRNA-positive cells detected by real-time polymerase chain reaction in node-negative breast cancer patients. J Clin Oncol 24:3756–3762, 2006.
42. Ignatiadis M, Xenidis N, Perraki M, et al: Different prognostic value of cytokertain-19 mRNA-positive circulating tumor cells according to estrogen receptor and HER2 status in early-stage breast cancer. J Clin Oncol 25:5194–5202, 2007.
43. Braun S, Vogl FD, Naume B, et al: A pooled analysis of bone marrow micrometastasis in breast cancer. N Engl J Med 353:793–802, 2005.
44. Janni W, Rack B, et al: Detection of micrometastatic disease in bone marrow: Is it ready for prime time? Oncologist 10: 480–492, 2005.
45. Klausner RD: The fabric of cancer cell biology—weaving together the strands. Cancer Cell 1:3–10, 2002.
46. Wiseman BS, Werb Z: Stromal effects on mammary gland development and breast cancer. Science 296:1046–1049, 2002.
47. Patocs A, Zhang L, Xu Y, et al: Breast-cancer stromal cells with TP53 mutations and nodal metastases. N Eng J Med 357: 2543–2551, 2007.
48. Allinen M, Beroukhim R, Cai L, et al: Molecular characterization of the tumor microenvironment in breast cancer. Cancer Cell 6:17–32, 2004.
49. Finak G, Bertos N, Pepin F, et al: Stromal gene expression predicts clinical outcome in breast cancer. Nat Med 14:518–527, 2008.
50. Yang NJ, Wechsler-Reya RJ: Hit 'em where they live: Targeting the cancer stem cell niche. Cancer Cell 11:3–5, 2007.
51. De Azambuja E, Cardoso F, de Castro G, et al: Ki-67 as prognostic markers in early breast cancer: A meta-analysis of published studies involving 12,155 patients. Br J Cancer 96:1504–13, 2007.
52. Shapiro G: Cyclin-dependent kinase pathways as targets for cancer treatment. J Clin Oncol 24:1770–1783, 2006.
53. Ellis MJ, Coop A, Singh B, et al: Letrozole is more effective neoadjuvant therapy than tamoxifen for ErbB1 and ErbB2-positive, estrogen receptor-positive primary breast cancer: Evidence from a phase III randomized trial. J Clin Oncol 19:3808–3816, 2001.
54. Smith IE, Dowsett M, Ebbs SR, et al: Neoadjuvant treatment of postmenopausal breast cancer with anastrozole, tamoxifen, or both in combination: The Immediate Preoperative Anastrozole, Tamoxifen, or Combined With Tamoxifen (IMPACT) multicenter double-blind randomized trial. J Clin Oncol 23:5108–5116, 2005.
55. Pritchard KI, Shepherd LE, O'Malley FP, et al: HER2 and responsiveness of breast cancer to adjuvant chemotherapy. N Engl J Med 354:2103–2111, 2006.
56. Dowsett M, Allred DC: Relationship between quantitative ER and PgR expression and HER2 stratus with recurrence in the ATAC trial. Presented at San Antonio Breast Cancer Symposium, San Antonio, TX, December 2006.
57. Dowsett M, Allred C, Knox J, et al: Relationship between quantitative estrogen and progesterone receptor expression and human epidermal growth factor receptor 2 (HER-2) status with recurrence in the Arimidex, Tamoxifen, Alone or in Combination Trial. J Clin Oncol 26:1059–1065, 2008.
58. McGrogan G, Rudolph P, de Mascarel I, et al: DNA topoisomerase IIa expression and the response to primary chemotherapy in breast cancer. Br J Cancer 89:666–671, 2003.
59. Martin RM, Munoz M, Albanell J, et al: Serial topoisomerase II expression in primary breast cancer and response to neoadjvuant anthracycline-based chemotherapy. Oncology 66:388–394, 2004.
60. Pritchard KI, Messersmith H, Elavathil L, et al: HER-2 and topoisomerase II as predictors of response to chemotherapy. J Clin Oncol 26:736–744, 2008.
61. Isola JJ, Tanner M, Holli K, et al: Amplification of topoisomerase II alpha is a strong predictor or response to epirubicin-based chemotherapy in HER-2/neu positive metastatic breast cancer. Proc Breast Cancer Res Treat 64:31, 2000 [abstract 21].
62. van't Veer LJ, Dai H, van de Vijver MJ, et al: Gene expression profiling predicts clinical outcome of breast cancer. Nature 415:530–536, 2002.

63. Sorlie T, Tibshirani R, Parker J, et al: Repeated observation of breast tumor subtypes in independent gene expression data sets. Proc Natl Acad Sci USA 100:8418–8423, 2003.

64. Carey LA, Perou CM, Livasy CA, et al: Race, breast cancer subtypes, and survival in the Carolina Breast Cancer Study. JAMA 295:2492–2502, 2006.

65. Andre F: DNA arrays as predictors of efficacy of adjuvant/neoadjuvant chemotherapy in breast cancer patients: Current data and issues on study design. Biochem Biophys Acta 1766:197–204, 2006.

66. Foulkes WD, Stefansson IM, Chappuis PO, et al: Germline *BRCA1* mutations and a basal epithelial phenotype in breast cancer. J Natl Cancer Inst 95:1482–1485, 2003.

67. Olopade OI, Grushko T. Gene-expression profiles in hereditary breast cancer. N Engl J Med 344:2028–2029, 2001.

68. Sotiriou C, Neo SY, McShane LM, et al: Breast cancer classification and prognosis based on gene expression profiles from a population-based study. Proc Natl Acad Sci USA 100:10393–10398, 2003.

69. Yu K, Lee CH, Tan PH, Tan P: Conservation of breast cancer molecular subtypes and transcriptional patterns of tumor progression across distinct ethnic populations. Clin Cancer Res 10:5508–5517, 2004.

70. Sorlie T, Wang Y, Xiao C, et al: Distinct molecular mechanisms underlying clinically relevant subtypes of breast cancer: Gene expression analyses across three different platforms. BMC Genomics 7:127, 2006.

71. van de Vijver MJ, He UD, van't Veer LJ, et al: A gene-expression signature as a predictor of survival in breast cancer. N Engl J Med 347:1999–2009, 2002.

72. Buyse M, Loi S, van't Veer L, et al: TRANSBIG Consortium. Validation and clinical utility of a 70-gene prognostic signature for women with node-negative breast cancer. J Natl Cancer Inst. 98:1183–1192, 2006.

73. Wang Y, Klijin JG, Zhang Y, et al: Gene-expression profiles to predict distant metastasis of lymph-node-negative primary breast cancer. Lancet 365:671–679, 2005.

74. Foekens JA, Atkins D, Zhang Y, et al: Multi-center validation of a gene expression-based prognostic signature in lymph node-negative primary breast cancer. J Clin Oncol 24:1665–1671, 2006.

75. Paik S, Shak S, Tang G, et al: A multigene assay to predict recurrence of tamoxifen-treated, node-negative breast cancer. N Engl J Med 351:2817–2826, 2004.

76. Paik S, Shak S, Tang G, et al: Multigene RT-PCR assay for predicting recurrence in node-negative breast cancer patients-NSABP studies B-20 and B-14. Breast Cancer Res Treat 82:A16, 2003.

77. Esteva FJ, Sahin AA, Cristofanilli M, et al: Prognostic role of a multigene reverse transcriptase-PCR assay in patients with node-negative breast cancer not receiving adjuvant systemic therapy. Clin Cancer Res 11:3315–3319, 2005.

78. Chang HY, Nuyten DS, Sneddon JB, et al: Robustness, scalability, and integration of a wound-response gene expression signature in predicting breast cancer survival. Proc Natl Acad Sci USA 102:3738–3743, 2005.

79. Glinsky GV, Berezovska O, Glinskii AB: Microarray analysis identifies a death-from-cancer signature predicting therapy failure in patients with multiple types of cancer. J Clin Invest 115:1503–1521, 2005.

80. Sotiriou C, Wirapati P, Loi S, et al: Gene expression profiling in breast cancer: Understanding the molecular basis of histologic grade to improve prognosis. J Natl Cancer Inst 98:262–272, 2006.

81. Loi S, Haibe-Kains B, Desmedt C, et al: Definition of clinically distinct molecular subtypes in estrogen receptor–positive breast carcinomas through genomic grade. J Clin Oncol 25:1239–1246, 2007.

82. Miller LD, Smeds J, George J, et al: An expression signature for p53 status in human breast cancer predicts mutation status, transcriptional effects, and patient survival. Proc Natl Acad Sci USA 102:13550–13555, 2005.

83. Chi JT, Wang Z, Nuyten DS, et al: Gene expression programs in response to hypoxia: Cell type specificity and prognostic significance in human cancers. PLoS Med 3:e47, 2006.

84. Fan C, Oh DS, Wessels L, et al: Concordance among gene-expression-based predictors for breast cancer. N Engl J Med 355:560–569, 2006.

85. Acharya CR, Hsu DS, Anders CK, et al: Gene expression signatures, clinicopathological features, and individualized therapy in breast cancer. JAMA 299:1574, 2008.

86. Paik S, Kim CY, Song YK, et al: Technology insight: Application of molecular techniques to formalin fixed paraffin embedded tissues from breast cancer. Nat Clin Pract Oncol 2:246–254, 2005.

87. Shi L, Reid LH, Jones WD, et al: MAQC Consortium. The MicroArray Quality Control (MAQC) project shows inter- and intraplatform reproducibility of gene expression measurements. Nat Biotechnol 24:1151–1161, 2006.

88. Jansen MP, Foekens JA, van Staveren IL, et al: Molecular classification of tamoxifen-resistant breast carcinomas by gene expression profiling. J Clin Oncol 23:732–740, 2005.

89. Bardou V, Arpino G, Elledge R, et al: Progesterone receptor status significantly improves outcome prediction over estrogen receptor status alone for adjuvant endocrine therapy in two large breast cancer databases. J Clin Oncol 21:1973–1979, 2003.

90. Clarke R, Liu MC, Bouker KB, et al: Antiestrogen resistance in breast cancer and the role of estrogen receptor signaling. Oncogene 22:7316–7339, 2003.

91. Osborne CK, Schiff R: Growth factor receptor cross-talk with estrogen receptor as a mechanism for tamoxifen resistance in breast cancer. Breast 12:362–367, 2003.

92. Jansen MP, Sieuwerts AM, Look MP, et al: HOXB13-to-IL17BR expression ratio is related with tumor aggressiveness and response to tamoxifen of recurrent breast cancer: A retrospective study. J Clin Oncol 25:662–668, 2007.

93. Ma XJ, Wang Z, Ryan PD, et al: A two-gene expression ration predicts clinical outcome in breast cancer patients treated with tamoxifen. Cancer Cell 5:607–616, 2004.

94. Wang Z, Dahiya S, Provencher H, et al: The prognostic biomarkers *HOXB13*, *IL17BR*, and *CHDH* are regulated by estrogen in breast cancer. Clin Cancer Res 13:6327–6334, 2007.

95. Jerevall PL, Brommesson S, Strand C, et al: Exploring the two-gene ratio in breast cancer-independent roles for *HOXB13* and *IL17BR* in prediction of clinical outcome. Breast Cancer 107:225–234, 2008.

96. Ma XJ, Hilsenbeck SG, Wang W, et al: The *HOXB13:IL17BR* expression index is a prognostic factor in early-stage breast cancer. J Clin Oncol 24:4611–4619, 2006.

97. Reid JF, Lusa L, De Cecco L, et al: Limits of predictive models using microarray data for breast cancer clinical treatment outcome. J Natl Cancer Inst 97:927–930, 2005.

98. Kok M, Linn SC, Van Laar RK, et al: Comparison of gene expression profiles predicting progression in breast cancer patients treated with tamoxifen. Breast Cancer Res Treat 113:275–283, 2009.

99. Simon R: Development and validation of therapeutically relevant multi-gene biomarker classifiers. J Natl Cancer Inst 97:866–867, 2005.

100. Ayers M, Symmans WF, Stec J, et al: Gene expression profiles predict complete pathologic response to neoadjuvant paclitaxel and fluorouracil, doxorubicin, and cyclophosphamide chemotherapy in breast cancer. J Clin Oncol 22:2284–2293, 2004.

101. Hess KR, Anderson K, Symmans W, et al: Pharmacogenomic predictor of sensitivity to preoperative paclitaxel and 5-fluorouracil, doxorubicin, cyclophosphamide chemotherapy in breast cancer. J Clin Oncol 24:4236–4244, 2006.

102. Folgueira MA, Carraro DM, Brentani H, et al: Gene expression profile associated with response to doxorubicin-based therapy in breast cancer. Clin Cancer Res 11:7434–7443, 2005.

103. Chang JC, Wooten EC, Tsimelzon A, et al: Gene expression profiling for the prediction of therapeutic response to docetaxel in patients with breast cancer. Lancet 362:362–369, 2003.

104. Chang JC, Wooten EC, Tsimelzon A, et al: Patterns of resistance and incomplete response to docetaxel by gene expression profiling in breast cancer patients. J Clin Oncol 23:1169–1177, 2005.

105. Potti A, Dressman HK, Bild A, et al: Genomic signatures to guide the use of chemotherapeutics. Nat Med 12:1294–1300, 2006.

106. Pustzai L: Markers predicting clinical benefit in breast cancer from microtubule-targeting agents. Ann Oncol 18(suppl 12):xii15–xii20, 2007.

107. Rouzier R, Rajan R, Wagner P, et al: Microtubule-associated protein tau: A marker of paclitaxel sensitivity in breast cancer. Proc Natl Acacd Sci USA 102:8315–8320, 2005.

108. Iwao-Koizumi K, Matoba R, Ueno N, et al: Prediction of docetaxel response in human breast cancer by gene expression profiling. J Clin Oncol 23:422–431, 2005.

109. Cobleigh MA, Tabesh B, Bittreman P, et al: Tumor gene expression and prognosis in breast cancer patients with 10 or more positive lymph nodes. Clin Cancer Res 11:8623–8631, 2005.

110. Gianni L, Zambetti M, Clark K, et al: Gene expression profiles in paraffin-embedded core biopsy tissue predict response to chemotherapy in women with locally advanced breast cancer. J Clin Oncol 23:7265–7277, 2005.

111. Bild AH, Yao G, Chang JT, et al: Oncogenic pathway signatures in human cancers as a guide to targeted therapies. Nature 439: 353–357, 2006.

112. Weinshilboum R: Inheritance and drug response. N Engl J Med 348:529–537, 2003.

113. Shurin SB, Nabel EG: Pharmacogenomics: Ready for prime time? N Engl J Med 358:1061–1063, 2008.

114. Desta Z, Ward BA, Soukhova NV, Flockhart DA: Comprehensive evaluation of tamoxifen sequential biotransformation by the human cytochrome P450 system in vitro: Prominent roles for CYP3A and CYP2D6. J Pharmacol Exp Ther 310:1062–1075, 2004.

115. Jin Y, Desta Z, Stearns V, et al: CYP2D6 genotype, antidepressant use, and tamoxifen metabolism during adjuvant breast caner treatment. J Natl Cancer Inst 97:30–39, 2005.

116. Borges S, Desta Z, Li L, et al: Quantitative effect of CYP2D6 genotype and inhibitors on tamoxifen metabolism: Implication for optimization of breast cancer treatment. Clin Pharmacol Ther 80:61–74, 2006.

117. Goetz MP, Knox SK, Suman VJ, et al: The impact of cytochrome P450 2D6 metabolism in women receiving adjuvant tamoxifen. Breast Cancer Res Treat 101:113–121, 2007.

118. Schroth W, Antoniadou L, Fritz, P, et al: Breast cancer treatment outcome with adjuvant tamoxifen relative to patient CYP2D6 and CYP2C19 genotypes. J Clin Oncol 25:5187–5193, 2007.

119. Wegman P, Elingarami S, et al: Genetic variants of CYP3A5, CYP2D6, SULT1A1, UGT2B15 and tamoxifen response in postmenopausal patients with breast cancer. Breast Cancer Res 9:R7, 2007.

120. Vaclavikova R, Nordgard SH, Alnaes GI, et al: Single nucleotide polymorphisms in the multidrug resistance gene 1 (ABCB1): Effects on its expression and clinicopathological characteristics in breast cancer patients. Pharmacogenet Genomics 18:263–273, 2008.

chapter 26

Risk Factors for Breast Carcinoma in Women with Proliferative Breast Disease

WILLIAM D. DUPONT | DAVID L. PAGE

The histology of benign breast biopsies is highly variable, and biopsied tissue may vary from the physiologically normal at one extreme to in situ carcinoma at the other. It thus made sense to subdivide these lesions into biologically meaningful categories and to attempt to determine the cancer risk associated with these different categories. This task has proved to be difficult, because the studies must be large, and there have been numerous classification schemes as there have been studies addressing this question. Many of these authors[1-6] have performed concurrent studies in which the malignant potential of benign lesions was judged by the frequency of their association with breast carcinoma in the same biopsy. The problem with such studies is that it is impossible to infer whether the implicated benign lesions are true precursor lesions for cancer, markers of risk elevation, or themselves a consequence of the malignancy. Thus, to prove that a benign lesion increases a woman's risk of breast cancer, it is necessary to establish a temporal relationship between the occurrence of the benign lesion and the later development of breast cancer. Several investigators have performed such studies, most notably Kodlin and colleagues,[7] Black and associates,[8] Hutchinson and coworkers,[9] and our own group studying the Nashville cohort.[10-19] In addition, other studies have assessed Page's histologic classification scheme in various cohorts of women using other pathologists.[20-23] These studies will be discussed later.

The other major challenge with studies of premalignant breast disease is that of establishing reproducible and biologically meaningful diagnoses. Our approach to this problem has been, first, through extensive pretesting, to devise a preliminary classification scheme that can distinguish between fine differences in breast morphology and cytology and yet be reproducible. This classification scheme was first evaluated[13] in 1978. After revision, it was then applied to more than 10,000 benign breast biopsies, and follow-up from a suitable sample of the biopsied women was obtained. Relative risk estimates associated with the different benign lesions were derived and compared. Our published benign disease categories represent groupings of preliminary classifications that are associated with consistent and clinically meaningful levels of cancer risk. These categories and the cancer risks associated with them have been endorsed by the College of American Pathologists.[24] The results of our studies are discussed in the next section. The relationship between our results and those of other investigators will be described subsequently.

Nashville Studies

We re-evaluated 10,366 consecutive benign breast biopsies performed between 1950 and 1968 at three hospitals in Nashville, Tennessee[10] (Table 26-1). These analyses indicated that 70% of women who undergo biopsy revealing benign breast tissue are not at increased risk for breast cancer. The remaining 30% of the 10,000 evaluated biopsies contained proliferative lesions. These lesions are characterized by at least moderate hyperplasia[25] and are associated with an approximate twofold increase in risk of breast cancer. The lesions within this disease category include, most prominently, hyperplasia of usual type (ductal) of moderate and florid degree as well as sclerosing adenosis and papillomas. Also constituting a minor component of this category are mild or poorly developed examples of atypical hyperplasia (AH). This latter category was created primarily to provide a clear lower boundary for the criteria needed to diagnose AH. Mild hyperplasia of usual type is excluded from the proliferative disease category because it is not associated

TABLE 26-1

Relative Risk of Breast Cancer in Women Who Have Undergone Benign Breast Biopsy

	No. of Women	No. of Cancers	Relative Risk*	95% Confidence Interval	P Value
All women	3303	134	1.5	1.3–1.8	<0.0001
Proliferative disease	1925	103	1.9	1.6–2.3	<0.0001
No proliferative disease	1378	31	0.89	0.62–1.3	0.51
Family history[†]	369	26	2.5	1.7–3.7	<0.0001
No family history	2934	108	1.4	1.2–1.7	0.0007
Proliferative disease and					
Family history	234	22	3.2	2.1–4.9	<0.0001
No family history	1691	81	1.7	1.4–2.2	<0.0001
Calcification	359	23	2.4	1.6–3.6	<0.0001
No calcification	1566	80	1.8	1.5–2.3	<0.0001
Age[‡] 20–45	1205	57	1.9	1.5–2.5	<0.0001
Age 46–55	563	35	1.9	1.3–2.6	0.0002
Age >55	157	11	2.2	1.2-4	0.007
No proliferative disease and					
Family history	135	4	1.2	0.43–3.1	0.78
No family history	1243	27	0.86	0.59–1.3	0.43
Calcification	174	4	0.80	0.30–2.1	0.66
No calcification	1204	27	0.90	0.62–1.3	0.59
Age 20–45	1025	23	0.99	0.66–1.5	0.96
Age 46–55	247	7	0.83	0.40–1.8	0.63
Age >55	106	1	0.30	0.04–2.2	0.21
Family history and					
Cysts	246	21	3	1.9–4.5	<0.0001
No cysts	123	5	1.6	0.65–3.7	0.32
No family history and					
Cysts	1808	73	1.5	1.2–1.9	0.0008
No cysts	1126	35	1.2	0.88–1.7	0.23

*Risk relative to women from Cutler and Young survey, adjusted for age at biopsy and length of follow-up. See Cutler SJ, Young JL (eds): Third national cancer survey: Incidence data. Publication no. (NIH) 75-787. Bethesda, MD, National Cancer Institute, 1975.
[†]Mother, sister, or daughter with breast cancer.
[‡]Age at benign breast biopsy.
Modified from Dupont WD, Page DL.[10] Follow-up was obtained on 3303 of these women, representing 84% of eligible subjects. This sample was weighted in favor of patients with proliferative disease. The median length of follow-up was 17 years.

with increased risk of cancer and thus is not considered a disease. Clinical correlates of proliferative disease are unproven except for dense mammographic patterns that are positively correlated with the presence of proliferative disease.[26]

The proliferative lesions can be further dichotomized into those with and without atypia. The former (AH) are characterized by meeting some but not all the criteria needed for a diagnosis of carcinoma in situ. These lesions are rare, having a prevalence of 4% in our consecutive series of benign biopsies, and are associated with a fourfold to fivefold increase in breast cancer risk. There are two morphologically distinct subtypes of AH: atypical lobular hyperplasia (ALH) and atypical ductal hyperplasia (ADH; see Chapter 8). However, women with these lesions have roughly comparable breast cancer risks.[14] Minor differences include a shorter average period between biopsy and invasive carcinoma diagnosis for ADH (8 years) than for ALH (12 years). There are

also differences in the age distribution,[14,22] with both types predominating in the perimenopausal period but with ALH even less common in younger and older women. Proliferative disease without atypia (PDWA) was associated with a 60% increase in risk of breast cancer (1.6 times) when compared with women from the Third National Cancer Survey and was associated with a 90% increase (1.9 times) when compared with women without such changes from our study. The College of American Pathologists Consensus Conference[24] stated that this slight elevation in risk ranged from 1.5 to 2 times that of the general population.

Tables 26-1 and 26-2 are adapted from Dupont and Page.[10] In reading these tables, it is important to bear in mind that the estimated relative risks may differ from their true values because of chance by the amount indicated in the 95% confidence intervals (CIs). The P values given in these tables are with respect to the null hypothesis that the true relative risk equals 1. Table 26-1 shows

TABLE 26-2

Relative Risk of Breast Cancer in Women with Proliferative Breast Disease

	No. of Women	No. of Cancers	Relative Risk*	95% Confidence Interval	*P* Value
Proliferative disease without atypia	1693	73	1.6	1.3–2	0.0001
Atypical hyperplasia	232	30	4.4	3.1–6.3	<0.0001
Calcification	533	27	1.8	1.3–2.7	0.001
Proliferative disease without atypia and					
Family history†	195	12	2.1	1.2–3.7	0.009
No family history	1498	61	1.5	1.2–1.9	0.002
Calcification	321	16	1.9	1.2–3.1	0.012
No calcification	1372	57	1.5	1.2–1.9	0.002
Atypical hyperplasia and					
Family history	39	10	8.9	4.8–17	<0.0001
No family history	193	20	3.5	2.3–5.5	<0.0001
Calcification	38	7	6.5	3.1–14	<0.0001
No calcification	194	23	4	2.7–6.1	<0.0001

*Risk relative to women from Cutler and Young survey, adjusted for age at biopsy and length of follow-up. See Cutler SJ, Young JL (eds): Third national cancer survey: Incidence data. Publication no. (NIH) 75-787. Bethesda, MD, National Cancer Institute, 1975.
†Mother, sister, or daughter with breast cancer.
Modified from Dupont WD, Page DL.[10]

the effect of family history, calcification, and age on the risk of breast cancer in women with and without proliferative disease. Study subjects with a mother, sister, or daughter who developed breast cancer were at 2.5 times the risk of women in the general population, whereas study subjects without such a history had only a 40% increase in risk of cancer. This 40% increase reflects the average of our entire study group. A family history of breast cancer had little effect on breast cancer risk in women without proliferative disease. However, in women with proliferative disease, a family history almost doubled the risk of breast cancer. This interaction is much stronger for AH (see Table 26-2). It must be noted, however, that in the Nurse's Health Study, Collins and colleagues[27] found that a positive family history of breast cancer only slightly increased the risk of breast cancer in women with PDWA and had no significant effect on the risk of breast cancer in women with AH. The presence of calcification was of some importance in women with proliferative disease, but it had no effect on risk of cancer in women lacking proliferative lesions.

The interaction between proliferative disease and age at biopsy is particularly interesting. Women with proliferative disease have approximately twice the risk of breast cancer compared with women of similar age from the general population regardless of whether they are in the premenopausal, perimenopausal, or postmenopausal age group. In contrast, the relative risk of breast cancer falls with increasing age in patients lacking proliferative disease, with postmenopausal patients having about one third the risk of postmenopausal women in general. This result suggests that women undergoing senile involution whose breasts lack any hyperplastic activity may be at reduced risk of developing breast cancer.

Table 26-2 shows how breast cancer risk varies in women with proliferative breast disease. Note the profound interaction between family history and AH.

Figure 26-1 shows the absolute risk of breast cancer associated with the disease categories discussed previously as a function of time since benign biopsy. These curves emphasize the considerable variation in cancer risk associated with these lesions. Patients with both AH and a first-degree family history have an incidence of breast cancer of about 20% in the first 15 years after biopsy. This level of risk is comparable to that of women with in situ carcinoma (see Chapter 83). Traditionally, all patients in our study cohort would have been diagnosed as having fibrocystic disease. It is clear from Figure 26-1 that this term has little prognostic value and should be replaced by more precise terminology. When an imprecise indication is useful, the term *fibrocystic change* may be preferred.

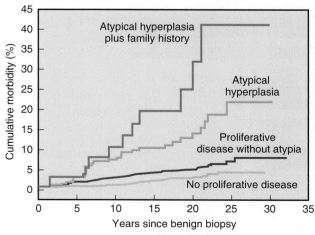

Figure 26-1 Proportion of patients who have developed invasive breast cancer as a function of time since their benign biopsy. (Adapted from Dupont WD, Page DL: Relative risk of breast cancer varies with time since diagnosis of atypical hyperplasia. Human Pathol 20:723–725, 1989.)

Evaluation of Page's Histologic Classification Scheme by Other Authors

Page's histologic classification scheme has been evaluated in four other studies.[20-23] Dupont and colleagues[20] studied women who underwent benign biopsy as part of the Breast Cancer Detection Demonstration Project (BCDDP). Page was not consulted during the pathology review of this study. London and associates[21] studied women from Harvard's Nurses Health Study, and Hartman and coworkers[23] conducted a cohort study of women diagnosed with benign breast disease at the Mayo Clinic between 1967 and 1991. The results of these studies are summarized in Figure 26-2. These studies have overlapping confidence intervals within each diagnostic category and are consistent, with AH being associated with a fourfold to fivefold elevation in risk of breast cancer, whereas PDWA approximately doubles the risk of breast cancer. The fact that other pathologists have found similar levels of the risk of breast cancer associated with these lesions supports the reproducibility and credibility of our findings.

Marshall and colleagues[22] have studied the difference in risk of breast cancer between women with ALH and ADH. The estimate of the relative risk of breast cancer in women with ALH was 5.3 (95% confidence interval [CI] 2.7–10.4), whereas for women with ADH this risk was 2.4 (95% CI 1.3–4.5). Although the estimated risk was higher for women with ALH than with ADH, the CIs are wide and these estimates are not significantly different. The researchers also observed a higher estimated relative risk for premenopausal women with ALH than for postmenopausal women with ALH.

Relationship between the Histologic Classification Schemes of Different Authors

The results of our studies should be compared with those of Kodlin and colleagues[7] and Hutchinson and associates.[9] Kodlin and colleagues use a scheme devised by Black and Chabon[28] that classifies lesions by their location in the breast and by their degree of proliferation. Black and Chabon's method of grouping lesions by location has not proved to be useful in distinguishing between different levels of risk of breast cancer, and those authors who have used their system have emphasized the component of this system that quantifies the degree of proliferation. This system consists of an atypia score in which 1 denotes normal epithelium, 2 denotes hyperplasia, 3 and 4 denote different degrees of atypia, and 5 denotes in situ carcinoma. The major results of the study by Kodlin and colleagues[7] are summarized in Table 26-3. This was a retrospective cohort study of women in a health maintenance organization. It is important to note that 11% of their patients had atypia scores of 3 or 4 as compared with 4% of our patients with AH. Thus, it is clear that the criteria for atypia in the Black-Chabon system are broader than those in our own. It would appear, however, that their grade 4 atypia is roughly comparable to our AH. As a group, the patients in Kodlin's cohort had a considerably higher risk of breast cancer than the women in our study.

TABLE 26-3

Summary of Results from Two Large Cohort Studies of Histologically Defined Benign Breast Disease

Histologic Diagnoses	No. of Patients	Relative Risk*
Kodlin[7]		
Entire group	2931	2.7
Black-Chabon atypia score 4	49	6
Black-Chabon atypia score 3	262	2.4
Black-Chabon atypia score 1–2	2092	2.3
Fibroadenoma	849	7
Adenosis or fibrosing adenosis	177	5
Intraductal papilloma	80	5
Hutchinson[9]		
Entire group	1356	2.2
Epithelial hyperplasia or papillomatosis	466	2.8
With atypia	33	2.9
Without atypia	433	2.8
With calcification[†]	102	5.3
Without calcification[†]	190	2.8
Fibroadenoma with fibrocystic disease	122	3.8

*Calculated with respect to the general population. Different external reference populations were used in each study.
[†]Women with main lesion type other than epithelial hyperplasia or papillomatosis were excluded.

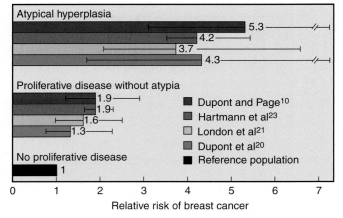

Figure 26-2 Estimated relative risks of breast cancer associated with atypical hyperplasia and proliferative disease without atypia that have been reported in the literature. The studies shown are those that have used Page's histologic criteria. These studies suggest that different pathologists can identify subgroups of patients with benign breast disease who have similar levels of breast cancer risk.

This discrepancy may be the result of several factors, including different selection biases between the studies.

Table 26-3 also shows the results of the retrospective cohort study by Hutchinson and coworkers.[9] In this study, as in Kodlin's and our own, the benign breast biopsies of the study patients were reanalyzed using a predefined classification scheme. The discussion of the classification scheme is brief, making it difficult to compare their results with those of other investigators. They found a threefold elevation in cancer risk associated with epithelial hyperplasia or papillomatosis. This risk was not appreciably affected by the presence or absence of atypia. They did find that calcification substantially increased the risk of breast cancer associated with epithelial hyperplasia or papillomatosis. This result is consistent with our finding of increased risk associated with calcification and proliferative disease.

Haagensen and associates[29] have reported an increased risk of breast cancer associated with cysts. This result is in partial agreement with our finding that the presence of cysts increased cancer risk in women with a first-degree family history of breast cancer. This association was not present in women without such a history (see Table 26-1). Dixon and colleagues[30] observed a modest elevation in risk of breast cancer in women with palpable cysts. The relative risk of breast cancer associated with cysts in this study was higher in premenopausal women than in postmenopausal women.

Complex Fibroadenoma and Proliferative Breast Disease

Fibroadenomas exhibit a wide range of cytologic and histologic patterns, with the histological component of these lesions varying from nonexistent through carcinoma in situ. Also, although fibroadenomas have been traditionally thought to be unrelated to risk of breast cancer, several authors have reported that women with these lesions have a mildly elevated risk of breast cancer.[9,31-35] This led us to investigate whether different histologic types of fibroadenomas were associated with different levels of breast cancer risk.[11] We obtained follow-up on 1835 patients from our Nashville study hospitals who were diagnosed with fibroadenoma between 1950 and 1968. These women represented 90% of eligible subjects. The histologic slides of study subjects were reclassified without knowledge of subsequent cancer outcome. The risk of breast cancer in patients who had had fibroadenomas was 2.17 times that of women from a sister-in-law control group. This risk increased to 3.1 in patients with complex fibroadenomas that contained either cysts, sclerosing adenosis, epithelial calcifications, or papillary apocrine changes. Risk of breast cancer was also elevated in patients whose adjacent parenchyma contained proliferative disease (Table 26-4). Risk of breast cancer was further enhanced in patients with a family history of a first-degree relative with breast cancer and either complex fibroadenoma or adjacent proliferative disease. These women had a cumulative 25-year incidence of breast cancer of about 20% (Fig. 26-3). Two thirds of study subjects had simple fibroadenomas and no family history of breast cancer. These patients did not have a significant elevation in risk of breast cancer compared with women from the general population. We have also studied the importance of ALH or ADH within fibroadenomas.[18] These findings are rare, being found in 0.8% of fibroadenomas. Atypia within fibroadenomas cannot be used to predict the presence of atypia in the adjacent parenchyma and does not impart a clinically meaningful elevation in risk of breast cancer over that associated with fibroadenoma alone.

TABLE 26-4

Relative Risk of Invasive Breast Cancer in Patients with Fibroadenoma

Risk Factor	No. of Women	No. of Cancers	Connecticut Controls Relative Risk*	Connecticut Controls 95% Confidence Interval	Sister-in-Law Controls Relative Risk*	Sister-in-Law Controls 95% Confidence Interval
All patients	1835	87	1.61	1.3–2	2.17	1.5–3.2
Internal diagnosis[†]						
Not complex	1413	58	1.42	1.1–1.8	1.89	1.3–2.9
Complex	422	29	2.24	1.6–3.2	3.10	1.9–5.1
External diagnosis[‡]						
No parenchyma	477	21	1.59	1–2.5	1.89	1.1–3.2
No proliferative disease (PD)	1177	51	1.48	1.1–1.9	2.07	1.4–3.2
PD without atypia	162	12	2.16	1.2–3.8	3.47	1.8–6.8
Atypical hyperplasia	19	3	4.77	1.5–15	7.29	2.2–24
Total PD	181	15	2.43	1.5–4	3.88	2.1–7.2

*Risks are relative to women from Connecticut and to sister-in-law controls. The Connecticut risks are adjusted for age at diagnosis, year of diagnosis, and length of follow-up. The sister-in-law risks are adjusted for age at diagnosis, length of follow-up, parity, age of first birth, and age of menarche. (The age of diagnosis for each sister-in-law was the age at which her matched ir-law's fibroadenoma was diagnosed.)
[†]Complex fibroadenomas contain either cysts, sclerosing adenosis, epithelial calcifications, or papillary apocrine change.
[‡]Diagnosis of parenchyma adjacent to the fibroadenoma.

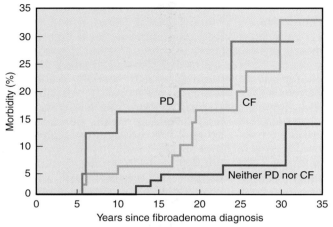

Figure 26-3 Cumulative incidence of invasive breast cancer in patients with fibroadenoma and a family history (FH) of a first-degree relative with breast cancer. In fibroadenoma patients with FH, women with complex fibroadenomas (CF) or adjacent proliferative disease (PD) had significantly greater cancer incidence than women without CF ($P = 0.004$) or PD ($P = 0.001$), respectively. The cumulative incidence after 25 years for women with FH and either CF or PD was about 20%. (Adapted from Dupont WD, Page DL, Parl FF, et al: Long-term risk of breast cancer in women with fibroadenoma. N Engl J Med 331:10–15, 1994. Copyright 1994 Massachusetts Medical Society. All rights reserved.)

The clinical implications of these results are most important in women with a family history of a first-degree relative with breast cancer. For these women, the presence of either adjacent proliferative disease or complex fibroadenomas adds to the magnitude of their risk of breast cancer. Although it is not appropriate to unduly concern young women with a family history of the disease, a diagnosis of complex fibroadenoma should be a further encouragement for regular mammographic surveillance by 35 or 40 years of age. Although it may occasionally be technically difficult, the inclusion of some adjacent parenchyma when fibroadenomas are surgically removed seems appropriate and will more often reduce anxiety than increase it. Women with noncomplex fibroadenomas who have neither adjacent

proliferative disease nor a family history of breast cancer are not at elevated risk of breast cancer. It should be emphasized that two thirds of patients with fibroadenoma have neither a complex lesion nor a family history, and they may be reassured by the knowledge that their risk of breast cancer is not appreciably affected by their tumor.

We believe that there is clinical value in defining *proliferative breast disease* to mean lesions that have been shown to be markers approaching a twofold to threefold elevation in risk of breast cancer. Using this definition, complex fibroadenomas should be included among the proliferative breast lesions.

Effect of Time since Biopsy on Risk of Breast Cancer

Most relative risk estimates from longitudinal studies are derived under the assumption that each patient's relative risk remains constant over time. It is possible, however, for the relative risk of an individual patient to vary as a function of either age or time since initial diagnosis. An example of such a change can be found in our studies of benign breast disease. We have previously reported that women who have undergone breast biopsy revealing AH have 5.3 times the risk of breast cancer of biopsied women who lacked proliferative disease and that the corresponding relative risk for women with PDWA is 1.9.[10] These results were obtained using a proportional hazards regression model that assumes that relative risk remains constant over time. Figure 26-4, however, shows an alternative analysis of these same data. The risk estimates were derived from a hazard regression model that uses time-dependent covariates.[36,37] Figure 26-4 shows that the breast cancer risk for women with both AH and PDWA is greatest in the first 10 years after benign breast biopsy. Women with PDWA who remain free of breast cancer for 10 years are at no greater risk than are women of similar age who do not have such a history. The relative risk of breast cancer in women with AH is halved if they remain free of breast cancer for 10 years after their initial biopsy.

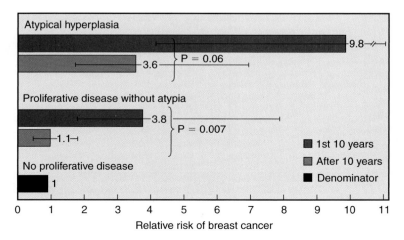

Figure 26-4 Relative risk of breast cancer in women with proliferative disease. Risks of patients with and without atypia are contrasted with risks of biopsied women who did not have proliferative disease. Relative risks of breast cancer drop substantially in women who remain free of breast cancer for 10 years following their proliferative disease biopsy. (From Dupont WD, Page DL: Relative risk of breast cancer varies with time since diagnosis of atypical hyperplasia. Human Pathol 20:723–725, 1989. Reprinted with permission.)

This supports the hypothesis that AHs are not obligate precursor lesions for breast cancer and that these lesions may progress to cancer, remain unchanged, or possibly regress over a substantial period. Their presence at time of biopsy may be best regarded as a marker of increased risk.

Krieger and Hiatt[32] have reported similar findings on the effect of time since biopsy on the risk of breast cancer. Women whose benign breast lesions had a Black-Chabon[28] score of 1 or 2 had a twofold elevation in risk of breast cancer that varied little with time since biopsy. For women with a Black-Chabon score of 4, however, relative risks of breast cancer of 3.5, 2.4, and 1.7 were reported for follow-up intervals of 0–17, 10–17, and 15–17 years, respectively.

The absolute risk for all the women in our study group[10] seems to be approximately evenly distributed over the 17-year period of follow-up (see Fig. 26-1). The knowledge that invasive carcinomas were fairly evenly distributed over this time, combined with the fact that approximately half the invasive carcinomas had occurred by year 10, would have led us to predict the finding just described. Thus, an approximately constant cancer incidence over a 17-year span, together with a rising age-specific incidence in women without proliferative disease (the denominator of the relative risk statistic), implies that a woman's relative risk of breast cancer must fall with increasing time since biopsy. Whether relative risk will continue to drop with further follow-up is, of course, yet to be determined. This time-dependent analysis does suggest that one should not presume the constancy of relative risk figures through an entire lifetime when making clinical decisions.

RADIAL SCAR

Jacobs and colleagues[38] studied the association between radial scars in benign breast biopsies and risk of breast cancer. They found that women with radial scars had 1.8 (95% CI 1.1–2.9) times the risk compared with women without radial scars. This risk increased to 3 (95% CI 1.7–5.5) in women with both radial scars and PDWA compared with women with neither lesion. In our cohort, we found that the relative risk of breast cancer associated with radial scar was 1.82 (95% CI 1.2–2.7) at 10 years.[39] Restricting the analysis to women older than 49 years of age increased the risk to 2.14 (95% CI 0.6–2.8). These risks decreased with increasing years of follow-up. Approximately 92% of women with radial scars also had proliferative disease, but radial scars were present in only 1.3% of biopsies without proliferative disease. Analyses stratifying relative risk with regard to proliferative disease found radial scars to minimally elevate the relative risk of subsequent breast cancer. Radial scars in the absence of proliferative disease are uncommon. Although the presence of radial scars in a benign breast biopsy mildly elevates risk of breast cancer, we believe that this risk can be largely attributed to the category of coexistent proliferative disease. In women with both radial scars and AH, recommendations for interventions beyond biopsy should be based on the extent of the AH.

HORMONAL REPLACEMENT THERAPY IN WOMEN WITH PROLIFERATIVE DISEASE

A question of great importance to women and their physicians is whether hormonal replacement therapy (HRT) can be safely given to women with a history of proliferative breast disease. This question has been studied by the authors[40] and by Byrne and colleagues.[41] Both of these studies found no evidence that risk of breast cancer in women with either PDWA or AH was further increased by taking HRT. Although these findings are reassuring, it must be noted that the power of both studies to detect a moderate elevation in risk due to this therapy was fairly low. Hence, these studies cannot rule out such an increase. Also, the majority of women in both studies took HRT for less than 5 years. Hence, the question of risk in these women associated with long-term HRT use cannot be adequately addressed.

It should also be noted that a clinical trial conducted by the Women's Health Initiative[42] found HRT to be associated with a relative risk of breast cancer of 1.26 (95% CI 1–1.59). In this trial, women were enrolled after the menopause. The average age at recruitment was 63 years, which raises questions about the external validity of this study in regard to perimenopausal women considering HRT for vasomotor symptoms. Therapy consisted of conjugated equine estrogens plus a progestin, which study subjects took for an average duration of 5.2 years. Risk of breast cancer was entirely restricted to women who had taken HRT prior to enrolling in this study. The relative risk of breast cancer in women with no prior HRT exposure was 1.06 (95% CI 0.81–1.38). Hence, the Women's Health Initiative provides no evidence that taking HRT for a few years to wean women from their endogenous estrogen increases risk of breast cancer. This study also did not address risk of breast cancer in women with a history of benign breast disease. However, in light of these results, it would be prudent for women with a history of AH to avoid taking HRT for more than 5 years.

REDUCED EXPRESSION OF TRANSFORMING GROWTH FACTOR-β TYPE II RECEPTORS IN WOMEN WITH PROLIFERATIVE DISEASE

We have studied the effect on breast cancer risk of reduced expression of the transforming growth factor-β (TGF-β) type II receptors (TβRII) in women with epithelial hyperplasia lacking atypia (EHLA).[19] We found that risk of breast cancer increased with decreasing expression of this receptor in women with these lesions. Women with EHLA and 25% to 75% TβRII-positive cells had 1.98 times the risk of breast cancer of women with EHLA and normal TβRII expression (more than 75% TβRII-positive cells). Women with EHLA and less than 25% TβRII-positive cells had 3.41 times the risk of breast cancer of women with EHLA and normal TβRII expression (test for trend $P = 0.008$). This finding is biologically plausible because the normal role of TGF-β is to down-regulate cellular proliferation. There is a reasonable hypothesis consistent with these results. Proliferative lesions that cannot "hear" this down-regulating TGF-β signal are more likely to progress to cancer than are lesions with normal TβRII expression that are at least aware of this signal.

REFERENCES

1. Foote FW, Stewart FW: Comparative studies of cancerous versus noncancerous breasts. Ann Surg 121:197–222, 1945.
2. Frantz VK, Pickren JW, Melcher GW, Auchingloss HJ: Incidence of chronic cystic disease in so-called "normal breasts." Cancer 4:762–783, 1951.
3. Jensen HM, Rice JR, Wellings SR: Preneoplastic lesions in the human breast. Science 191:295–297, 1976.
4. Kramer WM, Rush BF Jr: Mammary duct proliferation in the elderly. A histopathologic study. Cancer 31:130–137, 1973.
5. Sandison AT: An autopsy study of the adult human breast. National Cancer Institute Monograph No. 8, DHEW PHS. Washington, DC: US Government Printing Office, 1962.
6. Sasano N, Tateno H, Stemmermann GN: Volume and hyperplastic lesions of breasts of Japanese women in Hawaii and Japan. Prev Med 7:196–204, 1978.
7. Kodlin D, Winger EE, Morgenstern NL, Chen U: Chronic mastopathy and breast cancer. A follow-up study. Cancer 39:2603–2607, 1977.
8. Black MM, Barclay TH, Cutler SJ, et al: Association of atypical characteristics of benign breast lesions with subsequent risk of breast cancer. Cancer 29:338–343, 1972.
9. Hutchinson WB, Thomas DB, Hamlin WB, et al: Risk of breast cancer in women with benign breast disease. J Natl Cancer Inst 65:13, 1980.
10. Dupont WD, Page DL: Risk factors for breast cancer in women with proliferative breast disease. N Engl J Med 312:146–151, 1985.
11. Dupont WD, Page DL, Parl FF, et al: Long-term risk of breast cancer in women with fibroadenoma. N Engl J Med 331:10–15, 1994.
12. Jensen RA, Page DL, Dupont WD, Rogers LW: Invasive breast cancer risk in women with sclerosing adenosis. Cancer 64:1977–1983, 1989.
13. Page DL, Vander Zwaag R, Rogers LW, et al: Relation between component parts of fibrocystic disease complex and breast cancer. J Natl Cancer Inst 61:1055–1063, 1978.
14. Page DL, Dupont WD, Rogers LW, Rados MS: Atypical hyperplastic lesions of the female breast. A long-term follow-up study. Cancer 55:2698–2708, 1985.
15. Page DL, Kidd TE, Jr., Dupont WD, et al: Lobular neoplasia of the breast: Higher risk for subsequent invasive cancer predicted by more extensive disease. Hum Pathol 22:1232–1239, 1991.
16. Page DL, Salhany KE, Jensen RA, Dupont WD: Subsequent breast carcinoma risk after biopsy with atypia in a breast papilloma. Cancer 78:258–266, 1996.
17. Page DL, Dupont WD, Jensen RA: Papillary apocrine change of the breast: Associations with atypical hyperplasia and risk of breast cancer. Cancer Epidemiol Biomarkers Prev 5:29–32, 1996.
18. Carter BA, Page DL, Schuyler P, et al: No elevation in long-term breast carcinoma risk for women with fibroadenomas that contain atypical hyperplasia. Cancer 92:30–36, 2001.
19. Gobbi H, Dupont WD, Simpson JF, et al: Transforming growth factor-beta and breast cancer risk in women with mammary epithelial hyperplasia. J Natl Cancer Inst 91:2096–2101, 1999.
20. Dupont WD, Parl FF, Hartmann WH, et al: Breast cancer risk associated with proliferative breast disease and atypical hyperplasia. Cancer 71:1258–1265, 1993.
21. London SJ, Connolly JL, Schnitt SJ, Colditz GA: A prospective study of benign breast disease and the risk of breast cancer. JAMA 67:941–944, 1992.
22. Marshall LM, Hunter DJ, Connolly JL, et al: Risk of breast cancer associated with atypical hyperplasia of lobular and ductal types. Cancer Epidemiol Biomarkers Prev 6:297–301, 1997.
23. Hartmann LC, Sellers TA, Frost MH, et al: Benign breast disease and the risk of breast cancer [see comment]. N Engl J Med 353:229–237, 2005.
24. Fitzgibbons PL, Henson DE, Hutter RV: Benign breast changes and the risk for subsequent breast cancer: an update of the 1985 consensus statement. Cancer Committee of the College of American Pathologists. Arch Pathol Lab Med 122:1053–1055, 1998.
25. Page DL, Anderson TJ, Rogers LW: Epithelial hyperplasia. In Page DL, Anderson TJ (eds): Diagnostic histopathology of the breast. Edinburgh, Churchill Livingstone, 1987, pp 120–156.
26. Friedenreich C, Bryant H, Alexander F, et al: Risk factors for benign proliferative breast disease. Int J Epidemiol 29:637–644, 2000.
27. Collins LC, Baer HJ, Tamimi RM, et al: The influence of family history on breast cancer risk in women with biopsy-confirmed benign breast disease: Results from the Nurses' Health Study. Cancer 107:1240–1247, 2006.
28. Black MM, Chabon AB: In situ carcinoma of the breast. In Sommers SC (ed): Pathology annual. New York, Appleton-Century-Crofts, 1969, pp 185–210.
29. Haagensen CD, Bodian C, Haagensen DEJ: Breast cancer risk and detection. Philadelphia, WB Saunders, 1981.
30. Dixon JM, McDonald C, Elton RA, Miller WR: Risk of breast cancer in women with palpable breast cysts: A prospective study. Edinburgh Breast Group. Lancet 353:1742–1745, 1999.
31. Carter CL, Corle DK, Micozzi MS, et al: A prospective study of the development of breast cancer in 16,692 women with benign breast disease. Am J Epidemiol 128:467–477, 1988.
32. Krieger N, Hiatt RA: Risk of breast cancer after benign breast diseases. Variation by histologic type, degree of atypia, age at biopsy, and length of follow-up. Am J Epidemiol 135:619–631, 1992.
33. Levi F, Randimbison L, Te VC, La Vecchia C: Incidence of breast cancer in women with fibroadenoma. Int J Cancer 57:681–683, 1994.
34. McDivitt RW, Stevens JA, Lee NC, et al: Histologic types of benign breast disease and the risk for breast cancer. The Cancer and Steroid Hormone Study Group. Cancer 69:1408–1414, 1992.
35. Moskowitz M, Gartside P, Wirman JA, McLaughlin C: Proliferative disorders of the breast as risk factors for breast cancer in a self-selected screened population: Pathologic markers. Radiology 134:289–291, 1980.
36. Dupont WD, Page DL: Relative risk of breast cancer varies with time since diagnosis of atypical hyperplasia. Human Pathol 20:723–725, 1989.
37. Kalbfleisch JD, Prentice RL: The statistical analysis of failure time data, 2nd ed. New York, Wiley, 2002.
38. Jacobs TW, Byrne C, Colditz G, et al: Radial scars in benign breast-biopsy specimens and the risk of breast cancer. N Engl J Med 340:430–436, 1999.
39. Sanders ME, Page DL, Simpson JF, et al: Interdependence of radial scar and proliferative disease with respect to invasive breast carcinoma risk in patients with benign breast biopsies. Cancer 106:1453–1461, 2006.
40. Dupont WD, Page DL, Parl FF, et al: Estrogen replacement therapy in women with a history of proliferative breast disease. Cancer 85:1277–1283, 1999.
41. Byrne C, Schairer C, Wolfe J, Parekh N, et al: Mammographic features and breast cancer risk: Effects with time, age, and menopause status. J Natl Cancer Inst 87:1622–1629, 1995.
42. Rossouw JE, Anderson GL, Prentice RL, et al: Risks and benefits of estrogen plus progestin in healthy postmenopausal women: Principal results from the Women's Health Initiative randomized controlled trial. Jama 288:321–333, 2002.

chapter 27

Steroid Receptors in Breast Cancer

DOUGLAS YEE | DAVID POTTER

Estrogen Receptors in Breast Cancer

OVERVIEW

Estrogen is a steroid hormone, synthesized by ovaries and other tissues, that is essential for normal mammary development as well as lactation. Estrogen mediates its activities in target tissues by activating estrogen receptors, which exhibit transcriptional (genomic) and membrane localized (nongenomic) signaling activities. The transcriptional activity in targeted genes occurs in cooperation with coactivator proteins that interact directly or indirectly with estrogen responsive genes facilitating mammary tissue proliferation. The physiologic functions of estrogen signaling pathways are co-opted in breast cancer to promote cancer progression. There are two major receptors for estrogen of the nuclear hormone receptor family, ERα and ERβ. The majority of breast cancers, about 70%, expresses the estrogen receptor ERα, and immunohistochemical detection of ERα is predictive of response to hormonal therapy. ERα is cyclically regulated to the menstrual cycle in normal mammary tissue, but it is constitutively expressed in the most common subtypes of human breast cancer wherein it functions as a master regulator, promoting breast cancer growth and disease progression. In contrast, ERβ exhibits an overlapping, but distinct, tissue distribution of its pattern of expression in mammary tissue, cardiovascular tissue, the gastrointestinal tract, and bone. The role of ERβ in breast cancer is less well characterized. On the basis of extensive clinical trial data in the 1970s and since then, ERα has been developed clinically as classifier of breast cancers that respond to hormonal therapy. ERα can be targeted with selective estrogen receptor modulators (SERMs) such as tamoxifen that compete with estrogen and alter the conformation of the ligand-binding domain of the receptor. SERMs such as tamoxifen are effective in the metastatic and adjuvant settings, and tamoxifen itself has also been successful in chemoprevention of breast cancer in women at elevated risk of breast cancer. Although tamoxifen is effective in pre- and postmenopausal women, estrogen deprivation therapy is possible in postmenopausal women, because the majority of their estrogen is synthesized from androstenedione by aromatase. In postmenopausal women, available estrogen can be reduced by aromatase inhibitors (AIs), which block aromatase (CYP19) function, resulting in adjuvant effectiveness that exceeds tamoxifen, as measured in several large phase III clinical trials, including the Arimidex, Tamoxifen, Alone or in Combination (ATAC) trial. A third approach for hormonal therapy is exemplified by the antiestrogen drug fulvestrant, which promotes proteolytic degradation of ERα. The mechanisms by which inhibition of estrogen signaling in breast cancer affects growth and survival pathways are still poorly understood, despite a recent wealth of information on estrogen's classical genomic (transcription) and novel nongenomic (membrane-associated) signaling mechanisms. We discuss the strengths and limitations of current clinical approaches that target estrogen signaling pathways.

HISTORICAL BACKGROUND

In the mid-1890s, Dr. George T. Beatson presented a paper to the Edinburgh Medico-Chirurgical Society stating that oophorectomy in rabbits resulted in loss of lactation. This led to his hypothesis that lactation is controlled by the ovaries and that removal of the ovaries could potentially benefit patients with breast cancer. Based on his hypothesis, Dr. Beatson performed an oophorectomy on June 15, 1895 on a premenopausal patient with advanced, unresectable breast cancer with soft tissue recurrence. The patient showed clinical improvement, had a complete remission, and survived 4 years after the surgery. This finding was the first clinical evidence that breast cancer, rather than simply lactation, may be dependent on ovarian function.[1,2] Although the benefit of oophorectomy in some breast cancer patients was quickly confirmed by Dr. Stanley N. Boyd, with a case report[3] and a subsequent series of 46 premenopausal women with advanced breast cancer, the hormonal mechanism remained to be discovered.[4] In 1923, an ovarian hormone regulating mammary tissue, estrogen, was discovered by Drs. Edgar Allen and Edward Doisy.[5]

Nearly 40 years then passed, until Jensen and Jacobson synthesized radioactive estradiol (E2), leading to the discovery in rats that E2 localized to the uterus and vagina.[6] The observation of tissue specific localization of E2 led to the hypothesis that there is a specific receptor for estrogen. In 1966, the estrogen receptor (ER) was purified and characterized,[7] leading to the subsequent findings that breast tissue expresses ER[8] and some breast cancers contain ER.[9] Furthermore, E2 was linked to cellular proliferation and differentiation in normal tissues,[10,11] whereas growth of rat mammary carcinomas was found to be both E2 dependent and independent, suggesting that although E2 plays a role in mammary carcinoma growth, it is not required.[12] The concentration range under which hormone binding occurs varies depending on biologic conditions. E2 concentrations much lower than 10^{-12} M are capable of stimulating ER function; these are well below the concentrations that can be measured by generally available clinical assays.

With the understanding that E2 is synthesized from adrenal androstenedione, it was hypothesized that adrenalectomy would help patients with ER-expressing breast cancer, and in 1971 a study found supporting clinical evidence.[13] The utility of ER testing was subsequently established when investigators found that patients responding to tamoxifen exhibited higher levels of ER,[14,15] leading to the further study and refinement of endocrine therapy for ER-positive breast cancer in clinical trials during the past 40 years. Most notably, researchers demonstrated that 5 years of tamoxifen was effective for prevention of breast cancer recurrence when added to adjuvant chemotherapy in node-positive patients[16] and subsequently was effective as adjuvant therapy in node-negative patients (Trial NSAPB B14).[17] In a landmark breast cancer prevention study, tamoxifen exhibited efficacy as a preventative agent in patients with increased risk for breast cancer estimated by the Gail model, demonstrating proof of principle of chemoprevention in an "at risk" patient population (National Surgical Adjuvant Breast and Bowel Project [NSABP] P-1).[18] Aiding the development of prognostic models for hormonally responsive breast cancer was the discovery that ER controls the progesterone receptor (PR).[19] Although ER is predictive of response to hormonal therapy rather than prognostic, a prognostic risk model for recurrence in patients with ER-positive breast cancer receiving adjuvant tamoxifen has been developed; it incorporates, in part, gene expression of ER and PR, along with expression of a defined set of additional genes measured by real-time polymerase chain reaction (PCR) from paraffin block material.[20]

Expression of Estrogen Receptors in Breast Cancer

About 70% of breast cancers express ERα detectable by immunohistochemistry. The expression of ERα in breast cancer is constitutive, in contrast to the normal mammary epithelium, where proliferating cells fail to exhibit ER expression and ERα expression is confined to a small proportion of nonproliferating luminal epithelial cells.

Current information suggests that ER-expressing breast cancer cells can be held in a nonproliferative state by growth inhibitory proteins, including tumor growth factor-β (TGF-β) and p27.[21-23] The p27 protein is an inhibitor of cyclin-dependent protein kinases (CDKs) that regulate cell cycle progression. The mechanisms by which ERα expression increases during the evolution of breast cancer are unknown. About 21% of ERα-positive breast cancers exhibit amplification of the gene encoding ERα, ESR1, but this observation leaves the increased expression of ERα in the remaining ER-positive breast cancers unexplained.[24] Another mechanism may be related to caveolin-1 mutations, which are associated with ERα-positive breast cancer.[25] ERα-expressing mammary epithelial cells appear to undergo a growth pattern alteration during carcinogenesis, in which autocrine or paracrine growth stimulation removes inhibitory controls.

It has been hypothesized that ERα could play a role in the etiology of breast cancer under conditions of prolonged exposure to estrogens, such as those occurring with early menarche or late menopause,[26] obesity,[27,28] hormone replacement therapy, or increased circulating estrogen levels.[29] Prolonged exposure to E2 could lead to increased proliferation of mammary epithelial cells, increasing the risk of mutation events. Supporting this hypothesis, SERMs that bind to ER and inhibit function, such as tamoxifen or raloxifene, can decrease breast cancer risk. Tamoxifen decreased the risk of breast cancer in women at increased risk (NSABP P-1), and raloxifene also decreased breast cancer risk (NSABP P-2 or Study of Tamoxifen and Raloxifene [STAR] trial).[18,30,31] A second hypothesis is that high E2 levels lead to increased metabolism of E2 to carcinogenic derivatives, such as the reactive catechol 4-hydroxy-E2, which can damage DNA and lead to mutation.[32]

Molecular Cloning and Characterization of the Estrogen Receptors

There are two ubiquitous ERs, ERα and ERβ, but the relative abundance of each receptor determines, in part, the tissue specificity of their effector functions. The molecular era of estrogen biology began with the molecular cloning and sequencing of the ERα cDNA and its gene (ESR1)[33] (Fig. 27-1). ERα expression predominates over ERβ in mammary, uterine, cervical, and vaginal tissue. ERβ was cloned shortly after ERα and predominates in ovarian, lung, and vascular tissue.[34,35] In the brain and cardiovascular systems as well as in bone, ERα and ERβ are both expressed. ERα and ERβ exhibit dissociation constants for E2 of 0.1 and 0.4 nM, respectively,[36] measured by Scatchard analysis methods.[37] Both ERs exhibit E2-dependent DNA binding and mediate transcriptional regulation through interaction with estrogen-response elements (EREs) that may promote or inhibit transcription.

The two ERs exhibit overlapping, but distinct, biologic functions, best described by comparison of ERα and ERβ knockout (KO) mice.[38-40] Female ERα KO mice exhibit arrest of mammary development neonatally and do not

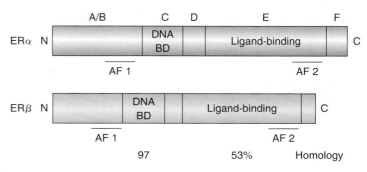

Figure 27-1 Structure of the estrogen receptors (ERs). The A/B domain contains the activator function region AF1. The C domain contains the DNA binding domain and is 97% homologous between ERα and ERβ. The D domain is a spacer. The E domain contains ligand-binding function and is 53% homologous between ERα and ERβ. The E domain also contains the activator region AF2. The F domain is a carboxyl-terminal domain.

undergo pubertal development and differentiation,[38] whereas female ERβ KO mice exhibit normal mammary development.[41] Female ERα KO mice are infertile and exhibit a hypoplastic uterus, cystic and hemorrhagic follicles, few ovarian granulosa cells, and no corpus luteum formation.[38,41] Female ERβ KO mice exhibit reduced fertility, a normal uterus, early atretic follicles, and decreased corpus luteum formation.[41] Bone formation is decreased in the female ERα KO mice[42] but increased in the ERβ KO mice.[43]

STRUCTURE OF ESTROGEN RECEPTORS

The two forms of the ER, ERα and ERβ, are encoded by different genes. ESR1 maps to chromosome 6q25.1, whereas ESR2 maps to 14q23.2. After translation, ERs are initially complexed with heat shock protein 90 (Hsp90); they then dimerize when exposed to estrogen. Dimerization can also be facilitated by DNA binding. ERα (ESR1) and ERβ (ESR2) may form homodimers or heterodimers. The six domains of ERα and ERβ are from N to C terminus: A/B containing transcription activating domain AF1; C containing the DNA binding domain; D, which is an interdomain region; E, which is a ligand-binding domain containing transcription activating domain AF2; and F, which contains the C-terminal domain (see Fig. 27-1). ERα exhibits regulatory phosphorylation sites at Ser106 (CDK2), Ser118 (ERK), Ser236 (PKA), and Tyr537 (Src family kinases), among others. Phosphorylation at Ser118, for example, allows interaction with the p68 RNA helicase coactivator, facilitating transcriptional activation.[44] ERβ exhibits regulatory phosphorylation sites at Ser124 (ERK) and Ser255 (Akt). ERα and ERβ exhibit high homology in the DNA-binding domain (97% homology) and moderate homology of the ligand-binding domain (60%) and AF2 (59%), but differ markedly in AF1 (19%). ERα and ERβ also exhibit a similar binding profile for E2, natural estrogen derivatives, and SERMs.[36] In addition to epidermal growth factor signaling, which can activate ER-mediated transcription through MAPKinase (ERK)-mediated ER phosphonylation,[45] the IGF pathway can also promote ER-mediated transcription.[46] Akt kinase can also promote genomic activity of the ER.[47]

Transcriptional Regulation by Estrogen Receptors

ERα recognizes a 13-base pair ERE consisting of inverted half site repeats characterized as 5′-RGGTCANNNTGACCY-3′ (R = purine, Y = pyrimidine) by recent studies using chromosomal immunoprecipitation in combination with tiled arrays.[48] The consensus sequence reflects the general concept that nuclear hormone receptors are homo- or heterodimers that bind to response elements that consist of half sites of direct or inverted repeats separated by spacers of variable length.[49] ERβ can interact with the same ERE, and the two ER subtypes can form heterodimers. The ERs can substitute for each other for some, but not all, functions as evidenced by studies of KO mice. In cells that express both subtypes, the ratio affects ER function.[49]

Ligand-dependent transcription activation mediated by ERα involves two distinct domains, activator function-1 (AF1) in the NH2-terminus and AF2 in the ligand-binding domain. The two AF domains interact synergistically. The AF2 domain contains a highly conserved amphipathic α-helix that interacts with coactivators to promote transcription.[50]

Genomic Estrogen Receptor Signal Transduction

Ligand-dependent activity of the ER is described by a model in which ERs are located primarily in the cytosol under conditions of low hormone concentration (Fig. 27-2). When hormone binding occurs, transcriptional activation becomes possible through folding of the ER to its active conformation, which can dimerize. The ER-ligand dimer complex dissociates from Hsp90 and translocates to the nucleus, where it binds to EREs in cis-acting enhancers or to repressors that contribute to the regulation of estrogen-responsive genes (see Fig. 27-2). The ER-ligand complex can therefore activate certain estrogen-regulated genes while suppressing others. ER dimers can interact directly with the ERE, but they can also sit piggyback on Fos/Jun (AP1) transcription factor heterodimers and promote transcription of AP1-regulated genes. A number of coactivators also participate in ER transcription, including NCoA-1 (SRC-1),[51] NCoA-2 (TIF-2, GRIP1),[52] and NCoA-3 (AIB1, ACTR, RAC3, p/CIP, TRAM-1),[53,54] which are members of the p160 steroid coactivator family. The closely related histone acetyltransferase (HAT) proteins CREB-binding protein (CBP) and/or p300 protein associate with the HAT PCAF and coactivator ACTR and acetylate histones in chromatin. The acetylation of histones on lysine residues helps promote an open, active conformation facilitating RNA polymerase II (pol II)–mediated transcription of E2-regulated genes. HAT activity overcomes the activity of

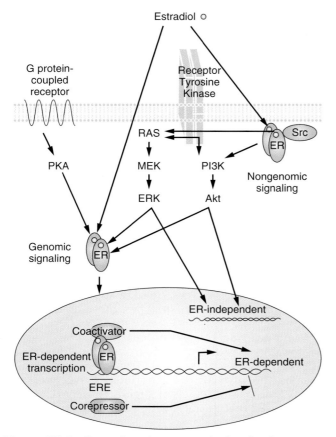

Figure 27-2 Genomic and nongenomic signaling by estrogen receptors (ERs). The ER can signal through genomic pathways by binding E2, followed by release from Hsp90 (not shown), dimerization, and translocation to the nucleus, where the hormone-receptor complex binds to the estrogen-response element (ERE). Depending on whether coactivators or corepressors are recruited, the complex may stimulate or inhibit transcription of ERE-regulated genes. Binding of tamoxifen alters the conformation of the receptor-hormone complex, leading to association with corepressors. Nongenomic signaling involves interaction between hormone-receptor complexes and signaling complexes at the inner leaflet of the plasma membrane, including those containing the nonreceptor tyrosine kinase Src. Growth factor receptors binding EGF (EGFR) and IGF (IGFR-1) also influence signaling of the ER. Signaling through the ERK (MAPK) pathway can directly phosphorylate and activate the ER. Independent of direct transcriptional effects, ER-mediated activation of ERK and Akt kinase at the plasma membrane can stimulate ER-independent gene expression.

histone deacetylases and thereby promotes chromatin activation for transcription. After initial identification of coactivators, it is unknown whether each coactivator is necessary and/or sufficient to interact with the ER to drive estrogen-regulated gene transcription. The need to characterize the roles of individual coactivators and their complexes led to the development of chromatin immunoprecipitation (ChIP), which gives a snapshot of the gene promoter complexes during the process of transcription.[55] This method involves the reversible cross-linking of proteins with formaldehyde, immunoprecipitation of chromatin, and PCR amplification of the immunoprecipitated DNA after reversal of cross-linking to identify which proteins are associated with the ERE.

ChIP analysis has led to new insights into the dynamic interaction of ERα and estrogen-regulated genes in breast cancer cells.[55] This method allowed identification of the time course of association of transcription factors with the ERα-driven promoters and discovery that estrogen-driven association with p160 coactivators occurs in a specific order. The association of the complex of factors was found to be cyclical, with initiation of the initial response peaking at 30 minutes, followed by a trough. A second peak occurs at 2 hours. Each cycle of ERα recruitment corresponds with a cycle of pol II recruitment. This result suggests that estrogen-directed transcription involves assembly and then reassembly of transcription factor complexes, promoting the formation of complexes, consistent with a model of resampling of the hormonal milieu. Associated with ERα are coactivator proteins that facilitate ligand-dependent ERα transcription or inhibition of transcription, indicating that ERα is associated with a specific program of gene expression. Coactivators that promote transcription include p300 and the p160 family coactivators, which along with the factor PBP, play central roles in the assembly of the ER transcription complex.[56–58] In genetic studies, recruitment of p160 is sufficient to initiate ER-mediated transcription.[59] The p160-p300-PBP complex acetylates histones, promoting an open, active chromatin conformation in the vicinity of the ERE. HAT activity is intrinsic to p300 as well as recruited PCAF and TAF250. Subsequently, coactivators CBP and PCAF are recruited and facilitate phosphorylation of the C-terminal domain (CTD) of pol II, promoting transcription. Once the CTD of pol II is phosphorylated, ER and p160 are released. The p300 factor is not required for subsequent cycles. Certain EREs recruit complexes that contain corepressors such as N-CoR and SMRT and not coactivators, resulting in repression of transcription (see Fig. 27-2). Furthermore, when tamoxifen binds ERα, promoter recruitment of the nuclear receptor corepressors N-CoR and SMRT occurs, suggesting that tamoxifen bound to ERα actively represses estrogen-regulated genes by inducing an ERα-corepressor complex (see Fig. 27-2).[55]

Estrogen Receptor Inhibition by Tamoxifen and Its Metabolites in Premenopausal Women

It was recently recognized that the tamoxifen metabolite 4-hydroxy-N-desmethyl-tamoxifen (endoxifen; Fig. 27-3) is likely to be responsible for most of the biologic activity of tamoxifen. Tamoxifen is metabolized to its active metabolites endoxifen and 4-hydroxy-tamoxifen primarily through two cytochrome P450–dependent pathways, which involve CYP2D6 and CYP3A4 (see Fig. 27-3).[60] The principal pathway of endoxifen biosynthesis is demethylation of tamoxifen to N-desmethyl-tamoxifen (endoxifen) by CYP3A4 followed by hydroxylation of N-desmethyl-tamoxifen to endoxifen by CYP2D6 (see Fig. 27-3). Endoxifen is the major metabolite of tamoxifen and is present in plasma at concentrations five to ten times

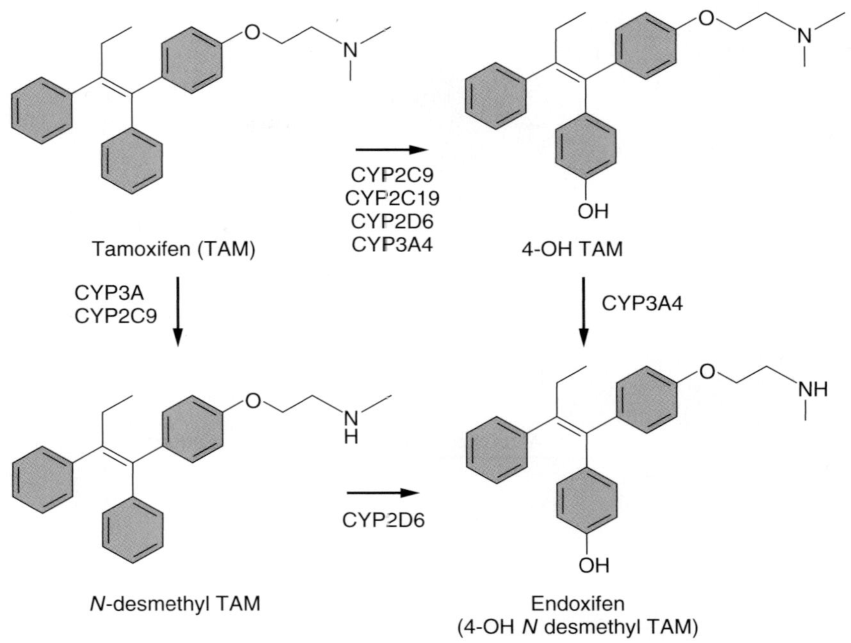

Figure 27-3 Tamoxifen metabolism to endoxifen and 4-hydroxy-tamoxifen. Endoxifen (4-OH-N-desmethyltamoxifen is the major metabolite of tamoxifen. The major route of metabolism is conversion of tamoxifen to N-desmethyl-tamoxifen (N-desmethyl TAM) by cytochrome P450 enzymes CYP3A and to a lesser extent, CYP2C9, followed by hydroxylation by CYP2D6. (Stearns V, Johnson MD, Rae JM, et al: Active tamoxifen metabolite plasma concentrations after coadministration of tamoxifen and the selective serotonin reuptake inhibitor paroxetine. J Natl Cancer Inst 95:1758, 2003.)

higher than 4-hydroxy-tamoxifen.[60] Endoxifen is therefore the most abundant of the active metabolites of tamoxifen.

Endoxifen exhibits potent antiestrogenic activity in vitro and clinically. Endoxifen and 4-hydroxy-tamoxifen exhibit similar higher affinity binding to ER in nuclear extracts[61] and similar inhibition curves for blockade of E2 stimulation of breast cancer lines, whereas tamoxifen is significantly less potent.[60] In studies of tamoxifen metabolism in women of known CYP2D6 genotype, investigators discovered that women carrying wild type CYP2D6 alleles metabolized tamoxifen to endoxifen, whereas women carrying mutant alleles were poor effectors of this conversion and experienced lower exposure to endoxifen.[60,62] Furthermore, when the CYP2D6 inhibitor paroxetine was coadministered with tamoxifen, metabolism of tamoxifen to endoxifen was greatly impaired. Together, these results strongly suggest that endoxifen and 4-hydroxy-tamoxifen account for most of the clinical activity of tamoxifen and that important consideration must be given to coadministered medications. Among antidepressant drugs, venlafaxine exhibits less interaction with tamoxifen than paroxetine in patients with a homozygous wild type CYP2D6 genotype, suggesting that certain selective serotonin reuptake inhibitors are less likely to interact with tamoxifen.[62]

Pharmacogenetics of tamoxifen metabolism has been found to be of significant clinical importance in outcomes of ER-positive breast cancer. In the North American population, genotypes *1, *3, *4, *5 and *6 are the most prevalent, exhibiting frequencies of 77.8%, 1.3%, 18%, 2.3%, and 0.63%, respectively.[62] Genotype *1 is wild type, *4 results in a splicing defect, *3 and *6 result in translation frame shifts, and *5 results in deletion of the entire CYP2D6 gene. It has recently been discovered that tamoxifen-treated women in a North Central Cancer Treatment Group clinical trial who exhibited a *4/*4 genotype had decreased disease-free survival ($P = 0.012$) and did not have moderate to severe hot flashes that were experienced by women who were heterozygous or homozygous for the wild type CYP2D6 allele.[63,64] Patients who fail to experience hot flashes on tamoxifen should have their medications checked for possible drug interactions, and they now can be genotyped for CYP2D6 polymorphisms that fail to metabolize tamoxifen to active metabolites.

E2 Synthesis and the Role of Aromatase Inhibitors in Postmenopausal Women

There are many natural and drug ligands for the estrogen receptors that exhibit different binding specificities and associated activities. The three most common estrogenic hormones are 17-β estradiol (E2), which exhibits 3- and 17-hydroxy moieties important for receptor interaction, estriol (E3), which is hydroxylated at the 16-position, and estrone, which exhibits a 17-keto moiety (Fig. 27-4A). E2 is the most abundant estrogen and interacts with ER through contacts at the 3-OH and 17-OH positions, as well as the critical aromatic ring. Estrone is converted to estrone sulfate, which is a long-lived derivative that forms a storage pool that can be converted to the more active E2. The classical ligand E2 exhibits a similar affinity for both receptors. Estrone binds preferentially to ERα, while E3 binds selectively to ERβ. A critical step in the synthesis of estrogens, particularly in postmenopausal women, is aromatase (CYP19) conversion of androstenedione to E2 or testosterone to estrone. Estrone and E2 are interconvertable by

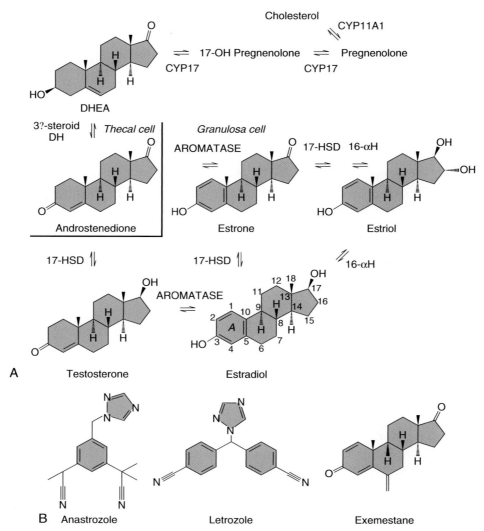

Figure 27-4 Estradiol synthesis in the ovary by aromatase and inhibition by aromatase inhibitors. **A,** The cytochrome P450 enzymes CYP11A1 and CYP17 facilitate conversion of cholesterol to dehydroepiandrosterone (DHEA) through the intermediates pregnenolone and 17-OH pregnenolone. In thecal cells, DHEA is converted to androstenedione by 3β-hydroxysteroid dehydrogenase (3β-steroid DH). Androstenedione crosses the basement membrane and enters granulosa cells, where it is converted by aromatase (CYP19) to estrone or by 17-hydroxysteroid dehydrogenase (17-HSD) to testosterone. Estrone is converted to estradiol (E2) by 17-HSD. Alternatively, testosterone is converted to E2 by CYP19. Through another pathway, estrone can be converted by 17-HSD and 16α-hydroxylase (16α-H) to estriol (E3). E3 can also be synthesized from E2 by 16α-H. **B,** CYP19 inhibitors (AIs) may be either nonsteroidal (anastrozole and letrozole) or steroidal (exemestane).

17-hydroxysteriod dehydrogenase (17-HSD). E3 can be synthesized from E2 by 16α-hydroxylase.

In premenopausal women, estrogen is synthesized primarily in the ovaries. Ovarian thecal cells and granulosa cells cooperate to produce estrogen. The thecal cells respond to luteinizing hormone (LH) and produce androstenedione (see Fig. 27-4A), which then crosses the basement membrane and enters granulosa cells, where it is processed to E2.[65,66] At the thecal cell, LH stimulates cyclic AMP second messenger, which induces transcription of mRNA encoding the enzymes CYP11A1, CYP17, and 3β-hydroxysteroid dehydrogenase (3β-steroid DH), which convert cholesterol to androstenedione.[67,68] The granulosa cell depends on CYP19 to convert androstenedione to estrone, which is then converted to E2 by 17-hydroxysteroid dehydrogenase (17-HSD).[69,70]

Follicle-stimulating hormone (FSH) increases cAMP in the granulosa cells, which promotes CYP19 mRNA expression.[71,72] In premenopausal women, most of the circulating E2 is produced by the ovaries, not by conversion of androgens to E2. CYP19 can be stimulated in the ovary by FSH and blocking CYP19 with AIs in functional ovaries is not effective, based on empiric clinical studies performed early in the course of development of these drugs.[73]

Although most E2 is synthesized in the ovaries in premenopausal women, extragonadal conversion of testosterone to E2 by CYP19 is the major source of E2 biosynthesis in postmenopausal women. Extragonadal tissues active in synthesis of E2 include adipose stromal cells and adrenal tissue. In extragonadal tissues, androstenedione is converted by 17-HSD to testosterone and subsequently by CYP19 to E2 (see Fig. 27-4A). In contrast to premenopausal women, AI inhibition is more effective in reducing circulating E2 levels in postmenopausal women. The AIs may be either nonsteroidal (anastrozole and letrozole) or steroidal (exemestane; see Fig. 27-4B).

In postmenopausal women, E2 deprivation by AIs has been successful in hormonal treatment of recurrent/metastatic disease and subsequently, in adjuvant hormonal therapy to prevent recurrence. When compared with tamoxifen in recurrent/metastatic breast cancer in postmenopausal patients in phase III trials, letrozole and anastrozole resulted in improved time to progression.[74,75] Currently, the most important use of AIs has been in the adjuvant setting, where anastrozole has been demonstrated to be superior to tamoxifen in the ATAC trial, in terms of recurrence-free survival in the 5-year as well as the 100-month follow-up analyses.[76,77] In one study, letrozole compared with placebo after the completion of 5 years of tamoxifen treatment significantly improved disease-free survival.[78,79] A major side effect of AIs is loss of bone mineral density and increased fracture rates.[76] Bone mineral density is monitored closely, and calcium and vitamin D supplementation are recommended (along with an oral bisphosphonate if indicated).

The Suppression of Ovarian Function Trial (SOFT) is an ongoing trial to determine whether AIs can be used in premenopausal women; it is testing tamoxifen, ovarian function suppression plus tamoxifen, or ovarian function suppression plus the AI exemestane. The primary end point is disease-free survival. Another trial is the Tamoxifen and Exemestane Trial (TEXT). In this trial, patients are started on ovarian function suppression with a gonadotropin-releasing hormone (GnRH) analog at the beginning of adjuvant therapy. Both trials use triptorelin as the GnRH analog to suppress ovarian function.

Selective Estrogen Receptor Modulator Inhibition of Estrogen Signaling

In contrast to E2, which is a full agonist, certain SERMs function as mixed agonists-antagonists. Triphenylethylene SERMs, such as tamoxifen (see Fig. 27-3) and toremifene (Fig. 27-5A), bind to ERα or ERβ. Tamoxifen exhibits agonist activity when bound to ERα in certain tissues, most importantly the uterus, thereby increasing risk of endometrial cancer. Simultaneous inhibitory effects of tamoxifen on the breast and growth-promoting effects on endometrial cancer have been demonstrated in an dual xenograft model.[80] These conflicting effects are likely through differential effects on ERα, because, when bound to ERβ, tamoxifen exhibits pure antagonist activity. Toremifene exhibits comparable efficacy to tamoxifen in metastatic breast cancer, has a favorable side-effect profile,[81] and has been approved for treatment of metastatic breast cancer. Because toremifene binds ERα and has agonist activity in uterine tissue, there are similar concerns as for tamoxifen about risks of endometrial cancer, although this issue is somewhat less concerning in the time frame of treatment for recurrent or metastatic disease.

The benzothiophene drug raloxifene binds selectively to ERα and does not act as an agonist in endometrial tissue; therefore, it does not raise the risk of endometrial cancer (see Fig. 27-5A). Raloxifene was observed to promote bone density.[82] The initial studies led to the STAR trial comparing raloxifene and tamoxifen in reducing the risk of invasive breast cancer.[31] Both SERMs were equally effective, but raloxifene exhibited a lower risk of thromboembolic events and cataracts. Raloxifene has been studied primarily in the postmenopausal setting and may increase E2 levels in premenopausal women. Studies of raloxifene in premenopausal women are ongoing.

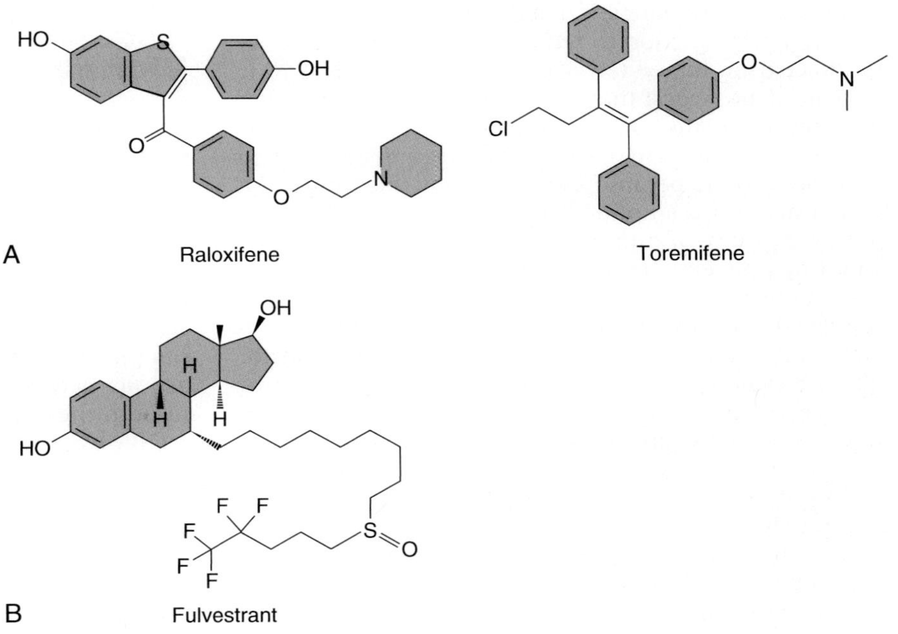

Figure 27-5 Selective estrogen receptor modulators (SERMs) of the benzothiophene and triphenylethylene classes and a full antagonist, fulvestrant. **A,** Raloxifene is a benzothiophene SERM that selectively binds estrogen receptor-α (ERα). Toremifene is a triphenylethylene SERM in the same class as tamoxifen. Toremifene binds ERα and ERβ. **B,** Fulvestrant is a full antagonist of the ER and induces proteasome-mediated proteolysis of the receptor.

A   Raloxifene

Toremifene

B   Fulvestrant

Fulvestrant is a pure antagonist in clinical use (ICI-182, 780; see Fig. 27-5B). Fulvestrant down-regulates the ER through proteosomal proteolysis.[83] Fulvestrant is administered monthly by injection of a depot formulation of the drug. Fulvestrant and exemestane exhibited equivalent activity in an advanced breast cancer study of postmenopausal women.[84] One challenge with fulvestrant has been determining an optimal dosing schedule in metastatic breast cancer.

Nongenomic Estrogen Receptor Signal Transduction

Although the mechanisms outlined in the classical genomic pathway are undoubtedly true, it is also clear that other mechanisms for ERα function also exist. First, estradiol binding of ERα not only initiates transcription, but it also appears that some genes are repressed in breast cancer cells by the "activated" ERα.[85,86] Second, ERα may also regulate breast cancer cells in a manner independent of its ability to act as a transcription factor. These "nongenomic" pathways have been documented in a number of model systems and may be relevant to breast cancer biology. For example, estradiol treatment of ERα-expressing breast cancer cells results in rapid activation of mitogen-activated protein kinase (MAPK; see Fig. 27-2).[87,88] MAPK is a key downstream target of many growth factor signaling pathways, suggesting that signaling events between growth factor and estrogen may overlap. Third, ERα can be found in the plasma membrane, cytoplasm, and mitochondria, as Levin and Pietras stated.[89] A role for membrane-associated ERα in the rapid action of estradiol signaling to MAPK has been shown.[90] In breast cancer cells, this plasma membrane ER is identical to nuclear ERα.[91] ERα may also participate in growth factor receptor signal transduction. In cells that have accommodated to survive in low concentrations of estradiol, such as seen during therapy with AIs, ERα can directly function as an adaptor protein in growth factor receptor signaling.[92] Finally, ERα and ERβ in the mitochondria function to reduce reactive oxygen species and have been linked to breast cancer cell survival.[93]

These data suggest that ERα functions in many different compartments of the breast cancer cell. These findings underline the relevance of targeting this protein in breast cancer, because the malignant phenotype can be affected by disruption of ERα function. However, given the ability of multiple pathways to affect ER function, this provides the breast cancer cell an opportunity to circumvent ERα inhibition. For example, there may be several ways by which growth factor signaling pathways could influence estrogen action. Growth factor receptor signaling pathways may affect the function of ERα as a transcription factor. In addition, ERα itself may be involved in signaling pathways activated by growth factor receptors (see Fig. 27-2). Modification of ERα by growth factor signaling events may also influence ERα function in the nucleus, cytoplasm, membrane, or mitochondrion. However, it remains a challenge to determine which of these functions is critical to the survival, growth, and metastasis of breast cancer cells.

Cross-Talk between Growth Factor Receptors and Estrogen Receptorα Function

One of the first observations suggesting that these two pathways are linked came from the observation that activation of the MAPK signaling pathway by epidermal growth factor resulted in phosphorylation of ERα at a serine residue important in its dimerization.[45] Subsequent studies have shown that a variety of growth factors activate ERα gene transcription in the absence of estradiol.[94-96] In addition to these ligand-independent pathways, many model systems have shown synergy between estradiol and growth factor activation. Thus, it is apparent that ERα function is influenced by other signaling events within a cell. Moreover, ERα-initiated gene transcription may occur in the traditional estrogen-mediated fashion or even in the absence of steroid hormones if other cellular inputs are active. Given the new molecular inhibitors of these growth factor signaling pathways, it would seem logical to combine ERα inhibitors with molecules that block growth factor signaling.

Perhaps the best characterized axis of growth factor signaling is represented by the epidermal growth factor receptor (EGFR) family. EGFR and HER2 have been linked to breast cancer biology, and some breast cancers express both ERα and EGFR signaling components. In a model of HER2 and ERα overexpression, it has been shown that the SERM fulvestrant in combination with the EGFR antagonist gefitinib disrupted growth in an animal model system. Similar preclinical data exist for tamoxifen and the HER2 tyrosine kinase inhibitor lapatinib[48] and tamoxifen and trastuzumab (anti-HER2 antibody).[97] Models of AI resistance have also shown a benefit for combining anti-EGFR strategies with endocrine therapy.[98,99]

Clinical Evidence for Estrogen Receptorα and Growth Factor Signaling Interaction

Are there clinical data supporting the idea that growth factors affect ERα function and outcome? In general, there is an inverse relationship between EGFR expression and ERα.[100-102] The inverse relationship between HER2 and ERα is not as strong as between EGFR and ERα, and a substantial number of patients show both ERα and HER2 expression.[103-106] Because HER2 expression could affect response to tamoxifen therapy, clinical samples have been examined to explore potential interactions between these two growth regulatory pathways in both the adjuvant and metastatic setting.

Newby and colleagues showed that patients who experienced progressive disease while taking tamoxifen were more likely to express either EGFR or HER2. Of the tamoxifen-insensitive patients, over half had expression of EGFR, HER2, or both, in the pretreatment specimens.[105] Patients who responded to tamoxifen rarely had expression of EGFR or HER2, suggesting that activated signaling through EGFR family members may be associated with de novo resistance to tamoxifen.

In the Naples/Grupo Universitario Napoletano 1 (GUN-1) trial, operable breast cancer patients were randomized to receive tamoxifen or no further therapy after primary treatment of the tumor. Elevated levels of HER2 measured by immunohistochemistry were associated with a relative lack of efficacy of adjuvant tamoxifen.[107] The number of women treated by this group is small, but for women with elevated HER2 treated with tamoxifen, there is a trend to an increased risk of recurrence compared with no treatment at all. The number of patients comprising the ERα/HER2-positive patients treated with tamoxifen was small, and a statistically significant effect for worse outcome was not evident. Similar results were found in a study that randomized ERα-positive patients to 2 years of tamoxifen versus placebo. In this study, HER2 expression was associated with little benefit from tamoxifen in operable breast cancer.[108] However, HER2 overexpression is not only associated with poor response to tamoxifen, as recent data from a large randomized trial (ATAC) have suggested—HER2 also identifies patients who have less benefit from either anastrozole or tamoxifen.[109]

In contrast, other studies have not shown that HER2 affects response to tamoxifen. Elledge and others retrospectively evaluated HER2 expression in patients enrolled on a cooperative group study who were treated with tamoxifen for metastatic disease. They showed that HER2 expression had no influence on tamoxifen response rate, time to treatment failure, or survival.[103] In an adjuvant study (Cancer and Leukemia Group [CALGB] 8541), patients were randomized to receive varying doses of cyclophosphamide, doxorubicin, and fluorouracil (CAF).[110] All ERα-positive patients also received tamoxifen. When this trial was analyzed for patients receiving additional hormonal therapy, there was no evidence of an adverse effect of HER2 expression for patients who received tamoxifen.[111] Knopp and associates reported results of a Danish randomized trial of tamoxifen adjuvant therapy.[112] In this report, there was no adverse effect of HER2 on outcome in women receiving tamoxifen.

Love and coworkers examined a different population group and showed that HER2 overexpression identifies favorable outcome to tamoxifen adjuvant therapy.[113] In this study, premenopausal women were subjected to oophorectomy and tamoxifen versus no therapy. As expected, HER2 by itself was a poor prognostic factor. Women who received adjuvant oophorectomy and tamoxifen had improved disease-free survival compared with women who had no detectable levels of HER2. The number of women analyzed was small, but this was the first study to show a better outcome with tamoxifen therapy for tumors overexpressing HER2.

Another way to examine the question about interaction between growth factor signaling and response to SERMs is in the neoadjuvant setting. Ellis and colleagues have reported the results of a randomized trial comparing letrozole to tamoxifen in the neoadjuvant setting.[114] This study confirmed an earlier trial[115] suggesting that tamoxifen was an inferior drug compared with letrozole for patients with overexpression of either EGFR or HER2.

As can be seen, there are conflicting data on the relevance of EGFR/HER2 to ERα inhibition, depending on whether the study was conducted in the metastatic, neoadjuvant, or adjuvant setting. There may be several reasons for this confusion. First, measurement of HER2 expression varies among centers.[116] A central review of specimens was not performed in all of the studies. Thus, it is possible that assay differences could account for the varying results. However, one study has suggested that the results were independent of the HER2 assay.[117] Second, many of the studies also included analysis of patients who had received both tamoxifen and chemotherapy. Because it is apparent that HER2 expression influences response to chemotherapy, these combined treatments add confounding factors. Formal tests for interaction among treatments, HER2 status, and ERα expression were not reported in many studies. Third, simple overexpression is used as a surrogate indicator for activation of post-HER2 signaling pathways. As noted previously, the signaling pathways engaged after growth factor receptor activation are complex. Overexpression alone cannot substitute for a more detailed analysis of signal transduction.

Clinical Trials Designed to Examine Interactions between Growth Factor Signaling and Estrogen Receptorα Inhibition

These data have led to the conduct of preclinical trials combining anti-EGFR inhibitors with antiestrogen strategies. Adding gefitinib to the AI anastrozole in the neoadjuvant setting had no discernible favorable effect in one study based on Ki-67 changes as the primary end point.[118] Another study adding gefitinib to anastrozole demonstrated a marked improvement of progression-free survival, the primary end point.[119] However, the related EGFR tyrosine kinase inhibitor erlotinib alone in the neoadjuvant setting disrupted several biomarkers associated with clinical benefit in ERα-positive tumors.[120] In metastatic disease, the combination of anastrozole plus trastuzumab was superior to anastrozole alone.[121] These apparent discrepant results might be explained by differences in preclinical model systems and the subsequent design of the clinical trial. Most preclinical models address acquired resistance to hormone therapy or rely on creation of cell lines designed to model resistance (e.g., by introducing HER2 in a cell line that does not normally express HER2). In contrast human clinical trials address de novo endocrine resistance. In addition, there are differences in the design of human clinical trials (SERMs vs. AIs; tyrosine kinase inhibitors vs. antibodies) that could account for these differences.

The identification of signaling pathways that impinge on ERα function may provide additional strategies to enhance response to hormonal manipulation. Inhibitors of growth factor receptors, either monoclonal antibodies or tyrosine kinase inhibitors, have been approved for treatment of cancer. Molecules that inhibit specific molecules important in signal transduction pathways (e.g., the mTOR inhibitor everolimus) are currently being examined in phase II and III clinical trials. The preclinical data suggest that combination therapy, including antigrowth factor signaling and anti-ERα strategies will prove superior to either one alone. Thus, the final chapter on inhibition of ERα functions is not yet written.

Progesterone Receptor and Breast Cancer

Progesterone is a steroid hormone synthesized by the ovaries that directs breast development and prepares the breast for lactation after pregnancy. Progesterone receptor (PR) expression is driven by ER transcriptional activation of the PR gene, and only about 5% of breast cancer is PR positive and ER negative. In contrast, about 30% of ER positive breast cancers fail to express PR. There are two hormone-binding PR isoforms, PR-A and -B, which are splicing variants and bind progesterone with high affinity. The PR-B isoform is full length (116 kDa), whereas the PR-A isoform lacks the N-terminal domain (94 kDa). Similar to the ER, there are AF domains, a DNA binding domain, and a hormone-binding domain. PR-A appears to have inhibitory activity, whereas PR-B has transcription activating activity. There is also a truncated PR-C isoform (60 kDa) that lacks classical transcriptional activity.

The role of PR in breast cancer etiology and progression is not well understood. The PR isoforms are induced transcriptionally by ERα in mammary epithelial cells and are indicative of ER function. It is therefore difficult to separate the function of PR from ER, but PR and ER KO mice have helped determine a concerted role for estrogen and progesterone in normal mammary development and differentiation. Because PR-/- mice fail to become pregnant, transplant of mammary tissue revealed that progesterone functions in a paracrine fashion to promote mammary epithelial growth and differentiation.[122] Estrogen and progesterone together promote ductal growth and side branching, which is augmented by growth hormones such as epidermal growth factor and insulin-like growth factor-I.[123,124]

The PR has unclear significance as a prognostic factor. Similar to ER, it may be best considered a predictive factor, because PR expression is closely linked to ER expression. Several studies have indicated that PR expression is a predictor of response to hormonal therapy. In Southwest Oncology Group (SWOG) study 8228, higher PR levels were associated with increased likelihood of response to tamoxifen and improved progression-free survival and overall survival.[125]

REFERENCES

1. Beatson GT: On the treatment of inoperable cases of carcinoma of the mamma. Suggestions for a new method of treatment with illustrative cases. Lancet ii:104, 1896.
2. Beatson GT: On the treatment of inoperable cases of carcinoma of the mamma. Suggestions for a new method of treatment with illustrative cases. Lancet ii:162, 1896.
3. Boyd S: On oophorectomy in the treatment of cancer. BMJ 2:890, 1897.
4. Boyd S: On oophorectomy in cancer of the breast. BMJ 2:1161, 1900.
5. Allen E, Doisy EA: An ovarian hormone: Preliminary report on its localization, extraction, and partial purification and action in test animals. JAMA 81:819, 1923.
6. Jensen EV, Jacobson HI: Basic guides to the mechanism of estrogen action. Recent Prog Horm Res 18:387, 1962.
7. Toft D, Gorski J: A receptor molecule for estrogens: Isolation from the rat uterus and preliminary characterization. Proc Natl Acad Sci USA 55:1574, 1966.
8. Deshpande N, Jensen V, Bulbrook RD: Accumulation of tritiated oestradiol by human breast tissue. Steroids 10, 1967.
9. Wittliff JL, Hilf R, Brooks WF Jr, et al: Specific estrogen-binding capacity of the cytoplasmic receptor in normal and neoplastic breast tissues of humans. Cancer Res 32:1983, 1971.
10. Oka T, Schimke RT: Interaction of estrogen and progesterone in chick oviduct development. I. Antagonistic effect of progesterone on estrogen-induced proliferation and differentiation of tubular gland cells. J Cell Biol 41:816, 1969.
11. Oka T, Schimke RT: Progesterone antagonism of estrogen-induced cytodifferentiation in chick oviduct. Science 163:83, 1969.
12. Turkington RW, Hilf R: Hormonal dependence of DNA synthesis in mammary carcinoma cells in vitro. Science 160:1457, 1968.
13. Fracchia AA, Farrow JH, Miller TR, et al: Hypophysectomy as compared with adrenalectomy in the treatment of advanced carcinoma of the breast. Surg Gynecol Obstet 133:241, 1971.
14. Kiang DT, Frenning DH, Goldman AI, et al: Estrogen receptors and responses to chemotherapy and hormonal therapy in advanced breast cancer. N Engl J Med 299:1330, 1978.
15. Kiang DT, Kennedy BJ: Tamoxifen (antiestrogen) therapy in advanced breast cancer. Ann Intern Med 87:687, 1977.
16. Fisher B, Redmond C, Brown A, et al: Treatment of primary breast cancer with chemotherapy and tamoxifen. N Engl J Med 305:1, 1981.
17. Fisher B, Costantino J, Redmond C, et al: A randomized clinical trial evaluating tamoxifen in the treatment of patients with node-negative breast cancer who have estrogen-receptor-positive tumors. N Engl J Med 320:479, 1989.
18. Fisher B, Costantino JP, Wickerham DL, et al: Tamoxifen for prevention of breast cancer: Report of the National Surgical Adjuvant Breast and Bowel Project P-1 Study. J Natl Cancer Inst 90:1371, 1998.
19. Horwitz KB, Koseki Y, McGuire WL: Estrogen control of progesterone receptor in human breast cancer: Role of estradiol and antiestrogen. Endocrinology 103:1742, 1978.
20. Paik S, Shak S, Tang G, et al: A multigene assay to predict recurrence of tamoxifen-treated, node-negative breast cancer. N Engl J Med 351:2817, 2004.
21. Harvat BL, Seth P, Jetten AM: The role of p27Kip1 in gamma interferon-mediated growth arrest of mammary epithelial cells and related defects in mammary carcinoma cells. Oncogene 14:2111, 1997.
22. Sgambato A, Doki Y, Schieren I, et al: Effects of cyclin E overexpression on cell growth and response to transforming growth factor beta depend on cell context and p27Kip1 expression. Cell Growth Differ 8:393, 1997.
23. Zugmaier G, Lippman ME: Effects of TGF beta on normal and malignant mammary epithelium. Ann NY Acad Sci 593:272, 1990.
24. Holst F, Stahl PR, Ruiz C, et al: Estrogen receptor alpha (ESR1) gene amplification is frequent in breast cancer. Nat Genet 39:655, 2007.
25. Li T, Sotgia F, Vuolo MA, et al: Caveolin-1 mutations in human breast cancer: Functional association with estrogen receptor alpha-positive status. Am J Pathol 168:1998, 2006.
26. Colditz GA: Epidemiology of breast cancer. Findings from the nurses' health study. Cancer 71:1480, 1993.
27. Hankinson SE, Willett WC, Manson JE, et al: Alcohol, height, and adiposity in relation to estrogen and prolactin levels in postmenopausal women. J Natl Cancer Inst 87:1297, 1995.
28. Huang Z, Willett WC, Colditz GA, et al: Waist circumference, waist:hip ratio, and risk of breast cancer in the Nurses' Health Study. Am J Epidemiol 150:1316, 1999.

29. Beral V: Breast cancer and hormone-replacement therapy in the Million Women Study. Lancet 362:419, 2003.

30. Fisher B, Costantino JP, Wickerham DL, et al: Tamoxifen for the prevention of breast cancer: Current status of the National Surgical Adjuvant Breast and Bowel Project P-1 study. J Natl Cancer Inst 97:1652, 2005.

31. Vogel VG, Costantino JP, Wickerham DL, et al: Effects of tamoxifen vs raloxifene on the risk of developing invasive breast cancer and other disease outcomes: The NSABP Study of Tamoxifen and Raloxifene (STAR) P-2 trial. JAMA 295:2727, 2006.

32. Han X, Liehr JG: Microsome-mediated 8-hydroxylation of guanine bases of DNA by steroid estrogens: Correlation of DNA damage by free radicals with metabolic activation to quinones. Carcinogenesis 16:2571, 1995.

33. Walter P, Green S, Greene G, et al: Cloning of the human estrogen receptor cDNA. Proc Natl Acad Sci USA 82:7889, 1985.

34. Kuiper GG, Enmark E, Pelto-Huikko M, et al: Cloning of a novel receptor expressed in rat prostate and ovary. Proc Natl Acad Sci USA 93:5925, 1996.

35. Mosselman S, Polman J, Dijkema R: ER beta: Identification and characterization of a novel human estrogen receptor. FEBS Lett 392:49, 1996.

36. Kuiper GG, Carlsson B, Grandien K, et al: Comparison of the ligand binding specificity and transcript tissue distribution of estrogen receptors alpha and beta. Endocrinology 138:863, 1997.

37. McGuire WL: Estrogen receptors in human breast cancer. J Clin Invest 52:73, 1973.

38. Iafrati MD, Karas RH, Aronovitz M, et al: Estrogen inhibits the vascular injury response in estrogen receptor alpha-deficient mice. Nat Med 3:545, 1997.

39. Korach KS: Insights from the study of animals lacking functional estrogen receptor. Science 266:1524, 1994.

40. Krege JH, Hodgin JB, Couse JF, et al: Generation and reproductive phenotypes of mice lacking estrogen receptor beta. Proc Natl Acad Sci USA 95:15677, 1998.

41. Couse JF, Curtis Hewitt S, Korach KS: Receptor null mice reveal contrasting roles for estrogen receptor alpha and beta in reproductive tissues. J Steroid Biochem Mol Biol 74:287, 2000.

42. Vidal O, Lindberg MK, Hollberg K, et al: Estrogen receptor specificity in the regulation of skeletal growth and maturation in male mice. Proc Natl Acad Sci USA 97:5474, 2000.

43. Windahl SH, Vidal O, Andersson G, et al: Increased cortical bone mineral content but unchanged trabecular bone mineral density in female ERbeta(-/-) mice. J Clin Invest 104:895, 1999.

44. Kato S: Estrogen receptor-mediated cross-talk with growth factor signaling pathways. Breast Cancer 8:3, 2001.

45. Kato S, Endoh H, Masuhiro Y, et al: Activation of the estrogen receptor through phosphorylation by mitogen-activated protein kinase. Science 270:1491, 1995

46. Lee AV, Weng CN, Jackson JG, et al: Activation of estrogen receptor-mediated gene transcription by IGF-I in human breast cancer cells. J Endocrinol 152:39, 1997

47. Stoica GE, Franke TF, Moroni M, et al: Effect of estradiol on estrogen receptor-alpha gene expression and activity can be modulated by the ErbB2/PI 3-K/Akt pathway. Oncogene 22:7998, 2003.

48. Carroll JS, Liu XS, Brodsky AS, et al: Chromosome-wide mapping of estrogen receptor binding reveals long-range regulation requiring the forkhead protein FoxA1. Cell 122:33, 2005.

49. Olefsky JM: Nuclear receptor minireview series. J Biol Chem 276:36863, 2001.

50. Hall JM, Couse JF, Korach KS: The multifaceted mechanisms of estradiol and estrogen receptor signaling. J Biol Chem 276: 36869, 2001.

51. Onate SA, Tsai SY, Tsai MJ, et al: Sequence and characterization of a coactivator for the steroid hormone receptor superfamily. Science 270:1354, 1995.

52. Voegel JJ, Heine MJ, Zechel C, et al: TIF2, a 160 kDa transcriptional mediator for the ligand-dependent activation function AF-2 of nuclear receptors. Embo J 15:3667, 1996.

53. Anzick SL, Kononen J, Walker RL, et al: AIB1, a steroid receptor coactivator amplified in breast and ovarian cancer. Science 277:965, 1997.

54. Chen H, Lin RJ, Schiltz RL, et al: Nuclear receptor coactivator ACTR is a novel histone acetyltransferase and forms a multimeric activation complex with P/CAF and CBP/p300. Cell 90:569, 1997.

55. Shang Y, Hu X, DiRenzo J, et al: Cofactor dynamics and sufficiency in estrogen receptor-regulated transcription. Cell 103:843, 2000.

56. Heery DM, Kalkhoven E, Hoare S, et al: A signature motif in transcriptional co-activators mediates binding to nuclear receptors. Nature 387:733, 1997.

57. Smith CL, Onate SA, Tsai MJ, et al: CREB binding protein acts synergistically with steroid receptor coactivator-1 to enhance steroid receptor-dependent transcription. Proc Natl Acad Sci USA 93:8884, 1996.

58. Zhu Y, Qi C, Jain S, et al: Amplification and overexpression of peroxisome proliferator-activated receptor binding protein (PBP/PPARBP) gene in breast cancer. Proc Natl Acad Sci USA 96:10848, 1999.

59. Yadav N, Lee J, Kim J, et al: Specific protein methylation defects and gene expression perturbations in coactivator-associated arginine methyltransferase 1-deficient mice. Proc Natl Acad Sci USA 100:6464, 2003.

60. Stearns V, Johnson MD, Rae JM, et al: Active tamoxifen metabolite plasma concentrations after coadministration of tamoxifen and the selective serotonin reuptake inhibitor paroxetine. J Natl Cancer Inst 95:1758, 2003.

61. Johnson MD, Zuo H, Lee KH, et al: Pharmacological characterization of 4-hydroxy-N-desmethyl tamoxifen, a novel active metabolite of tamoxifen. Breast Cancer Res Treat 85:151, 2004.

62. Jin Y, Desta Z, Stearns V, et al: CYP2D6 genotype, antidepressant use, and tamoxifen metabolism during adjuvant breast cancer treatment. J Natl Cancer Inst 97:30, 2005.

63. Goetz MP, Knox SK, Suman VJ, et al: The impact of cytochrome P450 2D6 metabolism in women receiving adjuvant tamoxifen. Breast Cancer Res Treat 101:113, 2007.

64. Goetz MP, Rae JM, Suman VJ, et al: Pharmacogenetics of tamoxifen biotransformation is associated with clinical outcomes of efficacy and hot flashes. J Clin Oncol 23:9312, 2005.

65. Armstrong DT, Weiss TJ, Selstam G, et al: Hormonal and cellular interactions in follicular steroid biosynthesis by the sheep ovary. J Reprod Fertil Suppl 30:143, 1981.

66. McNatty KP, Smith DM, Makris A, et al: The intraovarian sites of androgen and estrogen formation in women with normal and hyperandrogenic ovaries as judged by in vitro experiments. J Clin Endocrinol Metab 50:755, 1980.

67. Bogovich K, Richards JS: Androgen biosynthesis in developing ovarian follicles: Evidence that luteinizing hormone regulates thecal 17 alpha-hydroxylase and C17-20-lyase activities. Endocrinology 111:1201, 1982.

68. Rani CS, Payne AH: Adenosine 3′,5′-monophosphate-mediated induction of 17 alpha-hydroxylase and C 17-20 lyase activities in cultured mouse Leydig cells is enhanced by inhibition of steroid biosynthesis. Endocrinology 118:1222, 1986.

69. Makris A, Ryan KJ: Aromatase activity of isolated and recombined hamster granulosa cells and theca. Steroids 29:65, 1977.

70. McNatty KP, Makris A, Reinhold VN, et al: Metabolism of androstenedione by human ovarian tissues in vitro with particular reference to reductase and aromatase activity. Steroids 34:429, 1979.

71. Orly J, Sato G, Erickson GF: Serum suppresses the expression of hormonally induced functions in cultured granulosa cells. Cell 20:817, 1980.

72. Steinkampf MP, Mendelson CR, Simpson ER: Regulation by follicle-stimulating hormone of the synthesis of aromatase cytochrome P-450 in human granulosa cells. Mol Endocrinol 1:465, 1987.

73. Chung CT, Carlson RW: The role of aromatase inhibitors in early breast cancer. Curr Treat Options Oncol 4:133, 2003.

74. Milla-Santos A, Milla L, Portella J, et al: Anastrozole versus tamoxifen as first-line therapy in postmenopausal patients with hormone-dependent advanced breast cancer: A prospective, randomized, phase III study. Am J Clin Oncol 26:317, 2003.

75. Mouridsen H, Gershanovich M, Sun Y, et al: Phase III study of letrozole versus tamoxifen as first-line therapy of advanced breast cancer in postmenopausal women: Analysis of survival and update of efficacy from the International Letrozole Breast Cancer Group. J Clin Oncol 21:2101, 2003.

76. Forbes JF, Cuzick J, Buzdar A, et al: Effect of anastrozole and tamoxifen as adjuvant treatment for early-stage breast cancer: 100-month analysis of the ATAC trial. Lancet Oncol 9:45, 2008.

77. Howell A, Cuzick J, Baum M, et al: Results of the ATAC (Arimidex, Tamoxifen, Alone or in Combination) trial after completion of 5 years' adjuvant treatment for breast cancer. Lancet 365:60, 2005.

78. Goss PE, Ingle JN, Martino S, et al: Randomized trial of letrozole following tamoxifen as extended adjuvant therapy in recetor-positive breast cancer: Updated findings from NCIC CTG MA.17. J Natl Cancer Inst 97:1262, 2005.

79. Goss PE, Ingle JN, Martino S, et al: A randomized trial of letrozole in postmenopausal women after five years of tamoxifen therapy for early-stage breast cancer. N Engl J Med 349:1793, 2003.

80. Gottardis MM, Robinson SP, Satyaswaroop PG, et al: Contrasting actions of tamoxifen on endometrial and breast tumor growth in the athymic mouse. Cancer Res 48:812, 1988.

81. Gershanovich M, Garin A, Baltina D, et al: A phase III comparison of two toremifene doses to tamoxifen in postmenopausal women with advanced breast cancer. Eastern European Study Group. Breast Cancer Res Treat 45:251, 1997.

82. Shah A, Iversen P, Mitlak B: Clinically favorable effects of raloxifene on bone mineral density and serum lipids: Population assessment via bivariate analysis. Prim Care Update Ob Gyns 5:165, 1998.

83. Preisler-Mashek MT, Solodin N, Stark BL, et al: Ligand-specific regulation of proteasome-mediated proteolysis of estrogen receptor-alpha. Am J Physiol Endocrinol Metab 282:E891, 2002.

84. Chia S, Gradishar W, Mauriac L, et al: Double-blind, randomized placebo controlled trial of fulvestrant compared with exemestane after prior nonsteroidal aromatase inhibitor therapy in postmenopausal women with hormone receptor-positive, advanced breast cancer: Results from EFECT. J Clin Oncol 26:1664, 2008.

85. Charpentier AH, Bednarek AK, Daniel RL, et al: Effects of estrogen on global gene expression: identification of novel targets of estrogen action. Cancer Res 60:5977, 2000.

86. Seth P, Krop I, Porter D, et al: Novel estrogen and tamoxifen induced genes identified by SAGE (Serial Analysis of Gene Expression). Oncogene 21:836, 2002.

87. Improta-Brears T, Whorton AR, Codazzi F, et al: Estrogen-induced activation of mitogen-activated protein kinase requires mobilization of intracellular calcium. Proc Natl Acad Sci USA 96:4686, 1999.

88. Migliaccio A, Pagano M, Auricchio F: Immediate and transient stimulation of protein tyrosine phosphorylation by estradiol in MCF-7 cells. Oncogene 8:2183, 1993.

89. Levin ER, Pietras RJ: Estrogen receptors outside the nucleus in breast cancer. Breast Cancer Res Treat 108:351, 2008.

90. Razandi M, Pedram A, Greene GL, et al: Cell membrane and nuclear estrogen receptors (ERs) originate from a single transcript: studies of ERalpha and ERbeta expressed in Chinese hamster ovary cells. Mol Endocrinol 13:307, 1999.

91. Pedram A, Razandi M, Levin ER: Nature of functional estrogen receptors at the plasma membrane. Mol Endocrinol 20:1996, 2006.

92. Song RX, Barnes CJ, Zhang Z, et al: The role of Shc and insulin-like growth factor 1 receptor in mediating the translocation of estrogen receptor alpha to the plasma membrane. Proc Natl Acad Sci USA 101:2076, 2004.

93. Pedram A, Razandi M, Wallace DC, Levin ER: Functional estrogen receptors in the mitochondria of breast cancer cells. Mol Biol Cell 17:2125–2137, 2006.

94. Ignar-Trowbridge DM, Nelson KG, Bidwell MC, et al: Coupling of dual signaling pathways: Epidermal growth factor action involves the estrogen receptor. Proc Natl Acad Sci USA 89:4658, 1992.

95. Ignar-Trowbridge DM, Teng CT, Ross KA, et al: Peptide growth factors elicit estrogen receptor-dependent transcriptional activation of an estrogen-responsive element. Mol Endocrinol 7:992, 1993.

96. Lee AV, Weng CN, Jackson JG, et al: Activation of estrogen receptor-mediated gene transcription by IGF-I in human breast cancer cells. J Endocrinol 152:39, 1997.

97. Wang CX, Koay DC, Edwards A, et al: In vitro and in vivo effects of combination of Trastuzumab (Herceptin) and Tamoxifen in breast cancer. Breast Cancer Res Treat 92:251, 2005.

98. Jelovac D, Sabnis G, Long BJ, et al: Activation of mitogen-activated protein kinase in xenografts and cells during prolonged treatment with aromatase inhibitor letrozole. Cancer Res 65:5380, 2005.

99. Macedo LF, Sabnis G, Brodie A: Preclinical modeling of endocrine response and resistance: Focus on aromatase inhibitors. Cancer 112:679, 2008.

100. deFazio A, Chiew YE, Sini RL, et al: Expression of c-erbB receptors, heregulin and oestrogen receptor in human breast cell lines. Int J Cancer 87:487, 2000.

101. Klijn JG, Berns PM, Schmitz PI, et al: The clinical significance of epidermal growth factor receptor (EGF-R) in human breast cancer: A review on 5232 patients. Endocrinol Rev 13:3, 1992.

102. Wright C, Angus B, Nicholson S, et al: Expression of c-erbB-2 oncoprotein: A prognostic indicator in human breast cancer. Cancer Res 49:2087, 1989.

103. Elledge RM, Green S, Ciocca D, et al: HER-2 expression and response to tamoxifen in estrogen receptor-positive breast cancer: A Southwest Oncology Group Study. Clin Cancer Res 4:7, 1998.

104. Houston SJ, Plunkett TA, Barnes DM, et al: Overexpression of c-erbB2 is an independent marker of resistance to endocrine therapy in advanced breast cancer. Br J Cancer 79:1220, 1999.

105. Newby JC, Johnston SR, Smith IE, et al: Expression of epidermal growth factor receptor and c-erbB2 during the development of tamoxifen resistance in human breast cancer. Clin Cancer Res 3:1643, 1997.

106. Rudolph P, Olsson H, Bonatz G, et al: Correlation between p53, c-erbB-2, and topoisomerase II alpha expression, DNA ploidy, hormonal receptor status and proliferation in 356 node-negative breast carcinomas: Prognostic implications. J Pathol 187:207, 1999.

107. De Placido S, De Laurentiis M, Carlomagno C, et al: Twenty-year results of the Naples GUN randomized trial: Predictive factors of adjuvant tamoxifen efficacy in early breast cancer. Clin Cancer Res 9:1039, 2003.

108. Dowsett M, Houghton J, Iden C, et al: Benefit from adjuvant tamoxifen therapy in primary breast cancer patients according oestrogen receptor, progesterone receptor, EGF receptor and HER2 status. Ann Oncol 17:818, 2006.

109. Dowsett M, Allred C, Knox J, et al: Relationship between quantitative estrogen and progesterone receptor expression and human epidermal growth factor receptor 2 (HER-2) status with recurrence in the Arimidex, Tamoxifen, Alone or in Combination trial. J Clin Oncol 26:1059, 2008.

110. Thor AD, Berry DA, Budman DR, et al: erbB-2, p53, and efficacy of adjuvant therapy in lymph node-positive breast cancer. J Natl Cancer Inst 90:1346, 1998.

111. Berry DA, Muss HB, Thor AD, et al: HER-2/neu and p53 expression versus tamoxifen resistance in estrogen receptor-positive, node-positive breast cancer. J Clin Oncol 18:3471, 2000.

112. Knoop AS, Bentzen SM, Nielsen MM, et al: Value of epidermal growth factor receptor, HER2, p53, and steroid receptors in predicting the efficacy of tamoxifen in high-risk postmenopausal breast cancer patients. J Clin Oncol 19:3376, 2001.

113. Love RR, Duc NB, Havighurst TC, et al: Her-2/neu overexpression and response to oophorectomy plus tamoxifen adjuvant therapy in estrogen receptor-positive premenopausal women with operable breast cancer. J Clin Oncol 21:453, 2003.

114. Ellis MJ, Ma C: Letrozole in the neoadjuvant setting: The P024 trial. Breast Cancer Res Treat 105 Suppl 1:33, 2007.

115. Ellis MJ, Coop A, Singh B, et al: Letrozole is more effective neoadjuvant endocrine therapy than tamoxifen for ErbB-1- and/or ErbB-2-positive, estrogen receptor-positive primary breast cancer: Evidence from a phase III randomized trial. J Clin Oncol 19:3808, 2001.

116. Paik S, Bryant J, Tan-Chiu E, et al: Real-world performance of HER2 testing—National Surgical Adjuvant Breast and Bowel Project experience. J Natl Cancer Inst 94:852, 2002.

117. Nelson NJ: Can HER2 status predict response to cancer therapy? J Natl Cancer Inst 92:366, 2000.

118. Smith IE, Walsh G, Skene A, et al: A phase II placebo-controlled trial of neoadjuvant anastrozole alone or with gefitinib in early breast cancer. J Clin Oncol 25:3816, 2007.

119. Crisofanilli M, Valero V, Mangalik A, et al: A phase II multicenter, double-blind, randomized trial to compare anastrozole plus gefitinib with anastrozole plus placebo in postmenopausal women with hormone receptor-positive (HR+) metastatic breast cancer (MBC). J Clin Oncol 26:44S, 2008.

120. Guix M, Granja Nde M, Meszoely I, et al: Short preoperative treatment with erlotinib inhibits tumor cell proliferation in hormone receptor-positive breast cancers. J Clin Oncol 26:897, 2008.
121. Mackey JR, Kaufman B, Clemens M, et al: Trastuzmab prolongs progression-free survival in hormone-dependent and HER2-positive metastatic breast cancer. Breast Cancer Res Treat 100, 2006 [abstract 3].
122. Brisken C, Park S, Vass T, et al: A paracrine role for the epithelial progesterone receptor in mammary gland development. Proc Natl Acad Sci USA 95:5076, 1998.
123. Haslam SZ, Counterman LJ, Nummy KA: Effects of epidermal growth factor, estrogen, and progestin on DNA synthesis in mammary cells in vivo are determined by the developmental state of the gland. J Cell Physiol 155:72, 1993.
124. Ruan W, Monaco ME, Kleinberg DL: Progesterone stimulates mammary gland ductal morphogenesis by synergizing with and enhancing insulin-like growth factor-I action. Endocrinology 146:1170, 2005.
125. Ravdin PM, Green S, Dorr TM, et al: Prognostic significance of progesterone receptor levels in estrogen receptor-positive patients with metastatic breast cancer treated with tamoxifen: Results of a prospective Southwest Oncology Group study. J Clin Oncol 10:1284, 1992.

SECTION VIII

Molecular Biology of Breast Carcinogenesis

chapter 28

Molecular Oncology of Breast Cancer

**ANAMARIA IOAN* | MERIEME KLOBOCISTA* |
SHERIN SHIRAZI* | MICHAEL F. PRESS**

Introduction

The development of malignancies is a multistep process that occurs over time. Tumor development proceeds as a progression of a series of genetic changes, each potentially conferring a growth advantage for the cells (and their daughter cells), leading to progressive conversion of normal cells into cancer cells.[1] Normal cells have numerous pathways that regulate cell proliferation and cell death. These normal regulatory pathways are altered through mutations and natural selection to transform normal cells into malignant cells. Therefore, cancer cells lack normal functions that regulate cell growth and involution. Hanahan and Weinberg[1] have summarized the basic traits needed by cells to become cancerous. There are six acquired fundamental alterations in cell physiology that dictate malignant growth. They are self-sufficiency in growth signals, insensitivity to antigrowth signals, evasion of apoptosis (programmed cell death), infinite replicative potential, sustained angiogenesis, and tissue invasion and metastasis (Fig. 28-1). Understanding the physiology of malignancy provides new opportunities to develop biologic or targeted therapies that can disrupt these cancer-related growth pathways, providing new treatments for breast cancer.

NORMAL CELL CYCLE

The normal cell cycle[2] consists of five stages: G_0 (gap 0), G_1 (gap 1), S (synthesis), G_2 (gap 2) and M (mitosis; Fig. 28-2). The progression of cells through the various stages of the cell cycle is controlled by cyclins, cyclin-dependent kinases (CDKs), and CDK inhibitors. CDKs are expressed throughout the cell cycle, whereas cyclins (cyclins D, E, A, and B) are synthesized during specific stages of the cell cycle. The retinoblastoma susceptibility protein (pRb) is the restriction point for cell cycle progression. When hypophosphorylated, it forms

a tight bond with transcription factor E2F, disabling it. When ready for cell reproduction, quiescent cells are stimulated by external signals, growth factors, which activate a number of transduction pathways that ultimately lead to the synthesis of cyclin D. This in turn results in hyperphosphorylation of pRb, thus releasing its inhibitory bond on E2F, and allowing the cell to proceed through the G_1 restriction point. E2F then proceeds to the transcription of cyclin E and cyclin A and other proteins required for cell cycle progression. Cyclin E forms a complex with CDK2, which is involved in the G_1/S transition. Once in the S phase, DNA synthesis begins and cyclin A forms a complex with CDK2 allowing the cell to proceed to the M phase. In the M phase, cyclin B binds to CDK1 which activates the disintegration of the nuclear envelope and mitosis commences. Once the cells have divided, they can re-enter the cell cycle through G_1 or become quiescent (G_0).

The cell cycle is also composed of inhibitory components that are the CDK inhibitors. There are two classes of CDK inhibitors, the Cip/Kip family and the *INK4α/ ARF* locus (inhibitor of kinase 4/alternative reading frame). The Cip/Kip family is made up of p21, p27, and p57, which inhibit all CDKs. The *INK4α/ARF* locus encodes for proteins $p16^{INK4α}$ and $p14^{ARF}$, both of which inhibit the cyclin D–CDK4 complex, consequently inhibiting the phosphorylation of pRb and ultimately causing cell cycle arrest at G_1.

The cell cycle has two key checkpoints that permit policing the DNA replication product. The G_1/S transition checkpoint permits assessment of DNA damage. This process is mediated by p53. If DNA is damaged, the steps for DNA repair are activated. If the damage cannot be repaired, then the cell undergoes apoptosis. The G_2/M checkpoint monitors completion of DNA replication and the ability of the cell to undergo mitotic cell division. The purpose of the cell cycle control processes is to ensure that the daughter cells are normal. Cancer cells have acquired the ability to evade these regulatory processes so mitosis can proceed for the genetically altered daughter cells of cancer cells.

---

*Contributed equally and should be considered joint first authors.

Component	Acquired capability	Example of mechanism
	Self-sufficiency in growth signals	Activate H-Ras oncogene
	Insensitivity to antigrowth signals	Lose retinoblastoma suppressor
	Evading apoptosis	Produce IGF survival factors
	Limitless replicative potential	Turn on telomerase
	Sustained angiogenesis	Produce VEGF inducer
	Tissue invasion and metastasis	Inactivate E-cadherin

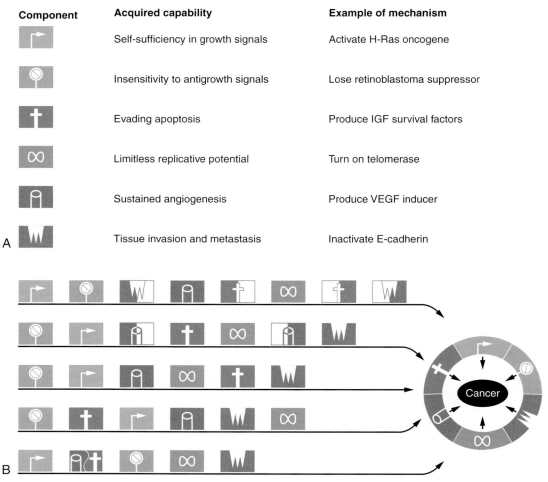

Figure 28-1 Acquired traits of cancer. The order in which somatic cells acquire various growth characteristics appears to be variable; however, acquisition of the full complement of these traits leads to cancer. IGF, insulin-like growth factor; VEGF, vascular endothelial growth factor. (Reproduced from Hanahan D, Weinberg RA: The hallmarks of cancer. Cell 100:57–70, 2000.)

HALLMARKS OF CANCER

Self-Sufficiency in Growth Signals

As discussed previously, a growth activation signal is required to proceed from a quiescent state into an active state. These signals are provided by various growth factors. Cancer cells maintain self-sufficiency in growth signals by the ability to synthesize their own growth factors, overexpress receptors, alter the structure of receptors, alter the type of receptors expressed favoring receptors that transmit growth signals, and alter the pathways in the cytoplasm that receive and process these signals. By synthesizing their own growth factors, cancer cells become independent from their normal microenvironment and produce growth factors that favor promotion of growth. Examples of growth factors known to play a role in breast cancer growth promotion are platelet-derived growth factor (PDGF), transforming growth factor-α (TGF-α), and estrogen. TGF-α binds to epidermal growth factor receptor (EGFR) and acts as a potent mitogen in breast cells.[3] Estrogen binds to estrogen receptors (ERs), promoting proliferation of epithelial cells in the breast. The ER is one of the most important

growth factor receptors identified in breast cancer. Overexpression of receptors also allows cancer cells to respond to levels of growth factors that would normally not elicit cell proliferation. The human EGFR type 2 (HER2) is the most important such receptor.[4] The human EGFR family of genes is involved in the regulation of normal breast growth and development.[5] The HER2 gene is amplified[6] and the protein is overexpressed in approximately 25% of invasive breast cancer, where it is associated with a poorer prognosis.[7] Alteration of receptor structure may facilitate ligand-independent signaling, which is seen in truncated versions of the EGFR that lack much of the extracellular domain. Some cancers alter the type of integrin expressed in such a way that integrins promoting growth are favored, permitting cells to activate the pathways that promote cell proliferation. The SOS-Ras-Raf-MAP kinase pathway is such a mitogenic pathway that promotes tumor growth. There are many ways in which cancer cells can initiate and promote their own growth. The preceding is a brief summary of a few of the mechanisms used by cancer cells, especially breast cancer cells, to provide self sufficiency in growth signals.

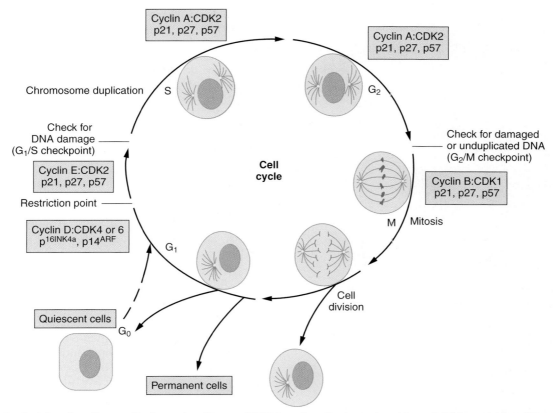

Figure 28-2 Activity of cyclins, cyclin-dependent kinases (CDKs), and cyclin-dependent kinase inhibitors during different phases of the cell cycle. (Redrawn from Kumar V, Abbas A, Fausto N: Robbins and Cotran: Pathologic basis of disease, 7th ed. Philadelphia, Elsevier, 2005. Copyright Elsevier 2005.)

Insensitivity to Antigrowth Signals

Growth inhibitory signals, like growth promoting signals, are located in the extracellular matrix and surfaces of nearby cells. They, too, act on transmembrane cell surface receptors to initiate intracellular signal transduction pathways that alter growth. Cells can be directed into a quiescent (G_0) phase from which they can emerge in the future, or they can be induced into a postmitotic state, which results in permanent differentiation of the cell. Cyclin, CDKs, and CDK inhibitors function to control cell cycle progression.[8] Cyclin D1 is expressed in atypical hyperplasias and ductal carcinoma in situ of the breast and overexpression of cyclins and CDKs are associated with impaired outcomes in breast cancer.[8] Many, if not all, antiproliferative signals channel through the retinoblastoma protein (pRb), p107, and p130. Transforming growth factor-β (TGF-β) is an antigrowth factor that prevents the disruption of the pRb circuit by preventing phosphorylation of pRb, thus inhibiting growth. It also suppresses expression of the *c-myc* gene, which regulates the G_1 cell cycle. Tumor cells can alter TGF-β responsiveness by decreasing the number of receptors that respond to TGF-β, or by altering the function of the receptors. The Smad4 protein that transduces the TGF-β signals to receptors in the cytoplasm can be eliminated through mutation in its encoding gene. Also, pRb can be affected through mutation of its gene.

Tumor cells avoid entering the irreversible, postmitotic differentiated state by overexpression of the *c-myc* oncogene, which increases Myc-Max complexes that impair differentiation and promote growth. By eluding the antigrowth function necessary for homeostasis, cancer cells are able to continue to grow, consequently expanding in numbers.

Evasion of Apoptosis

Both survival and death signals are required for apoptosis to transpire. Survival signals include insulin-like growth factor-1 (IGF-1), IGF-2, and interleukin-3 (IL-3). IGF-1 is required for cell cycle progression.[8] Death signals include the FAS ligand and tumor necrosis factor-α (TNF-α). These signals, when bound to their respective receptors, activate caspases 8 and 10, which trigger effector caspases downstream that execute apoptosis. Apoptosis can be triggered through either an extrinsic pathway, which involves transmembrane death receptors such as TNF receptor (Fig. 28-3), or the intrinsic pathway, which involves mitochondrial release of cytochrome C, which activates caspase 9. The intrinsic pathway is regulated by proapoptotic molecules Bak and Bax and antiapoptotic molecule Bcl-2.[8] The p53 protein can stimulate apoptosis through both intrinsic and extrinsic pathways. Tumor cells evade apoptosis

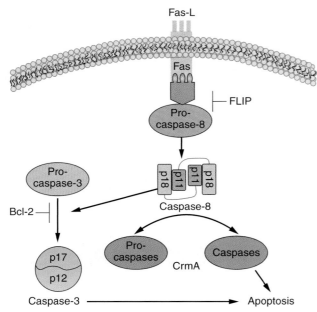

Fas-L

Fas

FLIP

Pro-
caspase-8

Pro-
caspase-3

p18 p11 p11 p18

Caspase-8

Bcl-2

Pro-
caspases

Caspases

CrmA

p17
p12

Caspase-3 ──────────────→ Apoptosis

Figure 28-3 Intrinsic pathway of apoptosis triggered by the Fas ligand (or tumor necrosis factor-α) to activate caspase 8, subsequently leading to apoptosis. (Fas Signaling Pathway, courtesy of Sigma-Aldrich Corporation, St. Louis, MO, USA.)

by mutating the pro- and antiapoptotic genes and *TP53* tumor suppressor gene; this activates the survival signaling pathways such as PI3 kinase-AKT/PKB pathway (phosphatidylinositol 3-kinase-serine/threonine/protein kinase b), increasing survival signals such as IGF-1, IGF-2, and IL-3, or by loss of the tumor suppressor gene phosphatase and tensin homolog deleted from chromosome 10 (PTEN) that moderates the AKT survival pathway. Carcinomas with *TP53* mutations are more likely to be highly invasive, poorly differentiated, and high-grade breast tumors. Loss of p53 function results in loss of cell cycle checkpoint control.[9]

Infinite Replicative Potential

Once cells have progressed through a limited number of generations, they become senescent. Stem cells, on the other hand, have unlimited replicative capabilities, making them more prone to mutations. To achieve unlimited replicative potential, cancer cells must maintain telomeres, specialized structures found at the end of chromosomes, which protect the chromosome ends against degradation. During each cell cycle, telomeric DNA is lost from the ends of every chromosome, and eventually the unprotected chromosomal ends partake in end-to-end chromosomal union, resulting in a cell crisis that ultimately leads to cell death. Cancer cells maintain telomere length by up-regulating expression of the enzyme telomerase, which adds nucleotide repeats (TTAGGG) to the ends of telomeric DNA,[10] or by activating one or more novel mechanisms called alternative lengthening of telomeres, which maintains telomeres.[11] Telomerase expression is common in breast cancer,

including preinvasive disease, and it is associated with lymphovascular invasion, nodal metastasis, and increased relapse rate.[8] Factors that affect telomerase expression include estrogen and progesterone, which stimulate telomerase activity, and tamoxifen, which inhibits it.[8] Inhibition of telomerase in breast cancer cells causes them to be more sensitive to topoisomerase inhibition, which in turn, generates sensitivity to anthracyclines.[8]

Sustained Angiogenesis

Growth, multiplication, function, and survival of cells require oxygen and nutrients, which are transported by blood vessels. This process requires a balance between initiation and inhibition of angiogenesis. Angiogenesis-initiating signals include vascular endothelial growth factor (VEGF) and fibroblast growth factor-1 (FGF-1) and FGF-2, which bind to tyrosine kinase receptors on cell membranes of endothelial cells. Tumors promote angiogenesis by altering the balance between initiation and inhibition of neovascularization. This is accomplished by altering gene transcription to increase expression of proangiogenesis signals such as VEGF and/or FGF and/or by down-regulating angiogenesis inhibitors such as thrombospondin-1. Much research has been undertaken in developing agents to target angiogenesis. Bevacizumab (Avastin)[12] is a humanized monoclonal antibody designed to inhibit angiogenesis by targeting VEGF. Bevacizumab has been approved for treatment of metastatic breast cancer and phase III clinical trials are evaluating its utility in the adjuvant treatment of breast cancer. Other antiangiogenesis agents are in development and early phase clinical trials.

Tissue Invasion and Apoptosis

Once cancer cells have grown and multiplied, it is time for them to seek new territory, where nutrients and space are abundant. Cell-to-cell adhesion molecules (CAMs), integrins, and proteases, such as matrix metalloproteinases, are affected in the process of invasion and metastasis. Connection between adjacent cells by E-cadherin (CAM) results in transmission of antigrowth signals, consequently acting as a suppressor of metastasis. In the majority of epithelial cancers, E-cadherin function is lost by mutation of the E-cadherin gene and transcriptional suppression or lysis of the extracellular cadherin domain. Alteration in integrin expression is also evident in cancer cells, allowing them to preferentially express integrins that aid in invasion and metastasis. Activation of matrix metalloproteinases, by up-regulating protease genes and down-regulating protease inhibitory genes, aids the process of metastasis by degrading the basement membrane of the tissue and adjacent stroma. Expression of matrix metalloproteinase 2 and 9 has been linked with the grade and stage of breast cancer.[8]

In general, these changes are acquired as somatic mutations during the life of the individual. Genomic instability has to be present for cancer cells to acquire these functions, for example, altering genetic transcription to increase expression of VEGF or telomerase, or mutation of key genes that control apoptosis.

Role of Endogenous Hormones in Breast Development and Carcinogenesis

Epidemiologic studies have shown that hormones play an important role in the pathogenesis of breast cancer. In general, exposure to hormones is believed to increase risk of breast cancer. Early menarche, late menopause, nulliparity, and delayed child bearing are all associated with increased breast cancer risk. Many studies on the biology of and the role of hormones on breast development have been performed on rodents. Estrogen and progesterone have a profound role in breast development, but there is an important role for pituitary hormones because ovarian hormones fail to promote proliferation and/or differentiation in hypophysectomized animals.[13] To understand the role of hormones on breast cancer, an understanding of the role of hormones in breast development and differentiation is helpful.

The mammary gland is composed of epithelial and mesenchymal components. The major functional unit of the mammary gland is the terminal ductal lobular unit. This terminal lobular structure is composed of the terminal breast ducts and the blind-ended ductules at the end of these terminal ducts. Most breast tumors arise in the terminal ductal lobular unit[14] and retain some of the morphologic and molecular biologic features of those cells. The ductal system is lined by luminal epithelial cells surrounded by myoepithelial cells that are in direct contact with the basement membrane. The majority of proliferating cells are found within the luminal epithelium,[14] and it is these dividing cells that are most prone to malignant transformation. Their growth is stimulated by the interaction of hormones with hormone receptors, especially ERs and progesterone receptors (PRs).

There are two types of ERs, the classical estrogen receptor (ERα) and the more recently identified ERβ. ERα is expressed in 15% to 30% of normal luminal epithelial cells and not at all in any of the other cell types.[15,16] ERβ is present in most luminal epithelium and myoepithelial cells as well as in some fibroblasts, endothelial cells, and lymphocytes.[17] Data suggest that ERα is the key mediator of the growth stimulatory effects of estrogen on the mammary gland.[14] ERα is expressed in infant, pubertal, and cycling adult breast.[18]

There are two types of PRs, PRA and PRB. PRA and PRB are expressed similarly to ERα in that they are expressed in a minority of cells throughout the luminal epithelium. They are concentrated in the terminal bud cells. They are not expressed in the myoepithelial or stromal cells.[15,19,20] PR expression is induced by estrogens at the transcriptional level and decreased by progestins at both the transcriptional and translational levels.[21] All the cells that express PR also contain ERα.[15]

Studies have shown that, in the normal human breast, proliferating cells contain neither ERα nor PRs.[15] The cells that contain these receptors are separate from, but adjacent to, the proliferating cells. This suggests that estrogen and/or progesterone controls proliferation of luminal epithelial cells indirectly through paracrine growth factors secreted by the epithelium.[14]

PRENATAL OR FETAL BREAST DEVELOPMENT

Mammary gland development is divided into several stages: prenatal (fetal), postnatal, pubertal, adult, and postmenopausal. Mammary glands are derived from mammary buds, which are ectodermal ingrowths along the mammary lines[20] that are present in 4-week-old embryos.[22] Both the male and female glands develop similarly in utero, unlike with rodent breast development.[23] Between 14 and 18 weeks of gestation, the mammary gland appears as an epithelial anlage resulting from the focal in-growth of the epidermis into the underlying mesenchyme. Subsequently, the breast bud starts to branch. Ductal morphogenesis occurs as the sprouts elongate and invade the mesenchymal tissue.[23] At 18 weeks, Bcl-2 expression is observed. This prevents apoptosis and permits expansion of the cell population.[24] During the second half of the fetal period, the areola and the nipple differentiate, and the mammary glands become canalized to form a rudimentary ductal system with lobular acini.[22] Ductal budding is under the influence of prolactin, acting as a sensitizer of cells to insulin, which promotes its mitogenic effect. Aldosterone promotes optimal differentiation of ductal buds. By 28 weeks, there are two distinct cell populations in the breast. The inner luminal cell population is separated from the basement membrane by an outer basal or myoepithelial layer.[23] The basal cells express EGFR and TGFα.[23] Bcl-2 is expressed in stromal cells, at this time, protecting them from apoptosis and permitting their expansion as future breast fibroblasts.[24] Basal, undifferentiated, or germinal cells are still seen at the end of the fetal period and have been interpreted as reserve cells for the renovation of the mammary epithelium. ERs are present in the fetal breast epithelium by the third trimester of pregnancy and PRs from term to 2 to 3 months after birth.[25]

POSTNATAL BREAST DEVELOPMENT

There are no identifiable morphologic differences in the development of the breasts in males and females.[23] Mammary glands are not fully developed and functional at birth. At birth, the ductal system opens onto the surface through the breast pit. With birth, there is a decline of prolactin, estrogen, and progesterone, which results in involution of the newborn breast.[22] Apocrine and cystic changes are observed similar to those seen in postmenopausal women.[23] By 2 years of age, all that remain are small ductal structures in a fibroblastic stroma. This is seen in both sexes until puberty.[23]

PUBERTAL BREAST DEVELOPMENT

The mammary gland undergoes a massive increase in proliferation during two stages, puberty and early pregnancy.[14] Ovarian secretion of estrogen increases as a response to the hypothalamic-pituitary secretion of gonadotrophins. Full differentiation of the gland requires insulin, cortisol, thyroxine, prolactin, and growth hormone.[26] Estrogen is required; however, alone it is inadequate to induce pubertal breast development.[27]

Several rodent studies, especially in mice in which the ERα gene had been knocked out, confirm that estrogen has an important role in breast development. The mammary glands of these mice consisted of rudimentary ducts without terminal end buds or alveolar buds,[28] and they could not be stimulated for further development with exogenous estrogen treatment. Furthermore, these glands were more resistant to tumor development.[28] In brief, estrogen stimulates ductal elongation.[29] The role of progesterone in mammary gland development, ascertained through mice models, is to promote lobuloalveolar development by stimulating terminal ductal lobular unit formation and expansion during puberty and pregnancy.[14] In PR knockout mice, mammary glands form ductal structures that lack lobular-alveolar components.[30]

Increase in growth hormone secretion occurring in adolescence increases the sensitization of mammary cells to the mitogenic effects of insulin. The terminal end buds undergo dichotomous branching, leading to smaller ducts and ductules,[31] and ultimately give rise to blind-ended ductules called acini. A collection of acini arising from one terminal duct and embedded in intralobular stroma is called a terminal ductal lobular unit, the functional unit of the breast.[23] The terminal ductal lobular unit is the site from which epithelial hyperplasia and carcinoma originate.[32] Once menarche is established, the mammary gland undergoes a cyclical increase in proliferation associated with the menstrual cycle, and the terminal ductal lobular units contain an increase in alveolar number with each successive cycle.[31] In the adult, nonlactating breast, epithelial proliferation is at its peak one week after ovulation (during the luteal phase), when levels of both estrogen and progesterone are high (Fig. 28-4).[33-35] This association suggests a role for hormonal stimulation in mitotic cell division, in both somatic and reserve or stem cells, thus increasing the chance of errors in DNA replication and repair, leading to carcinogenesis. The luminal cells account for more than 90% of the epithelial cell proliferation in the nonpregnant breast.[32] Significantly, more than 90% of breast carcinomas synthesize cytokeratins characteristic of the luminal phenotype, and more than 70% synthesize steroid receptors, indicating that the luminal cell type is the major target for breast tumorigenesis.[32]

ADULT BREAST DEVELOPMENT

The mammary gland becomes fully developed and attains complete structural and functional maturity at the time of pregnancy and lactation. Although there are limited data describing the changes that occur during pregnancy and lactation, available information suggests that the changes are similar to those seen in rodent breasts. There is an increase in the epithelial component to produce more terminal ductal lobular units containing large numbers of acini.[14] Increased levels of estrogen and progesterone during pregnancy lead to ductal and alveolar proliferation secondary to increased mitotic activity and formation of new alveoli. At this point, there is a transient increase in breast cancer risk, probably because of the increase in mitotic activity and potential for faulty DNA synthesis and accumulation of DNA

mutations. This may explain the effect of late first full-term pregnancy on breast cancer risk. With increasing age at parity, there is limited time, prior to menopause, to compensate for the increased rate of mitosis that occurs during pregnancy.[36] Human placental lactogen, present during gestation, results in increased protein and fluid secretion with consequent alveolar dilation. DNA content of the breast continues to increase during the late stages of pregnancy and early stage of lactation, which allows for the continued growth of the mammary gland.

Shortly after delivery, the levels of estrogen, progesterone, and human placental lactogen decrease. The decrease in estrogen and progesterone removes their inhibitory effect on prolactin in preparation for lactation. Once lactation is established, epithelial cells no longer proliferate. Final differentiation of the alveolar epithelial cells into a mature milk-secreting cell is accomplished by the gestational increase in estrogen and progesterone, combined with the presence of prolactin, but only after prior exposure to cortisol, growth hormone, thyroid hormone, and insulin.[20]

Once weaning has transpired the secretory luminal epithelial cells undergo apoptosis, the alveoli collapse and the mammary gland involutes to its pregestational state.[37] Even though the mammary gland regresses to a pregestational state, the ductal system of the parous mammary gland retains a more extensive framework of side-branching than the nulliparous gland.[13] The ability of the mammary gland to undergo proliferation and differentiation with each pregnancy gives rise to the concept of mammary stem cells as the critical reserve cell population for this renewal of the breast epithelial population.

POSTMENOPAUSAL BREAST REGRESSION

Successive rounds of pregnancy and involution are associated with an increase and subsequent decrease in both the size and the number of breast acini. The ducts are not involved in this process.[23] However, during postmenopausal involution, both the lobules and ducts are reduced in number (Fig. 28-5). The intralobular stroma is replaced by collagen. The glandular epithelium and the interlobular connective tissue are replaced by fat, leading to reduced mammographic density.[23] In the end, the few acini and ducts that remain are set in thin strands of collagen scattered throughout the fat.[23] Menopausal involution occurs because of a decrease in estrogen and progesterone. This in turn decreases the rate of mitosis, thus decreasing the rate of mutations in the breast epithelium.

STEM CELLS IN THE BREAST

Breast stem cells, an example of somatic stem cells, are totipotent cells that have the ability to self-renew as well as to differentiate into mammary epithelial cells. Stem cells have the ability to divide symmetrically, to produce two clonal stem cells, or asymmetrically, to produce one stem cell and one differentiated epithelial progenitor cell.[38] Studies suggest that cancer stem cells or their immediate progenitor cells may be the sites of initial mutation. This is in contrast to the traditional model that mutations develop and accumulate in somatic cells.[39,40] Somatic cells have a relatively short life span and thus a

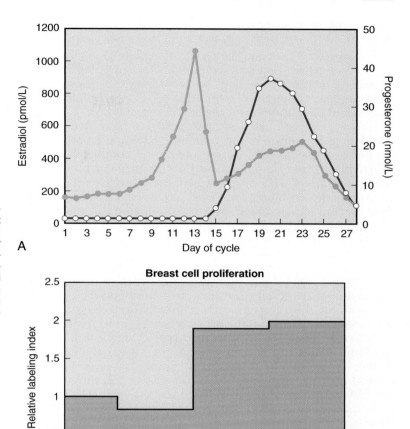

Figure 28-4 Comparison of the estrogen and progesterone levels throughout the menstrual cycle with breast cell proliferation during the menstrual cycle. Breast cell proliferation is increased from days 13 to 27 when higher levels of estrogen and progesterone are present. (Reproduced from Pike MC, Spicer DV, Dahmoush L, et al: Estrogens, progestogens, normal breast cell proliferation, and breast cancer risk. Epidemiol Rev 15:17–35, 1993; and from Anderson TJ, Ferguson DJ, Raab GM: Cell turnover in the "resting" human breast: Influence of parity, contraceptive pill, age and laterality. Br J Cancer 46:376–382, 1982.)

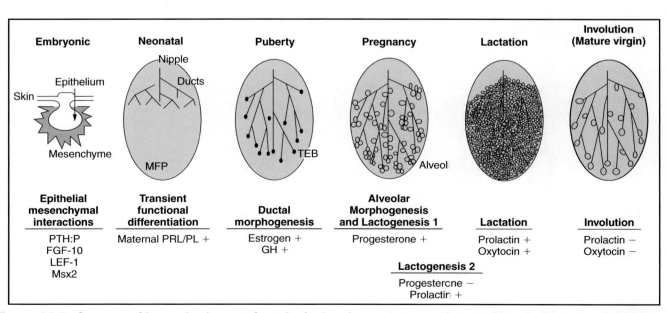

Figure 28-5 Summary of breast development from the fetal to the postmenopausal stages. Note the increase and subsequent decrease of the number of ducts and alveoli and degree of branching. (Reprinted from www.endotext.org, the free online endocrinology textbook.)

limited opportunity to acquire the multiple mutations required for tumor development.[40] In contrast, stem cells have a longer life span and can acquire the multiple mutations necessary for tumor development. With deregulated symmetric division, this could lead to clonal expansion of the mutated, cancerous stem cells.[38] This model has considerable implications for therapy in breast cancer.

Increased breast cancer risk is suggested to be related, not only to prolonged estrogen and progesterone action on breast epithelial cells, but to a failure to completely differentiate the mammary gland through pregnancy in young adulthood. This would explain the protective role of early parity on breast cancer risk. Russo and Russo[41] describe the development and differentiation of the breast from the perspective of four different types of lobules found in the breast. The breast tissue of normal cycling women contains the undifferentiated lobules, or type 1 lobules, whereas more differentiated lobules are referred to as type 2 and 3 lobules. The breast achieves its maximum development during pregnancy and lactation with the differentiation of lactating lobules, or type 4 lobules. After lactation, the breast regresses from a type 4 to type 3 lobule and retains this type of lobule until the fourth decade of life, after which time it undergoes further involution to type 2, and finally, to type 1. In contrast, the nulliparous breast contains a larger number of type 1 lobules. During menopause, both parous and nulliparous breasts contain predominantly type 1 lobules, but they are thought to be biologically different in these two groups. It is believed that the differentiation that occurs during pregnancy creates a specific genomic signature in the mammary gland that makes it resistant to carcinogenesis, specifically in the stem cells. Pregnancy shifts the stem cells from stem cells 1 (found in type 1 lobules in nulliparous breasts) to stem cells 2 (found in type 1 lobules in parous breasts), making them refractory to carcinogenesis.[41]

Important Molecular Markers in Current Clinical Management of Breast Cancer Patients

CLINICAL PERSPECTIVES RELATED TO BREAST CANCER DEVELOPMENT AND DISEASE PROGRESSION

Clinical studies have suggested that the natural history of breast cancer involves stepwise progression through defined clinical and pathologic stages.[42,43] Animal models demonstrate that this process begins with early proliferative changes in breast luminal epithelial cells located within the terminal duct lobule units, which can subsequently evolve into in situ and invasive carcinomas.[42,44] Accumulation of genetic and epigenetic alterations within various key pathways is hypothesized to account for this transition; this can be demonstrated in the modified Wellings-Jensen-Marcum model of breast cancer evolution (Fig. 28-6).[43,44] Despite this seemingly straightforward hypothesis, finding a network mechanism or pathway responsible for the progressively more malignant phenotype remains elusive. Instead, current scientific evidence indicates that breast cancer is rather a clinically heterogeneous and dynamic process with distinct clinical behavior attributed to characteristic molecular signatures.[45] Many complexities seem to arise early in the course of disease. In addition, important consideration must be given not only to somatic genetic changes that arise in the tumor but also to clinical issues related to the affected individual patient. As a result, determining individualized options for diagnosis, treatment, and subsequent surveillance of women affected by breast cancer has become a key objective in the modern multidisciplinary management of breast cancer as we enter into an era of increasingly more personalized cancer care.

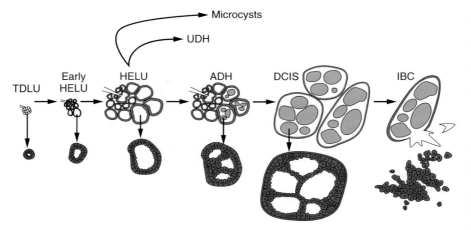

Figure 28-6 Modified Wellings-Jensen-Marcum model of breast cancer illustrating the evolution of infiltrating ductal carcinoma of the breast based almost entirely on evidence of histologic continuity. In this model, hyperplastic breast epithelial cells gradually enlarge normal terminal duct lobular units (TDLUs) to form hyperplastic enlarged lobular units (HELUs). HELUs then may differentiate to microcysts or progress to more complex lesions, including usual duct hyperplasia (UDH) and atypical ductal hyperplasia (ADH). Progression is believed to be slow and overall nonobligatory, with only a small portion of HELUs ever progressing to ADH or beyond. How this progression occurs is dictated by acquisition of both genetic and epigenetic abnormalities. DCIS, ductal carcinoma in situ; IBC, invasive breast cancer. (Redrawn from Wellings SR, Jensen HM, Marcum RG: An atlas of subgross pathology of the human breast with special reference to possible precancerous lesions. J Natl Cancer Inst 55:231–273, 1975; and from Lee S, Mohsin SK, Mao S, et al: Hormones, receptors, and growth in hyperplastic enlarged lobular units: Early potential precursors of breast cancer. Breast Cancer Res 8: R6, 2006.)

CURRENT RECOMMENDATIONS FOR MOLECULAR MARKERS IN ROUTINE CLINICAL USE

Extensive analysis of gene expression microarrays has shed light on possible genetic mechanisms that account for the diversity of biologic behaviors within breast cancer.[46-48] Although these promising advances continue, the importance of consistently measuring key molecular features such as ER and PR status, as well as evaluating HER2/*neu* gene amplification status remain paramount in routine treatment planning. In fact, currently, measurement of ER, PR, and HER2/*neu* are the only molecular prognostic and predictive factors that have been validated for routine use according to the 2007 National Cancer Center Network (NCCN) and American Society of Clinical Oncology (ASCO) guidelines.[49] Other measures such as tumor TNM stage, presence of lymphovascular space invasion, and histologic grade and subtype continue to be important predictors of clinical outcome. Gene expression profiling, pharmacogenomics, proliferative indices, and other molecular assays evaluating the presence of circulating tumor cells have not yet been determined to meet the level of validation necessary for use in routine clinical practice. Large prospective randomized trials are currently underway to evaluate the utility of these tools in everyday clinical practice. Additionally, individual risk is contingent on several lifetime events; therefore, clinical management of cancers must continue to take into account relevant reproductive, personal, and familial risk factors. A woman with a *BRCA* mutation or other high-risk factor, for example, should be managed in a different manner than a woman with low risk. Taking a precise reproductive, personal, and family cancer history, therefore, remains crucial in assessing the future risk of recurrence for an individual woman. It is also important to thoroughly evaluate the molecular biology of her cancer.

Estrogen Receptor

As a member of the steroid hormone receptor superfamily, ER is a ligand-dependent transcription factor, which controls a number of essential developmental and physiologic processes in humans. Estrogen interacts with its receptor in its predominant form, estradiol, to regulate growth and differentiation, as well as maintain homeostasis in normal breast epithelial cells. Estradiol is known to be a key hormone responsible for regulating many aspects of female development and reproductive physiology. Dysregulation of the normal endocrine axis has long been understood to be important in both the development and subsequent clinical behavior of breast cancer. Some studies suggest that a recapitulation of the essential roles that estrogen and progesterone play in normal mammary development may be important in the initiation of breast carcinogenesis.[50] Steroid hormones play an important role in breast tumorigenesis, and the role of the ER in this process has been well characterized in animal models as summarized previously.[51] Steroid hormone–mediated carcinogenesis is a complex process involving many growth factors and the interaction of many intracellular pathways. Variations in both genetic and epigenetic events within the estrogen pathway are believed to be crucial for initiation and progression of breast cancers.[52] Successful treatment of breast cancer is therefore intrinsically linked to accurate manipulation of the ER pathway and requires a greater understanding of the aberrations within this pathway that result in cancer.

The relationship between breast cancer and estrogen deprivation was initially documented in 1896 by Sir George Beatson, who reported regression of advanced breast cancer in women who underwent oophorectomy.[53] Epidemiologic studies have since consistently demonstrated a correlation between increased breast cancer risk and increased endogenous estrogen levels as described previously. Use of hormone replacement therapy (HRT) is also associated with an increased risk of breast cancer. This has been demonstrated in large prospective observational trials[54,55] in which the relative risk seems to increase with longer duration of HRT use; it increases after 5 years of use.

The predominant effects of estrogen are mediated through interaction with two receptor proteins, ERα and ERβ. These proteins are encoded by two genes located on chromosome 6q and on 14q, respectively. ERα and ERβ show substantial homology in the DNA binding domain but relatively little conservation in other domains such the aminoterminal A/B domain (Fig. 28-7).[56] The cDNA encoding ERα was isolated in 1986,[57,58] yet many features of its signaling pathway have yet to be characterized. In 1996, the cDNA encoding ERβ was isolated and characterized.[59] The role of ERβ in breast cancer, if any, is yet to be elucidated. The discussion, which follows, is focused on the role of ERα in breast cancer. The classical mechanism of action for estrogen's effect within a cell involves binding of 17β estradiol to ER located in the cell nucleus. This activated complex dimerizes and binds to estrogen-response elements (EREs) located upstream, which are subsequently transcribed. Resultant ERE-activated genes are capable of inhibiting apoptosis, altering gene expression and stimulating progression through the cell cycle. The ER signaling pathway may also engage in cross-talk with other intracellular mitogenic pathways (Fig. 28-8).

Transcription of ERα from the ESR1 gene is a complex process that is under the control of several distinct promoters,[60,61] which give rise to alternate transcripts. ER-mediated transcriptional activation of estrogen target genes is accomplished through direct hormonal interaction with the ER, with binding of activated ER dimers to an ERE in the promoter/enhancer region of the target gene. Activation of the target gene also involves ER-mediated recruitment of estrogen-related nuclear protein regulators known as coactivators and corepressors.[62] These nuclear coregulators facilitate transcription by interaction with transcription machinery proteins with some recruited coregulator proteins responsible for chromatin remodeling to facilitate binding of RNA polymerase (see Fig. 28-7). Histone acetylation accomplished through acetyl transferases, for example, correlates with a more actively transcribed state of chromatin resulting from its greater accessibility. Methylation of histones through recruitment of methyl transferases, on the other hand, favors more tightly coiled chromatin, which is less accessible to transcriptional machinery and therefore less expressed. Presently,

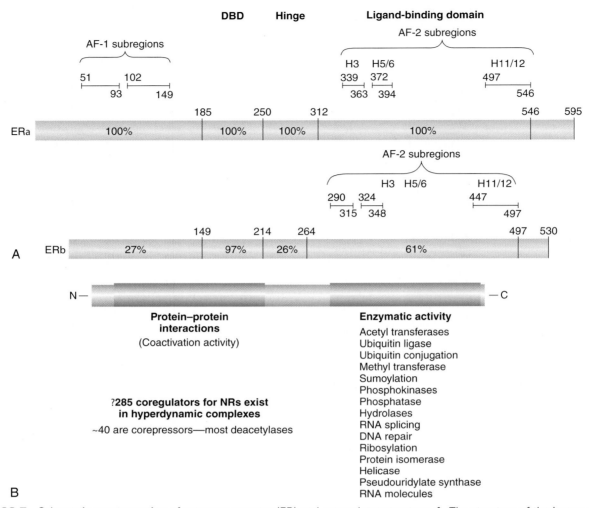

Figure 28-7 Schematic representation of estrogen receptor (ER) and coregulator structure. **A,** The structure of the known ERs with identified activating functions (AFs) that bind coactivators. Also identified are the DNA-binding domain (DBD) and the ligand-binding domain. **B,** Typical domain structure of a nuclear receptor (NR) coactivator is shown. There are two main domains: (1) a protein-protein interacting domain that binds other coactivators in the functional high-molecular-weight coactivator complex and (2) an enzymatic domain that either has intrinsic enzyme activity or binds a protein that has enzyme activity. (Reproduced from Jordan V, O'Malley B: Selective estrogen-receptor modulators and antihormonal resistance in breast cancer. J Clin Oncol 25:5815–5824, 2007.)

nuclear coactivators, such as nuclear coactivator 1 (NCOA1) and NCOA3, which acetylate histones, are under investigation as potential targets for therapy. From this perspective, histone deacetylase inhibitors could potentially play a therapeutic role in the treatment of some women with breast cancer. Alteration of these coactivators and corepressors may also play a significant role in alteration of gene expression leading to proliferative changes and carcinogenesis.

ER status of primary breast carcinoma is highly predictive of clinical benefit from endocrine therapy in both the adjuvant and metastatic settings in the treatment of women with breast cancer. Breast cancer patients with tumors that express ER are more likely to respond to hormone therapy,[63] and have a greatly improved prognosis when compared to women with ER negative cancers. Accurately measuring ER is of considerable importance, because it continues to be one of the strongest predictive factors of responsiveness to endocrine manipulative management. Additionally, for some subsets of women,

endocrine therapy alone may provide an excellent treatment response allowing them to forego additional cytotoxic therapy. In the last decade, large multinational prospectively randomized clinical trials have demonstrated the superiority of aromatase inhibitors over tamoxifen in postmenopausal women.[64,65] Recent trials also show that the benefits of prolonged estrogen deprivation continue for many years after completion of initial hormonal therapy with both a reduction in ipsilateral and contralateral breast cancers.[64,65] In addition, extending antihormonal treatment following completion of 5 years of tamoxifen therapy, results in a further reduction of the recurrence rate.[66] From this perspective, there is a need to more clearly define the role of steroid receptors and their respective pathways in the initiation, promotion and progression of breast cancer.

Although approximately two thirds of breast cancers are ER positive and responsive to estrogen, one third of cancers are ER negative. In ER-positive tumors, only 70% show clinical response to estrogen manipulation,

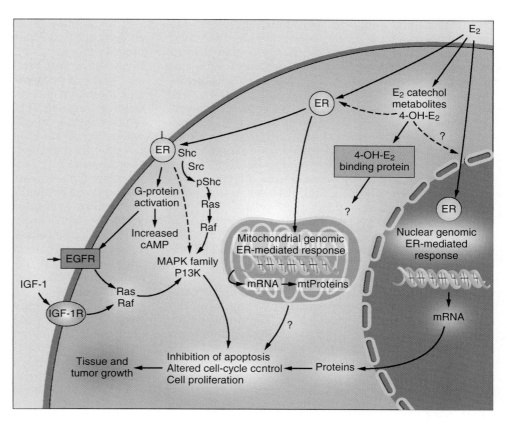

Figure 28-8 Estrogen receptor (ER) interaction with estrogen response elements and cross-talk with intracellular pathways. Dashed line *arrows* indicate putative pathways. CAMP, cyclic AMP; E2, estradiol; EGFR, epidermal growth factor receptor; IGF-1 insulin-like growth factor 1; IGF-1R, insulin-like growth factor 1 receptor; MAPK, mitogen-activated protein kinase; MPI3K, phosphoinositide 3 kinase; mtProteins, mitochondrial proteins; mRNA, messenger RNA; 4-OH-E₂, 4-hydroxyestradiol; pShc, phosphorylated Shc protein. (Redrawn from Yager JD, Davidson NE: Estrogen carcinogenesis in breast cancer. N Engl J Med 354:270–282, 2006. Copyright © 2006. Massachusetts Medical Society. All rights reserved.)

and a fraction of these ER-positive tumors go on to develop endocrine resistance. Progressive disease appears to correlate with hormone resistance over time, both in in vitro conditions and in clinical follow-up. It is unclear how this hormone resistance occurs. Loss of estrogen response and loss of the ER itself correlates with a more aggressive clinical course. Several important mechanisms may be involved in resistance to endocrine therapies. Epigenetic alteration of ER promoter through promoter/enhancer methylation of the ESR1 gene is hypothesized to be an important event in the development of ER-negative tumors.

Progesterone Receptor

Despite the long understanding that estrogen and progesterone are the hormones most responsible for proliferative effects in breast tissue, increasing epidemiologic data showing increased risks of breast cancer in women with long-term use of progestin-containing HRT regimens.[55] Progesterone has an essential role in breast maturation, and during pregnancy it is responsible for ductal branching and lobuloalveolar differentiation.[67] A clear role for progesterone has been documented in animal models, which show it plays a role in the induction, maintenance, and progression of a neoplastic phenotype.[68] ERs are important for regulating the expression of PRs, and recent animal studies in ER knockout mice confirm absence of PR expression as well.[51] In fact, colocalization studies show that all cells that are positive for PR also express ER.[69] As with ER, therapy aimed at blocking PR alone or in combination with other treatments

has become a potential therapeutic option.[70] Sixty percent of all invasive breast cancers express PR, and this expression is largely regarded as a marker of intact ER function.[42] Earlier studies indicate that the presence of PR may predict responsiveness to endocrine therapy in ER-positive patients.[71] However, now it is understood that loss of PR can occur through mechanisms that are independent of the ER pathway, including PR promoter methylation and loss of heterozygosity.

The PR, like ERα and ERβ, is a member of the nuclear receptor superfamily, which regulates the expression of target genes in response to ligand binding. The effects of progesterone are mediated through the intracellular receptor proteins PRA and PRB. These two proteins are produced from the same gene using two distinct translation initiation sites under the control of separate promoters.[72] In response to the binding of progesterone, the PR undergoes confirmation changes and dissociation from heat shock protein. Subsequent dimerization is followed by binding of the receptor to progesterone-response elements of progestin target genes. Binding to progesterone response elements is followed by coactivator recruitment and resultant transcription of target genes. Expression of PR in breast cancer tissue is associated with a higher probability of responsiveness to endocrine manipulative management.

HER2

The human epidermal growth factor receptor (HER) family of genes is important in the normal regulation of embryonic migration, epithelial cell growth, proliferation, and apoptosis. The epidermal growth factor receptor EGFR, or HER1, is the archetype for these transmembrane tyrosine kinase receptors that activate mitogenic downstream signaling pathways following binding to known ligands (Fig. 28-9). There are four members of the family: HER1, HER2, HER3, and HER4. Their role in breast cancer is the subject of considerable research interest. The most important of these in breast cancer is the HER2 (*neu*) oncogene, or *ERBB2* gene, which was originally identified from rat neuroglioblastomas and, subsequently, found to be distinct from the EGFR receptor.[73,74] Overexpression of HER2 in a stably transfected NIH/3T3 fibroblast cell line resulted in malignant transformation of these cells.[75] The HER2 gene was shown to be amplified and overexpressed in human breast and ovarian cancers as early as 1989.[76,77] HER2 amplification in breast cancer is associated with poor differentiation, a high proliferative rate, decreased expression of steroid hormone receptors, and an increased likelihood of having lymph node metastases.[7]

HER2 gene amplification is correlated with poor disease-free and overall survival.[7] Since the initial debate about the potential for HER2 gene amplification as a significant prognostic marker, its clinical significance has become widely accepted, and more attention is being paid to problems in clinical testing to identify women whose breast cancers have this alteration.[78] Survival analyses have repeatedly shown that the presence of the HER2 amplification or overexpression is more predictive of clinical outcome than all other clinical factors, with the exception of axillary lymph node status.[7,79,80] Although HER2 overexpression is correlated with increased proliferation, increased cell migration, increased invasion, and stimulation of angiogenesis, the detailed mechanisms stimulating changes in these biologic behaviors are under investigation.[5,81]

The HER2 membrane receptor protein mediates normal cellular signaling by forming heterodimers (or hetero-oligomers) with other members of the HER receptor family while cancer cells with HER2 overexpression mediate cellular signaling through either homodimerization (or homo-oligomerization) with itself or heterodimer formation. A normal cell has two copies of the HER2 gene with low expression of the gene protein product. When HER2 gene amplification is present in a cell, there is resultant greatly increased level of expression, referred to as pathologic overexpression of the HER2 protein on the cell surface leading to substantially higher concentrations of HER2 receptor on the cell membrane. Formation of HER2 heterodimers and homodimers results in activation of the intracellular tyrosine kinase domain of the receptor and phosphorylation of tyrosine residues located within the intracellular domain of HER2 protein. A series of adaptor proteins are recruited to these phosphorylated sites, and a complex set of intracellular signaling pathways is activated as a result.[12] This leads to constitutive activation of the ras/MAP kinase and PI3 kinase/AKT pathways, resulting in increased cell proliferation and survival with concomitant loss of apoptosis. HER2 itself and this signaling pathway are targeted by a series of new therapeutic agents.

Trastuzumab, a humanized monoclonal antibody recognizing the extracellular domain of HER2, has been approved for treatment of HER2-amplified/overexpressed breast cancer patients. The development of this therapeutic is a "proof of principle" confirming that tumors with specific molecular alterations can be successfully treated with tailored, targeted therapy. The primary mechanism by which the drug functions is not well understood, but it is widely agreed that binding of trastuzumab to the HER2 receptor disrupts the HER2-mediated signaling caused by overexpression. The antibody interaction with the receptor interferes with downstream signaling, turns off increased cell proliferation, and induces apoptosis. Another possible mechanism of trastuzumab action is through increased antibody–dependent cellular cytoxicity with activation of natural killer cells directed against cells with HER2 overexpression. Large trials have shown the efficacy of trastuzumab therapy both in advanced, metastatic disease,[82] as well as in earlier, nonmetastatic disease by the use of adjuvant treatment to decrease the risk of recurrence and death.[83,84] Although women with breast cancer have in the past been found to have a greater benefit from anthracycline-based chemotherapy,[85] this benefit is restricted to those women whose breast cancers have HER2 amplification/overexpression.[86-88] However, the use of anthracyclines in combination with trastuzumab is also associated with significantly greater toxicity, especially cardiac toxicity.[82-84] In addition, it has been suggested that inclusion of a second gene, the topoisomerase II-alpha gene, in the HER2 amplicon is primarily responsible for the incremental responsiveness to anthracycline chemotherapy. Topoisomerase II-alpha, the primary molecular target of anthracyclines, is expressed during the S phase of the cell cycle to resolve DNA topologic constraints that develop during DNA synthesis. Although the importance of TOP2A gene coamplification has not yet been established as clinically important, it has become increasingly important that accurate molecular testing is performed to determine the HER2 amplification/overexpression status,[78] so that women who have the alteration are correctly identified and most appropriately treated.[89]

Not all patients overexpressing HER2 show an initial response to trastuzumab therapy.[90] The number of responders is increased by concurrent use of selected cytotoxic chemotherapy agents in combination with trastuzumab. However, resistance to trastuzumab therapy remains an important issue. No naturally occurring receptor ligand has been identified to date for HER2. The conformation of the unoccupied HER2 receptor is the preferred dimerization partner for itself and for the other members of the HER family. Dimerization with HER1 or HER3 could play a role in the development of resistance to trastuzumab therapy.[81] Of those who do have a response, resistance may be seen within 12 months.

A second targeted therapeutic agent, lapatinib, is a tyrosine kinase inhibitor of both HER1 and HER2. Because of this dual kinase inhibitory activity, lapatinib is expected to be efficacious in a wider spectrum of women with breast cancer than those responsive to trastuzumab; in addition, it may be efficacious in some women who show resistance to trastuzumab. The initial

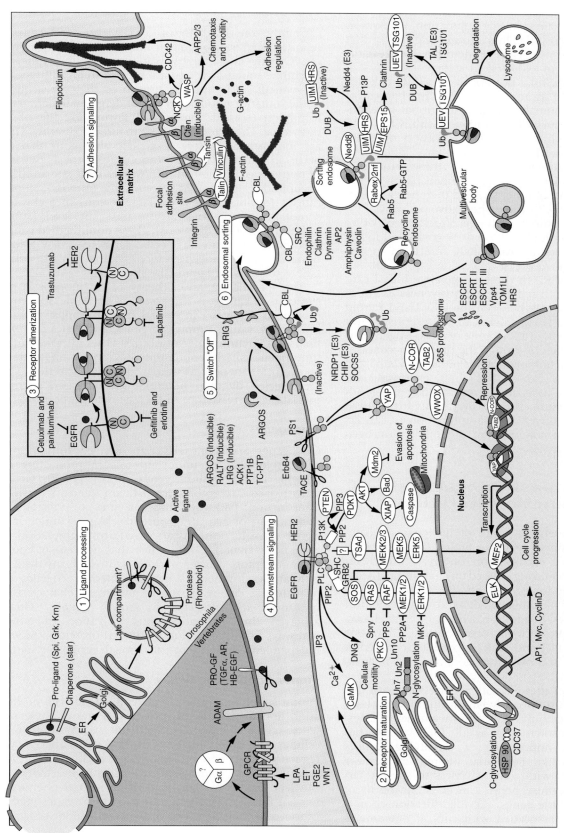

Figure 28-9 Overview of epidermal growth factor receptor signaling. (Modified from Yarden Y, Shilo BZ: SnapShot: EGFR signaling pathway. Cell 131:1018, 2007.)

phase III clinical trial of lapatinib in women with metastatic trastuzumab-resistant breast cancer has shown lapatinib to be efficacious in this population[91]; however, subsequent studies of this clinical trial have shown that lapatinib responsiveness is dependent on HER2 status and is independent of EGFR/HER1 status.[92]

Loss of the extracellular portion of the HER2 receptor has been implicated as another possible mechanism of resistance to trastuzumab therapy. Additional mechanisms for resistance include redundancy within the HER family pathways, which may permit evasion of HER2 therapeutic blockade through the Ras/MAP kinase and AKT/PI3 kinase pathways. Each of these molecular mechanisms for resistance to trastuzumab points to the potential importance of other targeted therapeutic agents that could interfere with these alternative pathways.

Although breast cancers with overexpression of HER2 have reduced expression of ER and PR compared to the nonamplified tumors, approximately one third to one half of HER2-amplified breast cancers do express ER.[93,94] Amplification of HER2 in these ER-positive breast cancers is associated with reduced responsiveness to endocrine therapy. Cross-talk between the HER2 and steroid hormone pathways is considered to be responsible for constitutive activation of ER in spite of antiestrogen therapy such as tamoxifen. Although the precise mechanism for this activation is unknown, ER is phosphorylated and activated in breast cancer cell lines expressing ER through a hormone-independent mechanism as a result of HER2 overexpression. These observations suggest that women with ER-positive, HER2-amplified breast cancers may benefit from a combination of both antiestrogen and anti-HER2 therapies.

Sporadic Breast Cancer and Somatic Genetic Alterations

Breast cancer represents a group of malignancies composed of numerous heterogeneous molecular genetic entities. The traditional classification of breast cancer for therapeutic decision making is based on anatomical disease attributes, including tumor size, microscopic histopathologic classification, histologic grade, and involvement of axillary lymph nodes. In addition, a few molecular characteristics, including presence or absence of steroid hormone receptors (ER and PR) and HER2 growth factor receptor gene amplification and overexpression, are used in treatment decisions.

Although each of these factors is correlated with disease progression, histologically similar tumors can have different clinical outcomes. The clinical impact of assessing single gene markers such as ER, PR, or HER2 has demonstrated the importance of classifying tumors according to particular molecular biomarkers because of their association with responsiveness to specific targeted therapies. Because breast cancer is the result of alterations in multiple genes, the identification of new molecular markers associated with clinical outcome is leading to the development of a new, improved approach to classification of breast carcinomas based on evaluation of multiple genes.

GENETIC ABNORMALITIES IN BREAST CANCER

Currently, the function of over a thousand genes is reported as affected by genetic modifications in breast cancer. Genetic alterations in cancers are either inherited (germline mutations) and are present in all cell types of the patient, including the tumor, or they are acquired in the somatic or body cells that undergo malignant transformation (somatic mutations) during the life of the individual. The latter are present in tumor cells only. There are four general classes of genetic alterations that can occur in cancers[95]: translocations (reciprocal exchange of portions of different chromosomes with one another), aneuploidy (alteration in chromosome number), amplifications (multiple repeats of large regions of a chromosome), and mutations at the base-pair level (substitutions, insertions, deletions). These noninherited genetic modifications involving specific genes may play a functional role in tumorigenesis by providing a growth advantage to the cells containing the alteration.

The somatic mutation theory of carcinogenesis presumes that cancer is the result of multiple sequential mutations occurring in several critical groups of genes: oncogenes, tumor suppressor genes, and genes responsible for the maintenance of normal DNA in cells. During tumorigenesis, cells containing these mutations undergo an evolutionary process similar to natural selection. They are selected by their potential for increased survival, metastasis, or resistance to therapeutic agents.

Oncogenes

Oncogenes are characteristically derived from normal genes that play an important role in promoting cell growth. Typically, these genes encode growth factors, growth factor receptors, downstream effectors of signal transduction pathways and enzymes responsible for metabolism of activating proteins. Normal function of signal transduction cascades requires stimulation by exogenous signaling molecules that activate receptors; these receptors trigger various pathways involved in cellular development. When activated, oncogenes can provide the cell with one of the main characteristics of cancer: self-sufficiency in growth signals.[1] This is achieved through endogenous activation of growth pathways from the level of a mutated protein to provide independence from exogenous growth regulatory signals.

Tumor Suppressor Genes

Tumor suppressor genes, in general, encode cell proliferation and differentiation proteins. Some of these proteins regulate entry to apoptosis when irreparable cellular damage occurs. Most of these genes are cell cycle regulators, such as retinoblastoma or p53, which prevent cells with DNA damage from proliferative activity that can lead to clonal expansion of an altered phenotype. Loss of function in the tumor suppressor genes enables cancer cells to acquire two of their basic traits: resistance to antigrowth signals and evasion of apoptosis.[1]

Mutations in oncogenes can lead to gain of function and alterations in tumor suppressor genes can lead to loss of function. These alterations may play a role in the cascade of molecular events that lead to cell immortality and to the accumulation of additional mutations.[96] Activation of oncogenes occurs by alteration of a single allele, inducing changes in quantity or quality of the protein to confer new growth characteristics for the cell. A gain in function may be accomplished through several different mechanisms: somatic mutation, gene amplification, translocations, or other genetic rearrangements. In the case of tumor suppressor genes, in general, both alleles are usually modified in order to interfere with the production of a protein that inhibits tumorigenesis. Inactivation of this group of genes is usually achieved by somatic mutation, combined with loss of heterozygosity or DNA methylation.

Genes involved in genomic stability regulate normal DNA replication and protect DNA from mutations that might occur during division or by the action of mutagens. Some of the classes of genes in this category regulate mismatch repair, nucleotide-excision repair, and base-excision repair genes.[97] Mutations in such genes lead to chromosomal instability, a well-known feature of cancer. According to mathematical models that calculate the contribution of chromosomal instability to tumorigenesis, it is presumed that chromosomal instability leads to increased accumulation of mutations in the genome of affected cells.[98] In cancer cells, chromosomal instability is the cause of multiple losses of DNA fragments leading to aneuploidy and loss of heterozygosity.[99] One of the results of genetic instability is loss of function of tumor suppressor genes by loss of heterozygosity, a common mechanism of gene inactivation. It occurs in normal cells with two different inherited copies of the same genes and inactivates both functional alleles through a succession of events. One allele is presumed to be altered by mutation, and the remaining normal allele may be lost by deletion of a large chromosomal area or by inactivation of the promoter through DNA methylation. During the process of DNA repair following these events, the mutated allele is duplicated, resulting in multiple defective copies of the gene and leading to the expression of only the abnormal protein.

SOMATIC MUTATIONS

P53 Tumor Suppressor

TP53 gene is mutated in breast cancers as well as in a variety of other cancers,[100] including carcinomas of the ovary, colon, lung, liver, and bladder. The gene is located on the short arm of chromosome 17 and encodes a 393–amino acid protein. It contains a transactivation domain, a DNA-binding domain, and a C-terminal oligomerization domain. The transcription factor p53 is involved in signaling pathways activated by cellular stress, which has an important role in inhibiting proliferation of damaged cells. It is activated by phosphorylation following DNA breaks[101] (Fig. 28-10) and is stabilized through post-translational modifications. After activation, p53 binds to specific DNA promoter sites and acts as a transcriptional activator of other genes involved in inhibition of the cell cycle, inhibition of blood vessel formation, stimulation of

apoptosis, and promotion of DNA repair.[101] The result is cell cycle arrest and DNA repair or, alternatively, in the case of irreparable DNA damage, apoptosis (see Fig. 28-10).

Approximately 2412 single nucleotide polymorphisms (SNPs) have been reported in *TP53*, most of which involve intronic regions of the gene. A clear role of SNPs in altering p53 function is not established, although the SNPs represent altered DNA sequences and might affect the stability of the protein product. One such example, a protein variant in p53, involves a polymorphism at residue 72. The presence of an arginine rather than a proline at codon 72 is associated with induction of apoptosis,[102] interaction with multiple transcription factors,[103] and increased turnover of the protein.[104] Germline mutations of *TP53* are associated with the Li-Fraumeni syndrome,[105] a familial disorder manifested by multiple tumors including soft tissue sarcomas, breast cancer and adrenal carcinoma.

The frequency of somatic mutations in p53 varies depending on the tumor type. Currently, approximately 2500 *TP53* mutations have been identified in breast tissue samples. In breast cancer, *TP53* mutations are reported in approximately 20% of cases and vary depending on the patient cohort analyzed[106] and on the stage of disease. Mutations in one allele are frequently associated with inactivation of the other allele by loss of heterozygosity in as many as 30% of the breast tumors.[107] In sporadic cancers there is one or, infrequently, more point mutations identified in the gene causing translation of a mutant, nonfunctional protein, which accumulates in the nucleus.[108] The accumulation of protein in the nucleus identified by immunohistochemistry (IHC) is correlated with the presence of mutations identified by direct DNA sequencing. However, there is not always a direct correlation between mutations in the gene and positive IHC staining. Some mutations may lead to a rapidly degraded mRNA or protein product that is not detectable. Most mutations arise in the DNA-binding domain and prevent the protein's activity as a transcription factor.[109] Also, deletions of the carboxyterminal domain prevent tetramerization and proper function of the protein.[110] Approximately 75% of *TP53* mutations are single nucleotide substitutions leading to substitution of a single amino acid. The majority of mutations involve substitutions of G-C base pairs into A-T sites (40%). These single amino acid substitutions are predominantly (approximately 85%) associated with positive nuclear p53 protein overexpression by IHC. The remaining 25% of mutations include insertions, deletions, and nonsense mutations. These are associated with p53 nuclear IHC immunostaining in only approximately 30% of cases.

Somatic mutations in p53 occur early in the progression of the disease and are identified in ductal carcinoma in situ alone as well as accompanied by invasive disease.[111] Mutations in *TP53* are associated with increasing tumor size and grade, as well as axillary lymph nodal metastases and recurrent tumors.[106] There is also a high frequency of TP53 mutations associated with *BRCA1/BRCA2* carriers.[112] This correlation suggests that defective DNA repair due to *BRCA1/BRCA2* might influence

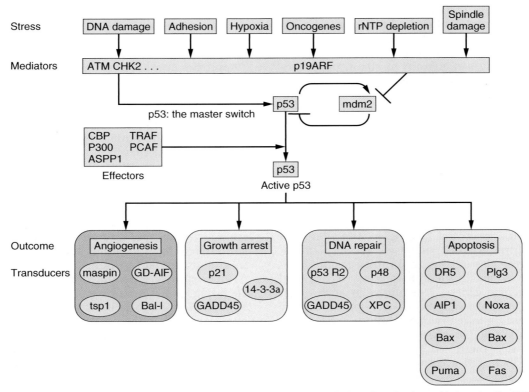

Figure 28-10 Schematic illustration showing the central role of p53 as a switch deciding the fate of injured cells. P53 is activated by mediators of stress, signaling pathways initiated by DNA damage, adhesion signals, hypoxia, action of oncogenes, rNTP depletion, or spindle damage. On activation it binds to DNA and regulates transcription of genes involved in inhibition of blood vessel formation, cell cycle inhibition, apoptosis, and DNA repair. The result is cell cycle arrest and DNA repair or, in case of increased damage, apoptosis. (Adapted from Vogelstein B, Lane D, Levine AJ: Surfing the p53 network. Nature 408:307–310, 2000.)

the development of *TP53* mutations in breast cancer.[17] *TP53* mutations are also correlated with a lack of ER or PR expression.[113]

The presence of *TP53* mutations is a prognostic marker in breast cancer[114] correlated with shorter disease-free and shorter overall survival in node-negative and node-positive patients. The correlation of p53 mutations with response to therapy has been rather controversial, in spite of the numerous published studies. Although tumors with certain mutations are reported to be resistant to chemotherapy,[109] an increased patient survival rate was observed in women with node-negative breast cancers and *TP53* mutations who were treated with local radiotherapy compared with women who had node-negative breast cancers having wild-type *TP53*.[115] These findings suggest that mutations of *TP53* have potential for treatment selection in breast cancer management.

Estrogen Receptorα Gene (ESR1) Mutations

Steroid hormone receptors, as previously discussed in this chapter, play an important role in the initiation, promotion and progression of breast cancer. The ER (ERα) is involved in the transcriptional regulation of numerous target genes responsible for cell growth, differentiation, and resistance to apoptosis.[56] ERα has been reported as mutated and amplified in some breast cancers. As described previously, approximately 70% of breast carcinomas are associated with ERα expression

determined by IHC.[116] It is difficult to evaluate the actual activity of ER in the tumors because multiple splice variants of ERα have been reported, including a constitutively active and a dominant negative isoform that might have an impact on the activity level of the receptor. In addition, somatic mutations have been described in the ESR1 gene in breast cancer patients, and some of these are suggested to play a role in tumorigenesis and in metastatic spread of primary tumors.[56] The ERα A86V mutation is predicted to lead to lower activity of the receptor. ERα K303R is hypothesized to give the receptor the ability to react to smaller concentrations of the stimulating hormone than the wild-type ERα. ERα 437Stop, identified only in metastatic breast cancers, may have an important role in the spread of the disease. Although mutations in the ERα gene could be clinically important, subsequent studies of ERα mutations have suggested that these mutations are much less frequent than originally reported, placing their clinical relevance in doubt.

GENE COPY NUMBER ABERRATIONS

Gene copy number aberrations are relatively common in human cancers, with approximately 50% of breast cancers considered "amplifying" in terms of genome-wide copy number assessment.[117] Gene amplification, an increased copy number of specific genes or chromosomal regions, is a pathologic change commonly associated with increased mRNA transcription and protein expression of affected genes.

Amplification of several regions in the breast cancer genome contain genes coding for oncogenes. For example, the chromosome 17q12 amplicon contains the HER2/neu gene, the 8q24 amplicon contains the *myc* gene, and the 11q13 amplicon contains the cyclin D1 gene, all of which are amplified and overexpressed in breast cancer.[118]

HER2/*neu*

HER2 is a well-known oncogene previously presented in this chapter as a breast cancer marker used for selection of patients for specific treatment options.[7] HER2 is also amplified in gynecologic cancers, such as ovarian and endometrial carcinomas, as well as in carcinomas of the stomach and salivary gland.[77,119–121] HER2 amplification is associated with a high recurrence rate and poor overall survival in each of these types of carcinomas.[77,79,119–121]

The gene, also known as HER2, NEU, or ERBB2, is one of the most studied genes in the field of breast cancer during the past 20 years. It encodes a 1255–amino acid protein, composed of an extracellular domain, a single transmembrane domain, and an intracellular region containing a tyrosine kinase domain as well as phosphorylation sites.[122] HER2 is an orphan receptor, normally activated by heterodimerization[123] with other members of the EGFR family (ERBB1/ERBB 3/ERBB 4)

after these family members are activated through binding of their respective extracellular ligands. The activated receptor complex interacts with a variety of proteins to activate selected signaling pathways. These interacting proteins include kinases such as Src, PLCγ, or PI3K; phosphatases such as Shp2; adaptor proteins such as Shc and Grb-2; and G-proteins such as Ras[124] (Fig. 28-11). Activation of the mitogen-activated protein kinase (MAPK) cascade through Grb-2, Shc, Sos, and Ras leads to activation of transcription factors involved in transcriptional activation of genes involved in cell proliferation. Activation of the PI3K (phosphoinositol-3-kinase) pathway is followed by activation of protein kinases B and C with induction of the NF-kB signaling pathway and inhibition of apoptosis and stimulation of cell cycle progression.[125] The JAK/STAT pathway, activated through c-Src, is associated with tumorigenic transformation of breast epithelial cells.[101]

HER2 gene amplification is associated with high levels of HER2 messenger RNA and p185^HER2 protein expression, referred to as pathologic overexpression.[77] When frozen tissues are used for analyses of HER2 copy number and expression, there is a direct one-to-one association of amplification with overexpression. Overexpression of HER2 leads to receptor homodimerization and autophosphorylation with enhanced function in the absence of ligand.[126] This unregulated stimulation of the HER2 pathway is associated with aggressive biologic behavior and an invasive phenotype. Protein overexpression is identified in clinical samples or archived

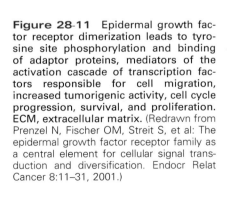

Figure 28-11 Epidermal growth factor receptor dimerization leads to tyrosine site phosphorylation and binding of adaptor proteins, mediators of the activation cascade of transcription factors responsible for cell migration, increased tumorigenic activity, cell cycle progression, survival, and proliferation. ECM, extracellular matrix. (Redrawn from Prenzel N, Fischer OM, Streit S, et al: The epidermal growth factor receptor family as a central element for cellular signal transduction and diversification. Endocr Relat Cancer 8:11–31, 2001.)

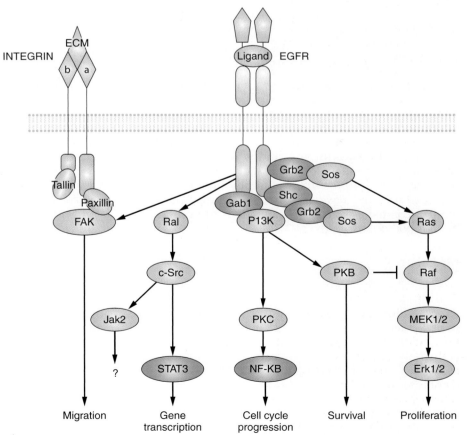

paraffin-embedded specimens by IHC using antibodies against HER2. Comparison of HER2 gene status with HER2 expression status in these clinical samples, using fluorescent in situ hybridization (FISH) and IHC leads, not infrequently, to discrepancies in HER2 classification by these methods. These differences are due primarily to problems of IHC related to tissue fixation and processing as well as antigen retrieval use in this assay method.[89,92,127] The use of an appropriate antibody with a high affinity for the fixed, paraffin-embedded protein is of major importance for the adequate identification of protein overexpression by immunohistochemistry.[89,128,129] It is equally important that the anti-HER2 antibody not require antigen retrieval during the IHC procedure to minimize false-positive results.[89,128,129] In contrast, assessment of HER2 gene amplification by FISH is relatively unaltered by tissue processing of clinical samples for paraffin embedding.[79,89,129] Microscopic detection of HER2 gene copy number by FISH involves the direct visualization of specific genes in the nuclei of tumor cells by hybridization of specific, fluorescently tagged probes having a sequence complementary to the gene of interest. The hybridization mixture contains specific HER2 probes labeled with an orange fluorophore as well as a probe specific to the chromosome 17 centromere, labeled by a different fluorescent color (green). The amplification rate is calculated by reporting the ratio of the average number of HER2 gene copies divided by the average number of chromosome 17 centromere copies in the scored tumor cell nuclei. Specimens with a HER2/CEP17 ratio greater than 2 are considered amplified. HER2 amplification and overexpression in breast cancer has important prognostic and treatment implications as summarized in the previous section.

Estrogen Receptor Gene Amplification

ER gene (ESR1) amplification has been reported in 20% of breast cancer cases.[130] ESR1 amplification is correlated with both high-level ER protein expression and increased responsiveness to tamoxifen therapy. ESR1 amplification has been identified in preneoplastic lesions as well as in advanced invasive tumors, and it is suggested to be an early genetic alteration in some breast cancers.[130] Although this is a potentially clinically important finding, several groups have not been able to reproduce the results, and there is active debate about the validity of these initial observations.[131–134]

Myc

Myc is a nuclear protein involved in transcriptional regulation of genes involved in cell growth and proliferation. Early studies using Southern blotting demonstrated that Myc is amplified and overexpressed in breast cancers and is associated with high tumor grade, high proliferative rate, early recurrence of disease, and death.[135] Although MYC and HER2 are on different chromosomes, there is a statistically significant association between MYC amplification and HER2 amplification in invasive ductal carcinomas as well as an association of both with a high proliferative rate.[136–138]

Treatment with chemotherapy is associated with a shorter disease-free survival than when either of the genes is amplified.[136, 139] The addition of trastuzumab to standard anthracycline-containing chemotherapy is associated with a markedly improved disease-free survival when HER2 and MYC are coamplified compared with amplification of HER2 alone.[139] Although these findings need confirmation, they suggest an important role for MYC in the regulation of apoptosis in breast cancer.

Cyclin D1

Cyclin D1 is a cell cycle regulatory protein that plays an important role in normal mammary gland development.[140] The gene encoding cyclin D1 is located on chromosome 11q13 and is amplified in approximately 20% of breast cancers, with amplified breast cancers showing a significant correlation with both lobular histology and with ER or PR positivity.[137] Cyclin D1 overexpression alone is not associated with malignant transformation in either cultured cells or in animal models. However, coexpression of cyclin D1 with c-Myc in mice is associated with the formation of malignant tumors having an aggressive phenotype.[141] Patients with two or more amplified loci, such as CCND1 and FGFR1, have a significant reduction in overall survival, indicating cooperative effects.[142] Cell cycle regulatory proteins represent attractive targets for development of novel therapeutic inhibitors. Some of these are already in early phase clinical trials.[143]

Amplification of Multiple Genes

Amplification and coamplification at different loci in different tumors has been analyzed and found to be indicative of the tumor phenotype as well as predictive for clinical evolution of the tumor.[136,137,142] Amplification of genes such as MDM2 has been correlated with poor survival in patients without nodal metastasis, whereas other genes such as cyclin D1 and EGFR are associated with poor prognosis in patients with metastatic disease.[142] The frequency of gene amplification and coamplification in breast cancer is also suggestive of chromosome instability and is viewed as a potential prognostic factor 1. The number of amplicons is correlated with shorter telomeres, suggesting that telomere dysfunction might play a role in chromosome stability and in the induction of gene number aberrations.[144,145]

An increase in gene copy number over large DNA regions, referred to as amplicons, has been described in breast cancer as in other cancers. This suggests that multiple genes in amplicons such as the 17q22-q24 amplicon and 20q11-q13 amplicon may be activated and could contribute to the disease process or in resistance to treatment.[146,147] Not all the genes in a given chromosomal region are consistently amplified. The size and extent of the amplicon is variable, and the number of genes included in a particular amplicon is variable among carcinomas.[146] The chromosome 17q22-24 (HER2) amplicon may contain a variable number of genes in this region of the chromosome, such as topoisomerase II-alpha (TOP2A), RARA,[148] or PPARB,[149] which are frequently coamplified with HER2 in breast cancer. Approximately 35% of breast cancers with HER2 amplification also have amplification of the TOP2A gene. Recent studies show that coamplification of HER2 and TOP2A is significantly correlated with response to anthracycline-containing chemotherapy.[150,151] TOP2A is well established as the primary target for anthracyclines, and its amplification is proposed as a potential marker for responsiveness to this type of chemotherapy.[150]

Amplifications on chromosome 20 can occur independently or concurrently in one to three regions: 20q11, 20q12, and 20q13.2.[152] There are numerous genes in these regions of chromosome 20 that represent good candidates for promoting cell immortality and that might contribute to tumor progression. These genes include the BCL-X gene, with a role in apoptosis; the transcription factor encoding gene (E2F); protein tyrosine phosphatase (PTPN1)[147]; and amplified breast cancer genes 1, 3, and 4 (AIB1, AIB3, and AIB4).[153] Although specific clinical roles for these genes have not been identified, the presence of multiple amplified genes in breast cancer is, in itself, a marker of a breast cancer class with a poor clinical outcome.[117]

GENOME-WIDE ASSESSMENT OF GENETIC ALTERATIONS

The completion of the human genome sequence project, the development of computational biology as well as new technological advances (sequencing technologies, microarrays) facilitate extensive genetic analyses of human cancers. The characterization of genetic alterations involved in human carcinogenesis has been more and more successful in the last few years, and a more comprehensive overview of the "genomic landscapes"[154] of human cancers has emerged (Figs. 28-12 and 28-13).

Whole Genome DNA Sequencing of Breast Cancers

A detailed sequence analysis of 11 breast and 11 colorectal cancers involving more than 18,000 genes revealed alterations in multiple genes, and these genes have been referred to as candidate cancer genes.[154–156] The authors identified approximately 80 different mutations occurring in the DNA-coding regions of each tumor and among those, less than 15 were considered to make an important contribution in driving the tumor phenotype. An overview of these mutation patterns suggests that the identification of specific pathways altered in cancer is also important in addition to the analysis of mutations in specific genes. Any of the multiple members of a given pathway can be targeted by mutation at various rates to confer a growth, survival, or expansion advantage for the cancer. In this study, there are 122 candidate cancer genes, with different roles, mutated in breast cancer. These genes are involved in regulation of cellular adhesion, signal transduction, transcriptional regulation, cellular transport, cellular metabolism, intracellular trafficking, and RNA metabolism.[156] The list of altered genes contains some well-known mutations frequently encountered in breast cancers, but it also contains many altered genes that occur relatively infrequently (i.e., in <5% of the cases). These less frequent but numerous mutations are hypothesized to provide the background on which the carcinoma is building its survival advantages.[154] These mutations occur in proteins from different families such as spectrins, zinc-finger proteins, signal transductions proteins, ankyrins, histone methyl transferases, cadherins, semaphorins, and DNA or RNA helicases.[155] Although multiple members of the same family may be involved in a specific signaling transduction pathway, the mutation of any single protein in a given pathway is probably sufficient to disturb the function of the pathway.[155] Interaction studies among these proteins show that more than half of them are involved in networks driven by TP53, BRCA1, PIK3R1, and NFKB. The identification of distinct protein domains that tend to be mutated in specific cancers is also of particular interest for the classification of mutations. Breast cancer mutations are identified more frequently in proteins containing domains such as extracellular epidermal growth factor–related domains, spectrin repeats, proline-rich regions, domains associated with ABC transporters, and actin-binding domains.[155] When put together, all the results create a coherent image of mutation patterns in breast cancer. Although there is variability among the proteins identified to be affected in different samples, most of them are members of the same pathways involved in cellular interaction, cell cycle control, DNA damage repair, and apoptosis (Fig. 28-14). This approach revealing mutagenesis patterns provides new insights into the process of cellular selection during tumorigenesis.

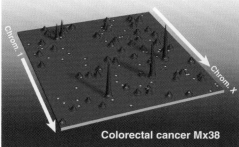
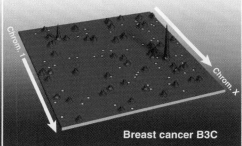

Figure 28-12 Genomic landscapes of colorectal and breast cancer. The 60 most competitive candidate cancer genes for each type of tumor are illustrated in purple. Chromosomes are pictured from Chromosome 1 in the back of the image toward chromosome X in the front of the image in the direction of the arrow. (Redrawn from Wood LD, Parsons DW, Jones S, et al: The genomic landscapes of human breast and colorectal cancers. Science 318:1108–1113, 2007.)

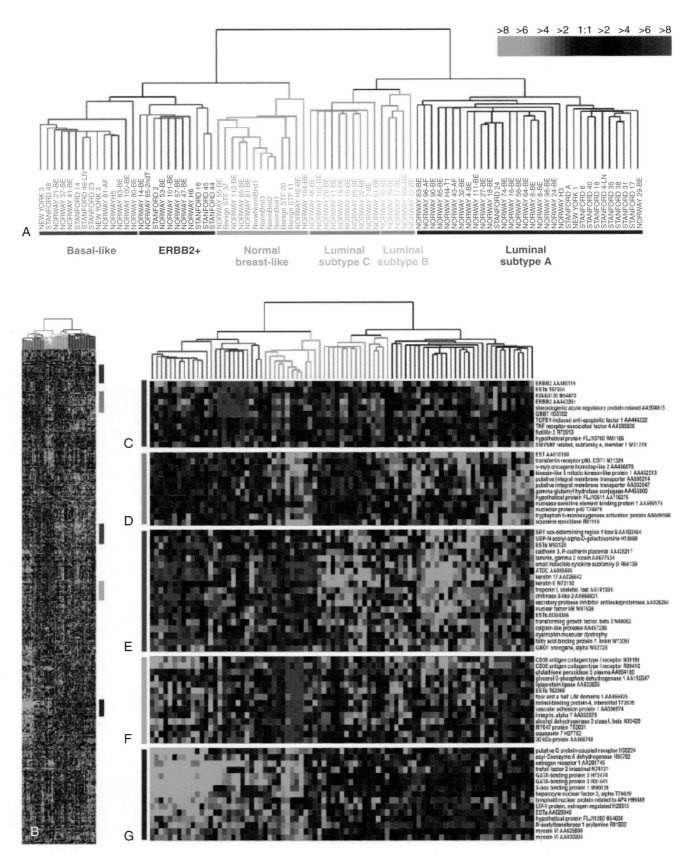

Figure 28-13 Expression array patterns of breast carcinomas. **A,** The breast cancer specimens are divided into subtypes based on differences in gene expression. These tumor subtypes are grouped as basal-like, ERBB2+, normal breast-like, and luminal clusters subdivided into luminal A, B, and C. **B,** Illustration of the scaled-down version of the diagram of clustered tumors according to the intrinsic set of genes. The colored bars to the right show the inset illustrated in **C–G**. These subtypes of breast cancers and the genes that define them are HER2-overexpression subtype (**C**), a group of cases not classified yet (**D**), basal epithelial set of genes (**E**), normal breast-defining genes (**F**), and luminal-type group of genes (**G**). (Reproduced from Sorlie T, Perou CM, Tibshirani R, et al: Gene expression patterns of breast carcinomas distinguish tumor subclasses with clinical implications. Proc Natl Acad Sci USA 98:10869–10874, 2001. Copyright 2001. National Academy of Sciences, USA.)

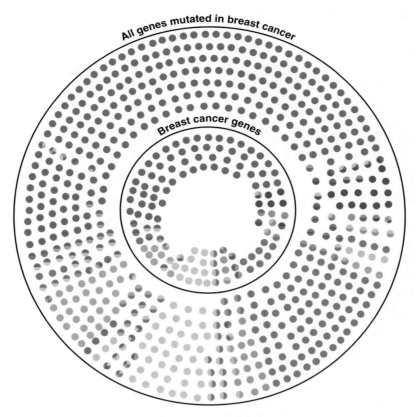

Functional annotation of mutated genes in breast cancer

All	Cancer		Label
0%	0%		RNA localization
11.51%	13.17%		Signal transduction
0.58%	0.00%		Stress response
0.79%	1.30%		DNA metabolism
1.24%	1.33%		Cell cycle
6.92%	5.70%		Transcription
1.87%	2.05%		Protein amino acid phosphorylation
9.84%	13.11%		Transport
0.96%	1.56%		DNA repair
2.20%	1.23%		RNA processing
2.60%	1.09%		Protein degradation
15.57%	11.84%		Metabolism
0.59%	0.41%		Carbohydrate metabolism
0.67%	0%		Protein biosynthesis
0.70%	2.05%		Protein amino acid dephosphorylation
1.95%	1.64%		Protein transport
3.47%	4.92%		Cell organization and biogenesis
0.20%	0.16%		DNA replication
0.14%	0.57%		DNA recombination
0.07%	0.16%		DNA damage response
38.12%	37.70%		Unknown

Figure 28-14 Functional categories of genes mutated in breast cancer. The color assigned to each category as well as the percentage of mutated genes belonging to each category are indicated on the right side panel. Each mutated gene is represented by a circle colored accordingly to the category of genes it belongs to. The center of the figure contains candidate cancer genes. (Reproduced from Lin J, Gan CM, Zhang X, et al: A multidimensional analysis of genes mutated in breast and colorectal cancers. Genome Res 17:1304–1318, 2007.)

Microarray-Based Methods for Analysis of Alterations

The use of whole genome approaches facilitates the identification of genetic differences between tumors and leads to the discovery of specific genes responsible for characteristic tumor behaviors. High-throughput techniques such as comparative genomic hybridization (CGH), cDNA expression microarrays, and analysis of SNPs are currently considered key for delivering relevant information leading to better individualized treatment strategies for breast cancer patient.[157–160]

Microarray-Based Comparative Genomic Hybridization

Microarray-based CGH provides a comprehensive genome-wide scanning method for changes in chromosome structure and in gene copy number. The principle of the method[160] is based on the capacity for complementary DNA sequences to hybridize competitively to one another. A microarray slide is spotted with a series of bacterial artificial chromosomes, which are DNA regions containing sequences of genes as they appear in chromosomes. These bacterial artificial chromosomes are arranged sequentially in such a way that they encompass the entire genome. DNA extracted from the frozen tumor samples and reference samples are labeled with specific fluorochromes. They are both mixed and hybridized to the microarray slide, and then the intensity of the fluorescent signal is translated into a ratio between the copy numbers of the sample and the normal genome. Although microarray-based CGH provides valuable information about DNA copy number across the entire genome, expression analysis of these genes requires the use of other methods.

Expression Microarrays

Expression arrays provide qualitative and quantitative information about gene transcription by analysis of messenger RNA extracted from a carcinoma. This method is based on a similar principle as that used for CGH.[157] RNA extracted from frozen tumor samples and reference samples is submitted to reverse transcription to create a complementary strand of DNA and subsequently double-stranded cDNA. The cDNAs are labeled with fluorescent tags; the sample cDNA is labeled with one fluorochrome and the normal reference cDNA is labeled with a fluorochrome of a different color. They are both mixed and hybridized on the microarray slide spotted with oligonucleotides or cDNA clones of the interrogated genes, representing as many as 20,000 expressed genes. After hybridization, each spot on the slide is scanned at the appropriate wavelengths for the two fluorochromes, and a signal intensity ratio is calculated for each gene, indicating which of the original RNA samples, tumor RNA or normal RNA, is more abundant.

After computerized analysis, the array data provides information about overexpression or loss of expression of genes in each test sample, compared to the reference sample and to other test samples. One way of detecting genetic patterns is by hierarchical clustering of the information, grouping together similar samples or similarly expressed genes (see Fig. 28-13). Data can also be processed by supervised clustering, using known information for categorizing the samples and comparing their genetic profile.[157]

ALTERED GENE EXPRESSION

Extensive gene expression profiling studies have been performed by several groups, leading to the definition of novel molecular subtypes of breast cancer and to new approaches for classification of breast cancers.[51,117,155,157,158,161–167] One of the landmark studies of this nature[165] is based on expression data for more than 8000 human genes. In this study, breast cancers were separated into four different categories: a group of breast cancers whose expression pattern resembles that of breast epithelial cells lining the ductal lumen or a luminal-like cluster of cases that expresses, among other characteristic genes, ER; a group of breast cancers whose expression pattern resembles that of breast reserve cells or basal myoepithelial cells, with this group referred to as basal-like showing an ER-negative, HER2-negative phenotype; a group of breast cancers whose expression pattern includes high expression of HER2, referred to as HER2-positive tumors; and a group of breast cancers showing a pattern of expression similar to normal ductal epithelium, referred to as the normal-like breast cancer. Additional studies unveiled further clinical characteristics, as well as new molecular subsets of these clusters, each with a different expression profile.[45] A set of 1753 genes has been used to define these molecular portraits.[45,165] Among these, a subset of 427 genes has been selected and presented as the "intrinsic set of genes" whose expression is used to characterize the molecular subsets. Luminal A–type breast cancers have the best prognosis among all categories. They express the ER gene along with a set of other receptors, enzymes, and transcription factors such as prolactin receptor, putative G protein–coupled receptor, acyl-CoA dehydrogenase, GATA–binding protein, FOXA1, and hepatocyte nuclear factor 3-alpha. Among luminal subsets, luminal A is a category of tumors with higher expression of genes implicated in estrogen-regulated signaling and fatty acid metabolism.

Luminal B breast cancers also express ER but have lower expression of ER and higher expression of genes associated with the basal or ERBB2 overexpressing tumors. Luminal C type carcinomas are associated with the highest relapse rate among luminal subtypes.

The basal-like breast cancer phenotype expresses genes implicated in cell cycle control, cell proliferation and differentiation, or protein phosphorylation.[47] This basal-like type of carcinoma is characterized by a myoepithelial pattern of gene expression including keratins 5 and 17, integrin-beta 1, laminin, and TGF-β.[165] Carcinomas in this group are associated with a poor prognosis. They also have the highest frequency of P53 gene mutations among all groups.

The carcinomas in the HER2-overexpressing group show coamplification of HER2 with other genes such as GRB7 located nearby on chromosome 17 and coordinately amplified as part of the HER2 amplicon. As expected, the HER2-overexpression group has a poor prognosis compared with the other expression groups.

The normal-like breast cancer group overexpresses genes that are also expressed in normal breast tissue, such as CD36 antigen, collagen type I receptor, glutathione peroxidase 3, integrin alpha 7, and aquaporin.

Additional studies involving breast cancer cell lines describe that the gene amplification and expression profiles identified in tumors are closely replicated in breast cancer cell lines.[163] Fifty-one breast cancer cell lines, each one with a different molecular profile, have been used to make this comparison between human tumor specimens and human breast cancer cell lines.[117,163] This represents a confirmation that breast cancer cell lines, although propagated in culture, maintain the similar molecular characteristics and behavior as the spectrum of breast carcinomas from which they arise.

Cell lines from specific molecular subtypes have distinct phenotypes such as specific morphology or capacity for invasion.[163] Luminal cells grown in culture prove to be more differentiated, more adherent and less invasive than other cell types. The genes overexpressed in this category, such as GATA3 and ERBB3, define a less aggressive phenotype than the category described for basal-like cells. Basal-like cell lines are divided in two groups, A and B. Between these two, the basal A type has the genomic signature corresponding to the basal-like carcinomas. This group is represented by less differentiated, more invasive cells that have a "mesenchymal-like appearance." The basal B group has a "stem-like" genetic signature that may correspond to the "triple negative" (ER negative, PR negative, HER2 not amplified) tumors that express genes such as CD44, CAV1/CAV2, and SPARC. The genetic profile of the HER2-overexpressing cell lines is not analyzed as a distinct group. Some of the HER2-positive cells are also ER positive, and these are included in the luminal cluster. Others share genetic features with cell lines in the basal A cluster.

COMPARATIVE GENOMIC HYBRIDIZATION

Genomic aberrations identified in breast carcinomas at the DNA level define specific subtypes of breast cancer within the molecular groups presented previously.[144,168,169] Combined information on gene expression profiles and on genome copy number abnormalities has been gathered in a series of papers using microarray analysis.[117,161,163,168] These data provide a complex association between the presence of genetic abnormalities in tumors, the classification based on gene expression profiles and the clinical outcome of patients.

Genomic regions of breast cancers frequently identified as high-level amplification areas involve chromosomes 8, 11, 12, 17, and 20. Amplification of genes at these locations such as HER2, cyclin D1, c-myc, and ZNF217 have been identified as having important roles in breast cancer pathogenesis and disease progression which has been confirmed by the use of complementary methods.[161] In addition, several regions are found as frequently coamplified such as 8q24 (locus for *c-myc* gene) and 20q13.[117] Within the amplified regions are 66 genes identified as having high-level amplification and are correlated with poor outcome. These genes, are considered to be good candidates to play important roles in the pathogenesis of breast cancer.[117] These 66 genes include genes encoding proteins involved in cellular signaling pathways, nucleic acid metabolism, and cell cycle progression. The 8p11 amplicon contains genes encoding an RNA-binding protein (LSM1), a receptor tyrosine kinase (FGFR1), a cell cycle regulator protein (TACC1), a serine-threonine kinase from the NF-kB pathway (IKBKB), and a DNA polymerase (POLB). The 11q13 amplicon contains not only cyclin D1 but a gene encoding a growth factor (FGF3). Other potentially interesting genes include a transcription regulator (PPARBP) on chromosome 17, an adaptor protein (GRB7) on chromosome 17, a transcription factor involved in the PI3K/Akt pathway (ZNF217) and a RNA-binding protein (REA1) on chromosome 20.[117] The breast cancer cell lines show similar genetic aberration profiles as the primary breast cancers, supporting the relevance of these abnormalities in the pathology of the disease.[163] These 66 genes are not only deregulated by high-level amplification but are considered to be potential targets for drugs.[117,163]

Clinical Applications of Multigene Assessment Methods

Although relatively new, genetic profiling of breast cancer has already been adapted for clinical use. Two tests, MammaPrint and Oncotype DX, are commercially available to aid oncologists in making treatment decisions. The tests assign patients to different risk groups based on the association of their breast cancer molecular profile and risk for metastatic recurrence or death from their disease. One limitation of these advanced diagnostic tools is that they were both developed for lymph node–negative patients, and, so far, there are no such tests available for lymph node–positive breast cancer patients. However, gene expression data have also been collected for the identification of a set of genes differentially expressed in primary tumors and nodal metastases. The expression level of these genes is used for classification of patients into two groups—a high- or low-risk of developing distant metastases within 3 to 4 years. This type of study may be used in the future for predicting clinical outcome of node-positive breast cancer patients.[51]

MAMMAPRINT

MammaPrint is a 70-gene prognostic marker panel used to identify young, node-negative breast cancer patients who are at high-risk or low-risk for recurrent or metastatic disease. Those women with high-risk disease are selected for treatment with chemotherapy, whereas those with low-risk disease may be spared treatment with chemotherapy. This approach identifies those women at risk for recurrent or metastatic disease who do not benefit significantly from chemotherapy and, thereby, can be used to reduce the number of patients that have such treatment.[170,171]

The set of 70 genes evaluated by MammaPrint were compiled based on data from expression microarray studies.[48,166] The 70 genes were selected from an initial set of 5000 genes following a three-step supervised clustering of tumors followed by several rounds of additional optimization, cross-validation, and testing on additional sets of tumors.[48,166,170] The selected genes were ranked using patients with known clinical outcomes and then adapted for clinical application. Ongoing research is exploring extending the use of MammaPrint to patients with one to three positive nodes at diagnosis,[172] and a prospective clinical trial is in progress to confirm the clinical utility of the assay.

This test requires a frozen sample of the tumor, which is used for RNA extraction and analysis of the tumor's gene expression profile. The interpretation of the profile is based on the concept that the metastatic potential of cancer is acquired early in tumor development and can be identified in the level of expression of certain genes in the tumor. A "good prognosis" or a "poor prognosis" has been associated with developing distant metastases within 5 years. The 70 genes selected for the Mamma-Print profile are involved in the regulation of cell cycle, invasion, and angiogenesis. Interestingly, the gene expression signature panel does not include genes well known as prognostic markers for breast cancer, such as ERα, PR, or HER2.

The Microarray in Node-Negative Disease May Avoid Chemotherapy (MINDACT) trial[173] was designed to prove that patients with a poor prognosis are the ones who benefit from receiving adjuvant therapy compared with the ones with a good prognosis. It is a large-scale prospective validation study involving 6000 patients who will be evaluated by both the new genomic test and the currently used clinicopathologic method. The patients identified as low risk for developing metastases by both methods will not receive adjuvant chemotherapy. Similarly, patients scored with both assessment methods as having a high risk of recurrence will be treated with adjuvant chemotherapy. The patients scored differently by the two methods will be randomly assigned to one of the treatment arms of the trial. Of particular interest are patients assessed with high risk of recurrence by the clinicopathologic method who are assigned to the arm containing no chemotherapy. The evaluation of these patients will show if the MammaPrint test is a better choice than currently used clinicopathologic criteria. Given the toxicity of chemotherapeutic agents it is important to correctly identify the patients that need treatment and spare the rest from the toxic effects of these drugs. This MammaPrint test may identify patients who are in danger of being overtreated as well as undertreated, and it is a potentially helpful genomic tool.

ONCOTYPE DX

Oncotype DX is a 21-gene expression assay of 16 known cancer related genes and 5 reference genes, which provides a recurrence score (0 to 100) using RNA extracted from formalin-fixed, paraffin-embedded tissue.[164] It assigns a recurrence score based on the evaluation of gene expression levels of several known markers of proliferation along with genes that are known to be important in breast cancer. The 21 genes considered in this test were selected from a list of 250 candidate genes compiled from data acquired through interrogation of expression microarrays with samples from breast cancer patients. The subset of genes was tested and validated on archival tissue samples from node-negative breast cancer patients in the National Surgical Adjuvant Breast and Bowel Project (NSABP) B-20 and B-14 clinical trials.

The assay measures the expression of the 16-gene profile in a given sample by reverse transcriptase–polymerase chain reaction (RT-PCR) and then normalizes to the expression of the panel of five reference genes. The 16 selected genes represent different functional groups. One group is composed of proliferation markers such as Ki67, survivin, and cyclin B1. A second functional group is composed of two genes involved in invasion, stromolysin 3 (MMP11) and cathepsin L2 (CSL2). The HER2 group contains the HER2 gene and the GRB7 gene, a growth factor receptor–binding protein located on chromosome 17 near the chromosomal site for HER2 gene. The estrogen group contains four members, including ER and PR. Three other proteins are included in the panel as separate prognostic markers, glutathione S-transferase M1 (GSTM1), cluster of differentiation 68 (CD68), and the BCL-2 binding protein BAG1.[164]

The recurrence score estimates low (<18), intermediate (18–31), or high risk (>31) of distant recurrence within 10 years in node-negative, ER-positive breast cancer patients treated with tamoxifen. The test also assesses the potential benefit of chemotherapy. Patients with a high recurrence score might benefit from adjuvant chemotherapy more than patients in other groups, and the patients in the low-risk group might not need chemotherapy.[174] Ongoing clinical validation trials such as Trial Assigning IndividuaLized Options for Treatment (Rx; TAILORx) will assess the benefit of adjuvant chemotherapy on women assigned to the intermediate risk group. These patients will be treated either with hormonal therapy and chemotherapy or with hormonal therapy alone.

All these achievements in molecular forecasting definitely add to the traditional methods of staging and prediction in breast cancer. Still, an optimal standardization of recurrence or outcome prediction based on the new molecular classification is difficult to achieve. The different clustering algorithms, the different number of samples taken into consideration, and the various subsets of genes used for clustering make it difficult to compare the results from the different multigene assay methods.

Hereditary Breast Cancer

All cancers are genetic in origin due to an accumulation of genetic errors that result in tumor formation. These genetic alterations may arise at the somatic level, as occurs in sporadic cancers, or may be inherited through the germline, in which case they are hereditary. Although approximately 20% of breast cancers may be associated with a familial inheritance pattern, only approximately 10% are currently considered hereditary, with inheritance of a known genetic alteration. Hereditary breast cancers are most frequently associated with an autosomal dominant pattern of inheritance. Of these, BRCA1 and BRCA2 are the most prevalent and well studied.

Presently there are at least eight additional genes with known germline mutations that are under study at this time.[175] These include mutations in p53, PTEN, CHEK2, ATM, NBS1, RAD50, BRIP1, and PALB2.

BRCA1 AND BRCA2

Intensive study of the high-penetrance genes, *BRCA1* and *BRCA2*, has revealed that the cancers associated with mutations in these two genes are genetically and morphologically distinct from one another, as well as different from breast carcinomas seen in sporadic disease.[176] These cancers are also different from those seen in other heritable syndromes. Cancers arising in women with germline mutations in *BRCA1/BRCA2* have distinct pathologic features and corresponding gene expression profiles that lead to further genetic alterations that are specifically involved in the development and progression of each of these cancers. BRCA1 tumors are more often high grade and more often ER negative and PR negative with lower rates of HER2 amplification.[177,178] BRCA2 tumors share more characteristics with sporadic cancers and may have more favorable features than BRCA1 tumors (Table 28-1).[176] It is hypothesized that the BRCA1 and BRCA2 proteins have an important function in maintaining genomic stability by promoting efficient and precise repair of DNA double strand breaks when they arise during cell replication.[179]

BRCA1

The breast cancer susceptibility 1 (*BRCA1*) gene was described in 1994 and is a classic tumor suppressor gene localized to chromosome 17q21.[180] The gene consists of 22 coding regions that are distributed over approximately 81 kb of genomic DNA on chromosome 17q21, and it encodes a 1863–amino acid protein.[180] More than 500 mutations have been described in this gene, spanning its entire coding sequence, with approximately 80% of these mutations encoding a truncated BRCA1 protein. Most of the mutations are single nucleotide insertion or deletion, loss-of-function, or frame shift alterations. BRCA1 protein functions as a gatekeeper in controlling gene transcription and regulating repair of DNA damage. The prevalence of *BRCA1* mutations has a strong association for particular ethnic populations with well-described "founder" mutations that are specific to each population. For example, there is a high prevalence of specific *BRCA1* mutations in Ashkenazi Jewish women who are found to have specific mutations in *BRCA1* (185delAG, 5382insC). Other specific *BRCA1* mutations have been identified in Dutch, Scandinavian, French-Canadian, and Belgian populations.[181,182]

BRCA1 functions together with a variety of associated proteins in repair of DNA double strand breaks, as may be observed during cell replication. Accurate repair mechanisms are vital to maintaining the integrity of the genome, and are accomplished in part by a protein complex termed BASC (BRCA1-associated genome surveillance complex).[183] This complex includes DNA damage sensors, tumor suppressors, and other signal transducers that are important in DNA repair, such as RAD51. When DNA damage occurs, there is an initial cellular signal that is important for recognition of the damaged DNA. Subsequent phosphorylation of BRCA1 protein results in recruitment of downstream repair kinases such as ATM, ATR, and CHK2, which is necessary for cell cycle arrest and repair of the damaged DNA.[184,185]

Repair of double strand breaks may occur by three mechanisms: nonhomologous end joining,[186] homologous recombination by gene conversion, and single strand annealing.[187] BRCA1 is associated with protein kinases ATM, ATR, and CHK2, which are integral to the repair of double strand breaks. ATM and ATR are both integral to the DNA repair process, because each phosphorylates downstream proteins, including BRCA1, which allows cell cycle arrest to take place with subsequent repair of DNA damage. Each kinase phosphorylates BRCA1 at different serine residues in response to varying forms of DNA damage.[184,188] ATM/ATR also mediates phosphorylation of CHK2, which in turn phosphorylates BRCA1 to allow for repair of double strand breaks.[184] BRCA1 plays a role in cell cycle arrest in response to DNA damage, by facilitating the ATM/ATR-mediated phosphorylation of p53, which is essential for G_1/S arrest with induction of p21.[189]

BRCA2

The breast cancer susceptibility type 2 gene (*BRCA2*) is composed of 27 coding exons spanning 84 kb on chromosome 13q12.3 and encodes a 3418-amino-acid protein (Table 28-2). Approximately 450 mutations have been described in the *BRCA2* gene distributed throughout the coding region from the initiation site to the termination site. Like *BRCA1*, particular *BRCA2* mutations have been identified in specific populations with

TABLE 28-1 Immunophenotype of *BRCA1/BRCA2* and Sporadic Tumors			
Antibodies	**BRCA1**	**BRCA2**	**Sporadic**
ER, PR	−	+	+
BCL-2, BAX	−	+	+
Cyclin D1	−	+	+
P16, p27, p21	−	+	+
RAD50	−	+	+
RAD51 (cytoplasm)	−	+	−
HER-2	−	−	+
CHEK2	+	+	−
RAD51 (nucleus)	+	−	+
P53, Ki-67	+	−	−
Cyclins (E, A, B1)	+	−	−
Skp2	+	−	−
CK5/6, 14, 17	+	−	−
EGFR, p-cadherin	+	−	−

Reproduced from Honrado E, Osorio A, Palacios J, et al: Pathology and gene expression of hereditary breast tumors associated with *BRCA1*, *BRCA2*, and *CHEK2* gene mutations. Oncogene 25: 5837–5845, 2006.

TABLE 28-2

Comparison of *BRCA1* and *BRCA2*

	BRCA1	BRCA2
Chromosome	17q21	13q12.3
Gene size	81 kb	84 kb
Protein size	1863 amino acids	3418 amino acids
Function	Tumor suppressor	Tumor suppressor
	Transcriptional regulation	Transcriptional regulation
	Role in DNA repair	Role in DNA repair
Mutations	>500 identified	450 identified
Mutations in population	Approximately 0.1%	Approximately 0.1%
Risk of breast cancer	60%–80%	60%–80%
Age at onset	Younger age (40s to 50s)	50 years
Families with breast cancer due to a single gene	52%	32%
Families with breast and ovarian cancer	81% (20%–40% risk)	14% (10%–20% risk)

Ashkenazi Jewish women having a specific 617delT mutation. Mutations in *BRCA2* are associated with early-onset breast cancer and bilateral disease. Families with inheritance of this mutant gene may also have men with breast cancer. BRCA2, like BRCA1, protein functions as a gatekeeper, controlling gene transcription and regulating repair of DNA damage. BRCA2 plays an important role both in the repair of DNA double strand breaks and also in maintaining genomic stability of cells progressing through mitosis. In the repair of double strand breaks via homologous recombination, BRCA2 functions closely with a DNA recombinase known as RAD51. BRCA2 regulates the function of RAD51 in this process and must bind to RAD51 in order for error-free homologous recombination to occur.[179] BRCA2 binds to RAD51 and transports it to areas of DNA damage, where RAD51 is released. Double strand breaks are repaired via RAD51-mediated nucleoprotein formation, and the physical interaction between BRCA2 and RAD51 is essential for error-free HR to take place.[179,190] BRCA2-deficient cells accumulate DNA damage because they do not form the RAD51 foci necessary for the repair of double strand breaks. There are also data to suggest that BRCA2 functions in the M-phase checkpoint in replicating cells undergoing mitosis. In cell culture, introducing antibodies that block either BRCA2 or an associated DNA-binding protein, BRAF35, stops mitosis.[191]

CHK2

CHK2 is a tumor suppressor gene that functions as an important signal transducer in response to DNA damage. This is an example of a less highly penetrant genetic defect that contributes to the pathogenesis of many hereditary and sporadic breast cancers. The human gene is on chromosome 22q12.1 and spans approximately 50 kilobases of genomic DNA with 14 exons. Activation of the CHK2 protein kinase occurs in response to DNA damage (e.g., in response to ionizing radiation or other causes of DNA double strand breaks).[192] It is initiated by ATM-mediated phosphorylation of the N-terminal regulatory domain of the CHK2 protein

that occurs exclusively at the sites of the DNA damage. This leads to activation of the kinase and interaction with a wide variety of downstream substrates, including proteins involved in cell cycle control and regulation such as Cdc25A, Pik3 kinase, and regulators of cell apoptosis. Defects in this pathway are associated with an approximate 23.8% lifetime risk of female breast cancer in women who are homozygous for 1100delC.[193] Varying risk is conferred for carriers of single copies of the allele.

Tumor Microenvironment

Although most of our focus has been on genetic alterations within the breast cancer cell, recent evidence has emerged that the tumor microenvironment composed of fibroblasts, myofibroblasts, and immune cells (including macrophages and endothelial cells) can exert profound effects on breast cancer progression and metastasis through paracrine signaling.[194–197] Several lines of evidence have demonstrated the contribution of altered stromal cells to primary tumor growth.[197, 198]

One line of evidence has indicated that genomic instability is not confined to just the carcinoma cells but can be exhibited by the stromal fibroblasts. Another line of evidence is that stromal cells themselves can be quite heterogeneous, with some subpopulations expressing tenascin and other subpopulations expressing smooth muscle actin. The types of molecules the stromal cells secrete, such as matrix metalloproteinases and tissue inhibitors of metalloproteinases, can also be quite heterogeneous.

The latest studies of the tumor microenvironment have focused on Pten, Rb/E2F, and ras/ets-2 pathways in the stromal fibroblasts/myofibroblasts. Ets-2 is a transcription factor that, when phosphorylated, turns on the expression of matrix metalloproteinases in stromal cells. Human breast cancers are quite heterogeneous in the expression of these stromal molecules and gene profiling of the tumor microenvironment may also lead to meaningful molecular classifications of breast cancer.

Conclusions

Molecular investigations of breast cancer have the potential to refine classification of the disease to better identify patients by clinical outcome, to improve selection of patients for therapy, and to identify potential new molecular targets for novel therapies (Fig. 28-15). The application of molecular methods is leading to the development of new complementary tools for predicting clinical outcome by combining the known clinical parameters with genetic determinants of the disease.

Figure 28-15 Correlation of copy number aberrations (CNAs) with gene-expression subtypes. Each row contains a chromosome location identified with a frequent aberration. Columns are represented by each subtype: lum A, lum B, ERBB2, and basal-like. Normal-like subtype was underrepresented and therefore is not shown. The lighter green fields show DNA loss, orange fields show DNA gain, and triangles show high-level amplifications. (Reproduced from Bergamaschi A, Kim YH, Wang P, et al: Distinct patterns of DNA copy number alteration are associated with different clinicopathological features and gene-expression subtypes of breast cancer. Genes Chromosomes Cancer 45:1033–1040, 2006.)

Cytobands	Lum A	Lum B	ERBB2	Basal-like
1p34.1–p34.2 (2)		▓		
1q12–p23.3 (8)	▓			▓
1q25.2	▓			▓
1q31.1	▓			▓
1q31.3	▓			▓
1q32.1	▓			▓
1q41	▓			▓
3p11.2		▓		▓
3q12.1–q12.3 (3)				▓
3q21.1				▓
4p15.2–p15.32 (3)				▓
4q31.22–q35.2 (12)				▓
5q11.1–q11.2 (2)				▓
5q12.1				▓
5q12.3–q14.2 (6)				▓
5q15				▓
5q21.1				▓
5q21.3				▓
5q22.1–q31.3 (9)				▓
6p12.1–p25.3 (18)				▓
6q22.33		Δ		
7p22.1–p22.2 (2)		Δ		
7q21.12				
7q22.1				
7q32.2–q34 (4)				
7q36.1–q36.3 (3)				
8q11.21		Δ		
8q11.23		▓ Δ		
8q12.1–q24.3 (24)		▓ Δ		
9q34.13		▓ Δ		
10p12.33–p15.3 (6)				▓
11p11.2				
12p12.3				
12q22				
14q22.1–q23.1 (4)				
15q22.2				
16p12.1–p12.2 (2)	▓			
16p13.2–p13.3 (2)	▓			
17q12–q21.2 (2)			Δ	
17q25.2–q25.3 (2)				▓
19q13.32–q13.33 (2)		Δ		
20p12.2		▓		
20q13.13–q13.33 (5)		▓ Δ		
21q22.12–q22.3 (4)				▓

□ Loss ▓ Gain Δ Amplification

REFERENCES

1. Hanahan D, Weinberg RA: The hallmarks of cancer. Cell 100: 57–70, 2000.
2. Kumar V, Abbas A, Fausto N: Robbins and Cotran: Pathologic basis of disease, 7th ed. Philadelphia, Elsevier, 2005.
3. Booth BW, Smith GH: Roles of transforming growth factor-alpha in mammary development and disease. Growth Factors 25: 227–235, 2007.
4. Lupu R, Cardillo M, Harris L, et al: Interaction between ERB-receptors and heregulin in breast cancer tumor progression and drug resistance. Sem Cancer Biol 6:135–145, 1995.
5. Yarden Y: Biology of HER2 and its importance in breast cancer. Oncology 61 Suppl 2:1–13, 2001.
6. Pauletti G, Godolphin W, Press MF, et al: Detection and quantitation of HER-2/neu gene amplification in human breast cancer archival material using fluorescence in situ hybridization. Oncogene 13:63–72, 1996.
7. Slamon DJ, Clark GM, Wong SG, et al: Human breast cancer: Correlation of relapse and survival with amplification of the HER-2/neu oncogene. Science 235:177–182,1987.
8. Sledge GW Jr, Miller KD: Exploiting the hallmarks of cancer: The future conquest of breast cancer. Eur J Cancer 39:1668–1675, 2003.
9. Keen JC, Davidson NE: The biology of breast carcinoma. Cancer 97(suppl 3):825–833, 2003.
10. Bryan TM, Englezou A, Gupta J, et al: Telomere elongation in immortal human cells without detectable telomerase activity. Embo J 14:4240–4248, 1995.
11. Bryan TM, Englezou A, Dalla-Pozza L, et al: Evidence for an alternative mechanism for maintaining telomere length in human tumors and tumor-derived cell lines. Nat Med 3:1271–1274, 1997.
12. Press MF, Lenz HJ: EGFR, HER2 and VEGF pathways: Validated targets for cancer treatment. Drugs 67:2045–2075, 2007.
13. Fendrick JL, Raafat AM, Haslam SZ: Mammary gland growth and development from the postnatal period to postmenopause: Ovarian steroid receptor ontogeny and regulation in the mouse. J Mammary Gland Biol Neoplasia 3:7–22, 1998.
14. Anderson E, Clarke RB: Steroid receptors and cell cycle in normal mammary epithelium. J Mammary Gland Biol Neoplasia 9:3–13, 2004.
15. Clarke RB, Howell A, Potten CS, et al: Dissociation between steroid receptor expression and cell proliferation in the human breast. Cancer Res 57:4987–4991, 1997.
16. Peterson OW HP, Van Deurs B: Frequency and distribution of estrogen receptor-positive cells in normal, nonlactating human breast tissue. Cancer Res 47:5745–5751, 1987.
17. Speirs V, Skliris GP, Burdall SE, et al: Distinct expression patterns of ER alpha and ER beta in normal human mammary gland. J Clin Pathol 55:371–374, 2002.
18. Bartow SA: Use of the autopsy to study ontogeny and expression of the estrogen receptor gene in human breast. J Mammary Gland Biol Neoplasia 3:37–48, 1998.
19. Bernstein L, Press MF: Does estrogen receptor expression in normal breast tissue predict breast cancer risk? J Natl Cancer Inst 90:5–7, 1998.
20. Speroff L: Role of progesterone in normal breast physiology. J Reprod Med 44(suppl 2):172–179, 1999.
21. Horowitz KB, Tung L, Takimoto GS: Novel mechanisms of antiprogestin action. J Steroid Biochem Mol Biol 53:9–17, 1995.
22. Salazar H, Tobon H, Josimovich JB: Developmental, gestational and postgestational modifications of the human breast. Clin Obstet Gynecol 18:113–137, 1975.
23. Howard BA, Gusterson BA: Human breast development. J Mammary Gland Biol Neoplasia 5:119–137, 2000.
24. Nathan B, Anbazhagan R, Clarkson P, et al: Expression of BCL-2 in the developing human fetal and infant breast. Histopathology 24:73–76, 1994.
25. Keeling JW, King G, Walker F: Oestrogen and progesterone receptors in fetal, infant and childhood mammary tissue. J Pathol 186:21A, 1998.
26. Kleinberg DL, Niemann W, Flamm E, et al: Primate mammary development. Effects of hypophysectomy, prolactin inhibition, and growth hormone administration. J Clin Invest 75:1943–1950, 1985.
27. Laron Z, Pauli R, Pertzelan A: Clinical evidence on the role of estrogens in the development of the breasts. Proc R Soc Edinb 95:13–22, 1989.
28. Bocchinfuso WP, Korach KS: Mammary gland development and tumorigenesis in estrogen receptor knockout mice. J Mammary Gland Biol Neoplasia 2:323–334, 1997.
29. Humphreys RC, Lydon JP, O'Malley BW, et al: Use of PRKO mice to study the role of progesterone in mammary gland development. J Mammary Gland Biol Neoplasia 2:343–354, 1997.
30. Lydon JP, DeMayo FJ, Funk CR, et al: Mice lacking progesterone receptor exhibit pleiotropic reproductive abnormalities. Genes Dev 9:2266–2278, 1995.
31. Russo J, Russo IH: Development of the human mammary gland. The mammary gland development, regulation, and function. New York, Plenum, 1987, pp 67–93.
32. Clarke RB, Anderson E, Howell A: Steroid receptors in human breast cancer. Trends Endocrinol Metab 15:316–323, 2004.
33. Anderson E, Clarke RB, Howell A: Estrogen responsiveness and control of normal human breast proliferation. J Mammary Gland Biol Neoplasia 3:23–35, 1998.
34. Anderson TJ, Ferguson DJ, Raab GM: Cell turnover in the "resting" human breast: Influence of parity, contraceptive pill, age and laterality. Br J Cancer 46:376–382, 1982.
35. Pike MC, Spicer DV, Dahmoush L, et al: Estrogens, progestogens, normal breast cell proliferation, and breast cancer risk. Epidemiol Rev 15:17–35, 1993.
36. Pike MC, Krailo MD, Henderson BE, et al: "Hormonal" risk factors, "breast tissue age" and the age-incidence of breast cancer. Nature 303:767–770, 1983.
37. Richert MM, Schwertfeger KL, Ryder JW, et al: An atlas of mouse mammary gland development. J Mammary Gland Biol Neoplasia 5:227–241, 2000.
38. Kakarala M, Wicha MS: Cancer stem cells: Implications for cancer treatment and prevention. Cancer J 13:271–275, 2007.
39. Dontu G, Al-Hajj M, Abdallah WM, et al: Stem cells in normal breast development and breast cancer. Cell Prolif 36(suppl 1): 59–72, 2003.
40. Spillane JB, Henderson MA: Cancer stem cells: A review. ANZ J Surg 77:464–468, 2007.
41. Russo J, Moral R, Balogh GA, et al: The protective role of pregnancy in breast cancer. Breast Cancer Res 7:131–142, 2005.
42. Allred DC, Mohsin SK, Fuqua SA: Histological and biological evolution of human premalignant breast disease. Endocr Relat Cancer 8:47–61, 2001.
43. Lee S, Mohsin SK, Mao S, et al: Hormones, receptors, and growth in hyperplastic enlarged lobular units: Early potential precursors of breast cancer. Breast Cancer Res 8:R6, 2006.
44. Wellings SR, Jensen HM, Marcum RG: An atlas of subgross pathology of the human breast with special reference to possible precancerous lesions. J Natl Cancer Inst 55:231–273, 1975.
45. Sorlie T, Perou CM, Tibshirani R, et al: Gene expression patterns of breast carcinomas distinguish tumor subclasses with clinical implications. Proc Natl Acad Sci USA 98:10869–10874, 2001.
46. Sorlie T: Molecular classification of breast tumors: Toward improved diagnostics and treatments. Methods Mol Biol 360:91–114, 2007.
47. Sorlie T, Wang Y, Xiao C, et al: Distinct molecular mechanisms underlying clinically relevant subtypes of breast cancer: Gene expression analyses across three different platforms. BMC Genomics 7:127, 2006.
48. van de Vijver MJ, He YD, van't Veer LJ, et al: A gene-expression signature as a predictor of survival in breast cancer. N Engl J Med 347:1999–2009, 2002.
49. Harris L, Fritsche H, Mennel R, et al: American Society of Clinical Oncology 2007 update of recommendations for the use of tumor markers in breast cancer. J Clin Oncol 25:5287–5312, 2007.
50. Coletta RD, Christensen K, Reichenberger KJ, et al: The Six1 homeoprotein stimulates tumorigenesis by reactivation of cyclin A1. Proc Natl Acad Sci USA 101:6478–6483, 2004.
51. Feng Y, Sun B, Li X, et al: Differentially expressed genes between primary cancer and paired lymph node metastases predict clinical outcome of node-positive breast cancer patients. Breast Cancer Res Treat 103:319–329, 2007.
52. Russo J, Russo IH: The role of estrogen in the initiation of breast cancer. J Steroid Biochem Mol Biol 102:89–96, 2006.

53. Beatson G: On the treatment of inoperable cases of carcinoma of the mamma: Suggestions for a new method of treatment with illustrative cases. Lancet 2:104–107, 1896.

54. Beral V: Breast cancer and hormone-replacement therapy in the Million Women Study. Lancet 362:419–427, 2003.

55. Rossouw JE, Anderson GL, Prentice RL, et al: Risks and benefits of estrogen plus progestin in healthy postmenopausal women: Principal results from the Women's Health Initiative randomized controlled trial. JAMA 288:321–333, 2002.

56. Herynk MH, Fuqua SA: Estrogen receptor mutations in human disease. Endocr Rev 25:869–898, 2004.

57. Green S, Walter P, Greene G, et al: Cloning of the human oestrogen receptor cDNA. J Steroid Biochem 24:77–83, 1986.

58. Greene GL, Press MF: Structure and dynamics of the estrogen receptor. J Steroid Biochem 24:1–7, 1986.

59. Mosselman S, Polman J, Dijkema R: ER beta: Identification and characterization of a novel human estrogen receptor. FEBS Letters 392:49–53, 1996.

60. Keaveney M, Klug J, Dawson MT, et al: Evidence for a previously unidentified upstream exon in the human oestrogen receptor gene. J Mol Endocrinol 6:111–115, 1991.

61. Piva R, Bianchi N, Aguiari GL, et al: Sequencing of an RNA transcript of the human estrogen receptor gene: Evidence for a new transcriptional event. J Steroid Biochem Mol Biol 46:531–538, 1993.

62. Smith CL, O'Malley BW: A key to understanding tissue specificity of selective receptor modulators. Endocr Rev 25:45–71, 2004.

63. Jordan VC, Wolf MF, Mirecki DM, et al: Hormone receptor assays: Clinical usefulness in the management of carcinoma of the breast. Crit Rev Clin Lab Sci 26:97–152, 1988.

64. Howell A, Cuzick J, Baum M, et al: Results of the ATAC (Arimidex, Tamoxifen, Alone or in Combination) trial after completion of 5 years' adjuvant treatment for breast cancer. Lancet 365:60–62, 2005.

65. Thurlimann B, Keshaviah A, Coates AS, et al: A comparison of letrozole and tamoxifen in postmenopausal women with early breast cancer. N Engl J Med 353:2747–2757, 2005.

66. Goss PE, Ingle JN, Martino S, et al: Randomized trial of letrozole following tamoxifen as extended adjuvant therapy in receptor-positive breast cancer: updated findings from NCIC CTG MA.17. J Natl Cancer Inst 97:1262–1271, 2005.

67. Conneely OM, Lydon JP: Progesterone receptors in reproduction: Functional impact of the A and B isoforms. Steroids 65:571–577, 2000.

68. Goepfert TM, McCarthy M, Kittrell FS, et al: Progesterone facilitates chromosome instability (aneuploidy) in p53 null normal mammary epithelial cells. Faseb J 14:2221–2229, 2000.

69. Clarke CL, Sutherland RL: Progestin regulation of cellular proliferation. Endocr Rev 11:266–301, 1990.

70. Klijn JG, Setyono-Han B, Foekens JA: Progesterone antagonists and progesterone receptor modulators in the treatment of breast cancer. Steroids 65:825–830, 2000.

71. Cui X, Schiff R, Arpino G, et al: Biology of progesterone receptor loss in breast cancer and its implications for endocrine therapy. J Clin Oncol 23:7721–7735, 2005.

72. Richer JK, Jacobsen BM, Manning NG, et al: Differential gene regulation by the two progesterone receptor isoforms in human breast cancer cells. J Biol Chem 277:5209–5218, 2002.

73. Coussens L, Yang-Feng T, Liao Y, et al: Tyrosine kinase receptor with extensive homology to EGF receptor shares chromosomal location with neu oncogene. Science 230:1132–1139, 1985.

74. Schechter AL, Hung MC, Vaidyanathan L, et al: The neu gene: An erbB-homologous gene distinct from and unlinked to the gene encoding the EGF receptor. Science 229:976–978, 1985.

75. Di Fiore P, Pierce J, Kraus M, et al: erbB-2 is a potent oncogene when overexpressed in NIH/3T3 cells. Science 237:178–182, 1987.

76. Slamon DJ: Proto-oncogenes and human cancers. N Engl J Med 317:955–957, 1987.

77. Slamon DJ, Godolphin W, Jones LA, et al: Studies of the HER-2/neu proto-oncogene in human breast and ovarian cancer. Science 244:707–712, 1989.

78. Wolff AC, Hammond ME, Schwartz JN, et al: American Society of Clinical Oncology/College of American Pathologists guideline recommendations for human epidermal growth factor receptor 2 testing in breast cancer. J Clin Oncol 25:118–145, 2007.

79. Press MF, Bernstein L, Thomas PA, et al: HER-2/neu gene amplification characterized by fluorescence in situ hybridization: Poor prognosis in node-negative breast carcinomas. J Clin Oncol 15:2894–2904, 1997.

80. Ross JS, Fletcher JA: The HER-2/neu oncogene in breast cancer: Prognostic factor, predictive factor, and target for therapy. Oncologist 3:237–252, 1998.

81. Yarden Y, Sliwkowski MX: Untangling the ErbB signalling network. Nat Rev Mol Cell Biol 2:127–137, 2001.

82. Slamon DJ, Leyland-Jones B, Shak S, et al: Use of chemotherapy plus a monoclonal antibody against HER2 for metastatic breast cancer that overexpresses HER2. N Engl J Med 344:783–792, 2001.

83. Piccart-Gebhart MJ, Procter M, Leyland-Jones B, et al: Trastuzumab after adjuvant chemotherapy in HER2-positive breast cancer. N Engl J Med 353:1659–1672, 2005.

84. Romond EH, Perez EA, Bryant J, et al: Trastuzumab plus adjuvant chemotherapy for operable HER2-positive breast cancer. N Engl J Med 353:1673–1684, 2005.

85. Gennari A, Pia Sormani M, Pronzato P, et al: HER2 status and efficacy of adjuvant anthracyclines in early breast cancer: A pooled analysis of randomized trials. J Natl Cancer Inst 100:14–20, 2008.

86. Moliterni A, Menard S, Valagussa P, et al: HER2 overexpression and doxorubicin in adjuvant chemotherapy for resectable breast cancer. J Clin Oncol 21:458–462, 2003.

87. Muss H, Thor A, Berry D, et al: c-erbB-2 expression and response to adjuvant therapy in women with node-positive early breast cancer. N Engl J Med 330:1260–1266, 1994.

88. Paik S, Bryant J, Park C, et al: erbB-2 and response to doxorubicin in patients with axillary lymph node-positive, hormone receptor-negative breast cancer. J Natl Cancer Inst 90:1361–1370, 1998.

89. Sauter G, Lee J, Bartlett J, et al: Guidelines for HER-2 testing: Biologic and methodologic considerations. J Clin Oncol 27:1323–1333, 2009.

90. Vogel C, Cobleigh M, Tripathy D, et al: Efficacy and safety of trastuzumab (Herceptin) as a single agent in first-line treatment of HER2-overexpressing metastatic breast cancer. J Clin Oncol 20:719–726, 2002.

91. Geyer CJ, Forster J, Lindquist D, et al: Lapatinib plus capecitabine for HER2-positive advanced breast cancer. N Engl J Med 355:2733–2743, 2006.

92. Press M, Finn R, Cameron D, et al: HER2 gene amplification, HER2 and EGFR mRNA and protein expression, and lapatinib efficacy in women with metastatic breast cancer. Clin Cancer Res 14:7861–7870, 2008.

93. Konecny G, Pauletti G, Pegram M, et al: Quantitative association between HER-2/neu and steroid hormone receptors in hormone receptor-positive primary breast cancer. J Natl Cancer Inst 95:142–153, 2003.

94. Lal P, Tan LK, Chen B: Correlation of HER-2 status with estrogen and progesterone receptors and histologic features in 3,655 invasive breast carcinomas. Am J Clin Pathol 123:541–546, 2005.

95. Lengauer C, Kinzler KW, Vogelstein B: Genetic instabilities in human cancers. Nature 396:643–649, 1998.

96. Blagosklonny MV: Molecular theory of cancer. Cancer Biol Ther 4:621–627, 2005.

97. Vogelstein B, Kinzler KW: Cancer genes and the pathways they control. Nat Med 10:789–799, 2004.

98. Michor F, Iwasa Y, Vogelstein B, et al: Can chromosomal instability initiate tumorigenesis? Semin Cancer Biol 15:43–49, 2005.

99. Nowak MA, Komarova NL, Sengupta A, et al: The role of chromosomal instability in tumor initiation. Proc Natl Acad Sci USA 99:16226–16231, 2002.

100. Hussain SP, Harris CC: Molecular epidemiology of human cancer: Contribution of mutation spectra studies of tumor suppressor genes. Cancer Res 58:4023–4037, 1998.

101. Karni R, Jove R, Levitzki A: Inhibition of pp60c-Src reduces Bcl-XL expression and reverses the transformed phenotype of cells overexpressing EGF and HER-2 receptors. Oncogene 18:4654–4662, 1999.

102. Dumont P, Leu J, Della Pietra Ar, et al: The codon 72 polymorphic variants of p53 have markedly different apoptotic potential Nat Genet 33:357–365, 2003.

103. Thomas M, Kalita A, Labrecque S, et al: Two polymorphic variants of wild-type p53 differ biochemically and biologically. Mol Cell Biol 19:1092–1100, 1999.

104. Storey A, Thomas M, Kalita A, et al: Role of a p53 polymorphism in the development of human papillomavirus-associated cancer. Nature 393:229–234, 1998.

105. Malkin D, Li FP, Strong LC, et al: Germ line p53 mutations in a familial syndrome of breast cancer, sarcomas, and other neoplasms. Science 250:1233–1238, 1990.

106. Borresen-Dale AL: TP53 and breast cancer. Hum Mutat 21:292–300, 2003.

107. Osborne RJ, Merlo GR, Mitsudomi T, et al: Mutations in the p53 gene in primary human breast cancers. Cancer Res 51:6194–6198, 1991.

108. Moll UM, Riou G, Levine AJ: Two distinct mechanisms alter p53 in breast cancer: Mutation and nuclear exclusion. Proc Natl Acad Sci USA 89:7262–7266, 1992.

109. Harris SL, Levine AJ: The p53 pathway: Positive and negative feedback loops. Oncogene 24:2899–2908, 2005.

110. Vogelstein B, Lane D, Levine AJ: Surfing the p53 network. Nature 408:307–310, 2000.

111. Lukas J, Niu N, Press MF: p53 mutations and expression in breast carcinoma in situ. Am J Pathol 156:183–191, 2000.

112. Olivier M, Hainaut P: TP53 mutation patterns in breast cancers: Searching for clues of environmental carcinogenesis. Semin Cancer Biol 11:353–360, 2001.

113. Ioakim-Liossi A, Karakitsos P, Markopoulos C, et al: p53 protein expression and oestrogen and progesterone receptor status in invasive ductal breast carcinomas. Cytopathology 12:197–202, 2001.

114. Fitzgibbons PL, Page DL, Weaver D, et al: Prognostic factors in breast cancer. College of American Pathologists Consensus Statement 1999. Arch Pathol Lab Med 124:966–978, 2000.

115. Jansson T, Inganas M, Sjogren S, et al: p53 Status predicts survival in breast cancer patients treated with or without postoperative radiotherapy: A novel hypothesis based on clinical findings. J Clin Oncol 13:2745–2751, 1995.

116. Hart LL, Davie JR: The estrogen receptor: More than the average transcription factor. Biochem Cell Biol 80:335–341, 2002.

117. Chin K, DeVries S, Fridlyand J, et al: Genomic and transcriptional aberrations linked to breast cancer pathophysiologies. Cancer Cell 10:529–541, 2006.

118. Kallioniemi A, Kallioniemi OP, Piper J, et al: Detection and mapping of amplified DNA sequences in breast cancer by comparative genomic hybridization. Proc Natl Acad Sci USA 91:2156–2160, 1994.

119. Press MF, Pike MC, Hung G, et al: Amplification and overexpression of HER-2/neu in carcinomas of the salivary gland: Correlation with poor prognosis. Cancer Res 54:5675–5682, 1994.

120. Ranzani GN, Pellegata NS, Previdere C, et al: Heterogeneous protooncogene amplification correlates with tumor progression and presence of metastases in gastric cancer patients. Cancer Res 50:7811–7814, 1990.

121. Saffari B, Jones LA, el-Naggar A, et al: Amplification and overexpression of HER-2/neu (c-erbB2) in endometrial cancers: Correlation with overall survival. Cancer Res 55:5693–5698, 1995.

122. Linggi B, Carpenter G: ErbB receptors: New insights on mechanisms and biology. Trends Cell Biol 16:649–656, 2006.

123. Zhang X, Gureasko J, Shen K, et al: An allosteric mechanism for activation of the kinase domain of epidermal growth factor receptor. Cell 125:1137–1149, 2006.

124. Prenzel N, Fischer OM, Streit S, et al: The epidermal growth factor receptor family as a central element for cellular signal transduction and diversification. Endocr Relat Cancer 8:11–31, 2001.

125. Biswas DK, Cruz AP, Gansberger E, et al: Epidermal growth factor-induced nuclear factor kappa B activation: A major pathway of cell-cycle progression in estrogen-receptor negative breast cancer cells. Proc Natl Acad Sci USA 97:8542–8547, 2000.

126. Chazin V, Kaleko M, Miller A, et al: Transformation mediated by the human HER-2 gene independent of the epidermal growth factor receptor. Oncogene 7:1859–1866, 1992.

127. Press MF, Sauter G, Bernstein L, et al: Diagnostic evaluation of HER-2 as a molecular target: An assessment of accuracy and reproducibility of laboratory testing in large, prospective, randomized clinical trials. Clin Cancer Res 11:6598–6607, 2005.

128. Press M, Hung G, Godolphin W, et al: Sensitivity of HER-2/neu antibodies in archival tissue samples: Potential source of error

129. Press M, Slamon D, Flom K, et al: Evaluation of HER-2/neu gene amplification and overexpression: Comparison of frequently used assay methods in a molecularly characterized cohort of breast cancer specimens. J Clin Oncol 20:3095–3105, 2002.

130. Holst F, Stahl PR, Ruiz C, et al: Estrogen receptor alpha (ESR1) gene amplification is frequent in breast cancer. Nat Genet 39:655–660, 2007.

131. Brown L, Hoog J, Chin S-F, et al: Correspondence to the editor: ESR1 gene amplification in breast cancer: A common phenomenon? Nat Genet 40:806–807, 2008.

132. Holst F, Stahl P, Hellwinkel O, et al: Correspondence in reply: ESR1 gene amplification in breast cancer: A common phenomenon? Nat Genet 40:810–812, 2008.

133. Reis-Filho J, Drury S, Lambros M, et al: Correspondence to the editor: ESR1 gene amplification in breast cancer: A common phenomenon? Nat Genet 40:809–810, 2008.

134. Vincent-Salomon A, Raynal V, Lucchesi C, et al: Correspondence to the editor: ESR1 gene amplification in breast cancer: A common phenomenon? Nat Genet 40:809, 2008.

135. Nass SJ, Dickson RB: Defining a role for c-Myc in breast tumorigenesis. Breast Cancer Res Treat 44:1–22, 1997.

136. Al-Kuraya K, Schraml P, Torhorst J, et al: Prognostic relevance of gene amplifications and coamplifications in breast cancer. Cancer Res 64:8534–8540, 2004.

137. Courjal F, Cuny M, Simony-Lafontaine J, et al: Mapping of DNA amplifications at 15 chromosomal localizations in 1875 breast tumors: Definition of phenotypic groups. Cancer Res 57:4360–4367, 1997.

138. Park K, Kwak K, Kim J, et al: c-myc amplification is associated with HER2 amplification and closely linked with cell proliferation in tissue microarray of nonselected breast cancers. Hum Pathol 36:634–639, 2005.

139. Kim C BJ, Horne Z, Geyer CE, Wickerham DL, et al: Trastuzumab sensitivity of breast cancer with co-amplification of HER2 and cMYC suggests pro-apoptotic function of dysregulated cMYC in vivo. San Antonio Breast Cancer Symposium, 2005.

140. Fantl V, Stamp G, Andrews A, et al: Mice lacking cyclin D1 are small and show defects in eye and mammary gland development. Genes Dev 9:2364–2372, 1995.

141. Wang Y, Thakur A, Sun Y, et al: Synergistic effect of cyclin D1 and c-Myc leads to more aggressive and invasive mammary tumors in severe combined immunodeficient mice. Cancer Res 67:3698–3707, 2007.

142. Cuny M, Kramar A, Courjal F, et al: Relating genotype and phenotype in breast cancer: An analysis of the prognostic significance of amplification at eight different genes or loci and of p53 mutations. Cancer Res 60:1077–1083, 2000.

143. Osborne C, Wilson P, Tripathy D: Oncogenes and tumor suppressor genes in breast cancer: Potential diagnostic and therapeutic applications. Oncologist 9:361–377, 2004.

144. Fridlyand J, Snijders AM, Ylstra B, et al: Breast tumor copy number aberration phenotypes and genomic instability. BMC Cancer 6:96, 2006.

145. Hackett JA, Feldser DM, Greider CW: Telomere dysfunction increases mutation rate and genomic instability. Cell 106:275–286, 2001.

146. Kauraniemi P, Kallioniemi A: Activation of multiple cancer-associated genes at the ERBB2 amplicon in breast cancer. Endocr Relat Cancer 13:39–49, 2006.

147. Tanner MM, Tirkkonen M, Kallioniemi A, et al: Independent amplification and frequent co-amplification of three nonsyntenic regions on the long arm of chromosome 20 in human breast cancer. Cancer Res 56:3441–3445, 1996.

148. Keith WN, Douglas F, Wishart GC, et al: Co-amplification of erbB2, topoisomerase II alpha and retinoic acid receptor alpha genes in breast cancer and allelic loss at topoisomerase I on chromosome 20. Eur J Cancer 29A:1469–1475, 1993.

149. Zhu Y, Qi C, Jain S, et al: Amplification and overexpression of peroxisome proliferator-activated receptor binding protein (PBP/PPARBP) gene in breast cancer. Proc Natl Acad Sci USA 96:10848–10853, 1999.

150. Arriola E, Rodriguez-Pinilla SM, Lambros MB, et al: Topoisomerase II alpha amplification may predict benefit from adjuvant

anthracyclines in HER2 positive early breast cancer. Breast Cancer Res Treat 106:181–189, 2007.

151. Tanner M, Isola J, Wiklund T, et al: Topoisomerase IIalpha gene amplification predicts favorable treatment response to tailored and dose-escalated anthracycline-based adjuvant chemotherapy in HER-2/neu-amplified breast cancer: Scandinavian Breast Group Trial 9401. J Clin Oncol 24:2428–2436, 2006.

152. Tanner MM, Tirkkonen M, Kallioniemi A, et al: Amplification of chromosomal region 20q13 in invasive breast cancer: Prognostic implications. Clin Cancer Res 1:1455–1461, 1995.

153. Guan XY, Xu J, Anzick SL, et al: Hybrid selection of transcribed sequences from microdissected DNA: Isolation of genes within amplified region at 20q11-q13.2 in breast cancer. Cancer Res 56:3446–3450, 1996.

154. Wood LD, Parsons DW, Jones S, et al: The genomic landscapes of human breast and colorectal cancers. Science 318:1108–1113, 2007.

155. Lin J, Gan CM, Zhang X, et al: A multidimensional analysis of genes mutated in breast and colorectal cancers. Genome Res 17:1304–1318, 2007.

156. Sjoblom T, Jones S, Wood LD, et al: The consensus coding sequences of human breast and colorectal cancers. Science 314:268–274, 2006.

157. Jeffrey SS, Fero MJ, Borresen-Dale AL, et al: Expression array technology in the diagnosis and treatment of breast cancer. Mol Interv 2:101–109, 2002.

158. Johnson N, Speirs V, Curtin NJ, et al: A comparative study of genome-wide SNP, CGH microarray and protein expression analysis to explore genotypic and phenotypic mechanisms of acquired antiestrogen resistance in breast cancer. Breast Cancer Res Treat 111:53–63, 2008.

159. Pusztai L, Mazouni C, Anderson K, et al: Molecular classification of breast cancer: Limitations and potential. Oncologist 11:868–877, 2006.

160. Reis-Filho JS, Simpson PT, Gale T, et al: The molecular genetics of breast cancer: The contribution of comparative genomic hybridization. Pathol Res Pract 201:713–725, 2005.

161. Chin SF, Wang Y, Thorne NP, et al: Using array-comparative genomic hybridization to define molecular portraits of primary breast cancers. Oncogene 26:1959–1970, 2007.

162. Hu Z, Fan C, Oh DS, et al: The molecular portraits of breast tumors are conserved across microarray platforms. BMC Genomics 7:96, 2006.

163. Neve RM, Chin K, Fridlyand J, et al: A collection of breast cancer cell lines for the study of functionally distinct cancer subtypes. Cancer Cell 10:515–527, 2006.

164. Paik S, Shak S, Tang G, et al: A multigene assay to predict recurrence of tamoxifen-treated, node-negative breast cancer. N Engl J Med 351:2817–2826, 2004.

165. Perou CM, Sorlie T, Eisen MB, et al: Molecular portraits of human breast tumours. Nature 406:747–752, 2000.

166. van 't Veer LJ, Dai H, van de Vijver MJ, et al: Gene expression profiling predicts clinical outcome of breast cancer. Nature 415:530–536, 2002.

167. Wang Y, Klijn JG, Zhang Y, et al: Gene-expression profiles to predict distant metastasis of lymph-node-negative primary breast cancer. Lancet 365:671–679, 2005.

168. Bergamaschi A, Kim YH, Wang P, et al: Distinct patterns of DNA copy number alteration are associated with different clinicopathological features and gene-expression subtypes of breast cancer. Genes Chromosomes Cancer 45:1033–1040, 2006.

169. Hicks J, Muthuswamy L, Krasnitz A, et al: High-resolution ROMA CGH and FISH analysis of aneuploid and diploid breast tumors. Cold Spring Harb Symp Quant Biol 70:51–63, 2005.

170. Buyse M, Loi S, van't Veer L, et al: Validation and clinical utility of a 70-gene prognostic signature for women with node-negative breast cancer. J Natl Cancer Inst 98:1183–1192, 2006.

171. Caldas C, Aparicio SA: The molecular outlook. Nature 415:484–485, 2002.

172. Tuma RS: Trial and error: Prognostic gene signature study design altered. J Natl Cancer Inst 97:331–333, 2005.

173. Cardoso F, Van't Veer L, Rutgers E, et al: Clinical application of the 70-gene profile: The MINDACT trial. J Clin Oncol 26:729–735, 2008.

174. Paik S, Tang G, Shak S, et al: Gene expression and benefit of chemotherapy in women with node-negative, estrogen receptor-positive breast cancer. J Clin Oncol 24:3726–3734, 2006.

175. Walsh T, King MC: Ten genes for inherited breast cancer. Cancer Cell 11:103–105, 2007.

176. Honrado E, Osorio A, Palacios J, et al: Pathology and gene expression of hereditary breast tumors associated with BRCA1, BRCA2 and CHEK2 gene mutations. Oncogene 25:5837–5845, 2006.

177. Foulkes WD, Metcalfe K, Sun P, et al: Estrogen receptor status in BRCA1- and BRCA2-related breast cancer: The influence of age, grade, and histological type. Clin Cancer Res 10:2029–2034, 2004.

178. Grushko TA, Blackwood MA, Schumm PL, et al: Molecular-cytogenetic analysis of HER-2/neu gene in BRCA1-associated breast cancers. Cancer Res 62:1481–1488, 2002.

179. Gudmundsdottir K, Ashworth A: The roles of BRCA1 and BRCA2 and associated proteins in the maintenance of genomic stability. Oncogene 25:5864–5874, 2006.

180. Miki Y, Swensen J, Shattuck-Eidens D, et al: A strong candidate for the breast and ovarian cancer susceptibility gene BRCA1. Science 266:66–71, 1994.

181. Huusko P, Paakkonen K, Launonen V, et al: Evidence of founder mutations in Finnish BRCA1 and BRCA2 families. Am J Hum Genet 62:1544–1548, 1998.

182. Peelen T, van Vliet M, Petrij-Bosch A, et al: A high proportion of novel mutations in BRCA1 with strong founder effects among Dutch and Belgian hereditary breast and ovarian cancer families. Am J Hum Genet 60:1041–1049, 1997.

183. Wang Y, Cortez D, Yazdi P, et al: BASC, a super complex of BRCA1-associated proteins involved in the recognition and repair of aberrant DNA structures. Genes Dev 14:927–939, 2000.

184. Cortez D, Wang Y, Qin J, et al: Requirement of ATM-dependent phosphorylation of brca1 in the DNA damage response to double-strand breaks. Science 286:1162–1166, 1999.

185. Kennedy RD, Quinn JE, Mullan PB, et al: The role of BRCA1 in the cellular response to chemotherapy. J Natl Cancer Inst 96:1659–1668, 2004.

186. Lieber MR, Ma Y, Pannicke U, et al: Mechanism and regulation of human non-homologous DNA end-joining. Nat Rev Mol Cell Biol 4:712–720, 2003.

187. van Gent DC, Hoeijmakers JH, Kanaar R: Chromosomal stability and the DNA double-stranded break connection. Nat Rev Genet 2:196–206, 2001.

188. Lee JS, Collins KM, Brown AL, et al: hCds1-mediated phosphorylation of BRCA1 regulates the DNA damage response. Nature 404:201–204, 2000.

189. Foray N, Marot D, Gabriel A, et al: A subset of ATM- and ATR-dependent phosphorylation events requires the BRCA1 protein. EMBO J 22:2860–2871, 2003.

190. Saeki H, Siaud N, Christ N, et al: Suppression of the DNA repair defects of BRCA2-deficient cells with heterologous protein fusions. Proc Natl Acad Sci USA 103:8768–8773, 2006.

191. Esashi F, Christ N, Gannon J, et al: CDK-dependent phosphorylation of BRCA2 as a regulatory mechanism for recombinational repair. Nature 434:598–604, 2005.

192. Bartek J, Lukas C, Lukas J: Checking on DNA damage in S phase. Nat Rev Mol Cell Biol 5:792–804, 2004.

193. Johnson N, Fletcher O, Naceur-Lombardelli C, et al: Interaction between CHEK2*1100delC and other low-penetrance breast-cancer susceptibility genes: A familial study. Lancet 366: 1554–1557, 2005.

194. Karnoub AE, Dash AB, Vo AP, et al: Mesenchymal stem cells within tumour stroma promote breast cancer metastasis. Nature 449:557–563, 2007.

195. Darbon JM: A new model of metastatic dissemination of breast cancer bringing into play mesenchymal stem cells. Bull Cancer 94:1035–1036, 2007.

196. Karnoub AE, Weinberg RA: Chemokine networks and breast cancer metastasis. Breast Dis 26:75–85, 2006–2007.

197. Azenshtein E, Luboshits G, Shina S, et al: The CC chemokine RANTES in breast carcinoma progression: Regulation of expression and potential mechanisms of promalignant activity. Cancer Res 62:1093–1102, 2002.

198. Kaminski A, Hahne JC, Haddouti el-M, et al: Tumour-stroma interactions between metastatic prostate cancer cells and fibroblasts. Int J Mol Med 18:941–950, 2006.

chapter 29

Stem Cells, the Breast, and Breast Cancer

MAX WICHA | SANFORD H. BARSKY

Overview

The cancer stem cell (CSC) hypothesis proposes that cancers arise from only certain types of cells within tissues. These select cells are termed tissue stem or progenitor cells. A second part of this hypothesis is that cancers are "driven" by cells with stem cell properties. The CSC hypothesis, however, is still somewhat controversial, and oncologists are split into two camps: believers and agnostics.

Believers contend that most malignancies (both liquid and solid) maintain the differentiation hierarchy of their tissue of origin. The bulk of cells that characterize cancers are differentiated progeny of CSCs, which arise from long-lived, self-renewing cells. These self-renewing stem cells may or may not be classic stem cells. In addition, the CSC, also thought of as the cancer-initiating (or reinitiating) cell, may or may not be derived from a transformed normal tissue stem cell. Believers also think that drug resistance of a cancer is a result of co-opting resistance mechanisms exhibited by its stem cell population and that initial treatment response is not reflected by the properties of its stem cells but rather by the properties of the majority population of proliferating cells. Our biologic high throughput assays, including gene profiling, assess the differentiated or proliferating cancer cell pool, not the CSCs.

Agnostics, on the other hand, maintain that the "mathematical support for the concept of stem cells is weak" and that "tumorigenic behavior might be a varying probabilistic potential of all tumor cells rather than quantal and deterministic feature of a minority of tumor cells." Evidence supporting the stem cell hypothesis is strong for leukemias but weaker for the solid cancers, including breast cancer. This is the result, in part, of the robustness of the specificity of CSC markers in leukemia and the ability to purify and sort subpopulations of cells and study their biology in the liquid malignancies. Evidence is weaker in the solid cancers, including breast cancer, because the stem cell markers that exist are not as robust and our ability to purify and sort subpopulations is more limited.

Stem Cells in the Normal Breast

Embryologic studies of the normal mammary gland indicate that stem cells in the mammary bud develop into early progenitors and then late progenitors, which then differentiate into either ductal epithelial cells or myoepithelial cells.[1-3] Ductal and alveolar epithelial cells express MUC1 and epithelial keratins, whereas myoepithelial cells express common acute lymphoblastic leukemia antigen (CALLA) and other keratins.[4,5] Ductal and alveolar epithelial cells are fundamentally different from myoepithelial cells. Ductal and alveolar epithelial cells can express hormonal receptors, can secrete casein, and can proliferate. Myoepithelial cells, in contrast, synthesize a basement membrane, do not express hormone receptors, and undergo only limited proliferation. Both cell lineages are thought to be derived from undifferentiated mammary stem cells. These normal mammary stem cells are $CD44^+$ and $CD24^-$, and they are capable of self-renewal and differentiation both in vitro and in vivo.[6] In fact, one obligate feature of stem cells is their dual ability to both self-renew as well as differentiate. In other words, stem cells must be able to undergo both symmetric cell division (into two daughter stem cells) and asymmetric division (into one daughter stem cell and one proliferating cell). Stem cells usually differentiate along several lines.[7-9] This ability is reflected in the property of multipotency (Fig. 29-1). So, for example, a normal mammary stem cell can differentiate into either a ductal or alveolar epithelial cell or myoepithelial cell. Certain tissue stem cells can occasionally exhibit evidence of pluripotency, the ability to differentiate along different germlines, or totipotency, the ability to differentiate into trophoblastic tissue. Embryonal stem cells can exhibit this latter property. The ability of mammary stem cells to exhibit evidence of "stemness" can be assayed in two-dimensional culture, three-dimensional culture, and in mice (Fig. 29-2). In in vitro assays, predetermined growth conditions with serum, growth factors, and Matrigel are used. One important in vitro property exhibited by mammary stem cells is the property of

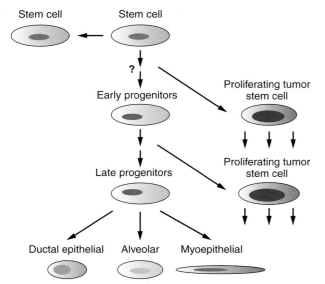

Figure 29-1   The breast stem cell property of multipotency is illustrated.

forming mammospheres,[10-12] tight aggregates of cells in suspension culture (Fig. 29-3). Single mammary stem cells also have the ability to exhibit alveolar and ductal morphogenesis in Matrigel (Fig. 29-4). In the developing normal breast, aldehyde dehydrogenase 1 (ALDH1)–positive stem cells, which are also thought to be estrogen receptor (ER) negative, are thought to generate ER-positive progeny.

MARKERS OF NORMAL STEM CELLS

Normal breast stem cells exhibit an immunocytochemical profile of $CD44^+/CD24^-/lin^-$. These markers are not very specific and their stem cell function is unknown. Another marker that has recently been used to define normal mammary stem cells is the enzyme ALDH.[13-15] This enzyme has shown increased activity in hematopoietic and neuronal stem/progenitor cells, and unlike CD44 and CD24, has shown to have functional role in stem cell differentiation. The activity of ALDH can easily be determined by an enzymatic assay termed the Aldefluor assay (Fig. 29-5), and a monoclonal antibody detecting the ALDH1 protein can also be used for immunodetection. Studies of normal breast have revealed that approximately 6% of the epithelial cells within the ductal-lobular units were positive for

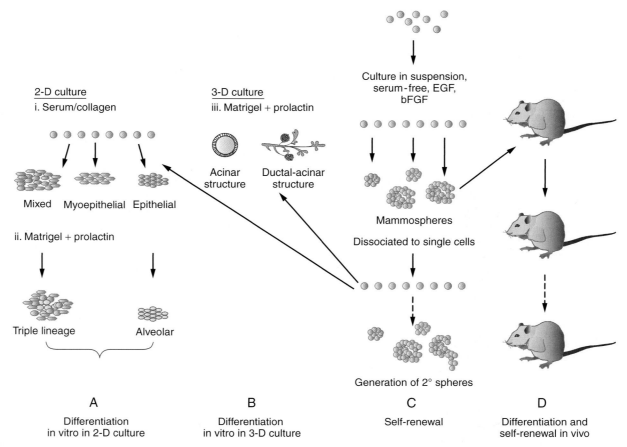

Figure 29-2   Different assays to measure "stemness."

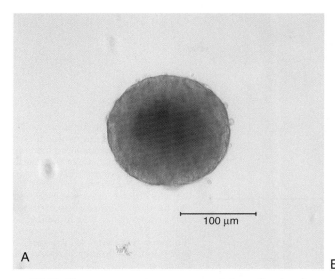
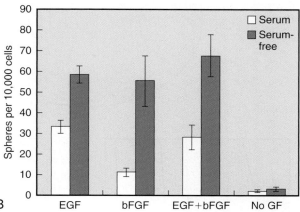

Figure 29-3 The mammosphere assay and its optimal culture conditions. Mammosphere culture was performed as previously described. Single cells were plated in ultralow attachment plates (Corning, Acton, Massachusetts) or plates coated with 1% agarose in PBS, at a density of 20,000 viable cells/mL in primary culture and 5000 cells/mL in subsequent passages. For mammosphere culture, cells were grown in a serum-free mammary epithelial basal medium (Cambrex Bio Science Walkersville, Inc, Walkerville, Maryland) supplemented with B27 (Invitrogen, Carlsbad, California), 20 ng/mL EGF (BD Biosciences, San Jose, California), antibiotic-antimycotic (100 unit/mL penicillin G sodium, 100 µg/mL streptomycin sulfate and 0.25 µg/mL amphotericin B), 20 µg/mL gentamicin, 1 ng/mL hydrocortisone, 5 µg/mL insulin and 100 µM beta-mercaptoethanol (GIBCO, Invitrogen) in a humidified incubator (10% CO_2: 95% air, 37 ° C for 7–10 days), as previously described.

Aldefluor.[16] Only Aldefluor-positive cells generated mammospheres in suspension culture (Fig. 29-6). In nonobese diabetic mice with severe combined immunodeficiency syndrome, only Aldefluor-positive cells formed ductal structures.

KEY SIGNALING PATHWAYS OF NORMAL STEM CELLS

A number of different signaling pathways have been implicated in normal stem cell self-renewal, maintenance of developmental potential, and proliferation. All of these signaling pathways have ligand activation of a membrane protein, which signals through the cytoplasm and activates transcription factors that regulate gene expression downstream. Key stem cell signaling pathways include hedgehog, notch, bmi-1, Wnt, and Pten pathways.[17–20] Hedgehog signaling is depicted in Figure 29-7. Hedgehog ligands, receptors, and transcription factors are expressed at higher levels in mammospheres in suspension (Fig. 29-8). Conversely, hedgehog signaling regulates mammary stem cell self-renewal, causing the number of

cells and mammospheres to increase (Fig. 29-9). Notch signaling via gamma secretase activation, NICD fragment generation, and downstream activation of bHLH genes (hes-1, hes-5, hey-1, hey-2; see Fig. 29-9) is also involved in mammosphere formation and increased number of cells and mammospheres (Fig. 29-10). The bmi-1 pathway is also involved in normal stem cell self-renewal. The evidence for this comes from RNA interference experiments where bmi-1 knockdown reduces the number of secondary mammospheres (Fig. 29-11). These signaling pathways do not operate in isolation but are thought to interact (Fig. 29-12). Other pathways are thought to be involved in the maintenance of developmental potential and the proliferating and differentiating potential of stem cells.

Stem Cells in Breast Cancer

Even though it is thought that human cancers and human breast cancers are monoclonal, it is well accepted that human cancers are quite heterogeneous in nature.

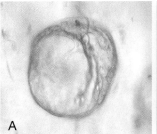
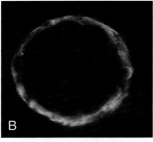
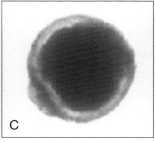
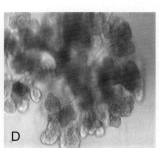

Figure 29-4 Alveolar and ductal morphogenesis from single cells in Matrigel culture. **A** and **B,** Alveolar morphology. **C,** Immunostaining for casein. **D,** Mixed; alveolar and ductal morphology.

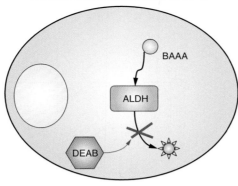

Aldefluor+ cells in normal breast epithelium

BAAA

ALDH

DEAB

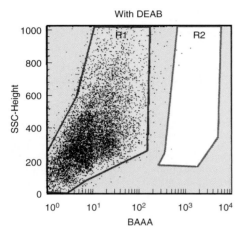

With DEAB

R1   R2

SSC-Height

1000
800
600
400
200
0

10^0 10^1 10^2 10^3 10^4
BAAA

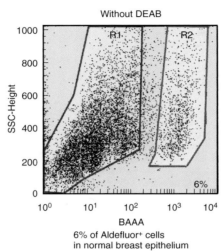

Without DEAB

R1   R2

SSC-Height

1000
800
600
400
200
0

6%

10^0 10^1 10^2 10^3 10^4
BAAA

6% of Aldefluor+ cells
in normal breast epithelium

Figure 29-5 The Aldefluor assay. Normal breast tissue from reduction mammoplasties was dissociated mechanically and enzymatically. Cells incubated with Aldefluor substrate (BAAA) and the aldehyde dehydrogenase (ALDH)–specific inhibitor DEAB were used to establish the baseline fluorescence of these cells (R1) and to define the Aldefluor-positive region (R2). Incubation of cells with Aldefluor substrate in the absence of DEAB induced a shift in BAAA fluorescence defining the Aldefluor-positive population.

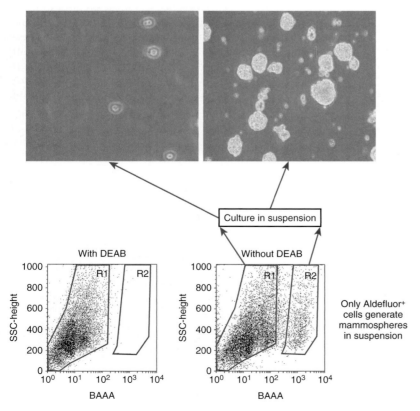

Culture in suspension

With DEAB

R1   R2

SSC-height

1000
800
600
400
200
0

10^0 10^1 10^2 10^3 10^4
BAAA

Without DEAB

R1   R2

SSC-height

1000
800
600
400
200
0

10^0 10^1 10^2 10^3 10^4
BAAA

Only Aldefluor+
cells generate
mammospheres
in suspension

Figure 29-6 Aldefluor-positive cells and mammosphere formation.

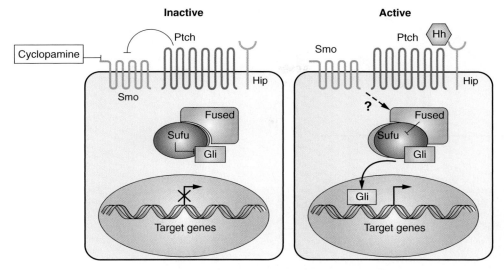

Figure 29-7 The hedgehog signaling pathway.

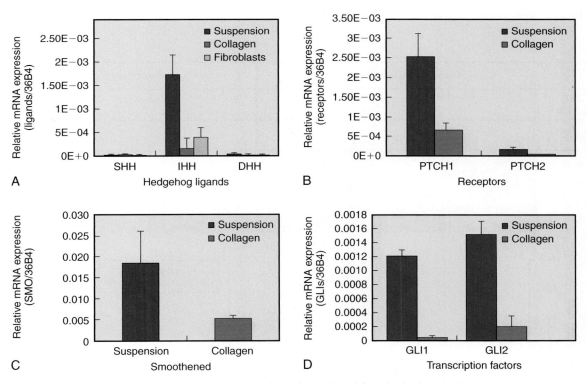

Figure 29-8 Increased expression of members of the hedgehog pathway.

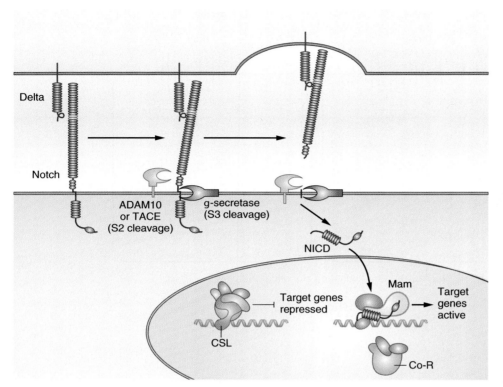

Figure 29-9 Notch signaling in normal breast stem cells.

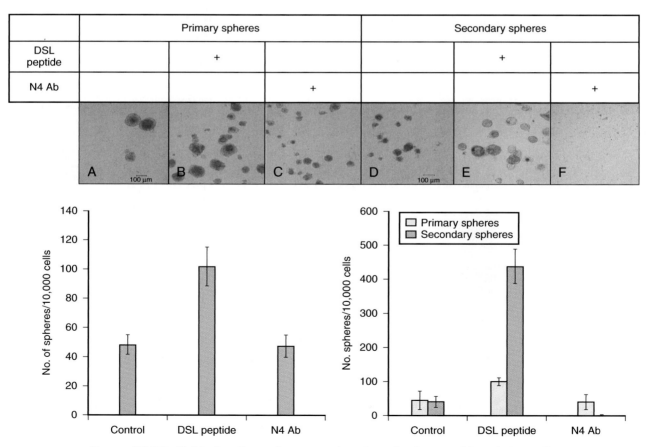

Figure 29-10 Notch signaling and mammosphere formation in normal breast stem cells.

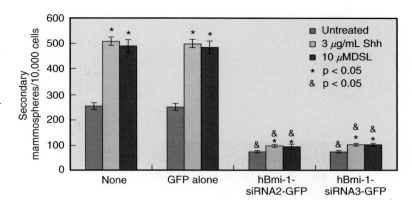

Figure 29-11 Effects of bmi-1 knockdown on secondary mammosphere generation.

It is this tumor cell heterogeneity that confounds successful attempts at therapy. Two models to explain tumor cell heterogeneity have evolved (Fig. 29-13). The first model is a stochastic model, proposing that cancer cells are inherently heterogeneous because of genomic instability but that most cells have the ability to proliferate and form new tumors. The second model, in contrast, is the CSC model, proposing that although cancer cells are heterogeneous, only rare CSCs have the ability to proliferate extensively and form new tumors.[21] The stochastic model governed our thinking about cancer over the past several decades, whereas the stem cell model has been gaining in popularity over the past 5 years.

Evidence supporting the stem cell model in breast cancer is based on studies with established human breast cancer cell lines that were sorted on the basis of putative stem cell markers such as $CD44^+/CD24^-/lin^-$, and those cells expressing the stem cell markers were highly tumorigenic in contrast to the cells lacking the stem cell markers[10] (Fig. 29-14). These experiments were repeated using a different stem cell marker, Aldefluor, but the results were the same: the Aldefluor-positive subpopulation was much more tumorigenic than the Aldefluor-negative population (Fig. 29-15). The agnostics argued, however, that what these experiments showed was simply that a subset of human tumor cells was able to grow better in an immunodeficient murine host and that this subset had nothing to do with "stemness" but simply had to do with factors such as membrane receptors that allowed these cells to grow better in a xenotransplant. It was argued that if one did the same experiment with a murine tumor in a syngeneic murine host that this differential tumorigenicity would not be observed. The believers countered with the argument that the stem cell subpopulation (i.e., the Aldefluor-positive subpopulation) could regenerate the tumor heterogeneity of the initial tumor—additional evidence of "stemness." The believers also argued that although there was little overlap between the

Figure 29-12 Interaction of key stem cell self-renewal pathways in normal breast stem cells.

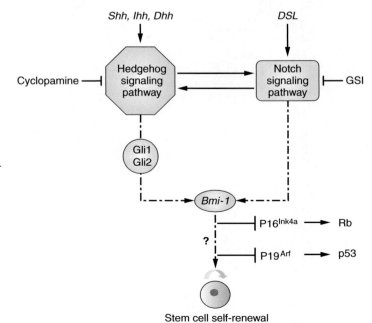

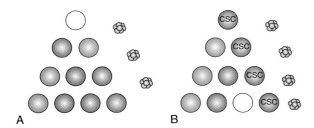

Figure 29-13 Models of tumor heterogeneity. **A,** Stochastic model: Cancer cells are heterogeneous, but most cells can proliferate extensively and form new tumors. **B,** Cancer stem cell model: Cancer cells are heterogeneous, and only rare cancer stem cells have the ability to proliferate extensively and form new tumors.

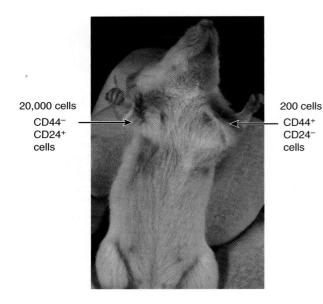

20,000 cells
CD44⁻
CD24⁺
cells

200 cells
CD44⁺
CD24⁻
cells

Figure 29-14 Enhanced tumorigenicity by human breast cancer "stem cells" identified by CD44⁺/CD24⁻.

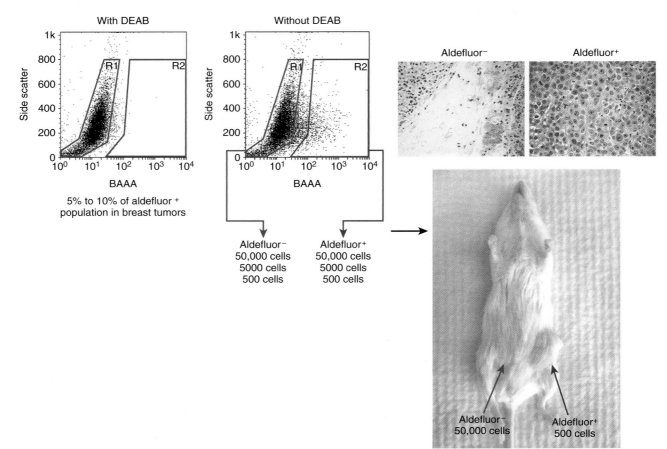

Figure 29-15 Select tumorigenicity by human breast cancer "stem cells" identified by Aldefluor positivity.

CD44$^+$/CD24$^-$ subpopulations and the Aldefluor-positive subpopulation, the small subpopulation that expressed both sets of markers had the shortest latency of all (Fig. 29-16). Other experiments showed that the Aldefluor-positive subset of cells in a number of different cell lines had increased invasive properties in vitro as well as increased ability to form hematogenous metastasis (Fig. 29-17).

MARKERS OF CANCER STEM CELLS

In addition to the expression of similar markers expressed by normal tissue stem cells, CSCs are thought to express embryonal stem cell markers. Common embryonal stem cell markers often expressed by CSCs include stellar, rex-1, nestin, and H19, as well as transcriptional factors, which include nuclear β-catenin, oct-4, nanog, and sox-2, determinants associated with the maintenance of the stem cell state of self-renewal and developmental potential in embryonal stem cells. These latter transcription factors have recently been found to be able to revert adult fibroblasts to an embryonal stem cell state.[22] It is not surprising, therefore, that these same transcription factors could regulate self-renewal and differentiation potential in the CSC subpopulation. An ever growing list of cancer stem markers is being described and characterized (Tables 29-1 to 29-3). It should be pointed out that the function of many of these markers is still not understood. One stem cell marker whose function is understood is the ATP-binding cassette transporter protein ABCG2.[23,24] This transporter enables stem cells to efflux lipophilic dyes such as Hoechst 33342 and gives rise to a population of cells that is termed the side population on flow cytometric analysis.[24] This transporter is also thought to efflux chemotherapeutic drugs from the stem cells and make them resistant to chemotherapy.

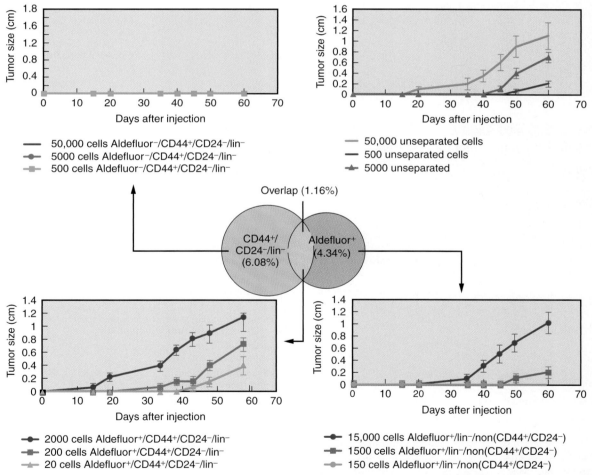

Figure 29-16 Overlap between the cell populations identified by the Aldefluor assay and the CD44$^+$/CD24$^-$/linphenotype in human breast tumors. Aldefluor-negative and -positive cells from three human breast tumor xenotransplants (MC1, UM1, UM2) were separated by FACS using the Aldefluor assay. In all experiments cells were first gated on PI-negative cells (viable cells) that represented 73.6 ± 1.8% of the total population. Cells were then fixed in RNA later, immunostained with a CD24-PE antibody, a CD44–APC antibody, and antibodies for lineage markers, labeled Pe-Cy5. In all the flow cytometry analyses cells were first gated on lin$^-$ markers that represented 12.3 ± 1.1% of the total population. These cell populations were gated out in the flow charts shown on the left side of the figure. The diagrams in the right side show the representation of the cell fractions defined by the Aldefluor and the CD44$^+$/CD24$^-$/lin$^-$ combined phenotype in the total tumor cell population (PI negative).

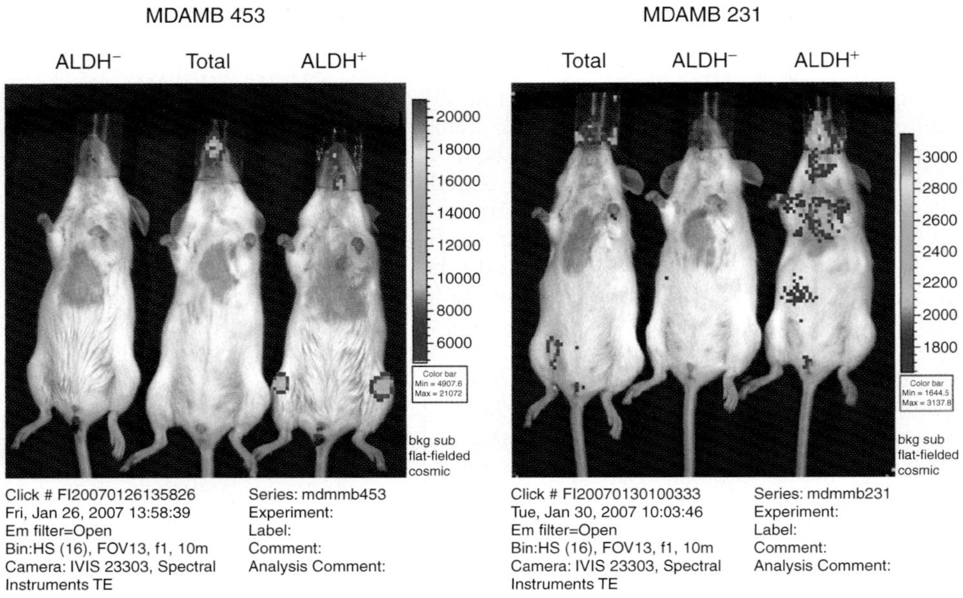

Figure 29-17 Metastasis of breast cancer stem cells. For luciferase gene transduction, 70% confluent cells were incubated overnight with a 1:3 precipitated mixture of lentiviral supernatants Lenti-LUC-VSVG (Vector Core, University of Michigan, Ann Arbor, Michigan) in culture medium. The following day the cells were harvested by trypsin/EDTA and subcultured at a ratio of 1:6. After 1 week incubation, luciferase expression was verified by adding 2 μL D-luciferin 0.0003% (Promega, Madison, Wisconsin) in the culture medium and counting photon flux by device camera system (Xenogen, Alameda, California). Six-week-old nonobese diabetic mice with severe combined immunodeficiency syndrome were anesthetized with 1.75% isoflurane/air anesthesia, and their left ventricles were injected with 50,000 or 100,000 cells (Aldefluor-positive, -negative, or unseparated) in 100 μL of sterile Dulbecco's PBS lacking Ca^{2+} and Mg^{2+}. After cell inoculations, the animals were screened for metastasis using bioluminescence. ALDH, aldehyde dehydrogenase.

TABLE 29-1

Normal and Embryonal Stem Cell Markers Expressed by Cancer Stem Cells*

Stem Cell Type	Molecular Marker	Significance
Embryonic stem cells (ES) or Pluripotent stem cells (PS)	Oct-4	Transcription factor essential for establishment and maintenance of undifferentiated PS
	Pax-6	Transcription factor expressed as ES differentiates into neuroepithelium
	Stellar	Specific marker of undifferentiated ES
	Alpha-fetoprotein (AFP)	Reflects endodermal differentiation of PS
	Rex-1	Specific marker of undifferentiated ES
	Germ cell nuclear factor (GCNF)	Transcription factor expressed by PS
	Sox-2	Transcription factor essential for establishment and maintenance of undifferentiated PS
	H19	Marker developmentally regulated in skeletal muscle, smooth muscle, and fetal liver
	Nanog	Transcription factor unique to PS; essential for establishment and maintenance of undifferentiated PS
Hematopoietic stem cells (HS)	CD34	Indicative of HS and EP
	c-kit	Cell surface receptor on bone marrow cell types that identifies HS and MS
	Stem Cell Antigen (Sca-1)	Indicative of HS and MS in bone marrow and blood
Mesenchymal stem and progenitor cells (MS)	Bone morphogenetic protein receptor (BMPR)	BMPR identifies early mesenchymal lineages (MS)
	Stro-1 antigen	Cell surface glycoprotein on subsets of bone marrow MS
Neural stem cells (NS)	CD133	Identifies NS and HS
	Nestin	Identifies NS
Endothelial progenitor cells (EP)	Fetal liver kinase-1 (Flk-1)	Cell surface receptor protein that identifies EP

*More resources are available on the National Institutes of Health website: http://stemcells.nih.gov/info/scireport/appendixE.asp.

TABLE 29-2

Cancer Stem Cell Markers Observed in Human Cancers

Human Cancer Type	Phenotypic Marker	Side Population
Leukemia	CD34$^+$/CD38$^-$, CD44$^+$	Yes
Breast cancer	CD44$^+$/CD24$^{-/low}$, spheroid formation	Not determined
Prostate cancer	CD44$^+$/$\alpha_2\beta_1$^{hi}/CD133$^+$, Sca-1$^+$	Not determined
Melanoma	CD20$^+$, spheroid formation	Yes
Brain cancer	CD133$^+$, neurospheroid formation	Not determined
Retinoblastoma	ABCG2$^+$, ALDH1 positive	Yes
Colon cancer	CD133$^+$	Not determined
	CD44$^+$/CD133$^+$/CD24$^{-/low}$, spheroid formation	No

TABLE 29-3

Summary of Stem Cell Properties Exhibited in Vitro by Cancer Stem Cells

	Stem Cell Properties Exhibited in Vitro
Stem cell–specific markers	Transcriptional determinants as well as specific markers (e.g., oct-4, sox-2, nanog, rex-1) known to be restricted to normal embryonal or tissue stem cells detected within cancer stem cells
Self-renewal and proliferation	Ability of single cancer stem cell to generate secondary spheroids (mammospheres) without initial cell aggregation/cell-cell contact; spheroids containing as few as 100 cells are fully tumorigenic.
Multipotency	Ability of single cancer stem cell cultured in Matrigel to manifest multipotency or differentiation

KEY SIGNALING PATHWAYS OF CANCER STEM CELLS

The same signaling pathways that exist in normal stem cells are thought to be important in CSCs. Key stem cell signaling pathways include hedgehog, notch, bmi-1, Wnt, and Pten pathways.[17-20] Evidence of the importance of these pathways in CSCs has been derived from experiments showing that the CSC subpopulation exhibiting enhanced tumorigenicity is the same population displaying pathway activation (Fig. 29-18). Because of these similarities between CSCs and normal stem cells (Fig. 29-19), it has been hypothesized that the cancer-initiating cell indeed is derived from the normal stem cell. If, in fact, this hypothesis is true and tissue stem cells are rare in tissues, this could explain the rareness of malignant transformation. In human breast cancer, for example, even in the setting of inherited breast cancer from BRCA1, where every cell of the breast would have

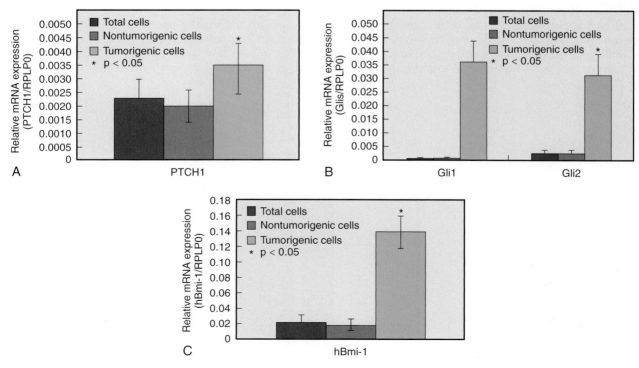

Figure 29-18   Hedgehog activation and bmi-1 expression in cancer initiating stem cells.

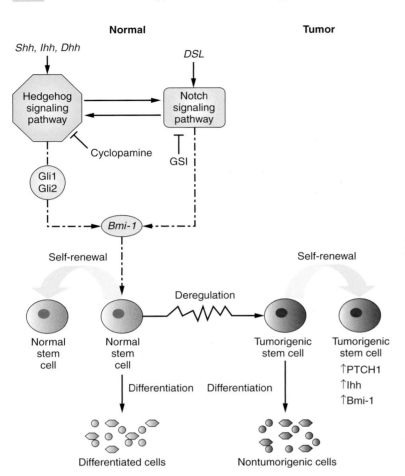

Figure 29-19 Hypothesis of cancer stem cell origin from normal stem cells.

this mutation, malignant transformation is still rare on a cellular basis. If any ductal epithelial cell could transform, then patients with BRCA1 should get thousands of cancers, but they get one or two. If only tissue stem cells can transform, and their numbers are few, then this would better support the clinical observations. Still, the evidence linking the tissue stem cell with the CSC is indirect at best.

Cells sorted on the basis of a stem cell marker (e.g., Aldefluor) express a stem cell "signature" on the basis of cDNA microarray analysis (Fig. 29-20). Unsupervised hierarchical clustering reveals expression of the hedgehog,

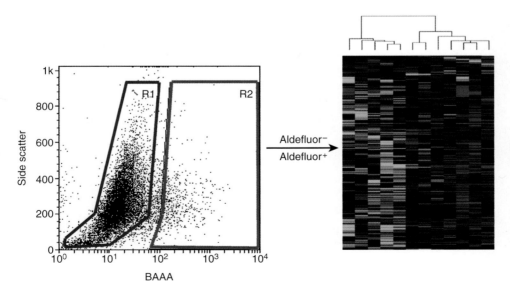

Figure 29-20 Stem cell gene signature.

notch, bmi-1, Wnt, and Pten pathways in sorted "stem" cells versus nonstem cells. Other evidence implicating key signaling pathways in breast cancer stem cells is the relationship of other key genes previously implicated in breast cancer pathogenesis to these pathways. The other key genes previously implicated in breast cancer pathogenesis include BRCA1, Her2/neu, and PTEN. BRCA1 is a gene in which a germline mutation can confer a 80% risk of breast cancer. In addition, the majority of BRCA1 cancers are "triple negative," and there is a significant expression of basal markers (CK5, 6). Methylation changes are thought to occur in BRCA1 in sporadic breast cancers. BRCA1 is thought to play a key role in mammary differentiation. As it turns out, BRCA1 has an important role also in stem cells. Gene knockdown of BRCA1 can increase the number of derived mammospheres and furthermore can increase the ALDH-positive subpopulation. In addition, BRCA1 knockdown can block the differentiation of stem cells into the late progenitors of ER-positive ductal and lobular epithelium. Therefore, BRCA1 is thought to interact with many of the pathways responsible for stem cell self-renewal. Her2/neu is amplified in 20% of breast cancers and is associated with a more aggressive clinical course. Her2/neu has been targeted by trastuzumab and lapatinib. As it turns out, Her2/neu overexpression in breast cancer cell lines increases the ALDH1 stem cell pool. PTEN is thought to be deleted in 40% of breast cancers and has been associated with Her2/neu resistance. PTEN knockdown also increases the stem cell phenotype and is also synergistic with Her2/neu overexpression in this regard. The interaction of these genes previously implicated in breast cancer pathogenesis with key stem cell signaling pathways, including hedgehog, notch, and bmi-1, is thought to regulate breast cancer stem cell self-renewal and differentiation (Fig. 29-21).

Epithelial-mesenchymal transition (EMT) is another pathway that has been implicated in breast cancer progression involving snail, slug, twist, E-cadherin, and β-catenin. Recently, it has been shown that breast cancer stem cells express the EMT pathway to an exaggerated degree, and conversely breast cancer cells undergoing EMT become stemlike.[25]

Can the Stem Cell Paradigm Shift Result in Improved Cancer Treatment and Survival?

To begin to answer this question, we first need to examine the evidence that CSCs exist in actual human breast cancers. Recent studies have observed CD44$^+$/CD24$^-$ and ALDH1+ in tissue microarrays of human breast cancer (Fig. 29-22). Recent studies have also shown that an increased population of stem cells exist in certain types of breast cancer.[26,27] Of special note in this regard is inflammatory breast cancer,[28,29] which is especially rich in cells expressing a stem cell phenotype. Other studies have shown that human breast cancers expressing a stem cell signature exhibit a decreased overall survival.[30] Recent work using human breast cancer core biopsies obtained before and after chemotherapy confirmed that conventional chemotherapy did not eliminate the tumorigenic subpopulation of CD44$^+$/CD24$^-$ cells, which were enriched after chemotherapy. Expression profiling revealed up-regulation of the notch pathway in the CD44$^+$/CD24$^-$ cells. Specifically MAML2, Jagged 2, and HES1 were up-regulated. Developmental genes (e.g., ARID1B) and transcriptional factors were especially important in embryonic development. Beta-catenin, a key regulator of both normal mammary and breast cancer development, was also up-regulated. The study concluded that a small subpopulation of cells with tumorigenic potential is intrinsically resistant to chemotherapy and that these cells have the property of stem cells. The significance of these findings was that the stem cell signature increased after treatment. This validated the clinical importance of breast cancer stem cells in breast cancer treatment.

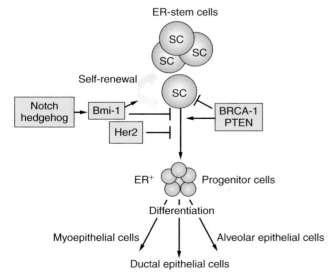

Figure 29-21 Interaction of breast cancer pathogenesis genes with stem cell genes. ER, estrogen receptor.

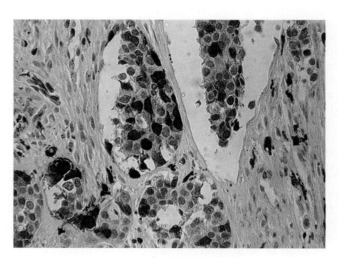

Figure 29-22 LDH1 positivity in human breast carcinoma.

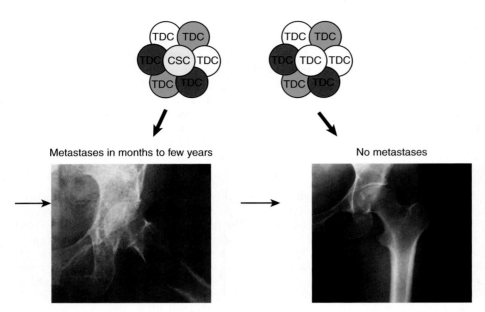

Figure 29-23 Cancer stem cell (CSC) metastatic determination in circulating tumor cells and disseminated tumor cells. TDC, terminally differentiated cell.

If larger prospective studies emerge that support this notion—that stem cells exist but that they are inherently resistant to chemotherapy—then many things previously unexplained may suddenly have explanations. For example, the circulating tumor cells (CTCs) and disseminated tumor cells (DTCs) in the bone marrow and lymph nodes that exist in many patients with "early stage" breast cancer has been a bit of an enigma.[31,32] What is their significance on outcome? Some patients do very well and others do not. It may be that the stem cell composition of the CTC or DTC clump may well determine outcome. If the CTCs and DTCs are passively disseminated in some instances and contain no CSCs, they may not self-renew and may remain dormant. On the other hand, if they have actively disseminated and contain CSCs, they may exhibit clonogenic potential and become metastatic (Fig. 29-23).

The implications of breast CSCs in therapeutics and how we gauge the effectiveness of therapy is vast. Tumor regression in preclinical models and phase II clinical trials may be an inadequate end point. Because many cancers, including breast cancer, initially go into a complete remission, only to subsequently relapse and show no improvement in overall survival, it may well be that the measure we are using to reflect response is inaccurate and inadequate. We may be observing a response in the proliferating compartment but not in the stem cell compartment, the latter of which is the major determinant of survival. Effective therapies then need to target specifically CSCs (Fig. 29-24). Of course, we need to spare normal stem cells in the gut and bone marrow. The pathways involved in self-renewal of CSCs may provide new and specific therapeutic targets. The notch pathway, for example, has specifically been targeted in emerging clinical trials.[33]

Many questions are still unanswered. Our overall classification of breast cancer is based on the overall appearance of the tumor and its overall molecular signature.

Selective gene profiling, including the 21-gene, the 70-gene, and the 76-gene profiles (Oncotype DX, MammaPrint, and multicenter profiles), are also based on profiling of the entire tumor and not the minor stem cell subpopulation. Both our prognostic and predictive markers such as ER, progesterone receptor, and Her-2/neu are also based on the overall tumor and not on the rare stem cell population. But if the rare stem cell population governs overall survival, then why is our analysis of the whole tumor useful at all? If the stem cell signature is "bad" from a chemotherapeutic standpoint, then why are germ cell tumors that express an embryonal stem cell

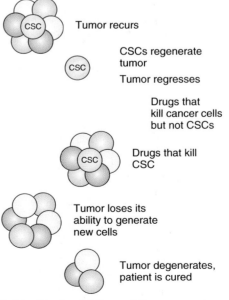

Tumor recurs

CSCs regenerate tumor

Tumor regresses

Drugs that kill cancer cells but not CSCs

Drugs that kill CSC

Tumor loses its ability to generate new cells

Tumor degenerates, patient is cured

Figure 29-24 The implications of the cancer stem cell (CSC) paradigm shift.

signature so sensitive to chemotherapy? These questions notwithstanding, the stem cell paradigm shift holds promise of improved cancer treatment and survival.

REFERENCES

1. Boecker W, Moll R, Dervan P, et al: Usual ductal hyperplasia of the breast is a committed stem (progenitor) cell lesion distinct from atypical ductal hyperplasia and ductal carcinoma in situ. J Pathol 198:458–467, 2002.
2. Shackleton M, Vaillan F, Simpson KJ, et al: Generation of a functional mammary gland from a single stem cell. Nature 439: 84–88, 2006.
3. Stingl J, Eaves CJ, Kuusk U, et al: Phenotypic and functional characterization in vitro of a multipotent epithelial cell present in the normal adult human breast. Differentiation 63:201–213, 1998.
4. Stingl J, Eirew P, Ricketson I, et al: Purification and unique properties of mammary epithelial stem cells. Nature 439:993–999, 2006.
5. Villadsen R, Fridriksdottir AJ, Ronnov-Jessen L, et al: Evidence for a stem cell hierarchy in the adult human breast. J Cell Biol 177: 87–101, 2007.
6. Kuperwasser C, Chavarria T, Wu M, et al: Reconstruction of functionally normal and malignant human breast tissues in mice. Proc Natl Acad Sci USA 101:4966–4971, 2004.
7. Phillips TM, McBride WH, F Pajonk: The response of CD24(/low)/CD44+ breast cancer-initiating cells to radiation. J Natl Cancer Inst 98:1777–1785, 2006.
8. Al Hajj M, Wicha MS, Benito-Hernandez A, et al: Prospective identification of tumorigenic breast cancer cells. Proc Natl Acad Sci USA 100:3983–3398, 2003.
9. Ginestier C, Hur MH, Charafe-Jauffret E, et al: ALDH1 is a marker of normal and malignant human mammary stem cells and a predictor of poor clinical outcome. Cell Stem Cell 1:555–567, 2007.
10. Wicha MS, Liu S, Dontu G: Cancer stem cells: An old idea—a paradigm shift. Cancer Res 66:1883–1890, 2006.
11. Christgen M, Ballmaier M, Bruchhardt H, et al: Identification of a distinct side population of cancer cells in the Cal-51 human breast carcinoma cell line. Mol Cell Biochem 306:201–221, 2007.
12. Ho MM, Ng AV, Lam S, Hung JY: Side population in human lung cancer cell lines and tumors is enriched with stem-like cancer cells. Cancer Res 67:4827–4833, 2007.
13. Chute JP, Muramoto GG, Whitesides J, et al: Inhibition of aldehyde dehydrogenase and retinoid signaling induces the expansion of human hematopoietic stem cells. Proc Natl Acad Sci USA 31: 11707–11712, 2006.
14. Hess DA, Meyerrose TE, Wirthlin L, et al: Functional characterization of highly purified human hematopoietic repopulating cells isolated according to aldehyde dehydrogenase activity. Blood 104: 1648–1655, 2004.
15. Pearce, DJ, Taussig D, Simpson C, et al: Characterization of cells with a high aldehyde dehydrogenase activity from cord blood and acute myeloid leukemia samples. Stem Cells 23:752–760, 2005.
16. Dontu G, Abdallah WM, Foley JM, et al: In vitro propagation and transcriptional profiling of human mammary stem/progenitor cells. Genes Dev 17:1253–1270, 2003.
17. Molofsky AV, Pardal R, Morrison SJ: Diverse mechanisms regulate stem cell self-renewal. Curr Opin Cell Biol 16:700–707, 2004.
18. Androutsellis-Theotokis A, Leker RR, Soldner F, et al: Notch signalling regulates stem cell numbers in vitro and in vivo. Nature 442:823–826, 2006.
19. Politi K, Feirt N, Kitajewski J: Notch in mammary gland development and breast cancer. Semin Cancer Biol 14:341–347, 2004.
20. Dontu G, Jackson KW, et al: Role of notch signaling in cell-fate determination of human mammary stem/progenitor cells. Breast Cancer Res 6:R605–R615, 2004.
21. Reya T, Morrison SJ, Clarke MF, Weissman IL: Stem cells, cancer, and cancer stem cells. Nature 414:105–111, 2001.
22. Takahashi K, Tanabe K, Ohnuki M, et al: Induction of pluripotent stem cells from adult human fibroblasts by defined factors. Cell 131:1–12, 2007.
23. Kondo T, Setoguchi T, Taga T: Persistence of a small subpopulation of cancer stem-like cells in the C6 glioma cell line. Proc Natl Acad Sci USA 101:781–787, 2004.
24. Wang J, Guo LP, Chen LZ, et al: Identification of cancer stem cell-like side population cells in human nasopharyngeal carcinoma cell line. Cancer Res 67:3716–3772, 2007.
25. Mani SA, Guo W, Liao MJ, et al: The epithelial-mesenchymal transition generates cells with properties of stem cells. Cell 133: 704–715, 2008.
26. Kondo T: Stem cell-like cancer cells in cancer cell lines. Cancer Biomarkers 3:245–250, 2007.
27. Lobo NA, Shimono Y, Qian D, Clarke MF: The biology of cancer stem cells. Annu Rev Cell Dev Biol 23:675–699, 2007.
28. Bertucci F, Finetti P, Rougemont J, et al: Gene expression profiling for molecular characterization of inflammatory breast cancer and prediction of response to chemotherapy. Cancer Res 64: 8558–6855, 2004.
29. Xiao Y, Ye Y, Yearsley K, et al: The lymphovascular embolus of inflammatory breast cancer expresses a stem cell-like phenotype. Am J Pathol 173:561–574, 2008.
30. Glinsky GV, Berezovska O, Glinskii AB: Microarray analysis identifies a death-from-cancer signature predicting therapy failure in patients with multiple types of cancer. J Clin Invest 115: 1503–1521, 2005.
31. Riethdorf S, Pantel K: Disseminated tumor cells in bone marrow and circulating tumor cells in blood of breast cancer patients: Current state of detection and characterization. Pathobiology 75: 140–148, 2008.
32. Nagrath S, Sequist LV, Maheswaran S, et al: Isolation of rare circulating tumour cells in cancer patients by microchip technology. Nature 450:1235–1239, 2007.
33. Yamaguchi N, Oyama T, Ito E, et al: Notch3 signaling pathway plays crucial roles in the proliferation of erbB2-negative human breast cancer cells. Cancer Res 68:881–1888, 2008.

Concepts and Mechanisms of Breast Cancer Metastasis

JANET E. PRICE

Once breast cancer has been diagnosed, the most important question is whether the cancer is confined to the breast or has spread to distant sites. The prognosis for recurrence and death after treatment of primary breast cancer is related to the disease stage and the presence of axillary lymph node metastases at the time of diagnosis. The general understanding of the pathogenesis of metastasis has increased considerably in the past three decades, but comparable improvements in the treatment of metastatic disease have, for the most part, not yet been realized. The majority of the deaths of women with breast cancer result from the growth of metastases that are nonresponsive to therapy, and a major obstacle to the successful treatment of metastatic disease is that the cancer cells in primary and secondary tumors are biologically heterogeneous.[1,2] The development of more effective therapies for metastatic breast cancer should be based on a better understanding of the mechanisms responsible for the spread of cells from the breast to distant sites, plus an appreciation of the consequences of tumor heterogeneity. This chapter discusses some of the recent findings on mechanisms of metastasis that are relevant to metastatic breast cancer.

Pathogenesis of Metastasis

To establish metastases in distant organs, cancer cells must complete a sequence of steps, each of which may be described as rate limiting (Fig. 30-1). Failure to complete any of the steps will abort the process. The cells that do survive may represent selected populations of cells, and numerous experimental studies have shown that the cells recovered from metastases have enhanced metastatic capabilities when compared with the original populations of cells. The metastatic potential depends on intrinsic properties of the tumor cells, and their interactions with elements of the tissue environment. The essential steps in the formation of a metastasis are essentially similar for all solid tumors and consist of the following:

- *Proliferation* of the tumor cells, supported by growth factors from the tissue environment (paracrine growth) or from the tumor cells themselves (autocrine growth). Overexpression of the tyrosine kinase receptors, such as the epidermal growth factor receptor (EGFR) and *c-erbB-2*/HER2/*neu*, may confer a growth advantage, and some breast cancer cells are reported to overexpress and respond to transforming growth factor (TGF)-α in an autocrine manner.
- *Neovascularization* or *angiogenesis* is necessary for the continued growth of a tumor of greater than 1 to 2 mm^3. This is made possible by new blood vessel growth, promoted by angiogenic factors released by both tumor cells and local stromal tissues. The balance between angiogenic promoters and inhibitors controls the establishment of a new capillary network, originating from surrounding vessels.
- Some tumor cells show reduced or no expression of cohesive molecules, contributing to increased *motility*, and therefore increasing the likelihood of detachment and movement away from the primary tumor.
- *Invasion* from the primary tumor is a complex process involving destruction of basement membranes and connective tissues, adhesion and motility in response to paracrine or autocrine motility factors.
- Distant metastasis requires the entry of cancer cells into blood or lymphatic vessels, potentially leading to *dissemination* throughout the body as single cells or emboli.
- The emboli can *arrest* in draining lymph nodes or organ capillary beds and may adhere to the endothelial cells or to exposed subendothelial basement membrane.
- Some of the cells *extravasate*, using similar mechanisms as those for invasion of the vessels; however,

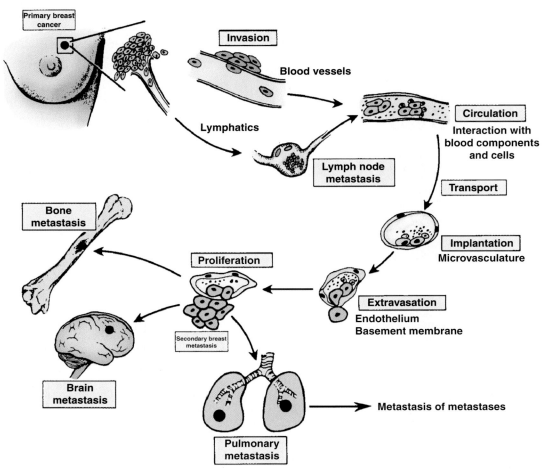

Figure 30-1   The pathogenesis of breast cancer metastasis. The process of breast cancer metastasis is sequential and requires that metastatic cells complete all steps of the highly selective events.

extravasation is not required, because some cancer cells can proliferate actively within the vessel lumen.

- *Growth* in the new organ site, as for the original primary tumor, is dependent on responses to paracrine or autocrine factors, and establishment of a vascular network. Once established, a metastatic lesion can itself serve as the source of more metastases (i.e., the phenomenon of "*metastasis of metastases*").

The time course of the events of metastasis can vary greatly. The survival of cells in the circulation may be relatively brief; experimental studies using various methods of labeling cancer cells that were then injected into appropriate host animals have shown that the cells can reach a potential metastasis site within minutes. However, once established in a distant site, the growth rates of different metastases are highly variable. The risk of recurrence in patients with breast cancer is highest in the first 2 years after diagnosis and initial treatment, but some metastases can remain dormant for many years after apparently successful treatment.[3] The mechanisms underlying the dormancy are not known, although experimental studies suggest that this may be linked to the control of angiogenesis.[4]

ANGIOGENESIS AND METASTASIS

Angiogenesis is required for the growth of primary and metastatic tumors.[5] The angiogenic process is mediated by factors released by malignant and normal cells in the microenvironment that can promote or inhibit the outgrowth of endothelial cells from established vessels. The capillary sprouts arise from the division of microvascular endothelial cells and migration of cells toward the source of the angiogenic molecules, requiring invasion and penetration of the stromal tissues. Endothelial cells undergoing sprouting express matrix-degrading proteases, including those of the matrix metalloproteinase family (MMP) and urokinase plasminogen activator (uPA). Molecules that inhibit MMP activity have been found to have antiangiogenic activity and be capable of impeding tumor growth and metastasis in preclinical models.[6] Counting the numbers and density of microscopic blood vessels in sections of breast cancer specimens has been used as a measure of angiogenesis,[7] using antibodies against endothelial markers such as factor VIII–related antigen, CD34, CD105, and the integrin heterodimer $\alpha v\beta 3$ to identify the new blood vessels. Increased microvessel density is associated with a poor prognosis in the majority of published reports.[8]

Breast cancer cells can release a variety of angiogenic factors, including members of the fibroblast growth factor family (FGF-1 and FGF-2), vascular endothelial growth factors (VEGF), platelet-derived endothelial cell growth factor (PD-ECGF, also known as *thymidine phosphorylase*), interleukin (IL)-8, angiopoietins, platelet-derived growth factors (PDGF), and TGF-α and TGF-β.[9–13] Normal cells within the tissue environment, such as endothelial cells, epithelial cells, mast cells and leukocytes, can also release proangiogenic factors. Macrophage infiltration into invasive breast cancers can be elevated in the highly angiogenic tumors[14] with the tumor-associated macrophages (TAMs) clustered in areas of central necrosis. TAMs can release angiogenic factors such as VEGF and tumor necrosis factor (TNF)-α and proteolytic enzymes that activate profactors or factors sequestered in the extracellular matrix.[15] The appearance of necrosis in angiogenic tumors may result from the growth of the tumor cells outpacing the ingrowth of new blood vessels. Hypoxic conditions, resulting from focal ischemia, can upregulate expression of a variety of genes that may contribute to malignant progression, including angiogenic factors such as VEGF and IL-8.[16]

Members of the VEGF family (A, B, C, and D) are commonly reported as important angiogenic factors associated with poor prognosis for patients with breast cancer.[17,18] VEGF-A, present in four major isoforms resulting from alternate splicing, binds and activates VEGFR-2 tyrosine kinase receptors on endothelial cells. There are some reports also of VEGF-receptors on breast cancer cells, suggesting an autocrine mechanism promoting growth, motility, and invasion.[19] VEGF-B binds to the VEGFR-1 tyrosine kinase receptor, and in endothelial cells this has been shown to increase the expression and activity of uPA and plasminogen activator (PAI)-1.[20] In a study of VEGF-B levels in breast tissues, there was no significant relationship between presence of the factor and tumor vascularity, but there was a significant relationship with the numbers of lymph nodes with metastases.[17] VEGF-B may contribute to cancer progression by a role in the regulation of matrix degradation and cell adhesion of endothelial cells undergoing angiogenesis and vascular remodeling.[20] VEGF-C and VEGF-D have been associated with lymphangiogenesis, and both factors bind to the lymphatic endothelial cell receptor VEGFR-3. VEGF-C is a growth factor for lymphatic vascular endothelium and stimulates lymphangiogenesis in chorioallantoic membrane assays. Measurements of VEGF-C RNA in tissue specimens have shown a correlation with metastasis to lymph nodes of patients with breast cancer.[21] Experimental studies demonstrated that introduction of VEGF-C into cancer cell lines resulted in increased intratumor lymphangiogenesis and promoted the growth and metastasis of the xenografts in immunodeficient mice.[22] VEGF-D also promotes tumor lymphangiogenesis and metastatic spread of experimental tumors via lymphatics.[23] Assessing the degree of lymphangiogenesis in cancer specimens has been problematic because of poor availability of reagents to identify lymphatic-specific markers. Markers used in recent reports include antibodies recognizing podoplanin, LYVE-1, and Prox-1.[18,24] Significant associations have been reported between angiogenic cytokine expression, lymphatic vessel density, and lymph node metastases, notably for VEGF-C, suggesting that these factors contribute to the malignant progression of breast cancer through promotion of lymphangiogenesis.[25]

The importance of angiogenesis for cancer progression has led to the development of therapies targeting either the angiogenic factors or receptors responding to the factors.[26] An antibody to VEGF, bevacizumab, when used in combination with paclitaxel has been shown to prolong the progression-free survival of women with metastatic breast cancer.[27]

Angiogenesis is determined by the balance between promoters and inhibitors of new blood vessel growth. A variety of endogenous antiangiogenic molecules have been identified, including angiostatin, endostatin, thrombospondin (TSP1), interferon-α, and IL-12.[28] In normal tissues, an inhibitory influence may predominate, and the activation of an "angiogenic switch" may be required for the further growth of the cancer cells, or to allow release from a dormant state.[4] Systemic administration of angiostatin, a fragment of plasminogen, was shown to restrict the growth and metastasis of human and rodent cancers in experimental models and induce dormancy of micrometastatic foci.[29] In a transgenic mouse model of pancreatic carcinogenesis, a key component of the angiogenic switch was MMP-9, acting potentially through increased proteolytic release of VEGF-A sequestered in extracellular matrix.[30] In the MMTV-PyMT transgenic model of mammary tumorigenesis, there is evidence that tumor-associated macrophages are essential for regulating the angiogenic switch and promoting malignant progression of the tumors.[31]

INVASION

Breast cancer cell invasion through the basement membranes of ducts and lobules can result in cells entering vascular and lymphatic vessels. The penetration of basement membranes and connective tissues of the breast is mediated by the synthesis of degradative enzymes, by normal and neoplastic cells in the microenvironment.[6,32] There are four major groups of proteases: (1) MMPs, collagenases, gelatinases, stromelysins; (2) cysteine proteases (cathepsin B, H, L); (3) aspartyl proteases (cathepsin D); and (4) serine proteases (i.e., plasminogen activators [uPA, tPA] and the activated product plasmin). Several inhibitory molecules have been identified, including the tissue inhibitors of metalloproteinase (TIMP-1, TIMP-2, and TIMP-3) and PAI-1 and PAI-2. Proteolytic activity represents a balance between the proteolytic enzymes, activators of the enzymes (e.g., membrane-type MMPs) and the inhibitory molecules. The expression of proteases is normally under the control of cytokines and growth factors such as PDGF, TGF-β, amphiregulin, EGF interferons, IL-4, and IL-6. Estrogen and progesterone can also regulate proteolytic enzyme expression and the invasive potential of breast cancer cells.[33]

Data from in vitro and experimental studies provide evidence for the role of two MMPs that degrade the collagen type IV of basement membranes, MMP-2 and

MMP-9, in invasion and metastasis. Metastatic clones of heterogeneous tumors often express elevated levels of these enzymes, and the introduction of an inhibitory molecule can reduce invasive and metastatic ability. TIMP-1 can bind to and inhibit the activity of MMP-9, and TIMP-2 complexes with the latent and active forms of MMP-2. The expression levels of MMP-2, MMP-3, and MMP-9, uPA, and TIMP-1 and TIMP-2 were found to be elevated in breast cancer samples compared with normal tissue, and the total proteolytic activity was higher in the neoplastic samples.[34] Whereas protease production by tumor cells is implicated in invasion, many proteases are also produced by stromal cells, in addition to the malignant epithelial cells. The net increase in protease activity in tumor tissue samples may be a function of induction of stromal cell expression of the proteases, in response to tumor-derived factors such as cytokines and extracellular matrix metalloprotease inducer (EMMPRIN).[35,36] Immunolocalization of different components of the MMP system point to the important role of the membrane-type MMPs (MT1, MT2 and MT3-MMP) as activators of MMP-2 and facilitating the invasion and clinical progression of invasive breast cancers.[37] Invasive lobular cancers were shown to express more abundant MMP-9 than invasive ductal cancers, and colocalization of MT1-MMP and MMP-2 in both types of invasive cancer was significantly associated with the presence of lymph node metastases.[38]

The contributions of the MMP system and uPA system to tumor progression go beyond the dissolution of barriers constraining cancer cell invasion. In addition to the degradation of ECM and basement membranes, other actions of proteases include cleavage and activation of growth factors (e.g., latent TGF-β) and other factors that act as angiogenic factors (VEGF-C and two forms of PDGF [C and D]), which are activated or have enhanced binding to receptors after proteolytic activation.[6,39,40] Release and activation of the factors can have an impact on the growth of tumors, increasing local availability of growth factors to tumor cells and to stromal cells, including the endothelial cells forming the new blood supply essential for continued tumor growth.

CELL-TO-CELL COHESION AND MOTILITY

Most tumor cells possess the cytoplasmic machinery that is necessary for active locomotion, and increased tumor cell motility is preceded by a loss of cell-to-cell cohesion. Members of the cadherin family of cell surface glycoproteins are essential for cell-cell adhesion and maintenance of tissue integrity.[41] Cadherins are linked to the actin cytoskeleton via association with the cytoplasmic catenins α, β, and γ. β-Catenin is also involved in the Wnt-1 signaling pathway and gene transcription through interactions with the TCF-1/LEF transcription factor.[42] For many epithelial cancers, the loss of contact is associated with the loss of expression of one of the cadherin family members, E-cadherin. In experimental studies, the enforced expression of E-cadherin in highly malignant cells has been shown to reduce or inhibit invasive and metastatic abilities.[43,44] Analyses of breast cancers show that loss or reduced expression of E-cadherin

and catenins can correlate with a poor prognosis.[45] The gene encoding E-cadherin is located on chromosome 16q22.1, an area of frequent loss of heterozygosity in sporadic breast cancers. Loss of E-cadherin is more common in specimens of lobular carcinoma than ductal carcinoma; specimens of this type of breast cancer can show heterogeneous protein expression. For the lobular types, loss of E-cadherin expression has been linked to loss of heterozygosity and somatic mutation in the remaining allele. No such mutations have been reported in ductal carcinomas (or cell lines derived from ductal tumors), and reduced expression is thought to be due to epigenetic changes, including promoter hypermethylation or repression by the Snail family of transcription factors.[41,46] Loss of E-cadherin expression is considered a hallmark of epithelial-mesenchymal transition (EMT). There is increasing interest in the contribution of this phenomenon to cancer invasion and metastasis, because the changes in cell adhesion and migration of metastatic cells are similar to what is seen in developmental EMT.[47] However, the contribution of EMT to metastatic progression remains controversial, and events defining the transition are not easily documented in clinical specimens.[48] The transcription factors, including Snail family members, bHLH and ZEB factors, which regulate expression of E-cadherin and other EMT-related genes, also regulate additional genes that may contribute to the growth or survival of malignant cells.[49] Abnormal expression of Snail factors has been reported in breast cancer specimens,[50] and high Snail expression was linked in one study with shorter overall survival in women with metastatic disease.[51] In contrast to what is seen with most breast cancers, E-cadherin expression is reported to be maintained in inflammatory breast cancer,[52] showing therefore an exception to the more general observation of loss of this adhesion molecule and poor prognosis for breast cancers.[53]

Tumor cell motility is an active process dependent on the release of motility-promoting factors and activation of receptors. Motility and migration of normal and malignant cells can be promoted by cytokines released by other cells in the tissue environment or by the cancer cells.[54] Autocrine motility factor (AMF) is a protein produced by malignant cells that binds to its own surface receptor and can stimulate motility and metastatic properties in experimental systems. Elevated expression of AMF and its receptor AMFR was associated with shorter patient survival in women with breast cancer.[55] Heregulin treatment of HER2-expressing breast cancer cells stimulated AMF expression, and treatment with Herceptin blocked this increase.[56]

Another factor that promotes motility is hepatocyte growth factor (HGF), which binds to c-met, a member of the tyrosine kinase family of cell surface receptors. Higher expression of c-met has been reported as an independent predictor of decreased survival for women with invasive ductal breast carcinoma.[57] HGF is released by mesenchymal/stromal cells, as well as epithelial cells. There are reports of coexpression of HGF, activators and inhibitors of this factor, and the c-met receptor in breast carcinomas, suggesting a potential autocrine mechanism of promoting motility.[58] Signaling through c-met has also been associated with enhanced survival from DNA-damaging agents and increased angiogenesis, hence contributing to survival of the metastatic cells.[57]

Chemokine receptors have been identified as potential players in determining patterns of breast cancer metastasis. Chemokines, cytokine-like proteins, and their G-protein–coupled receptors promote motility and direct the homing of hematopoietic cells; experimental data suggest that tumor cells can use similar mechanisms. The chemokine receptors CXCR4 and CXCR7 were found on breast cancer tissues and cell lines, and some reports have linked higher expression of these receptors with increased metastasis.[59,60] The respective ligands CXCL12 and CCL21 were detected at highest levels in organs where breast cancer cells can form metastases, such as bone marrow, lymph nodes, and lung. Treatment with an antibody to CXCR4 blocked motility and invasion in vitro and metastasis of human breast cancer cells to lymph nodes and lungs of mice with severe combined immunodeficiency syndrome.[61] Thus interfering with chemokine receptors, and blocking the cancer cell interaction with organ-derived chemokines, may be another approach for inhibiting metastasis.

CELL-TO-CELL ADHESION

Adhesion of tumor cells to other tumor cells (homotypic adhesion) or other cell types (heterotypic adhesion) are considered essential steps in the formation of metastases. Experimental studies have shown that the arrest of tumor emboli is more efficient than the arrest of single cells in capillary networks of organs such as the lungs.[62] Numerous molecules that can facilitate heterotypic adhesions and adhesion to extracellular matrix have been identified, and they can be classified into the general categories of cadherins, selectins, immunoglobulin-like cell adhesion molecules, and integrins. Aberrant or dysregulated expression of many of these have been reported in breast and other epithelial cancers.[63-65] The initial binding of tumor cells to capillary endothelial cells under flow conditions is primarily mediated by selectin molecules, followed by more stable integrin-mediated binding and subsequent migration through the subendothelial basement membrane. Aberrant expression of integrins has been proposed as a possible therapeutic target (e.g., the $\alpha v\beta 3$ integrin on cancer cells, mature osteoclasts, and angiogenic endothelial cells with a monoclonal antibody or peptide antagonists) against the integrin heterodimer to potentially inhibit both tumor and stromal cells.[66,67] There is also increasing evidence that altered expression of cell adhesion molecules has an impact not only on the adhesive interactions of malignant cells but also on signal transduction pathways important for cell survival, proliferation, and differentiation.[65] Notably, focal-adhesion kinase (FAK), found at sites of integrin clustering, is considered an important mediator of growth factor signaling and cell migration.[68] Increased FAK expression and activity is associated with poor disease prognosis in various cancer types, and FAK has been shown in a rodent model of mammary tumor metastasis to be required for lung metastasis.[69]

LYMPHATIC METASTASIS

In the process of invasion from the primary lesion and through infiltration and expansion in the surrounding tissues, tumor cells can penetrate small lymphatic vessels. The spread of tumor cells via the lymphatics has been documented and studied for centuries. The presence of breast cancer cells in axillary lymph nodes has very high prognostic significance, yet until recently surprisingly little was known about the mechanisms of lymphatic metastasis.[25] The introduction of reagents to reliably identify lymphatic endothelial cells has facilitated the detection of tumor-induced lymphangiogenesis, and experimental studies have identified VEGF-C and VEGF-D as mediators of interactions between tumor cells and lymphatic endothelial cells.[70] The enforced expression of either factor in experimental tumors was shown to increase lymphangiogenesis in the tumors and promote lymphatic metastasis.[22,23] Once inside the lymphatics, tumor cells or emboli may be passively transported to arrest either in the first lymph node downstream or bypass to more distal nodes. The microenvironment of the lymph nodes is a rich source for growth factors and chemokines that can promote tumor motility, survival, or growth. Experimental studies with rodent or rabbit tumors illustrated that lymph nodes can act as physical barriers to tumor cells traveling in lymphatics. However, tumor cells have also been found in venous effluent and lymphatic efferent vessels of lymph nodes with metastases. Hence, the lymph node metastases might be the source of hematogenous or further lymphatic spread.[71] Hellman has proposed a "spectrum hypothesis," describing breast cancer as a spectrum of heterogeneous diseases, with increasing propensity to metastasize as tumors become more malignant through clinical evolution. His hypothesis proposes that the presence of lymph node metastases serves both as a marker of prognosis and as a source of additional metastases.[72] The fact that lymphadenectomy does not affect overall survival may be a reflection of the systemic nature of the disease once lymph node metastasis has occurred. The use of sentinel lymph node biopsy as a staging procedure for breast cancer can reduce unnecessary axillary lymph node dissection and associated morbidity in women with negative sentinel nodes.[73] However, a report has associated lymphangiogenesis within metastasis-positive sentinel nodes with metastatic involvement of nonsentinel nodes, supporting a hypothesis that sentinel nodes are involved in further metastatic dissemination.[74] As the mechanisms underlying lymphatic metastasis are elucidated, possible therapeutic interventions to prevent or restrict lymphatic metastasis may be realized.[25]

HEMATOGENOUS METASTASIS

For hematogenous metastasis, tumor cells must survive transport in the circulation, arrest and form adhesions in small vessels and capillaries, and extravasate by invading through the vessel wall; however, hematogenous metastasis is considered an inefficient process that eliminates most cells in the circulation.[75] The survival of a few cells may represent the selection of preexisting subpopulations of cells endowed with the properties required to form metastases.[76] With the advent of sensitive detection methods, the presence of circulating tumor cells is being proposed as an additional source of prognostic information. Although one report described most circulating breast cancer cells as apoptotic,[77] others have found viable cells in the peripheral blood of patients with breast cancer.[78] The number of circulating cells in pretreatment samples was found to be an independent predictor of survival of women with metastatic breast cancer.[79]

Death of cells within the circulation has been attributed to simple mechanical factors, most notably turbulence. Factors that contribute to the survival of cells in the circulation may include the propensity to form either homotypic, or heterotypic aggregates with normal cells such as platelets or lymphocytes.[80,81] Components of the blood clotting pathway may also contribute to the metastatic process by trapping cells in capillaries or facilitating adherence of cells to vessel walls. Circulating tumor cells can be thromboplastic, and increased coagulability is commonly observed in patients with advanced cancers. There is good experimental evidence that fibrinolytic agents and inhibitors of platelet aggregation, such as prostacyclin, can reduce or inhibit hematogenous metastases in rodent models. However, clinical studies have yet to provide similarly convincing evidence that anticoagulant agents can effectively prevent or reduce blood-borne metastases.[82]

Once in the microcirculation, the metastatic cells interact with cells of the vascular endothelium. The interaction may begin as nonspecific lodging of the tumor cell or emboli, followed by formation of adhesions mediated by cell surface molecules such as selectins and integrins, recognizing ligands on the endothelial cells and the subendothelial matrix.[83,84] Once bound to endothelial cells, tumor cells elicit endothelial cell retraction, resulting in the exposure of the basement membrane.[85] There is increasing evidence of phenotypic heterogeneity in capillary endothelial cells isolated from different organs as well as of endothelial cells populating tumors and metastases. The identification of "vascular addresses" by phage display techniques has been used to target therapy to lung metastases in experimental models.[86] Endothelial cell heterogeneity may also be a determinant of organ specific metastasis, with tumor cells expressing a certain repertoire of cell surface molecules being more likely to arrest and extravasate in capillaries of organ with a particular vascular address.[87]

Extravasation of arrested tumor cells is thought to occur by mechanisms similar to those responsible for local invasion and release into the circulation. Tumor cells can penetrate the endothelial basement membrane or follow extravasating lymphocytes. Alternatively, the tumor cells can proliferate within the vessel and ultimately destroy the normal structure.[88] The invasion, survival, and growth of tumor cells in the metastatic site can be in response to factors present in the tissue or organ. Metastatic tumor cells can recognize and respond to organ-specific factors, whereas nonmetastatic counterparts fail to respond.[62] An example of one such factor

is CXCL12, the ligand for CXCR4, an important factor for promoting metastatic cell homing to sites with high levels of the chemokine.[89]

Recent developments in imaging technology have provided some further insights into steps of hematogenous metastasis. Fluorescent labeling of tumor cells was used to show that the rate of intravasation at the site of primary implanted tumors distinguished metastatic from poorly metastatic rat mammary tumor cells, identifying this step as critical in determining the metastatic potential of these tumors.[90] Chambers and colleagues[91] included plastic microspheres with the test cell inoculum to develop an accounting technique, and they have shown that the survival of tumor cells within the circulation and arrest in the microcirculation is not such an inefficient process as has been previously proposed. The data from the in vivo videomicroscopy using transplantable rodent tumors suggests that survival, arrest, and extravasation of metastatic and nonmetastatic or poorly metastatic cells in mouse liver is equally likely. However, after extravasation, few of the poorly metastatic cells proliferate to form metastatic lesions; many cells persist in the liver, yet remain dormant.[91] Elimination of extravasated cells that do not become dormant may be the result of apoptosis. In vivo videomicroscopy was used in another study to follow the fate of intravenously injected cells and showed that many of these cells underwent apoptosis in the lungs of the recipient animals within 24 to 48 hours.[92] The new imaging techniques may help revise or refine the general understanding of different steps in the process of metastasis.[75]

METASTASIS-RELATED GENES

Considering that the metastatic process should be viewed as a sequence of different events, it is not surprising that a variety of genes have been nominated as key players in determining the metastatic phenotype of breast cancer cells. Examples of breast cancer metastasis-associated genes include growth factor receptors (HER2/*neu* and EGFR), angiogenic factors, adhesion molecules such as E-cadherin, and degradative enzymes that will facilitate invasion. An experimental approach used by many investigators is the identification of genes differentially expressed in metastatic versus nonmetastatic counterparts, using rodent or human tumor cells. A key point is that for optimal comparative analyses, the tumor samples should be isogenic (i.e., clones or variants of a single tumor) and vary only in the capacity for metastasis.[93-95] Table 30-1 shows examples of genes that have been implicated in the metastasis of breast cancer and for which there is experimental evidence for a potential mechanism to promote or reduce metastatic progression. For some of these, measurements of protein in patient samples have been associated with the prognosis. Table 30-2 identifies four genes found to have metastasis-suppressing activity in in vivo models of breast cancer.[96] Clinical studies have shown support for the involvement of these in breast cancer progression, although there have been some conflicting reports on the role of *KiSS1*, possibly related to the estrogen receptor (ER) status of the breast cancers.[97] A concept

TABLE 30-1

Genes associated with Breast Cancer Metastasis

Gene	Origin	Known or Proposed Mechanism	Clinical Observations	References
S100A4	Upregulated in metastatic mammary tumors	Regulator of the cytoskeleton	Expression correlated with poor prognosis	See footnotes[a]
MTA-1	Differentially expressed in metastatic rat mammary tumors	Gene regulation	Gene present in node positive breast cancers	See footnotes[b]
Osteopontin	Increased expression in metastatic clones of rat and human breast cancer	Extracellular phosphoprotein; interactions with integrins; protection from macrophage-mediated killing	Elevated plasma levels associated with poor prognosis	See footnotes[c]
bcl-2	Introduction into breast cancer cells conferred metastatic ability	Inhibitor of apoptosis	Expression associated with lymph node metastasis	See footnotes[d]
maspin	Reduced expression in cancer cells	Serine protease inhibitor	Reduced expression in metastatic breast cancer	See footnotes[e]
Twist-1	Differentially expressed in metastatic mammary tumor clones	Transcriptional regulator	Expressed in bone marrow micrometastases of breast cancer patients	See footnotes[f]
CXCR4	Increased expression in metastatic breast cancer cell lines	Chemokine receptor	Elevated expression in metastatic cancers	See footnotes[g]

[a]Rudland PS, Platt-Higgins A, Renshaw C, et al: Prognostic significance of the metastasis-inducing protein S100A4 (p9Ka) in human breast cancer. Cancer Res 60:1595–1603, 2000; and Platt-Higgins AM, Renshaw C, West CR, et al: Comparison of the metastasis-inducing protein S100A4 (p9Ka) with other prognostic markers in human breast cancer. Int J Cancer (Pred Oncol) 89:198–208, 2000.

[b]Nawa A, Nishimori K, Lin P, et al: Tumor metastasis-associated human MTA1 gene: Its deduced protein sequence, localization, and association with breast cancer cell proliferation using antisense phosphorothioate oligonucleotides. J Cell Biochem 79:202–212, 2000; and Martin MD, Fischbach K, Osborne CK, et al: Loss of heterozygosity events impeding breast cancer metastasis contain the MTA1 gene. Cancer Res 61: 3578–3580, 2001.

[c]Singhal H, Bautista DS, Tonkin KS, et al: Elevated plasma osteopontin in metastatic breast cancer associated with increased tumor burden and decreased survival. Clin Cancer Res 3:605–611, 1999; and Feng B, Rollo EE, Denhardt DT: Osteopontin (OPN) may facilitate metastasis by protecting cells from macrophage NO-mediated cytotoxicity: Evidence from cell lines down-regulated for OPN expression by a targeted ribozyme. Clin Exp Metastasis 13:453–462, 1995.

[d]Sierra A, Castellsague X, Escobedo A, et al: Bcl-2 with loss of apoptosis allows accumulation of genetic alterations: A pathway to metastatic progression in human breast cancer. Int J Cancer 89:142–147, 2000; and Del BD, Biroccio A, Leonetti C, Zupi G: Bcl-2 overexpression enhances the metastatic potential of a human breast cancer cell line. FASEB J 11: 947–953, 1997.

[e]Maass N, Teffner M, Rosel F, et al: Decline in the expression of the serine proteinase inhibitor maspin is associated with tumor progression in ductal carcinomas of the breast. J Pathol 195:321–326, 2001; and Sheng S, Carey J, Seftor EA, et al: Maspin acts at the cell membrane to inhibit invasion and motility of mammary and prostatic cancer cells. Proc Natl Acad Sci USA 93:11669–11674, 1996.

[f]Yang J, Mani SA, Donaher JL, et al: Twist, a master regulator of morphogenesis, plays an essential role in tumor metastasis. Cell 117: 927–939, 200; and Watson MA, Ylagan LR, Trinkaus KM, et al: Isolation and molecular profiling of bone marrow micrometastases identifies TWIST1 as a marker of early tumor relapse in breast cancer patients. Clin Cancer Res 13:5001–5009, 2007.

[g]Kato M, Kitayama J, Kazama S, Nagawa H[59]; Cabioglu N, Yazici MS, Arun B, et al[60]; and Müller A, Homey B, Soto H, et al.[61]

emerging from studies of metastasis suppression is that of suppression of the growth and development of cells arrested in the metastatic site.[98] If so, this points to new approaches for checking the growth of metastases, which have disseminated before diagnosis and treatment of the primary tumor, by introducing agents that can reproduce the action of the suppressor gene product but with less systemic toxicity than standard antineoplastic drugs.

Further information about what regulates the metastasis-associated and the metastasis suppressor genes may identify ways to modify their expression. For example, promoter methylation can silence gene expression, and exposure of human breast cancer cells to the DNA methylation inhibitor 5-aza-2′-deoxycytidine has been reported to increase expression of nm23 and suppress cell motility.[99]

MicroRNA (miRNA) is now recognized as an important class of gene regulatory molecules, targeting mRNA for cleavage or translational repression. MiRNAs can act as oncogenes by inhibition of tumor suppressors, or through interference in pathways controlling differentiation or apoptosis.[100] A recent report suggested a role for miRNA in the regulation of metastasis, showing high expression of miR-10b in metastatic breast cancer cells and linking mi-R10b with Twist-1 and RhoC, two genes previously reported to promote the metastatic potential of breast cancer.[101] The analysis of germline polymorphisms in different mouse strains adds another factor that may regulate the outcome of metastasis.[102] Hunter and associates found significant variation in the metastatic ability of transgenic mammary tumors driven by polyoma middle-T antigen in different strains of mice, and they identified SIPA1 as one gene that can regulate metastatic efficiency in this model. A further study by these authors using analysis of leukocyte DNA from breast cancer patients showed that SIPA1 germline polymorphisms were associated with aggressive disease,[103] suggesting

		TABLE 30-2		

Genes with Metastasis-Suppressing Function in Breast Cancer

Gene	Origin	Known or Proposed Mechanism	Clinical Observations	References
Nm23	Differentially expressed, lost in metastatic melanoma cells.	Control of cell cycle progression; protein phosphorylation; transcription.	Reduced expression; absence correlated with poor prognosis.	See footnotes[a]
KAI1	Chromosome hybrid studies; suppressor of prostate cancer metastasis.	Tetraspanin; suggested roles in aggregation, motility, invasion.	Reduced expression in invasive breast cancers.	See footnotes[b]
KiSS1	Chromosome hybrid studies; suppressor of melanoma and breast cancer metastasis.	Ligand for G-protein coupled receptor, inhibits invasion.	Loss of KiSS1 expression in malignant tumors	See footnotes[c]
BRMS1	Isolated in metastasis-suppressed chromosome hybrids of breast cancer cells.	Mediates gap junctional cell-cell communication; suppressed motility.	Reduced BRMS1 expression associated with poor prognosis	See footnotes[d]

[a]Hennessy C, Henry JA, May FEB, et al: Expression of the antimetastatic gene nm23 in human breast cancer: An association with good prognosis. J Natl Cancer Inst 83:281–285, 1991; and Freije JMP, MacDonald NJ, Steeg PS: Differential gene expression in tumor metastasis: Nm23. Curr Top Microbiol Immunol 213:215–232, 1996.

[b]Dong JT, Lamb PW, Rinker-Schaeffer CW, et al: KAI1, a metastasis suppressor gene for prostate cancer on human chromosome 11p.11.2. Science 268:884–886, 1995; Yang X, Wei L, Tang C, et al: KAI1 protein is down-regulated during the progression of human breast cancer. Clin Cancer Res 6: 3424–3429, 2000; and Bandyopadhyay S, Zhan R, Chaudhuri A, et al: Interaction of KAI1 on tumor cells with DARC on vascular endothelium leads to metastasis suppression. Nat Med 12:933–938, 2006.

[c]Harms JF, Welch DR, Miele ME: KISS1 metastasis suppression and emergent pathways. Clin Exp Metastasis 20:11–18, 2003; and Marot D, Bieche I, Aumas C, et al.[97]

[d]Seraj MJ, Samant RS, Verderame MF, Welch DR: Functional evidence for a novel human breast carcinoma metastasis suppressor, BRMS1, encoded at chromosome 11q13. Cancer Res 60: 2764–2769, 2000; and Zhang Z, Yamashita H, Toyama T, et al: Reduced expression of the breast cancer metastasis suppressor 1 mRNA is correlated with poor prognosis in breast cancer. Clin Cancer Res 12:6410–6414, 2006.

that genetic factors in addition to gene aberrations in the malignant cells might influence the outcome of metastasis.

Patterns of Metastasis

CLINICAL AND AUTOPSY FINDINGS

Clinical observations have shown that some cancers have a marked preference for metastasis in specific organs that is not necessarily related to the vascular anatomy, rate of blood flow, or the numbers of tumor cells that may arrive in the organ. In 1889, Stephen Paget published an analysis of 735 autopsy records from women with breast cancer, and the nonrandom pattern of visceral metastases suggested that the process was not a result of chance but rather that certain tumor cells ("seeds") had an affinity for the milieu provided by certain organs ("soils").[104] Animal studies have demonstrated that the formation and anatomical locations of metastases are determined by host factors and tumor cell properties,[105] and the results have been proposed as experimental examples of Paget's seed and soil hypothesis.[61]

The use of peritoneovenous shunts in patients with intransigent malignant ascites provided an opportunity to study factors affecting metastatic spread in humans. The published studies on 29 patients with different primary tumors (the most common was ovarian carcinoma) reported that the peritoneovenous shunts provided good palliation with minimal complications. Autopsy findings from 15 patients showed that the shunts did not promote widespread systemic metastasis;

in only eight were metastases found in extra-abdominal organs, and in seven there was no evidence of metastasis. These results suggest that even though the tumor cells were introduced into the circulation, micrometastases formed only in some sites, or did not form at all.[94] The interpretation that the outcome of tumor cell dissemination is determined by both tumor cells and normal organ factors, as originally proposed by Paget,[104] may be correct.

INFLUENCE OF THE ORGAN ENVIRONMENT ON METASTASIS: EXPERIMENTAL ANALYSES

Paget's hypothesis that the soil can determine whether metastases form, in combination with attributes of the metastatic cells, has been tested in various experimental rodent tumor systems, or using human tumors transplanted into immunodeficient animals. Tracking the hematogenous distribution of radiolabeled tumor cells injected into suitable hosts has shown that cells reach the microvasculature of most organs sampled; however, the proliferation of the cells occurs only in some organs.[94] Some recent data from studies of metastasis suppressor genes suggest that one mechanism may be growth arrest of cells in the microenvironment of the sites of metastasis, even though the growth of the primary tumor is not restricted.[98]

A model used for testing the seed and soil hypothesis was developed by Hart and Fidler using the B16 murine melanoma. The intravenous injection of these cells into syngeneic mice resulted in the growth of tumors in the lungs and also in fragments of ovary or lung previously grafted into the quadriceps femoris of the host mice. In contrast, no tumors formed in control grafts of kidney or at sites of surgical trauma. When radiolabeled cells were injected, and the distribution patterns monitored, there were no differences between distribution to legs grafted with lung compared with the control grafts.[105] Thus the lungs (grafts or intact) provided a receptive organ for the proliferation of the tumor cells that reached these sites. The model of engrafting different tissues has been used to study aspects of organ-specific metastasis of human tumor cells, with grafts of human fetal tissue placed in mice with severe combined immunodeficiency syndrome.[106,107] Injection of human prostate or lung tumors resulted in species- and tissue-specific patterns of metastasis, therefore providing systems for studying the tissue interactions involved in growth of human tumors in human tissues, which may not be readily simulated with culture techniques. For example, the technique allowed analysis of mechanisms involved in the preferential homing of human prostate cancer cells to grafts of fetal bone but not to grafts of lung or intestine.[107] In vitro experiments have provided some insight into organ selectivity by analyzing adhesion and/or growth of different tumors to cells or factors isolated from different organs. A model of human breast cancer cell interactions in tissue cultures revealed that cells isolated from primary tumors or tumor-involved lymph nodes bound preferentially to bone marrow stromal cells rather than to mammary fibroblasts, whereas epithelial cells isolated from benign or normal breast tissues revealed no preference for adhesion to the stromal cells.[108] Lymphatic stromal cells were found to promote the growth of breast cancer cells, and insulin-like growth factor I and epidermal growth factor were identified as two of the key growth regulating factors.[109] In contrast, analysis of muscle cell–conditioned medium identified adenosine as one of the active components restricting tumor cell growth, possibly accounting for the low incidence of metastasis in striated muscle.[110] The findings from these different studies provide further support for the hypothesis that elements within the organ microenvironment can modulate neoplastic proliferation and may therefore play a role in determining the distribution of metastases.[94]

Mechanisms of tumor growth modulation may be related to the homeostatic processes that control normal cell replication and regulate organ growth and repair. Metastatic tumor growth in areas of injury and wound repair has been documented clinically and in a number of experimental systems. One example is the promotion of mammary tumor metastases in the livers of rats following trauma to this organ, with no metastases seen in the noninjured animals.[111] In vitro assays have demonstrated that media from cultures of resorbing bones contain factors capable of modulating normal osteoblasts and also stimulating the proliferation of rodent and human breast tumor cells.[112] These results can be interpreted as the local effects of wound healing (which include neovascularization and tissue remodeling) being subverted to support the growth of cancer cells in the organ or tissue, possibly in a state of dormancy or slow proliferation since arrest in the site before the local injury.

The common sites for breast cancer metastasis, in addition to regional lymph nodes, are lung, liver, brain and bone, with this last site being the most commonly involved. As many as 80% of women with metastatic breast cancer may develop bone metastases.[113] Many of these are lytic lesions, and a variety of growth factors and cytokines released by cancer cells have been shown to promote the activation of osteoclasts, the cells primarily responsible for bone destruction. The destruction of bone is thought to release factors that may in turn promote the growth of cancer cells, creating a "vicious cycle."[114] Inhibitors of bone resorption, such as the bisphosphonates, can reduce the skeletal morbidity in women with advanced breast cancer. The mechanism is thought to be primarily through impeding osteoclastic bone resorption. However, some experimental reports have suggested a direct inhibitory action of bisphosphonates on metastatic cells, preventing adhesion or inhibiting the activation of MMPs.[115] Analyses of clinical specimens and experimental metastatic systems have been used to delineate factors that contribute to the promotion of breast cancer metastasis in bone. One example is parathyroid hormone–related protein (PTHrP), which was identified as a factor responsible for hypercalcemia associated with malignancy. A commonly used experimental model for bone metastasis is the injection of cancer cells into the left ventricle of the heart of rodents, which can result in distribution of tumors in many organs, including bone. This model was used to demonstrate that antibodies to PTHrP reduced the extent of human breast cancer bone metastases, and that TGF-β released from the matrix of resorbing bone can promote the expression of PTHrP by the cancer cells. Compromising the TGF-β receptor function in the cells reduced their potential for bone metastasis.[116] Thus, interfering with components of the "vicious cycle" that promotes bone destruction resulted in a reduction in bone metastasis. The effect of the local microenvironment may be highly significant for bone metastases. PTHrP expression was high in the samples of breast cancer bone metastases, yet an analysis of expression in the primary tumors did not find a correlation between PTHrP and the incidence of bone metastasis or the survival of breast cancer patients, suggesting that this measurement was not a predictor of risk for bone metastasis.[117] Instead, the experimental findings may point to microenvironmental regulation of a factor that promotes osteoclast activation and bone destruction and can enhance the growth of the breast cancer cells in the bone.

A model of tumor cell dissemination in immunodeficient mice was used to generate populations of a human breast cancer cell line with different metastatic abilities and expression array analyses performed to determine the gene expression profiles characteristic of cells metastasizing to lungs or bone. A gene expression signature defined in cells with high lung metastatic potential (in mice) was also found in primary human breast cancers with high risk of metastasis to lungs.[118] The results reflect the underlying heterogeneity in metastatic potential of cells from an individual breast cancer and provide more detailed information about the molecular mechanisms underlying organ-specific metastasis.[95]

Within a tumor mass, individual cells are exposed to different microenvironments, as a function of the anatomical site, and to differences in concentrations of nutrients and oxygen growth factors, among other factors.[16] Microenvironmental factors are thought to have a major impact on the sensitivity of cancer cells to therapy, and hypoxia and low extracellular pH are two of these that have been studied extensively. Cells in chronically hypoxic cancers are growth inhibited and considered likely to be resistant to most anticancer drugs. Low extracellular pH can have the same effect on cell proliferation and thus compound the potential effects of chemotherapy drugs. In addition, there is increasing awareness that exposure to the stresses of hypoxia and low extracellular pH can alter gene expression in tumor cells, inducing expression of genes that can promote the survival of the cells, such as angiogenic or antiapoptotic factors.[119,120] Clinical observations suggest that responses of breast cancer metastases to chemotherapy are influenced by the anatomical location of the lesions, possibly related to differences in microenvironmental stresses.[121,122] Differential sensitivity to antineoplastic treatment of metastases in different locations may be a function of heterogeneity of the tumor population, with different clones metastasizing to different organs. However, the influence of the organ environment cannot be ignored. The results from experimental tumor models have demonstrated that the same tumor implanted in different organs can have different responses to a chemotherapeutic agent. The sensitivity of mouse mammary tumor cells to different chemotherapy agents was assessed in vivo, comparing response in subcutaneous tumors with responses of cells in bone marrow, spleen, lungs, liver, and brain. The subcutaneous tumors were generally sensitive, whereas cells in liver and brain were less sensitive to alkylating agents. Sensitivity of cells in the bone marrow was variable for the different drugs tested, but addition of an antiangiogenic combination (TNP-470/ minocycline) markedly increased killing of the bone marrow metastases by cyclophosphamide.[123] Thus the microenvironment may contribute to the chemotherapy sensitivity of disseminated cancer cells, and altering an aspect of the normal stroma (in this example, the vascular supply) can have an impact on the response to chemotherapy. Understanding the impact of the microenvironment on sensitivity to different forms of therapy may identify important ways to improve the efficiency of eliminating metastatic cells.[124]

The microenvironment of cancers consists of many different cell types, including fibroblasts, lymphocytes, endothelial cells, macrophages, and neutrophils. Serial analysis of gene expression was applied to breast cancer specimens to define gene expression profiles of in situ and invasive cancer cells and corresponding stromal cells. Dramatic gene expression changes were noted in all cell types, including mediators of epithelial-stromal interactions, such as the chemokines CXCL12 and CXCL14.[125] Bone marrow–derived mesenchymal stem cells are reported to be recruited to the stroma of tumors, an ability that may be exploited to deliver antitumor agents.[126] Recruitment of mesenchymal stem cells to tumors, as well as secretion of the chemokine CCL5 to stimulate motility and invasion of human breast cancer

cells growing in immunodeficient mice, illustrates the contribution of stromal-tumor interactions in promoting metastasis.[127] Several steps in the sequence of metastasis involve the same mechanisms used for tissue homing by normal trafficking lymphocytes.[61]

The concept of specialized niches that can regulate normal hematopoietic stem cell differentiation also appears to apply to metastasis. In vivo imaging was used to demonstrate that niches in mouse bone marrow, characterized by expression of E-selectin and CXCL12, promoted engraftment of leukemia cells.[128] Primary tumors can release factors that can prime distant organs to create "premetastatic" niches, for example, by remodeling vasculature in sentinel lymph nodes.[129] Hematopoietic progenitor cells expressing VEGFR-1 have been found clustered in lymph nodes of women with breast cancer. In experimental models, the formation of clusters of these cells precedes the arrival of metastatic cancer cells, and inhibition of VEGFR-1 prevented formation of the premetastatic niches.[130] Identifying the mediators of tumor-stromal interactions and factors that form premetastatic niches, notably chemokines and receptors, can offer new avenues of therapy or chemoprevention by targeting the microenvironment.[131]

Biologic Diversification and Heterogeneity of Metastatic Cancers

There is a large body of literature supporting the concept that individual cancers are composed of diverse cell populations that are heterogeneous for a wide variety of characteristics, and that the heterogeneous expression patterns are passed on to progeny cells, at least for several generations. A number of factors, including microenvironmental factors, may modulate gene expression in different tumor cells.[132] One aspect of tumor heterogeneity is the ability of one tumor cell population to influence the properties of others within the same tumor, in such a way as to modify growth rates, metastatic properties and sensitivity to chemotherapeutic agents.[1,133,134] Cellular heterogeneity is not unique to transformed cells, and normal cells and tissues can be heterogeneous for a wide variety of properties. However, the degree of cellular heterogeneity is often more pronounced in the malignant population than in the counterpart benign or normal tissue. Serial analysis of gene expression was applied to normal and malignant breast specimens, and one observation was that the normal cells had the least variable gene expression profiles. In contrast, a high degree of diversity was found in the malignant tumor samples, although there were few genes universally up-regulated in all tumors.[135]

EVOLUTION OF HETEROGENEOUS NEOPLASMS

Most naturally occurring and induced neoplasms develop from the transformation and proliferation of single cells. Even in tumors in which the progeny of a single cell have diversified to heterogeneous cellular phenotypes, evidence of a clonal origin still exists. Clinical and histologic observations of tumors suggested to Foulds that tumors undergo a series of changes during the course of the disease.[136] For example, a mammary tumor that was initially diagnosed as benign can over a period of many months or years evolve into a malignant tumor. To explain the process of tumor evolution and progression, Nowell suggested that acquired genetic variability within developing clones of tumors, combined with host selection pressures, can bring about the emergence of new clonal sublines of increased growth autonomy or malignancy.[137] Tumor heterogeneity may emerge because individual neoplasms display various rates of phenotypic diversification, yielding different combinations of cellular phenotypes. A benign tumor may be expected to show relatively less diversification when compared with a more malignant counterpart.[138] Studies with clonally derived populations of rodent tumors have shown that certain neoplasms had altered rates of phenotypic diversification, and *phenotypic drift* or *dynamic heterogeneity* are terms used to describe changes in tumor cell properties, especially metastatic ability, which may occur more rapidly than predicated from gradual selection of diversified clones.[76]

One question addressed using clones of rodent and human tumors is whether metastatic variants have a growth advantage over nonmetastatic cells, such that over time the metastatic clones would constitute the majority of cells in a tumor. One experimental approach used exploited the random integration of introduced foreign DNA molecules in the tumor cell genome as a way of generating clones with unique genetic tags, which were identified by Southern blotting. Mixed populations of tagged breast tumor cells were implanted in recipient mice and metastases recovered and analyzed to identify clones. The results from several studies showed that one or a few "growth dominant" clones emerged in both the primary and metastatic tumors.[139] A clinical study of clonality in breast cancer specimens used DNA ploidy analyses and immunohistochemistry for HER2 expression to assess heterogeneity. The results indicated that clonal majorities may be identified in metastases and that these clones can also be detected in the primary tumors,[140] providing an example of selection of clones in metastatic tumors but not the complete dominance seen in experimental systems. This may be a function of the different ways of identifying the clones; a study of clonality of prostate tumors used *p53* mutations and found evidence of limited clonal expansion in the primary tumor, yet significant clonal growth of cells with *p53* mutations in metastases.[141] However, mutations in *p53* can have significant impact on the malignant phenotype and have been linked to increased risk of relapse and metastasis in breast cancer.[142,143] The difference between using a "tag" that can modulate tumor cell phenotype, rather than an inert marker such as used in the experimental studies, may be one reason for the apparent disparity in outcomes.

MOLECULAR HETEROGENEITY OF HUMAN BREAST CANCER

The development of genomic technologies and bioinformatics has provided the means to identify the expression patterns of thousands of genes and proteins in breast cancer specimens. Expression array techniques have confirmed the high level of heterogeneity within and between different breast cancers. The study by Perou and colleagues[144] described distinct molecular phenotypes among the group of breast cancers sampled. Five major subtypes were defined: basal-like, luminal A, luminal B, HER2-positive/ER–negative, and normal breastlike. Survival analyses on a subcohort of patients with locally advanced breast cancer that had received similar treatment showed different outcomes for patients with tumors classified into these different groups, with poor prognosis for patients with basal-like cancers and a better outcome for patients with luminal A-type cancers.[145] ER status has been a major distinguishing factor in the clinical management of breast cancer for decades. The recognition of further subtypes of breast cancer may provide additional insight into tumor heterogeneity and appropriate choices of therapy.[146,147] Expression array analyses have been used to define poor-prognosis gene signatures, with the goal of identifying the breast cancer patients who will benefit most from adjuvant chemotherapy.[148,149] Analyses of gene expression data from different studies can also provide additional insight into the pathobiology of breast cancer, because the molecular signatures include genes involved in various biologic processes, including angiogenesis, matrix remodeling, cell signaling, proliferation, and apoptosis.[147,150,151]

Recent advances in stem cell biology have stimulated a revived interest in cancer stem cells.[152] One possible explanation for the molecular heterogeneity seen in human breast cancers is the transformation of mammary stem cells or of early progenitor cells, resulting in cancers with the distinct phenotypes, such as the basal or luminal subtypes.[153,154] Alternatively, subtype specific genetic or epigenetic events and clonal evolution may be responsible for the heterogeneity. The two explanations are not necessarily mutually exclusive, and the origin and clinical consequences of cancer heterogeneity continue to be active areas of research.[2]

GENETIC AND EPIGENETIC INSTABILITY

The accumulation of genetic changes underlies malignant transformation and progression and the development of heterogeneity within tumor cell populations.[155] Evidence for the linkage of genetic alterations and malignant progression of tumors has come from examination of gross chromosomal alterations.[156,157] In mouse tumor models, mitotic errors and rates of spontaneous mutations were increased in highly metastatic cells as compared with low or nonmetastatic clones.[158] As tumors progress to the metastatic stage, chromosomal alterations and karyotypic anomalies can become more complex.[159] Evidence from loss-of-heterozygosity analyses revealed that genetic changes are relatively rare in hyperplastic breast epithelial cells, yet the incidence increases in premalignant lesions, with further increases in ductal carcinoma in situ. Shared loss-of-heterozygosity profiles between synchronous ductal carcinoma in situ and invasive breast cancer showed that the in situ neoplasms are a precursor of the invasive disease.[138] A similar conclusion was reached from studies using comparative genomic hybridization.[156]

Epigenetic modifications can also contribute to the high rates of cellular diversity found in many malignant populations. The epigenetic changes may be a function of various mechanisms, including DNA methylation, nucleosome remodeling, histone modifications, or other mechanisms that may be responsive to tumor microenvironments.[132,160,161] Methylation-specific polymerase chain reaction assays were used to show extensive methylation in the regulatory region of the estrogen receptor-α gene in ER-negative breast cancer specimens and cell lines. Some of the ER-positive samples also showed methylation in the promoter, resulting in phenotypic heterogeneity that may result in ER-positive tumors recurring as ER-negative tumors.[162] Hypermethylation of various genes, including E-cadherin, ER-α, ER-β, the tumor suppressor p16, and DNA repair gene MGMT, has been reported in human breast cancer specimens, and silencing of multiple genes was associated with reduced patient survival.[163,164]

ORIGIN OF BIOLOGIC DIVERSITY IN METASTASES

Metastases proliferating in the same or different organs can exhibit heterogeneity in a variety of characteristics such as capacity for further metastatic spread, hormone receptor expression, growth rates, and responses to chemotherapy.[1,62] Classic experimental studies have shown that metastasis is a clonally selective process. One of these used x-irradiation of tumor cells to induce random chromosome breaks and rearrangements, generating unique karyotypic patterns that served to identify different clones. When mixed populations were injected into mice and metastases recovered, the karyotype analyses showed that the majority of the metastases were the result of the outgrowth of single clones.[76] Analyses of breast cancer specimens have shown clonality in metastases[159,165,166] yet also that some metastases develop additional genetic abnormalities, reflecting continuing diversification of the metastatic population by genetic and epigenetic mechanisms to create intralesional heterogeneity. The potential for different clonal origins of different metastases from a single primary tumor, plus the continued generation of heterogeneity in the different metastases, may contribute to differences in responses to therapy.

Findings from gene expression array analyses showing similar expression patterns in primary tumors and matched metastases have challenged the concept that metastases are seeded by rare or selected subpopulations from the primary tumor.[167,168] However, the array results represent the average gene expression signatures in RNA extracted from tissues (including stromal elements), which may obscure differential expression of key genes that may regulate the metastatic ability of minor populations of tumor cells. Different investigators have used microarray analyses to identify distinct cellular clones with different metastatic ability isolated from individual tumors. Notably, reports of gene signatures characteristic of metastatic ability to different organs in immunodeficient mice provides evidence of intratumor heterogeneity, as well as the multigenic nature of metastasis.[94,95,169]

The cancer stem cell concept is also relevant to metastasis, and this is an area of current research interest. Wicha and colleagues first identified and characterized CD44+/CD24−/low populations of cells from breast cancer specimens, which had remarkable tumorigenic potential in immunodeficient mice.[170] Molecular characterization of CD44+ and CD24+ cells in breast cancer specimens has revealed that the former population expressed many stem cell markers and showed more aggressive tumor behavior. The different cell types from individual tumors were found to be clonally related but not always identical, supporting a concept of clonal evolution towards heterogeneity.[171] CD44+ populations of tumor cell lines are generally considered to be enriched in tumorigenic and metastatic progenitor cells,[172] yet only a subset of the CD44+/CD24− populations from human breast cancer cell lines were able to form experimental metastases.[173] Theoretically, successful metastatic cells would need the self-renewal ability of stem or progenitor cells, although not all stem cells may be capable of completing all steps of the metastatic process. Recent insights into interactions between cancer cells and the premetastatic niche suggest that microenvironmental factors could dictate the fate of disseminating metastatic stem cells.[174] As more is discovered about the phenotype of cancer stem cells, their significance to metastasis and whether the cells can be targeted for therapy may be revealed.

Conclusions

Metastasis of breast cancer is a complex process that appears to depend on both unique tumor cell phenotypes and normal host factors, and it should be interpreted in the context of the "seed and soil" hypothesis presented by Stephen Paget in 1889. In breast and other cancers, the contributions of regional lymph nodes and distant organ sites to the pathogenesis of metastasis have been recognized. Clinical and experimental data indicate that specific cellular mechanisms exist for tumor cell arrest and implantation, invasion, survival, and growth of metastatic cells in different organs. An important aspect of malignancy is the genetic and phenotypic instability of individual tumor cells and their ability to undergo diversification to form heterogeneous populations. Distinct originating cells (stem cells) and genetic and epigenetic events driving malignant transformation are two nonmutually exclusive explanations for the intra- and inter-heterogeneity of human breast cancers. A major obstacle to successful clinical management of established metastases may well be the diversification and heterogeneity resulting from continuing malignant progression. A better understanding of the molecular mechanisms regulating the process of breast cancer metastasis and of the complex interactions between the metastatic cells and the organ environment provides a rational foundation for the design of more effective therapies for different cancers and new options for clinical management of metastatic cancer.

REFERENCES

1. Heppner GH: Cancer cell societies and tumor progression. Stem Cells 11:199–203, 1993.
2. Polyak K: Breast cancer: Origins and evolution. J Clin Invest 117:3155–3163, 2007.
3. Demicheli R, Abbattista A, Miceli R, et al: Time distribution of the recurrence risk for breast cancer patients undergoing mastectomy: Further support about the concept of tumor dormancy. Breast Cancer Res Treat 41:177–185, 1996.
4. Naumov GN, Akslen LA, Folkman J: Role of angiogenesis in human tumor dormancy: Animal models of the angiogenic switch. Cell Cycle 5:1779–1787, 2006.
5. Folkman J: Role of angiogenesis in tumor growth and metastasis. Semin Oncol 29:15–18, 2002.
6. Chang C, Werb Z: The many faces of metalloproteases: Cell growth, invasion angiogenesis and metastasis. Trends Cell Biol 11:S35–S43, 2001.
7. Weidner N, Folkman J: Tumor vascularity as a prognostic factor in cancer. Important Adv Oncol 26:167–190, 1996.
8. Gasparini G: Clinical significance of determination of surrogate markers of angiogenesis in breast cancer. Crit Rev Oncol/Hematol 37:97–114, 2001.
9. Coltrera MD, Wang J, Porter PL, Gown AM: Expression of platelet-derived growth factor B-chain and the platelet-derived growth factor receptor β subunit in human breast tissue. Cancer Res 55:2703–2708, 1995.
10. De Larco JE, Wuertz BRK, Rosner KA, et al: A potential role for interleukin-8 in the metastatic phenotype of breast carcinoma cells. Am J Pathol 158:639–646, 2001.
11. De Jong JS, van Diest PJ, van der Valk P, Baak JPA: Expression of growth factors, growth inhibiting factors, and their receptors in invasive breast cancer. I. An inventory in search of autocrine and paracrine loops. J Pathol 184:44–52, 1998.
12. Brown LF, Guidi AJ, Schnitt SJ, et al: Vascular stroma formation in carcinoma in situ, invasive carcinoma, and metastatic carcinoma of the breast. Clin Cancer Res 5:1041–1056, 1999.
13. Currie MJ, Gunningham SP, Han C, et al: Angiopoietin-1 is inversely related to thymidine phosphorylase expression in human breast cancer, indicating a role in vascular remodeling. Clin Cancer Res 7:918–927, 2001.
14. Leek RD, Landers RJ, Harris AL, Lewis CE: Necrosis correlates with high vascular density and focal macrophage infiltration in invasive carcinoma of the breast. Br J Cancer 79:991–995, 1999.
15. Yu JL, Rak JW: Inflammatory and immune cells in tumour angiogenesis and arteriogenesis. Breast Cancer Res 5:83–88, 2003.
16. Chaudary N, Hill RP: Hypoxia and metastasis in breast cancer. Breast Dis 26:55–64, 2007.
17. Gasparini G, Pozza F, Harris AL: Evaluating the potential usefulness of new prognostic and predictive indicators in node-negative breast cancer patients. J Natl Cancer Inst 85:1206–1219, 1993.
18. Mohammed RAA, Green A, El-Shikh S, et al: Prognostic significance of vascular endothelial cell growth factors-A, -C and -D in breast cancer and their relationship with angio- and lymphangiogenesis. Br J Cancer 96:1092–1100, 2007.
19. Price DJ, Miralem T, Jiang S, et al: Role of vascular endothelial growth factor in the stimulation of cellular invasion and signaling of breast cancer cells. Cell Growth Differ 12:129–135, 2001.
20. Olofsson B, Korpelainen E, Pepper MS, et al: Vascular endothelial growth factor B (VEGF-B) binds to VEGF receptor-1 and regulates plasminogen activator activity in endothelial cells. Proc Natl Acad Sci USA 95:11709–11714, 1998.
21. Kurebayashi J, Otsuki T, Kunisue H, et al: Expression of vascular endothelial growth factor (VEGF) family members in breast cancer. Jpn J Cancer Res 90:977–981, 1999.
22. Skobe M, Hawighorst T, Jackson DG, et al: Induction of tumor lymphangiogenesis by VEGF-C promotes breast cancer metastasis. Nat Med 7:92–198, 2001.
23. Stacker SA, Caesar C, Baldwin ME, et al: VEGF-D promotes the metastatic spread of tumor cells via the lymphatics. Nat Med 7:186–191, 2001.
24. an den Eynden GG, Van der Auwera I, Van Laere SJ, et al: Comparison of molecular determinants of angiogenesis and lymphangiogenesis in lymph node metastases and in primary tumours of patients with breast cancer. J Pathol 213: 56–64, 2007.
25. Eccles SA, Paon L, Steeman J: Lymphatic metastasis in breast cancer: Importance and new insights into cellular and molecular mechanisms. Clin Exp Metastasis 24: 619–636, 2007.
26. Folkman J: Tumor angiogenesis: Therapeutic implications. N Engl J Med 285:1182–1186, 1971.
27. Miller K, Wang M, Gralow J, et al: Paclitaxel plus bevacizumab versus paclitaxel alone for metastatic breast cancer. N Engl J Med 357:2666–2676, 2007.
28. Hagedorn M, Bikfalvi A: Target molecules for anti-angiogenic therapy: From basic research to clinical trials. Crit Rev Oncol/Hematol 34:89–110, 2000.
29. O'Reilly MS, Holmgren L, Chen C, Folkman J: Angiostatin induces and sustains dormancy of human primary tumors in mice. Nat Med 2:689–692, 1996.
30. Bergers G, Brekken R, McMahon G, et al: Matrix metalloproteinase-9 triggers the angiogenic switch during carcinogenesis. Nat Cell Biol 2:737–744, 2000.
31. Lin EY, Pollard JW: Tumor-associated macrophages press the angiogenic switch in breast cancer. Cancer Res 67:5064–5066, 2007.
32. Liotta LA, Kohn EA: The microenvironment of the tumour-host interface. Nature 411:375–379, 2001.
33. Van den Brule F, Engel J, Stetler-Stevenson WG, et al: Genes involved in tumor invasion and metastasis are differentially modulated by estradiol and progestin in human breast cancer cells. Int J Cancer 52:653–657, 1992.
34. Garbett EA, Reed MW, Brown NJ: Proteolysis in human breast and colorectal cancer. Br J Cancer 81:287–293, 1999.
35. Heppner KJ, Matrisian LM, Jensen RA, Rodgers WH: Expression of most matrix metalloproteinase family members in breast cancer represents a tumor-induced host reponse. Am J Pathol 149: 273–282, 1996.
36. Sun J, Hemler ME: Regulation of MMP-1 and MMP-2 production through CD147/extracellular matrix metalloproteinase inducer interactions. Cancer Res 61:2276–2281, 2001.
37. Ueno H, Nakamura H, Inoue M, et al: Expression and tissue localization of membrane-types 1,2, and 3 matrix metalloproteinases in human invasive breast cancer. Cancer Res 57:2055–2060, 1997.
38. Jones JL, Glynn P, Walker RA: Expression of MMP-2 and MMP-9, their inhibitors, and the activator MT1-MMP in primary breast carcinomas. J Pathol 189:161–168, 1999.
39. Bergsten E, Uutela M, Li X, et al: PDGF-D is a specific, protease-activated ligand for the PDGF b-receptor. Nat Cell Biol 3: 512–516, 2001.
40. Li X, Ponten A, Aase K. et al: PDGF-C is a new protease-activated ligand for the PDGF a-receptor. Nat Cell Biol 2:302–309, 2000.
41. Berx G, Van Roy F: The E-cadherin/catenin complex: An important gatekeeper in breast cancer tumorigenesis and malignant progression. Breast Cancer Res 3:289–293, 2001.
42. Gumbiner BM: Signal transduction by b-catenin. Curr Opin Cell Biol 7:634–640, 1995.
43. Meiners S, Brinkmann V, Naundorf H, Birchmeier W: Role of morphogenetic factors in metastasis of mammary carcinoma cells. Oncogene 16:9–20, 1998.
44. Vleminckx K, Vakaet L, Mareel M, et al: Genetic manipulation of E-cadherin expression by epithelial tumor cells reveals an invasion suppressor role. Cell 66:107–119, 1991.
45. Bukholm IK, Nesland JM, Karensen R, et al: E-cadherin and α-, β- and γ-catenin protein expression in relation to metastasis in human breast carcinoma. J Pathol 185:262–266, 1998.
46. Graff JR, Gabrielson E, Fujii H, et al: Methylation patterns of the E-cadherin 5′ CpG island are unstable and reflect the dynamic, heterogeneous loss of E-cadherin expression during metastatic progression. J Biol Chem 275:2727–2732, 2000.
47. Thompson EW, Newgreen DF, Tarin D: Carcinoma invasion and metastasis: A role for epithelial-mesenchymal-transition? Cancer Res 65:5991–5995, 2005.
48. Tarin D, Thompson EW, Newgreen DF: The fallacy of epithelial mesenchymal transition in neoplasia. Cancer Res 65:5996–6000, 2005.
49. Peinado H, Olmeda D, Cano A: Snail, ZEB and bHLH factors in tumour progression: An alliance against the epithelial phenotype? Nat Rev Cancer 7:415–428, 2007.
50. Martin TA, Goyal A, Watkins G, Jiang WG: Expression of the transcription factors Snail, Slug and twist and their clinical significance in human breast cancer. Ann Surg Oncol 12:1–9, 2005.

51. Elloul S, Elstrand MB, Nesland JM, et al: Snail, Slug and Smad-interacting protein 1 as novel parameters of disease aggressiveness in metastatic ovarian and breast carcinoma. Cancer 103:1631–1643, 2005.

52. Kleer CG, van GK, Merajver SD: Persistent E-cadherin expression in inflammatory breast cancer. Mod Pathol 14:458–464, 2001.

53. Tomlinson JS, Alpaugh ML, Barsky SH: An intact overexpressed E-cadherin/α,β-catenin axis characterizes the lymphovascular emboli of inflammatory breast carcinoma. Cancer Res 61:5231–5241, 2001.

54. Arihiro K, Oda H, Kaneko M, Inai K: Cytokines facilitate chemotactic motility of breast carcinoma cells. Breast Cancer 7:221–230, 2000.

55. Jiang WG, Raz A, Douglas-Jones A, Mansel RE: Expression of autocrine motility factor (AMF) and its receptor AMFR, in human breast cancer. J Histochem Cytochem 54:231–241, 2006.

56. Talukder AH, Bagheri-Yarmand R, Williams RRE, et al: Antihuman epidermal growth factor receptor 2 antibody herceptin inhibits autocrine motility factor (AMF) expression and potentiates antitumor effects of AMF inhibitors. Clin Cancer Res 8:3285–3289, 2002.

57. Tuck A, Park M, Sterns EE, et al: Coexpression of hepatocyte growth factor and receptor (Met) in human breast carcinoma. Am J Pathol 148:225–232, 1996.

58. Parr C, Watkins G, Mansel RE, Jiang WG: The hepatocyte growth factor regulatory factors in human breast cancer. Clin Cancer Res 10:202–211, 2004.

59. Kato M, Kitayama J, Kazama S, Nagawa H: Expression pattern of CXC chemokine receptor-4 is correlated with lymph node metastasis in human invasive ductal carcinoma. Breast Cancer Res 5:144–150, 2003.

60. Cabioglu N, Yazici MS, Arun B, et al: CCR7 and CXCR4 as novel biomarkers predicting axillary lymph node metastasis in T1 breast cancer. Clin Cancer Res 11:5686–5693, 2005.

61. Müller A, Homey B, Soto H, et al: Involvement of chemokine receptors in breast cancer metastasis. Nature 410:50–56, 2001.

62. Fidler IJ: Critical determinants of metastasis. Semin Cancer Biol 12:89–96, 2002.

63. Felding-Habermann B: Integrin adhesion receptors in tumor metastasis. Clin Exp Metastasis 20:203–213, 2003.

64. Kannagi R, Izawa M, Koike T, et al: Carbohydrate-mediated cell adhesion in cancer metastasis and angiogenesis. Cancer Sci 95:377–384, 2004.

65. Cavallaro U, Christofori G: Cell adhesion and signalling by cadherins and Ig-CAMs in cancer. Nat Rev Cancer 4:118–132, 2004.

66. Engleman VW, Nickols GA, Ross FP, et al: A peptidomimetic antagonist of the avb3 integrin inhibits bone resorption in vitro and prevents osteoporosis in vivo. J Clin Invest 99:2284–2292, 1997.

67. Mulgrew K, Kineer K, Yao X-T, et al: Direct targeting of αvβ3 integrin on tumor cells with a monoclonal antibody, AbegrinTM. Mol Cancer Ther 5:3122–3129, 2006.

68. McLean GW, Carragher NO, Avizienyte E, et al: The role of focal-adhesion kinase in cancer—a new therapeutic opportunity. Nat Rev Cancer 5:505–515, 2005.

69. van Nimwegen MJ, Verkoeijen S, van Buren L, et al: Requirement for focal adhesion kinase in the early phase of mammary adenocarcinoma lung metastasis formation. Cancer Res 65:4698–4706, 2005.

70. Karpanen T, Alitalo K: Lymphatic vessels as targets of tumor therapy? J Exp Med 194:F37–F42, 2001.

71. Fisher B: The evolution of paradigms for the management of breast cancer: A personal perspective. Cancer Res 52:2371–2383, 1992.

72. Hellman S: Karnofsky Memorial Lecture. Natural history of small breast cancers. J Clin Oncol 12:2229–2234, 1994.

73. Veronesi U, Paganelli G, Viale G, et al: Sentinel-lymph-node biopsy as a staging procedure in breast cancer: Update of a randomised controlled study. Lancet Oncol 7:983–990, 2006.

74. Van den Eynden GG, Vandenberghe MK, van Dam P-JH, et al: Increased sentinel lymph node lymphangiogenesis is associated with nonsentinel axillary lymph node involvement in breast cancer patients with a positive sentinel node. Clin Cancer Res 13:5391–5397, 2007.

75. Bockhorn M, Jain RK, Munn LL: Active versus passive mechanisms in metastasis: Do cancer cells crawl into vessels, or are they pushed? Lancet Oncol 8:444–448, 2007.

76. Talmadge JE: Clonal selection of metastasis within the life history of a tumor. Cancer Res 67:11471–11475, 2007.

77. Mehes G, Witt A, Kubista E, Ambros PF: Circulating breast cancer cells are frequently apoptotic. Am J Pathol 159:17–20, 2001.

78. Alix-Panabières C, Müller V, Pantel K: Current status in human breast cancer micrometastasis. Curr Opin Oncol 19:558–563, 2007.

79. Cristofanilli M, Budd GT, Ellis MJ, et al: Circulating tumor cells, disease progression, and survival in metastatic breast cancer. N Engl J Med 351:781–791, 2004.

80. Yu Y, Merlino G: Constitutive c-met signaling through a nonautocrine mechanism promotes metastasis in a transgenic transplantation model. Cancer Res 62:2951–2956, 2002.

81. Liotta LA, Saidel MG, Kleinerman J: The significance of hematogenous tumor cell clumps and the metastatic process. Cancer Res 36:889–894, 1976.

82. Niers TMN, Klerk CPW, DiNisio M, et al: Mechanisms of heparin induced anti-cancer activity in experimental cancer models. Crit Rev Oncol/Hematol 61:195–207, 2007.

83. Kramer RH, Gonzales R, Nicolson GL: Metastatic cells adhere preferentially to extracellular matrix of endothelial cells. Int J Cancer 26:639–645, 1980.

84. Cheng HC, Abdel-Ghany M, Elble RC, Pauli BU: Lung endothelial dipeptidyl peptidaseIV promotes adhesion and metastasis of rat breast cancer cells via tumor surface associated fibronectin. J Biol Chem 273:24207–24215, 1998.

85. Nicolson GL: Metastatic tumor cell interactions with endothelium, basement membrane and tissue. Curr Opin Cell Biol 1:1009–1019, 1989.

86. Kolonin M, Pasqualini R, Arap W: Molecular addresses in blood vessels as targets for therapy. Curr Opin Chem Biol 5:308–313, 2001.

87. Langley RR, Ramirez KM, Tsan RZ, et al: Tissue-specific microvascular endothelial cell lines from H-2Kb-tsA58 mice for studies of angiogenesis and metastasis. Cancer Res 63:2971–2976, 2003.

88. Al-Mehdi AB, Tozawa K, Fisher AB, et al: Intravascular origin of metastasis from the proliferation of endothelium-attached tumor cells: A new model for metastasis. Nat Med 6:100–102, 2000.

89. Muller A, Homey B, Soto H, et al: Involvement of chemokine receptors in breast cancer metastasis. Nature 410:50–56, 2001.

90. Wyckoff JB, Jones JG, Condeelis JS, Segall JE: A critical step in metastasis: In vivo analysis of intravasation at the primary tumor. Cancer Res 60:2504–2511, 2000.

91. Chambers AF, Naumov GN, Vantyghem SA, Tuck AB: Molecular biology of breast cancer metastasis: Clinical implications of experimental studies on metastatic inefficiency. Breast Cancer Res 2:400–407, 2000.

92. Wong CW, Lee A, Shientag L, et al: Apoptosis: An early event in metastatic inefficiency. Cancer Res 61:333–338, 2001.

93. Kluger HM, Chelouche Lev D, Kluger Y, et al: Using a xenograft model of human breast cancer metastasis to find genes associated with clinically aggressive disease. Cancer Res 65:5578–5587, 2005.

94. Tarin D: New insights into the pathogenesis of breast cancer metastasis. Breast Dis 26:13–25, 2006.

95. Kang Y, Siegel PM, Shu W, et al: A multigenic program mediating breast cancer metastasis to bone. Cancer Cell 3:537–549, 2003.

96. Rinker-Schaeffer CW, O'Keefe JP, Welch DR, Theodorescu D: Metastasis suppressor proteins: Discovery, molecular mechanisms, and clinical application. Clin Cancer Res 12:3882–3889, 2006.

97. Marot D, Bieche I, Aumas C, et al: High tumoral levels of Kiss1 and G-protein-coupled receptor 54 expression are correlated with poor prognosis of estrogen-receptor positive breast tumors. Endocr Rel Cancer 14:691–702, 2007.

98. Welch DR, Steeg PS, Rinker-Schaeffer CW: Molecular biology of breast cancer metastasis. Genetic regulation of human breast carcinoma metastasis. Breast Cancer Res 2:408–416, 2001.

99. Hartsough MT, Clare SE, Mair M, et al: Elevation of breast carcinoma Nm23-H1 metastasis suppressor gene expression and reduced motility by DNA methylation inhibition. Cancer Res 61:2320–2327, 2001.

100. Lowery AJ, Miller N, McNeill RE, Kerin MJ: MicroRNAs as prognostic indicators and therapeutic targets: Potential effects on breast cancer management. Clin Cancer Res 14:360–365, 2008.

101. Ma L, Teruya-Feldstein J, Weinberg RA: Tumour invasion and metastasis initiated by microRNA-10b in breast cancer. Nature 449:682–688, 2007.
102. Hunter K: Host genetics influence tumour metastasis. Nat Rev Cancer 6:141–146, 2006.
103. Crawford NPS, Ziogas A, Peel DJ, et al: Germline polymorphisms in SIPA1 are associated with metastasis and other indicators of poor prognosis in breast cancer. Breast Cancer Res 8:R16, 2006.
104. Paget S: The distribution of secondary growths in cancer of the breast. Lancet 1:571–573, 1889.
105. Fidler IJ: The pathogenesis of cancer metastasis: The "seed and soil" hypothesis revisited. Nat Rev Cancer 3:453–458, 2003.
106. Shtivelman E, Namikawa R: Species-specific metastasis of human tumor cells in the severe combined immunodeficiency mouse engrafted with human tissue. Proc Natl Acad Sci USA 92:4661–4665, 1995.
107. Nemeth JA, Harb JF, Barroso U, et al: Severe combined immuno-deficient-hu model of human prostate cancer metastasis to human bone. Cancer Res 59:1987–1993, 1999.
108. Brooks B, Bundred N, Howell A, et al: Investigation of mammary epithelial cell-bone marrow stroma interactions using primary human cell culture as a model of metastasis. Int J Cancer 73:690–696, 1997.
109. LeBedis C, Chen K, Fallavollita L, et al: Peripheral lymph node stromal cells can promote growth and tumorigenicity of breast carcinoma cells through the release of IGF-1 and EGF. Int J Cancer 100:2–8, 2001.
110. Bar-Yehuda S, Barer F, Volfsson L, Fishman P: Resistance of muscle to tumor metastases: A role for α3 adenosine receptor agonists. Neoplasia 3:125–131, 2001.
111. Fisher B, Fisher ER: Experimental evidence in support of the dormant cell. Science 130:918–919, 1959.
112. Manishen WJ, Sivananthan K, Orr FW: Resorbing bone stimulates tumor cell growth. A role for the host microenvironment in bone metastasis. Am J Pathol 123:39–45, 1986.
113. Coleman RE: Management of bone metastases. Oncologist 5:463–470, 2000.
114. Guise TA, Kozlow WK, Heras-Herzig A, et al: Molecular mechanisms of breast cancer metastases to bone. Clin Breast Cancer 5:S46–S53, 2005.
115. Boissier S, Ferreras M, Peyruchaud O, et al: Bisphosphonates inhibit breast and prostate carcinoma cell invasion, an early event in the formation of bone metastases. Cancer Res 60:2949–2954, 2000.
116. Yin JJ, Selander K, Chirgwin JM, et al: TGF-b signaling blockade inhibits PTHrP secretion by breast cancer cells and bone metastases development. J Clin Invest 103:197–206, 1999.
117. Henderson MA, Danks JA, Moseley JM, et al: Parathyroid hormone-related protein production by breast cancers, improved survival and reduced bone metastases. J Natl Cancer Inst 93:234–237, 2000.
118. Minn AJ, Gupta GP, Siegel PM, et al: Genes that mediate breast cancer metastasis to lung. Nature 436:518–524, 2005.
119. Graeber TJ, Osmanian C, Jacks T, et al: Hypoxia-mediated selection of cells with diminished apoptotic potential in solid tumors. Nature 379:88–91, 1996.
120. Maxwell PH, Dachs GU, Gleadle JM, et al: Hypoxia-inducible factor-1 modulates gene expression in solid tumors and influences both angiogenesis and tumor growth. Proc Natl Acad Sci USA 94:8104–8109, 1997.
121. Kamby C, Ejlertsen B, Andersen J, et al: The pattern of metastases in human breast cancer. Influence of systemic adjuvant therapy and impact on survival. Acta Oncol 27:715–719, 1988.
122. Pusztai L, Asmar L, Smith TL, Hortobagyi GN: Relapse after complete response to anthracycline-based combination chemotherapy in metastatic breast cancer. Breast Cancer Res Treat 55:1–8, 1999.
123. Holden SA, Emi Y, Kakeji Y, et al: Host distribution and response to antitumor alkylating agents of EMT-6 tumor cells from subcutaneous tumor implants. Cancer Chemother Pharmacol 40:87–93, 1997.
124. Sausville EA: The challenge of pathway and environment-mediated drug resistance. Cancer Metastasis Rev 20:117–122, 2001.
125. Allinen M, Beroukhim R, Cai L, et al: Molecular characterization of the tumor microenvironment in breast cancer. Cancer Cell 6:17–32, 2004.
126. Klopp AH, Spaeth EL, Dembinski JL, et al: Tumor irradiation increases the recruitment of circulating mesenchymal stem cells into the tumor microenvironment. Cancer Res 67:11687–11695, 2007.
127. Karnoub AE, Dash AB, Vo AP, et al: Mesenchymal stem cells within tumour stroma promote breast cancer metastasis. Nature 449:557–563, 2007.
128. Sipkins DA, Wei X, Wu JW, et al: In vivo imaging of specialized bone marrow endothelial microdomains for tumour engraftment. Nature 435:969–973, 2005.
129. Qian C-N, Berghuis B, Tsarfaty G, et al: Preparing the "soil": The primary tumor induces vasculature reorganization in the sentinel lymph node before the arrival of metastatic cancer cells. Cancer Res 66:10365–10376, 2008.
130. Psaila B, Kaplan RN, Port ER, Lyden D: Priming the "soil" for breast cancer metastasis: The pre-metastatic niche. Breast Disease 26:65–74, 2007.
131. Radisky ES, Radisky DC: Stromal induction of breast cancer: Inflammation and invasion. Rev Endocr Metab Disord 8:279–287, 2007.
132. Park CC, Bissell MJ, Barcellos-Hoff MH: The influence of the microenvironment on the malignant phenotype. Mol Med Today 6:324–329, 2000.
133. Jouanneau J, Moens G, Bourgeois Y, et al: A minority of carcinoma cells producing acidic fibroblast growth factor induces a community effect for tumor progression. Proc Natl Acad Sci USA 91:286–290, 1994.
134. Martorana AM, Zheng G, Crowe TC, et al: Epithelial cells up-regulate matrix metalloproteinases in cell within the same mammary carcinoma that have undergone an epithelial-mesenchymal transition. Cancer Res 58:4970–4979, 1998.
135. Porter DA, Krop IE, Nasser S, et al: A SAGE (serial analysis of gene expression) view of breast tumor progression. Cancer Res 61:5697–5702, 2001.
136. Foulds L: Neoplastic development. London, Academic Press, 1975.
137. Nowell PC: The clonal evolution of tumor cell populations. Science 194:23–28, 1976.
138. O'Connell P, Pekkel V, Fuqua SAW, et al: Analysis of loss of heterozygosity in 399 premalignant breast lesions at 15 genetic loci. J Natl Cancer Inst 90:697–703, 1998.
139. Kerbel RS: Growth dominance of the metastatic cancer cell: Cellular and molecular aspects. Adv Cancer Res 55:87–132, 1990.
140. Marks JR, Humphrey PA, Wu K, et al: Overexpression of p53 and HER2/neu proteins as prognostic markers in early stage breast cancer. Ann Surg 219:332–341, 1994.
141. Stapleton AMF, Timme TL, Gousse AE, et al: Primary human prostate cancer cells harboring p53 mutations are clonally expanded in metastases. Clin Cancer Res 3:1389–1397, 1997.
142. Silvestrini R, Daidone MG, Benini E, et al: Validation of p53 accumulation as a predictor of distant metastasis at 10 years of follow-up in 1400 node-negative breast cancers. Clin Cancer Res 2:2007–2013, 1996.
143. van Slooten HJ, van de Vijver MJ, Borresen AL, et al: Mutations in exons 5–8 of the p53 gene, independent of their type and location, are associated with increased apoptosis and mitosis in invasive breast carcinoma. J Pathol 189:504–513, 1999.
144. Perou CM, Sorlie T, Eisen MB, et al: Molecular portraits of human breast tumours. Nature 406:747–752, 2000.
145. Sorlie T, Perou CM, Tibshirani R, et al: Gene expression patterns of breast carcinomas distinguish tumor subclasses with clinical implications. Proc Natl Acad Sci USA 98:10869–10874, 2001.
146. Loi S, Piccart M, Sotiriou C: The use of gene-expression profiling to better understand the clinical heterogeneity of estrogen receptor positive breast cancers and tamoxifen resistance. Crit Rev Oncol/Hematol 61:187–194, 2007.
147. Morris SR, Carey LA: Gene expression profiling in breast cancer. Curr Opin Oncol 19:547–551, 2007.
148. van't Veer LJ, Dai H, van de Vijver MJ, et al: Gene expression profiling predicts clinical outcome of breast cancer. Nature 415:530–536, 2002.

149. Dunstan CR, Felsenberg D, Seibel MM: Therapy insight: The risks and benefits of bisphosphonates for the treatment of tumor-induced bone disease. Nat Clin Pract Oncol 4:42–55, 2007.

150. Nuyten DSA, van de Vijver MJ: Gene expression signatures to predict the development of metastasis in breast cancer. Breast Dis 26:149–156, 2007.

151. Yu JX, Sieuwerts AM, Zhang Y, et al: Pathway analysis of gene signatures predicting metastasis of node-negative primary breast cancer. BMC Cancer 7:182, 2007.

152. Wicha MS, Liu S, Dontu G: Cancer stem cells: An old idea—a paradigm shift. Cancer Res 66:1883–1890, 2006.

153. Dontu G, Al-Ashry D, Wicha MS: Breast cancer, stem/progenitor cells and the estrogen receptor. Trends Endocrinol Metab 15: 193–197, 2004.

154. Stingl J, Caldas C: Molecular heterogeneity of breast carcinomas and the cancer stem cell hypothesis. Nat Rev Cancer 7:791–799, 2007.

155. Wood LD, Parsons DW, Jones S, et al: The genomic landscapes of human breast and colorectal cancers. Science 318:1109–1113, 2007.

156. Teixeira MR, Pandis N, Heim S: Cytogenetic clues to breast carcinogenesis. Genes Chromosomes Cancer 33:1–16, 2002.

157. Kittiniyom K, Gorse KM, Dalbegue F, et al: Allelic loss on chromosome band 18p11.3 occurs early and reveals heterogeneity in breast cancer progression. Breast Cancer Res 3:192–198, 2001.

158. Cifone MA, Fidler IJ: Increasing metastatic potential is associated with increasing genetic instability of clones isolated from murine neoplasms. Proc Natl Acad Sci USA 78:6949–6952, 1981.

159. Pandis N, Teixeira MR, Adeyinka A, et al: Cytogenetic comparison of primary tumors and lymph node metastases in breast cancer patients. Genes Chromosomes Cancer 22:122–129, 1998.

160. Jones PA, Baylin SB: The epigenomics of cancer. Cell 128: 683–692, 2007.

161. Bernardino J, Roux C, Almeida A, et al: DNA hypomethylation in breast cancer: An independent parameter of tumor progression? Cancer Genet Cytogenet 97:83–89, 1997.

162. Lapidus RG, Nass SJ, Butash KA, et al: Mapping of ER gene CpG island methylation by methylation-specific polymerase chain reaction. Cancer Res 58:2515–2519, 1998.

163. Buerger H, Simon R, Schafer KL, et al: Genetic relation of lobular carcinoma in situ, ductal carcinoma in situ, and associated invasive carcinoma of the breast. Mol Pathol 53:118–121, 2000.

164. Munot K, Bell SM, Lane S, et al: Pattern of expression of genes linked to epigenetic silencing in human breast cancer. Hum Pathol 37:989–999, 2006.

165. Symmans WF, Liu J, Knowles DM, Inghirami G: Breast cancer heterogeneity: Evaluation of clonality in primary and metastatic lesions. Hum Pathol 26:210–216, 1994.

166. Kuukasjarvi T, Karhu R, Tanner M, et al: Genetic heterogeneity and clonal evolution underlying development of asynchronous metastasis in human breast cancer. Cancer Res 57:1597–1604, 1997.

167. Ramaswamy S, Ross KN, Lander ES, Golub TR: A molecular signature of metastasis in primary solid tumors. Nat Genet 33:49–54, 2003.

168. Weigelt B, Hu Z, He Z, et al: Molecular portraits and 70-gene prognosis signature are preserved throughout the metastatic process of breast cancer. Cancer Res 65: 155–9158, 2005.

169. Minn AJ, Kang Y, Serganova I, et al: Distinct organ-specific metastatic potential of individual breast cancer cells and primary tumors. J Clin Invest 115:44–55, 2005.

170. Al-Hajj M, Wicha MS, Benito-Hernandez A, et al: Prospective identification of tumorigenic breast cancer cells. Proc Natl Acad Sci USA 100:3983–3988, 2003.

171. Shipitsin M, Campbell LL, Argani P, et al: Molecular definition of breast tumor heterogeneity. Cancer Cell 11: 59–273, 2007.

172. Patrawala L, Calhoun T, Schneider-Broussard R, et al: Highly purified CD44+ prostate cancer cells from xenograft human tumors are enriched in tumorigenic and metastatic progenitor cells. Oncogene 25:1696–1708, 2006.

173. Sheridan C, Kishimoto H, Ruchs RK, et al: CD44+/CD24− breast cancer cells exhibit enhanced invasive properties: An early step necessary for metastasis. Breast Cancer Res 8:R59, 2006.

174. Sleeman AP, Cremers N: New concepts in breast cancer metastasis: Tumor initiating cells and the microenvironment. Clin Exp Metastasis 24:707–715, 2007.

chapter 31

Gene Therapy for Breast Cancer

THERESA V. STRONG | DAVID T. CURIEL

Although the treatment of breast cancer has improved significantly over the past decades, locoregional recurrence and disseminated disease still represent formidable challenges for conventional therapies. The field of gene therapy is rapidly developing and has greatly expanded the opportunities for new breast cancer treatments. Defined as the introduction of genetic material for the treatment of disease, gene therapy was originally envisioned primarily for the correction of inherited genetic defects. To date, however, gene therapy has found more extensive application in the treatment of malignant disease, with approximately two thirds of all gene therapy clinical trials targeting cancer. This comes from several realizations. First, it has been appreciated that breast cancer, like other cancers, develops through the progressive accumulation of alterations in specific genes, resulting in abnormal cell growth and invasion. These genetic abnormalities can be corrected or altered via the introduction of therapeutic genes. Second, many limitations of current gene therapy approaches pose less of a challenge in their application to the treatment of cancer. Most notably, difficulties in maintaining long-term gene expression are obviated for most approaches to gene therapy for cancer, because transgene expression of a limited duration can achieve therapeutic effect. Finally, a better understanding of the molecular pathology of tumors, including the underlying molecular changes in tumor cells and interactions of the tumor with the microenvironment, has led to identification of new therapeutic targets that can be manipulated through gene therapy.

Based on these concepts, numerous approaches to gene therapy for breast cancer have been considered, each targeting different points in the cancer progression pathway. Given that conventional therapies for early-stage breast cancer are generally effective, gene therapy approaches have focused on three clinical scenarios. One is the treatment of advanced, widely disseminated disease, for which conventional therapy is inadequate. A second potential target population is women who have responded favorably to conventional therapy but are at high risk for recurrence. In this case, gene therapy strategies designed to eliminate micrometastatic disease

with low toxicity may be considered. Finally, gene therapy has been applied to breast cancer in conjunction with bone marrow transplantation therapy. Some of the approaches evaluated to date seek to alter or kill the tumor cells directly, whereas others attempt to alter the tumor environment. This chapter will review the basic concepts of gene therapy as they apply to the treatment of breast cancer. Although many of these therapeutic strategies are still in preclinical development, clinical evaluation has been initiated for selected approaches. An updated listing of approved gene therapy clinical trials is available through the National Institutes of Health/Food and Drug Administration Genetic Modification Clinical Research Information System (GeMCRIS) database (http://www4.od.nih.gov/oba/RAC/GeMCRIS/GeMCRIS.htm).

Gene Therapy Strategies

STRATEGIES TO ACCOMPLISH GENE THERAPY FOR BREAST CANCER: TARGETING THE TUMOR CELL

In considering gene therapy for breast cancer, a critical issue is the choice of therapeutic gene. Unlike colon cancer, where a well-defined accumulation of genetic aberrations leads to progressively more aggressive disease,[1] the genetic alterations leading to breast cancer are apparently more diverse, and suggest that at the genetic level, breast cancer is not a single disease. Molecular profiling of breast tumors has begun to delineate discrete molecular subtypes of breast cancer, including luminal A, luminal B, HER2+/estrogen receptor–negative and basal-like.[2] A better understanding of the underlying genetic changes contributing to the development of each of these subtypes will be pivotal in designing more specific, targeted approaches that will allow for individualized therapy. Until that goal is fully achieved, gene therapy approaches have focused on a number of mutations found to be common in breast cancer. Inherited or somatic genetic changes in tumor suppressor genes, oncogenes, growth factor receptors, DNA repair

TABLE 31-1		
Gene Therapy Strategies for Breast Cancer		
Approach	**Rationale**	**Examples (ref. nos.)**
Mutation compensation	Targets specific gene mutations to restore normal growth or induce apoptosis	4,6,33
Molecular chemotherapy	Local conversion of a prodrug into a toxic drug to kill tumor cells	34
Viral oncolysis	Tumor-specific viral replication and lysis	16,23
Genetic immunotherapy	Stimulates host immune system to recognize and eliminate tumor cells	30–32
Anti-angiogenic	Ablates the ability of the tumor to establish a blood supply	14–16
Metastasis suppression	Interrupts the process of tumor cell dissemination and growth at distant sites	17–19
Bone marrow chemoprotection	Protects normal cells from high-dose chemotherapy	20
Bone marrow purging	Eliminates contaminating tumor cells for autologous bone marrow transplant	21,22

enzymes, and/or cell signaling molecules lead to low or high risk carcinomas in situ, and additional changes involving genes important in invasive and angiogenesis promote metastatic spread. These tumor-specific genetic alterations can be targeted through approaches that include mutation compensation, molecular chemotherapy, and viral oncolysis (or virotherapy; Table 31-1).

Mutual Compensation

Mutation compensation aims to correct the genetic defects that contribute to the malignant phenotype. Such correction may be accomplished by replacing the function of tumor suppressor genes, ablating the function of a dominant oncogene, or interfering with dysregulated signal transduction pathways. For inactive tumor suppressor genes, one logical approach is the replacement of the deficient gene. A well-studied example of this in breast cancer is the replacement of the p53 gene (gene name *TP53*),[3] the most commonly altered tumor suppressor gene in human cancers. Replacement of p53 in deficient tumor cells leads to reversion of the malignant phenotype and/or induction of apoptosis. For dominant oncogenes or dysregulated signaling proteins, it is possible to abrogate the function of the encoded proteins at many levels. Perhaps the best-studied molecule in this respect is the product of the HER2/neu gene (gene name *ERBB2*), which is overexpressed in approximately 30% of breast tumors and is associated with a poor prognosis. Degradation of the mRNA encoding this oncogene and interference with protein translation can be promoted through the use of specific, antisense oligonucleotides[4]; but practical application of the technology and idiosyncrasies in the effects of specific antisense molecules have posed a challenge in this field. Short interfering RNA (siRNA) and short hairpin RNA (shRNA) have emerged over the past several years as promising new technologies to specifically ablate expression of target oncogenes. These short ($\approx$22 nucleotides) RNA molecules exploit existing cellular mechanisms to interfere with target mRNA by promoting degradation and/or interfering with translation. Application of this technology to breast cancer therapeutics has not yet reached the clinic,[5] but preclinical studies have validated the ability of siRNA directed toward the *ERBB2* mRNA to attenuate tumor growth.[6] At the protein level, expression of intracellular antibodies against *ERBB2* promotes degradation of the protein and induces apoptosis in *ERBB2* expressing cells.[7] Although mutation compensation is straightforward and many preclinical studies have demonstrated the utility of these strategies, significant obstacles remain for these approaches to achieve therapeutic efficacy in the clinical setting. Chief among these is the theoretical need to correct the deficit in all tumor cells to achieve a therapeutic effect. So-called "quantitative transduction" of the tumor cells is elusive, and to date no vectors for gene delivery have been able to achieve this goal. Another significant limitation stems from the accumulated genetic changes found in highly malignant cells, which may not be amenable to correction by the introduction a single therapeutic gene.

Molecular Chemotherapy

As a method to overcome some of the practical limitations of mutation compensation, the concept of molecular chemotherapy, or "suicide" gene therapy, has also been explored. The premise of this approach is to restrict the toxic effects of a chemotherapeutic drug specifically to tumor cells by mediating conversion of a systemically delivered prodrug into a toxic metabolite within the tumor cells, as directed by an expressed transgene.[8] Molecular chemotherapy strategies may offer an advantage compared with most mutation compensation approaches in that nearby tumor cells that did not receive the transgene may also be affected by the toxin, the so-called "bystander effect." Many prodrug systems exist, but the most studied method to accomplish tumor cell killing in this way uses the thymidine kinase gene from the herpes simplex virus (HSV-TK). Expression of this gene in mammalian cells in not harmful, but allows conversion of the relatively nontoxic nucleoside analog, ganciclovir, to a phosphorylated form which incorporates into the cellular DNA, inhibits DNA synthesis and RNA polymerase, and leads to cell death. For this and other molecular chemotherapy approaches to be successful, transgene expression must be confined to the tumor cells, and thus appropriately targeted gene delivery and expression is critical.

Viral Oncolysis

As the field of gene therapy has advanced, it has become apparent that first-generation, replication-incompetent viral vectors lack the ability to achieve quantitative transduction of tumors, limiting their therapeutic efficacy. To overcome this limitation, conditionally replicative viruses have been investigated.[9,10] These viruses are engineered such that they can replicate within genetically aberrant cancer cells, resulting in specific, intratumoral viral propagation. Replication in normal cells is absent or attenuated. The therapeutic effect may be achieved solely as a result of virus-driven tumor cell lysis, or it may be augmented by the addition of a therapeutic transgene, such as an immunostimulatory cytokine. These oncolytic vectors, derived from a number of different naturally occurring viruses, have shown promise in preclinical and some early clinical trials for other tumor types. Additional modifications to the vectors to enhance tumor specificity, intratumoral spread, and immune response evasion promise to further improve the potential of this approach.

STRATEGIES TO ACCOMPLISH GENE THERAPY FOR BREAST CANCER: TARGETING THE TUMOR ENVIRONMENT

Genetic Immunotherapy

Rather than directly targeting the growth promoting genetic changes inherent in the cancerous cell, a variety of gene therapy strategies focus instead on manipulating the tumor microenvironment, including stromal cells, extracellular matrix, and immune cells, to limit tumor growth or promote the destruction of the tumor cells. *Genetic immunotherapy* refers to gene transfer strategies designed to recruit the patient's immune system to identify and destroy aberrant tumor cells, by virtue of tumor associated antigens expressed in the tumor cell.[11] It has long been apparent that tumor cells possess some degree of immunogenicity, and, furthermore, tumors use a variety of strategies to evade detection by the host immune system. Immunotherapy seeks to stimulate the immune response to the tumor cells, and genetic immunotherapy approaches use gene transfer technology to achieve this end. Immunotherapy potentially addresses a central issue in the management of women with breast cancer—the development of relatively nontoxic therapies designed to eliminate micrometastatic disease and prevent disease recurrence. Thus, breast cancer vaccines developed to date have been primarily therapeutic rather than preventive in nature and will likely find their application in the setting of minimum residual disease. Perhaps more so than other gene therapy approaches, the success of genetic immunotherapy strategies will depend on a sophisticated understanding of how best to integrate gene therapy with conventional therapies, including cytotoxic chemotherapy.[12] Notably, a better understanding of the role of regulatory T cells has led to a realization of the potential for chemotherapeutic approaches to relieve tumor immunosuppression mechanisms and synergize with active immunotherapy.[13]

Two general strategies have been used for breast cancer immunotherapy. Nonspecific genetic immunotherapy uses transfer of immunomodulatory genes such as cytokines and costimulatory molecules to overcome immunologic tolerance to tumors and promote tumor rejection. Gene transfer can be accomplished ex vivo, using either autologous or allogeneic breast tumor cells, which are inactivated prior to reinfusion of the cancer vaccine or in vivo by delivering immunostimulatory genes to the tumor. This approach does not require knowledge of the tumor antigens expressed in a particular tumor. In contrast, active specific immunotherapy uses in situ immunization with defined antigen(s) to elicit a specific antitumor immune response. Advances in the identification and characterization of tumor antigens relevant to breast cancer have expanded the possible target antigens for this approach.

Anti-angiogenic Gene Therapy

The growth of tumors is dependent on the process of angiogenesis, which establishes the tumor blood supply. Preclinical studies suggest that interfering with the factors necessary to establish appropriate blood flow to the tumor effectively inhibits tumor growth.[14,15] Several proteins, including angiostatin, endostatin, and soluble vascular-endothelial growth factor receptor may act to inhibit tumor cell growth when administered. Clinically, gene therapy offers some advantages compared to protein-based therapy. Long-term expression of the therapeutic gene offered by some vectors permits a continuous, endogenous source of the protein. Furthermore, because the protein is synthesized in vivo, stability is improved compared with protein produced in vitro. In its optimal form, this approach requires a vector capable of directing long-term expression of the transgene, with the ability to regulate the level of transgene expressed. Alternative approaches seek to downregulate the expression of proangiogenic factors; for example, the use of shRNA against interleukin-8.[16]

GENE THERAPY TO INHIBIT TUMOR METASTASES

Tumor cell dissemination and growth at distant sites is the key process that contributes significantly to morbidity and mortality in patients with breast cancer. Driven by a better understanding of the biologic factors directing the stepwise events of metastasis, gene therapy strategies are being developed to interrupt this cascade. In preclinical studies, the rationale of inducing the expression of metastasis suppressor genes,[17] promoting expression of tissue inhibitors of matrix metalloproteinases,[18] or knocking down expression of metastasis promoting genes, such as CXCR4,[19] has been validated.

GENE THERAPY IN CONJUNCTION WITH BONE MARROW TRANSPLANT

Gene therapy has been applied to breast cancer autologous bone marrow transplantation in two ways (see Table 31-1). One of the first applications of gene therapy for breast cancer was the transduction of normal cells in the bone marrow with a protective gene (e.g., the multidrug resistance gene) to mitigate the myelosuppressive effects of high-dose chemotherapy.[20] In a second application, viral vectors that specifically transduce and kill tumor cells have been used to purge bone marrow cells of contaminating tumor cells.[21,22]

Vectors for Gene Transfer

Once a general strategy and therapeutic gene have been determined, a second consideration for all gene therapy protocols is the choice of vector to most effectively deliver the gene. There is a vast array of choices, and these continue to expand as new vectors are characterized, modified, or synthesized to achieve more efficacious gene delivery. Gene transfer vectors generally fall into two classes, viral and nonviral; each with its advantages and disadvantages. Because the primary focus of breast cancer gene therapy is targeting and eliminating metastatic disease, the ideal gene transfer vector would possess the following attributes: (1) stability in vivo to allow intravenous delivery; (2) ability to target gene transfer to the desired cells (e.g., disseminated breast tumor cells) while leaving normal cells unaltered; (3) ability to transfer large genes with the appropriate regulatory sequences; (4) ability to direct sufficiently prolonged expression of the therapeutic transgene; (5) ability to replicate autonomously or integrate at a defined chromosomal site; and finally, (6) lack of stimulation of unwanted host immune response that might interfere with transgene expression. Nonviral gene delivery systems have advantages in that they have low toxicity and may not elicit immune responses; however, they are generally inefficient in their ability to deliver the genes, and transgene expression is transient. Viral vectors, having evolved to deliver their nucleic acids into cells, are generally much more efficient than nonviral methods but suffer from other limitations, including preexisting immune responses that may interfere with gene transduction, induction of antivector immune responses that limit the ability to repetitively dose, and potential safety concerns including recombination with wild type virus. Chimeric vectors combine features of different nonviral and/or viral components to achieve the desired gene delivery profile. Finally, mesenchymal stem cells have been used as a cellular delivery vehicle for gene therapy vectors.[23]

A summary of gene therapy vectors explored for use in breast cancer therapy is found in Table 31-2. Unfortunately, none of these vectors yet meets the criteria for the ideal, and thus a major focus in the field of gene therapy has been the development of novel or modified vectors toward this end. Considerable progress has been made, including the development of vectors that target tumor cells specifically,[24-26] express their genes only in recipient tumor cells by virtue of tumor specific promoters, evade the immune response, and replicate specifically in tumor cells.[27-29]

Breast Cancer Gene Therapy: Clinical Experience

Evaluation of gene therapy in the clinical setting is still in its nascency. Of the wide range of tumor types that have been the subject of experimental gene therapies,

---

TABLE 31-2

Gene Delivery Systems in Preclinical or Clinical Development for Breast Cancer

Method	Advantages	Disadvantages
Nonviral		
Liposomes	Nonimmunogenic, repeated delivery possible	Inefficient gene delivery
Naked nucleic acids	Easy to prepare, limited immunogenicity	Inefficient gene delivery
Conjugates	Targeted delivery, flexible design,	Unstable, inefficient
Nanoparticles	Targeted delivery, flexible design, penetrability	Potential toxicity incompletely characterized
Mesenchymal stem cells	Cellular delivery of viral or nonviral vectors	Labor intensive and expensive
Viral		
Adenovirus	Comparatively efficient gene delivery, targeted	Transient, immunogenic, preexisting antibodies
Retrovirus	Long-term expression	Risk of insertional mutagenesis, transduces dividing cells only
Lentivirus	Long-term expression, transduces nondividing cells	Risk of insertional mutagenesis
Poxvirus	Robust, short-term expression for immunotherapy	Immunogenic, repeat dosing limited
Adeno-associated virus	Long-term expression, nonpathogenic	Small insert size, difficult preparation
Herpes simplex virus	Efficient in vivo, large insert size	Not completely characterized
Reovirus	Specific oncolysis in cells with activated Ras pathway	Clinical profile not yet known
Chimeric vectors	May improve targeting, long-term expression	Not fully developed

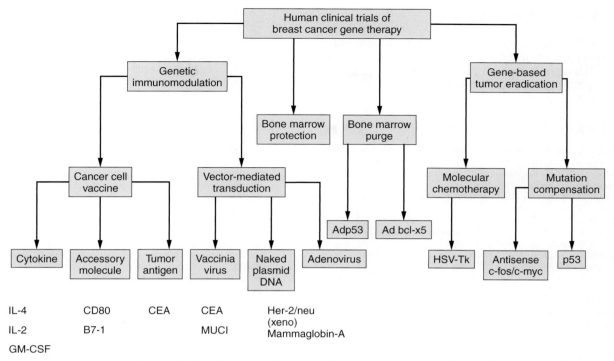

Figure 31-1 Human clinical trials of breast cancer gene therapy.

breast cancer tumors have represented a prominent proportion. At the present juncture, these trials have primarily been phase I trials, designed to evaluate dose-related toxicity as a primary end point (Fig. 31-1). Thus, whereas clinical responses may be evaluated, this is not the primary intention of such trials. In some instances, surrogate end points have provided key insight into the induction of a biologic effect, suggesting therapy and/or highlighting the issues related to the basic pharmacology of effective gene delivery.

The evaluation of clinical trials for breast cancer has paralleled the field evolution of cancer gene therapy in general. Thus, the majority of breast cancer gene therapy trials to date have used genetic immunotherapy approaches against either defined tumor antigens, such as MUC-1 or carcinoembryonic antigen,[30,31] or non-specific genetic immunotherapy using gene-modified autologous or allogeneic breast cancer cells.[32]

The subsequent evolution of vectors to achieve a level of in vivo transduction capacity led to the development of a set of approaches based on in situ modification of tumor. Largely applied for locoregional disease, these strategies were designed to deliver either corrective genes to the tumor (e.g., p53)[33] or to induce the local ability to convert prodrug into antitumor metabolite (such as HSV-tk).[34] Again, it was the development of vectors with enhanced in vivo delivery capacity, such as adenovirus, that made these interventions possible. Ultimately, however, it has become clear that the requirements for effective gene delivery in the context of in situ therapy could not be met by existing adenovirus-based vectors. Furthermore, no vector within the available repertoire was capable of the in vivo cell selective transduction required for application of these approaches for metastatic disease.

The overall lessons of the human breast cancer clinical trials have highlighted the safety and tolerability of the gene therapy approach. Nonetheless, the lack of index of clinical activity to date has also been apparent. Data obtained in these trials, however, have made it clear that ineffective gene delivery constitutes the basis of this limited clinical activity. Thus, the clinical experience has served to better define the limitations of current gene therapy strategies and vectors, providing the basis for the development of the next generation of gene therapy vectors. Vectors with improved gene delivery and specific targeting will be needed for therapeutic efficacy to become a reality.[35]

Conclusions

Advances in cancer treatment have significantly improved clinical outcome, but no single therapeutic intervention has yet proven effective for all breast cancer. Gene therapy offers promise to expand and complement the current arsenal of therapies that can be applied to breast cancer. In fact, gene therapy is likely to find its most useful clinical application in combination with conventional therapeutic approaches; acting to sensitize tumor cells, increase the specificity of toxins to the tumor cells, or, in combination with chemotherapy, manipulate the immune response to promote a favorable outcome. In the coming years, the development of advanced generation gene delivery vectors should enhance the ability to target the appropriate cells and achieve optimal transgene expression, allowing gene therapy to reach its full potential and offering new hope to those with breast cancer.

Acknowledgments

The authors acknowledge the support of the United States Army Medical Research and Materiel Command Breast Cancer Research Program, Award number 07-1-0369 (TVS) and NIH grant P50CA086306 (DTC).

REFERENCES

1. Fearon ER, Vogelstein B: A genetic model for colorectal tumorigenesis. Cell 61:759–767, 1990.
2. Morris SR, Carey LA: Molecular profiling in breast cancer. Rev Endocr Metab Disord 8:185–198, 2007.
3. Obermiller PS, Tait DL, Holt JT: Gene therapy for carcinoma of the breast: Therapeutic genetic correction strategies. Breast Cancer Res 2:28–31, 2000.
4. Roh H, et al: HER2/neu antisense targeting of human breast carcinoma. Oncogene 19:6138–6143, 2000.
5. Storvold GL, et al: siRNA: A potential tool for future breast cancer therapy? Crit Rev Oncog 12:127–150, 2006.
6. Urban-Klein B, et al: RNAi-mediated gene-targeting through systemic application of polyethylenimine (PEI)-complexed siRNA in vivo. Gene Ther 12:461–466, 2005.
7. Curiel, DT: Gene therapy for carcinoma of the breast: Genetic ablation strategies. Breast Cancer Res 2:45–49, 2000.
8. Vassaux, G, Lemoine NR: Gene therapy for carcinoma of the breast: Genetic toxins. Breast Cancer Res 2:22–27, 2000.
9. Ring CJ: Cytolytic viruses as potential anti-cancer agents. J Gen Virol 83(Pt 3):491–502, 2002.
10. Gomez-Navarro J, Curiel DT: Conditionally replicative adenoviral vectors for cancer gene therapy. Lancet Oncol 1:148–158, 2000.
11. Strong TV: Gene therapy for carcinoma of the breast: Genetic immunotherapy. Breast Cancer Res 2:15–21, 2000.
12. Prendergast GC, Jaffee EM: Cancer immunologists and cancer biologists: Why we didn't talk then but need to now. Cancer Res 67:3500–3504, 2007.
13. Gallimore A, Godkin A: Regulatory T cells and tumour immunity—observations in mice and men. Immunology 123:157–163, 2008.
14. Chen QR, et al: Liposomes complexed to plasmids encoding angiostatin and endostatin inhibit breast cancer in nude mice. Cancer Res 59:3308–3312, 1999.
15. Sauter BV, et al: Adenovirus-mediated gene transfer of endostatin in vivo results in high level of transgene expression and inhibition of tumor growth and metastases. Proc Natl Acad Sci USA 97:4802–4807, 2000.
16. Yoo JY, Kim JH, Kim J, et al: Short hairpin RNA-expressing oncolytic adenovirus-mediated inhibition of IL-8: Effects on antiangiogenesis and tumor growth inhibition. Gene Ther 15:635–651, 2008.
17. Steeg PS, et al: Metastasis suppressor genes: Basic biology and potential clinical use. Clin Breast Cancer 4:51–62, 2003.
18. Lee YK, et al: Suppression of distant pulmonary metastasis of MDA-MB 435 human breast carcinoma established in mammary fat pads of nude mice by retroviral-mediated TIMP-2 gene transfer. J Gene Med 7:145–157, 2005.
19. Liang Z, et al: Silencing of CXCR4 blocks breast cancer metastasis. Cancer Res. 65:967–971, 2005.
20. Cowan KH, et al: Paclitaxel chemotherapy after autologous stem-cell transplantation and engraftment of hematopoietic cells transduced with a retrovirus containing the multidrug resistance complementary DNA (MDR1) in metastatic breast cancer patients. Clin Cancer Res 5:1619–1628, 1999.
21. Seth P, et al: Adenovirus-mediated gene transfer to human breast tumor cells: An approach for cancer gene therapy and bone marrow purging. Cancer Res 56:1346–1351, 1996.
22. Wu A, et al: Biological purging of breast cancer cells using an attenuated replication-competent herpes simplex virus in human hematopoietic stem cell transplantation. Cancer Res 61:3009–3015, 2001.
23. Stoff-Khalili MA, et al: Mesenchymal stem cells as a vehicle for targeted delivery of CRAds to lung metastases of breast carcinoma. Breast Cancer Res Treat 105:157–167, 2007.
24. Campos SK, Barry MA: Current advances and future challenges in adenoviral vector biology and targeting. Curr Gene Ther 7:189–204, 2007.
25. Sandrin V, et al: Targeting retroviral and lentiviral vectors. Curr Top Microbiol Immunol 281:137–178, 2003.
26. Lavigne MD, Górecki DC: Emerging vectors and targeting methods for nonviral gene therapy. Expert Opin Emerg Drugs 11:541–557, 2006.
27. Glasgow JN, et al: Transductional targeting of adenovirus vectors for gene therapy. Cancer Gene Ther 13:830–844, 2006.
28. Gomez-Navarro J, Curiel DT, Douglas JT: Gene therapy for cancer. Eur J Cancer 35:2039–2057, 1999.
29. Vähä-Koskela MJ, et al: Oncolytic viruses in cancer therapy. Cancer Lett 254:178–216, 2007.
30. Acres B: Cancer immunotherapy: Phase II clinical studies with TG4010 (MVA-MUC1-IL2). J BUON(suppl 1):S71–S75, 2007.
31. Marshall JL, et al: Phase I study of sequential vaccinations with fowlpox-CEA(6D)-TRICOM alone and sequentially with vaccinia-CEA (6D)-TRICOM, with and without granulocyte-macrophage colony-stimulating factor, in patients with carcinoembryonic antigen-expressing carcinomas. J Clin Oncol 23:720–731, 2005.
32. Stewart AK, et al: Adenovector-mediated gene delivery of interleukin-2 in metastatic breast cancer and melanoma: Results of a phase 1 clinical trial. Gene Ther 6:350–363, 1999.
33. Cristofanilli M, et al: A nonreplicating adenoviral vector that contains the wild-type p53 transgene combined with chemotherapy for primary breast cancer: Safety, efficacy, and biologic activity of a novel gene-therapy approach. Cancer 107:935–944, 2006.
34. Singh S, et al: Toxicity assessment of intratumoral injection of the herpes simplex type I thymidine kinase gene delivered by retrovirus in patients with refractory cancer. Mol Ther 4:157–160, 2001.
35. Waehler R, Russell SJ, Curiel DT: Engineering targeted viral vectors for gene therapy. Nat Rev Genet 8:573–587, 2007.

chapter 32

Angiogenesis in Breast Cancer

MAI N. BROOKS | M. JUDAH FOLKMAN

Tumor Angiogenesis: Biologic Basis

PREVASCULAR PHASE

When a new primary tumor first arises, it is usually not vascularized. In this prevascular state, tumor volume is less than a few cubic millimeters. External in situ carcinomas of the skin, cervix, and oral mucous membranes, which can be observed directly, are usually thin and flat because their expansion is limited by the diffusion of nutrients and oxygen from normal vessels that lie beneath the epithelial layer. Thus, a new melanoma is separated from capillary vessels in the dermis, which are already occupied by normal cells. The prevascular stage of an internal tumor, such as carcinoma in situ of the breast, can usually be seen only with microscopic examination (Fig. 32-1). These tumor cells are also usually separated from host microvessels by a basement membrane. From experimental studies, we know that these prevascular lesions exist in a steady state of tumor cell proliferation balanced by cell death.[1] Externally located prevascular tumors may remain in this state for months to years, but we do not know about internal lesions. The onset of neovascularization, however, can be relatively sudden and is called the *angiogenic switch*.[2,3]

SWITCH TO THE ANGIOGENIC PHENOTYPE

The appearance of a thin layer of new periductal vessels may be the first evidence of neovascularization of in situ breast carcinoma (see Fig. 32-1). Experimental studies of spontaneous tumors in mice, especially in transgenic mice, reveal that the angiogenic switch is a discrete event that develops during progressive stages of tumorigenesis, beginning with the premalignant stage in these mouse models (Fig. 32-2).[4] The stages are similar to those in human carcinoma of the cervix, in which the onset of angiogenesis occurs during the premalignant dysplastic stage.[5] In contrast, breast cancer and other cancers are already at the in situ stage when neovascularization appears. Nevertheless, in both animal and human tumors, neovascularization usually develops before the emergence of invasive malignancy. In the 1970s, before the discovery of angiogenic proteins, increased angiogenic activity was demonstrated in breast tissue that progressed from a preneoplastic to a neoplastic stage.[6]

Increased expression of the angiogenic proteins vascular endothelial growth factor (VEGF)[7] or basic fibroblast growth factor (bFGF)[8] and of the angiogenic mediators thymidine phosphorylase[9] and tissue factor[10] has been reported in human breast cancer. VEGF mRNA and protein levels are dramatically upregulated by human mammary fibroblasts in response to hypoxia.[11] Thus, mammary stromal cells may play a role in the angiogenic phenotype in breast cancer. Also, bFGF and other angiogenic proteins can be mobilized from storage sites in the extracellular matrix in breast cancer.[12] Expression of VEGF in node-negative breast cancers has prognostic significance.[13] However, it should be emphasized that because the angiogenic activity of a tumor is the sum total of positive and negative regulators of angiogenesis, it would not be expected that quantification of a single angiogenic factor in tumor tissue would uniformly provide prognostic information.

The switch to the angiogenic phenotype also is understood as a shift in the net balance between positive regulators of angiogenesis (e.g., bFGF, VEGF) and negative regulators of angiogenesis (e.g., thrombospondin-1, 16-kD prolactin, interferon (IFN)-α, IFN-β, platelet factor 4, angiostatin, endostatin, and others such as interleukin (IL)-12.[14] Macrophages and other host cells may contribute to the angiogenic switch in breast cancer.[15] However, the genetic control of these regulators has begun to be elucidated.[16] For example, an angiogenesis inhibitor, thrombospondin-1, may be under the control of the *p53* tumor-suppressor gene[17]; induction of wild-type *p53* in glioblastoma cells releases an angiogenesis inhibitor[18]; VEGF is in part under the control of the *VHL* suppressor gene and also the *p53* suppressor gene[19]; and activation of oncogenes such as *RAS*, *RAF*, *FOS*, *SV₄OT* antigen, and others appears to be involved in production of angiogenic factors by tumor cells. The positive regulators of angiogenesis that are overexpressed in breast cancer must overcome a variety of negative regulators, some of which are produced by myoepithelial

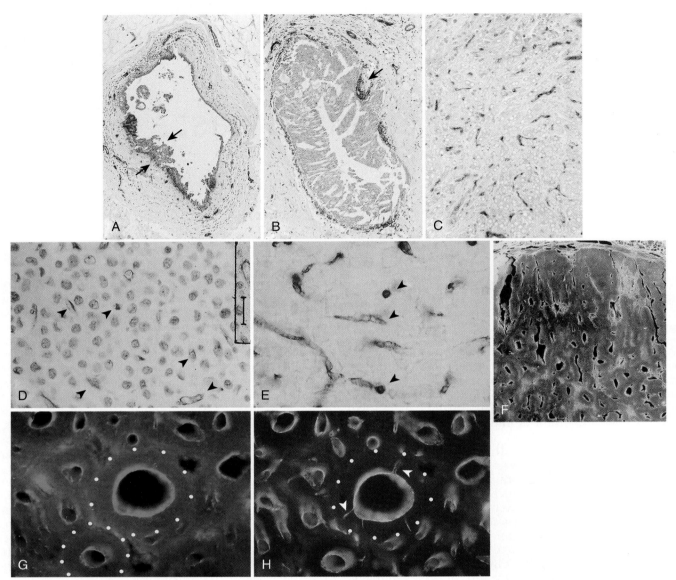

Figure 32-1 Human breast cancer. **A**, Large breast duct partially lined by ductal carcinoma in situ *(right arrow)* and intense angiogenesis in the immediately adjacent periductal breast stroma. Brown staining microvessels (antibody to von Willebrand factor) are indicated by the *left arrow*. Note the absence of angiogenesis in the areas of breast stroma adjacent to portion of duct lined with benign duct epithelium. **B**, Large breast duct filled with carcinoma in situ and surrounded by new microvessels in the periductal breast stroma. *Arrow* indicates invasion of microvessels through basement membrane of the duct, accompanied by invasion of tumor cells into the periductal stroma. **C**, Invasive ductal carcinoma showing area of highest density of microvessels. **D**, Higher power of invasive human breast carcinoma (4-μm section). Microvessels (brown stained with antibody to CD31) are indicated by *arrowheads*. **E**, A 50-μm-thick confocal microscopy section showing microvessels in three dimensions *(arrowheads)* surrounded by tumor cells that fill the intercapillary space. **F–H**, Cross-sections of breast cancer in mice showing the microcylinders of tumor cells that surround each microvessel. The 100-μm thickness of these tumor microcylinders is within the range of the oxygen diffusion limit. Scanning electron microscope view of 100-μm Vibratome section of a subcutaneous MCa-IV mouse breast tumor with the skin at the top (**F**). Blood vessels appear as black holes emptied of blood and preserved in an open state by vascular perfusion of fixative. Pale necrotic regions surround perivascular rings of tumor tissue that are approximately 100 μm thick. (Original magnification 25×; a 10-mm scale bar would equal 400 μm.) Large and small thin-walled blood vessels in MCa-IV mouse breast tumor labeled by vascular perfusion of green (FITC) fluorescent lectin staining (**G**, green) and CD31-immunoreactivity viewed by Cy3 fluorescence (**H**, *gold*). Like the lectin, CD31-immunoreactivity defines the luminal surface of the vessels but, unlike the lectin, it also labels tiny sprouts, which have no apparent lumen because they have CD31-immunoreactivity but no lectin staining. Sprouts *(white arrowheads)* about 1 μm in diameter radiate from the vessel lining into the 100-μm-thick perivascular ring of tumor tissue (outlined by *white dots*). Vessels preserved in open state by vascular perfusion of fixative. (**A**, From Weidner N, Semple JP, Welch WR, Folkman J: Tumor angiogenesis correlates with metastasis in invasive breast carcinoma. N Engl J Med 324:1–8, 1991; **F–H**, Courtesy of Donald M. McDonald, University of California, San Francisco.)

cells that surround ducts.[20] These inhibitors include thrombospondin-1, bFGF soluble receptor, and tissue inhibitor of metalloproteinase-1 (TIMP-1).

Normal cells that have been transformed to neoplastic cells are not usually angiogenic at the outset. Experimental studies of spontaneous tumors in transgenic mice reveal that the angiogenic switch is a discrete event that develops during progressive stages of tumorigenesis, beginning with the premalignant stage in these mouse models.[2] By the time most human tumors are detected, for example, with

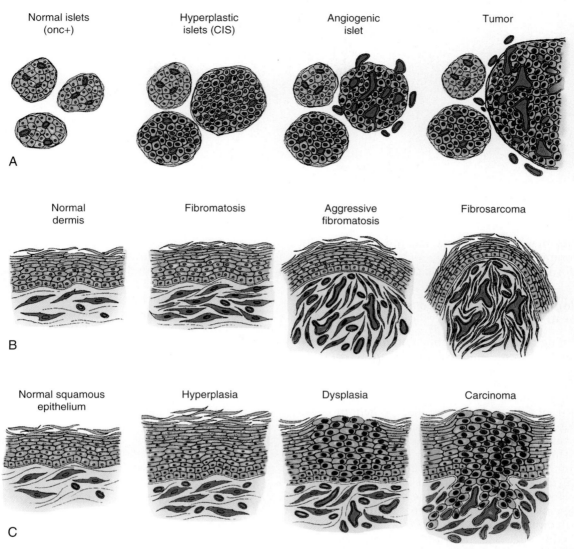

Figure 32-2   Histologic representations of the switch to the angiogenic phenotype. **A,** Islet cell carcinoma in transgenic RIP-Tag mice. **B,** Fibrosarcoma in transgenic mice. **C,** Human cervical carcinoma. CIS, carcinoma in situ. (**A** and **B,** Adapted from Hanahan D, Folkman J: Patterns and emerging mechanisms of the angiogenic switch during tumorigenesis. Cell 86:353, 1996; **C,** Adapted from Hanahan D, Folkman J: Patterns and emerging mechanisms of the angiogenic switch during tumorigenesis. Cell 86:353, 1996; and Smith-McCune KK, Weidner N: Demonstration and characterization of the angiogenic properties of cervical dysplasia. Cancer Res 54:800, 1994.)

mammography, neovascularization has usually occurred. However, most human tumors arise without angiogenic activity, exist in situ without neovascularization for months to years, and then switch to an angiogenic phenotype. Therefore, the angiogenic phenotype appears after the expression of the malignant phenotype in most primary tumors. For certain human tumors such as carcinoma of the cervix, the preneoplastic stage of dysplasia becomes neovascularized before the malignant tumor appears.[5] This sequence of events also occurs in certain spontaneously arising tumors in animals. At least four mechanisms of the angiogenic switch have been identified in both human tumors and spontaneous tumors in mice.

Prevascular Tumors Recruit Their Own Blood Supply

This is the most common mechanism of the angiogenic switch. Approximately 95% of human cancers are

carcinomas that originate as microscopic in situ lesions in an avascular epithelial layer separated by a basement membrane from underlying vasculature in the dermis or submucosa, respectively. The basement membrane is not only a physical barrier but also a molecular barrier to migrating endothelial cells. For example, tumstatin, a potent inhibitor of endothelial cell migration and proliferation, is found in collagen IV.[21] After the basement membrane has been breached by new vessel sprouts, tumor cells form multiple cell layers around each new capillary blood vessel. The radius of these microcylinders is restricted to the oxygen diffusion limit for a given tumor type as originally defined by Thomlinson and Gray.[22] For example, for a human melanoma, the oxygen diffusion limit is approximately 85 μ. Beyond that distance from a capillary blood vessel, virtually all tumor cells are apoptotic (or necrotic). Within that radius, most tumor cells are viable (Fig. 32-3). For a prostate carcinoma, the oxygen diffusion limit is approximately

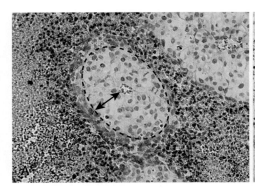 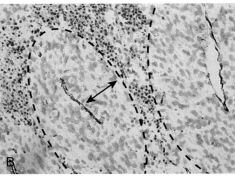

Figure 32-3 **A,** Cuff of live tumor cells around a microvessel in a human melanoma growing in a mouse with severe combined immunodeficiency syndrome has an average radius of 85 μ *(arrow)*. The appearance of an ellipsoid is due to the way the section is cut. **B,** Cuff of rat prostate cancer cells around a microvessel has an average radius of 110 μ *(arrow)*. (From Folkman J, Kalluri R: Tumor angiogenesis. In Kufe DW, Pollock RE, Weichselbaum RR, et al [eds]: Cancer medicine, 6th ed. Hamilton, Ontario, Decker, 2003.)

110 μ; and it may be greater for certain tumors, such as for a chondrosarcoma or a tumor in which *p53* is mutated or absent. However, it would rarely exceed 200 μ.

Circulating Endothelial Stem Cells Participate in Tumor Angiogenesis

It is becoming clear that circulating endothelial progenitor cells derived from bone marrow can be recruited to the vascular bed of tumors and contribute to tumor growth.[23] VEGF is elaborated by a variety of tumor signals through both VEGFR-1 (Flt-1) and VEGFR-2 (Flt-1) on endothelial cells and can mobilize progenitor endothelial cells into the circulation, where they are recruited into the vascular bed of certain tumor types, but not others.[24] The current view is that microvascular endothelial cells in the vascular bed of a tumor may be recruited both from the local neighborhood and from the bone marrow. However, the ratio of these endothelial cells from different sources may differ by tumor type.[25] Although lymphomas may recruit the majority (>90%) of their endothelial cells from the bone marrow, other tumors (e.g., breast cancer) recruit vascular endothelial cells both from the local neighborhood and to a lesser extent from the bone marrow. In contrast, in prostate cancer, most endothelial cells are recruited locally, and very few are derived from bone marrow. The ratios of bone marrow–derived endothelium and local endothelium have not yet been elucidated for most tumors. This phenomenon has certain implications. First, the efficacy of conventional chemotherapy may eventually be shown to correlate with the percentage of bone marrow–derived endothelial cells in a tumor. Second, during conventional chemotherapy administered at maximum tolerated dose, the off-therapy intervals necessary to rescue bone marrow may result in a surge of progenitor endothelial cells, which could traffic to the tumor. Third, certain angiogenesis inhibitors may suppress the release of bone marrow–derived progenitor endothelial cells. For example, angiostatin targets progenitor endothelial cells,[26] endostatin induces apoptosis in circulating endothelial cells in tumor-bearing mice,[27] and thalidomide decreases circulating endothelial cells by tenfold in multiple myeloma.[28]

Circulating VEGF may be one of the angiogenic signals by which tumors can recruit endothelial cells from bone marrow. Subcutaneously implanted collagen gels embedded with VEGF are invaded by endothelial cells from bone marrow and from the local neighborhood.[24] VEGF serum concentrations closely correlate with platelet counts in cancer patients.[29] VEGF is stored, transported, and released from platelets. Furthermore, it has been reported that platelet counts have prognostic significance for cancer patients; higher platelet counts correlate with a worse prognosis.[30] Therefore, it is possible that for those types of tumors that recruit bone marrow–derived endothelial cells, communication from tumor to bone marrow may be mediated in part by the VEGF in circulating platelets. According to Pinedo and colleagues,[30] "these results do not at this time have a direct impact on clinical cancer therapy." However, he emphasizes that "oncologists should be aware of a potential role for platelets in cancer growth" and in tumor angiogenesis.

Nonendothelial Host Cells May Contribute to the Angiogenic Switch by Amplifying Tumor Angiogenesis

In addition to recruiting vascular endothelium from the host, certain tumors may also attract mast cells, macrophages, and inflammatory cells.[31] These cells can amplify tumor angiogenesis by releasing proangiogenic molecules such as bFGF or by releasing metalloproteinases, which can mobilize VEGF and other angiogenic proteins.[32] Tumor angiogenesis and tumor growth are significantly diminished in mice deficient in metalloproteinase-9.[33] Certain tumor cells may also trigger host stromal cells in the tumor bed to overexpress the angiogenic protein VEGF.[34] This is a novel mechanism of amplification of the angiogenic phenotype once it has been initiated.

Vessel Co-option and Vascular Mimicry

In certain metastases (e.g., in the mouse brain), tumor cells exit from microvessels in the target organ, encircle these vessels, cause the endothelial cells to undergo apoptosis, and finally induce neovascular sprouts from neighboring vessels. This process, called co-option, may represent an intermediate or alternative step in the switch to the angiogenic phenotype.[35] In vascular mimicry, the tumor cells dedifferentiate into an endothelial phenotype and make tubelike structures.[36]

In summary, the hypothesis that all malignancies are angiogenesis dependent and that antiangiogenic therapy may control tumor growth appears to be true for all of these mechanisms of angiogenic switching.

PERSISTENCE OF NONANGIOGENIC TUMOR CELLS IN THE VASCULARIZED TUMOR

After a nonangiogenic microscopic in situ carcinoma has become neovascularized, the tumor still contains a significant proportion of tumor cells that have not switched.[37] Vascularized human primary tumors appear to contain a mixture of angiogenic and nonangiogenic tumor cells. The nonangiogenic tumor cells can be isolated from a human tumor removed at surgery by implanting numerous tiny pieces (1 mm^3) of tumor into the subcutaneous dorsum of mice with severe combined immunodeficiency syndrome or by implanting cultured human tumor cells. Although a few tumors grow to a palpable and visible size (100 to >1000 mm^3) within a few weeks and a few others appear after several months, most human tumor transplants remain invisible in the majority of mice, a phenomenon called "no take." However, on opening the skin of these mice, one invariably finds a tiny (<0.5 to 1 mm^3) whitish avascular or poorly vascularized tumor that is transplantable, contains proliferating and apoptotic tumor cells, but does not expand or metastasize. A few of these nonangiogenic dormant tumors have spontaneously become angiogenic after 1 month or more, depending on the tumor type, and have then grown. In contrast, others (e.g., osteosarcoma) have remained nonangiogenic and dormant up to 3 years after being transplanted to new mice every 8 months.[38] Some tumor types that remain nonangiogenic can be rapidly switched to the angiogenic phenotype through transfection with the *ras* oncogene, which significantly increases tumor cell production of VEGF and decreases thrombosponsin-1 production.[38] Furthermore, nonangiogenic tumor cells can be labeled with green fluorescent protein and mixed 1:1 with angiogenic tumor cells that are not labeled. The resulting large neovascularized tumor that grows rapidly contains tiny (<0.5 mm^3) green nonangiogenic colonies dispersed throughout. When the nonangiogenic green tumor cells are mixed with a decreasing fraction of angiogenic tumor cells, there is a long latent period of 1 month or more before neovascularized tumors arise. The latent period appears to be the time required for the angiogenic tumor cells to accumulate to a threshold population sufficient to recruit new blood vessels for the whole tumor. Once neovascularization has occurred, spontaneous metastases may appear in the lung (depending on the tumor type). Nonangiogenic tumor cells form microscopic nonangiogenic metastases.

These studies indicate that a nonangiogenic, dormant primary tumor may not shed tumor cells into the circulation. Once it switches to the angiogenic phenotype, it may then shed both angiogenic and nonangiogenic tumor cells into the circulation. The nonangiogenic tumor cells may be the source of microscopic metastases, which are capable of remaining dormant for prolonged periods. It has also been reported that in some instances, tumor cells may remain dormant as solitary cells.[39]

ONSET OF NEOVASCULARIZATION PERMITS EXPANSION OF TUMOR MASS, INVASION, AND METASTASIS

Expansion of Tumor Mass

As new capillaries are induced to sprout from preexisting capillaries and venules, tumor cells grow around them. Three or more concentric layers of tumor cells may encircle a single capillary tube. The replication of new capillaries, each supporting a microcylinder of tumor cells, permits rapid expansion of tumor mass. A segment of capillary tube formed by a single endothelial cell can support 5 to 50 tumor cells, based on the finding that a gram of tumor contains approximately 20 million endothelial cells and 108 to 109 tumor cells.[40] A large breast carcinoma of 1 cm^3 or greater may appear white or pale on gross examination and thus is often assumed to be avascular. However, microscopic examination reveals a fine vascular network interspersed with tumor cells. The microvessels are often difficult to see on a routine 4-μm-thick paraffin section, because their lumina are compressed. However, if endothelial cells are highlighted with antibody to von Willebrand factor or to CD34, the microvessels are more readily visualized. Furthermore, if the thickness of the histologic section is increased to 50 μm, it is possible to see microvessels projecting in three dimensions, and each vessel is surrounded by a microcylinder of three to four layers of tumor cells.

The stimulation of tumor cell growth after the onset of neovascularization is usually ascribed to perfusion of the tumor cells by new blood flow, which delivers oxygen and nutrients and removes catabolites. A paracrine effect of endothelial cells on tumor cell growth may be equally important.[41] In vitro studies reveal that tumor cells grow preferentially around capillary tubes despite the absence of flow.[42] Endothelial cells also produce growth and survival factors such as insulin-like growth factor-I (IGF-I), bFGF, platelet-derived growth factor (PDGF-BB), heparin-binding epithelial growth factor (HB-EGF), and granulocyte-macrophage colony-stimulating factor. Because a neovascularized tumor is flooded with growth factors and survival factors, complete blockade of neovascularization by an angiogenesis inhibitor could result in disappearance of growth factors, survival factors, or both. In animal and human tumors, the induction of angiogenesis correlates with a significant decrease in apoptosis (by as much as sevenfold in mice).[43] Nevertheless, in these tumors the proliferation rate of tumor cells remains equivalently high in the prevascular and in the vascularized tumor (up to 40% by bromo-deoxy-uridine [BrdU]). This pattern is observed in a variety of tumor types. It indicates that tumor expansion after neovascularization may depend mainly on a decrease in apoptosis. Analogous systems are found in *MYC*-dependent lymphoma cells or in fibroblasts with dysregulated *MYC* expression. Both cell types grow in the presence of IGF-I or IGF-II, respectively, but die when these factors are withdrawn.[44]

Although the absence of angiogenesis prevents expansion of tumor mass beyond a microscopic size of a few millimeters, the presence of angiogenesis is necessary but not sufficient for expansion of tumor mass. Some benign tumors, such as adrenal adenoma, may lack the proliferative capacity to match their high angiogenic activity. Conversely, the rate of expansion of a tumor mass can be regulated independently of tumor cell proliferation. Some human tumors (e.g., prostate and breast cancer) grow slowly for years and then seem to shift to a rapid rate of expansion of tumor mass. Neglected breast cancers that have attained a large size may slow their growth, possibly from diminished angiogenic activity. Experimental evidence for this idea comes from murine fibrosarcoma cells transfected with the angiogenesis inhibitor angiostatin.[45] Inoculation of mice with transfected cells that express increasing levels of angiostatin yields tumors that grow slowly (i.e., 77% inhibition of tumor growth compared with nontransfected tumor cells in the same period). Furthermore, because it is now clear that tumor burden can inhibit angiogenesis, the slowing of certain tumors as they increase in size could be attributable in part to angiogenic mechanisms.[46,47]

Invasion

Tumor invasion may be facilitated by neovascularization. Although microinvasion may be observed in a carcinoma in situ of the breast before it has become neovascularized (i.e., a thin file of tumor cells breaches the basic membrane of a duct filled with tumor), invasion into adjacent connective tissue occurs along a broad front and tumor cords follow the path of newly generated blood vessels after neovascularization.[48] Microvascular endothelial cells under the stimulus of angiogenic proteins (e.g., bFGF, VPF/VEGF) increase their expression of proteolytic enzymes (e.g., collagenase IV), which contribute to the invasiveness of endothelial cells and tumor cells.[49] The ability of growing capillaries to liquefy extracellular matrix is clearly illustrated by the following experiment. India ink (containing carbon particles of approximately 200 Å) is injected into a rabbit cornea so that the ink is trapped in a square corneal pocket, like a tattoo, between a tumor implant and the vascular bed at the limbal edge of the cornea.[50] As new blood vessels are attracted into the cornea by the tumor, they first encounter the India ink. India ink is dispersed only from the inferior border of the pocket, coincident with dissolution of the corneal matrix by the neovascular front. The superior border of the India ink, contiguous to the avascular tumor, remains intact. Only after the tumor has become neovascularized is it capable of invading the corneal pocket and dispersing all of the India ink. In the absence of neovascularization, India ink remains sharply demarcated in the corneal pocket. This result suggests that the proteolytic activity produced by proliferating capillary blood vessels may enhance invasion of endothelial cells into extracellular matrix but may also contribute to the invasiveness of tumor cells. Therefore, antiangiogenic therapy could inhibit tumor invasion. Conversely, certain protease inhibitors are antiangiogenic.[51] However, some protease inhibitors may also decrease the enzymatic release of angiogenesis inhibitors (e.g.,

angiostatin, endostatin, tumstatin). When human skin grafted to immunodeficient mice was inoculated with human breast cancer cells, the resulting tumors became vascularized by human blood vessels. When the animals were injected with antibody against $\alpha_v\beta_3$ integrin on the human endothelial cells, angiogenesis was inhibited, but so was tumor invasiveness, despite the fact that the tumor cells lacked the $\alpha_v\beta_3$ receptor.[52]

Metastasis

Experimental and clinical evidence suggest that the process of metastasis is also angiogenesis dependent.[53] For a tumor cell to metastasize successfully, it must breach several barriers and be able to respond to specific growth factors. Tumor cells must gain access to the vasculature in the primary tumor, survive the circulation, arrest in the microvasculature of the target organ, exit from this vasculature, grow in the target organ, and induce angiogenesis. Thus, angiogenesis appears to be necessary at both the beginning and end of the metastatic cascade.

In experimental animals, tumor cells are generally found in the circulation only after a primary tumor has become vascularized.[54] The number of cells shed from the primary tumor correlates with the density of vessels in the primary tumor and with the number of lung metastases observed subsequently. Tumor cells can enter the circulation by penetrating through proliferating capillaries whose basement membranes are fragmented and leaky. Increasing tumor angiogenesis has also been correlated with increased tumor cell shedding into the circulation in human tumors. Furthermore, angiogenic factors from tumors (bFGF and VEGF) induce plasminogen activator and collagenases in proliferating endothelial cells and contribute to the degradation of basement membranes.[55] Other evidence that metastasis is angiogenesis dependent is based on the suppression of metastatic growth in mice treated with endothelial-specific angiogenesis inhibitors, such as angiostatin or endostatin. The metastases remain dormant at a microscopic size. Dormancy occurs despite the fact that the angiogenesis inhibitors have no inhibitory effect on the tumor cells in vitro. In these animals, microscopic dormant metastases are harmless, and the mice appear perfectly healthy for as long as the inhibitor is administered (up to 2 to 10 months).[56] In another animal tumor model, lung metastases remain nonangiogenic and avascular, even after the original primary tumor has been removed. These mice are healthy for as long as they have been observed, or almost half their normal life span. The dormant, nonangiogenic metastases can be induced to grow at any time through local trauma to the chest or systemic administration of transforming growth factor (TGF) (J. Folkman and M. O'Reilly, personal communication). Correlative clinical data also suggest that metastatic potential may depend on the intensity of angiogenesis. Neovascularization can be quantified in human tumors by staining histologic sections with an antibody to von Willebrand factor, an endothelial cell marker. This method also reveals a significant direct correlation between the highest density of microvessels in a histologic section of invasive breast cancer and the occurrence of future metastases.[48]

Angiogenesis Progression

Rak and colleagues[16] proposed the term *angiogenic progression* in a hypothesis that states that "a stepwise accumulation of genetic alterations during tumor progression is likely to be paralleled by a stepwise increase in angiogenic competence of tumor cells." Angiogenesis and neoplastic progression have also been linked in animal tumors. For example, a primary breast cancer may produce one angiogenic protein, for example VEGF, but subsequent metastases may produce up to six angiogenic proteins.[57] In the advanced stages of breast cancer or other malignancies, the clinical picture is one of new metastases that parasitize the circulation and that appear ever more frequently at decreasing intervals.

Angiogenesis in Human Breast Cancer

ANGIOGENIC FACTORS IN BODY FLUIDS

Serum tumor markers for breast cancer used in the clinic include cancer antigen (CA) 15-3, carcinoembryonic antigen (CEA), and CA 27-29. All have low sensitivity and specificity; thus, they are unhelpful in detecting early breast cancer.[58] Numerous peptides associated with breast malignant transformation have been extensively investigated in the blood of patients with breast cancer and compared with control healthy women. Individually, none of the markers thus far has been sensitive or specific enough to detect early breast cancer. However, it is possible that future combinations of certain protein levels in the blood may be useful. Because the process of angiogenesis plays a critical role in breast tumor growth, there has been much interest in the possible use of several angiogenic factors or inhibitors as biomarkers. In population studies, angiogenic factors are significantly elevated in cancer patients, in comparison with normal controls. However, overlap values between cancer and normal groups have made it difficult to diagnose breast tumor early at an individual basis,[59] although bFGF may have the best sensitivity and specificity.[60] The same may apply to cytokines, such as IL-6 and tumor necrosis factor-α,[61] hepatocyte growth factor,[62] and others.[63]

It is possible that the level of angiogenic factor(s) may be useful for prognostic purposes or for monitoring therapeutic response. Treatment of breast cancer has resulted in decreasing plasma VEGF, Tie-2, and angiopoietin-1.[64] The growth factor bFGF has been reported to increase the predictive value of the conventional marker CA 15-3 in response to chemotherapy of advanced breast cancer.[65] High levels of plasma TIMP-1 predicts survival in women with metastatic breast cancer,[66] whereas low serum levels of promatrix metalloproteinase 2 correlate with aggressive behavior in operable breast cancer.[67] Preoperative E-selectin levels also correlate with advanced stage.[68] Plasma prolactin concentrations are reported to associate with an increased risk of postmenopausal breast cancer.[69] Also, circulating IGF-I and IGF-binding protein (IGFBP-3) are positively associated with breast cancer risk in older women but not in younger women.[70] Of interest, circulating endothelial cells have also been reported to decrease with treatment.[71]

Breast cancer arises from the epithelial cells that line the ductal/lobular systems of the milk ducts. Therefore, it makes sense that examination of this ductal system or analysis of its secretions may reveal signs of early cancer. It appears that many breast-related molecules exist at a higher concentration in nipple fluid than in blood. Although unlike blood, nipple fluid is not universally available, it can be elicited in nearly all premenopausal women and in the majority of older women. Potential areas of usefulness include early detection of breast cancer risk or breast cancer, as well as monitoring and/or predicting preventive therapy.[72] Certain angiogenic peptides have emerged as potential tumor markers in nipple aspirate fluid. The growth factor bFGF was found by our group to be significantly elevated in nipple fluid from cancerous breasts.[73] At a cutoff level of 250 pg/mL, sensitivity is 79%, specificity 83%, and accuracy 66%.[74] The results are not influenced by race, age, menopausal status, or hormone use. This finding was confirmed by others to have a sensitivity of 90% to 94% and a specificity of 69% to 97%.[75] Among several tested, nipple-fluid bFGF was the best predictive tumor marker.[76] Other angiogenic candidates include HER2,[77] IGFBP-3,[78] and urokinase-type plasminogen activator.[79]

QUANTIFICATION OF INTRATUMORAL MICROVESSEL DENSITY

Weidner and associates[48] first reported that quantification of microvessel density in breast cancer was an independent prognostic indicator of metastatic risk and mortality. Microvessels were highlighted in histologic sections by staining with an antibody to von Willebrand factor. In subsequent studies, other endothelial markers have been used, such as CD31.[80] Without such endothelial markers, microvessels are often difficult to visualize in the standard histologic section, which is cut at 4-μm thickness. This is in part because of the closure of some vessels by compressive interstitial pressures.

Weidner and colleagues also found that microvessels were not homogeneously distributed, but that there were areas of increased microvessel density. Quantification of the number of vessels in these areas gave the best predictive values for overall survival. It is critical to choose the invasive components of breast cancer specimens.[81] Areas of highest microvessel density (vascular hotspots) are selected by scanning a tumor section at low magnification (10–100×). A generous section through the middle of the tumor (which includes the tumor periphery) is selected for microvessel analysis. Vascular hotspots are encountered predominantly at the peripheral tumor margin. A higher magnification (approximately 200–400×) is then used to count individual stained microvessels. When microvessels are counted in a field, it is not necessary to identify the lumen or red cells in a vessel, and a cutoff caliber size is not used. Both single cell sprouts and larger vessels are included in the counts. Even if distinct clusters give the impression of being part of one larger vessel transected by the plane of the tissue section more than once, they are counted as separate microvessels. Averaging counts of all the vessels in a section does not correlate with clinical outcome, but quantification of hotspots does. In more than 3200 cases worldwide of breast cancer assessed for angiogenic activity, 80% of the studies that included multivariant analysis found that angiogenesis is a significant prognostic indicator of overall survival.[82] Intratumoral microvessel density is a prognostic indicator in patients who are lymph node negative, and this may be an important use for this method. This method has been successful in the majority of reports for a variety of other tumors from many centers worldwide.[83]

Most studies reveal that the higher the microvessel count in areas of highest vessel density, the lower the overall survival. The decreased survival is generally related to increased metastatic risk. Possible biologic explanations for this correlation include the following:

- Increasing microvessel density provides an increased vascular surface area for cells to escape from the primary tumor into the main circulation.
- Because of the clonal origin of metastases, a primary tumor containing a high proportion of angiogenic malignant cells is more likely to generate metastases that are already angiogenic when they arrive at the target tissue.[84]
- Some tumor cells produce multiple angiogenic factors compared with others and thus have a higher probability of rapid tumor growth.[57]
- Certain angiogenic factors such as bFGF and VEGF also upregulate production of metalloproteinases

by endothelial cells and increase the possibility that tumor cells enter the circulation.

- Endothelial cells in the vascular bed of a tumor release cytokines that can facilitate metastasis. For example, IL-6 produced by endothelial cells is a motility factor for breast cancer cells and may facilitate their escape from a vascularized tumor into the circulation.[85]
- There are also confounding biologic factors that could explain some reports that find no prognostic value for microvessel density. For example, mouse experiments reveal that tumor burden can influence angiogenesis at a remote site.[46,47]

Although microvessel density is a useful prognostic indicator of metastatic risk in many tumors, it may not be a good indicator of therapeutic efficacy for several reasons. In normal tissues, the degree of vascularization and oxygen/nutrient demand are tightly coupled. In tumors, however, the degree of vascularization and tumor growth are loosely coupled, or even uncoupled. This may be because in tumor cells, expression of angiogenic factors, such as VEGF, are no longer regulated by oxygen concentration. During tumor regression under antiangiogenic therapy, microvessel density may decrease if capillary dropout exceeds tumor cell dropout (autolysis), increase if tumor cell dropout exceeds capillary dropout, or remain the same if disappearance of capillaries and tumor cells parallel each other. Mice bearing human osteosarcomas were treated with endostatin until there was more than a 50% inhibition of tumor growth (Fig. 32-4).[86] Despite the fact that this drug inhibited growth of both treated tumors depicted, the intensity of

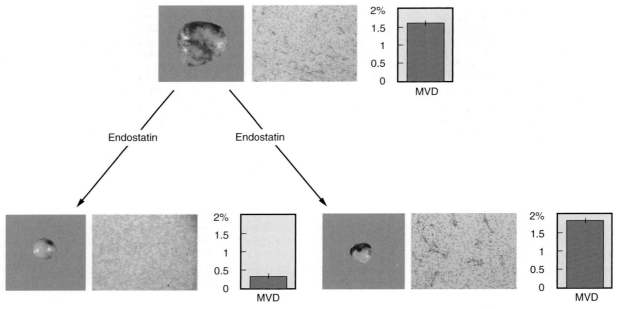

Figure 32-4 Human osteosarcomas growing in immunodeficient mice were treated with endostatin. Endostatin significantly inhibited tumor growth. Despite the fact that endostatin inhibited both treated tumors depicted here, the intensity of vascularization after treatment differed significantly between the tumors. Microvascular density (MVD) was quantified over the entire histologic section rather than over vascular hotspots to avoid the effects of heterogeneity of vascularization in the tissue sample. Sections were scored by imaging as many microscopic fields at 200× as necessary to cover the entire section. MVD dropped sharply in one treated tumor but rose slightly in the second, yet both tumors were equivalently reduced in size by the treatment relative to control. (Modified from Hlatky L, Hahnfeldt P, Folkman J: Clinical application of antiangiogenic therapy: Microvessel density, what it does and doesn't tell us. J Natl Cancer Inst 94:883, 2002.)

vascularization after treatment differed significantly between the tumors. Microvascular density was quantified over the entire histologic section rather than over vascular hotspots to avoid the effects of heterogeneity of vascularization in the tissue sample. Microvascular density dropped sharply in one treated tumor but rose slightly in the second, yet both tumors were equivalently reduced in size by the treatment relative to control. Thus, detection of a decrease in microvessel density during treatment with an angiogenesis inhibitor suggests that the agent is active. However, the absence of a drop in microvessel density does not indicate that the agent is ineffective.[87] Understanding this distinction between the usefulness of microvessel density as a prognostic indicator of future metastatic risk or mortality in contrast to its problematic status as a predictor of therapeutic efficacy is important in the design of clinical trials of angiogenesis inhibitors. Biopsies of tumors or lymph nodes for microvessel density, before or after antiangiogenic therapy, may not be useful. Furthermore, selecting patients for such clinical trials on the basis of whether their tumor is highly vascularized also appears to be unnecessary. In fact, experimental studies show that a given dose of an angiogenesis inhibitor is more effective in poorly vascularized tumors. Highly vascularized tumors require larger doses.[88]

DORMANT BREAST CANCER

It is not uncommon for a patient with node-negative breast cancer to remain asymptomatic for 10 to 12 years and then experience the sudden appearance of metastases. This phenomenon, called *tumor dormancy*, can be defined as microscopic disease in which there is no expansion of tumor mass.[89] There has been no satisfactory explanation for this long-term dormancy, and it is not clear where the tumor cells resided or whether they were proliferating or quiescent. Different explanations include the following: (1) the tumor cells could be in a prolonged G_0 state, removed from the cell cycle; (2) the cells could be immunologically suppressed[90]; (3) tumor cells could be dormant because of hormone withdrawal[91]; (4) tumor cells could be proliferating continuously, but take years to produce a tumor of the size that can be detected clinically[3]; or (5) expansion of microscopic metastases could be constrained throughout the dormant period but undergo a sudden change from a resting microtumor to an enlarging tumor mass within a year or less of the time of first clinical detection. The results reported by Demicheli and coworkers[92] best fit this model. They show that the mean rate of growth of the metastatic tumor, once it has grown beyond the dormant stage and has been detected clinically, is similar from one patient to another and is independent of the length of the dormant period. This model of tumor dormancy most closely resembles experimental models of blocked angiogenesis.[43] Murine lung metastases were held dormant at a microscopic size for as long as their angiogenesis was completely blocked by the administration of angiostatin. In these animals, proliferating tumor cells are balanced by apoptotic tumor cells. A provocative finding is that inhibition of angiogenesis significantly increases tumor cell apoptosis but has no effect on the high rate of tumor cell proliferation. Subsequent reports confirm that angiogenesis and apoptosis are inversely correlated, whereas tumor cell proliferation is independent of angiogenesis.[93]

Patients with locally advanced breast cancer who have no detectable metastases may develop rapid growth of metastases after removal of the large breast tumor. A possible explanation for this observation is that tumor burden can suppress tumor growth.[94] A suggested mechanism for this phenomenon comes from the recent discovery that increasing mass of a primary tumor inhibits angiogenesis at remote sites and that this process is mediated by angiostatin.[46] The inhibition of metastatic growth by a primary tumor may be only one pattern of a group of common patterns of presentation of metastases, some of which are observed in patients with breast cancer. Four common patterns and a rare pattern of metastatic presentation have been proposed.

The first pattern, in which metastases grow after removal of the primary tumor, is analogous to a mouse model of Lewis lung carcinoma in which lung metastases remain microscopic while a primary tumor is present (and generating angiostatin) but grow rapidly within 5 days after the primary tumor is removed.[46]

The second pattern, in which metastases grow concomitantly with the primary tumor, is analogous to a mouse model of a subclone of Lewis lung carcinoma in which the primary tumor does not suppress its lung metastases and does not generate detectable levels of angiostatin in the circulation.[46]

The third pattern, known to oncologists as the occult primary, could be based on metastatic cells that outgrow the primary tumor and suppress its angiogenesis. This is speculation, and there are no animal models, with the possible exception of one report, in which metastatic cells were seeded in the lungs, followed later by implantation of a subcutaneous tumor, whose growth was inhibited.[95]

The fourth pattern, in which metastases remain dormant for years following removal of the primary tumor, is observed in breast cancer, colon cancer, Ewing's sarcoma, and many other tumor types. Again, the mechanism of this prolonged dormancy is unknown. However, recent reports indicate that once metastases become clinically detectable, they display a similar rate of growth that is independent of the number of years of dormancy.[92] This observation is consistent with a model of microscopic dormant metastases that do not expand until sometime within a year of becoming clinically detectable. It can be speculated that these metastases originated from cells that were not angiogenic but underwent the switch to the angiogenic phenotype before becoming clinically detectable. No animal model has been reported. However, Folkman has demonstrated a B16 melanoma in C57Bl/6 mice in which dormant, nonangiogenic lung metastases of less than 0.1 to 0.2 mm diameter are found as late as 6 months after removal of the primary tumor in otherwise healthy mice. This is one fourth the normal life span of these animals (J. Folkman and M. O'Reilly, personal communication). A study of nonangiogenic tumor cells that escape from the primary tumor and the mechanism by which their metastases switch to the angiogenic phenotype may be a fruitful area of research.

A fifth pattern of metastatic presentation is occasionally observed, for example, when removal of a renal cell carcinoma is followed by regression of lung metastases. One can speculate that the metastases may have been dependent on high production of circulating angiogenic factors (and possibly other growth factors) from the primary tumor. In renal cell carcinomas, high tumor levels of bFGF correlate with high mortality.[96] In fact, we found that 10% of patients with a wide spectrum of malignancies had abnormally elevated levels of bFGF in their serum, and 37% of 950 patients had abnormally elevated levels of bFGF in urine.[97]

The clinical presentations of metastases are discussed here in terms of angiogenic mechanisms, because this approach offers a plausible unifying explanation for the different patterns that oncologists see in their cancer patients. The similarity of animal models to human patterns of metastasis presentation does not prove that angiogenic control of metastatic growth is responsible for the behavior of metastases in cancer patients. These mechanisms have yet to be demonstrated in human cancer. However, clinicians who are aware of them may be able to uncover evidence that supports or rejects the hypothesis.

Principles of Antiangiogenic Therapy in the Clinic

Certain guidelines are emerging from laboratory and clinical experience that may be helpful in the design of protocols for antiangiogenic therapy in breast cancer, as well as in other types of cancer. A goal of antiangiogenic therapy is to regress a focus of proliferating microvessels, that is to restore a local area of migrating and proliferating endothelial cells to their normal resting state. When used in cancer therapy, antiangiogenic therapy differs from cytotoxic chemotherapy, in which the objective is to kill as many tumor cells as possible in the shortest possible time with the maximum tolerated dose. Antiangiogenic therapy is usually administered for prolonged periods, without interruption, at the highest effective dosage that does not cause toxicity. It is neither necessary nor efficacious to discontinue an angiogenesis inhibitor at intervals, as is done for cytotoxic therapy. For example, infants with life-threatening hemangiomas have been treated daily for 9 months to 1 year with IFN-α)[98] Low-dose daily IFN-α (3 million U/m²/day for children or 3 million U/day for adults), which inhibits production by tumors of the proangiogenic protein bFGF, has been administered for 8 months to 1 year to patients with recurrent high-grade giant cell tumors of the mandible and maxilla.[99] This treatment has resulted in complete regression that has remained durable for up to 6 years' follow-up. Stable disease can also be a goal of antiangiogenic therapy. In clinical trials of endostatin, some patients with metastatic disease who self-inject the drug subcutaneously every day have had stable disease for years. Tumor growth is arrested. The patients

regain weight, strength, and hair. There has been virtually no toxicity.[100] Tumor arrest may be a better term than stable disease for this condition, because stable disease induced by conventional cytotoxic chemotherapy is often limited by eventual acquired drug resistance, is associated with the side effects of chemotherapy, and connotes probable failure of conventional cytotoxic chemotherapy.

DIRECT AND INDIRECT ANGIOGENESIS INHIBITORS

In designing a clinical trial for antiangiogenic therapy of cancer, especially breast cancer, it is helpful to understand that angiogenesis inhibitors can be either direct or indirect (Fig. 32-5).

Direct angiogenesis inhibitors such as vitaxin,[101] angiostatin, endostatin, 2-methoxyestradiol, combretastatin, NM-3, thrombospondin, ultra-low-dose continuous paclitaxel,[102] and others prevent vascular endothelial cells from proliferating and migrating. Alternatively, these inhibitors increase the endothelial survival in response to a spectrum of proangiogenic proteins, including VEGF, bFGF, IL-8, PDGF, and platelet-derived endothelial cell growth factor (PD-ECGF). Direct angiogenesis inhibitors are the least likely to induce acquired drug resistance, because they target genetically stable endothelial cells rather than unstable mutating tumor cells.[103] Tumors in mice treated with antiangiogenic therapy did not develop drug resistance.[104]

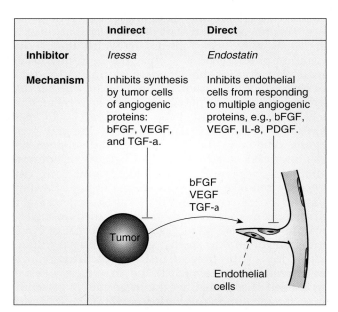

	Indirect	**Direct**
Inhibitor	*Iressa*	*Endostatin*
Mechanism	Inhibits synthesis by tumor cells of angiogenic proteins: bFGF, VEGF, and TGF-a.	Inhibits endothelial cells from responding to multiple angiogenic proteins, e.g., bFGF, VEGF, IL-8, PDGF.

Figure 32-5 Types of angiogenesis inhibitors. Direct angiogenesis inhibitors are less likely to induce acquired drug resistance because they inhibit endothelial cells in the tumor bed from responding to a wide spectrum of proangiogenic proteins from tumor or from stroma. In contrast, indirect angiogenesis inhibitors block an oncogene expressed by the tumor, a tumor cell product, or the receptor for that product. This block permits the emergence of mutants producing proangiogenic proteins that might not be antagonized by the indirect angiogenesis inhibitor. (See text for abbreviations.) (From Folkman J, Kalluri R: Tumor angiogenesis. In Kufe DW, Pollock RE, Weichselbaum RR, et al [eds]: Cancer medicine, 6th ed. Hamilton, Ontario, Decker, 2003.)

Figure 32-6 Production of proangiogenic proteins by human tumors. High-grade giant cell tumors and angioblastomas produce mainly bFGF as their angiogenic stimulator. In contrast breast cancers produce a spectrum of different angiogenic proteins. (See text for abbreviations.) (From Relf M, LeJune S, Scott PA, et al: Expression of the angiogenic factors vascular endothelial growth factor, acidic and basic fibroblast growth factor, tumor growth factor beta-1, platelet-derived endothelial cell growth factor, placenta growth factor, and pleiotrophin in human primary breast cancer and its relation to angiogenesis. Cancer Res 57:963–969, 1997.)

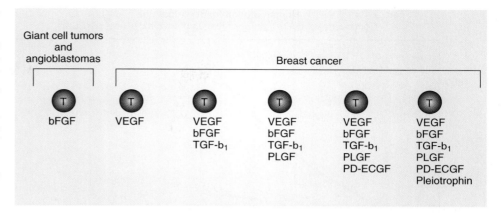

TREATMENT CONSIDERATIONS

Low Toxicity

Indirect angiogenesis inhibitors generally inhibit expression of a tumor cell product, neutralize the tumor product itself, or block its receptor on endothelial cells. Examples include: (1) EGF tyrosine kinase inhibitors, which block production of the proangiogenic proteins VEGF, bFGF, and TGF-α (e.g., gefitinib [Iressa], erlotinib HCl [Tarceva], cetuximab [Erbitux]); (2) an antibody that neutralizes VEGF (e.g., bevacizumab [Avastin]); or (3) inhibitors of VEGF receptors on endothelium (e.g., PTK787, ZD6474, SU11248). For indirect angiogenesis inhibitors, it may be important to know in advance if the tumor is producing one or more of the angiogenic proteins that are counteracted by the angiogenesis inhibitor(s) (Fig. 32-6). Therefore, it may be valuable to stratify patients who are receiving an indirect angiogenesis inhibitor, analogous to the selection of patients who receive trastuzumab (Herceptin) or tamoxifen. Also, indirect angiogenesis inhibitors are susceptible to acquired drug resistance as the tumor cells undergo mutation and produce angiogenic proteins not covered by the indirect angiogenesis inhibitor. Presumably, drug resistance is less likely to occur with the use of direct angiogenesis inhibitors, because they prevent endothelial cells from responding to a wide range of proangiogenic factors.

TREATMENT CONSIDERATIONS

Low Toxicity

Most angiogenesis inhibitors are not toxic to highly replicating cells such as those in the gut, bone marrow, bladder, or skin. In fact, the more selective an angiogenesis inhibitor is for endothelial cells, the less likely it is to cause diarrhea, bone marrow suppression, and hair loss. Delayed wound healing and contraception[105] are two side effects common to some angiogenesis inhibitors. Of course, there may be side effects unrelated to the anti-endothelial activity of these inhibitors. For example, when TNP-470 is administered at levels higher than its effective dosage, side effects may develop in the central nervous system, and this was also observed in preclinical animal studies. This toxicity has now been eliminated in tumor-bearing mice through a modification of TNP-470 in which the drug is conjugated to a polymer, hydroxypropyl methacrylamide, so that it no longer enters the

cerebrospinal fluid. In contrast, angiostatin and endostatin are specific inhibitors of endothelial proliferation and have no effect on a wide spectrum of other cell types tested up. Nor do they have any effect on resting, nonproliferating endothelial cells. No significant toxicity of any kind from these inhibitors has been detected in animals to date, and these drugs are both safe in phase I/II clinical trials so far.[106]

Continuous versus Bolus Dosing

Experimental studies in tumor-bearing animals have shown that continuous dosing of an angiogenesis inhibitor is approximately tenfold more effective than bolus dosing.[107] For example, continuous administration of endostatin by a micro-osmotic Alzet pump implanted into the peritoneal cavity caused regression of human tumors in mice, whereas the same amount of endostatin given as an intraperitoneal dose as a bolus every 24 hours did not regress the same tumor (Fig. 32-7). These experiments indicate that if endothelial cells in a tumor bed are constantly exposed to proangiogenic proteins issuing from adjacent tumor cells, then to counter this stimulation with antiangiogenic therapy requires the continual presence of an angiogenesis inhibitor (or inhibitors) in the lumen. In a sense, the angiogenesis inhibitor is titrated against the total amount of proangiogenic activity from a tumor during the therapeutic attack against the tumor.

Common Misperceptions about Antiangiogenic Therapy

Certain common misperceptions about the mechanisms of angiogenesis and about antiangiogenic therapy may be problematic in the design of protocols for clinical trials. For example, it is often assumed that tumors that are avascular or poorly vascularized cannot be treated with an angiogenesis inhibitor. This assumption originates from observations of gross specimens of tumors, some of which appear to be highly vascularized, whereas others are pale or white and appear not to be vascularized. In fact, the gross appearance of a tumor, whether it is observed before or after it has been removed from the patient, does not accurately reflect the intensity of

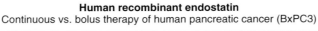

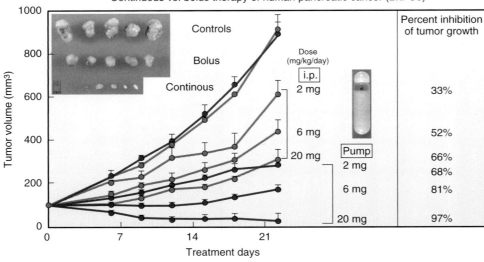

Figure 32-7 Demonstration in tumor-bearing mice that continuous infusion (*red lines*) of endostatin is approximately 10 times more effective than single daily bolus injection (*blue lines*). Continuous infusion leads to tumor regression, whereas bolus injection of the same dose does not. (From Folkman J, Kalluri R: Tumor angiogenesis. In Kufe DW, Pollock RE, Weichselbaum RR, et al [eds]: Cancer medicine, 6th ed. Hamilton, Ontario, Decker, 2003.)

neovascularization at the microscopic level. Virtually all tumors that are of clinically detectable size (>2 to 3 mm) are neovascularized. In principle, they are treatable with an angiogenesis inhibitor, although some tumors may be greater producers of angiogenic activity than others and require higher dosages of an angiogenesis inhibitor. In experimental animals, poorly vascularized, more slowly growing bladder cancers responded to a given dose of angiogenesis inhibitors with greater efficacy than did highly vascularized, rapidly growing tumors. Furthermore, antiangiogenic therapy may also be used to maintain the dormancy of microscopic metastases that are not neovascularized.

Another common misperception is that large, established tumors cannot be treated with an angiogenesis inhibitor, presumably because the vessels would no longer be growing or would be mature. Even in large tumors, endothelial cells in the new microvessels in a tumor bed have a high turnover rate compared with endothelial cells in quiescent microvessels outside the tumor.[108] Most tumor microvessels consist of thin-walled capillary tubes with or without pericytes but with little or no smooth muscle. After an angiogenic stimulus is removed from the rabbit cornea, neovessels involute and disappear within 1 to 2 weeks. However, the preexisting or established vessels in the sclera at the limbal edge of the cornea remain intact. These vessels may be equivalent to the arterial and venous feeder vessels of a tumor. It is not yet known whether some tumors may produce a combination of proangiogenic proteins that can produce mature, stabilized microvessels, which may not be as susceptible to certain angiogenesis inhibitors.

It is often assumed that only malignant tumors are treatable with antiangiogenic therapy. However, both benign and malignant tumors can be angiogenic. For example, a prostate gland enlarged by benign prostatic hypertrophy is neovascularized. Adrenal adenomas are benign but highly angiogenic tumors. Also, in children, benign hemangiomas and a benign giant cell tumor of

the mandible have regressed completely with IF-α therapy. One can speculate that certain slow-growing benign tumors, such as fibromas and neurofibromas, may be candidates for antiangiogenic therapy, especially because this form of therapy does not depend on a large pool of proliferating tumor cells.

Another common misperception is that antiangiogenic therapy should not be used before chemotherapy because an angiogenesis inhibitor closes blood vessels and thus reduces access to a chemotherapeutic drug. Just the opposite is true. First, Teicher and colleagues[109] have shown that antiangiogenic therapy increases flow and oxygen delivery as well as drug delivery to a tumor. Second, during inhibition of angiogenesis by either angiostatin or endostatin, apoptosis of tumor cells increased threefold to sevenfold but tumor cell proliferation remained high. These data argue that after a bulky tumor is reduced to a small tumor of microscopic size by antiangiogenic therapy, the residual tumor population should remain sensitive to cytotoxic chemotherapy. The mechanism by which antiangiogenic therapy would increase drug delivery and blood flow to a tumor as reported by Teicher is not clear but may be based on the lowering of interstitial pressure as a tumor becomes unpacked by capillary dropout.[110]

It is important to distinguish antiangiogenic from antivascular therapy.[111] Antivascular therapy, for example, with combretastatin, which can bring about rapid regression of large bulky tumors, depends on occlusion of tumor vasculature, in part by desquamation of endothelial cells into the lumen. Some scientists have assumed that the efficacy of antiangiogenic therapy would be limited by tumor cells that are p53 deficient and/or hypoxic. However, there is considerable evidence to the contrary.[112] In fact, at least two angiogenesis inhibitors, 2-methoxyestradiol and endostatin, have been demonstrated to downregulate expression of hypoxia inducible factor-1α, thus overriding tumor cell response to hypoxia.[113]

There is also confusion about whether radiotherapy can be used in combination with antiangiogenic therapy because of the notion that antiangiogenic therapy might decrease oxygen delivery to a tumor and lead to radioresistance. However, Teicher and associates[114] have reported that antiangiogenic therapy potentiates radiotherapy and increases tumor oxygenation in tumor-bearing animals, at least during the initial stages of antiangiogenic therapy.

It has been assumed that leukemia, called the liquid tumor, would not be dependent on angiogenesis. In fact, it has been reported that the bone marrow in human leukemia is highly angiogenic, with up to a sevenfold increase in microvessel density in acute lymphoblastic leukemia of children compared with nonleukemic bone marrows ($P < 0.0001$).[115] Confocal microscopy reveals that leukemic tumor cells in the marrow are configured as microcylinders around capillary vessels, not unlike the configuration of microcylinders of tumor cells around new microvessels in solid tumors, for example, in breast cancer (see Fig. 32-1).

CERTAIN CONVENTIONAL DRUGS MAY ALSO INHIBIT ANGIOGENESIS

Steiner[116] showed in 1992 that of 17 cytotoxic drugs tested in the chick embryo, only Adriamycin and its analogs or etoposide specifically inhibited angiogenesis. Mitoxantrone inhibited angiogenesis to a lesser extent. It has been demonstrated that paclitaxel (Taxol) inhibits angiogenesis in animals below the cytotoxic dose.[117] Of interest is that although paclitaxel is usually administered for metastatic breast cancer once every 3 weeks for approximately six to seven such cycles, scattered reports exist of patients treated for 20 cycles or more who have stable disease. Drug resistance does not appear to have developed in these patients. A possible explanation is that the tumor compartment may have become drug resistant but the endothelial cell compartment has not.

Vascular endothelial cells in the tumor bed are the first to be exposed to chemotherapy. However, conventional cytotoxic chemotherapy is usually administered at a maximum tolerated dose, followed by treatment-free intervals to allow recovery of bone marrow and gastrointestinal tract cells. Therefore, during treatment-free intervals, endothelial cells are untreated. Browder and coworkers[118] showed that by administering cyclophosphamide at more frequent intervals and at lower dosages, apoptosis of endothelial cells in the tumor bed preceded tumor cell apoptosis by 4 to 5 days. At these close intervals, the cytotoxic drug was converted to an angiogenesis inhibitor (i.e., *antiangiogenic chemotherapy*). It was effective even when the tumor was made completely resistant to cyclophosphamide. Others confirmed this result with different cytotoxic agents, and the term *metronomic therapy* was introduced.[119]

These two terms do not have precisely the same meaning. Antiangiogenic chemotherapy signifies that the target of the chemotherapy is microvascular endothelium in the tumor bed. Metronomic therapy indicates that the schedule of administration is at regular intervals. A recent in vitro study showed that ultra-low picomolar concentrations of paclitaxel, administered continuously, inhibited endothelial cell proliferation (Table 32-1).[102] This study suggests the possibility that prolonged ultra-low dosages of paclitaxel, or even sustained-release subcutaneous dosing of paclitaxel, could be used in cancer patients whose tumor had become resistant to dosing every 3 weeks or weekly. These results might also help explain why some patients who receive long-term maintenance or even palliative chemotherapy have stable disease beyond the time that the tumor would have been expected to develop drug resistance. Patients with slow-growing cancers who are on antiangiogenic scheduling of chemotherapy involving continuous infusion of 5-fluorouracil, weekly paclitaxel,[120] or daily oral etoposide[121] have shown an improved outcome, despite the fact that in some of these patients the tumors had already become drug resistant to conventional chemotherapy.

Tamoxifen inhibits the growth of human microvascular endothelial cells and induces apoptosis in these cells in vitro. It also inhibits angiogenesis in the chick embryo in vivo.[122] Thus, it is possible that some part of the antitumor effect of tamoxifen is related to its antiangiogenic activity, however weak this activity may be relative to other angiogenesis inhibitors. Thalidomide, a discontinued drug, has also been found to suppress tumor angiogenesis.[123]

Celecoxib, a cyclooxygenase-2 inhibitor used in the management of arthritis; rosiglitazone, a PPAR-gamma ligand used in type 2 late-onset diabetes; and zoledronate, a bisphosphonate used to treat osteoporosis, have recently been reported to inhibit angiogenesis.[124–126] Celecoxib also mobilizes endostatin from platelets and increases the blood level of endostatin. In the future, it is possible that celecoxib, rosiglitazone, and zoledronate may be administered chronically in cancer, as they now are administered for non-neoplastic diseases. One can also speculate that these types of relatively nontoxic drugs could be used as a platform of antiangiogenic therapy to which other agents could be added.

TABLE 32-1

Inhibition of Human Microvascular Endothelial Cell Proliferation by Chemotherapeutics*

Compounds	IC$_{50}$ (pM)
Paclitaxel	0.1
5-Fluorouracil	5000
Camptothecin	10,000
Doxorubicin	100,000
Cisplatin	5,000,000

*Human microvascular endothelial cells were grown in 96-well plate with EGM2 medium containing growth factors and fetal bovine serum (FBS). The cells were incubated with compounds at various concentrations for 3 days before MTS reagents were used to quantify the live cells. The IC$_{50}$ (concentration to achieve 50% of maximum inhibition) was the average of three independent experiments.
Modified from Wang J, Lou P, Lesniewski R, Henkin J: Paclitaxel at ultra low concentrations inhibits angiogenesis without affecting cellular microtubule assembly. Anticancer Drugs 14:13–19, 2003.

CLINICAL TRIALS

There are at least 45 angiogenic inhibitors in clinical development. Only one has recently been approved by the U.S. Food and Drug Administration (FDA) for breast cancer therapy. Bevacizumab (Avastin), a humanized monoclonal antibody against VEGF, is the first marketed angiogenesis inhibitor. It was approved by the FDA in 2003 for colorectal cancer and in 2006 for non–small cell lung cancer. Before its recent accelerated market approval by the FDA for advanced breast cancer in the United States, bevacizumab was allowed to be used as first-line therapy for metastatic breast cancer in Europe.[127] A prospective randomized clinical trial involved capecitabine and bevacizumab versus capecitabine alone in metastatic breast cancer that has been already treated with taxane and anthracycline, and it did not meet primary end point of progression-free survival.[128] Subsequently, a phase III study conducted by the Eastern Oncology Cooperative Group (ECOG) compared paclitaxel with or without bevacizumab in metastatic patients who have not received chemotherapy. Analysis of this trial, E2100, showed prolonged progression-free survival but not overall survival.[129] There was more morbidity in the combination treatment group, including hypertension, proteinuria, headache, cerebrovascular ischemia, and infection. Other clinical trials in metastatic breast cancer have begun to test combination of bevacizumab with other chemotherapeutic agents such as protein-bound paclitaxel (Abraxane)[130] and cyclophosphamide.[131]

The National Institutes of Health (NIH) Clinical Trial website lists 85 studies using Avastin in breast cancer (www.clinicaltrials.gov). Two ECOG trials, E2104 and E5103, will assess bevacizumab as adjuvant therapy in addition to chemotherapy for node-positive cancer.[132] Other clinical trials evaluate the combination of Avastin with other targeted therapies such as trastuzumab[133] or erlotinib.[134] Data from multiple trials show that the toxicities of bevacizumab appear manageable.[135] These include grade 3 hypertension in 15% to 20%, asymptomatic proteinuria in 5%, and postoperative healing complications in 25%. Occasional hemorrhages in colon and lung cancers are related to bulky disease located near blood vessels.

Aflibercept is a soluble VEGFR recombinant decoy receptor, using the "Trap" technology.[136] It is administered intravenously in phase III for non–small cell lung cancer and ovarian cancer. Adverse events are similar to bevacizumab, including hypertension and proteinuria.[137] It is in phase II testing for breast cancer as monotherapy for patients who have previously received taxane and/or anthracycline (clinicaltrials.gov). Cediranib (Recentin) is an oral drug that inhibits VEGF1, VEGF2, and VEGF3 tyrosine kinases.[138] It is in phase III clinical trials for renal cell cancer, colorectal cancer, and glioblastoma multiforma. Its late-stage study in non–small cell lung cancer was halted because of toxicity concerns. In breast cancer, it is in phase II testing in combination with fulvestrant (Faslodex) versus fulvestrant alone in hormone-sensitive postmenopausal women (clinicaltrials.gov).

Sorafenib (Nexavar) is an oral multikinase inhibitor that targets VEGFRs, PDGFR, KIT, Flt-3, RET, and colony stimulating factor-1 (CSF-1).[139] It has been approved for gastrointestinal stromal tumors, renal cell cancer, and hepatocellular carcinoma. Its phase III trial in non–small cell lung cancer did not meet the primary end point of improved overall survival. Sorafenib showed activity as a single agent in heavily pretreated patients with refractory metastatic breast cancer in phase II.[140] The NIH Clinical Trial web site lists 19 studies using sorafenib in breast cancer. Sunitinib (Sutent) is an oral multi-kinase inhibitor that targets VEGFRs, PDGFR and the MAPK pathway. It is FDA approved for renal cell cancer. A sunitinib-paclitaxel combination was well tolerated in a phase I study for first-line treatment of advanced breast cancer.[141] Sunitinib is in a phase III trial with paclitaxel versus bevacizumab and paclitaxel as first-line therapy for advanced breast cancer, as well as in another with capecitabine as second-line treatment. Both sorafenib and sunitinib share many common toxicities, including hand-foot skin reaction, skin rash, hypertension, and esophagitis/gastritis.[142]

Pazopanib inhibits VEGF11 and VEGF13, PDGFR, and KIT tyrosine kinases.[143] It is administered orally in phase III trials for inflammatory breast cancer, ovarian cancer, and renal cell cancer.[144] In breast, pazopanib is tested with lapatinib (Tykerb; Her2 inhibitor) versus lapatinib alone in Her2 positive inflammatory cancer cases that have failed prior chemotherapy with or without trastuzumab. Another randomized trial assesses whether the addition of pazopanib to Tykerb would improve outcome in Her2-positive patients whose tumors can be removed by surgery (clinicaltrials.gov). Other multikinase inhibitors include vatalanib and vandetanib (Zactima). Vatalanib suppresses VEGF-1, VEGF-2, and VEGF-3; PDGFR; c-kit; and cFMS;[145] and vandetanib interferes with VEGF-1, VEGF-2, and VEGF-3; PDGFR; c-kit; Src; and Abl. In a phase II clinical trial, vandetanib did not demonstrate significant efficacy as monotherapy for patients with refractory metastatic breast cancer.[146]

Many ongoing phase I/II clinical trials are testing agents that target tumor angiogenesis via mechanisms different from those mentioned previously. These include angiostatin in non–small cell lung cancer and endostatin[147] in neuroendocrine tumor and melanoma. An extensive list includes inhibitors of integrin, integrin receptor, thrombospondin-1, superoxide dismutase, urokinase plasminogen activator, cadherin-5, CXCR4 chemokine, CD49b, Tek receptor, Flt-3 tyrosine kinase, hypoxia-inducible factor-1, EIF protein kinase, chloride channel, aminopeptidase, EpCAM, and the S100A4 receptor.[148]

Conclusions and Future Directions

This review of the role of angiogenesis in breast cancer is based on principles of the angiogenic process that have been elucidated in the laboratory and are being translated to clinical application, not only in breast cancer but also in other neoplastic and non-neoplastic diseases. Angiogenesis research is nearly 40 years old and can be divided into four periods of development. The 1970s were devoted mainly to the development of methods to study blood vessel growth in vitro and in vivo. The 1980s saw the discovery of molecules that mediate angiogenesis, including inducers and inhibitors of angiogenesis. Proof of principle demonstrated that tumor growth is angiogenesis dependent. In the 1990s, a first generation of angiogenesis inhibitors entered clinical trials, and genetic proofs that tumors are angiogenesis dependent were reported. In the first decade of the 21st century, these drugs are being approved for the treatment of various cancers. These new antiangiogenic molecules could stop tumor growth but may not induce tumor regression like cytotoxic agents. Therefore, it is very important to design regimens that would optimize their unique activity with existing standard chemotherapies. Similarly, the currently required demonstration of overall survival improvement in advanced metastatic cancer cases may need to be more flexible to allow oncology patients to reap the benefits of four decades of angiogenesis research.

Acknowledgments

This chapter is dedicated to the memory of Dr. Judah Folkman, the pioneer of angiogenesis research, an exceptional teacher and devoted physician.[149]

REFERENCES

1. Gimbrone MA Jr, Leapman SB, Cotran RS, Folkman J: Tumor dormancy in vivo by prevention of neovascularization. J Exp Med 136:261–276, 1972.
2. Hanahan D, Folkman J: Patterns and emerging mechanisms of the angiogenic switch during tumorigenesis. Cell 86:353–364, 1996.
3. Folkman J, Watson K, Ingber D, Hanahan D: Induction of angiogenesis during the transition from hyperplasia to neoplasia. Nature 339:58–61, 1989.
4. Hanahan D, Christofori G, Naik P, Arbeit J: Transgenic mouse models of tumor angiogenesis: The angiogenic switch, its molecular controls, and prospects for preclinical therapeutic models. Eur J Cancer 32A:2386–2393, 1996.
5. Smith-McCune KK, Weidner N: Demonstration and characterization of the angiogenic properties of cervical dysplasia. Cancer Res 54:800–804, 1994.
6. Brem SS, Jensen HM, Gullino PM: Angiogenesis as a marker of preneoplastic lesions of the human breast. Cancer 41:239–244, 1978.
7. Yoshiji H, Gomez DE, Shibuya M, Thorgeirsson UP: Expression of vascular endothelial growth factor, its receptor, and other angiogenic factors in human breast cancer. Cancer Res 56:2013–2016, 1996.
8. McLeskey SW, Zhang L, Kharbanda S, et al: Fibroblast growth factor overexpressing breast carcinoma cells as models of angiogenesis and metastasis. Breast Cancer Res Treat 39:103–117, 1996.
9. Toi M, Hoshina S, Taniguchi T, et al: Expression of platelet-derived endothelial cell growth factor/thymidine phosphorylase in human breast cancer. Int J Cancer 64:79–82, 1995.
10. Contrino J, Hair G, Kreutzer DL, Rickles FR: In situ detection of tissue factor in vascular endothelial cells: Correlation with the malignant phenotype of human breast disease. Nat Med 2:209–215, 1996.
11. Hlatky L, Tsionou C, Hahnfeldt P, Coleman CN: Mammary fibroblasts may influence breast tumor angiogenesis via hypoxia-induced vascular endothelial growth factor up-regulation and protein expression. Cancer Res 54:6083–6086, 1994.
12. Briozzo P, Badet J, Capony F, et al: MCF7 mammary cancer cells respond to bFGF and internalize it following its release from extracel lular matrix: A permissive role of cathepsin D. Exp Cell Res 194:252–259, 1991.
13. Gasparini G, Toi M, Gion M, et al: Prognostic significance of vascular endothelial growth factor protein in node-negative breast carcinoma, J Natl Cancer Inst 89:139–147, 1997.
14. Folkman J: Clinical applications of research on angiogenesis. N Engl J Med 333:1757–1763, 1995.
15. Dong Z, Kumar R, Yang X, Fidler IJ: Macrophage-derived metalloelastase is responsible for generation of angiostatin in Lewis lung carcinoma. Cell 88:801–810, 1997.
16. Rak J, Filmus J, Finkenzeller G, et al: Oncogenes as inducers of tumor angiogenesis. Cancer Metastasis Rev 14:263–277, 1995.
17. Dameron KM, Volpert OV, Tainsky MA, Bouck N: Control of angiogenesis in fibroblasts by p53 regulation of thrombospondin-1. Science 265:1582–1584, 1994.
18. Van Meir EG, Polverini PJ, Chazin VR, et al: Release of an inhibitor of angiogenesis upon induction of wild type p53 expression in glioblastoma cells, Nat Genet 8:171–176, 1994.
19. Wizigmann-Voos S, Breier G, Risau W, Plate KH: Up regulation of vascular endo thelial growth factor and its receptors in von Hippel-Lindau disease- associated and sporadic hemangioblastomas. Cancer Res 55:1358–1364, 1995.
20. Nguyen M, Lee MC, Wang JL, et al: The human myoepithelial cell expresses a multifaceted anti-angiogenic phenotype. Oncogene 19:3449–3459, 2000.
21. Maeshima Y, Manfredi M, Reimer C, et al: Identification of the anti-angiogenic site within vascular basement membrane-derived tumstatin. J Biol Chem 276:15240–15248, 2001.
22. Thomlinson R, Gray L: The histological structure of some human lung cancers and the possible implications for radiotherapy. Br J Cancer 9:539–549, 1955.
23. Gao D, Nolan DJ, Mellick AS, et al: Endothelial progenitor cells control the angiogenic switch in mouse lung metastasis. Science 319:195–198, 2008.
24. Lyden D, Hattori K, Dias S, et al: Impaired recruitment of bonemarrow-derived endothelial and hematopoietic precursor cells blocks tumor angiogenesis and growth. Nat Med 7:1194–1201, 2001.
25. Rafii S, Lyden D: Cancer. A few to flip the angiogenic switch. Science 319:163–164, 2008.
26. Ito H, Rovira II, Bloom ML, et al: Endothelial progenitor cells as putative targets for angiostatin. Cancer Res 59:5875–5877, 1999.
27. Monestiroli S, Mancuso P, Burlini A, et al: Kinetics and viability of circulating endothelial cells as surrogate angiogenesis marker in an animal model of human lymphoma. Cancer Res 61:4341–4344, 2001.
28. Bertolini F, Mingrone W, Alietti A, et al: Thalidomide in multiple myeloma, myelodysplastic syndromes and histiocytosis: Analysis of clinical results and of surrogate angiogenesis markers. Ann Oncol 12:987–990, 2001.
29. Verheul HM, Hoekman K, Luykx-de Bakker S, et al: Platelet: Transporter of vascular endothelial growth factor. Clin Cancer Res 3:2187–2190, 1997.
30. Pinedo HM, Verheul HM, D'Amato RJ, Folkman J: Involvement of platelets in tumour angiogenesis? Lancet 352:1775–1777, 1998.
31. Polverini PJ, Leibovich SJ: Induction of neovascularization in vivo and endothelial proliferation in vitro by tumor-associated macrophages. Lab Invest 51:635–642, 1984.
32. Fang J, Shing Y, Wiederschain D, et al: Matrix metalloproteinase-2 is required for the switch to the angiogenic phenotype in a tumor model. Proc Natl Acad Sci USA 97:3884–3889, 2000.
33. Bergers G, Brekken R, McMahon G, et al: Matrix metalloproteinase-9 triggers the angiogenic switch during carcinogenesis. Nat Cell Biol 2:737–744, 2000.
34. Fukumura D, Xavier R, Sugiura T, et al: Tumor induction of VEGF promoter activity in stromal cells. Cell 94:715–725, 1998.
35. Holash J, Maisonpierre PC, Compton D, et al: Vessel cooption, regression, and growth in tumors mediated by angiopoietins and VEGF. Science 284:1994–1998, 1999.
36. Hillen F, Griffioen AW: Tumour vascularization: Sprouting angiogenesis and beyond. Cancer Metastasis Rev 26:489–502, 2007.
37. Achilles EG, Fernandez A, Allred EN, et al: Heterogeneity of angiogenic activity in a human liposarcoma: A proposed mechanism for "no take" of human tumors in mice. J Natl Cancer Inst 93:1075–1081, 2001.
38. Udagawa T, Fernandez A, Achilles EG, et al: Persistence of microscopic human cancers in mice: Alterations in the angiogenic balance accompanies loss of tumor dormancy. FASEB J 16:1361–1370, 2002.
39. Cameron MD, Schmidt EE, Kerkvliet N, et al: Temporal progression of metastasis in lung: Cell survival, dormancy, and location

dependence of metastatic inefficiency. Cancer Res 60:2541–2546, 2000.

40. Folkman J: The influence of angiogenesis research on management of patients with breast cancer. Breast Cancer Res Treat 36:109–118, 1995.

41. Hamada J, Cavanaugh PG, Miki K, Nicolson GL: A paracrine migration-stimulating factor for metastatic tumor cells secreted by mouse hepatic sinusoidal endothelial cells: Identification as complement component C3b. Cancer Res 53:4418–4423, 1993.

42. Nicosia RF, Tchao R, Leighton J: Interactions between newly formed endothelial channels and carcinoma cells in plasma clot culture. Clin Exp Metastasis 4:91–104, 1986.

43. Holmgren L, O'Reilly MS, Folkman J: Dormancy of micrometastases: Balanced proliferation and apoptosis in the presence of angiogenesis suppression. Nat Med 1:149–153, 1995.

44. Evans GI: Old cells never die, they just apoptose. Trends Cell Biol 4:191–192, 1994.

45. Cao Y, O'Reilly MS, Marshall B, et al: Expression of angiostatin cDNA in a murine fibrosarcoma suppresses primary tumor growth and produces long-term dormancy of metastases. J Clin Invest 101:1055–1063, 1998.

46. O'Reilly MS, Holmgren L, Shing Y, et al: Angiostatin: A novel angiogenesis inhibitor that mediates the suppression of metastases by a Lewis lung carcinoma. Cell 79:315–328, 1994.

47. O'Reilly MS, Boehm T, Shing Y, et al: Endostatin: An endogenous inhibitor of angiogenesis and tumor growth. Cell 88:277–285, 1997.

48. Weidner N, Semple JP, Welch WR, Folkman J: Tumor angiogenesis correlates with metastasis in invasive breast carcinoma. N Engl J Med 324:1–8, 1991.

49. Liotta LA, Steeg PS, Stetler-Stevenson WG: Cancer metastasis and angiogenesis: An imbalance of positive and negative regulation, Cell 64:327–336, 1991.

50. Smolin G, Hyndiuk RA: Lymphatic drainage from vascularized rabbit cornea. Am J Ophthalmol 72:147–151, 1971.

51. Wojtowicz-Praga S, Low J, Marshall J: Phase I trial of a novel matrix metalloproteinase inhibitor, batimastat (BB-94), in patients with advanced cancer. Invest New Drugs 14:193–202, 1996.

52. Brooks PC, Strömblad S, Klemke R, et al: Anti-integrin alpha v beta 3 blocks human breast cancer growth and angiogenesis in human skin. J Clin Invest 96:1815–1822, 1995.

53. Ellis LM, Fidler IJ: Angiogenesis and breast cancer metastasis. Lancet 346:388–390, 1995.

54. Dvorak HF, Nagy JA, Dvorak JT, Dvorak AM: Identification and characterization of the blood vessels of solid tumors that are leaky to circulating macromolecules. Am J Pathol 133:95–109, 1988.

55. Kalebic T, Garbisa S, Glaser B, Liotta LA: Basement membrane collagen: Degradation by migrating endothelial cells. Science 221:281–283, 1983.

56. O'Reilly MS, et al: Angiostatin induces and sustains dormancy of human primary tumors in mice. Nature Med 2:689–692, 1996.

57. Relf M, Lejeune S, Scott PA, et al: Expression of the angiogenic factors vascular endothelial growth factor, acidic and basic fibroblast growth factor, tumor growth factor beta-1, platelet-derived endothelial cell growth factor, placenta growth factor, and pleiotrophin in human primary breast cancer and its relation to angiogenesis. Cancer Res 57:963–969, 1997.

58. Harris L, Fritsche H, Mennel R, et al: American Society of Clinical Oncology 2007 update of recommendations for the use of tumor markers in breast cancer. J Clin Oncol 25:5287–5312, 2007.

59. Nguyen M: Angiogenic factors as tumor markers. Invest New Drug 15:29–37, 1997.

60. Granato AM, Nanni O, Falcini F, et al: Basic fibroblast growth factor and vascular endothelial growth factor serum levels in breast cancer patients and healthy women: Useful as diagnostic tools? Breast Cancer Res 6:R38–R45, 2004.

61. Bozcuk H, Uslu G, Samur M, et al: Tumour necrosis factor-alpha, interleukin-6, and fasting serum insulin correlate with clinical outcome in metastatic breast cancer patients treated with chemotherapy. Cytokine 27:58–65, 2004.

62. Eichbaum MH, de Rossi TM, Kaul S, et al: Serum levels of hepatocyte growth factor/scatter factor in patients with liver metastases from breast cancer. Tumour Biol 28:36–44, 2007.

63. Dehqanzada ZA, Storrer CE, Hueman MT, et al: Assessing serum cytokine profiles in breast cancer patients receiving a HER2/ neu vaccine using Luminex technology. Oncol Rep 17:687–694, 2007.

64. Caine GJ, Stonelake PS, Lip GY, Blann AD: Changes in plasma vascular endothelial growth factor, angiopoietins, and their receptors following surgery for breast cancer. Cancer Lett 248:131–136, 2007.

65. Granato AM, Frassineti GL, Giovannini N, et al: Do serum angiogenic growth factors provide additional information to that of conventional markers in monitoring the course of metastatic breast cancer? Tumour Biol 27:302–308, 2006.

66. Lipton A, Ali SM, Leitzel K, et al: Elevated plasma tissue inhibitor of metalloproteinase-1 level predicts decreased response and survival in metastatic breast cancer. Cancer 109:1933–1939, 2007.

67. Kuvaja P, Talvensaari-Mattila A, Pääkkö P, Turpeenniemi-Hujanen T: Low serum level of pro-matrix metalloproteinase 2 correlates with aggressive behavior in breast carcinoma. Hum Pathol 37:1316–1323, 2006.

68. Sheen-Chen SM, Eng HL, Huang CC, Chen WJ: Serum levels of soluble E-selectin in women with breast cancer. Br J Surg 91:1578–1581, 2004.

69. Tworoger SS, Eliassen AH, Sluss P, Hankinson SE: A prospective study of plasma prolactin concentrations and risk of premenopausal and postmenopausal breast cancer. J Clin Oncol 25:1482–1488, 2007.

70. Baglietto L, English DR, Hopper JL, et al: Circulating insulin-like growth factor-I and binding protein-3 and the risk of breast cancer. Cancer Epidemiol Biomarkers Prev 16:763–768, 2007.

71. Fürstenberger G, von Moos R, Lucas R, et al: Circulating endothelial cells and angiogenic serum factors during neoadjuvant chemotherapy of primary breast cancer. Br J Cancer 94:524–531, 2006.

72. Brooks MN: Will the analysis of nipple fluid and breast cells be useful in the clinical care of the breast patient? Women's Oncol Rev 3:179–186, 2003.

73. Liu Y, Wang JL, Chang H, et al: Breast cancer diagnosis with nipple fluid bFGF. Lancet 356:567, 2000.

74. Sartippour MR, Zhang L, Lu M, et al: Nipple fluid basic fibroblast growth factor in breast patients. Cancer Epidemiol Biomarkers Prev 4:2995–2998, 2005.

75. Hsiung R, Zhu W, Klein G, et al: High basic fibroblast growth factor levels in nipple aspirate fluid are correlated with breast cancer. Cancer J 8:308–310, 2002.

76. Sauter ER, Wagner-Mann C, Ehya H, Klein-Szanto A: Biologic markers of breast cancer in nipple aspirate fluid and nipple discharge are associated with clinical findings. Cancer Detect Prev 31:50–58, 2007.

77. Kuerer HM, Thompson PA, Krishnamurthy S, et al: High and differential expression of HER-2/neu extracellular domain in bilateral ductal fluids from women with unilateral invasive breast cancer. Clin Cancer Res 9:601–605, 2003.

78. Sauter ER, Chervoneva I, Diamandis A, et al: Prostate specific antigen and insulin like growth factor binding protein-3 in nipple aspirate fluid are associated with breast cancer. Cancer Detect Prev 26:149–157, 2002.

79. Qin W, Zhu W, Wagner-Mann C, et al: Association of uPA, PAT-1, and uPAR in nipple aspirate fluid (NAF) with breast cancer. Cancer J 9:293–301, 2003.

80. Horak ER, Leek R, Klenk N, et al: Angiogenesis, assessed by platelet/endothelial cell adhesion molecule antibodies, as indicator of node metastases and survival in breast cancer. Lancet 340:1120–1124, 1992.

81. Vermeulen PB, Gasparini G, Fox SB, et al: Quantification of angiogenesis in solid human tumours: An international consensus on the methodology and criteria of evaluation. Eur J Cancer 32A:2474–2484, 1996.

82. Gasparini G: Clinical significance of the determination of angiogenesis in human breast cancer: Update of the biological background and overview of the Vicenza studies. Eur J Cancer 32A:2485–2493, 1996.

83. Weidner N, Folkman J: Tumor vascularity as a prognostic factor in cancer. In DeVita VT Jr, Hellman S, Rosenberg SA (eds): Important advances in oncology. Philadelphia, Lippincott-Raven, 1996.

84. Kerbel RS, Waghorne C, Korczak B, et al: Clonal dominance of primary tumors by metastatic cells: Genetic analysis and biological implications. Cancer Surv 7:597–629, 1988.

85. Tamm I, Kikuchi T, Cardinale I, Krueger JG: Cell-adhesion–disrupting action of interleukin 6 in human ductal breast carcinoma cells. Proc Natl Acad Sci USA 91:3329–3333, 1994.

86. Folkman J: Angiogenesis-dependent diseases. Semin Oncol 28:536–542, 2001.

87. Hlatky L, Hahnfeldt P, Folkman J: Clinical application of antiangiogenic therapy: Microvessel density, what it does and doesn't tell us. J Natl Cancer Inst 94:883–893, 2002.

88. Beecken WD, Fernandez A, Joussen AM, et al: Effect of anti-angiogenic therapy on slowly growing, poorly vascularized tumours in mice. J Natl Cancer Inst 93:382–387, 2001.

89. Meltzer A: Dormancy and breast cancer. J Surg Oncol 43:181–188, 1990.

90. Wheelock EF, Weinhold KJ, Levich J: The tumor dormant state. Adv Cancer Res 34:107–140, 1981.

91. Noble RL, Hoover L: A classification of transplantable tumors in Nb rats controlled by estrogen from dormancy to autonomy. Nature Med 35:2935–2941, 1975.

92. Demicheli R, Terenziani M, Valagussa P, et al: Local recurrences following mastectomy: Support for the concept of tumor dormancy. J Natl Cancer Inst 86:45–48, 1994.

93. Wu J: Apoptosis and angiogenesis: Two promising tumor markers in breast cancer. Anticancer Res 16:2233–2239, 1996.

94. Prehn RT: The inhibition of tumor growth by tumor mass. Cancer Res 51:2–4, 1991.

95. Yuhas JM, Pazmino NH: Inhibition of subcutaneously growing line 1 carcinomas due to metastatic spread. Cancer Res 34:2005–2010, 1974.

96. Nanus DM, Schmitz-Dräger BJ, Motzer RJ, et al: Expression of basic fibroblast growth factor in primary human renal tumors: Correlation with poor survival. J Natl Cancer Inst 85:1597–1599, 1993.

97. Nguyen M, Watanabe H, Budson AE, et al: Elevated levels of an angiogenic peptide, basic fibroblast growth factor, in the urine of patients with a wide spectrum of cancers. J Natl Cancer Inst 86:356–361, 1994.

98. Ezekowitz RA, Mulliken JB, Folkman J: Interferon alfa-2a therapy for life-threatening hemangiomas of infancy. N Engl J Med 326:1456–1463, 1992.

99. Kaban LB, Troulis MJ, Ebb D, et al: Antiangiogenic therapy with interferon alpha for giant cell lesions of the jaws. J Oral Maxillofac Surg 60:1103–1111, 2002.

100. Whitworth A: Endostatin: Are we waiting for Godot? J Natl Cancer Inst 98:731–733, 2006.

101. Gutheil JC, Campbell TN, Pierce RR, et al: Targeted antiangiogenic therapy for cancer using Vitaxin: A humanized monoclonal antibody to the integrin $\alpha v \beta 3$. Clin Cancer Res 6:3056–3061, 2002.

102. Wang J, Lou P, Lesniewski R, Henkin J: Paclitaxel at ultra low concentrations inhibits angiogenesis without affecting cellular microtubule assembly. Anticancer Drugs 14:13–19, 2003.

103. Kerbel RS: Inhibition of tumor angiogenesis as a strategy to circumvent acquired resistance to anticancer therapeutic agents. Bioessays 13:31–36, 1991.

104. Boehm T, Folkman J, Browder T, O'Reilly MS: Antiangiogenic therapy of experimental cancer does not induce drug resistance. Nature 390:404–407, 1997.

105. Klauber N, Rohan RM, Flynn E, D'Amato RJ: Critical components of the female reproductive pathway are suppressed by the angiogenesis inhibitor AGM-1470. Nature Med 3:443–446, 1997.

106. Offodile R, Walton T, Lee M, et al: Regression of metastatic breast cancer in a patient treated with the anti-angiogenic drug TNP-470. Tumori 85:51–53, 1999.

107. Kisker O, Becker CM, Prox D, et al: Continuous administration of endostatin by intraperitoneally implanted osmotic pump improves the efficacy and potency of therapy in a mouse xenograft tumor model. Cancer Res 61:7669–7674, 2001.

108. Denekamp J: Vascular attack as a therapeutic strategy for cancer, Cancer Metastasis Rev 3:267–282, 1990.

109. Teicher BA, Dupuis NP, Robinson MF, et al: Antiangiogenic treatment (TNP-470/Minocycline) increases tissue levels of anticancer drugs in mice bearing Lewis lung carcinoma. Oncol Res 27:237–243, 1995.

110. Jain R: Barriers to drug delivery in solid tumors. Sci Am 271:58–65, 1994.

111. Huang X, Molema G, King S, et al: Tumor infarction in mice by antibody-directed targeting of tissue factor to tumor vasculature. Science 275:547–550, 1997.

112. Browder T, Folkman J, Hahnfeldt P, et al: Antiangiogenic therapy and p53. Science 297:471a, 2002.

113. Kieran MW, Folkman J, Heymach J: Angiogenesis inhibitors and hypoxia. Nat Med 9:1104–1105, 2003.

114. Teicher BA, Dupuis N, Kusomoto T, et al: Antiangiogenic agents can increase tumor oxygenation and response to radiation therapy. Radiat Oncol Invest 2:269–276, 1995.

115. Perez-Atayde AR, Sallan SE, Tedrow U, et al: Spectrum of tumor angiogenesis in the bone marrow of children with acute lymphoblastic leukemia. Am J Pathol 150:815–821, 1997.

116. Steiner R: Angiostatic activity of anticancer agents in the chick embryo chorioallantoic membrane (CHE-CAM) assay. In Steiner R, Weisz P, Langer R (eds): Angiogenesis: Key principles-science-technology-medicine. Basel, Switzerland, Birkhauser Verlag, 1992.

117. Belotti D, Vergani V, Drudis T, et al: The microtubule-affecting drug paclitaxel has antiangiogenic activity. Clin Cancer Res 2:1843–1849, 1996.

118. Browder T, Butterfield CE, Kräling BM, et al: Antiangiogenic scheduling of chemotherapy improves efficacy against experimental drug-resistant cancer. Cancer Res 60:1878–1886, 2000.

119. Hanahan D, Bergers G, Bergsland E: Less is more, regularly: Metronomic dosing of cytotoxic drugs can target tumor angiogenesis in mice. J Clin Invest 105:1045–1047, 2000.

120. Gabra H, Cameron DA, Lee LE, et al: Weekly doxorubicin and continuous infusional 5-fluorouracil for advanced breast cancer. Br J Cancer 74:2008–2012, 1996.

121. Neskovic-Konstantinovic ZB, Bosnjak SM, Radulović SS, Mitrović LB: Daily oral etoposide in metastatic breast cancer. Anticancer Drugs 7:543–547, 1996.

122. Gagliardi A, Collins DC: Inhibition of angiogenesis by antiestrogens. Cancer Res 53:533–555, 1993.

123. Nguyen M, Tran C, Barsky S, et al: Thalidomide and chemotherapy combination: Preliminary results of preclinical and clinical studies. Int J Oncol 10:965–969, 1997.

124. Kishi K, Petersen S, Petersen C, et al: Preferential enhancement of tumor radioresponse by a cyclooxygenase-2 inhibitor. Cancer Res 60:1326–1331, 2000.

125. Panigrahy D, Singer S, Shen LQ, et al: PPARgamma ligands inhibit primary tumor growth and metastasis by inhibiting angiogenesis. J Clin Invest 110:923–932, 2002.

126. Wood J, Bonjean K, Ruetz S, et al: Novel antiangiogenic effects of the bisphosphonate compound zoledronic acid, J Pharmacol Exp Ther 302:1055–1061, 2002.

127. Scott LJ: Bevacizumab: In first-line treatment of metastatic breast cancer. Drugs 67:1793–1799, 2007.

128. Miller KD, Chap LI, Holmes FA, et al: Randomized phase III trial of capecitabine compared with bevacizumab plus capecitabine in patients with previously treated metastatic breast cancer. J Clin Oncol 23:792–799, 2005.

129. Miller K, Wang M, Gralow J: Paclitaxel plus bevacizumab versus paclitaxel alone for metastatic breast cancer. N Engl J Med 357:2666–2676, 2007.

130. Link JS, Waisman JR, Nguyen B, Jacobs CI: Bevacizumab and albumin-bound paclitaxel treatment in metastatic breast cancer. Clin Breast Cancer 7:779–783, 2007.

131. Dellapasqua S, Bertolini F, Bagnardi V, et al: Metronomic cyclophosphamide and capecitabine combined with bevacizumab in advanced breast cancer. Evidence of activity of an antiangiogenic treatment. J Clin Oncol 26:4899–4905, 2008.

132. Salter JT, Miller KD: Antiangiogenic agents in breast cancer. Cancer Invest 25:518–526, 2007.

133. Pegram MD, Yeon C, Ku NC, et al: Phase I combined biological therapy of breast cancer using two humanized monoclonal antibodies directed against HER2 proto-oncogene and vascular endothelial growth factor (VEGF). Breast Cancer Res Treat 88(suppl 1):3039, 2004.

134. Rugo HS, Didder MN, Scott JH, et al: Circulating endothelial cell (CEC) and tumor cell (CTC) analysis in patients (pts) receiving bevacizumab and erlotinib for metastatic breast cancer (MBC). Breast Cancer Res Treat 88(suppl 1):3088, 2004.

135. Hayes DF, Miller K, Sledge G: Angiogenesis as targeted breast cancer therapy. Breast 16(suppl 2):S17–S19, 2007.

136. Holash J, Davis S, Papadopoulos N, et al: VEGF-Trap: A VEGF blocker with potent antitumor effect. Proc Natl Acad Sci 99: 11393–11398, 2002.

137. Tew WP, Colombo N, Ray-Coquard I, et al: VEGF-Trap for patients (pts) with recurrent platinum-resistant epithelial ovarian cancer (EOC): Preliminary results of a randomized, multicenter phase II study. J Clin Oncol 25(18S):5508, 2007.

138. Brandsma D, van den Bent MJ: Molecular targeted therapies and chemotherapy in malignant gliomas. Curr Opin Oncol 19: 598–605, 2007.

139. Chow LQ, Eckhardt SG: Sunitinib: From rational design to clinical efficacy. J Clin Oncol 25:884–896, 2007.

140. Bianchi GV, Loibl S, Zamagni C, et al: Phase II multicenter trial of sorafenib in the treatment of patients with metastatic breast cancer. Am Soc Clin Oncol Breast Cancer Symp, abstract 164, 2007.

141. Kozloff M, Chuang E, Roy J, et al: Preliminary results of a phase I study of sunitinib plus paclitaxel for first-line treatment of advanced breast cancer. Am Soc Clin Oncol Breast Cancer Symp, abstract 163, 2007.

142. Porta C, Paglino C, Imarisio I, Bonomi L: Uncovering Pandora's vase: The growing problem of new toxicities from novel anti-cancer agents. The case of sorafenib and sunitinib. Clin Exp Med 7:127–134, 2007.

143. Kumar R, Knick VB, Rudolph SK, et al: Pharmacokinetic-pharmacodynamic correlation from mouse to human with pazopanib, a multikinase angiogenesis inhibitor with potent antitumor and antiangiogenic activity. Mol Cancer Ther 6:2012–2021, 2007.

144. Hutson TE, Davis ID, Machiels JP, et al: Pazopanib (GW786034) is active in metastatic renal cell carcinoma (RCC): Interim results of a phase II randomized discontinuation trial (RDT). J Clin Oncol 25(18S):3031, 2007.

145. Scott EN, Meinhardt G, Jacques C, et al: Vatalanib: The clinical development of a tyrosine kinase inhibitor of angiogenesis in solid tumours. Expert Opin Investig Drugs 16:367–379, 2007.

146. Miller KD, Trigo JM, Wheeler C, et al: A multicenter phase II trial of ZD6474, a vascular endothelial growth factor receptor-2 and epidermal growth factor receptor tyrosine kinase inhibitor, in patients with previously treated metastatic breast cancer. Clin Cancer Res 11:3369–3376, 2005.

147. Folkman J: Antiangiogenesis in cancer therapy—endostatin and its mechanisms of action. Exp Cell Res 312:594–607, 2006.

148. Folkman J: Angiogenesis: An organizing principle for drug discovery? Nat Rev Drug Discov 6:273–286, 2007.

149. Klagsbrun M, Moses MA: Obituary: M. Judah Folkman (1933–2008). Nature 451:781, 2008.

chapter 33

Immune Recognition of Breast Cancer

VY PHAN | MARY L. DISIS | HAILING LU

The mechanism by which breast cancer cells are recognized immunologically is similar to the way a pathogen would be detected by immune system cells. There are a variety of proteins expressed in breast tumors that are capable of inducing immunity. Unfortunately, the endogenous breast cancer specific immune response, elicited by exposure to the tumor, is not capable of preventing tumor outgrowth in most patients with breast cancer. Understanding the primary reasons for immune system failure is crucial in the development of effective immune based therapies for the treatment of breast cancer.

Basics of Immune Recognition of Breast Cancer

The basic components required for the generation of an effective tumor-specific immune response include the presence of immunogenic proteins or tumor antigens, antigen-presenting cells (APCs), a variety of immune effector cells, and cytokines.

ADAPTIVE VERSUS INNATE IMMUNITY

In general, immune effectors belong to one of two broad classes of immune response: adaptive or innate immunity. Specifically, adaptive immunity occurs as an adaptation to pathogenic infection. It can consist of humoral, that is antibody responses, which are mediated by B lymphocytes that develop in the bone marrow, or cellular responses, which are mediated by T lymphocytes that develop in the thymus. B and T cells can be found in at least three stages of differentiation: (1) "naive" cells, which are matured cells that have left the bone marrow or thymus and are circulating in the lymphatic system but have not yet encountered their cognate antigen; (2) "effector" cells, which are those that have been activated by their cognate antigen and are actively involved in the process of pathogen destruction; and (3) "memory" cells, which are the antigen-specific cells that persist long-term after the infection and go on to develop "immunologic memory," thus enabling a rapid

elimination of the pathogen should a subsequent infection occur. Memory T cells consist of two subtypes: central memory T cells and effector memory T cells, and they can be either CD4+ or CD8+.[1,2] In breast cancer, collaboration of both humoral and cellular immunity and human epidermal growth factor receptor-2 (HER2)/*neu*, for example, is required for efficient tumor protection in rodent models of breast cancer; neither response is sufficient to mediate an antitumor response on its own.[3]

Unlike adaptive immunity, innate immunity defends the host against pathogenic organisms in a nonspecific manner. The innate immune system represents the first line of defense against pathogens but does not confer long-lasting or protective immunity to the host, and the cells of the innate immune system do not directly recognize antigens. Cells of the innate immune system include natural killer cells, mast cells, eosinophils, and basophils.[4] As well, they include phagocytic cells, namely neutrophils, macrophages, and dendritic cells (DCs). DCs are regarded as the most potent of the APCs.[5] Collectively, the cells of innate immunity function to activate T cells through the process of antigen presentation, recruit immune cells to sites of infection and inflammation via cytokine production, and/or activate the complement cascade to identify the pathogen and promote clearance of dead cells or antibody complexes.[4] Innate immune cells can respond to specific pathogens and tumors through toll-like receptors (for review, see Trinchieri and Sher[6]), which recognize a wide variety of pathogen-associated molecular patterns.

With regard to T cells, there are several types that can be distinguished, simplistically, into subsets based on their distinct function in antitumor immunity. CD8+ cytotoxic T lymphocytes (CTLs) are those cells that are capable of killing target tumor cells (e.g., via Fas ligand-mediated and perforin-dependent mechanisms); cancer immunotherapy has traditionally been aimed at activating these cells. CD4+ helper T cells (Th) cells are those cells that secrete cytokines to provide "help" to CTLs and B cells. Helper type 1 cells (Th1) secrete predominantly interferon (IFN)-γ, tumor necrosis factor (TNF)-α, and interleukin (IL)-2; helper type 2 cells

(Th2) secrete IL-4, IL-5, IL-6, and IL-10. In addition, there are regulatory T cells (Tregs),[7] which secrete IL-10 and transforming growth factor (TGF)-β, and Th17 cells, which secrete IL-17.[8,9] Tregs inhibit the function of tumor-specific CD4+ and CD8+ effector T cells,[7,10] and much interest has been paid to naturally occurring Tregs (CD4+CD25+FOXP3+), although there are many other types. Th17 cells are a newly identified subset of CD4+ T cells involved in several inflammatory diseases;[8,9] their role in tumor immunity is still undefined.[11] Other subsets of T cells include γδ T cells[12] and natural killer T cells.[13]

DIRECT ANTIGEN PRESENTATION VERSUS CROSS-PRESENTATION

Tumor cell recognition by T cells is first mediated by the interaction of T cell receptors on the surface of T cells with peptides bound to major histocompatibility complex (MHC) molecules on the surface of APCs, such as DCs (Fig. 33-1). This is termed "signal 1." Two other signals are needed for T-cell activation. Signal 2 is elicited via costimulation of T cells through binding, for example, of costimulatory molecules (B7-1, B7-2) on DCs to CD28 on T cells (see Fig. 33-1), and signal 3 comes from cytokines secreted by DCs (e.g., IL-12), which aid in sustaining the T cell–mediated antitumor response. Altogether, these signals promote activation, proliferation, and maturation of CD8+ T cells, also referred to as CTLs. Signal 1 alone is thought to promote naive T-cell inactivation by anergy (lack of reaction), deletion,

or development of a regulatory T-cell fate, thus leading to "tolerance."[14] Signal 2 (costimulation) is required along with signal 1 for the induction of immunity. Signal 3 (cytokines) is also important because it affects the fate of T-cell differentiation—that is, into a Th1, Th2, or CTL effector T cell.[14]

There are two modes of antigen presentation that can lead to T-cell recognition of tumor antigens. In the first, direct antigen presentation (i.e., direct priming of T cells), the tumor cell serves as the APC to present peptide/MHC directly to T cells[15] (see Fig. 33-1). The second mode of antigen presentation occurs when tumor antigens (from apoptotic or necrotic tumor cells), tumor-derived heat shock proteins, or tumor-derived exosomes are phagocytosed by APCs and presented in the context of their MHC class I or II to CTLs or Th. This process is referred to as cross-presentation (i.e., cross-priming of T cells)[15-17] (see Fig. 33-1).

DENDRITIC CELLS

Of the APCs, DCs are the most potent and serve as the critical link between adaptive and innate immunity.[5] DCs originate in the bone marrow and then migrate in the circulatory system, traveling to specific sites of the body where they act as sentinels for the immune system. DC migration is regulated in response to chemokines, which guide them to sites of inflammation. Following capture of antigen at the tumor sites, DCs become activated and migrate to the draining lymph nodes. In the process, they mature and upregulate MHC class II,

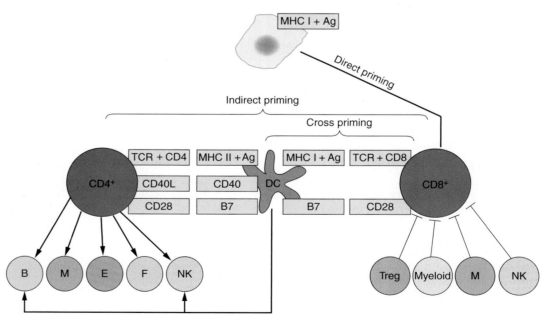

Figure 33-1 Interaction between dendritic cells (DCs), T cells, and other immune cells in the generation of a tumor antigen-specific immune response. Direct priming by a tumor cell happens infrequently due to low or absent expression of major histocompatibility complex (MHC) class I and costimulatory molecules on the tumor cell. However, T-cell activation can occur via cross-priming by DCs, the most potent antigen-presenting cells. MHC-peptide complexes on DCs interact with receptors on T cells (signal 1). Engagement of costimulatory molecules (e.g., B7) on DCs with accessory molecules (e.g., CD28) on T cells provides costimulation of T cells (signal 2). Interaction of CD40 on DCs with its ligand, CD40L, on CD4+ T cells matures and activates DCs, enabling production of cytokines (signal 3), which subsequently activates CD4+ and CD8+ T cells. Indirect priming of CD8+ T cell can occur via cytokine support by CD4+ T cells.

costimulatory molecules, and adhesion molecules.[5] In the lymph nodes, DCs present the processed antigens in the context of MHC class I or II to CD8+ or CD4+ T cells, respectively, inducing their activation, proliferation, and maturation. DCs not only stimulate CD4+ and CD8+ T cells, but they can also directly stimulate B cells[18] and natural killer cells[19] (see Fig. 33-1). The process of CTL activation may be inhibited by CD4+ CD25+FOXP3+ Tregs,[7] GR1+CD11b+ myeloid suppressor cells,[20] macrophages, and natural killer cells[21] (see Fig. 33-1).

By understanding the basics of immune recognition, we can begin to dissect the immune response specific to breast cancer and reasons for failure of immune surveillance in most patients with breast cancer.

Breast Cancer Antigens

The mechanism by which normal self proteins become tumor antigens is not completely clear. However, some of the most common breast cancer associated antigens can be separated into specific categories based on structural abnormalities or characteristic expression patterns (Table 33-1).

OVEREXPRESSED ANTIGENS

These antigens are expressed at low levels in normal tissues but are markedly overexpressed in malignant cells. For example, HER2/*neu* is a 185-kDa protein that is a member of the epithelial cell growth factor receptor family. This protein is expressed at basal levels in a variety of normal tissues. The protein is overexpressed in approximately 30% of patients with breast cancer. Both T cell and antibody immunity to HER2/*neu* can be detected in patients with breast cancer.[22,23] We have recently shown that antibodies are associated with the extent of protein overexpression in primary tumor.[24] Other breast cancer antigens that fall in this category include cyclin B1 and survivin.[25,26]

DIFFERENTIATION ANTIGENS

Differentiation antigens refer to antigens normally only seen at particular phases of differentiation of a cell type. For breast cancer, NY-BR-1 is a differentiation antigen of the mammary gland. It is expressed in normal breasts, testes, and 80% of breast cancers.[27] CTL clones recognizing NY-BR-1 epitopes have been isolated from patients with breast cancer, suggesting its role of a potential target for T cell–based therapy.[28] Carcinoembryonic antigen (CEA) is also a differentiation antigen. It is expressed exclusively in normal colonic epithelium and approximately 50% of breast cancers.[29] CEA was one of the first immunotherapy targets studied in breast cancer.

MUTATED ANTIGENS

An example of a tumor antigen resulting from gene mutation and that has been shown to be immunogenic in many types of cancer, including breast, ovarian, and colorectal, is p53, an approximately 53-kDa nuclear phosphoprotein that acts as a tumor suppressor. Anti-p53 antibodies have been detected in the serum from various patients with various types of cancer, including early stage.[30,31] Another mutated antigen is mutated epidermal growth factor receptor (EGF-RvIII), which results from an 801-bp deletion within the extracellular domain of wild-type EGF-R; this antigen is expressed by breast carcinomas but not by normal breast tissues.[32] EGF-RvIII is expressed both on the surface and in the cytoplasm of tumor cells. Patients with breast cancer specifically recognize EGF-RvIII with an overall immune response rate of 50%. The humoral and cellular immune responses correlate with EGF-RvIII expression by the tumors.[32]

CANCER-TESTIS ANTIGENS

Cancer-testis antigens have restricted expression pattern. In normal tissue, the expression is restricted to the testis and ovary, but there is a wider expression in cancer. NY-ESO-1, a cancer-testis antigen, is expressed in various human cancers, including melanoma, breast cancer, bladder cancer, prostate cancer, and hepatocellular carcinoma.[33] In patients with breast cancer, NY-ESO-1 mRNA was detected in 42% of cancer specimens.[34] More than 30 clinical trials have been initiated worldwide to evaluate the therapeutic use of NY-ESO-1.[35] Other cancer-testis antigens include MAGE, SCP-1, and SSX.[27,36,37]

The discovery of specific breast cancer–associated proteins that elicit immune responses in patients has allowed for a closer examination of breast cancer specific immunity and the identification of potential defects in the endogenous immune response.

TABLE 33-1 Common Breast Cancer Antigens	
Category	**Tumor Antigens**
Overexpressed antigens	HER-2/*neu*
	Cyclin B1
	Survivin
Differentiation antigens	NY-BR-1
	CEA
Mutated antigens	p53
	EGF-R
Cancer-testis antigens	NY-ESO-1
	MAGE
	SCP-1
	SSX

Endogenous Immune Responses Directed against Breast Cancer

Both cellular and humoral immune responses to a variety of breast cancer antigens have been documented in patients with breast cancer, including early-stage disease.[22,23] For example, high-titer antibody responses to

HER-2/*neu* ($\geq$1:100) have been detected in these patients (12 of 107, 11%).[23] Antibodies to cyclin B1 have also been detected in patients with breast cancer. High level of serum antibody was related to high expression of cyclin B1 in tumor.[38] Furthermore, tumor-infiltrating lymphocytes (TILs) have been isolated from breast cancer tissue, and the TILs can recognize autologous tumor cells in vitro by secreting cytokines and exhibiting MHC-restricted CTL activity.[39] It is now recognized that preexisting tumor-specific immunity coexists with established cancer; therefore, immunity is not protective against disease progression.

It has been demonstrated that the magnitude and affinity of the breast cancer–specific T-cell response is low, and the phenotype of the cells is not appropriate to create an inflammatory tissue destructive environment.[40] Using peripheral blood mononuclear cells from 13 patients with ovarian and breast cancer patients, we compared cytomegalovirus (CMV) and influenza-specific T-cell responses, by intracellular cytokine staining, to T cells specific for HER2, CEA, and MAGE-3 in the same patients. The magnitude of the tumor antigen–specific T-cell responses was markedly lower than CMV- or flu-specific T cell responses. Furthermore, the tumor antigen–specific T cells secreted only minimal levels of type I cytokines, IFN-γ, and TNF-α, in response to antigenic stimulation compared with CMV and flu responses in the same donors.[40]

In summary, endogenous immune response to multiple tumor antigens can be detected in patients with breast cancer. The preexistent immunity, however, is ineffective in controlling cancer growth due to defects in effector T-cell responses as well as an immunosuppressive microenvironment.

Role of the Immune Microenvironment in Limiting the Breast Cancer–associated Immune Response

The inability of existent immunity in controlling tumor growth may be a result of immune suppression and tolerance to self antigens. Mechanisms of immune evasion have been elucidated and will aid in the development of more effective immune-based therapies for breast cancer.

TOLERANCE LIMITS BREAST CANCER IMMUNITY

Humans own natural defenses preventing the development of autoimmunity also limit their ability to respond to growing cancers. Tregs (CD4+CD25+FOXP3+) represent a small fraction of the overall CD4$^+$ T-cell population and mediate immunosuppression through cell-cell contact and release of inhibitory cytokines, IL-10 and TGF-β.[41] Tregs are increased in the peripheral blood and in the tumor microenvironment in patients with cancer.[42,43] They suppress the immune response to the "self" tumor antigens expressed by the tumor and, thus,

facilitate tumor growth.[44,45] Treg numbers are significantly higher in in situ and invasive breast carcinomas than in the normal breast, and numbers are significantly higher in invasive tumors than in ductal carcinoma in situ. High numbers of Tregs were identified both in patients with ductal carcinoma in situ at increased risk for relapse and in patients with invasive tumors with both shorter relapse-free and overall survival.[46]

CHRONIC INFLAMMATION IN BREAST CANCER

In recent years, there has been increasing awareness of the paradoxical role of the immune system (for review, see de Visser, Eichten, and Coussens[47]). In breast neoplasia, the outcome of an immune response is dependent on the type of immune response elicited—acute or chronic.[48] Acute activation of tumor-directed immune responses involving CTLs appear to protect better against tumor development. On the other hand, chronic activation of humoral immunity, Th2 cells, and innate inflammatory cells (e.g., macrophages) appears to promote tumor development and disease progression (Fig. 33-2).

In breast cancer, adaptive immune cells, such as B lymphocytes, are recognized to exert antitumor immune responses via their secretion of antigen-specific immunoglobulin, and there is a suggestion that chronic activation of B cells may, conversely, potentiate development of breast carcinoma.[49] It is thought that accumulation of antibodies in afflicted tissues can induce chronic activation of innate immune cells via activation of Fc receptors and activation of the complement system, thereby resulting in tissue damage.[49] In patients, it has been seen that during breast carcinogenesis, mature B cells can be found in secondary lymphoid tissues as well as in tumor-associated stroma.[50] Compared with healthy patients without evidence of cancer, the sentinel (draining) lymph nodes of patients with breast cancer were enriched for populations of proliferating and mature B lymphocytes.[50] More importantly, the percentages of B cells present in sentinel and auxiliary lymph nodes, and their maturation status, correlated with increases in stage and total tumor burden.[51]

In theory, the interaction of the tumor and the immune system during immunosurveillance should lead to enhancement of tumor cell recognition and thus, eradication; however, this is not always the case. Sometimes, the interaction of the tumor and immune system can result in "immunoediting," which can lead to promotion of tumor growth (for review, see Dunn, Old, and Schreiber[52]). The term *cancer immunoediting* refers to any tumor alteration or sculpting that the tumor undergoes in response to immunosurveillance.[52] This sculpting can range from an amino acid substitution in a tumor-associated protein to an epithelial to mesenchymal transition, accompanied with antigen loss.[53] Tumors have various other mechanisms of inducing immune suppression. These include down-regulation/loss of MHC class I and impairment of antigen processing/presentation machinery,[15] activation of negative costimulatory signals in the tumor microenvironment (e.g., CTLA-4/B7),[54] induction of cell killing (e.g., tumor

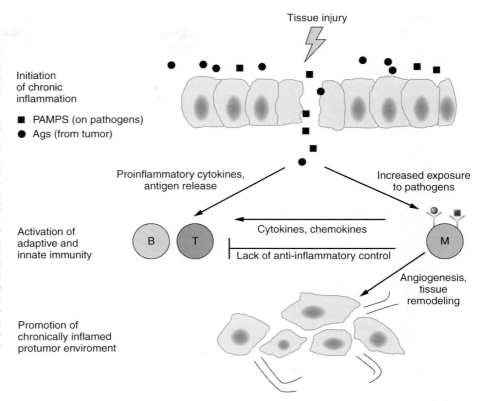

Figure 33-2 The induction and promotion of chronic inflammation in the tumor environment spurred by excessive activation of the innate immune response. Breakdown of the epithelial layer resulting from tissue injury, such as from pathogenic insult or aberrant cancer cell growth, releases pathogen-associated molecular patterns (PAMPs; e.g., heat shock protein) or tumor antigens that activate both adaptive and innate immunity. Secretion of proinflammatory cytokines and chemokines, along with release of antigens from host cells undergoing necrosis or apoptosis, facilitates recruitment of the adaptive immune cells (B and T lymphocytes) via innate immune cells (such as macrophages, M). These innate immune cells are excessively activated by increased exposure to PAMPs and secrete reactive oxygen species, among other molecules, which contribute to the chronic inflammation. Furthermore, macrophages can induce tissue remodeling and angiogenesis, promoting and enabling a tumorigenic microenvironment.

necrosis factor–related apoptosis-inducing ligand [TRAIL]) of TRAIL-R+ T lymphocytes,[55] and loss of responsiveness to key cytokines (e.g., IFN-γ).[56]

Summary and Future Directions

In summary, over the past decade our understanding of immune recognition in breast cancer has greatly improved. We know breast cancer is immunogenic and that tolerance to self antigens is a major mechanism of how breast cancers evade the immune system. Substantial evidence exists that the tumor microenvironment modulates breast cancer–specific immunity to decrease potential clinical efficacy. Several mechanisms of this modulation have been identified, and therapies are being developed that will correct preexisting immune defects.

REFERENCES

1. Fazilleau N, McHeyzer-Williams LJ, McHeyzer-Williams MG: Local development of effector and memory T helper cells. Curr Opin Immunol 19:259–267, 2007.
2. Klebanoff CA, Gattinoni L, Restifo NP: CD8+ T-cell memory in tumor immunology and immunotherapy. Immunol Rev 211:214–224, 2006.
3. Orlandi F, Venanzi FM, Concetti A, et al: Antibody and CD8+ T cell responses against HER2/neu required for tumor eradication after DNA immunization with an Flt-3 ligand fusion vaccine. Clin Cancer Res 13:6195–6203, 2007.
4. Schmitz F, Heit A: Protective cancer immunotherapy: What can the innate immune system contribute? Expert Opin Biol Ther 8:31–43, 2008.
5. Steinman RM: Dendritic cells: Understanding immunogenicity. Eur J Immunol 37(suppl 1):S53–S60, 2007.
6. Trinchieri G, Sher A: Cooperation of toll-like receptor signals in innate immune defence. Nat Rev Immunol 7:179–190, 2007.
7. Sakaguchi S: Naturally arising CD4+ regulatory T cells for immunologic self-tolerance and negative control of immune responses. Annu Rev Immunol 22:531–56, 2004.
8. Mangan PR, Harrington LE, O'Quinn DB, et al: Transforming growth factor-beta induces development of the T(H)17 lineage. Nature 441:231–234, 2006.
9. Nurieva R, Yang XO, Martinez G, et al: Essential autocrine regulation by IL-21 in the generation of inflammatory T cells. Nature 448:480–483, 2007.
10. Chaput N, Darrasse-Jeze G, Bergot AS, et al: Regulatory T cells prevent CD8 T cell maturation by inhibiting CD4 Th cells at tumor sites. J Immunol 179:4969–4978, 2007.
11. Kryczek I, Wei S, Zou L, et al: Cutting edge: Th17 and regulatory T cell dynamics and the regulation by IL-2 in the tumor microenvironment. J Immunol 178:6730–6733, 2007.
12. Beetz S, Marischen L, Kabelitz D, Wesch D: Human gamma delta T cells: Candidates for the development of immunotherapeutic strategies. Immunol Res 37:97–111, 2007.
13. Hong C, Park SH: Application of natural killer T cells in antitumor immunotherapy. Crit Rev Immunol 27:511–525, 2007.
14. Reis E, Sousa C: Dendritic cells in a mature age. Nat Rev Immunol 6:476–483, 2006.
15. Jensen PE: Recent advances in antigen processing and presentation. Nat Immunol 8:1041–1048, 2007.
16. Rock KL, Shen L: Cross-presentation: Underlying mechanisms and role in immune surveillance. Immunol Rev 207:166–183, 2005.
17. Shen L, Rock KL: Priming of T cells by exogenous antigen cross-presented on MHC class I molecules. Curr Opin Immunol 18:85–91, 2006.
18. Jego G, Pascual V, Palucka AK, Banchereau J: Dendritic cells control B cell growth and differentiation. Curr Dir Autoimmun 8:124–139, 2005.
19. Cooper MA, Fehniger TA, Fuchs A, et al: NK cell and DC interactions. Trends Immunol 25:47–52, 2004.

20. Nagaraj S, Gabrilovich DI: Myeloid-derived suppressor cells. Adv Exp Med Biol 601:213–223, 2007.

21. Bhardwaj N: Harnessing the immune system to treat cancer. J Clin Invest 117:1130–1136, 2007.

22. Disis ML, Calenoff E, McLaughlin G, et al: Existent T-cell and antibody immunity to HER-2/neu protein in patients with breast cancer. Cancer Res 54:16–20, 1994.

23. Disis ML, Pupa SM, Gralow JR, et al: High-titer HER-2/neu protein-specific antibody can be detected in patients with early-stage breast cancer. J Clin Oncol 15:3363–3367, 1997.

24. Goodell V, Waisman J, Salazar LG et al: Level of HER-2/neu protein expression in breast cancer may affect the development of endogenous HER2/neu-specific immunity. Mol Cancer Ther 7:449–454, 2008.

25. Egloff AM, Vella LA, Finn OJ: Cyclin B1 and other cyclins as tumor antigens in immunosurveillance and immunotherapy of cancer. Cancer Res 66:6–9, 2006.

26. Andersen MH, Pedersen LO, Capeller B, et al: Spontaneous cytotoxic T-cell responses against survivin-derived MHC class I-restricted T-cell epitopes in situ as well as ex vivo in cancer patients. Cancer Res 61:5964–5968, 2001.

27. Jager D, Unkelbach M, Frei C, et al: Identification of tumor-restricted antigens NY-BR-1, SCP-1, and a new cancer/testis-like antigen NW-BR-3 by serological screening of a testicular library with breast cancer serum. Cancer Immun 2:5, 2002.

28. Wang W, Epler J, Salazar LG, Riddell SR: Recognition of breast cancer cells by CD8+ cytotoxic T-cell clones specific for NY-BR-1. Cancer Res 66:6826–6833, 2006.

29. Hodge JW: Carcinoembryonic antigen as a target for cancer vaccines. Cancer Immunol Immunother 43:127–134, 1996.

30. Lubin R, Zalcman G, Bouchet L, et al: Serum p53 antibodies as early markers of lung cancer. Nat Med 1:701–702, 1995.

31. Trivers GE, De Benedetti VM, Cawley HL, et al: Anti-p53 antibodies in sera from patients with chronic obstructive pulmonary disease can predate a diagnosis of cancer. Clin Cancer Res 2:1767–1775, 1996.

32. Purev E, Cai D, Miller E, et al: Immune responses of breast cancer patients to mutated epidermal growth factor receptor (EGF-RvIII, Delta EGF-R, and de2-7 EGF-R). J Immunol 173:6472–6480, 2004.

33. Chen YT, Scanlan MJ, Sahin U, et al: A testicular antigen aberrantly expressed in human cancers detected by autologous antibody screening. Proc Natl Acad Sci USA 94:1914–1918, 1997.

34. Sugita Y, Wada H, Fujita S, et al: NY-ESO-1 expression and immunogenicity in malignant and benign breast tumors. Cancer Res 64:2199–2204, 2004.

35. Gnjatic S, Nishikawa H, Jungbluth AA, et al: NY-ESO-1: Review of an immunogenic tumor antigen. Adv Cancer Res 95:1–30, 2006.

36. Rentzsch C, Kayser S, Stumm S, et al: Evaluation of pre-existent immunity in patients with primary breast cancer: Molecular and cellular assays to quantify antigen-specific T lymphocytes in peripheral blood mononuclear cells. Clin Cancer Res 9:4376–4386, 2003.

37. Scanlan MJ, Gout I, Gordon CM, et al: Humoral immunity to human breast cancer: Antigen definition and quantitative analysis of mRNA expression. Cancer Immun 1:4, 2001.

38. Suzuki H, Graziano DF, McKolanis J, Finn OJ: T cell-dependent antibody responses against aberrantly expressed cyclin B1 protein in patients with cancer and premalignant disease. Clin Cancer Res 11:1521–1526, 2005.

39. Baxevanis CN, Dedoussis GV, Papadopoulos NG, et al: Tumor specific cytolysis by tumor infiltrating lymphocytes in breast cancer. Cancer 74:1275–1282, 1994.

40. Inokuma M, dela Rosa C, Schmitt C, et al: Functional T cell responses to tumor antigens in breast cancer patients have a distinct phenotype and cytokine signature. J Immunol 179:2627–2633, 2007.

41. Chen ML, Pittet MJ, Gorelik L, et al: Regulatory T cells suppress tumor-specific CD8 T cell cytotoxicity through TGF-beta signals in vivo. Proc Natl Acad Sci USA 102:419–424, 2005.

42. Curiel TJ, Coukos G, Zou L, et al: Specific recruitment of regulatory T cells in ovarian carcinoma fosters immune privilege and predicts reduced survival. Nat Med 10:942–949, 2004.

43. Liyanage UK, Moore TT, Joo HG, et al: Prevalence of regulatory T cells is increased in peripheral blood and tumor microenvironment of patients with pancreas or breast adenocarcinoma. J Immunol 169:2756–2761, 2002.

44. Fecci PE, Mitchell DA, Whitesides JF, et al: Increased regulatory T-cell fraction amidst a diminished CD4 compartment explains cellular immune defects in patients with malignant glioma. Cancer Res 66:3294–3302, 2006.

45. Turk MJ, Guevara-Patino JA, Rizzuto GA, et al: Concomitant tumor immunity to a poorly immunogenic melanoma is prevented by regulatory T cells. J Exp Med 200:771–782, 2004.

46. Bates GJ, Fox SB, Han C, et al: Quantification of regulatory T cells enables the identification of high-risk breast cancer patients and those at risk of late relapse. J Clin Oncol 24:5373–5380, 2006.

47. de Visser KE, Eichten A, Coussens LM: Paradoxical roles of the immune system during cancer development. Nat Rev Cancer 6:24–37, 2006.

48. DeNardo DG, Coussens LM: Inflammation and breast cancer. Balancing immune response: Crosstalk between adaptive and innate immune cells during breast cancer progression. Breast Cancer Res 9:212, 2007.

49. Tan TT, Coussens LM: Humoral immunity, inflammation and cancer. Curr Opin Immunol 19:209–216, 2007.

50. Whitford P, George WD, Campbell AM: Flow cytometric analysis of tumour infiltrating lymphocyte activation and tumour cell MHC class I and II expression in breast cancer patients. Cancer Lett 61:157–164, 1992.

51. Morton BA, Ramey WG, Paderon H, Miller RE: Monoclonal antibody-defined phenotypes of regional lymph node and peripheral blood lymphocyte subpopulations in early breast cancer. Cancer Res 46:2121–2126, 1986.

52. Dunn GP, Old LJ, Schreiber RD: The three Es of cancer immunoediting. Annu Rev Immunol 22:329–360, 2004.

53. Knutson KL, Lu H, Stone B, et al: Immunoediting of cancers may lead to epithelial to mesenchymal transition. J Immunol 177:1526–1533, 2006.

54. Hodi FS: Cytotoxic T-lymphocyte-associated antigen-4. Clin Cancer Res 13:5238–5242, 2007.

55. Xu J, Zhou JY, Wu GS: Tumor necrosis factor-related apoptosis-inducing ligand is required for tumor necrosis factor alpha-mediated sensitization of human breast cancer cells to chemotherapy. Cancer Res 66:10092–10099, 2006.

56. Dunn GP, Koebel CM, Schreiber RD: Interferons, immunity and cancer immunoediting. Nat Rev Immunol 6:836–848, 2006.

chapter 34

Immunology and the Role of Immunotherapy in Breast Cancer: Human Clinical Trials

WILLIAM E. GILLANDERS I PETER S. GOEDEGEBUURE I TIMOTHY J. EBERLEIN

Breast Cancer Immunotherapy in Perspective

Ever since Paul Ehrlich's seminal studies of the immune system and his proposed use of antibodies as "magic bullets," there has been considerable interest in the use of the immune system to treat cancer. The remarkable success of trastuzumab, a humanized monoclonal antibody that acts on the HER2/neu receptor, dramatically underscores the potential to harness the exquisite specificity of the immune system for the treatment of breast cancer.[1-3] After two decades of skepticism, antibody therapy for breast cancer is now so successful that it is no longer considered by many to be immunotherapy. The National Cancer Institute PDQ registry of cancer clinical trials currently lists 178 active clinical trials of antibody therapy in breast cancer. The rationale, indications and evolving role of antibody therapy in breast cancer is addressed in detail in separate chapters of this text.

Other forms of breast cancer immunotherapy such as vaccine, cytokine, and adoptive T-cell therapy have not enjoyed the same prominent success as antibody therapy. However, the past two decades have been witness to impressive advances in basic and translational immunology. These advances suggest that vaccine, cytokine, and adoptive T-cell therapy may soon be integrated into the clinical arena. Specific advances include (1) the definition of breast cancer antigens at the molecular level; (2) an improved understanding of the interplay between the innate and adaptive immune systems; (3) an understanding of the complex costimulatory signaling networks required for, and limiting T-cell activation; and (4) the recent characterization of the impact of the tumor microenvironment on the development of regulatory networks and concomitant inhibition of antitumor immune responses.

It is commonly believed that breast cancer is not immunogenic. The relative difficulty of successfully culturing autologous breast cancer cells and antigen-specific T cells in vitro has contributed to this general belief and limited progress in the identification of breast cancer antigens. Although breast cancer is perceived to be less immunogenic than melanoma or renal cell cancer, there is increasing evidence that the immune system can recognize breast cancer. Spontaneous regression of primary breast cancers has been described,[4] and the presence of immune infiltrates in primary breast cancers has been associated with clinical outcome.[5,6] Crosstalk between the immune system and primary breast cancers is clearly evident in the increased prevalence of regulatory T cells[7,8] and immature myeloid cells[9,10] observed in patients with breast cancer. Finally, there is clear evidence of preexisting immune responses to several breast cancer antigens, including HER2/neu,[11-14] MUC1,[15] and mammaglobin-A.[16-19]

The reality is that breast cancer may in fact be ideally suited for exploring the potential of vaccine therapy in patients with minimal residual disease.[20-22] Most patients with breast cancer are diagnosed with locoregional disease and are typically rendered disease-free by standard treatment modalities. With the success of standard therapies, relapse typically occurs years after diagnosis and treatment,[23] providing a window of opportunity to generate effective antitumor immune responses.

It should come as no surprise that the number of human breast cancer immunotherapy trials has increased dramatically in the past 5 years. In addition to the antibody therapy trials mentioned previously, the National Cancer Institute Physician Data Query registry of cancer clinical trials currently lists 27 active clinical trials of vaccine therapy, 8 trials of interleukin (IL) therapy, and 20 trials of adoptive cell therapy. In this chapter, we will review some of the most relevant ongoing trials in an effort to highlight important trends in this dynamic and rapidly changing field of research.

Vaccine Therapy

BREAST CANCER ANTIGENS AND PRELIMINARY VACCINE TRIALS

Breast cancer vaccines have generated considerable enthusiasm and remain an area of intense research interest.[24-26] After all, the successful development of vaccines for viral disease was one of the most significant medical achievements of the 20th century, and vaccines have had an enormous impact on human health. Breast cancer vaccines have proven to be safe and well tolerated with minimal side effects, and they can be administered in an outpatient setting. Breast cancer vaccines have been designed to elicit both cellular and humoral immunity. At the most basic level, "cellular vaccines" are designed to stimulate CD8 T cells, and "humoral vaccines" are designed to stimulate CD4 T cells and B cells, resulting in an antibody response. A major advance in basic immunology was the recognition that T cells do not recognize antigens in their native form but rather as peptide fragments bound to major histocompatability molecules. Although the identification of breast cancer antigens was initially limited by the relative difficulty in culturing autologous breast cancer cells and antigen-specific T cells in vitro, a number of breast cancer antigens have now been successfully identified.[27] Important breast cancer antigens include HER2/neu, MUC1, human telomerase reverse transcriptase, p53, and mammaglobin-A.

HER2/neu is a 185-kD transmembrane glycoprotein receptor with tyrosine kinase activity. HER2/neu overexpression is present in 20% to 30% of primary breast cancers and is associated with poor prognosis. This antigen has been successfully targeted in phase I clinical trials of peptide vaccines in patients with advanced or metastatic disease.[28,29] The peptide vaccines were able to elicit HER2/neu-specific immune responses in peripheral blood, but no objective clinical responses were observed. MUC1 is a membrane-bound glycoprotein that is overexpressed and aberrantly glycosylated in breast cancers.[15] Vaccination with peptides derived from this antigen are very effective at eliciting antibody responses in patients with advanced disease, although it is not clear if an effective CD8 T-cell response can be elicited.[30-32] No clear evidence of a clinical benefit has been demonstrated. Human telomerase reverse transcriptase (hTERT) is overexpressed in breast and other cancers,[33] and it contributes to the neoplastic phenotype.[34] A recent phase I clinical trial in patients with metastatic breast cancer confirms that hTERT peptide vaccination can successfully elicit CD8 T-cell responses, but no objective clinical responses were observed by Response Evaluation Criteria in Solid Tumors (RECIST) criteria.[35]

DEFINING A NEW PARADIGM FOR VACCINE DEVELOPMENT

To date, the majority of breast cancer vaccine trials have been performed in patients with metastatic disease. This is easy to understand because many of these trials represent the first human trials of novel biologic therapeutics with unknown side-effects. As such, these preliminary trials represent an appropriate and ethical balance between safety and potential clinical efficacy. Unfortunately, the results of cancer vaccines in patients with metastatic cancers (including breast cancer) have been disappointing, and some authors have advocated a fundamental reassessment of vaccine therapy. In a recent review of cancer vaccine trials of 440 patients at the National Cancer Institute, Rosenberg and colleagues noted that the objective clinical response rate by standard RECIST criteria was only 2.6%.[36] These results suggest that profound changes are required in the clinical development of cancer vaccines.

There is considerable evidence to suggest that generation of an effective antitumor immune response will be more difficult in patients with metastatic cancers.[37] Metastatic breast cancer is no exception. Specifically, metastatic breast cancer is associated with defects in T-cell activation and function,[38] as well as in dendritic cell function.[39,40] Furthermore, metastatic breast cancer is characterized by genomic instability and is more likely to be associated with antigen-loss variants through the selective pressures of immunoediting.[41] Finally, there is evidence that metastatic breast cancer is associated with an increase in the prevalence of regulatory T cells[7,8] and immature myeloid cells[9,10] in the peripheral blood and in the tumor microenvironment, and these cells are capable of inhibiting endogenous or elicited antitumor immune responses. For these reasons, it is likely that breast cancer vaccine therapy will be more successful in patients with "minimal residual disease" to prevent disease recurrence than in patients with metastatic breast cancer. For example, patients with breast cancer and node-positive disease or high-risk node-negative disease might be excellent candidates for vaccine therapy after multimodality treatment with surgery, chemotherapy, and radiation therapy. These patients typically have no gross evidence of disease but are at high-risk for disease recurrence. These issues have recently resulted in a fundamental reassessment of the development paradigm for cancer vaccines, with an emphasis on early assessment of vaccine efficacy in an appropriate clinical context.[42]

BREAST CANCER VACCINES IN MINIMAL RESIDUAL DISEASE

Recently, investigators at the University of Washington and Walter Reed Army Medical Center have independently demonstrated the potential clinical efficacy of breast cancer vaccines in patients with minimal residual disease. Coveler and associates at the University of Washington recently evaluated whether or not adjuvant therapies for breast cancer, including endocrine therapy, bisphosphonates, and trastuzumab (which are often administered for several years after surgery, standard chemotherapy, and radiation therapy), have an impact on the response to cancer vaccines.[20] Studies of 36 patients undergoing active immunization with a HER2/neu peptide vaccine[43] demonstrate that these adjuvant breast cancer therapies did not limit the development of immunity as shown by immune monitoring. Peoples and coworkers have recently reported on the combined results of two clinical trials of a HER2/neu peptide vaccine designed to prevent disease recurrence in patients with node-positive and high-risk node-negative breast cancer.[21,22] In these studies, all eligible patients were enrolled. HLA-A2 and HLA-A3 patients were vaccinated (n = 101), whereas all other patients were followed prospectively as controls (n = 85). The peptide vaccine was safe and well tolerated, with evidence of antigen-specific immune responses observed by immune monitoring and delayed type hypersensitivity responses. Of particular note, a planned analysis performed at 18 months median follow-up demonstrated that vaccination is associated with a significant improvement in disease-free survival. The recurrence rate in the vaccinated group was 5.6%, compared with 14.2% in the observation group ($P = 0.04$). Taken together, these studies confirm the clinical potential of vaccine therapy in patients with breast cancer who have minimal residual disease and suggest that a randomized phase III clinical trial of a HER2/neu peptide vaccine would be appropriate.

Breast Cancer Vaccines in Evolution

In the past two decades, considerable progress has been made in understanding the complex regulatory and signaling networks that control the immune system. It is becoming increasing clear that CD8 T-cell responses are tightly regulated, presumably to avoid deleterious autoimmune responses. Three important mechanisms that regulate CD8 T-cell responses and are currently being targeted in human clinical trials are described in detail later in the chapter. Targeting these networks has the potential to significantly enhance the efficacy of breast cancer vaccine therapy.

ENHANCING T-CELL COSTIMULATION

Costimulation is a critical component of T-cell activation. T-cell activation is dependent on two signals: the first signal is provided by T-cell receptor interaction with specific antigen, and the second signal is provided by engagement of costimulatory molecules on the surface of the T cell. CD28 is a costimulatory molecule that is constitutively expressed on T cells. CD28 engagement by CD80 or CD86 on professional antigen-presenting cells promotes T-cell activation, proliferation, and IL-2 production.[44] In the absence of this costimulatory signal, T cells are induced into a state of unresponsiveness.[45] Expression of CD80 and CD86 is generally limited to professional antigen-presenting cells: dendritic cells, macrophages, and activated B cells. Most epithelial cells and epithelial tumors do not express CD80 or CD86,

and this may explain in part why breast cancers fail to elicit effective antitumor immune responses. Given the critical importance of costimulation in initiating an effective immune response, investigators have explored strategies to enhance CD28 engagement and T-cell costimulation. One strategy to enhance costimulation is through the use of dendritic cell vaccines, because mature dendritic cells naturally express high levels of the costimulatory molecules CD80 and CD86.

Dendritic cells are potent antigen-presenting cells and are thought to be uniquely responsible for the induction of primary immune responses and the establishment of immunologic memory.[46] The discovery of conditions for in vitro culture and expansion of dendritic cells has opened new avenues for vaccine design,[47] and preclinical models confirm the potential of dendritic cells to generate protective antitumor immunity.[48] Avigan and colleagues recently reported the results of a phase I trial of a cellular vaccine prepared by fusing autologous tumor cells and dendritic cells in patients with metastatic breast and renal cancers.[49] Fusion vaccines were successfully generated for 16 patients with breast cancer, and 10 of these patients were successfully vaccinated. No dose-limiting toxicities were observed, and immune monitoring documented the generation of strong cellular immune responses. Two of the ten patients achieved objective clinical responses. Czerniecki and associates reported that vaccination with dendritic cells pulsed with HER2/neu HLA class I and II peptides were able to successfully generate HER2/neu-specific T-cell responses in patients with ductal carcinoma in situ (DCIS).[50] Seven of 11 patients also showed measurable decreases in residual DCIS confirming the potential efficacy of this strategy. Investigators at H. Lee Moffitt Cancer Center and the University of Nebraska are currently conducting a phase I/II clinical trial of p53-infected dendritic cells in patients with p53-overexpressing stage II or III breast cancer based on their earlier work in patients with lung cancer.[51,52] This study explores the potential of vaccine therapy in combination with chemotherapy. Finally, in a closely related strategy, Guckel and coworkers recently initiated a phase I/II clinical trial based on a CD80-transfected, HER2/neu-overexpressing breast cancer cell line. In proof-of-principle studies, this allogeneic cellular vaccine was able to successfully induce specific interferon-γ release following vaccination in the first two patients enrolled.[53] Taken together, these studies confirm the importance of effective costimulation in generating antitumor immune responses and represent a viable alternative to peptide-based vaccines.

PREVENTING T-CELL INHIBITION: CTLA4 BLOCKADE

Cytotoxic T lymphocyte antigen 4 (CTLA4) is a CD28-family receptor that plays an integral role in inhibiting primary T-cell responses. CTLA-4 is homologous to CD28 but has a much higher affinity for the costimulatory molecules CD80 and CD86 than CD28.[54] Although CTLA4 is not expressed on resting T cells, it is upregulated following T-cell activation. CTLA4 activation interferes with IL-2 production and interrupts cell cycle progression, inhibiting proliferation of activated T cells.[55,56] In preclinical studies, targeting this molecule has resulted in a dramatic improvement in antitumor immunity.[57,58] There is evidence to suggest that overexpression of CTLA4, or similar inhibitory molecules, may contribute to cancer immune evasion. Czerniecki and colleagues recently demonstrated that CTLA4 is overexpressed in breast cancer–specific T cells in patients with DCIS,[50] and similar findings have been reported in other malignancies.[59]

Phan and associates targeted CTLA4 in patients with metastatic melanoma.[60] Ipilimumab is a fully humanized anti-CTLA4 monoclonal antibody capable of blocking CTLA4 engagement with CD80 and CD86. Administration of this antibody in conjunction with a melanoma peptide vaccine was associated with objective cancer regression in three of 14 patients. CTLA4 blockade also resulted in autoimmune manifestations. Additional studies have been performed in patients with metastatic prostate cancer[61] or following vaccine failure[62] with promising results. The company Medarex has recently completed a phase II trial of ipilimumab in 33 patients with metastatic breast cancer.[63] Although the results of this study are not yet available, targeting CTLA4 and checkpoint blockade represents an attractive strategy for enhancing the immune response to breast cancer, and breast cancer vaccines.

TARGETING REGULATORY T CELLS

Regulatory T cells are a specialized subpopulation of T cells that help to maintain immune homeostasis and protect against autoimmune disease. Regulatory T cells are characterized by coexpression of CD4, CD25, and Foxp3, and are capable of directly suppressing immune effector cells. Liyanage and coworkers have demonstrated that the prevalence of regulatory T cells is increased in the peripheral blood and primary tumors of patients with breast cancer,[7] and this observation has been independently confirmed.[8] This increased prevalence of regulatory T cells in patients with metastatic breast cancer may explain why antitumor immune responses are attenuated in these patients and why cancer vaccines have limited efficacy in this clinical context. Several strategies are currently under evaluation in human clinical trials designed to specifically target regulatory T cells in patients with breast cancer.

One strategy to target regulatory T cells is an engineered fusion protein combining IL-2 and diphtheria toxin (denileukin diftitox, or ONTAK). This molecule is capable of specifically targeting regulatory T cells through the IL-2 receptor (CD25). Dannull and colleagues recently demonstrated that ONTAK administration significantly reduced the number of regulatory T cells in patients with metastatic renal cell carcinoma.[64] Regulatory T cell depletion and dendritic cell vaccination was associated with a significant increase in antitumor immune responses compared to vaccination alone. Investigators at the University of Washington have confirmed the potential role of ONTAK therapy in breast cancer. In preclinical studies, ONTAK significantly enhanced antitumor immune responses in HER2/neu transgenic mice.[65] Based on these studies, a phase I/II trial of ONTAK in patients with advanced, refractory breast cancer has been initiated.[66] Twenty patients with progressive or relapsed disease will be treated with up to six courses of ONTAK to assess the safety of this biologic therapy and its ability to specifically deplete regulatory T cells in patients with breast cancer.

A second strategy to target regulatory T cells is to use standard vaccine therapies in combination with chemotherapy. Investigators at Johns Hopkins University have demonstrated that regulatory T cells are particularly sensitive to chemotherapy, particularly cyclophosphamide.[67] In preclinical studies, these investigators demonstrated that cyclophosphamide administration prior to peptide vaccination selectively depletes regulatory T cells, enhancing antigen-specific T-cell responses. Based on these studies, a phase I clinical trial of an allogeneic granulocyte-macrophage colony-stimulating factor–secreting breast cancer vaccine given in a combination with cyclophosphamide and doxorubicin chemotherapy has been initiated.[68] This study will test the hypothesis that specifically timed administration of chemotherapeutic agents can be used to deplete regulatory T cells and enhance the efficacy of a cellular breast cancer vaccine.

Cytokine Therapy

Cytokines are small peptides that are central to the function of the immune system. Cytokines provide a mechanism for immune cells to communicate with each other, and they are integrally involved in most immune responses. The precise function of individual cytokines can be difficult to define because of the considerable redundancy and pleiotropism among cytokines. Cytokines have been successfully used for cancer immunotherapy. IL-2 was the first cytokine to be discovered, and this cytokine is critical to the growth, differentiation, and survival of T cells. IL-2 has been successfully used and is currently approved by the U.S. Food and Drug Administration (FDA) for the treatment of melanoma and renal cell carcinoma. Although IL-2 therapy has not been used extensively in breast cancer,[69] investigators are now exploring the potential role of IL-2—as in the context of peripheral blood stem cell transplantation. Although controversial, peripheral blood stem cell transplantation in combination with high-dose chemotherapy has been investigated for the treatment of high-risk breast cancer.[70] Investigators have now combined immunotherapy with high-dose chemotherapy to facilitate tumor cell killing. In a phase III randomized multicenter trial, eligible patients were treated with autologous bone marrow transplantation with or without immunotherapy.[71] Patients randomized to the immunotherapy arm received cells that were incubated with IL-2 and then received low-dose IL-2 following transplantation. In this well-controlled study, there was no significant difference in disease-free or overall survival between the two treatment arms. However, the study did not meet accrual goals, and it is possible that a trend toward improved overall survival may have reached statistical significance if the study had met accrual goals.

Adoptive T-Cell Therapy

For the purposes of this review, adoptive T-cell therapy, also known as passive immunotherapy, is the transfusion of autologous T cells into patients with cancer. Currently there are no FDA-approved adoptive cell therapies for cancer. However, this is an area of intense research interest, and recent progress in improved culture systems, adoptive transfer into lymphodepleted hosts, and the potential to effectively target regulatory T cells suggest that in the future adoptive cell therapies may find an important role in the clinic. One issue specific to breast cancer that may have limited investigation of adoptive T-cell therapy for this disease is the relative difficulty to generate breast cancer–specific T-cell populations. Tumor-infiltrating lymphocytes (TILs) were one of the first successful adoptive cell therapies for cancer and have had considerable success in melanoma and renal cell carcinoma. Although immunohistochemical analyses appear to confirm the presence of TILs in primary breast cancers,[72] attempts to generate populations of TILs suitable for adoptive cell therapy have had only limited success.[73] However, with the identification of breast cancer antigens and improved culture techniques, considerable progress has been made in this field, and there are now several clinical trials ongoing.

Bernhard and associates recently reported preliminary results of adoptive T-cell therapy with HER2/neu-specific T cells in patients with metastatic breast cancer.[74] HER2/neu-specific T cells were generated ex vivo by stimulating peripheral blood mononuclear cells with peptide-loaded dendritic cells. Immune monitoring, diagnostic imaging, and immunohistochemical analyses demonstrated that the T cells accumulated in the liver and bone marrow following adoptive transfer. Although the cells were not able to penetrate solid metastases, disseminated tumor cells in the bone marrow disappeared following therapy. Additional studies are currently ongoing studying the role of adoptive T-cell therapy either in patients with metastatic disease[75,76] or in the context of high-dose chemotherapy and peripheral blood stem cell transplantation.[77] In the future, adoptive T-cell therapy for breast cancer may be used in combination with lymphodepletion, a strategy that has been particularly effective in melanoma.[78]

Summary

- Antibody therapy represents a dramatic success of breast cancer immunotherapy.
- Breast cancer antigens have been identified and appear to be excellent candidates for vaccine therapy.
- Targeting patients with minimal residual disease represents a new paradigm in vaccine development with preliminary clinical trials suggesting increased efficacy.
- Concomitant targeting of the regulatory and signaling pathways limiting immune responses in patients with metastatic breast cancer may improve vaccine therapy.

REFERENCES

1. Joensuu H, Kellokumpu-Lehtinen PL, Bono P, et al: Adjuvant docetaxel or vinorelbine with or without trastuzumab for breast cancer. N Engl J Med 354:809, 2006.
2. Piccart-Gebhart MJ, Procter M, Leyland-Jones B, et al: Trastuzumab after adjuvant chemotherapy in HER2-positive breast cancer. N Engl J Med 353:1659, 2005.
3. Romond EH, Perez EA, Bryant J, et al: Trastuzumab plus adjuvant chemotherapy for operable HER2-positive breast cancer. N Engl J Med 353:1673, 2005.
4. Challis GB, Stam HJ: The spontaneous regression of cancer. A review of cases from 1900 to 1987. Acta Oncol 29:545, 1990.
5. Aaltomaa S, Lipponen P, Eskelinen M, et al: Lymphocyte infiltrates as a prognostic variable in female breast cancer. Eur J Cancer 28A:859, 1992.
6. Marrogi AJ, Munshi A, Merogi AJ, et al: Study of tumor infiltrating lymphocytes and transforming growth factor-beta as prognostic factors in breast carcinoma. Int J Cancer 74:492, 1997.
7. Liyanage UK, Moore TT, Joo HG, et al: Prevalence of regulatory T cells is increased in peripheral blood and tumor microenvironment of patients with pancreas or breast adenocarcinoma. J Immunol 169:2756, 2002.
8. Wolf AM, Wolf D, Steurer M, et al: Increase of regulatory T cells in the peripheral blood of cancer patients. Clin Cancer Res 9:606, 2003.
9. Almand B, Clark JI, Nikitina E, et al: Increased production of immature myeloid cells in cancer patients: A mechanism of immunosuppression in cancer. J Immunol 166:678, 2001.
10. Almand B, Resser JR, Lindman B, et al: Clinical significance of defective dendritic cell differentiation in cancer. Clin Cancer Res 6:1755, 2000.
11. Disis ML, Calenoff E, McLaughlin G, et al: Existent T-cell and antibody immunity to HER-2/neu protein in patients with breast cancer. Cancer Res 54:16, 1994.
12. Disis ML, Knutson KL, Schiffman K, et al: Pre-existent immunity to the HER-2/neu oncogenic protein in patients with HER-2/neu overexpressing breast and ovarian cancer. Breast Cancer Res Treat 62:245, 2000.
13. Disis ML, Pupa SM, Gralow JR, et al: High-titer HER-2/neu protein-specific antibody can be detected in patients with early-stage breast cancer. J Clin Oncol 15:3363, 1997.
14. Peoples GE, Goedegebuure PS, Smith R, et al: Breast and ovarian cancer-specific cytotoxic T lymphocytes recognize the same HER2/neu-derived peptide. Proc Natl Acad Sci USA 92:432, 1995.
15. von Mensdorff-Pouilly S, Snijdewint FG, Verstraeten AA, et al: Human MUC1 mucin: A multifaceted glycoprotein. Int J Biol Markers 15:343, 2000.
16. Jaramillo A, Majumder K, Manna PP, et al: Identification of HLA-A3-restricted CD8+ T cell epitopes derived from mammaglobin-A, a tumor-associated antigen of human breast cancer. Int J Cancer 102:499, 2002.
17. Jaramillo A, Narayanan K, Campbell LG, et al: Recognition of HLA-A2-restricted mammaglobin-A-derived epitopes by CD8+ cytotoxic T lymphocytes from breast cancer patients. Breast Cancer Res Treat 88:29, 2004.
18. Narayanan K, Jaramillo A, Benshoff ND, et al: Response of established human breast tumors to vaccination with mammaglobin-A cDNA. J Natl Cancer Inst 96:1388, 2004.
19. Tanaka Y, Amos KD, Fleming TP, et al: Mammaglobin-A is a tumor-associated antigen in human breast carcinoma. Surgery 133:74, 2003.
20. Coveler AL, Goodell V, Webster DJ, et al: Common adjuvant breast cancer therapies do not inhibit cancer vaccine induced T cell immunity. Breast Cancer Res Treat, 2008.
21. Peoples GE, Gurney JM, Hueman MT, et al: Clinical trial results of a HER2/neu (E75) vaccine to prevent recurrence in high-risk breast cancer patients. J Clin Oncol 23:7536, 2005.
22. Peoples GE, Holmes JP, Hueman MT, et al: Combined clinical trial results of a HER2/neu (E75) vaccine for the prevention of recurrence in high-risk breast cancer patients: U.S. Military Cancer Institute Clinical Trials Group Study I-01 and I-02. Clin Cancer Res 14:797, 2008.

23. Day RS, Shackney SE, Peters WP: The analysis of relapse-free survival curves: Implications for evaluating intensive systemic adjuvant treatment regimens for breast cancer. Br J Cancer 92:47, 2005.

24. Curigliano G, Spitaleri G, Dettori M, et al: Vaccine immunotherapy in breast cancer treatment: Promising, but still early. Expert Rev Anticancer Ther 7:1225, 2007.

25. Emens LA, Reilly RT, Jaffee EM: Breast cancer vaccines: Maximizing cancer treatment by tapping into host immunity. Endocr Relat Cancer 12:1, 2005.

26. Mittendorf EA, Peoples GE, Singletary SE: Breast cancer vaccines: Promise for the future or pipe dream? Cancer 110:1677, 2007.

27. Disis ML: Immunologic targets for breast cancer. Breast Dis 15:83, 2002.

28. Knutson KL, Schiffman K, Cheever MA, et al: Immunization of cancer patients with a HER-2/neu, HLA-A2 peptide, p369-377, results in short-lived peptide-specific immunity. Clin Cancer Res 8:1014, 2002.

29. Murray JL, Gillogly ME, Przepiorka D, et al: Toxicity, immunogenicity, and induction of E75-specific tumor-lytic CTLs by HER-2 peptide E75 (369-377) combined with granulocyte macrophage colony-stimulating factor in HLA-A2+ patients with metastatic breast and ovarian cancer. Clin Cancer Res 8:3407, 2002.

30. Gilewski T, Adluri S, Ragupathi G, et al: Vaccination of high-risk breast cancer patients with mucin-1 (MUC1) keyhole limpet hemocyanin conjugate plus QS-21. Clin Cancer Res 6:1693, 2000.

31. Karanikas V, Hwang LA, Pearson J, et al: Antibody and T cell responses of patients with adenocarcinoma immunized with mannan-MUC1 fusion protein. J Clin Invest 100:2783, 1997.

32. Reddish M, MacLean GD, Koganty RR, et al: Anti-MUC1 class I restricted CTLs in metastatic breast cancer patients immunized with a synthetic MUC1 peptide. Int J Cancer 76:817, 1998.

33. Kim NW, Piatyszek MA, Prowse KR, et al: Specific association of human telomerase activity with immortal cells and cancer. Science 266:2011, 1994.

34. Hahn WC, Counter CM, Lundberg AS, et al: Creation of human tumour cells with defined genetic elements. Nature 400:464, 1999.

35. Domchek SM, Recio A, Mick R, et al: Telomerase-specific T-cell immunity in breast cancer: Effect of vaccination on tumor immunosurveillance. Cancer Res 67:10546, 2007.

36. Rosenberg SA, Yang JC, Restifo NP: Cancer immunotherapy: Moving beyond current vaccines. Nat Med 10:909, 2004.

37. Finn OJ: Cancer vaccines: Between the idea and the reality. Nat Rev Immunol 3:630, 2003.

38. Finke J, Ferrone S, Frey A, et al: Where have all the T cells gone? Mechanisms of immune evasion by tumors. Immunol Today 20:158, 1999.

39. Gervais A, Leveque J, Bouet-Toussaint F, et al: Dendritic cells are defective in breast cancer patients: A potential role for polyamine in this immunodeficiency. Breast Cancer Res 7:R326, 2005.

40. Pockaj BA, Basu GD, Pathangey LB, et al: Reduced T-cell and dendritic cell function is related to cyclooxygenase-2 overexpression and prostaglandin E2 secretion in patients with breast cancer. Ann Surg Oncol 11:328, 2004.

41. Dunn GP, Bruce AT, Ikeda H, et al: Cancer immunoediting: From immunosurveillance to tumor escape. Nat Immunol 3:991, 2002.

42. Hoos A, Parmiani G, Hege K, et al: A clinical development paradigm for cancer vaccines and related biologics. J Immunother 30:1, 2007.

43. Disis ML, Schiffman K, Guthrie K, et al: Effect of dose on immune response in patients vaccinated with an her-2/neu intracellular domain protein-based vaccine. J Clin Oncol 22:1916, 2004.

44. Linsley PS, Brady W, Grosmaire L, et al: Binding of the B cell activation antigen B7 to CD28 costimulates T cell proliferation and interleukin 2 mRNA accumulation. J Exp Med 173:721, 1991.

45. Schwartz RH: A cell culture model for T lymphocyte clonal anergy. Science 248:1349, 1990.

46. Banchereau J, Steinman RM: Dendritic cells and the control of immunity. Nature 392:245, 1998.

47. Inaba K, Inaba M, Romani N, et al: Generation of large numbers of dendritic cells from mouse bone marrow cultures supplemented with granulocyte/macrophage colony-stimulating factor. J Exp Med 176:1693, 1992.

48. Mayordomo JI, Zorina T, Storkus WJ, et al: Bone marrow-derived dendritic cells pulsed with synthetic tumour peptides elicit protective and therapeutic antitumour immunity. Nat Med 1:1297, 1995.

49. Avigan D, Vasir B, Gong J, et al: Fusion cell vaccination of patients with metastatic breast and renal cancer induces immunological and clinical responses. Clin Cancer Res 10:4699, 2004.

50. Czerniecki BJ, Koski GK, Koldovsky U, et al: Targeting HER-2/neu in early breast cancer development using dendritic cells with staged interleukin-12 burst secretion. Cancer Res 67:1842, 2007.

51. United States National Cancer Institute: Vaccine therapy with either neoadjuvant or adjuvant chemotherapy and adjuvant radiation therapy in treating women with p53-overexpressing stage II or stage III breast cancer. http://clinicaltrials.gov/ct2/show/NCT00082641. Accessed March, 2008.

52. Antonia SJ, Mirza N, Fricke I, et al: Combination of p53 cancer vaccine with chemotherapy in patients with extensive stage small cell lung cancer. Clin Cancer Res 12:878, 2006.

53. Guckel B, Stumm S, Rentzsch C, et al: A CD80-transfected human breast cancer cell variant induces HER-2/neu-specific T cells in HLA-A*02-matched situations in vitro as well as in vivo. Cancer Immunol Immunother 54:129, 2005.

54. Linsley PS, Greene JL, Brady W, et al: Human B7-1 (CD80) and B7-2 (CD86) bind with similar avidities but distinct kinetics to CD28 and CTLA-4 receptors. Immunity 1:793, 1994.

55. Krummel MF, Allison JP: CTLA-4 engagement inhibits IL-2 accumulation and cell cycle progression upon activation of resting T cells. J Exp Med 183:2533, 1996.

56. Walunas TL, Bakker CY, Bluestone JA: CTLA-4 ligation blocks CD28-dependent T cell activation. J Exp Med 183:2541, 1996.

57. Chambers CA, Kuhns MS, Egen JG, et al: CTLA-4-mediated inhibition in regulation of T cell responses: mechanisms and manipulation in tumor immunotherapy. Annu Rev Immunol 19:565, 2001.

58. Leach DR, Krummel MF, Allison JP: Enhancement of antitumor immunity by CTLA-4 blockade. Science 271:1734, 1996.

59. Woo EY, Yeh H, Chu CS, et al: Cutting edge: Regulatory T cells from lung cancer patients directly inhibit autologous T cell proliferation. J Immunol 168:4272, 2002.

60. Phan GQ, Yang JC, Sherry RM, et al: Cancer regression and autoimmunity induced by cytotoxic T lymphocyte-associated antigen 4 blockade in patients with metastatic melanoma. Proc Natl Acad Sci USA 100:8372, 2003.

61. Small EJ, Tchekmedyian NS, Rini BI, et al: A pilot trial of CTLA-4 blockade with human anti-CTLA-4 in patients with hormone-refractory prostate cancer. Clin Cancer Res 13:1810, 2007.

62. O'Mahony D, Morris JC, Quinn C, et al: A pilot study of CTLA-4 blockade after cancer vaccine failure in patients with advanced malignancy. Clin Cancer Res 13:958, 2007.

63. United States National Cancer Institute: Study of MDX-010 in stage IV breast cancer. http://clinicaltrials.gov/ct2/show/NCT00083278. Accessed March, 2008.

64. Dannull J, Su Z, Rizzieri D, et al: Enhancement of vaccine-mediated antitumor immunity in cancer patients after depletion of regulatory T cells. J Clin Invest 115:3623, 2005.

65. Knutson KL, Dang Y, Lu H, et al: IL-2 immunotoxin therapy modulates tumor-associated regulatory T cells and leads to lasting immune-mediated rejection of breast cancers in neu-transgenic mice. J Immunol 177:84, 2006.

66. United States National Cancer Institute: Denileukin diftitox in treating patients with advanced breast cancer that did not respond to previous treatment. http://clinicaltrials.gov/ct2/show/NCT00425672. Accessed March, 2008.

67. Ercolini AM, Ladle BH, Manning EA, et al: Recruitment of latent pools of high-avidity CD8(+) T cells to the antitumor immune response. J Exp Med 201:1591, 2005.

68. Emens LA, Armstrong D, Biedrzycki B, et al: A phase I vaccine safety and chemotherapy dose-finding trial of an allogeneic GM-CSF-secreting breast cancer vaccine given in a specifically timed sequence with immunomodulatory doses of cyclophosphamide and doxorubicin. Hum Gene Ther 15:313, 2004.

69. Rosenberg SA, Yang JC, White DE, et al: Durability of complete responses in patients with metastatic cancer treated with high-dose interleukin-2: Identification of the antigens mediating response. Ann Surg 228:307, 1998.

70. Peters WP, Ross M, Vredenburgh JJ, et al: High-dose chemotherapy and autologous bone marrow support as consolidation after standard-dose adjuvant therapy for high-risk primary breast cancer. J Clin Oncol 11:1132, 1993.

71. Isaacs C, Slack R, Gehan E, et al: A multicenter randomized clinical trial evaluating interleukin-2 activated hematopoietic stem cell transplantation and post-transplant IL-2 for high risk breast cancer patients. Breast Cancer Res Treat 93:125, 2005.

72. Georgiannos SN, Renaut A, Goode AW, et al: The immunophenotype and activation status of the lymphocytic infiltrate in human breast cancers, the role of the major histocompatibility complex in cell-mediated immune mechanisms, and their association with prognostic indicators. Surgery 134:827, 2003.

73. Schwartzentruber DJ, Solomon D, Rosenberg SA, et al: Characterization of lymphocytes infiltrating human breast cancer: specific immune reactivity detected by measuring cytokine secretion. J Immunother 12:1, 1992.

74. Bernhard H, Neudorfer J, Gebhard K, et al: Adoptive transfer of autologous, HER2-specific, cytotoxic T lymphocytes for the treatment of HER2-overexpressing breast cancer. Cancer Immunol Immunother 57:271, 2008.

75. United States National Cancer Institute: A phase I study of infusion of HER-2/neu specific t cells in patients with advanced stage HER-2/neu expressing cancers who have received a HER-2/neu vaccine. http://clinicaltrials.gov/ct2/show/NCT00228358. Accessed March 2008.

76. United States National Cancer Institute: Treatment of stage IV breast cancer with OKT3 x Herceptin armed activated T Cells, low dose IL-2, and GM-CSF (phase I/II). http://clinicaltrials.gov/ct2/show/NCT00027807. Accessed March 2008.

77. United States National Cancer Institute: Treatment of stage IIIB or IV breast cancer or other solid tumors with activated T cells, low dose IL-2, and GM-CSF after peripheral blood stem cell transplant (pilot phase II). http://clinicaltrials.gov/ct2/show/NCT00020722. Accessed March 2008.

78. Dudley ME, Wunderlich JR, Robbins PF, et al: Cancer regression and autoimmunity in patients after clonal repopulation with anti-tumor lymphocytes. Science 298:850, 2002.

SECTION IX

Screening and Diagnosis of Breast Disease

Examination Techniques: Roles of the Physician and Patient in Evaluating Breast Disease

MEHRA GOLSHAN

In 2007, the estimated incidence of breast cancer was 178,000 cases of invasive breast cancer and nearly 60,000 cases of ductal carcinoma in situ (DCIS).[1] There are more than 2.4 million breast cancer survivors in the United States. Even more commonly, women present to their physician or surgeon for evaluation of breast findings, and the vast majority of the findings are not breast carcinoma. The goal of early detection and diagnosis has been to improve overall outcome and overall survival. To this end, several strategies exist to help in early detection of breast cancer, including breast self-examination, clinical breast examination, imaging, and biopsy.

Breast Self-Examination

Breast self-examination (BSE) is no longer a recommendation of the American Cancer Society, although the society states that its potential use should be discussed along with risk and benefits for a woman starting in her 20s. The U.S. Preventive Service Task Force (USPSTF) in 2002 decided that the data is insufficient to recommend for or against BSE. Women should be aware of how their breast looks and feels and report changes to their health care provider immediately. The limitations of breast cancer self-screening are based largely on a study of 266,000 female factory workers in Shanghai, China. One group was instructed in BSE, and the control group was given instructions about lower back pain. Neither group had routine conventional breast imaging or clinical examination. In both cohorts, the size of the tumor and mortality for breast cancer was similar, whereas a higher rate of benign breast biopsies was seen in the BSE group.[2] In another study of 27,421 women enrolled in a health plan in the Pacific Northwest, 75%

reported performing BSE, with 27% being reported as having performed an adequate examination. Participants ultimately diagnosed with breast cancer were significantly less likely to report performing BSE. Tumor size and stage were also not association with the performance of BSE.[3]

With this in mind, the discussion should be made about the limitations and potential benefits of BSE. Women who are comfortable with BSE should have a systematic and monthly approach to looking at and examining their own breasts. Instruction may first include a discussion of risk factors for development of breast cancer with a patient, including patient age, family history (both paternal and maternal) for breast and ovarian cancer, menarche, menopause, obesity, alcohol consumption, and hormone replacement. During this discussion, mention should be made of the fact that most early-stage breast cancers do not produce symptoms. The most common sign is a painless mass. The technique of BSE should be reviewed with a health professional. The importance of noticing changes to the contour of the breast and possible development of swelling, dimpling, nipple retraction, skin thickening, and nipple discharge along with identifying a palpable finding should be brought to the attention the health care provider—along with the caveat that most findings will not be cancer. In the premenopausal setting, a lump that develops may be normal and appear and disappear with the menstrual cycle. A lump that persists past one or two cycles should be brought to the attention of a health care provider. A lump that persists for more than a few weeks in the postmenopausal setting should also be brought to a care provider's attention.

The actual technique of BSE varies but should include the woman looking at herself in a full-length mirror, with her arms to her side, then over her head, and then to her side with flexion against the side to look for symmetry, dimpling, and retraction (Fig. 35-1). It should be noted that most women have a slight asymmetry in breast size, and this should be considered normal. A progressive change in size, whether an increase or decrease, in one breast should be brought to the attention of the health care provider. A BSE should also be performed lying down with the arm over the head to allow the breast tissue to splay out evenly over the chest The examination should be taught with using two or three fingers using a circular approach of light, moderate, and deep pressure going over the entire breast from the clavicle to the inframammary fold, laterally to the latissimus, medially to the sternum, and also including the low axilla. The entire breast should be examined either in a spoke-wheel fashion or vertical/horizontal blind or circular method, covering the entire surface area (Fig. 35-2). The timing of the BSE should be monthly, usually 1 week after menses in the premenopausal woman and on a set day of the month in the postmenopausal setting.

Clinical Breast Examination

The role of clinical breast examination has a stronger foundation in the early detection of breast carcinoma. The American Cancer Society recommends that a woman in her 20s or 30s with average risk for breast cancer should receive a clinical breast examination as part of her regular health examination at least every 3 years. Once a woman turns 40 the recommendation is yearly, along with a yearly mammogram; preferably the clinical examination should take place shortly before the noninvasive screening. The USPSTF in 2002 concluded that evidence was inconclusive for or against clinical breast examination to be performed alone without mammography; however, there was benefit when it was performed in conjunction with breast imaging.

The technique of breast examination should include a thorough inspection and palpation of the entire breast and the draining lymph node–bearing areas. The physician should stand in front of the gowned patient. In a manner that allows for minimal disrobement of the

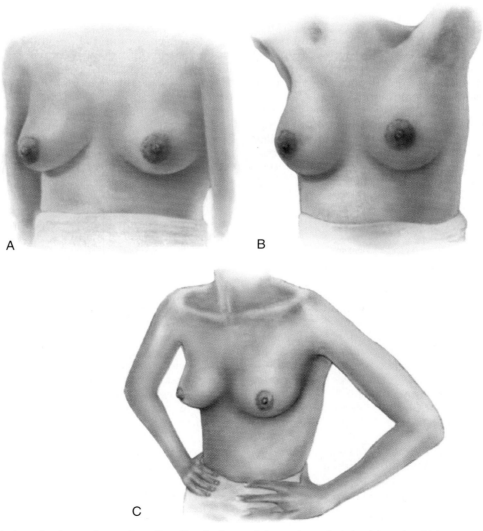

Figure 35-1 Technique for breast inspection. Standing in front of the patient, the physician should inspect the patient with the patient's arms at the sides (**A**), arms straight up in the air (**B**), and hands on hips (**C**).

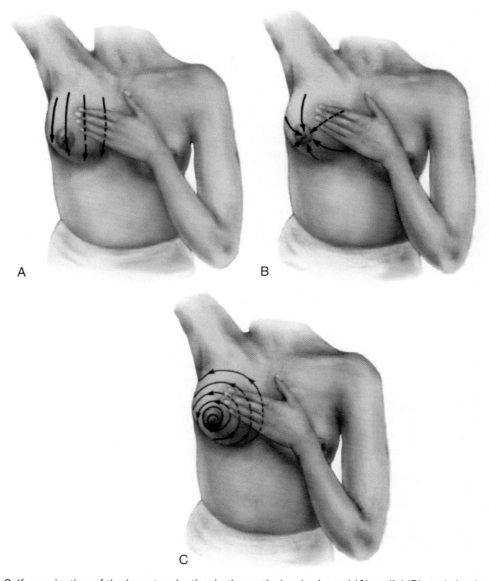

Figure 35-2 Self-examination of the breast; palpation in the vertical or horizontal (**A**), radial (**B**), and circular directions (**C**).

patient, both breasts should be inspected with the patient's arms by her side, with her hands over her head, and followed by the arms to her side with contraction of the pectoralis major muscle. Notes should be taken with regard to size, shape, and symmetry of the breasts. Attention should be made to any changes to the skin, including indentation, protrusions, or skin thickening. The nipple should be inspected for retraction or erosions. Palpation of the breast should be done both in the sitting and supine position. The entire breast should be examined from the clavicle to the rectus sheath insertion, medially to the sternum, and laterally to the latissimus. The palpation may again be in the spoke/wheel, vertical/horizontal blind, or circular fashion with the pads of the fingers using three degrees of pressure: light, moderate, and deep. The nipple and areola should be manipulated to identify nipple discharge. Fluid that is brown or black may undergo guaiac testing, looking for breakdown products of hemoglobin. Bloody nipple discharge also should be noted, with a description of the location of the offending duct. A detailed written description, which may also include a diagram or photograph, may be useful for objective reporting in the patient's progress notes. Special attention should be made to the lymph nodes in the sitting position. With one arm supporting the woman's hand, the other hand examines the axilla. The supraclavicular and infraclavicular lymph nodes are best examined from behind with the woman in a seated position. Lymph nodes that measure greater than 1 cm in diameter or that are fixed or matted should be noted.

If a mass is found, a tape measure or caliper is used to estimate its size in two dimensions. The location should be either drawn on a diagram or referenced to a clock time and measured in centimeters from the nipple in a radial fashion. For a woman who presents with a palpable lump, the detailed history should include length of time present, whether pain is associated with the mass, whether the lump changed in size since identification, and in a premenopausal woman, whether the mass changes after the menses.

Nipple discharge that is spontaneous or the result of mild manual compression should be noted. Whether the discharge is unilateral and from a single duct or multiple ducts and whether it is bilateral should be noted. The color of the discharge should also be noted, and the Hemoccult test should be performed at the time of examination. Discharge that is bilateral, multiductal, and milky, clear, or green or bluish in color is almost always benign. As many as 50% to 80% of women in their reproductive years may elicit discharge, and 7% of women referred for surgical evaluation have nipple discharge as their primary complaint.[4,5] Discharge that is unilateral and bloody or guaiac-positive has a risk of malignancy of approximately 20% to 25%; however, the vast majority is caused by benign entities such as papillomas.

At the time of clinical breast examination, risk factors for breast cancer should be reviewed with the patient, including history of breast and ovarian cancer on the maternal and paternal sides. It is estimated that 5% to 10% of carcinomas diagnosed in the United States result from an inherited predisposition to breast and ovarian cancer, the vast majority being BRCA1 and BRCA2 mutations.[6] Age of menarche, menopause, and parity should be determined.[7] The use of exogenous estrogen and/or progesterone in the premenopausal setting, and more importantly, the postmenopausal setting should be ascertained.[8] Previous personal history of carcinoma and breast biopsy should be detailed, if possible, to determine whether the previous biopsy specimen contained atypia.[9] Age is the most important risk factor for breast carcinoma; currently, a women living in the United States has a 12.3% chance of developing breast carcinoma.[10] A women's body habitus is also important; specifically, postmenopausal obesity has been linked to increasing risk of breast cancer.[11] With the widespread obesity in the United States, strategies to lower weight should be discussed with the patient. Intensive physical activity has been linked to decreased risk of developing breast carcinoma.[12] Along with obesity, excessive or more than moderate alcohol consumption also increases the risk of development of breast carcinoma. All these issues should be discussed with a patient at the time of clinical breast examination for a palpable complaint.[13] Once a palpable complaint has been examined or at the time of a women's clinical breast examination, non-invasive testing can be initiated. In the screening or surveillance setting, mammography is recommended as a baseline between the 35 and 40 years of age and yearly thereafter as long as the woman is healthy. Screening imaging may include breast magnetic resonance imaging (MRI) in the high-risk setting.

Imaging Modalities

Mammography has been shown in numerous randomized and population-based studies to help in early detection of carcinoma, patient outcome, and survival.[14]

Despite these trials, there have been some who suggest otherwise based on a meta-analysis of a few of the trials.[15] A more comprehensive meta-analysis and the vast majority of the major organizations who comment on cancer screening and detection agree that regular screening mammography should be a part of women's routine health care.[16] In general, mammography should be performed at the same center where films can be serially compared for changes. Expertise in breast imaging is important. A screening mammogram can detect more than 80% of all breast carcinomas in women without symptoms. Imaging is more accurate in the postmenopausal setting, although, with the use of digital mammography, there has been improvement in the younger woman with dense breasts.[17] Although widespread screening mammography has been in place in the United States for several decades now, a recent review from 2004 revealed that only 58% of women older than 40 years of age had a mammogram within the past year.[18] To allay the fears of a woman, it should be noted that the dose of radiation is low and the variability of equipment and imaging interpretation has decreased. In the diagnostic setting, it is paramount for the ordering physician to provide the radiologist or breast imaging center with all appropriate information on the location and size of the mass or abnormality.

Ultrasound should be used in the diagnostic setting or to work up an abnormality during the screening process. The widespread implementation of whole breast ultrasound screening in the United States has not been successful because of the large amount of time needed to perform the test and operator variability in expertise of the technique. A large American College of Radiology Trial (ACRIN 6666) is reviewing the addition of whole breast ultrasound in the high-risk screening setting.[19] Focused ultrasound is a valuable tool for the workup of a palpable complaint or mass identified by mammography. Ultrasound is particularly useful in the premenopausal setting of dense breasts, in evaluating for an underlying abnormality. Increasingly, surgeons are becoming more adept at the use of the technique in the office as an adjunct to physical examination, and care must be taken in terms of training, qualification, and interpretation before a surgeon implements this in his or her practice. In this respect, the American Society of Breast Surgeons and the American College of Surgeons have taken a leading role in the establishment of guidelines and standards in the use of ultrasound by the surgeon.

Contrast-enhanced breast MRI is a highly sensitive test with moderate specificity. In the screening population, its use can be justified in the high-risk setting as an adjunct but not a substitute to mammography. Women who have an inherited predisposition to breast and ovarian cancer, Li-Fraumeni syndrome, Cowden syndrome, lifetime risk of breast cancer of 20% to 25%, history of mantle radiation, or a first-degree relative with an inherited predisposition to breast carcinoma without self-testing are likely to benefit from the addition of breast MRI.[20] In the woman at moderate risk for breast carcinoma based on family history, atypical ductal hyperplasia, atypical lobular hyperplasia, lobular carcinoma in situ, or a lifetime risk of breast cancer of

15% to 20%, the risks and benefits of breast MRI should be discussed before recommending this as a screening tool. Of note should be the possibility of findings on MRI that will lead to additional imaging, the majority of which will be biopsy-proven benign.[21] Breast MRI should be performed by dedicated breast imagers using at least a 1.5-Tesla magnet, preferably with a dedicated breast coil and breast biopsy capability. Breast MRI in the diagnosed cancer patient may present unique possibilities of aid in the workup of a known cancer; there may also be additional benign biopsies, additional imaging, and unknown clinical benefit in terms of outcome and survival.[22] In fact, in a recent review from the University of Pennsylvania, the use of breast MRI at the time of initial diagnosis did not improve outcome in cases of breast-conserving therapy.[22]

Other techniques of breast imaging in the evaluation of breast diseases are under study, with limited benefit to date. Some groups have used scintimammography, the use of a breast-specific gamma camera to measure radiotracer uptake of abnormal breast tissue by using technetium sestamibi, with some success as an adjunct to mammography.[23] However, its widespread use has yet to be validated by prospective randomized trials or widespread availability. Breast tomosynthesis, the acquisition of three-dimensional digital image data, has also been explored in small numbers with promising results, although this has not received approval from the U.S. Food and Drug Administration.[24] Positron emission tomography with or without computed tomography is being studied but has not been shown to be of benefit in the screening or early detection of breast carcinoma.[25]

Invasive Diagnostic Procedures

Once an abnormality has been identified either by imaging or physical examination, the technique known as image-guided biopsy, freehand core biopsy, or fine needle aspiration biopsy (FNAB) has become the standard of care. The use of surgical open or wire-localized excisional or incisional biopsy should be used as a last resort when FNAB or core biopsy has failed. Surgical biopsy can also be considered for the uncommon imaging finding not amenable to image-guided biopsy either too close to the nipple, skin, or chest wall. FNAB requires dedicated and expertise in cytopathology and when applicable provides high degree of sensitivity and specificity.[26] In the cases of breast carcinoma cell blocks may be performed to characterize estrogen receptor (ER), progesterone receptor (PR), and HER2/neu receptor status. The technique of FNAB is also particularly useful in axillary lymph node evaluation under ultrasound guidance, when the diagnosis of breast carcinoma is made to rule out metastatic involvement.[27] More frequently, needle core biopsy is performed and its diagnostic accuracy and concordance with surgical excision is outstanding; this can be performed under stereotactic, ultrasound, or MRI guidance. The concordance with surgical excisional biopsy specimen is high, between 91% and 100%; sensitivity is 85% to 100%, and specificity is 96% to 100%.[28] In the modern era with larger biopsy

devices and the use of vacuum-assisted and en bloc resection devices, the concordance rates will only improve and in certain circumstances obviate the need for surgical resection. Another advantage is the decreased number of surgical procedures required for definitive therapy when a diagnosis of breast carcinoma is made. A study at the Brigham and Women's Hospital showed that women who underwent image-guided core biopsy had 1.25 surgical procedures as opposed to 2.01 in those who underwent wire-localized excisional biopsy for diagnosis.[29] Caveats to the core biopsy under image guidance include its occasional inability to target or adequately sample the lesion. More importantly, some image-guided diagnoses will be upstaged at the time of surgical excision, specifically atypical hyperplasia to ductal carcinoma in situ or ductal carcinoma in situ to invasive breast cancer.[30,31] Also, when a benign result is obtained, concordance to imaging or examination finding should be made. In cases of radiologic-pathologic discordance excision is mandatory. For example, a mass felt on examination or seen on breast imaging revealing epithelial hyperplasia is not concordant and requires surgical excision. Some surgical groups may also perform freehand core biopsy with a high rate of accuracy, whereas others find that image-guided core biopsy yields a higher rate of accuracy.[32,33]

Surgical excisional biopsy, either under image guidance or palpation guidance, should be performed as a diagnostic procedure only on rare occasions. Examples include (1) patient preference for surgical excision no matter the imaging finding or core biopsy finding, or (2) failed, nondiagnostic, or discordant core biopsy or FNAB. The surgical biopsy is a safe surgical procedure with outstanding results; however, it does leave a scar on the woman's breast, and if the results prove to be carcinoma, further surgery is necessary. With an easily palpable finding, surgical excisional biopsy without image guidance may proceed under local or regional anesthesia. Surgical incision planning is important for cosmetic purposes and the possibility of reoperation or eventual mastectomy if a carcinoma is identified. In general, circumareolar incisions provide outstanding cosmesis when excessive tunneling is not necessary, and curvilinear incisions along Langer's lines also provide reasonable cosmesis in most cases. In general, radial incisions should be avoided but may be considered for lesions at the 6 o'clock position and occasionally for 3 and 9 o'clock abnormalities. For lesions that are not easily palpable, wire localization either under mammographic, ultrasound, or MRI guidance is necessary. Initially described by Bolmgrem in 1977, stereotaxic or mammographic guidance has become a standard of care with high accuracy.[34,35] Ultrasound guidance provides another opportunity for wire placement and is often a simpler technique that can be performed quickly especially for a mass lesion.[36] With the advent of contrast-enhanced breast MRI for screening and diagnostic evaluation, abnormalities are identified that may not be correlated by mammography and ultrasound. It is imperative that a center that offers this test has the capability to perform biopsies under either wire guidance and/or needle core.[21,37]

Any nipple discharge, whether bloody or guaiac-positive, requires surgical evaluation and intervention in nearly all cases. The evaluation of the breast should include physical examination and mammography. Ultrasound evaluation of the retroareolar ductal system may also be helpful. The use of ductogram in centers with expertise with the diagnostic test is also helpful; specifically, lesions may be identified that can be preoperatively marked by methylene blue injection or wire guidance to help identify the abnormality and limit the extent of resection of the terminal ductal unit.[38] Other groups have found contrast-enhanced breast MRI to be more helpful in identifying underlying lesions in patients with suspicious nipple discharge.[39] More complex and expensive modalities include ductoscopy, where a fiberoptic camera (diameters ranging from 0.4 to 0.8 mm) is inserted into the offending duct either in the operating room or outpatient setting and abnormalities may be identified that can either be biopsied or resected. However, studies currently do not support its routine use, and its benefits over other more readily available and conventional techniques have yet to be proven.[40,41]

Over the past decades, extensive progress has been made in the modalities available for the evaluation of breast disease and early detection of breast carcinoma. These changes have vastly improved patient outcome and survival.

REFERENCES

1. Jemal A, Siegel R, Ward E, et al: Cancer statistics, 2007. CA Cancer J Clin 57:43–46, 2007.
2. Thomas DB, Gao DL, Ray RM, et al: Randomized trial of breast self-examination in Shanghai: Final results. J Nat Cancer Inst 94:1445–1457, 2002.
3. Tu SP, Reisch LM, Taplin SH, et al: Breast self examination: Self-reported frequency, quality, and associated outcomes. J Cancer Educ 21:175–181, 2006.
4. Isaacs JH: Other nipple discharge. Clin Obstet Gynecol 37:898–902, 1994.
5. Santen RJ, Mansel R: Benign breast disorders. N Engl J Med 353:275–285, 2005.
6. Nusbaum R, Vogel KJ, Ready K: Susceptibility of breast cancer: Hereditary syndromes and low penetrance genes. Breast Dis 27:21–50, 2006–2007.
7. Clavel-Chapelon L, Gerber M: Reproductive factors and breast cancer risk. Do they differ according to age at diagnosis? Breast Cancer Res Treat 72:107–115, 2002.
8. Chlebowski RT, Hendrix SL, Langer RD, et al: Influence of estrogen plus progestin on breast cancer and mammography in healthy postmenopausal women: The Women's Health Initiative Randomized Trial. JAMA 289:3242–3253, 2003.
9. Degnim AC, Visscher DW, Berman HK, et al: Stratification of breast cancer risk in women with atypia: A Mayo cohort study. J Clin Oncol 25:2671–2677, 2007.
10. Osteen R: Breast cancer. In Lenhard RE, Osteen RT, Gansler T (eds): Clinical oncology. Atlanta GA, American Cancer Society, 2001, 251–268.
11. Reeves GK, Pirie K, Beral V, et al: Cancer incidence and mortality in relation to body mass index in the Million Women Study: Cohort study. BMJ 335:1134, 2007.
12. Dallal CM, Sullivan-Halley J, Ross RK, et al: Long-term recreational physical activity and risk of invasive and in situ breast cancer: The California teachers study. Arch Intern Med 167:408–415, 2007.
13. Key J, Hodgson S, Omar RZ, et al: Meta-analysis of studies of alcohol and breast cancer with consideration of the methodological issues. Cancer Causes Control 17:759–777, 2006.
14. Smith RA, Duffy SW, Gabe R, et al: The randomized trials of breast cancer screening: What have we learned? Radiol Clin North Am 42:793–806, 2004.
15. Olsen O, Gotzsche PC: Screening for breast cancer with mammography. Cochrane Database Syst Rev 4:CD001877, 2001.
16. Humphrey LL, Helfand M, Chan BK, Woolf SH: Breast cancer screening: A summary of the evidence for the U.S. Preventive Services Task Force. Arch Intern Med 137:347–360, 2002.
17. Pisano ED, Hendrick RE, Yaffe MJ, et al: Diagnostic accuracy of digital versus film mammography: Exploratory analysis of selected population subgroups in DMIST. Radiology 246:376–383, 2008.
18. Behavioral Risk Factor Surveillance System Public Use Data 2004, National Center for Chronic Disease Prevention and Health Promotion, Centers for Disease Control and Prevention, 2005.
19. Berg WA: Rationale for a trial of screening breast ultrasound: American College of Radiology Imaging Network (ACRIN) 6666. AJR Am J Roentgenol 180:1225–1228, 2003.
20. Saslow D, Boetes C, Burke W, et al: American Cancer Society guidelines for breast screening with MRI as an adjunct to mammography. CA Cancer Clin J 57:75–89, 2007.
21. Javid SH, Carlson JW, Garber JE, et al: Breast MRI wire-guided excisional biopsy: Specimen size as compared to mammogram wire-guided excisional biopsy and implications for use. Ann Surg Oncol 14:3352–3358, 2007.
22. Solin LJ, Orel SG, Hwang WT, et al: Relationship of breast magnetic resonance imaging to outcome after breast-conservation treatment with radiation for women with early-stage invasive breast carcinoma or ductal carcinoma in situ. J Clin Oncol 26:386–391, 2008.
23. Brem RF, Michener KH, Zawistowski G: Approaches to improving breast cancer diagnosis using a high resolution, breast specific gamma camera. Phys Med 21:17–1, 2006.
24. Park JM, Franken EA, Garg M, et al: Breast tomosynthesis: Present considerations and future applications. Radiographics 27:S231–S240, 2007.
25. Rosen EL, Eubank WB, Mankoff DA: FDG PET, PET/CT, and breast cancer imaging. Radiographics 27:S215–S229, 2007.
26. Choi YD, Choi YH, Lee JH, et al: Analysis of fine needle aspiration cytology of the breast: A review of 1,297 cases and correlation with histologic diagnoses. Acta Cytol 2004;48:801–806.
27. Koelikker SL, Chung MA, Mainero MB, et al: Axillary lymph nodes: US-guided fine-needle aspiration for initial staging of breast cancer—correlation with primary tumor size. Radiology 246:81–89, 2008.
28. Rakha EA, Ellis IO: An overview of assessment of prognostic and predictive factors in breast cancer needle core biopsy specimens. J Clin Pathol 60:1300–1306, 2007.
29. Smith DN, Christian R, Meyer JE: Large-core needle biopsy of nonpalpable breast cancers. The impact on subsequent surgical excisions. Arch Surg 132:256–259, 1997.
30. Darling ML, Smith DN, Lester SC, et al: Atypical ductal hyperplasia and ductal carcinoma in situ as revealed by large-core needle breast biopsy: Results of surgical excision. AJR Am J Roentgenol 175:1341–1346, 2001.
31. Houssami N, Ciatto S, Ellis I, Ambrogetti D: Underestimation of malignancy of breast core-needle biopsy: Concepts and precise overall and category-specific estimates. Cancer 109:487–495, 2007.
32. Agarwal T, Patel B, Rajan P, et al: Core biopsy versus FNAC for palpable breast cancers. Is image guidance necessary? Eur J Cancer 39:52–56, 2003.
33. Shah VI, Raju U, Chitale D, et al: False-negative core needle biopsies of the breast: An analysis of clinical, radiologic, and pathologic findings in 27 consecutive cases of missed breast cancer. Cancer 97:1824–1831, 2003.
34. Bolmgren J, Jacobson B, Nordenstrom R: Stereotaxic instrument for needle biopsy of the mammary. Am J Roentgenol 129:121–125, 1977.
35. Gent HJ, Sprenger E, Dowlatshahi K: Stereotaxic needle localization and cytological diagnosis of occult breast lesions. Ann Surg 204:580–584, 1986.
36. Rissanen TJ, Makarainen HP, Kiviniemi HO, Suramo II: Ultrasonographically guided wire localization of nonpalpable breast lesions. J Ultrasound Med 13:183–188, 1994.
37. Liberman L, Mason G, Morris EA, Dershaw DD: Does size matter? Positive predictive value of MRI-detected breast lesions as a function of lesion size. AJR Am J Roentgenol 186:426–430, 2006.

38. Cabioglu N, Hunt KK, Singletary SE, et al: Surgical decision making and factors determining a diagnosis of breast carcinoma in women presenting with nipple discharge. J Am Coll Surg 196:354–364, 2003.

39. Morrogh M, Morris EA, Liberman L, et al: The predictive value of ductography and magnetic resonance imaging in the management of nipple discharge. Ann Surg Oncol 14:3369–3377, 2007.

40. Grunwald S, Heyer H, Paepke S, et al: Diagnostic value of ductoscopy in the diagnosis of nipple discharge and intraductal proliferations in comparison to standard methods. Onkologie 30:243–248, 2007.

41. Sauter E: Breast cancer detection using mammary ductoscopy. Future Oncol 1:385–393, 2005.

chapter 36

Breast Imaging

LAWRENCE W. BASSETT | **JANE W. LEE** |
CHRISTOPHER P. HSU

Breast imaging includes all of the diagnostic imaging methods used to detect and diagnose diseases of the breast. The most commonly used breast imaging procedure is mammography, defined as an x-ray examination of the breasts. Since the first report on mammography in the United States in the 1930s, mammography has undergone striking technologic improvements that have improved its sensitivity and accuracy.[1] Quality assurance procedures have also improved mammography in the United States.[2] In addition, standardized reporting has been developed to improve the communication of the results of mammography and appropriate management recommendations.[3]

The two major types of mammography are screening mammography and diagnostic mammography. *Screening mammography* is used to detect unexpected breast cancer in asymptomatic women. *Diagnostic mammography* is used to evaluate the breasts of patients with symptoms, such as a lump or nipple discharge. Mammography is also used to guide interventional procedures of the breast, including preoperative needle localization, needle aspiration, core needle biopsy (CNB), and ductography.[4-8]

Breast ultrasonography, the use of sonic energy to produce an image of the breast, is the next most commonly used modality for diagnostic imaging of the breast. In the past, the use of ultrasonography has primarily been restricted to differentiating benign from solid masses.[9] However, ultrasonography is increasingly being used to guide fine-needle aspiration, CNB, and preoperative needle localization of suspicious-looking solid masses.[4,10] In addition, high-resolution ultrasonography has been useful in the differentiation of benign and malignant solid masses.[11]

Digital mammography is a modern modality gaining increasing popularity for its usefulness in detecting and diagnosing breast diseases. In contrast to conventional screen-film mammography, digital mammography is an electronic method of recording breast images on computers instead of hard copy films. The main advantage of digital mammography is unlimited contrast resolution. This is of particular benefit in women with radiographically dense breasts, women younger than 50 years of age, and premenopausal or perimenopausal women.[12] Currently, digital mammography is being used for screening mammograms, diagnostic workups, and image-guided interventional procedures.

Magnetic resonance imaging (MRI) has also rapidly progressed over the past several years and has now become a valuable tool in evaluating benign and malignant breast lesions. Because MRI uses variable pulse sequences with postprocessing capabilities, it can provide three-dimensional evaluation of the extent of breast lesions, including multifocality, multicentricity, and bilaterality of breast carcinoma.[13] Ultimately, the goal is to provide further assistance in both staging and treatment options.

Other modalities used in the diagnosis of breast diseases include ductography and radionuclide imaging. Diagnostic imaging also has a role in identifying or documenting metastases to other organs in appropriate patients with breast cancer.[14]

Mammography

SCREENING MAMMOGRAPHY: GUIDELINES AND CONTROVERSIES

Breast cancer is the most common noncutaneous malignancy in women, and in recent years, has accounted for 30% of new cancer cases in American women.[15] Each year, approximately 185,000 new cases of breast cancer are diagnosed and about 45,000 women die of this disease.[16] The risk of developing breast cancer increases with age, with women older than 40 years of age being at greatest risk. Although multiple risk factors have been identified, three fourths of women who develop the disease have no special risk factors other than increasing age.[17] The benefit of screening mammography for women older than 50 years of age is universally accepted.[18,19] Breast cancer death rates from 1989 to 1998 have fallen in every age and racial group of women, and this is largely attributable to mammographic screening.[20]

In randomized controlled trials, noncompliance in the study group, and contamination in the control group are necessary tradeoffs to avoid self-selection and length-bias sampling. However, this results in dilution of the data and an underestimation of the real benefit of screening.

Recently, it has been proposed that reductions in breast cancer mortality after the introduction of screening are primarily related to improvements in therapeutic modalities.[21,22] It has been suggested that only one third of the recent reduction in breast cancer mortality in the United Kingdom is a result of screening mammography, with the balance attributable to advances in therapy.[23] However, in a 2002 Swedish screening trial, Tabár and colleagues compared breast cancer mortality rates in counties with screening versus counties without screening. This eliminated the effects of advances in therapy. They found a 30% reduction in breast cancer mortality in counties that offered screening versus counties without screening. When they compared women who actually underwent breast cancer screening with those who underwent mammography, the mortality reduction was 45%.[19] Therefore, screening mammography has the potential to reduce breast cancer mortality by at least 45% and perhaps even more.

SCREENING FOR WOMEN 40 TO 49 YEARS OF AGE

Since 1993, multiple meta-analyses of the eight randomized controlled trials have been performed, each demonstrating further effectiveness of screening mammography for women 40 to 49 years of age. Excluding data from National Breast Screening Study-1, Smart and coworkers[24] in 1995 demonstrated a statistically significant 23% breast cancer mortality reduction for women 40 to 49 years of age.

In 1996, results of a nonrandomized, population-based study in Uppsala, Sweden, supported the screening of women younger than 50 years.[25] Although actual mortality rate reduction data were not used, this program found 7-year survival rates of 92% and 87% for cancers detected both at screening and between screening in women younger than 50 years of age and those older than 50 years of age, respectively. This can be compared with the 7-year survival rate of 70% for patients with breast cancer in the general Swedish population.

PERFORMING THE EXAMINATION

To have the greatest possible impact, screening mammography must be widely used. Therefore, screening should be performed as efficiently as possible and at the lowest possible cost. For example, it has been recommended that mammography screening be done in high volume settings where the radiologic technologist performs as many examinations as can be done properly each day and the interpreting physician batch-reads the films later in the day.[26,27] The U.S. General Accounting Office has studied costs and quality in mammography and concluded that high-volume performance sites are more likely to provide higher quality examinations at lower cost.[28]

For screening mammography, two views of the breast are performed: the mediolateral oblique (MLO) and the craniocaudal (CC). The MLO is the most effective single view, because it includes the greatest amount of breast tissue and is the only whole-breast view to include all of the upper-outer quadrant and axillary tail (Figs. 36-1 and 36-2).[29] Compared with the MLO, the CC view provides better visualization of the medial aspect of the

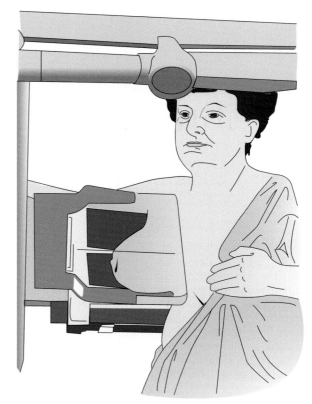

Figure 36-1   Positioning of a woman for mediolateral oblique view.

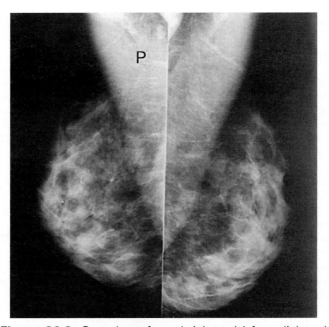

Figure 36-2   Properly performed right and left mediolateral oblique mammograms. Note the large amount of pectoral muscle (P) shown, which ensures that a large amount of the breast tissue and axilla are included in the image. The breasts should be viewed back-to-back as shown here to identify asymmetries in fibroglandular tissue distribution.

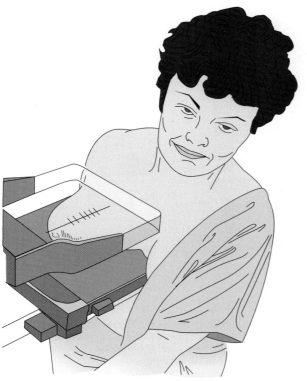

Figure 36-3 Positioning of woman for craniocaudal view.

breast and better image detail, because greater compression of the breast is usually possible (Figs. 36-3 and 36-4).[30]

The importance of proper breast compression during mammography cannot be overemphasized. The compression device (1) holds the breast still and thereby prevents motion unsharpness, (2) brings objects closer to

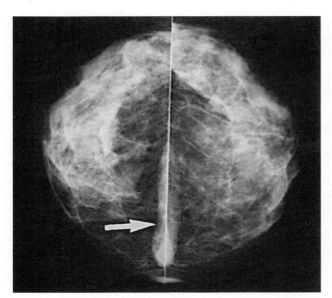

Figure 36-4 Properly performed right and left craniocaudal mammograms. When placed on the viewbox, the lateral aspect of the breasts is placed at the top, and the breasts are viewed back-to-back as shown here. Note pectoral muscle *(arrow)* visualized near the chest wall at the medial aspects of the breasts.

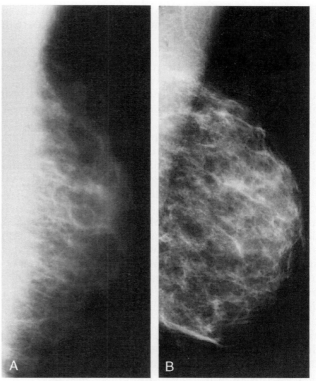

Figure 36-5 Importance of compression is shown in these inadequately compressed (**A**) and properly compressed (**B**) films of the same breast. Compression prevents blurring by holding structures still and bringing them closer to the film, and it evens out the thickness of the breast so that details can be seen in both the thicker tissues near the chest wall and the thinner superficial tissues.

the film and reduces blur, (3) separates overlapping tissues that might obscure underlying lesions, and (4) decreases the radiation dose of mammography by making the breast less thick (Fig. 36-5). Although breast compression may be uncomfortable, if properly performed, it is rarely painful.[31] Few women avoid mammograms because of the discomfort of compression.[32]

DIAGNOSTIC MAMMOGRAPHY

Diagnostic mammography, also called *consultative* or *problem-solving mammography,* is indicated when there are clinical findings such as a palpable lump or abnormal results on a screening examination that require additional imaging. The diagnostic examination is usually tailored to the clinical findings of the individual patient or a specific screening abnormality.[26] The interpreting physician directly supervises the performance of diagnostic mammography.

Performing the Examination

If the standard MLO and CC views have not been performed as part of a recent screening examination, the diagnostic examination should also begin with these two views. If there is a palpable mass, the presence and location of the mass should be communicated to the mammography facility by the referring health care provider at the time the examination is scheduled.

The mammography facility usually confirms the clinical findings with the patient at the time of the patient's examination.

The radiologic technologist or the interpreting physician palpates the mass and places a radiopaque BB (lead marker) directly over it before the mammograms are performed. The palpation of a reported lump by the radiologic technologist or interpreting physician is termed a *correlative breast examination*, which should not be considered a substitute for a complete clinical breast examination by the patient's referring health care provider. On the mammograms, the BB will indicate the exact location of any palpable findings (Fig. 36-6).

In addition to the MLO and CC views, the diagnostic examination may include a variety of additional mammographic views that are intended to better localize or define the nature of abnormalities.[33-37] The most commonly used additional views are the 90-degree lateral and spot compression views. The 90-degree lateral is used along with the CC view to triangulate the exact location of an abnormality. Spot compression can be done in any projection. It involves the use of a small compression device placed directly over an abnormal area (Figs. 36-7 and 36-8). The smaller compression device allows for greater compression over the area of interest and displaces overlying tissues that could obscure the lesion. Magnification technique is often combined with spot compression to better resolve the margins of masses and calcifications. Other additional

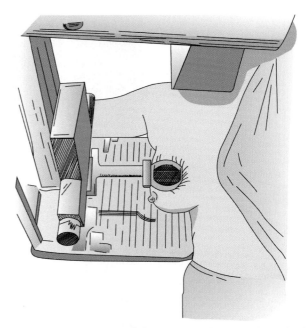

Figure 36-7 Positioning of the breast for spot compression views. The small spot compression device achieves greater compression over a localized area of interest and displaces adjacent breast tissue away from the area.

projections include rolled, cleavage, and axillary tail views. Ultrasonography is also commonly used during diagnostic examinations.

Mammography before Biopsy of a Suspicious Palpable Mass

For women older than 30 years of age, diagnostic mammography should be performed even when a biopsy is planned for a palpable breast lump. The purpose of mammography prior to the scheduled biopsy is to (1) better define the nature of the palpable abnormality, (2) detect unexpected lesions in the ipsilateral or contralateral breast, and (3) identify an extensive intraductal component of a palpable invasive carcinoma (Fig. 36-9).

DIGITAL MAMMOGRAPHY

Digital mammography is a type of mammography that records the radiographic image electronically in a digital format rather than directly onto film. The image is kept in a digital format in a computer and can be either displayed on a florescent monitor or transferred to a hard copy (film). It is hoped that digital mammography will eventually solve many of the problems inherent in film mammography, such as limited contrast, film storage, and lost films.[38]

Potential advantages of digital studies are unlimited contrast resolution, computer-aided diagnosis, and teleradiology (the ability to rapidly transmit the images over long distances).[39] Computer-aided diagnosis refers to the use of a computer to assist in interpretation by scanning images for abnormalities or using artificial

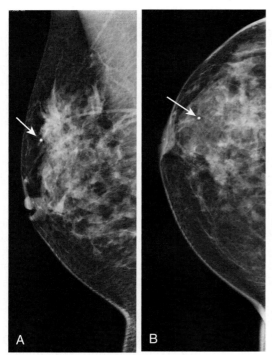

Figure 36-6 Mammograms of a 37-year-old woman with a palpable mass. **A**, Mediolateral oblique view. Radiopaque lead "BB" *(arrow)* was placed directly over the palpable mass just before the mammograms were performed. **B**, Close-up of craniocaudal view shows a subtle architectural distortion *(arrow)* posterior to the BB.

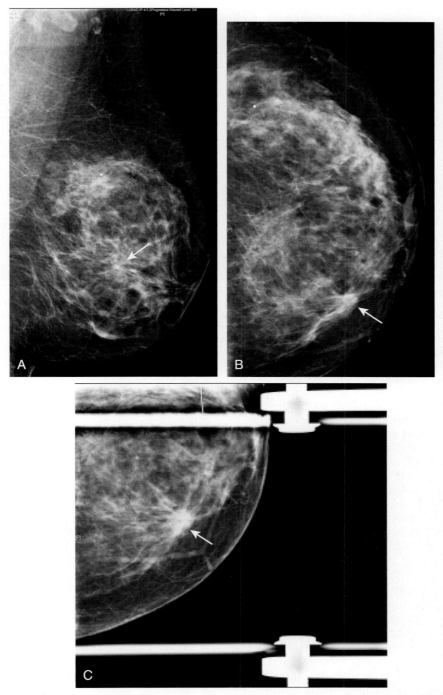

Figure 36-8 Left carcinoma in a woman. Left mediolateral oblique view (**A**) and left craniocaudal view (**B**) show a suspicious architectural distortion in the left breast (*arrows*). **C**, Spot compression magnification view reveals that the left breast mass has an irregular shape (*arrow*) with spiculations associated with architectural distortion.

intelligence to determine the probability of malignancy.[40–42] The ability of teleradiography to send digital images over long distances opens the possibilities for greater access to previous studies and consultations with experts.[43]

Although conventional screen-film mammography is still more commonly used, digital mammography has gained increasing popularity. Approximately 20% of mammography units are digital.

STANDARDIZED TERMINOLOGY FOR MAMMOGRAPHIC REPORTS

The American College of Radiology Breast Imaging Reporting and Data System (BI-RADS) was devised to standardize mammographic terminology, reduce confusing interpretations, and facilitate outcome monitoring.[3,44] BI-RADS uses a standardized lexicon to facilitate the uniformity of mammography reports from different radiology facilities.

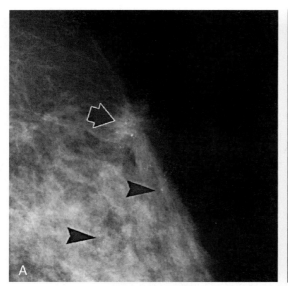
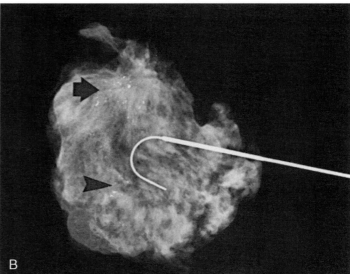

Figure 36-9 Invasive cancer with extensive intraductal carcinoma component in a woman with a palpable mass. **A,** Close-up of upper breast revealed a spiculated mass *(arrow)* at the site of the palpable mass. The mass contained multiple calcifications of varying size and shape. Additional clusters of calcifications *(arrowheads)* were identified extending into the tissue adjacent to the mass. **B,** Specimen radiograph verifies excision of the spiculated mass *(arrow)* and several clusters of calcifications *(arrowhead)* outside of the mass. Pathologic examination revealed invasive ductal carcinoma with extensive intraductal component.

The standardized mammography report also includes an overall assessment of the probability of malignancy that is incorporated in an impression at the end of every mammography report. The inclusion of a Final Assessment is required by the federal Mammography Quality Standards Act (MQSA). There are six assessment categories, each associated with a management recommendation. Only BI-RADS categories 1, 2, and 0 should be used for screening mammograms. BI-RADS category "0"—"Incomplete Assessment" identifies cases in which additional imaging is needed before a final assessment can be made. Once the additional imaging is accomplished, the case is assigned one of the six "Final Assessment" categories (Table 36-1). The inclusion of the Final Assessment in the "Impression" of every mammography report eliminates equivocation by the interpreter or misunderstanding by the referring health care provider as to the significance of the findings and the management recommendation. The Final Assessment also facilitates the follow-up and tracking of patients, because each Final Assessment category is associated with one specific follow-up recommendation. The most recent edition of BI-RADS (2003) now includes mammography, breast ultrasound, and breast MRI.[45]

NORMAL MAMMOGRAPHIC FINDINGS

There is a wide range of appearances of the normal breast on mammography with regard to size, shape, and breast tissue composition. Breast tissue composition can range from almost all fat to extremely dense fibroglandular tissue, and this composition directly relates to the sensitivity of mammography. Because breast cancers are radiodense, radiolucent fat (dark gray to black on mammograms) provides an excellent background on which to detect small cancers, but dense fibroglandular tissue (white on mammograms) can obscure breast cancers.

In the BI-RADS system, the breast tissue composition is divided into four categories (Fig. 36-10): (1) The breast is almost entirely fat; (2) there are scattered islands of fibroglandular densities that could obscure lesions on mammography; (3) the breast tissue is heterogeneously

	TABLE 36-1	
Mammography: Final Assessment Categories		
Category	Assessment	Description and Recommendation
1	Negative	Routine screening. There is nothing about which to comment.
2	Benign finding	Routine screening. This is a definitely benign finding.
3	Probably benign finding	Very high probability of benignity; short-term follow-up is recommended to establish stability.
4	Suspicious-looking abnormality	Not characteristic but has reasonable probability of malignancy; biopsy should be considered.
5	Highly suggestive of malignancy	Very high probability of malignancy; appropriate action shoud be taken.
6	Known cancer	Appropriate action should be taken.

Modified from the American College of Radiology Breast Imaging Reporting and Data System (BI-RADS).

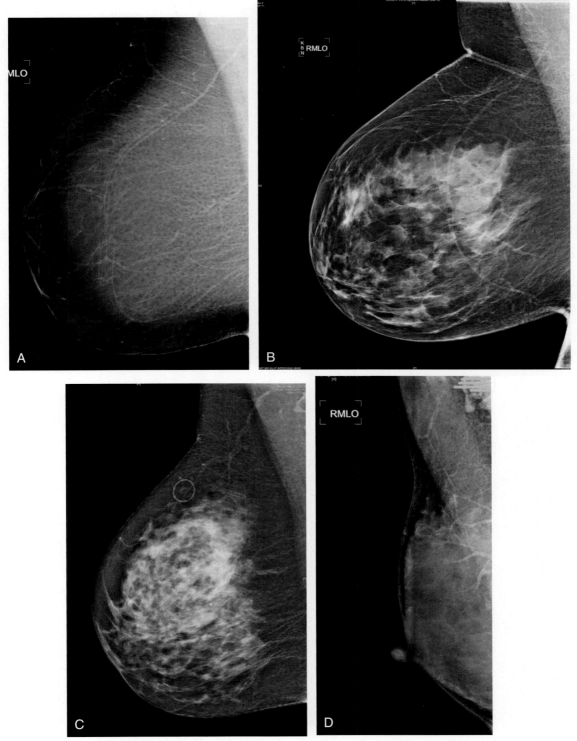

Figure 36-10 Four categories of mammographic breast tissue composition. **A**, The breast tissue is almost all fatty. **B**, There are scattered islands of fibroglandular tissue that could obscure a lesion on mammography. **C**, The breast is heterogeneously dense. This may lower the sensitivity of mammography. **D**, The breast is extremely dense, which lowers the sensitivity of mammography.

dense, which may lower the sensitivity of mammography; and (4) the breast tissue is extremely dense, which lowers the sensitivity of mammography.[3] Because young women tend to have more fibroglandular tissue, their breasts are usually more radiopaque than those of older women. However, it is important to understand that there is a wide variation in breast tissue density among women of the same age. Some young women have almost completely fatty breasts, and some older women have extremely dense breasts.

During pregnancy the breasts increase in density. An increase in density has also been associated with exogenous hormone therapy in some postmenopausal women.[46]

ABNORMAL MAMMOGRAPHIC FINDINGS

Masses and calcifications are the most common abnormalities encountered on mammograms, and the radiographic features of these abnormalities are important clues to their etiology. In the standardized mammography report, the descriptors used for masses and calcifications indicate the likelihood of malignancy. Other significant findings include new or evolving lesions, bilaterally asymmetric distribution of the fibroglandular tissue, architectural distortion, skin thickening or retraction, nipple retraction, and axillary node enlargement.

Masses

A *mass* can be defined as a space-occupying lesion that is seen on at least two mammographic projections. Masses are described by their shape, margins, and density. The

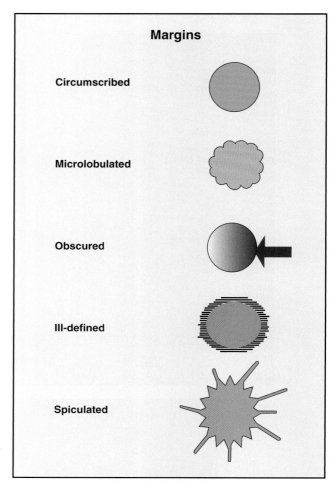

Figure 36-12 Standardized terminology for the margins of masses.

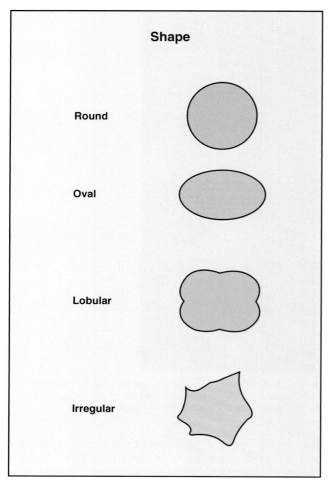

Figure 36-11 Standardized terminology for the shape of masses.

shape can be round, oval, lobulated, or irregular (Fig. 36-11). Oval and round masses are usually benign. An irregular shape suggests a greater likelihood of malignancy.

The *margins* of masses are also an important indicator of the likelihood of malignancy.[47] Margins can be described as circumscribed, microlobulated (multiple tiny lobulations), obscured (partially hidden by adjacent tissue), indistinct, or spiculated (Fig. 36-12). *Circumscribed* margins favor a benign etiology, with the likelihood of malignancy being very low, probably less than 2%.[48–50] Ultrasonography is used to establish whether a solitary circumscribed mass is cystic or solid. If it is cystic, no further workup is needed. If it is solid, magnification mammography may be required to confirm that all of the margins of a solid mass are truly circumscribed. A solitary circumscribed solid mass is usually managed with a 6-month follow-up to establish that it is stable (not growing). If it is stable, continued mammographic surveillance is recommended for at least 2 years.[51,52] The presence of multiple circumscribed masses is even stronger evidence of benignity, suggesting cysts, fibroadenomas, or benign intramammary lymph nodes,[37] and follow-up in 1 year is usually sufficient.

Microlobulated margins increase the likelihood of malignancy.[49] If the mass is directly adjacent to fibroglandular tissue of similar density, the margin may be *obscured*, in which case spot compression is used in an attempt to show the margins of the mass more completely.[34] The finding of indistinct margins suggests a possibility of malignancy. A mass with *spiculated* margins has lines radiating from its border and is highly suggestive of malignancy. An area of spiculation without any associated mass is called an *architectural distortion.*

The *density* of a mass also provides a clue as to its etiology. In general, benign masses tend to be lower in density than malignant masses. Malignant masses tend to have high radiodensity compared with benign masses or surrounding normal breast tissue. However, the density of a mass is not always a reliable sign as to whether it is benign or malignant.[53]

A variety of findings associated with masses may provide additional clues to their etiology. For example, calcifications in a mass often provide definitive information. The calcifications of fibroadenomas tend to be large and dense; these calcifications may be in the center or on the rim of the fibroadenoma. Fine, granular calcifications may be found in benign or malignant masses. Other findings that may be associated with a mass include skin retraction, nipple retraction, and skin thickening.

Calcifications

Calcium is a silver-white, bivalent, metallic element of the alkaline-earth group. Calcification is the deposition of calcium salts in tissues. In the breast, calcification usually occurs in the form of calcium hydroxyapatite or tricalcium phosphate.[54] In standardized terminology, calcifications are divided into three general groups: those that are typically benign, those that are indeterminate, and those that have a higher probability of malignancy. Typically, benign calcifications can be identified by their mammographic features and include skin, vascular, coarse, large rodlike, round, eggshell, and milk of calcium types (Fig. 36-13). *Intermediate* calcifications and those having a *higher probability of malignancy* can be described as amorphous or indistinct; pleomorphic or heterogeneous; or fine, linear, and branching (casting; Fig. 36-14).

Calcifications are also characterized by their distribution. *Grouped or clustered calcifications* include more than five calcifications in a small area (<2 cm^3) and can be benign or malignant. *Linear* calcifications are distributed in a line that may have small branch points. *Segmental* calcifications are distributed in a duct and its branches. *Regional* calcifications occur in a larger volume of breast tissue and not necessarily in a ductal distribution. *Diffuse/ scattered* calcifications are distributed randomly throughout the breast and are almost always benign.

BENIGN MASSES

Fibroadenomas are the most common masses in women younger than 30 years of age. Mammographically, fibroadenomas appear as round, oval, or lobulated masses

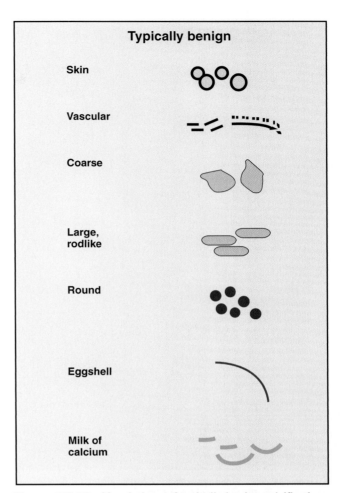

Figure 36-13 Morphology of typically benign calcifications.

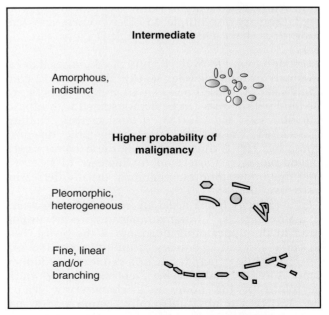

Figure 36-14 Morphology of indeterminate calcifications and calcification with a higher probability of malignancy.

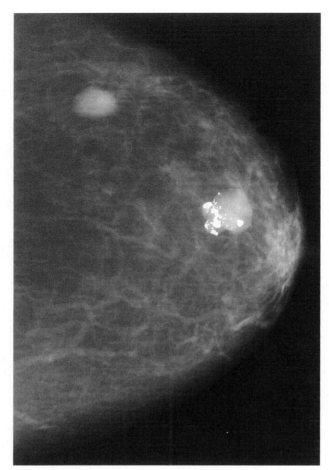

Figure 36-15 Fibroadenoma. Craniocaudal mammogram reveals a lobular, circumscribed mass with typically benign coarse calcifications of fibroadenoma. The oval circumscribed mass proved to be a fibroadenoma based on core needle biopsy.

with circumscribed margins (Figs. 36-15 to 36-17). They may be solitary or multiple. In older women, they tend to develop characteristic coarse calcifications (see Fig. 36-17).

Cysts are round to oval, circumscribed masses that can be solitary or multiple (Fig. 36-18). They are most commonly seen in women between 40 and 50 years of age. The fluid within cysts can be demonstrated with ultrasonography (see Fig. 36-18). If characteristic findings of cysts are present, the ultrasonographic diagnosis approaches 100%, thus eliminating the need for aspiration or biopsy.[55] Cysts tend to fluctuate in size over serial mammographic examinations, usually decreasing in size over time.[56]

Intramammary lymph nodes are commonly discovered on mammograms.[38] Intramammary nodes are usually found in the upper outer quadrant of the breast, near the axilla, and can be solitary or multiple. The indentation of the hilum may result in a reniform, or kidney, shape. A central radiolucency, representing fat within the hilum of the node, is a characteristic feature (Fig. 36-19). On ultrasonography, lymph nodes may have a highly echogenic center—a pathognomonic sign for intramammary lymph nodes.

Lipofibroadenoma, sometimes called a *hamartoma of the breast*, is another benign breast mass with characteristic radiographic features.[57] The mass contains a combination of fatty and soft tissue densities surrounded by a fibrous capsule (Fig. 36-20). The proportion of fatty and parenchymal tissue components can vary; thus, the lesion may be relatively radiolucent or radiodense.

Lipomas have a typical mammographic appearance. The lipoma is radiolucent and surrounded by a visible, thin fibrous capsule. Lipomas are always benign and

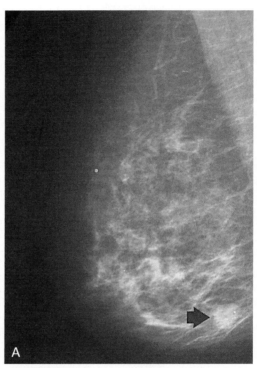

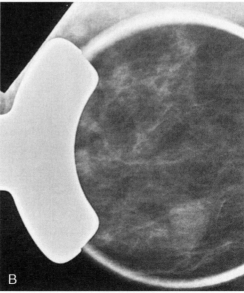

Figure 36-16 Fibroadenoma. **A,** Mediolateral oblique mammogram shows a round to oval mass *(arrow)* in the inferior aspect of the breast with a solitary calcification. **B,** Spot compression and magnification views show that the margins of the mass are circumscribed. Core biopsy revealed fibroadenoma.

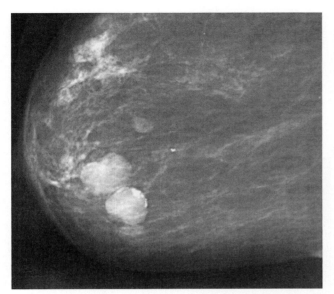

Figure 36-17   Multiple fibroadenomas. There are several lobulated, circumscribed masses. One of the masses shows the typically benign coarse, rim calcifications of a fibroadenoma.

usually found incidentally on mammography, although they occasionally may be palpable. In the fatty breast it may be difficult to determine whether a finding is a lipoma or normal fatty tissue.

Post-traumatic fat necrosis may manifest as a mass, calcifications, or both.[58] The mass associated with fat necrosis is usually a round to oval, radiolucent lipid cyst (Figs. 36-21 and 36-22). Often the wall of the cyst calcifies (see later discussion). Occasionally the fibrosis associated with post-traumatic fat necrosis results in an irregular, spiculated scar that can mimic malignancy.

Postsurgical hematomas are usually round to oval and dense (Fig. 36-23). They may rapidly increase in size immediately after surgery, but they resolve slowly.

Although ultrasonography may show an anechoic interior in the early stages of development, the hematoma will later show a mixture of cystic and solid components.

Postsurgical scars may show an irregular shape and spiculated margins, a mammographic appearance similar to that of invasive carcinomas (Fig. 36-24). Adjacent skin thickening and retraction also mimic the findings of an advanced breast cancer. Hence, knowledge of previous surgeries and their location is extremely important when interpreting mammograms.

Baseline mammograms are usually performed 6 months to 1 year after surgery.[59] Unlike carcinomas, scars tend to decrease in size over interval examinations, change their shape and appearance on mammograms taken in different projections, and be nonpalpable or barely palpable despite a relatively large size on mammograms.

Radial scars are benign lesions that are said to occur in approximately 1 in 1000 screening mammograms.[60] These scars, which occur in the absence of previous surgery, are a subject of controversy among pathologists, with nine different names having been given to them (e.g., infiltrating epitheliosis, benign sclerosing ductal proliferation). Radial scar best describes the mammographic appearances: relatively long spicules emanating from a center that may be radiolucent (Fig. 36-25). Calcifications may or may not be present.

It is important to differentiate radial scar from invasive carcinoma, which is also characterized by spiculations. Unlike carcinoma, radial scar is neither palpable nor associated with skin thickening or retraction. Although the radiolucent center of radial scars is an important clue to the correct diagnosis, excisional biopsy is needed to rule out malignancy with certainty.[61]

BENIGN CALCIFICATIONS

Skin (dermal) calcifications are secondary to dermatitis or residue from deodorants. They are usually located near

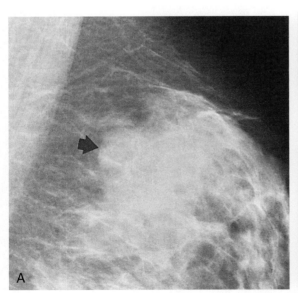
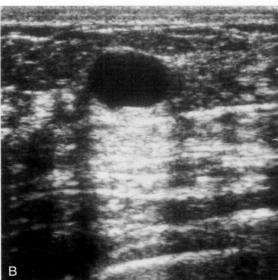

Figure 36-18   Cyst. **A,** Close-up of a mediolateral oblique mammogram shows a mass with circumscribed posterior margins *(arrow)* and obscured anterior margins. **B,** Ultrasonography revealed that the mass has a circumscribed border, anechoic interior (no interior echoes), and enhancement of echoes posterior to the mass.

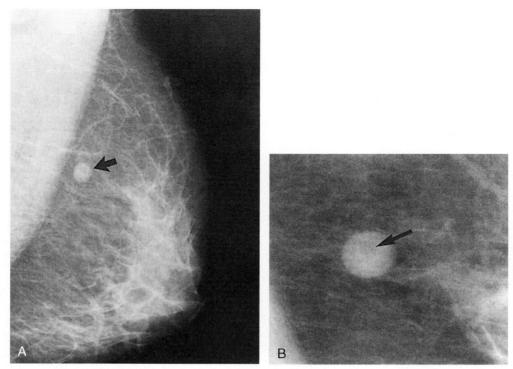

Figure 36-19 Intramammary lymph node. **A,** Mediolateral oblique mammogram reveals a small oval mass *(arrow)* in the postero-superior aspect of the breast. **B,** Spot compression-magnification view shows a central radiolucency *(arrow),* which is characteristic of an intramammary lymph node.

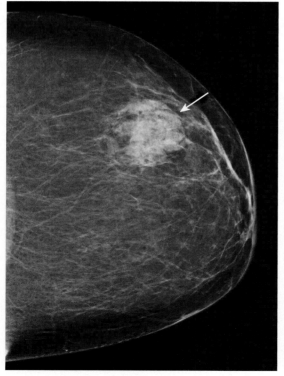

Figure 36-20 Lipofibroadenoma. Craniocaudal mammogram shows a mass *(arrow)* composed of radiolucent fat and soft tissue densities.

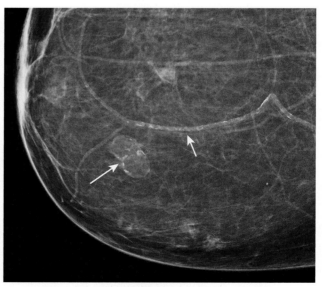

Figure 36-21 Fat necrosis. Close-up of mammogram shows typical lipid-filled cyst with calcification of fibrous capsule *(long arrow).* Elsewhere, there are vascular calcifications *(short arrow).*

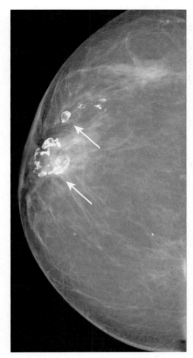

Figure 36-22 Fat necrosis. Multiple calcifying lipid cysts *(arrows)*.

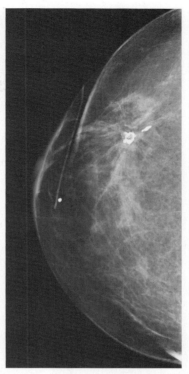

Figure 36-23 Postsurgical changes, including fat necrosis. A 66-year-old woman had a biopsy of a palpable mass. Pathologic examination revealed infiltrating ductal carcinoma. Right craniocaudal follow-up examination revealed postoperative changes.

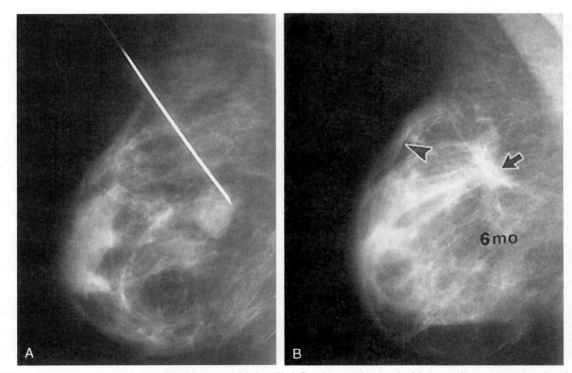

Figure 36-24 Postsurgical scar. A 50-year-old woman had an ill-defined mass detected with screening mammography. An excisional biopsy preceded by needle localization was scheduled. **A,** Mediolateral mammogram during localization procedure shows the tip of the needle positioned immediately posterior to the mass. Biopsy revealed invasive carcinoma. **B,** Mediolateral mammogram 6 months after surgery shows a spiculated mass *(arrow)* and skin thickening *(arrowhead)* at the surgical site.

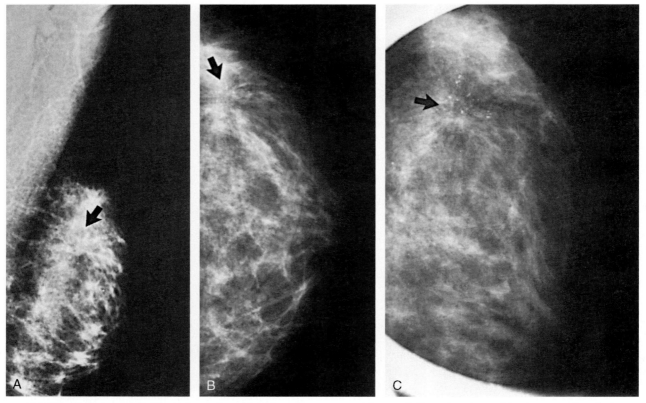

Figure 36-25 Radial scar. **A,** The left craniocaudal view shows an architectural distortion *(arrow)* in the outer hemisphere with multiple spicules emanating from a radiolucent center. **B** and **C,** Magnification views.

the skin on at least one of the mammographic views.[62] The calcifications are usually low in density, often with a central radiolucency.[37] If the dermal origin of the calcifications is not certain, maneuvers are performed to direct the x-ray beam tangential to the portion of the skin containing the calcifications (Fig. 36-26). The tangential view can prove that calcifications are in the skin, eliminating the need for a biopsy.

Vascular calcifications are characterized by linear, parallel calcifications, referred to as a *railroad track configuration* (Fig. 36-27). The calcifications are said to be more common in women with diabetes, but in fact, they are commonly seen in women with no history of diabetes.[63]

Fibroadenoma calcifications are usually coarse. The calcifications are usually centrally placed, are arranged in "popcorn" configuration (see Fig. 36-27), or may be positioned on the rim of the fibroadenoma (see Fig. 36-17). However, when calcifications occur within the ducts of the fibroadenoma, they may be indistinguishable from those of malignancy, and a biopsy may be necessary.

Secretory calcifications, or the calcifications of duct ectasia, involve the intermediate and larger ducts of the breast. Most women with this condition are asymptomatic. Although the exact cause of duct ectasia is uncertain, the calcifications are quite characteristic. The calcifications are usually thick and solid, representing calcium deposits in the benign secretions within dilated

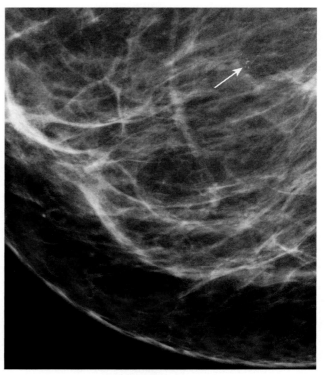

Figure 36-26 Skin calcifications. Multiple punctuate calcifications were identified as skin calcifications *(arrow)*.

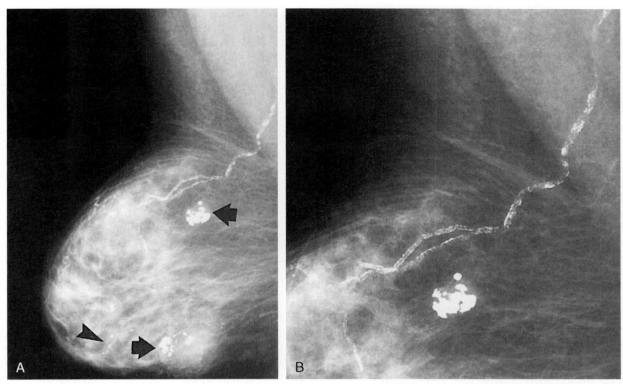

Figure 36-27 Typically benign calcifications. **A,** Right mediolateral oblique view shows prominent vascular calcifications, calcification in two degenerating fibroadenomas *(arrows)* and benign secretory calcifications *(arrowhead).* **B,** Close-up shows typical "railroad track" vascular calcifications and "popcorn" calcifications of fibroadenoma.

ducts (Fig. 36-28). They are often bilateral and in the subareolar location. A unilateral, segmental distribution of duct ectasia manifesting as calcification may be confused with comedo carcinoma, because both may show linear and branching configurations. Unlike comedo carcinoma, the calcifications of duct ectasia are solid, smooth, continuous rods, often more than 1 mm in diameter and more widely spaced than comedo carcinoma calcifications. In addition, the calcifications of duct ectasia usually do not branch.[64]

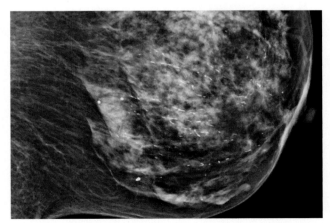

Figure 36-28 Typically benign calcifications. Secretory calcifications of duct ectasia. Unlike the calcifications of ductal carcinoma in situ, these calcifications are solid, rodlike, and relatively well separated and rarely show branching.

Post-traumatic fat necrosis calcifications usually develop within the fibrous walls of developing lipid cysts. In the early stages of development, they may be confused with malignant calcifications, but with time, they take on a characteristic eggshell configuration around the lipid-filled cysts (see Figs. 36-21 and 36-22).[58,65] These lesions are commonly found at the location of a previous biopsy, providing a further clue to their etiology.

Milk of calcium is free-floating calcium within cysts, usually tiny cysts. The mammographic features of this condition are pathognomonic; similar to the sediment at the bottom of a cup of tea, they change their appearance with different radiographic projections.[66] These gravity-dependent calcifications appear as amorphous and round or ovoid smudges on craniocaudal projections (Fig. 36-29). However, they are sharp and linear to crescent-shaped on 90-degree lateral views (see Fig. 36-29). Milk of calcium does not require a biopsy, but carcinoma may arise nearby, in which case the calcifications should be inspected carefully to rule out coexistent carcinoma.

MALIGNANT MASSES

The most common malignant breast mass is invasive breast carcinoma. The mass of invasive carcinoma is typically irregular in shape, indistinct or spiculated on its margin, and high in radiographic density compared with normal parenchymal tissue (Fig. 36-30). The mass may contain pleomorphic calcifications. Less commonly, the

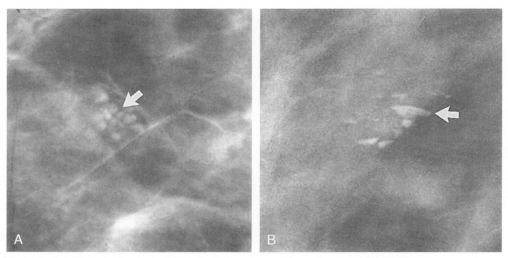

Figure 36-29 Typically benign calcifications. Milk of calcium detected on the screening mammograms of a 41-year-old woman. **A**, Close-up of craniocaudal view shows a cluster of amorphous, round calcifications *(arrow)*. **B**, Close-up of 90-degree lateral view demonstrates layering of the gravity-dependent calcifications *(arrow)*.

mass is circumscribed. There are several subtypes of invasive cancer, with the different histologic types differing in prognoses.[67]

Invasive Ductal Carcinoma, Not Otherwise Specified

The most common carcinoma, the not otherwise specified (NOS) type, usually presents as a mass. Most of these masses have the irregular shape, indistinct or spiculated margins, and high radiographic density characteristic of malignancy (Figs. 36-31 and 36-32; see Fig. 36-30). Although most NOS-type carcinomas have indistinct or spiculated margins, they occasionally have partially

circumscribed margins (Fig. 36-33). Spot compression-magnification films usually reveal indistinct margins at some portion of the boundary of an otherwise circumscribed carcinoma. Approximately 40% of invasive ductal carcinomas of the NOS type are associated with malignant calcifications.

Tubular Carcinomas

Tubular carcinomas grow very slowly and are usually small when they are first detected on mammographic screening. They have an excellent prognosis relative to the NOS-type cancers. Other than a characteristically small size, they have the mammographic features of the usual NOS type of

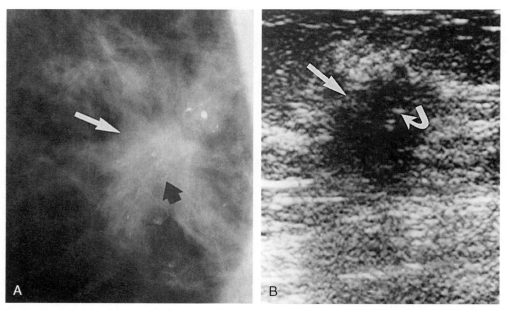

Figure 36-30 Typical invasive carcinoma. **A**, Close-up of mammogram showing typical invasive carcinoma mass, manifested by irregular shape, spiculated margins *(white arrow)*, high radiographic density, and numerous calcifications of varying size and shape *(black arrow)*. **B**, Ultrasonography shows that the mass *(straight arrow)* has an irregular shape, ill-defined margins, and low-level heterogeneous echoes within it. The bright echoes *(curved arrow)* within the mass represent calcifications.

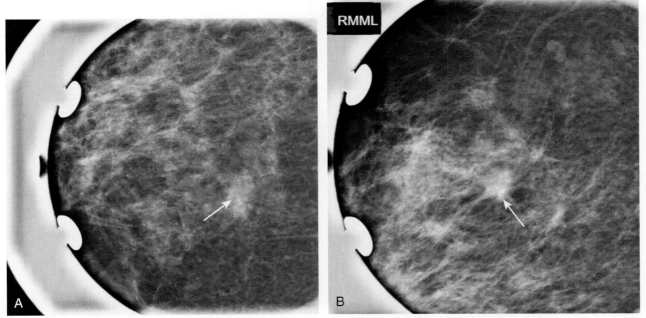

Figure 36-31   Invasive ductal carcinoma. **A** and **B,** Spot magnification views show a round, speculated mass *(arrows)*, approximately the same density as the surrounding fibroglandular tissue.

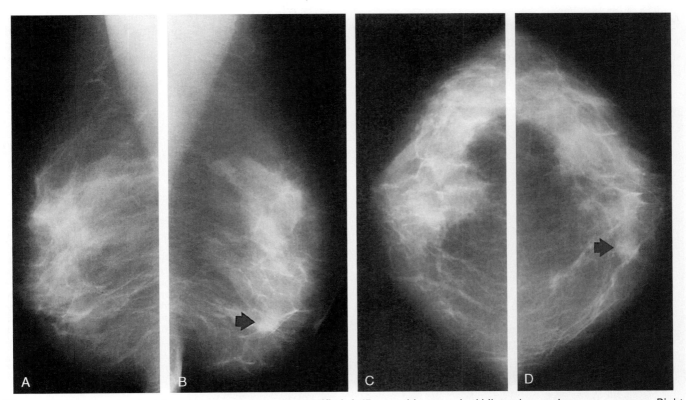

Figure 36-32   Invasive ductal carcinoma, not otherwise specified. A 47-year-old woman had bilateral screening mammograms. Right (**A**) and left (**B**) mediolateral oblique views and right (**C**) and left (**D**) craniocaudal views show a 1.5-cm round, spiculated mass *(arrows)*, approximately the same density as the surrounding fibroglandular tissue, in the lower inner quadrant of the left breast.

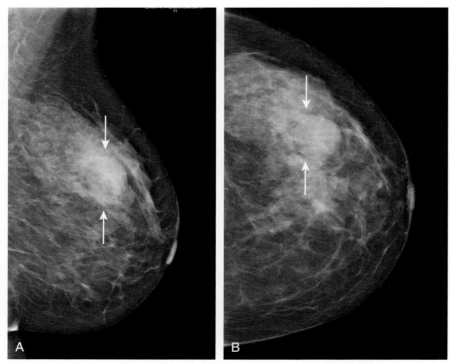

Figure 36-33 Circumscribed carcinoma. Left mediolateral oblique (**A**) and craniocaudal (**B**) views show a lobular, circumscribed mass *(arrows)*. Biopsy revealed invasive ductal carcinoma.

invasive breast carcinoma: irregular shape, spiculated margins, and high radiographic density (Fig. 36-34).[68]

Medullary Carcinomas

Medullary carcinomas are often oval or lobulated in shape and frequently have circumscribed margins (Fig. 36-35).[69] In addition to their benign-appearing mammographic features, the clinical findings may also mimic a benign lesion and they have a tendency to occur in younger women. This combination of features results in delayed diagnosis of many medullary carcinomas. Necrosis, cavitation, and bleeding may result in a rapid increase in lesion size; the presence of fluid within the tumor can be identified with ultrasonography (Fig. 36-36).

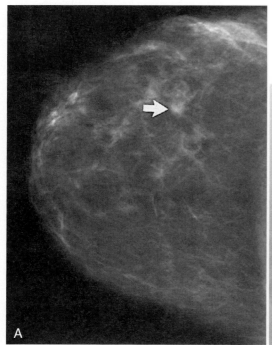

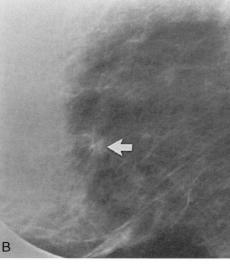

Figure 36-34 Tubular carcinoma. A 48-year-old woman had screening mammograms. **A**, Right craniocaudal view shows irregular density *(arrow)* in the outer hemisphere. **B**, Spot compression-magnification view in mediolateral projection confirms the presence of a small spiculated mass *(arrow)*. Biopsy revealed tubular carcinoma.

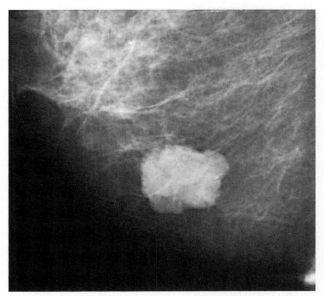

Figure 36-35 Medullary carcinoma. A 39-year-old woman felt a mass in her right breast. On palpation the mass was freely movable. Close-up of mediolateral oblique mammogram reveals a lobular mass with circumscribed margins. Biopsy revealed medullary carcinoma.

Colloid Carcinomas

Also called mucinous carcinomas, colloid carcinomas often show relatively circumscribed margins, but portions of the margin are usually microlobulated or indistinct (Fig. 36-37). Because of their compressibility, colloid carcinomas commonly may have radiographic density similar to that of normal fibroglandular tissue.

Invasive Papillary Carcinoma

Invasive papillary carcinoma, a rare invasive cancer, may appear as a solitary, circumscribed nodule or as a multinodular pattern.[70]

Intracystic Carcinoma

Adenocarcinoma arising from the wall of a cyst is a rare lesion.[71] If the tumor is totally intracystic, the cancer is non-invasive and the prognosis is excellent. The most common histologic type is papillary adenocarcinoma. The mass is often large and circumscribed on mammography. Ultrasonography may show both fluid and solid components. The solid portions often surround the central fluid-filled portion, or the solid components may project from a portion of the wall of the cyst into the center of the fluid.

Invasive Lobular Carcinoma

Invasive lobular carcinoma can appear as a mass with an irregular shape and spiculated or ill-defined margins on mammograms (Fig. 36-38). However, it is not uncommon for mammograms of invasive lobular carcinoma to show only a poorly defined asymmetric density (see Fig. 36-38), an architectural distortion (Fig. 36-39), or no recognizable abnormal findings.[72] Because they are often difficult to appreciate on mammography or palpation, even when relatively advanced in size, invasive lobular carcinomas are sometimes referred to as "sneaky" cancers.[73,74] They also have a higher rate of bilaterality than other carcinomas.

Breast Metastases from Extramammary Malignancies

Metastatic foci to the breast from extramammary sites are uncommon. Metastases to the breast can originate from a variety of primary sites.[75] The patient invariably has a known history of the extramammary malignancy before the mammographic examination. Metastatic melanoma is the largest reported source of metastases to the breast. The metastatic lesions usually have a round shape and indistinct margins (Fig. 36-40). Most metastatic foci to the breast are solitary lesions, although multiple masses may be seen occasionally (Fig. 36-41).[76]

Figure 36-36 Medullary carcinoma. A 41-year-old woman felt a movable mass in the upper outer quadrant of her left breast. A diagnostic mammogram was ordered. **A,** Left mediolateral oblique view shows an oval mass under the radiopaque BB, which was placed over the palpable mass. **B,** Ultrasonography reveals a lobulated mass with a thick wall surrounding an anechoic fluid-filled center *(arrow)*. Biopsy revealed medullary carcinoma with central hemorrhagic necrosis.

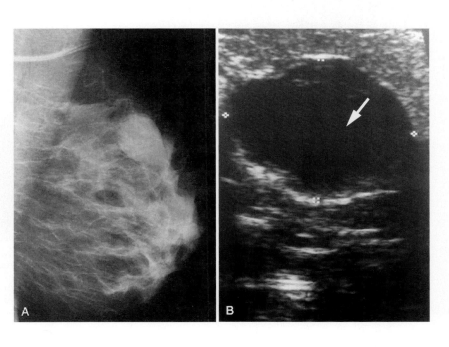

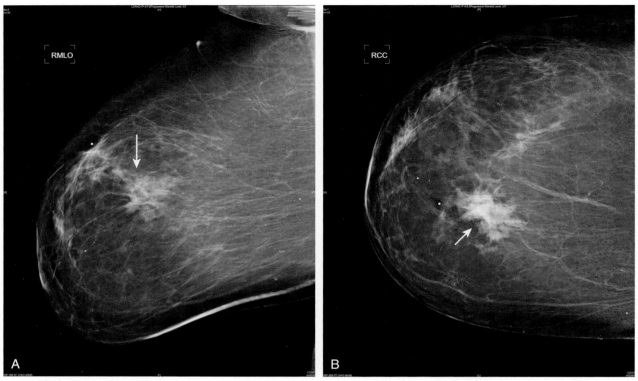

Figure 36-37 Colloid (mucinous) carcinoma. Right mediolateral oblique (**A**) and right craniocaudal (**B**) views demonstrated an irregular shape *(arrows)* with microlobulations and speculated margins. Multiple lobulations seen are typical of mucinous carcinoma, which was confirmed on biopsy.

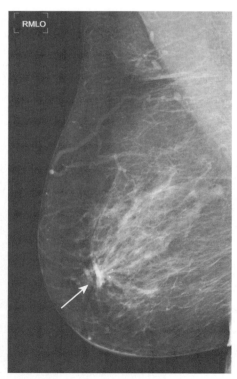

Figure 36-38 Invasive lobular carcinoma. A 76-year-old woman with a breast lump that is becoming harder and smaller. There is nipple retraction *(arrow)* and architectural distortion. Biopsy revealed a 5-cm invasive lobular carcinoma.

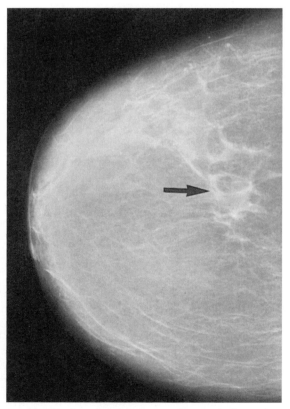

Figure 36-39 Invasive lobular carcinoma. Left craniocaudal view from screening mammograms reveals an architectural distortion *(arrow)* in the right breast. Palpation of the area failed to reveal any abnormality. Core needle biopsy revealed invasive lobular carcinoma.

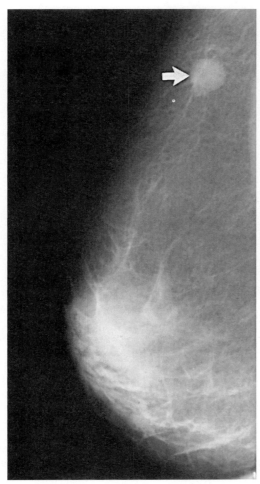

Figure 36-40 Lung carcinoma metastatic to the breast. A 54-year-old woman with a known history of lung carcinoma noticed a mass *(arrow)* in the superior aspect of her right breast. Mammograms revealed a solitary, round, ill-defined mass at the site of the palpable abnormality. Biopsy revealed metastatic carcinoma.

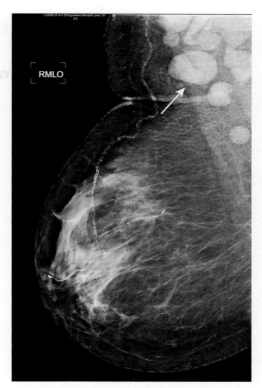

Figure 36-41 Multiple round, soft-tissue density masses seen in the axilla *(arrow)*. This patient had lymphoma.

MALIGNANT CALCIFICATIONS

Calcifications associated with breast cancer are dystrophic; they are deposited in abnormal tissue, not as a result of elevated levels of calcium or phosphate in the blood. Malignant calcifications may occur with or without the presence of a mass, and they are typically grouped or clustered; pleomorphic (varying in size and shape; Figs. 36-42 and 36-43); fine, linear, and branching (Figs. 36-44 and 36-45) and numerous. The greater the number of calcifications in a cluster, the greater the likelihood of malignancy, with a group containing fewer than five calcifications being unlikely to represent malignancy.[77] The distribution of the calcifications can be linear, linear and branching, or segmental.

Ductal Carcinoma in Situ

Ductal carcinoma in situ (DCIS), or intraductal carcinoma, is a precursor to invasive breast cancer, which on microscopic examination does not yet show clear evidence of stromal invasion.[78–80] Before the widespread

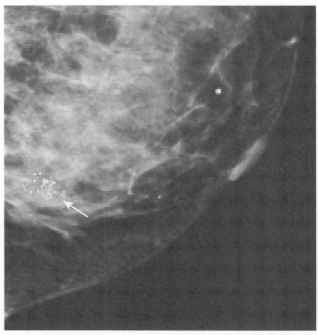

Figure 36-42 Noncomedo ductal carcinoma in situ. Multiple calcifications detected on screening mammography. Close-up of the calcifications reveals clustered calcifications *(arrow)* that vary in size and shape. Biopsy revealed noncomedo carcinoma.

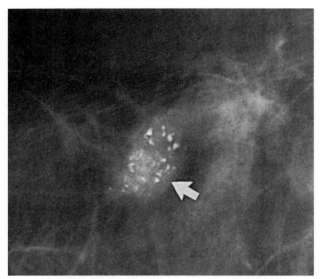

Figure 36-43 Noncomedo carcinoma. Suspicious calcifications were detected on the screening mammograms of a 60-year-old woman. Close-up of calcifications reveals that the calcifications are numerous, clustered, pleomorphic (varying in size and shape), and associated with a soft tissue density *(arrow)*. Biopsy revealed noncomedo ductal carcinoma in situ with surrounding inflammatory response.

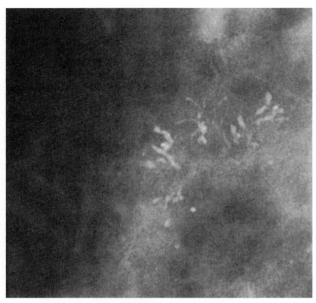

Figure 36-44 Comedo ductal carcinoma in situ. Fine, linear, and branching calcifications of comedo carcinoma.

use of mammography, DCIS represented less than 5% of newly detected breast cancers.[81] Today, DCIS makes up approximately 30% of newly detected breast cancers, with most DCIS cases being detected with screening mammography. Approximately 75% of DCIS cases are detected because of mammographically visible calcifications.

A major breakthrough in knowledge about DCIS occurred when Holland and coworkers[82,83] described their mastectomy specimen findings. They concluded

that DCIS typically is distributed within a single lobe of a duct system without intervening areas of normal tissue. This observation was contrary to the then-popular concept of a multifocal origin of breast cancer and was more consistent with the fact that breast cancer recurrences are usually in the region of the original tumor.[64,84] DCIS includes a spectrum of lesions, and individual cases do not have the same propensity for eventual invasion and metastasis.

Several classification systems have been developed based on the extent of the lesion, clinical findings, and histologic features. The most commonly used

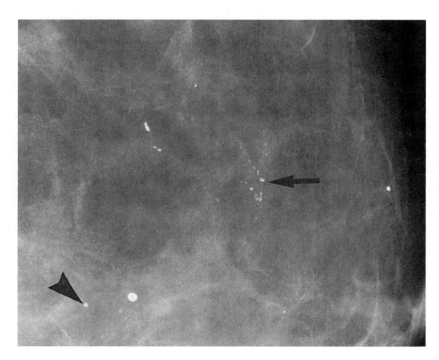

Figure 36-45 Comedo ductal carcinoma in situ. The cluster of calcifications *(arrow)* is composed of multiple fine, granular calcifications (compare with the solid, rodlike calcifications of duct ectasia in Fig. 36-30) and the benign punctuate calcification below *(arrowhead)*.

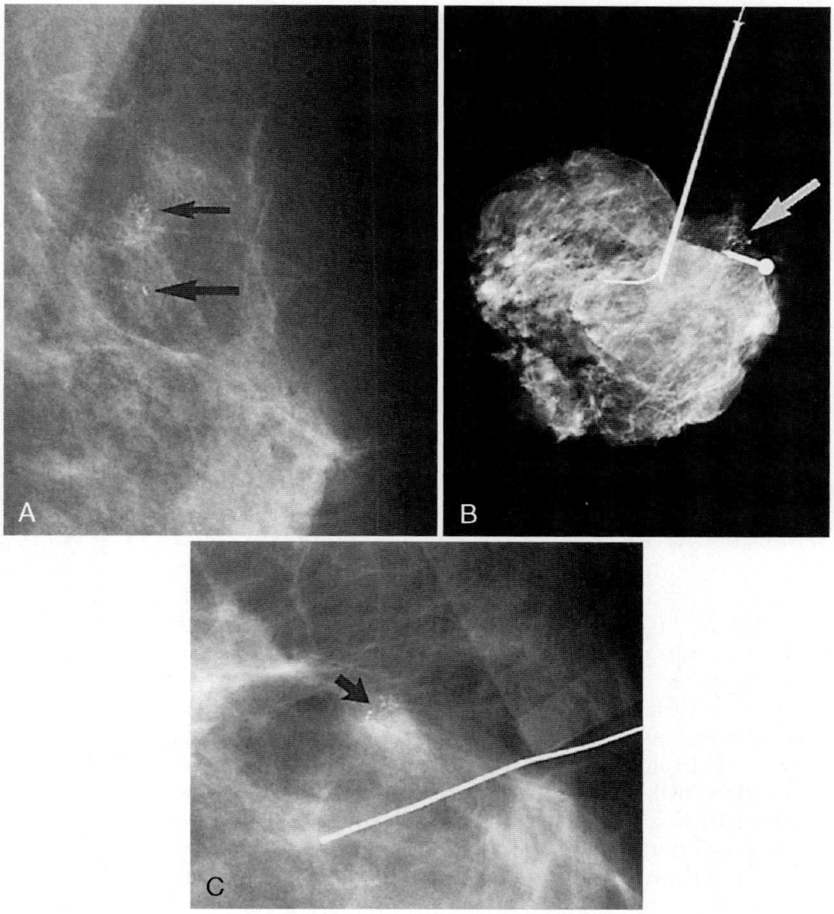

Figure 36-46 Residual noncomedo ductal carcinoma in situ (DCIS) following lumpectomy. **A,** The barely visible calcifications *(arrows)* are numerous, tiny, and pleomorphic. **B,** Specimen radiography following wire localization verifies the presence of calcifications at the edge of the excised tissue *(arrow)*. Histologic examination revealed micropapillary DCIS with clear margins. **C,** Preradiotherapy magnification mammograms of the surgical site revealed residual calcifications *(arrow)* in the breast. (The radiopaque wire was placed on the surface of the breast to mark the surgical site.) Reexcision following wire localization revealed micropapillary DCIS.

classification system divides DCIS into two major types: the more aggressive comedo carcinoma and the more indolent noncomedo carcinoma. In excised specimens containing comedo carcinoma, the involved ducts typically extrude a thick material resembling a comedone. Today, aggressive malignant cytologic features, such as the degree of nuclear atypia, are considered more important than the presence of central lumen necrosis in the histologic diagnosis of comedo carcinoma.[78] In fact, DCIS is often intermediate in the degree of malignant cytologic features or intermixed, and the prognosis depends on the prevalent nuclear grade. Micropapillary and cribriform DCIS are the most common histologic subtypes of noncomedo DCIS. The visible calcifications of comedo carcinoma closely match the actual extent of the lesion, but noncomedo carcinoma may be considerably more extensive than suggested by its calcifications.

The calcifications of comedo carcinoma usually occur in the central debris of ducts involved by tumor cells undergoing necrosis. As a result, the morphology of the calcifications of comedo carcinoma is typically fine, linear, and branching, suggesting casting of the duct system[85,86] (see Figs. 36-44 and 36-45). The calcifications of noncomedo carcinoma represent dystrophic laminated calcifications in intraductal cellular debris or calcified secretions in the cribriform spaces of noncomedo DCIS. These granular calcifications are fine

particles characterized by variable size and shape (Fig. 36-46; and see Figs. 36-42 and 36-43). However, radiographic features are not always reliable in differentiating between comedo and noncomedo carcinoma.[87]

In slightly more than 10% of DCIS cases, a soft tissue mass can also be seen on mammograms (see Fig. 36-43). This soft tissue mass is a manifestation of a solid mass of tumor cells or associated inflammation, edema, and fibrosis at the periphery of involved ducts.[88] Table 36-2 shows the approximate frequency of the most common radiographic manifestations of DCIS. Less common manifestations of DCIS include asymmetry; dilated retroareolar ducts; an ill-defined, rounded tumor; architectural distortion; and a developing density.

TABLE 36-2

Mammographic Manifestations of Ductal Carcinoma in Situ

Mammographic Finding	Frequency (%)
Calcifications alone	75
Calcifications plus soft tissue density	10
Soft tissue abnormality alone	10
No mammography findings	5

Invasive Cancer with Extensive Intraductal Component

Invasive tumors are classified as being extensive intraductal component (EIC) positive if they are predominately intraductal with small areas of invasion or predominantly invasive with one of the following conditions: (1) DCIS fills nonobliterated ducts within the invasive cancer, or (2) there is DCIS in the tissue adjacent to the invasive tumor[83] (see Fig. 36-9).

The significance of the EIC-positive designation is the greater incidence of local recurrence of breast cancer after surgical excision and radiotherapy. One study reported the incidence of recurrence for EIC-positive cases to be approximately 25% at 5 years compared with 6% for EIC-negative cases.[89] This report verifies observations of others that the presence of EIC in DCIS is a marker for widespread residual tumor after excision.[81,82,90–93] If all of the EIC is successfully removed, the local recurrence rate is similar to that of tumors without EIC.

Mammography plays an important role in the management of EIC-positive tumors. First, mammographic wire localization is essential before the surgical excision. If the purpose of the localization procedure is to excise all of the lesion for segmental resection before radiotherapy and not just to take a sample for diagnostic purposes, multiple localization wires may be used to bracket the full extent of the lesion.[94] At the time of surgical excision of DCIS, a specimen radiograph should always be performed (see Fig. 36-46). However, it should be borne in mind that specimen radiography is not an adequate tool to ensure that malignant calcifications have been completely removed.[95]

Traditionally, it is the pathologist's responsibility to determine whether the margins of a resected tissue are free of tumor. However, the complex branching of the breast ductal system may lead to errors regarding whether the intraductal tumor has been completely removed (Fig. 36-47; and see Fig. 36-46). Therefore, it is important that in cases with extensive DCIS manifested by calcifications, mammography be performed after surgery and before radiotherapy to look for residual malignant calcifications.[94,96]

To minimize the discomfort associated with mammographic compression, the pretherapy mammograms are delayed until just before radiotherapy, usually 3 to 5 weeks after surgery. At our institution, postsurgical preradiotherapy examination is performed with a wire over the surgical site. In addition to standard views, microfocus magnification views are performed over the scar (see Fig. 36-46). If the preradiotherapy mammograms disclose residual calcifications, a re-excision is performed after mammographically guided wire localization (see Fig. 36-47). Most re-excisions performed for residual calcifications at the lumpectomy site reveal residual carcinoma.[97] If only a few calcifications remain, re-excision is not always performed, but it is still important to know the number and location of these calcifications so that they are not mistaken for recurrent tumor on follow-up mammograms.

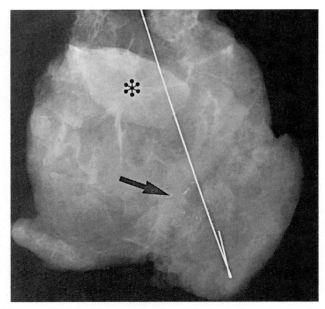

Figure 36-47 Specimen radiograph following wire localization of residual calcifications *(arrow)* of comedo carcinoma. Preradiotherapy mammograms had demonstrated these calcifications adjacent to the postsurgical hematoma *(asterisk)*.

INDIRECT SIGNS OF BREAST CANCER

Mammographic evidence of malignancy can be divided into primary, secondary, and indirect signs. *Primary signs* include a mass and calcifications. *Secondary signs*, such as skin thickening and retraction, are usually evident on clinical breast examination. When seen on mammograms they are usually associated with an advanced cancer. *Indirect or subtle signs* are associated with nonpalpable breast cancers and include bilaterally asymmetric breast tissue, new or evolving asymmetry, architectural distortion, and abnormal axillary lymph nodes. These indirect signs have been reported to be the only evidence of malignancy in up to 20% of mammographically detected cancers.[98]

Asymmetry

This indirect sign refers to a relative increase in the volume of fibroglandular tissue in one breast compared to the corresponding area in the contralateral breast. Because asymmetric breast tissue usually is a normal variation, the asymmetry should not be considered significant unless it is associated with suspect clinical or mammographic features. If there is a question as to the nature of a localized region of asymmetrical breast tissue, spot compression views can be used to determine if the asymmetric breast tissue is normal overlapping fibroglandular tissue. Magnification views might also disclose an underlying mass, clustered calcifications, or an architectural distortion associated with the asymmetry, findings that could justify biopsy (Fig. 36-48). Ultrasonography is generally not useful for evaluating an area of asymmetry.[99] Asymmetrical breast tissue in the axilla

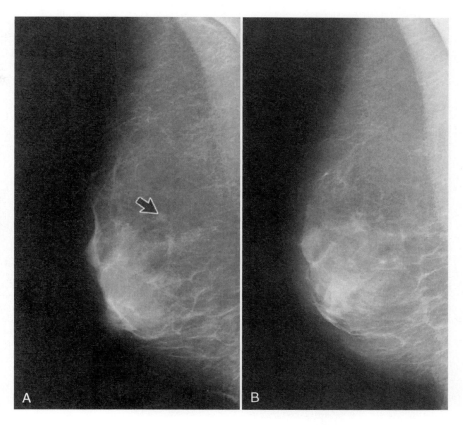

Figure 36-48 Neodensity. Right mediolateral oblique screening mammogram (**A**) of a 45-year-old woman revealed a small density *(arrow)*, which was not present on screening mammograms performed 1 year earlier (**B**). Biopsy revealed mucinous carcinoma.

is a common normal variant, which should not be mistaken for a significant abnormality.[100]

New or Evolving Asymmetry

Because the breasts of postmenopausal women are expected to undergo involution, the appearance of a new or developing asymmetry should be considered a possible sign of breast cancer in this group.[101] By definition, detection of a developing asymmetry requires access to previous mammograms (Fig. 36-49).[102] A "developing asymmetry" is one that was present at least in retrospect on a previous examination but was smaller and perhaps not recognized as significant. If a new or developing asymmetry has mammographic features that could represent a cyst, sonography or needle aspiration should be performed. If the existence of a simple cyst is proved by either method, and the cyst matches the site of the mammographic abnormality, no further workup is necessary.

Tissue densities caused by hormone replacement therapy can usually be differentiated from a new asymmetry associated with breast cancer. The new fibroglandular tissue caused by exogenous hormone therapy is usually present bilaterally and in several areas of the same breast. If there is a solitary new asymmetry in a woman on hormone replacement therapy, it may be difficult to

rule out breast cancer. In this situation, it may be useful to stop hormone replacement therapy for 2 to 3 months. If the asymmetry persists, biopsy should be considered.

Architectural Distortion

An architectural distortion may be the earliest sign of breast carcinoma (see Fig. 36-39). Architectural distortions can also be associated with surgical scars (see Fig. 36-24) and radial scars (see Fig. 36-25). Because postsurgical scarring can also result in distortions of the parenchyma, it is important to be aware of the location of any previous surgeries.[103] Some radiologists find it useful before performing mammograms for the radiologic technologist to place a wire directly over surgical scars to mark the exact site of the scar.[59]

Abnormal Axillary Lymph Nodes

Axillary lymph nodes are commonly seen on the MLO view. Normal nodes tend to be oval or kidney-shaped with a central radiolucency (hilar fat; Fig. 36-50). Abnormal nodes are more likely to be round, dense in the center, and larger than 2 cm (Fig. 36-51).[104] However, small nodes, even with central radiolucency, can harbor early metastases. Thus, mammography cannot be considered a substitute for axillary lymph node dissection.

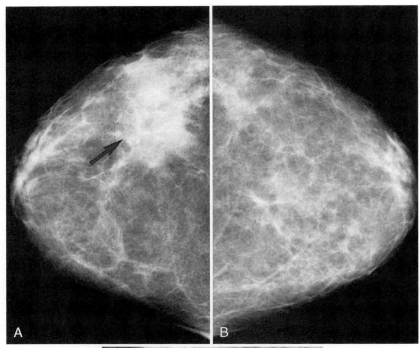

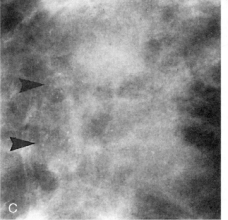

Figure 36-49 Asymmetric density. **A** and **B**, Craniocaudal mammograms from the screening examination of a 48-year-old woman revealed an asymmetric density *(arrow)* in the right breast. **C**, Magnification mammogram revealed multiple calcifications *(arrowheads)* associated with the asymmetric density. Biopsy revealed invasive ductal carcinoma, not otherwise specified.

SPECIAL SITUATIONS

Inflammatory Carcinoma

Inflammatory carcinoma is a clinical diagnosis based on the findings of an inflamed breast, which may feel hot and heavy to the patient. Inflammatory carcinoma is associated with diffuse skin thickening on mammography and overall increased breast density. The differentiation of mastitis from carcinoma with lymphangitic spread (inflammatory carcinoma) may be difficult. In both conditions, the primary lesion may be completely obscured by edema. In this situation, abscess may be excluded mammographically only if typical branching malignant calcifications are present. In general, the diagnosis of inflammatory carcinoma is made clinically unless the mammogram reveals an obvious malignancy.

Generalized skin thickening may also be associated with an abscess, progressive systemic sclerosis, obstruction of the superior vena cava, pemphigus, nephrotic syndrome, congestive heart failure, lymphoma, lymphatic extension from contralateral breast carcinoma, or changes secondary to radiotherapy.

Paget's Disease

Paget's disease of the nipple and areola is an uncommon condition in which malignant cells from intraductal or invasive ductal carcinoma migrate to the nipple skin, resulting in a clinical presentation of a chronic, moist, scaly, or erythematous eruption, with symptoms of itching, burning, oozing, or bleeding. These clinicopathologic changes in the nipple are pathognomonic of the early clinical presentation of breast carcinoma. A palpable or mammographically visible mass may or may not be present. The prognosis of a woman with Paget's disease of the nipple depends on the nature of the underlying carcinoma. Usually the underlying tumor is intraductal, and the patient has an excellent prognosis. Subareolar calcifications of DCIS are sometimes present.

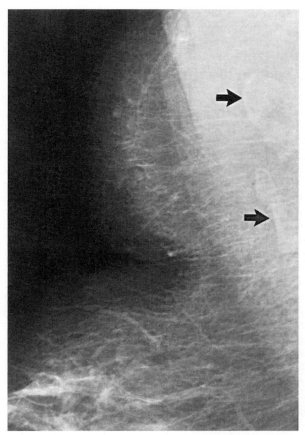

Figure 36-50 Normal axillary nodes. Close-up of mediolateral oblique mammogram shows normal axillary nodes *(arrows)* with oval shapes and radiolucent fatty centers.

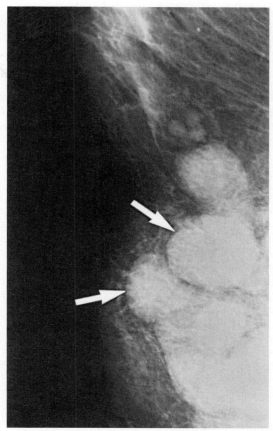

Figure 36-51 Abnormal lymph nodes. Close-up of mediolateral oblique mammogram shows large, round, dense axillary lymph nodes *(arrows)*. Biopsy revealed metastatic adenocarcinoma from an unknown primary.

POSITIVE PREDICTIVE VALUE OF MAMMOGRAPHY FOR BREAST CANCER

The positive predictive value is defined here as the number of cancers found at biopsy divided by the number of biopsies performed. This statistic is also known as the true-positive biopsy rate (or yield). In literature, the true-positive biopsy rates for mammographically detected abnormalities are reported from 10% to 40%.[6,48,49,105–107] In the past, rates as low as 10% were considered appropriate to maximize the number of early cancers detected by screening mammography.[108] However, concern over excessive numbers of false-positive mammograms leading to unnecessary investigations and surgical interventions has kept many referring physicians from ordering mammography screening.[109] Furthermore, the biopsies performed after screening can become the major cost associated with breast cancer screening with mammography.[110] Radiologists are being encouraged to audit their own practices to determine their true-positive rates, false-negative biopsy rates, and other measures of effectiveness.[111–113] Desirable positive predictive value rates in published literature based on abnormal mammogram findings are in the range of 25% to 40%.[114]

Other Breast Imaging Techniques

BREAST ULTRASONOGRAPHY

In the early 1950s, the breast was one of the first organs to be examined by ultrasonography.[115] Later, a number of ultrasonographers developed equipment especially for breast imaging.[116,117] After encouraging results, some ultrasonographers advocated the method for breast cancer screening, suggesting it was as effective as mammography.[116–119] Subsequent investigators could not reproduce these results and found that ultrasonography was inferior to mammography for the detection of early breast cancer masses.[120,121] In addition, ultrasonography could not reliably detect microcalcifications, the hallmark of intraductal carcinoma. Nonetheless, ultrasonography was very accurate in the diagnosis of cysts, eliminating the need for about 20% of the biopsies that had been performed in the past.[55]

Ultrasound was eventually recognized to be an important adjunct to mammography, but its role was primarily limited to determining whether nonpalpable masses were cystic or solid.[9,122,123] With the evolution of ultrasonographic technology, including the introduction of higher-resolution transducers and imaging protocols tailored for the breast, there has been a renewed interest in expanding the role of ultrasonography for the evaluation of breast diseases. Ultrasonography is an excellent method for guiding some interventional procedures.[4,124,125] Although ultrasonography is not recommended for breast cancer screening, there are reliable ultrasonographic criteria that can differentiate benign versus malignant solid masses.[11] In some practices, it is used to identify occult multicentric or bilateral disease in women with a mammographically or clinically evident breast carcinoma.[125] These newer roles for ultrasonography have not yet been widely accepted.[126]

Benign Masses

Criteria for differentiating benign from malignant solid masses with ultrasonography are of special interest. Ultrasonographic features suggesting benignity include absence of any malignant findings; ellipsoid shape or "parallel" (a length along the plane of the breast which is greater than the height of the mass); thin, echogenic pseudocapsule (circumscribed margins); hyperechogenicity (bright ultrasound echoes); homogeneous internal echoes; and enhanced echoes distal to the mass (Fig. 36-52).[11] Masses in this category consist of simple and mildly complicated cysts as well as benign solid masses, such as fibroadenomas. Since ultrasound is predominantly used in conjunction with diagnostic mammography, the findings of both are correlated for concordance.

Malignant Masses

Features in favor of malignancy include an irregular shape, indistinct margins, spiculation, microlobulation, "not parallel" to the surface of the breast (a height which is greater than the width of the lesion in the plane of the breast), hypoechogenicity, and shadowing (attenuation of echoes distal to the mass; Figs. 36-53 and 36-54).

Ultrasound can also be used to evaluate the integrity of silicone breast implants.[127] However, it is not as accurate as MRI for detecting implant ruptures.[128]

MAGNETIC RESONANCE IMAGING

The first reports of MRI for the evaluation of breast cancer were in the mid-1980s; they focused on breast tissue characterization using T1-weighted and T2-weighted images.[129] These early investigations were disappointing. In 1986, Heywang and coworkers first applied the use of MRI contrast agents to improve differentiation of benign from malignant lesions.[130,131] The results were encouraging; most malignant tumors showed enhancement, and most benign tumors did not. Numerous other investigators have confirmed the value of MRI with contrast agents.[132,133] Clinical investigations show a range of sensitivities from 88% to 100%.[134,135] However, the specificity of MRI may be relatively low, because many benign lesions show contrast enhancement.[131,132,136]

Two different methods for performing MRI of the breast for the assessment of breast tumors with gadolinium enhancement have emerged: (1) two-dimensional, medium resolution imaging during gadolinium enhancement and (2) three-dimensional high resolution imaging after gadolinium enhancement. Proponents of the two-dimensional approach believe that the most useful information concerning breast lesions is the time course of gadolinium enhancement; malignant tumors enhance more rapidly and more intensely than benign tumors. However, some investigators have shown an overlap in the enhancement patterns of malignant and benign tumors. Those advocating high-resolution three-dimensional imaging believe that it is more effective because whole-breast images are obtained, allowing for the detection of multicentric lesions. Furthermore, with three-dimensional whole-breast imaging, it is not necessary

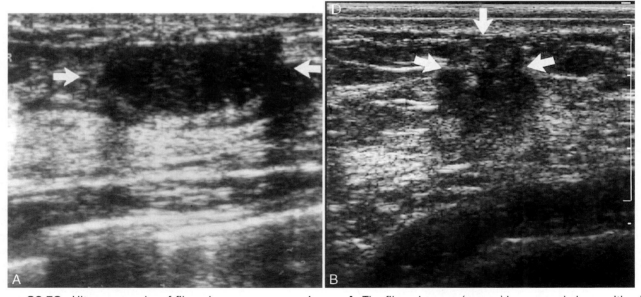

Figure 36-52   Ultrasonography of fibroadenoma versus carcinoma. **A,** The fibroadenoma *(arrows)* has an oval shape with width greater than height, circumscribed margins, and homogeneous low-level echoes. **B,** The invasive carcinoma *(arrows)* has an irregular shape, ill-defined margins, and heterogeneous echogenicity.

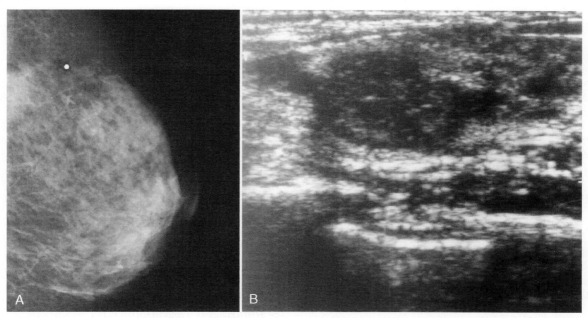

Figure 36-53 Ultrasonography of carcinoma. A 60-year-old woman felt a firm mass in her left breast. **A,** Mammogram shows a poorly defined density posterior to radiopaque BB placed at the site of the palpable mass. **B,** Ultrasonography shows a lobulated, partially ill-defined mass with heterogeneous low-level echoes. Biopsy revealed invasive ductal carcinoma.

to know the site of the abnormality prior to beginning the examination.

The potential advantages of MRI of the breast include (1) no ionizing radiation; (2) no limitations from breast density; (3) ability to localize lesions only seen on only one mammographic projection; (4) better characterization of lesions as benign or malignant; (5) improved

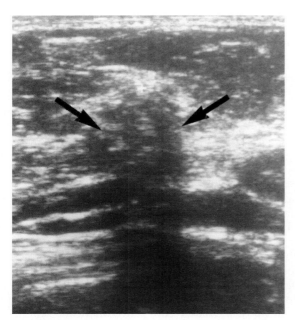

Figure 36-54 Ultrasonography of carcinoma. A 46-year-old woman noted a mass in her left breast. Mammograms were negative. Ultrasonography showed an irregular, poorly defined mass *(arrows)* with low-level internal echoes. Note the marked posterior echo attenuation ("posterior shadowing"). Biopsy revealed invasive ductal carcinoma.

evaluation of the extent of tumors, including multiple foci; and (6) surveillance of the postlumpectomy breast, which can be difficult to evaluate mammographically.

There are also a number of disadvantages associated with MRI: (1) cost; (2) unreliable depiction of microcalcifications; (3) lack of standardization of MRI sequences and methodologies used to image breast tumors; and (4) inability of some patients to complete an MRI scan because of claustrophobia or indwelling metal devices, such as pacemakers and aneurysm clips.

When evaluating breast disease with MRI, one should assess breast lesions with both dynamic imaging as well as high-resolution temporal and spatial imaging. If the breast tumor demonstrates contrast enhancement, then the morphology of the enhancement should be determined in a similar fashion of assessing the morphology of a breast lesion on mammography.

Typical Benign Findings

Benign breast lesions have been reported and described in the literature.[13,130–152] Classically, a benign breast tumor demonstrates a nonenhancing or slowly homogeneous enhancing kinetic curve pattern. In addition, the morphology of a benign tumor is also similar to that in mammography and ultrasound; tumors are typically round or oval with smooth, well-circumscribed, and well-defined margins. In addition, dark internal septations on MRI confer a more benign morphology. Fibroadenomas in postmenopausal women classically demonstrate a slow or nonenhancing round or oval mass with smooth, circumscribed margins. In a study of 57 patients, a 95% negative predictive value was reported[153] if nonenhancing internal septations were visualized within a morphologically benign appearing mass; nonenhancing septations seen within an irregular mass with spiculated margins suggest malignancy.

With regard to enhancement patterns, benign entities may demonstrate non-masslike regional or diffuse enhancement, homogeneous slow persistent enhancement, or no enhancement on MRI. However, that is not to say that benign tumors may not demonstrate rapid initial contrast enhancement. In fact, in our experience, some lymph nodes, almost all phyllodes tumors, and even occasional fibroadenomas (Fig. 36-55), especially those in younger women, have demonstrated rapid initial contrast enhancement. Furthermore, if the findings are symmetric in both breasts in a mirror-image pattern, it more likely represents a benign process.

Typical Malignant Findings

Malignant breast tumors have also been well described and evaluated in the literature. Again, both the morphology of the lesion and the enhancement pattern must be assessed. Classically, malignant breast tumors are identified as irregular masses with irregular or spiculated margins. This corresponds to their appearance on mammography.[135] But similar to the pitfalls in mammography, numerous breast cancers also appear as round or oval masses with smooth, circumscribed margins.[153]

With regard to dynamic enhancement patterns, breast cancers classically demonstrate rapid initial contrast rise with washout on delayed MRI. What this means is that the initial rate of rise of the kinetic curve can increase to levels three times its initial start point within 90 to 120 seconds of injection. It has also been reported that tumors with rim enhancement confer a higher suspicion for malignancy, with a positive predictive value of 86%.[153-155] With regard to washout, what this means is that there is marked decrease of the kinetic curve after 3 to 5 minutes during the delayed portion of the dynamic scan. Although the washout pattern has a high positive predictive value for malignancy, it certainly is not pathognomonic. Benign entities, such as lymph nodes and some fibroadenomas, have demonstrated the rapid washout pattern (Fig. 36-56).

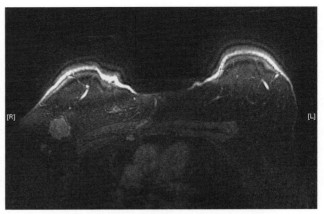

Figure 36-56 Magnetic resonance imaging scan of a breast carcinoma. Irregular bordered mass in the right axilla was found on pathology to be carcinoma.

Standardized Terminology for Magnetic Resonance Imaging Reports

Like the lexicon used to standardize mammography reports from different radiology facilities, the same format was applied to breast MRI, defined as the American College of Radiology BI-RADS. It includes terminology, imaging techniques, breast composition, evaluation of morphologic and kinetic curve patterns, impression, and recommendation. The lesion type, significant findings, and kinetic curve analysis are synthesized to arrive at the MR BI-RADS "Final Assessment." Identical to mammography assessment categories, they are: 0—Incomplete assessment; 1—Negative; 2—Benign findings; 3—Probably benign findings; 4—Suspicious abnormality; 5—Highly suggestive of malignancy; and 6—Known carcinoma (see Table 36-1).

Current Clinical Practice for Magnetic Resonance Imaging

The current guidelines for the application of breast MRI include the following: (1) imaging the augmented breast; (2) presurgical evaluation of the tumor size, extent of disease, and additional lesions (to assess multifocality, multicentricity, and bilaterality); (3) post–breast conserving-surgery and radiotherapy surveillance for residual or recurrent disease; (4) searching for unknown primary breast malignancy in a patient with malignant axillary lymphadenopathy; (5) further evaluation for inconclusive or negative mammography and ultrasound with suspicious clinical findings; (6) evaluation of tumor response to neoadjuvant chemotherapy; and (7) evaluation of nipple discharge.[156,157] Screening is recommended for women with BRCA1 and BRCA2 genetic mutation(s). In March 2007, the American Cancer Society guideline panel reviewed new evidence on MRI-based scientific studies published in peer-reviewed journals. The new recommendations include breast MRI screening for women with a risk of breast cancer of 20% to 30% and greater.[158]

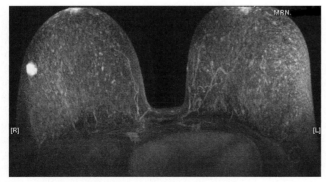

Figure 36-55 Magnetic resonance imaging scan of a fibroadenoma. Smooth bordered oval lesion in the right lateral breast was found on pathology to be a fibroadenoma. There are dark internal septations on the shown T2-weighted images.

DUCTOGRAPHY (GALACTOGRAPHY)

Ductography is the injection of contrast medium into the lactiferous ducts in an attempt to preoperatively determine the nature, location, and extent of lesions causing serous or bloody discharge. A serous or bloody discharge from the nipple may be caused by an intraductal papilloma (Fig. 36-57), "fibrocystic changes," duct ectasia, or carcinoma. Although bloody nipple discharge is usually associated with benign conditions, approximately 15% of cases are secondary to carcinoma.[159] Ductography is not useful in cases with discharge from multiple orifices, or with milky or greenish discharge.

During the procedure, the duct that is discharging is cannulated, and a small volume of water-soluble contrast material is injected. Mammograms are then taken in two projections, preferably with magnification mammography technique. When a filling defect is demonstrated, the ductogram may be repeated shortly before surgery using a mixture of methylene blue dye and contrast material. The blue dye identifies the abnormal duct, and the contrast medium verifies that the duct contains the filling defect.[160]

Ductography is effective in showing the cause of the discharge in almost all cases. Only half of the carcinomas demonstrated by filling defects on ductography are evident on conventional mammograms, and cytology is

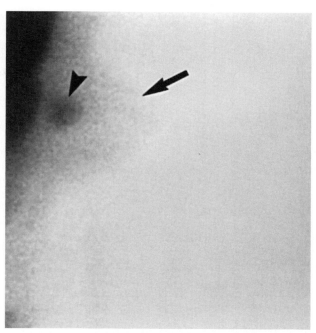

Figure 36-58 Sestamibi radionuclide imaging of the breast *(arrow)* reveals intense radionuclide uptake at the site of a breast carcinoma *(arrowhead)*. (Courtesy of Iraj Khalkhali, MD, Los Angeles, CA.)

even more unreliable in identifying malignant cells in the fluid from these cancers.[159]

Some surgeons believe that preoperative ductography allows them to do less radical surgery for serous or bloody nipple discharge.[161] Other surgeons prefer to go directly to solitary or major duct excision for bloody nipple discharge.

RADIONUCLIDE IMAGING

Another area of active investigation involves radionuclide scanning of the breast after the injection of radionuclide-labeled substances that concentrate in breast tumors. For example, tumor uptake has been identified on positron emission tomography after the injection of fluorine-18 2-deoxy-2-fluoro-D-glucose.[162] This agent also accumulates in axillary nodes, thus potentially indicating nodal status without surgery. Other investigators are scanning the breasts after the injection of ^{99m}Tc-sestamibi (2-methoxy isobutyl isonitril; Fig. 36-58).[163,164] Sestamibi has been reported to have a high sensitivity and high negative predictive value for breast carcinoma. The high negative predictive value of this agent could make it an important adjunct to mammography by potentially reducing the number of biopsies performed for benign findings. Additional studies are needed to determine cost-effectiveness and sensitivity and specificity in actual clinical populations.

Imaging-Guided Interventional Procedures

A variety of interventional procedures are guided by imaging. The most common of these is preoperative needle localization of nonpalpable lesions prior to

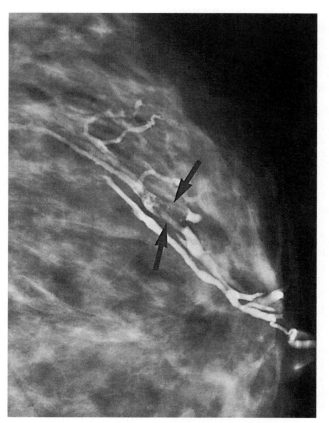

Figure 36-57 Ductogram demonstrating solitary papilloma. A 50-year-old woman presented with bloody discharge from the left nipple. A ductogram revealed a filling defect *(arrows)* in the discharging duct system. Surgery revealed a benign solitary papilloma at the site of the defect.

excisional biopsy. Fine needle aspiration cytology (FNAC) and CNB of the breast can also be performed under imaging guidance. In addition, ductography has been used in many practices for the purpose of determining the etiology of unilateral bloody or serous nipple discharge.

PREOPERATIVE NEEDLE LOCALIZATIONS

Imaging-guided needle localization is indicated prior to the surgical excision of any nonpalpable mammographic lesion. The purpose of needle localization is to ensure removal of a clinically occult lesion with the smallest possible breast deformity. Some variations on the needle localization method include: (1) a direct needle approach in which the tip of a hypodermic needle is inserted as close as possible to the mammographic abnormality and left in place when the patient goes to surgery (see Fig. 36-24A),[165] (2) a "spot" method in which methylene blue dye is injected into the breast tissue through a needle positioned near the mammographic abnormality,[166] and (3) a needle-wire method in which a malleable wire with a barbed or round end is positioned at the site of the abnormality (see Figs. 36-46B and 36-47).[167-169] The needle-wire method is most commonly used today.

The preoperative localization procedure begins with an evaluation of the abnormality that should include imaging in two orthogonal projections, usually craniocaudal and 90-degree lateral views. Using the initial films, the location of the lesion and the most appropriate approach to the lesion are determined. A mammogram is performed, with compression sustained while the film is being processed. Using the first film as a guide, the location of the lesion relative to a radiopaque alphanumeric grid or holes in the compression device is determined.

The needle is introduced through the skin and advanced to the approximate depth of the lesion. A second mammogram is performed to determine whether the needle is close enough to the lesion. If the needle placement is satisfactory, the modified compression plate is released. An orthogonal view is performed to evaluate the depth of the needle tip relative to the lesion. If the needle tip is too proximal or distal, the depth of the needle tip is adjusted. Once the needle tip is in the desired location, the wire is advanced through the needle until it is firmly in place. In the author's practice, the tip of the wire is positioned slightly posterior and distal to the lesion. The patient is sent to surgery either with the needle removed and a barbed-tip hookwire identifying the site of the lesion or with the needle anchored in place by a J-wire.

Specimen Radiography

Immediately after the surgeon has excised the biopsy specimen, radiographs of the specimen should be performed to verify that the nonpalpable lesion has been removed (see Fig. 36-46B).[170-172] In addition, specimen radiography can help the pathologist focus the histologic examination on the suspect area.

Immediately after inspection of the specimen radiograph and prior to sending the specimen to pathology, a pin or 25-gauge needle is inserted into the specimen at the exact site of the lesion. A second specimen radiograph with the pin or needle in place at the site of the lesion is sent to the pathologist along with the specimen. Methods for improving the quality of specimen radiographs include compression of the specimen and magnification mammography.[173] If the suspect lesion is not identified in the specimen radiograph, removal of more tissue is usually indicated.

Lesions containing microcalcifications deserve special consideration. The importance of mentioning the presence of the calcifications in the pathology report should be communicated to pathologists interpreting the breast biopsy. There are two reasons why microcalcifications present in the specimen radiograph might not be mentioned in the pathology report. First, the calcifications might not be seen by the pathologist because they are not in the sectioned tissue. Re-evaluation of other sections of the remaining tissue by the pathologist is warranted. Second, calcium oxalate calcifications may not be seen easily with hematoxylin-eosin staining, although they can be appreciated with polarized light.[174] If additional sections and polarized light fail to show calcifications in the histologic sections, radiography of the histologic paraffin blocks may disclose the location of the missing calcifications.[175] Additional sectioning can then be performed. Calcifications may also be lost during the preparation of the specimen; however, a review of the tissue specimens or the paraffin blocks should reveal some remaining calcifications.[176]

IMAGING-GUIDED NEEDLE BIOPSY

It is estimated that some 500,000 to 1,000,000 breast biopsies are performed each year in the United States.[48] This statistic translates to somewhere between 400,000 to 700,000 benign breast biopsies. In addition to tremendous costs, false-positive biopsies lead to unnecessary morbidity and are a barrier to women participating in breast-cancer screening projects.[109] Imaging-guided needle biopsy offers an attractive alternative to surgical biopsy for mammographically-detected abnormalities. Needle biopsy is generally less expensive than surgery, results in less morbidity, and leaves no scar. But is it accurate enough to replace surgery? In Europe, FNAC has reduced the costs of screening programs by greatly reducing the number of excisional biopsies performed.[177] Although FNAC has been less successful in the United States, CNB of the breast is gaining acceptance in many practices.

Needle biopsy of occult lesions can be guided by stereotactic mammography or ultrasonography. The modality chosen to guide the needle biopsy depends on (1) which technique best depicts the abnormality, (2) the location of the lesion within the breast, and (3) the operator's preferences. Stereotaxis uses the principle of triangulation to ascertain the exact location of an abnormality based on the shift in its position observed on two images taken at different angles off of the midline.[178] Stereotactic equipment includes add-on devices that are mounted on mammography units and dedicated stereotactic biopsy tables. With the add-on devices, the patient usually sits up during the procedure. Following the needle biopsy, the add-on stereotactic device is removed, and the mammography unit can be used for screening and diagnostic examinations. Using the dedicated stereotactic tables, the patient lies prone during the procedure with the breast suspended through an opening in the table. The dedicated tables are more expensive and can only be used for biopsy or localization procedures.

FINE NEEDLE ASPIRATION CYTOLOGY

FNAC of nonpalpable breast lesions has been very successful in some practices in the United States and Canada[4,179,180]; however, the method has not gained wide acceptance in these countries. Obstacles to the use of FNAC for mammographically detected abnormalities have included inadequate numbers of skilled cytopathologists to promote and validate the procedure, the variability in reported accuracy from one institution to another, the high rates of insufficient samples, the requirement for extremely accurate needle placement, and the medicolegal environment.[181,182] Even if adequate specimens are obtained with FNAC, a definitive diagnosis is not always possible, and it cannot differentiate in situ carcinoma from invasive breast carcinoma.

In some practices, high rates of insufficient specimens have been the major limitation to the use of FNAC for nonpalpable lesions, with insufficient rates as high as 54% reported.[183–186] Methods that can improve the results of FNAC for nonpalpable lesions include (1) more vigorous sampling of lesions, (2) onsite evaluation of specimens by a cytopathologist or a cytotechnologist, (3) exclusive use of stereotactic or ultrasound guidance for nonpalpable lesions, (4) a stereotactic equipment calibration program to ensure accurate targeting of lesions, and (5) verification of initial needle placement by stereotactic images prior to sampling the lesion.[181] Unfortunately, some of these methods also increase the cost of performing FNAC.

CORE NEEDLE BIOPSY

Several investigators believe that CNB of the breast is superior to FNAC because (1) the interpretation can be rendered by pathologists who do not have special training in cytopathology, (2) insufficient specimens are unusual, (3) it can usually differentiate in situ from invasive carcinoma, and (4) it can more completely characterize lesions.[8,187] CNB of the breast can be guided by stereotactic mammography or ultrasonography.

Vacuum-Assisted Devices

Limitations of traditional automated Tru-Cut (ATC) CNB include cases with insufficient samples to make a definitive diagnosis and problem histologies, such as a typical ductal hyperplasia and radial scar, where excisional biopsy is needed to rule out associated malignancy.[188–191] Vacuum-assisted devices (VADs) have been developed to improve tissue sampling by obtaining larger and more intact samples with only one insertion of the biopsy needle.[192] The most important contribution of VADs has been in the evaluation of calcifications, where cases of sampling errors or indeterminate pathology results are problematic. VAD tissue acquisition devices are available in 14 and 11 gauge sizes. Comparisons with ATC show improvements in most aspects, including few insufficient samples and discordant pathology. However, larger sample size has not reduced the incidence of carcinoma in situ found at excisional biopsy following a core biopsy diagnosis of atypical ductal hyperplasia (ADH).[193] VADs have recently been made available for ultrasound-guided biopsy. The exact benefits of ultrasound-guided biopsy remain to be determined.

Indications for Core Biopsy

Whereas there is general agreement that CNB is indicated when mammographic findings are suspect for malignancy (BI-RADS category 4), there are differences of opinion about the use of CNB for abnormalities that are probably benign (category 3) and highly suggestive of malignancy (category 5). Some investigators have asserted that probably benign lesions are good candidates for CNB, because needle biopsy of these lesions might uncover breast cancers when they are smaller and have a better prognosis.[194] However, the expected yield of breast cancers from cases with probably benign findings is very low.[50, 52] One recent report suggests that submitting the large number of women with probably benign findings to needle biopsy would undermine efforts to reduce the costs of screening mammography and could actually increase the overall costs of screening.[195] In the author's practice, CNB for probably benign findings is limited to those women who are too anxious to wait for a follow-up examination to confirm benignity. Only 2% of CNBs have been performed for probably benign findings, and none of these have revealed carcinoma.

Some investigators believe that CNB is inappropriate for lesions that are highly suggestive of malignancy. An example would be an irregular, spiculated, dense mass. Because malignancy is almost certain with such as a mass, the surgeon may choose to discuss treatment options with the patient based on the imaging findings and proceed directly to one-stage surgery. The one-stage procedure for nonpalpable masses that are highly suggestive of malignant lesions would include excision of the lesion, frozen section to confirm the diagnosis of malignancy, and definitive surgery once the frozen section is shown to be positive for cancer.

The one-stage operation reduces costs by eliminating a separate biopsy for tissue diagnosis.[196] Nevertheless, some surgeons routinely perform a two-stage procedure for lesions that are mammographically highly suggestive of malignancy. After a separate biopsy to confirm the diagnosis, these surgeons discuss treatment options with the patient and schedule definitive surgery. CNB is cost effective for lesions that are highly suggestive of malignancy only if a two-stage procedure is planned.

Analysis of Data and Management of Cases

It is important that physicians performing CNB collect and analyze their results in order to evaluate the effectiveness of the procedure. This means determining the number of true-positive, false-positives, true-negatives, and false-negatives. A true-positive CNB result is one that is interpreted to be intraductal or invasive carcinoma at CNB and confirmed to be either of these at subsequent surgery. A false-positive CNB is one that is incorrectly interpreted as showing carcinoma, and carcinoma is not found at excisional biopsy. Long-term follow-up is usually required to verify true negatives, but the exact length of follow-up required to verify a true negative is not yet standardized. Some investigators define long term follow-up as 1-year, whereas others define it as 2 years.

High risk lesions, such as lobular carcinoma in situ (LCIS) and ADH, are considered benign for statistical and medical audit purposes.[103,104] However, many physicians recommend open biopsy after CNB diagnosis of LCIS or ADH.[197] If ADH is diagnosed on CNB, an excisional biopsy is recommended because of the difficulty in differentiating ADH from intraductal carcinoma on the basis of a CNB.[198] In reported series, 50% of cases originally interpreted as ADH at CNB have turned out to be intraductal carcinoma at excisional biopsy.[198,199]

There are some contraindications to CNB. Certain mammographic findings indicate a condition best managed by complete excision. For example, if calcifications are few in number and not tightly clustered, CNB sampling errors are highly likely to occur. There are also limitations related to the location of the lesion or the size of the breast. A lesion very close to the skin or located in a very small breast may not be suitable for CNB because of the required throw of the needle. It may not be possible to visualize lesions adjacent to the chest wall on a stereotactic biopsy unit. If these lesions are not depicted on ultrasonography, they require excisional biopsy.

Staging and Follow-Up of Women with Breast Cancer

FOLLOW-UP OF THE CONSERVATIVELY TREATED BREAST

Follow-up evaluation after initial treatment with breast-conservation surgery, with or without adjuvant systemic therapy, consists of a mammogram prior to starting radiation therapy.[200] The preradiotherapy mammogram is most useful for women with extensive in situ (intraductal carcinoma) or the invasive carcinoma that coexists with an extensive intraductal component; these pathologic variants are often detectable by visible calcifications mammographically (Fig. 36-59).[85] Preoperative mammography and specimen radiography performed at the time of surgery are essential to document that calcifications were present and that calcifications were indeed removed. However, specimen radiography is not reliable in determining whether all of the tumor has been removed.[95]

It has been recommended that mammograms be performed at 6-month intervals for 2 years after lumpectomy and radiotherapy and annually thereafter.[59,201] On mammograms, recurrent carcinoma can be manifested by a

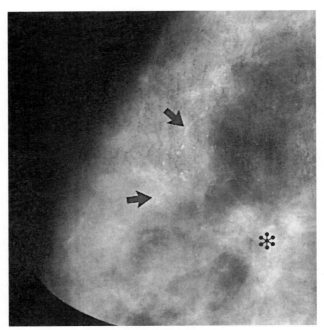

Figure 36-59 Recurrent breast carcinoma. Close-up of mammogram performed 3 years after lumpectomy shows calcifications (*arrows*) near the intramammary surgical scar (*asterisk*).

mass or calcifications (see Fig. 36-59). The importance of 6-month interval mammography is not universally accepted. More clinical investigation is needed to determine if annual mammography would be sufficient.[202]

FOLLOW-UP AFTER MASTECTOMY

For patients who are treated with mastectomy, routine imaging follow-up involves annual mammography of the contralateral breast. Mammography of the mastectomy site is not felt to have clinical utility since it does not increase the detection of locally recurrent disease.[203]

EVALUATION OF METASTASES FROM BREAST CANCER

The most common sites for distant metastases from breast carcinoma are the skeleton, lung, liver, and brain.[204,205] Several imaging examinations are available that can potentially identify metastases to these organs. Surveys of patients with breast cancer indicate that most of these patients prefer an intensive follow-up to detect asymptomatic disease, including metastases.[206] Surveys of physicians who take care of patients with breast cancer indicate that most of these physicians also favor intensive surveillance programs of patient with breast cancer who are asymptomatic.[207] However, for purposes of cost-effectiveness, there should be a reasonable anticipated yield and an expected effect on patient management and outcome when imaging examinations are ordered on asymptomatic patients with breast cancer.

Several large population-based studies have revealed that metastatic workups for stage I or stage II breast cancer are not cost-effective because of the low yield of the examination as well as the lack of a proven effect on management or survival.[208-210] The author's current policy is to limit imaging workups for metastatic disease to women with stage III carcinoma, in which (1) the tumor is greater than 5 cm and there are movable ipsilateral positive axillary nodes, (2) the invasive tumor is associated with positive ipsilateral axillary nodes fixed one to another or to other structures, or (3) the tumor has direct extension to the chest wall or skin.[208] These women receive a bone scan, chest radiographs, and, if liver function tests are abnormal, imaging of the liver.

Skeletal Metastases

Radionuclide scanning is more effective than conventional radiography for the detection of skeletal metastases because radionuclide scans have higher sensitivity and can survey the entire skeleton in one examination (Fig. 36-60).[211] Despite the low yield of bone scans in asymptomatic women with stage I or stage II breast carcinoma, many clinicians have continued to recommend baseline bone scans on the basis that they could be useful for comparison with subsequent scans performed if symptoms develop or if abnormal results are later obtained on a routine scan.[212] Routine baseline bone scans are unlikely to be useful in stage I or stage II disease in view of (1) the small number of patients who will later have positive scans and (2) evidence from long-term clinical trials indicating that earlier detection of metastases does not reduce overall mortality.[213-216] Furthermore, several studies have reported false-positive scans as a problem encountered when screening for metastases in asymptomatic patients.[216]

In the author's practice, ^{99m}Tc-diphosphonate whole-body radionuclide scans are performed on symptomatic patients or asymptomatic patients with stage III disease. Although bone scans are sensitive for the detection of

metastases, many benign conditions can result in abnormal scans. Correlation of clinical, radionuclide, and radiographic findings is important when imaging studies are performed. Therefore, unless the bone-scan findings are definitive for metastases, radiographs should be performed of symptomatic regions or localized areas of abnormal isotope accumulation. Breast metastases to the skeleton may show unusual radiographic manifestations, and it is important to be aware of these findings in order to avoid an incorrect diagnosis (Figs. 36-61 to 36-65). MRI can be useful when the findings of radionuclide scans and radiographs are discordant or indeterminate (Fig. 36-66).[217]

Lung Metastases

Because of its relatively low cost when compared to the other imaging modalities, conventional chest radiography is the most reasonable approach to (1) detection of unsuspected disease, (2) serve as a baseline for monitoring, and (3) be used for routine follow-up.[218] Signs of metastatic breast carcinoma include pulmonary nodules, adenopathy, lymphangitic spread, and pleural masses or effusions (Figs. 36-67 and 36-68). High-resolution computed tomography (CT) is the method of choice to evaluate equivocal findings on chest radiography and to identify additional nodules in positive cases (see Fig. 36-68).[219]

Investigators have questioned the use of routine chest radiography to detect intrathoracic metastases in asymptomatic patients with breast cancer, especially those with stage I disease, despite the relatively low cost of chest radiography. One problem is the low yield of routine chest radiographs in patients with stage I disease, reported at less than 0.5% in asymptomatic women who had routine chest x-rays after the diagnosis of stage I breast carcinoma.[213] Another problem is that

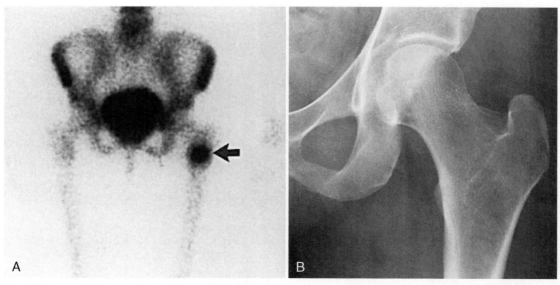

Figure 36-60 High sensitivity of radionuclide scans. Radionuclide scan was performed in a woman with diagnosed stage III breast carcinoma. **A**, ^{99m}Tc radionuclide bone scan shows abnormal area of intense radionuclide uptake *(arrow)* in the proximal left femur. Additional intense radionuclide activity in the bladder and iliac wings is normal. **B**, Radiograph shows no evidence of a lesion in the femur. Needle biopsy confirmed metastasis.

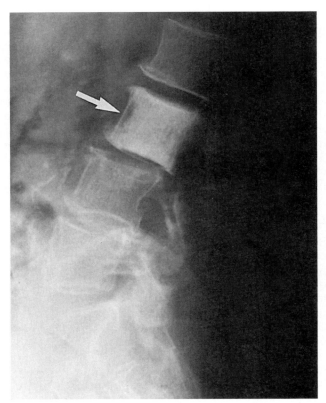

Figure 36-61   Blastic metastasis *(arrow)* to spine from breast carcinoma. "Ivory vertebrae" can also be seen in Paget's disease, lymphoma, and hemangioma.

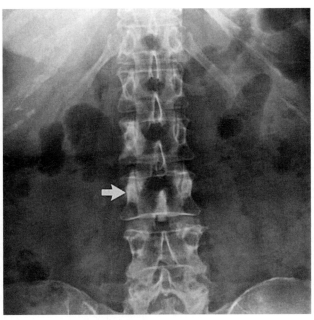

Figure 36-62   Breast cancer blastic metastasis *(arrow)* to pedicle of L3.

false-positive results from chest radiographs can lead to expensive diagnostic workups.[220,221] Two large randomized control studies failed to show a significant outcome benefit when routine chest radiography was used to detect metastases earlier in women of various stages of carcinoma.[209,213]

Liver Metastases

Both radionuclide scanning and ultrasonography have been used to detect liver metastases. Although liver metastases are not as common as lung or bone metastases, they are associated with a worse prognosis.[205] To be detected reliably by ^{99m}Tc-sulfur colloid liver scans, metastases generally must be greater than 2 cm in size.[222] Ultrasonography can also identify liver metastases 2 cm or larger, and it is often used to localize these lesions for biopsy or fine needle aspiration cytology.[223,224]

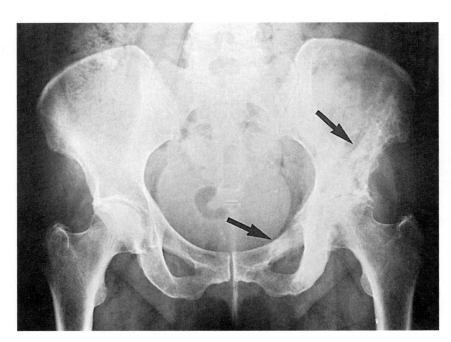

Figure 36-63   Mixed lytic and blastic metastases *(arrows)* to the left pelvis in a woman with breast cancer who was complaining of pain in the left hip.

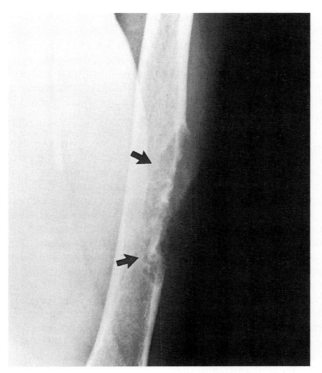

Figure 36-64 Lytic expansile cortical metastasis *(arrows)* in the femur of a woman with breast cancer. Metastases usually involve the medullary canal, and this is an unusual finding that can occur with breast cancer.

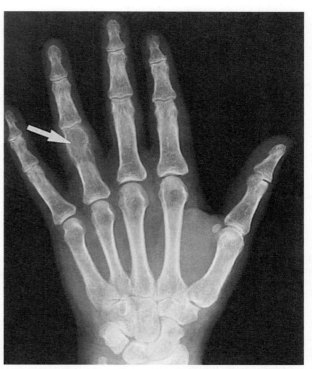

Figure 36-65 Lytic breast cancer metastasis *(arrow)* to proximal phalanx of hand. It is unusual for metastases to occur in the hands or feet, locations that suggest breast, lung, or renal carcinoma.

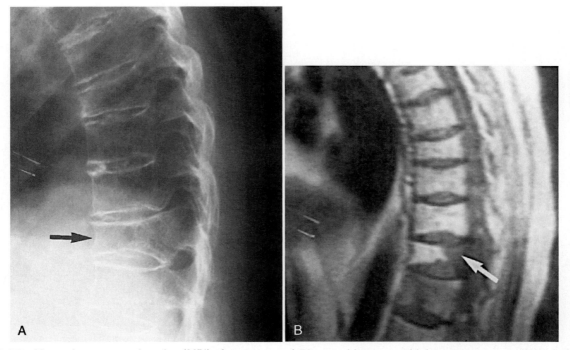

Figure 36-66 Magnetic resonance imaging (MRI) of metastases. A 70-year-old woman with breast cancer complained of back pain. **A,** Lateral radiograph of the thoracic spine reveals a compressed vertebra *(arrow)*, which could be due to osteoporosis or metastasis. **B,** Sagittal T1-weighted MRI reveals loss of normal high-signal intensity of the bone marrow in the posterior aspect of the compressed vertebra *(arrow)*, which is indicative of a metastatic lesion.

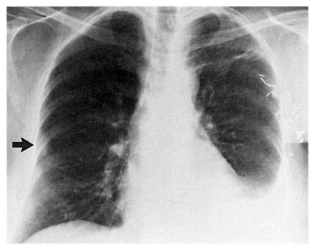

Figure 36-67 Chest radiograph of a woman with metastatic breast carcinoma shows metallic clips from previous left axillary node dissection, scarring of the left upper lobe, malignant left pleural effusion, and right pleural metastasis (arrow).

As with screening for bone and lung metastases, the yield of screening for liver metastases with radionuclide scans or ultrasonography is low. In one retrospective study of 234 asymptomatic patients with breast carcinoma at various stages, preoperative radionuclide liver scanning identified metastases in only 1% of cases.[225] Furthermore, in that study, 8 of 11 positive scans were eventually determined to be false positive. Another study showed that the yield for detecting metastases using radionuclide scans or ultrasonography was less than 0.5%.[213] Large randomized control studies have also failed to show a benefit from screening for liver metastases with ultrasonography.[209,210]

CT and MRI are more sensitive than radionuclide imaging or ultrasonography in the detection of liver metastases.[226] CT scans of the liver should be taken both before and after intravenous contrast injection, because some breast metastases may show up on one but not the other (Figs. 36-69 and 36-70). There is no evidence in the literature that routine imaging of the liver with either CT or MRI has clinical utility in asymptomatic patients with breast carcinoma.

Brain Metastases

Breast cancer is second only to lung carcinoma as a cause of intracerebral and orbital metastases, but few patients have brain metastases at the time of diagnosis of breast cancer, especially when the tumor is detected at stage I or II.[227,228] In CT examinations, brain metastases may be nodular or ring-shaped, single, or multiple. Brain metastases are usually associated with extensive edema and show varying amounts of enhancement with intravenous contrast agents.[229] One review of breast cancer patients at all stages having radionuclide brain scanning and CT found that imaging studies failed to identify brain metastases in the absence of neurologic symptoms.[230]

Because of its greater sensitivity, MRI has largely replaced CT for the detection and evaluation of brain lesions.[231] Contrast-enhanced MRI further increases the number of suspected cerebral metastases that can be detected.[227] Contrast-enhanced MRI has also proved superior to double-dose delayed CT for detection of brain metastases.[232] Despite these improvements in the sensitivity of imaging modalities for the detection of cerebral metastases, there are no studies suggesting any usefulness in routine imaging with any modality for the detection of cerebral metastases in asymptomatic women with breast carcinoma.

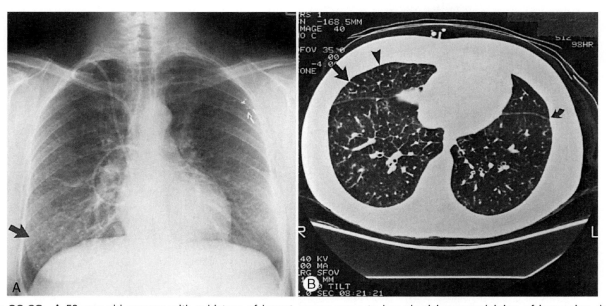

Figure 36-68 A 52-year-old woman with a history of breast cancer came to her physician complaining of increasing dyspnea. **A,** A chest radiograph in the hospital revealed changes from previous axillary node dissection and mild reticulation of the lungs, most conspicuous in the right lung base (arrow). **B,** High-resolution computed tomography, performed to evaluate for possible lymphangitic spread of breast cancer, shows prominence of the interlobular septae (curved arrow) and centrilobular interstitium (arrowhead). There is also subtle beading of the interfissural surfaces (arrow). These changes were considered diagnostic for lymphangitic carcinomatosis.

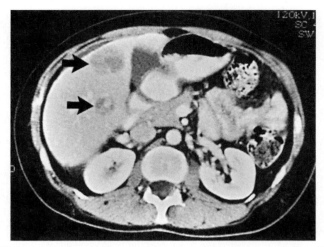

Figure 36-69 A 40-year-old woman with diagnosed stage III breast carcinoma had abnormal liver function tests. Intravenous contrast-enhanced computed tomography image of the liver shows two hypodense lesions *(arrows)* from metastatic breast carcinoma.

QUALITY-OF-LIFE ISSUES

One large randomized control study investigated quality of life issues related to surveillance for metastatic disease in breast cancer patients.[210] The results suggested that type of follow-up (i.e., intensive surveillance vs. routine clinical management) does not affect various dimensions of health-related quality of life. These dimensions include overall health and quality-of-life perception, emotional well-being, body image, social functioning, symptoms, and satisfaction with care. These parameters were almost identical between intensive and clinical-only surveillance groups. No comparison differences in any of the dimensions of quality-of-life issues were statistically significant between the two groups. Nonetheless, more than 70% of the breast cancer subjects said they wanted to be seen frequently by a physician and undergo diagnostic tests even if they were free of symptoms. This preference for intensive surveillance was not affected by whether the patient had been assigned to the intensive or minimalist follow-up regimen. Education of both physicians and patients seems to be an issue of extreme importance in order to provide cost-effective follow-up management of patients with breast cancer.

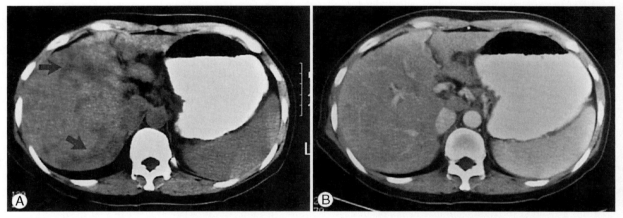

Figure 36-70 A 53-year-old woman with stage III breast carcinoma had abnormal liver function tests. **A,** Precontrast computed tomography (CT) scan of the liver shows inhomogeneous hypodense zones *(arrows)* caused by metastatic breast carcinoma. **B,** Intravenous contrast-enhanced CT scan of same patient. The vascular metastases were masked by the contrast agent.

REFERENCES

1. Bassett LW, Gold RH, Kimme-Smith C: History of the technical development of mammography in syllabus. In Haus AG, Yaffe MJ (eds): RSNA categorical course in physics, Oak Brook, IL, Radiological Society of North America, 1994.
2. Hendrick RE: Quality assurance in mammography: Accreditation, legislation, and compliance with quality assurance standards. Radiol Clin North Am 30:243, 1992.
3. American College of Radiology: Breast imaging reporting and data system (BI-RADS™), Reston, VA, American College of Radiology, 1993.
4. Fornage BD, Coan JD, David CL: Ultrasound-guided needle biopsy of the breast and other interventional procedures. Radiol Clin North Am 30:167, 1992.
5. Homer MJ: Localization of nonpalpable breast lesions: Technical aspects and analysis of 80 cases. AJR Am J Roentgenol 140:807, 1983.
6. Homer MJ, Smith TH, Safaii H: Prebiopsy needle localization. Radiol Clin North Am 30:139, 1992.
7. Jackson VP, Bassett LW: Stereotactic fine-needle aspiration biopsy for nonpalpable breast lesions. AJR Am J Roentgenol 154:1196, 1990.
8. Parker SH, et al: Stereotactic breast biopsy with a biopsy gun. Radiology 176:741, 1990.
9. Bassett LW, et al: Automated and hand-held breast ultrasound: Effect on patient management. Radiology 165:103, 1987.
10. Fornage BD: Percutaneous biopsies of the breast: State-of-the-art. Cardiovasc Intervent Radiol 14:29, 1991.

11. Stavros AT, et al: Solid breast nodules: Use of sonography to distinguish between benign and malignant lesions. Radiology 196:123, 1995.

12. Pisano ED et al: Diagnostic performance of digital versus film mammography for breast cancer screening. N Engl J Med 353: 1773–1783, 2005.

13. Heywang SH, et al: MR of the breast: Histopathologic correlation. Eur J Radiol 3:175–183, 1987.

14. Rosen EL, Eubank WB, Mankoff DA: FDG PET, PET/CT, and breast cancer imaging. Radiographics 27(suppl 1):S215, 2007.

15. Shen Y, Zelen M: Screening sensitivity and sojourn time from breast cancer early detection clinical trials: Mammograms and physical examinations. J Clin Oncol 19:3490, 2001.

16. Parker SL, et al: Cancer statistics, 1996. CA Cancer J Clin 65:5, 1996.

17. Seidman H, Stellman SD, Mushinski MH: A different perspective on breast cancer risk factors: Some implications for the nonattributable risk. CA Cancer J Clin 32:301, 1982.

18. Fletcher SW, et al: Report of the International Workshop on Screening for Breast Cancer. J Natl Cancer Inst 85:1644, 1993.

19. Tabár L, et al: Reduction in mortality from breast cancer after mass screening with mammography: Randomised trial from the Breast Cancer Screening Working Group of the Swedish National Board of Health and Welfare, Lancet 1:829, 1985.

20. Howe HL, et al: Annual report to the nation on the status of cancer (1973 through 1998), featuring cancers with recent increasing trends. J Natl Cancer Inst 93:824, 2001.

21. Baum M: Screening mammography re-evaluated. Lancet 355:751, 2000.

22. Peto R, et al: UK and USA breast cancer deaths down 25% in year 2000 at ages 20–69 years. Lancet 355:1822, 2000.

23. Blanks RG, et al: Effect of NHS breast screening programme on mortality from breast cancer in England and Wales, 1990–8: Comparison of observed with predicted mortality. BMJ 321:665, 2000.

24. Smart CR, et al: Benefit of mammography screening in women ages 40–49 years. Cancer 75:1619, 1995.

25. Thurfjell EL, Lindgren JAA: Breast cancer survival rates with mammographic screening: Similar favorable survival rates for women younger and those older than 50 years. Radiology 201:421, 1996.

26. American College of Radiology (ACR): Standards for the performance of diagnostic mammography and problem-solving breast evaluation [adopted by the ACR Council 1994] in ACR Digest of Official Actions. Reston, VA, American College of Radiology, 1994.

27. Sickles EA, et al: Mammographic screening: How to operate successfully at low cost. Radiology 160:95, 1986.

28. General Accounting Office: Screening mammography: Low cost services do not compromise quality. Washington, DC, General Accounting Office, 1990.

29. Bassett LW, Gold RH: Breast radiography using the oblique projection. Radiology 149:585, 1983.

30. Helvie MA, et al: Breast thickness on routine mammograms: Effect on image quality and radiation dose. AJR Am J Roentgenol 163: 1371, 1994.

31. Jackson VP, Lex AM, Smith DJ: Patient discomfort during screen-film mammography. Radiology 168:421, 1988.

32. Stomper PC, et al: Is mammography painful: A multicenter patient study. Arch Intern Med 148:521, 1988.

33. American College of Radiology Committee on Quality Assurance in Mammography: Mammography quality control. Reston, VA, American College of Radiology, 1992.

34. Berkowitz JE, Gatewood MB, Gayler BW: Equivocal mammographic findings: Evaluation with spot compression. Radiology 171:369, 1989.

35. Faulk RM, Sickles EA: Efficacy of spot compression-magnification and tangential views in mammographic evaluation of palpable breast masses. Radiology 185:87, 1992.

36. Feig SA: Importance of supplementary mammographic views to diagnostic accuracy. AJR Am J Roentgenol 151:40, 1988.

37. Feig SA: Breast masses: Mammographic and sonographic evaluation. Radiol Clin North Am 30:67, 1992.

38. Feig SA, Yaffe M: Digital imaging systems. In Basset LW et al (eds): Diagnosis of diseases of the breast. Philadelphia, WB Saunders, 1996.

39. Fajardo LL, et al: Detection of breast abnormalities on teleradiology transmitted mammograms. Invest Radiol 25:1111, 1990.

40. Thurfjell EL, Lernevall KA, Taube AAS: Benefit of independent double reading in a population-based mammography screening program. Radiology 191:241, 1994.

41. Vyborny CJ: Can computers help radiologists read mammograms? Radiology 191:315, 1994.

42. Vyborny CJ, Giger ML: Computer vision and artificial intelligence in mammography. AJR Am J Roentgenol 162:699, 1994.

43. Shtern F: Digital mammography and related technologies: A perspective from the National Cancer Institute. Radiology 183:629, 1992.

44. D'Orsi CJ, Kopans DB: Mammographic feature analysis. Semin Roentgenol 28:204, 1993.

45. American College of Radiology: Breast imaging reporting and data system (BI-RADS), 4th ed. Reston, VA, American College of Radiology, 2003.

46. McNicholas MM, et al: Pain and increased mammographic density in postmenopausal women. AJR Am J Roentgenol 163:311, 1994.

47. Gold RH, Montgomery CK, Rambo ON: Significance of margination of benign and malignant infiltrative mammary lesions: Roentgenologic-pathologic correlation. AJR Am J Roentgenol 118: 881, 1973.

48. Hall FM, et al: Nonpalpable breast lesions: Recommendations for biopsy based on suspicion of carcinoma at mammography. Radiology 167:353, 1988.

49. Moskowitz M: The predictive value of certain mammographic signs in screening for breast cancer. Cancer 51:1007, 1983.

50. Sickles EA: Nonpalpable, circumscribed, noncalcified solid breast masses: Likelihood of malignancy based on lesion size and age of patient. Radiology 192:439, 1994.

51. Brenner RJ, Sickles EA: Acceptability of periodic follow-up as an alternative to biopsy for mammographically detected lesions interpreted as probably benign, Radiology 171:645, 1989.

52. Sickles EA: Periodic mammographic follow-up of probably benign lesions: Results in 3,184 consecutive cases. Radiology 179:463, 1991.

53. Jackson VP, et al: Diagnostic importance of radiographic density of noncalcified breast masses: Analysis of 91 lesions. AJR Am J Roentgenol 157:25, 1991.

54. Lanyi M: Pathogenesis, pathophysiology, and composition of breast calcifications. In Lanyi M (ed): Diagnosis and differential diagnosis of breast calcifications, New York, Springer-Verlag, 1986.

55. Hilton SV, et al: Real-time breast sonography: Application in 300 consecutive patients. AJR Am J Roentgenol 147:479, 1986.

56. Brenner RJ, et al: Spontaneous regression of interval benign cysts of the breast. Radiology 193:365, 1994.

57. Crothers JG, et al: Fibroadenolipoma of the breast. Br J Radiol 48:191, 1985.

58. Bassett LW, Gold RH, Mirra JM: Nonneoplastic breast calcifications in lipid cysts: Development after excision and primary irradiation. AJR Am J Roentgenol 138:335, 1981.

59. Mendelson EB: Evaluation of the postoperative breast. Radiol Clin North Am 30:107, 1992.

60. Tabár L, Dean PB: Stellate lesions. In Tabár L, Dean PB (eds): Teaching atlas of mammography. New York, Thieme Stratton, 1985.

61. Orel SG, et al: Radial scar with microcalcifications: Radiologic-pathologic correlation. Radiology 183:479, 1992.

62. Kopans DB, Meyer JE, Grabbe J: Dermal deposits mistaken for breast calcifications. Radiology 149:592, 1983.

63. Sickles EA, Galvin HB: Breast arterial calcifications in association with diabetes mellitus: Too weak a correlation to have clinical utility. Radiology 171:577, 1989.

64. Bassett LW: Mammographic analysis of calcifications. Radiol Clin North Am 30:93, 1992.

65. Bassett LW, Gold RH, Cove HC: Mammographic spectrum of traumatic fat necrosis: The fallibility of "pathognomonic" signs of carcinoma. AJR Am J Roentgenol 130:119, 1978.

66. Sickles EA, Abele JS: Milk of calcium within tiny benign breast cysts. Radiology 141:655, 1981.

67. World Health Organization: Histological typing of breast tumors, vol 2. Geneva, World Health Organization, 1981.

68. Leibman AJ, Lewis M, Kruse B: Tubular carcinoma of the breast. AJR Am J Roentgenol 160:263, 1993.

69. Meyer JE, et al: Medullary carcinoma of the breast: Mammographic and US appearance. Radiology 170:79, 1989.
70. Mitnick JS, et al: Invasive papillary carcinoma of the breast: Mammographic appearance. Radiology 177:803, 1990.
71. Czernobilsky B: Intracystic carcinoma of the female breast. Surg Gynecol Obstet 124:93, 1967.
72. Helvie MA, et al: Invasive lobular carcinoma: Imaging features and clinical detection. Invest Radiol 28:202, 1993.
73. Hilleran DJ, et al: Invasive lobular carcinoma: Mammographic findings in a 10-year experience. Radiology 178:149, 1991.
74. Sickles EA: The subtle and atypical mammographic features of invasive lobular carcinoma. Radiology 178:25, 1991.
75. Toombs BD, Kalisher L: Metastatic disease to the breast: Clinical, pathologic, and radiographic features. AJR Am J Roentgenol 129: 673, 1977.
76. Bohman LG, et al: Breast metastases from extramammary malignancies. Radiology 144:309, 1982.
77. Powell RW, McSweeney MB, Wilson C: X-ray calcifications as the only basis for breast biopsy. Ann Surg 197:555, 1983.
78. Page DL, Anderson TJ (eds): Diagnostic histopathology of the breast. Edinburgh, Churchill Livingstone, 1987.
79. Betsill WL, et al: Intraductal carcinoma: Long-term follow-up after treatment by biopsy alone. JAMA 239:1863, 1978.
80. Page DL, et al: Intraductal carcinoma of the breast: Follow-up after biopsy only. Cancer 49:751, 1982.
81. Lagios MD: Duct carcinoma in situ. Surg Clin North Am 70:853, 1990.
82. Holland R, et al: The presence of an extensive intraductal component following a limited resection correlates with prominent residual disease in the remainder of the breast. J Clin Oncol 8:113, 1990.
83. Holland R, et al: Clinical practice: Extent distribution, and mammographic/histological correlations of breast ductal carcinoma in situ. Lancet 335:519, 1990.
84. Paulus DD: Conservative treatment of breast cancer: Mammography in patient selection and follow-up. AJR Am J Roentgenol 143:483, 1984.
85. Dershaw DD: Mammography in patients with breast cancer treated by breast conservation (lumpectomy with or without radiation). AJR Am J Roentgenol 164:309, 1995.
86. Dershaw DD, Abramson A, Kinne DW: Ductal carcinoma in situ: Mammographic findings and clinical implications. Radiology 170:411, 1989.
87. Stomper PC, Connolly JL: Ductal carcinoma in situ of the breast: Correlation between mammographic calcifications and tumor subtype. AJR Am J Roentgenol 159:483, 1992.
88. Kinkel K, et al: Focal areas of increased opacity in ductal carcinoma in situ of the comedo type: Mammographic-pathologic correlation. Radiology 192:443, 1994.
89. Boyages J, et al: Factors associated with local recurrence as a first site of failure following the conservation treatment of early breast cancer. Recent Results Cancer Res 115:92, 1989.
90. Eberlein TJ, et al: Predictors of local recurrence following conservative breast surgery and radiation therapy: The influence of tumor size. Arch Surg 125:771, 1990.
91. Osteen RT, et al: Early breast cancer: Predictors of breast recurrence for patients treated with conservative surgery and radiation therapy. Radiother Oncol 19:29, 1990.
92. Schnitt SJ, et al: Pathologic findings on reexcision of the primary site in breast cancer patients considered for treatment by primary radiation therapy. Cancer 59:675, 1987.
93. Vicini FA, et al: Recurrence in the breast following conservative surgery and radiation therapy for early-stage breast cancer. J Natl Cancer Inst Monogr 11:33, 1992.
94. Stomper PC, Margolin FR: Ductal carcinoma in situ: The mammographer's perspective. AJR Am J Roentgenol 162:585, 1994.
95. Graham RA, et al: The efficacy of specimen radiography in evaluating the surgical margins of impalpable breast carcinoma. AJR Am J Roentgenol 162:33, 1994.
96. Lagios MD, et al: Duct carcinoma in situ: Relationship of extent of noninvasive disease to the frequency of occult invasion, multicentricity, lymph node metastases, and short term treatment failures. Cancer 50:1309, 1982.
97. Gluck BS, et al: Microcalcifications on postoperative mammograms as an indicator of adequacy of tumor excision. Radiology 188:469, 1993.
98. Sickles EA: Mammographic features of 300 consecutive nonpalpable breast cancers. AJR Am J Roentgenol 146:661, 1986.
99. Kopans DB, et al: Asymmetric breast tissue. Radiology 171:639, 1989.
100. Adler DD, Rebner M, Pennes DR: Accessory breast tissue in the axilla. Radiology 163:709, 1987.
101. Sickles EA: The spectrum of breast asymmetries: Imaging features, work-up, management. Radiol Clin North Am 45:765, 2007.
102. Bassett LW, Shayestehfar B, Hirbawi I: Obtaining previous mammograms for comparison: Usefulness and costs. AJR Am J Roentgenol 163:1083, 1994.
103. Bassett LW, et al: Clinical Practice Guideline No 13. AHCPR Publication No. 95-0632. Rockville, MD, Agency for Health Care Policy and Research, Public Health Service, US Department of Health and Human Services, 1994.
104. Kalisher L, Chu AM, Peyster RG: Clinicopathological correlation of xeroradiography in determining involvement of metastatic axillary nodes in female breast cancer. Radiology 121:333, 1976.
105. Gisvold JJ, et al: Breast biopsy: A comparative study of stereotaxically guided core and excisional techniques. AJR Am J Roentgenol 162:815, 1994.
106. Meyer JE, et al: Occult breast abnormalities: Percutaneous preoperative needle localization. Radiology 50:335, 1984.
107. Rasmussen OS, Seerup A: Preoperative radiographically guided wire marking of nonpalpable breast lesions. Acta Radiol Diagn (Stockh) 25:13, 1984.
108. Moskowitz M: Impact of a priori medical decisions on screening for breast cancer. Radiology 171:605 1989.
109. Howard J: Using mammography for cancer control: An unrealized potential. CA Cancer J Clin 33:33, 1987.
110. Cyrlak D: Induced costs of low-cost screening mammography. Radiology 68:661, 1988.
111. Linver MN, et al: The mammography audit: A primer for the mammography quality standards act (MQSA). AJR Am J Roentgenol 165:19, 1995.
112. Murphy WA, Destouet JM, Monsees BS: Professional quality assurance for mammography screening programs. Radiology 175:319, 1990.
113. Sickles EA, et al: Medical audit of a rapid-throughput mammography screening practice: Methodology and results of 27,114 examinations. Radiology 175:323, 1990.
114. Linver MN: The medical audit: Statistical basis of clinical outcomes analysis. In Bassett LW, Jackson VP, Fu KL, Fu YS (eds): Diagnosis of disease of the breast. 2005, pp 135–148.
115. Wild JJ, Neal D: The use of high-frequency ultrasonic waves for detecting changes of texture in the living tissue. Lancet 1:655, 1951.
116. Jellins J, et al: Ultrasonic gray scale visualization of breast disease. Ultrasound Med Biol 1:393, 1975.
117. Kobayashi T: Diagnostic ultrasound in breast cancer: Analysis of retrotumorous echo patterns correlated with sonic attenuation by cancerous connective tissue. J Clin Ultrasound 7:471, 1979.
118. Cole-Beuglet C, et al: Ultrasound mammography: A comparison with radiographic mammography. Radiology 139:693, 1981.
119. Cole-Beuglet C, et al: Ultrasound analysis of 104 primary breast carcinomas classified according to histopathologic type. Radiology 147:191, 1983.
120. Kopans DB, Meyer JE, Lindfors KK: Whole-breast ultrasound imaging: Four-year follow-up. Radiology 157:505, 1985.
121. Sickles EA, Filly RA, Callen PW: Breast cancer detection with sonography and mammography: Comparison using state of the art equipment. AJR Am J Roentgenol 140:843, 1983.
122. Feig SA: The role of ultrasound in a breast imaging center. Semin Ultrasound CT MR 10:90, 1989.
123. Sickles EA, Filly RA, Callen PW: Benign breast lesions: Ultrasound detection and diagnosis. Radiology 151:467, 1984.
124. Evans WP: Fine-needle aspiration cytology and core biopsy of nonpalpable breast lesions. Curr Opin Radiol 4:130, 1992.
125. Gordon PB, Goldenberg LS: Malignant breast masses detected only by ultrasound: A retrospective review. Cancer 76:626, 1995.

126. Jackson VP: Management of solid breast nodules: What is the role of sonography? Radiology 196:14, 1995.

127. DeBruhl ND, et al: Silicone breast implants: US evaluation. Radiology 189:95, 1993.

128. Gorczyca DP, et al: Silicone breast implant ruptures in an animal model: Comparison of mammography, MR imaging, US and CT. Radiology 190:227, 1994.

129. Turner DA, Alcorn FS, Adler YT: Nuclear magnetic resonance in the diagnosis of breast cancer. Radiol Clin North Am 26:673, 1988.

130. Heywang SH, et al: MR imaging of the breast using gadolinium-DTPA. J Comput Assist Tomogr 10:199, 1986.

131. Heywang-Kobrunner SH: Contrast-enhanced MRI of the breast—overview after 1250 patient examinations. Electromedica 2:43, 1993.

132. Harms SE, et al: Fat-suppressed three-dimensional MR imaging of the breast. Radiographics 13:247, 1993.

133. Kaiser WA, Zeitler E: MR imaging of the breast: Fast imaging sequences with and without Gd-DTPA, Radiology 170:681, 1989.

134. Lewis-Jones HG, Whitehouse GH, Leinster SJ: The role of MRI in the assessment of local recurrent breast carcinoma. Clin Radiol 43:197, 1991.

135. Orel SG, et al: Suspicious breast lesions: MR imaging with radiologic-pathologic correlation. Radiology 190:485, 1994.

136. Harms SE, et al: MR imaging of the breast with rotating delivery of excitation off resonance: Clinical experience with pathologic correlation. Radiology 186:493, 1993.

137. Alcorn FS, et al: Magnetic resonance imaging in the study of the breast. Radiographics 5:631, 1985.

138. Heywang SH, et al: MR imaging of the breast using gadolinium-DTPA. J Comput Assist Tomogr 10:199, 1986.

139. Heywang SH, et al: MR imaging of the breast with Gd-DTPA: Use and limitations. Radiology 171:9, 1989.

140. Heywang-Kobrunner SH: Contrast-enhanced magnetic resonance imaging of the breast. Invest Radiol 29:94, 1994.

141. Heywang-Kobrunner SH: Contrast-enhanced MRI of the breast—overview after 1250 patient examinations. Electromedica 2:43, 1993.

142. Heywang-Kobrunner SH, et al: Contrast-material enhanced MRI of the breast in patients with postoperative scarring and silicon implants. J Comput Assist Tomogr 14:348, 1990.

143. Heywang-Kobrunner SH, et al: Contrast-enhanced MRI of the breast after limited surgery and radiation therapy. J Comput Assist Tomogr 17:891, 1993.

144. Kaiser WA: MRM promises earlier breast cancer diagnosis. Diagn Imaging Int 11:44, 1992.

145. Merchant TE, et al: Clinical magnetic resonance spectroscopy of human breast disease. Invest Radiol 26:1053, 1991.

146. Murphy WA, Gohagan JK: Breast. In Stark DD, Bradley WG Jr (eds): Magnetic resonance imaging. St. Louis, MO, Mosby, 1987, pp 861–886.

147. Partain CL, et al: Magnetic resonance imaging of the breast: Functional T1 and three-dimensional imaging. Cardiovasc Intervent Radiol 8:292, 1986.

148. Pierce WB, et al: Three-dimensional gadolinium-enhanced MR imaging of the breast: Pulse sequence with fat suppression and magnetization transfer contrast. Radiology 181:757, 1991.

149. Revel D, et al: Gd-DTPA contrast enhancement and tissue differentiation in MR imaging of experimental breast carcinoma. Radiology 158:319, 1986.

150. Rubens D, et al: Gadopentetate dimeglumin-enhanced chemical-shift MR imaging of the breast. AJR 157:267, 1991.

151. Stelling CB, et al: Prototype coil for magnetic resonance imaging of the female breast. Radiology 154:457, 1985.

152. Hochman, MG, et al: Fibroadenomas: MR imaging appearances with radiologic-histopathologic correlation. Radiology 204:123, 1997.

153. Nunes LW, Schnall MD, Orel SG: Update of breast MR imaging architectural interpretation model. Radiology 219:484, 2001.

154. Sherif H, Mahfouz AE, Oellinger H, et al: Peripheral washout sign on contrast-enhanced MR images of the breast. Radiology 205:209, 1997.

155. Matsubayashi R, Matsuo Y, Edakuni G, et al: Breast masses with peripheral rim enhancement on dynamic contrast-enhanced MR images: Correlation of MR findings with histologic features and expression of growth factors. Radiology 217:841, 2000.

156. Harms SE, et al: Technical report of the International Working Group on Breast MRI. J Magn Reson Imaging 10:979, 1999.

157. Kneeshaw PJ, Turnbull LW, Drew PJ: Current applications and future direction of MR mammography. Br J Cancer 88:4, 2003.

158. Saslow D, et al: American Cancer Society guidelines for breast screening with MRI as an adjunct to mammography. CA Cancer J Clin 57:75, 2007.

159. Tabár L, Dean PB, Péntek Z: Galactography: The diagnostic procedure of choice for nipple discharge. Radiology 149:31, 1983.

160. Threatt B, Appleman HD: Mammary duct injection. Radiology 108:71, 1973.

161. Cardenosa H, Doudna C, Eklund GW: Ductography of the breast: Technique and findings. AJR Am J Roentgenol 162:1081, 1994.

162. Adler LP, et al: Evaluation of breast masses and axillary lymph nodes with (F-18) 2-deoxy-2-fluoro-D-glucose PET. Radiology 187:743 1993.

163. Khalkhali I, et al: Scintimammography: The complementary role of Tc-99m sestamibi prone breast imaging for the diagnosis of breast carcinoma. Radiology 196:421, 1995.

164. Khalkhali I, et al: Prone scintimammography in patients with suspicion of carcinoma of the breast. J Am Coll Surg 178:491, 1994.

165. Threatt B, et al: Percutaneous needle localization of clustered microcalcifications prior to biopsy. AJR Am J Roentgenol 121:829, 1974.

166. Egan JF, Sayler CB, Goodman MJ: A technique for localizing occult breast lesions. CA Cancer J Clin 26:32, 1976.

167. Homer MJ: Nonpalpable breast lesion localization using a curved-end retractable wire. Radiology 157:259, 1985.

168. Kopans DB, Meyer JE: Versatile spring hookwire breast lesion localizer. AJR Am J Roentgenol 138:586, 1982.

169. Kwasnik EM, Sadowsky NL, Vollman RW: An improved system for surgical excision of needle-localized nonpalpable breast lesions. Am J Surg 154:476, 1987.

170. Bauermeister DE, Hall MH: Specimen radiography: A mandatory adjunct to mammography. Am J Clin Pathol 59:782, 1973.

171. Gallager HS: Breast specimen radiography: Obligatory, adjuvant and investigative. Am J Clin Pathol 64:759, 1975.

172. Stomper PC, et al: Efficacy of specimen radiography of clinically occult noncalcified breast lesions. AJR Am J Roentgenol 151:43, 1988.

173. D'Orsi CJ: Management of the breast specimen. Radiology 194:297, 1995.

174. Surratt JT, Monsees BS, Mazoujian G: Calcium oxalate microcalcifications in the breast. Radiology 181:141, 1991.

175. Rebner M, et al: Paraffin tissue block radiography: Adjunct to breast specimen radiography. Radiology 173:695, 1989.

176. D'Orsi CJ, et al: Breast specimen microcalcification: Radiographic validation and pathologic-radiologic correlation. Radiology 280:396, 1991.

177. Azevado E, Svane G, Aver G: Stereotactic fine needle biopsy in 2594 mammographically-detected nonpalpable lesions. Lancet 1:1033, 1989.

178. Hendrick RE, Parker SH: Stereotaxic imaging in syllabus: RSNA categorical course in physics. Chicago, Radiological Society of North America, 1993.

179. Gordon PB, Goldenberg SL, Chan NH: Solid breast lesions: Diagnosis with US-guided fine-needle aspiration biopsy. Radiology 189:573, 1993.

180. Mitnick J, et al: Stereotaxic localization for fine-needle aspiration breast biopsy. Arch Surg 126:1137, 1991.

181. Hayes MK, et al: Mammographically-guided fine-needle aspiration cytology of the breast: Reducing the rate of insufficient specimens. AJR Am J Roentgenol 167:381, 1996.

182. Masood S: Occult breast lesions and aspiration biopsy: A new challenge. Diagn Cytopathol 9:613, 1993.

183. Helvie MA, et al: Radiographically guided fine-needle aspiration of nonpalpable breast lesions. Radiology 174:657, 1990.

184. Jackson VP: The status of mammographically-guided fine needle aspiration biopsy of nonpalpable breast lesions. Radiol Clin North Am 30:139, 1992.

185. Layfield L, et al: Mammographically guided fine-needle aspiration biopsy of nonpalpable breast lesions. Cancer 68:2007, 1991.

186. Löfgren M, Andersson I, Lindholm K: Stereotactic fine-needle aspiration for cytologic diagnosis of nonpalpable breast lesions. AJR Am J Roentgenol 154:1191, 1990.
187. Elvecrog EL, Lechner MC, Nelson MJ: Nonpalpable breast lesions: Correlation of stereotaxic large-core needle biopsy and surgical biopsy results. Radiology 188:453, 1993.
188. Bassett LW, et al: Stereotactic breast CNB: Report of the Joint Task Force of ACT, ACS, COAP. CA Cancer J Clin 166:341, 1997.
189. Brenner RJ, et al: Percutaneous CNB: Effect of operator experience and number of samples on accuracy. AJR Am J Roentgenol 166: 341, 1996.
190. Dershaw DD, et al: Nondiagnostic stereo CNB: Results of rebiopsy. Radiology 204:485, 1996.
191. Jackman RJ, et al: Atypical ductal hyperplasia diagnosed at stereotactic breast biopsy: Improved reliability with 14-guage, directional, vacuum-assisted biopsy. Radiology 204:485, 1997.
192. Parker SH, Klaus AJ: Performing CNB with a directional, vacuum-assisted biopsy instrument. Radiographics 17:1233, 1997.
193. Philpotts LE, et al: Comparison of rebiopsy rates after stereotactic core needle biopsy of the breast with 11-G vacuum suction probe vs. 14-G automatic gun. AJR Am J Roentgenol 172:683, 1999.
194. Parker SH: When is core biopsy really core? Radiology 185:641, 1991.
195. Lindfors KK, Rosenquist CJ: Needle core biopsy guided with mammography: A study of cost-effectiveness. Radiology 190:217, 1994.
196. Scanlon EF: The case for and against two-step procedures for the surgical treatment of breast cancer. Cancer 53:677, 1984.
197. Reynolds HE: Core needle biopsy of challenging benign breast conditions: A comprehensive literature review. AJR Am J Roentgenol 174:1245, 2000.
198. Jackman RJ, et al: Stereotaxic large-core needle biopsy of 450 nonpalpable breast lesions with surgical correlation in lesions with cancer or atypical hyperplasia. Radiology 193:91, 1994.
199. Liberman L, et al: Atypical ductal hyperplasia diagnosed at stereotaxic core biopsy of breast lesions: An indication for surgical biopsy. AJR Am J Roentgenol 164:1111, 1995.
200. Love SM, McGuigan KA, Chap L: The Revlon/UCLA Breast Center practice guidelines for the treatment of breast disease. Cancer J 2:2, 1996.
201. Winchester DP, Cox JD: Standards for breast-conservation treatment. CA Cancer J Clin 42:134, 1992.
202. Orel SG, et al: Breast cancer recurrence after lumpectomy and irradiation: Role of mammography in detection. Radiology 183:201, 1992.
203. Fajardo LL, Roberts CC, Hunt KR: Mammographic surveillance of breast cancer patients: Should the mastectomy site be imaged? AJR Am J Roengentol 161:953, 1993.
204. Jain S, et al: Patterns of metastatic breast cancer in relation to histologic type, Eur J Cancer 29:2155, 1993.
205. Patanaphan V, Salazar OM, Risco R: Breast cancer: Metastatic patterns and their prognosis. South Med J 81:1109, 1988.
206. Muss HB, et al: Perceptions of follow-up care in women with breast cancer. Am J Clin Oncol 14:55, 1991.
207. Loomer L, et al: Postoperative follow-up of patients with early breast cancer. Cancer 67:55, 1991.
208. American Joint Committee on Cancer: Manual for staging cancer. Philadelphia, JB Lippincott, 1992.
209. Del Turco MR, et al: Intensive diagnostic follow-up after treatment of primary breast cancer. JAMA 271:1593, 1994.
210. Impact of follow-up testing on survival and health-related quality of life in breast cancer patients: A multicenter randomized controlled trial—The GIVIO investigators, JAMA 271:1587, 1994.
211. O'Mara RE: Bone scanning in osseous metastatic disease. JAMA 229:1915, 1974.
212. Khansur T, et al: Evaluation of bone scan as a screening work-up in primary and local-regional recurrence of breast cancer. Am J Clin Oncol 10:167, 1987.
213. Ciatto S, et al: Preoperative staging of primary breast cancer: A multicenter study. Cancer 61:1038, 1988.
214. Coleman RE, Rubens RD, Fogelman I: Reappraisal of the baseline bone scan in breast cancer. J Nucl Med 29:1045, 1988.
215. Kunkler IH, Merick MV, Rodger A: Bone scintigraphy in breast cancer: A nine-year follow-up, Clin Radiol 36:279, 1985.
216. McNeill BJ, et al: Preoperative and follow-up bone scans in patients with primary carcinoma of the breast, Surg Gynecol Obstet 147:745, 1978.
217. Bassett LW, Giuliano AE, Gold RH: Staging for breast carcinoma. Am J Surg 157:250, 1989.
218. Loprinzi CL: It is now the age to define the appropriate follow-up of primary breast cancer patients. J Clin Oncol 12:881, 1994.
219. Schaner EG, et al: Comparison of computed tomography and conventional whole lung tomography in detecting pulmonary nodules: A prospective radiologic-pathologic study. AJR Am J Roentgenol 131:51, 1978.
220. Didolkar MS, et al: Accuracy of roentgenograms of the chest in metastases to the lungs. Surg Gynecol Obstet 144:903, 1977.
221. Vestergaard A et al: The value of yearly chest x-ray in patients with stage I breast cancer. Eur J Cancer Clin Oncol 25:687, 1989.
222. Bernardino ME, et al: Diagnostic approaches to liver and spleen metastases. Radiol Clin North Am 20:469, 1982.
223. Friedman ML, Esposito FS: Comparison of CT scanning and radionuclide imaging in liver disease. CRC Crit Rev Diagn Imaging 14:143, 1980.
224. Yeh H, Rabinowitz JG: Ultrasonography and computed tomography of the liver. Radiol Clin North Am 18:321, 1980.
225. Weiner SN, Sachs SH: An assessment of positive liver scanning in patients with breast cancer. Arch Surg 113:126, 1978.
226. Ferrucci JT: Leo G. Rigler lecture: MR imaging of the liver. AJR Am J Roentgenol 147:1103, 1986.
227. Russell EJ, et al: Multiple cerebral metastases: Detectability with Gd-DTPA-enhanced MR imaging. Radiology 165:609, 1987.
228. Weisberg LA: The computed tomographic findings in intracranial metastases due to breast carcinoma. Comput Radiol 10:297, 1986.
229. Bentson JR, Steckel RJ, Kagan AR: Diagnostic imaging in clinical cancer management: Brain metastases. Invest Radiol 23:335, 1988.
230. Khansur T, et al: Preoperative evaluation with radionuclide brain scanning and computerized axial tomography of the brain in patients with breast cancer. Am J Surg 155:232, 1988.
231. Brant-Zawadzki M: MR imaging of the brain. Radiology 166:1, 1988.
232. Davis PC, et al: Diagnosis of cerebral metastases. AJNR Am J Neuroradiol 12:293, 1991.

chapter 37

Interval Breast Cancer: Clinical, Epidemiologic, and Biologic Features

STANLEY LIPKOWITZ | LOUISE A. BRINTON | JOHN E. NIEDERHUBER

Interval Breast Cancer: Definition of the Problem

Since 1990, the mortality due to breast cancer has been declining in the United States. In 1991, the death rate was 32.69 per 100,000 women, but in 2003, it fell to 25.19 per 100,000 women.[1] The continuing decrease in mortality from breast cancer has been attributed to early detection resulting from screening, improved adjuvant therapy, and more recently to decreases in the incidence due to lowered rates of usage of hormone replacement therapy.[2,3] Mammographic screening for breast cancer has become the established standard of care for women older than 50 years of age. Large randomized trials and meta-analyses have demonstrated that screening reduces breast cancer mortality by as much as 20% to 40% in women 50 to 79 years of age and to a lesser extent in women 40 to 49 years of age.[4-9] In the United States, approximately 50% of women older than 40 years of age undergo screening mammography at least every 2 years, and recent analyses have estimated that screening mammography accounts for approximately half of the decrease in mortality due to breast cancer.[2,10] Based on this, the absolute benefit of screening has been estimated as a 15% (range, 7% to 23%) reduction in breast cancer mortality.[2]

Interval breast cancers, defined as breast cancers that are detected after a negative mammographic screening and before the subsequent scheduled screening mammogram, are a major problem for breast cancer screening. Data from various trials suggest that the interval cancers represent between approximately 20% to 30% of all breast cancers found in a screened population.[8,11] In the first large randomized trial, the Health Insurance Plan of New York (HIP) study, 63 interval cancers were found out of a total of 190 cancers in the screened group (33%).[6] In the Swedish two-county screening trial, 104 interval breast cancers (including in situ cancers) were found out of a total of

465 cancers in the screened population (22%). In the Canadian National Breast Cancer Screening Studies (CNBSS)-1 and CNBSS-2, 186 interval breast cancers (including in situ cancer) were found out of a total of 766 cancers in the screened population (24%).[8] In the breast cancer screening programs in Malmö, Sweden (including the Malmö Mammographic Screening Trial and the population-based Malmö Mammographic Screening Program [MMSP]), the frequency of interval breast cancer was 16% to 17%.[12] A meta-analysis of interval breast cancers detected in published international studies found that interval cancers account for approximately 24% of the overall cancers (range, 15.7% to 27.5%).[13]

Several factors affect the incidence of interval cancers. An interval cancer may have been missed on the reading of the initial mammogram. Interval cancers have been classified as those in which the tumor had been overlooked (observer error), those in which the tumor was outside the imaging field (technical error), those in which review revealed slight abnormalities that were insufficient to prospectively classify as suspected malignancy (unrecognized sign), and true interval cancers.[14,15] True interval cancers, then, are those that are not seen on the screening mammogram (even retrospectively) but present clinically before the next mammogram. Observer errors have been documented in a number of clinical screening trials. In the Swedish two-county screening trial, 104 of 465 cancers that were found in the screened population during the first 7 years of screening presented as interval cancers.[11] Of the 104, 10 were ductal carcinoma in situ and were excluded from further analysis. A blinded radiographic review found that only six cancers (6%) had been missed on the prior screen. Thus, there were 88 true interval cancers in the screened population (19% of the total cancers in the screened population).[11] Other analyses have found that the proportion of interval cancers that were missed varies from 4% to as high as 56%.[16-18] Technical errors also account for a proportion of interval cancers. A recent study found that the odds of interval breast cancer detection increased more than two-fold if the positioning of the mammogram was inadequate.[19]

Overall, true interval breast cancers represent between 35% to 70% of the interval cancers found between mammograms in screening trials.[14,15,20–22] Although the exact occurrence of true interval breast cancers among all cancers is difficult to assess precisely, because not all studies have re-evaluated the mammograms from these patients, the cited studies suggest that it is between 10% and 20%. As will be discussed later, these true interval cancers are biologically distinct from the cancers that are found by mammographic screening and are likely to account for a disproportionate fraction of breast cancer mortality.

Another factor affecting the incidence of interval breast cancer is the length of the interval between screening mammograms. For example, in the Stockholm study, the planned interval was 24 months. There were 22 interval cancers and 8 true interval cancers in the first year after the initial screening mammogram, and there were 38 interval cancers and 23 true interval cancers in the second year after the initial mammogram. A trend toward increasing percentages of true interval cancers of all interval cancers was also seen in a population of patients screened every 36 months in West Sussex, United Kingdom.[23] There were 45 interval cancers and 9 true interval cancers in the first year after the initial screening mammogram, 88 interval cancers and 30 true interval cancers in the second year after the initial screening mammogram, and 97 interval cancers and 39 true interval cancers in the third year after the initial screening mammogram. Similarly, a recent analysis of the screened population of the United Kingdom National Health Service Breast Screening Programme (NHSBSP) demonstrated increasing frequency over time of interval breast cancers in the 3 years after a screening mammogram.[24] These observations support the use of shorter intervals for breast cancer screening and have led to the recommendations for annual screening.[25,26]

There are several possible reasons a true interval cancer may not be detected by routine mammographic screening. One is the inability of mammograms to detect interval cancers given certain characteristics of these tumors. Analysis of interval cancers in the Malmö mammographic screening trial and the Breast Cancer Detection Demonstration Project (BCDDP) screening project at the Ellis Fischel Cancer Hospital found that a high proportion of the patients with interval breast cancers had mammographic patterns (i.e., high mammographic density) that are more likely to obscure early diagnosis.[27,28] A similar observation has been found in a recent study of patients who underwent screening mammography in the Group Health Cooperative of Puget Sound.[19,29] In this study, 51% of the patients with interval breast cancer had high mammographic density compared with 24% of the patients with screen-detected cancers.[19] However, the interpretation of these observations is complicated by a lack of understanding of the biologic underpinnings of high breast density as a risk factor for the development of breast cancer (reviewed in Vachon

and colleagues[30] and discussed later). In addition, the Malmö mammographic screening trial found that 15% of the interval cancers were lobular cancers and 38% were invasive comedo carcinoma, medullary, or mucinous cancers.[27] Breast cancers with these histologies frequently lack calcifications and are difficult to image at an early stage. Thus, a fraction of the interval breast cancers may be ones that are not imaged well by mammography.

The NHSBSP screening program described previously demonstrated increasing frequency of interval breast cancers with time in the 3 years after a screening mammogram (115, 170, and 226 interval cancers, respectively) and then a dramatic decrease in year 4 after the initial screen (27 interval cancers).[24] The screening interval in this study was 3 years, suggesting that the decrease in interval breast cancers in the fourth year was the result of detection by the screening at the third year of a significant fraction of cancers that otherwise would have been classified as interval cancers. Evaluation of 57 true interval cancers in the NHSBSP found only 8 (14%) with a negative mammogram at the time of clinical presentation of the cancer.[31] A larger study found that 53 of 317 (17%) true interval breast cancers were radiographically occult at the time of diagnosis.[32] Thus, although some of the interval cancers may be difficult to detect by mammography, many truly appear in the interval between screenings. This suggests that the growth rate of interval cancers is higher than cancers detected by mammographic screening. The doubling time of mammographically detectable breast tumors has been determined by analyses of tumors present on sequential mammograms. In 1963, Gershon-Cohen, Berger, and Klickstein reported 18 patients who had not undergone immediate biopsy until two or more mammograms had been obtained.[33] These data and an additional case from the Ellis Fischel Cancer Hospital were used to calculate a median observed doubling time of 120 days for mammographically detected breast cancer (range, 23 to 209 days).[34] Another study evaluated 23 screen-detected tumors that retrospectively had evidence of the tumor on a prior mammogram and estimated the mean doubling time for these tumors as 325 days (range, 109 to 944 days).[35] The largest study reported 147 breast cancers that had been imaged with 388 serial mammograms before definitive treatment was undertaken.[36] The observation time in this study ranged from 2 months to 11 years (average, 27 months). Measured tumor volume doubling times were an average of 212 days (range, 44 to 1869 days). From these observations, the authors concluded that the smallest lesion detectable with mammography would be 1 to 2 mm in diameter (about 20 doublings).[36] The doubling time of the interval cancers cannot be measured using similar techniques because, by definition, they are not present on the initial mammogram. The absence of the true interval breast cancers on the screening mammogram and their clinical appearance either by examination or mammogram in the interim between screening mammograms allows the authors of a number of papers to infer that these are rapidly growing tumors.[20,22,35,37–41] As will be discussed in the following section, a variety of biologic indices of cell proliferation are consistent with this inference.

Epidemiologic, Clinical Features, and Outcomes of Interval Breast Cancer Compared with Screen-Detected Breast Cancer

It is clear from a number of reports that the relative proportion of interval cancers is higher among younger women.[42-44] Less is known about other epidemiologic predictors. One report indicated that taller women and those with histories of either artificial menopause or benign breast disease were more likely to develop interval cancers.[42] As previously noted, women with highly dense breasts are also more likely to develop interval cancers.[45-47] Studies have also identified that menopausal hormone therapy is positively associated with the risk of developing an interval cancer (reviewed in Banks[48] and Hofvind and colleagues[49]). This could reflect masking of tumors by increased breast density (because hormone use increases density), although at least one study has identified that hormone use and breast density have independent effects on interval cancers.[46] It is also possible that hormone use affects interval cancers either (1) through increased proliferation or more rapid tumor growth or (2) increased surveillance in hormone users.[49] Further studies are needed to distinguish between these alternative hypotheses.

Comparisons of the clinical features between interval breast cancers and screen-detected breast cancers have demonstrated that tumors in the former condition have features suggestive of a more aggressive phenotype. Early observations on small numbers of interval cancers suggested that these cancers were a subset of cancers with a rapid doubling time too short to be detected by routine mammograms and that these interval tumors were more likely to be metastatic at the time of diagnosis compared with screen-detected breast cancers.[22,35,50] A more systematic analysis of interval breast cancer found in the BCDDP of the University of Medicine and Dentistry of New Jersey compared 21 true interval breast cancers with 64 cancers detected on the initial screening mammogram and 35 cancers detected on the second screening mammogram.[39] In this study, they found that the frequency of nodal involvement was higher in the interval cancers compared with those detected either on the first or second screening mammogram (68% vs. 30% and 33%, respectively). The interval breast cancers were more likely to present as stage II or III disease than the screen-detected cancers (48% vs. 29% and 31%, respectively). Finally, the patients diagnosed with interval breast cancer were more likely to be younger than 50 years of age (52% vs. 30% and 34%, respectively). A similar analysis of the Utrecht DOM screening project of the Netherlands found that true interval cancers had a higher frequency of nodal involvement than screen-detected cancers (52.6% vs. 26.8%), were more likely to be advanced stage (58.9% vs. 34%), and were more likely to be estrogen receptor (ER) negative (35.3% vs. 25.6%).[51] This study did not find a difference between the age of the patients with true interval breast cancer and screen-detected breast cancer. In the West Sussex study, interval cancers were found more often than screen-detected

cancers to be greater than 2 cm (31% vs. 19%) and to have positive axillary nodal metastases (46% vs. 28%).[23] In the NHSBSP, interval breast cancers were more likely to be invasive than screen-detected cancers (96% vs. 76%), have larger median sizes (1.95 cm vs. 1.48 cm), be grade 3 (51% vs. 16%), have vascular invasion (34% vs. 14%), and have an intermediate or poor Nottingham prognostic index (61% vs. 37%).[31] A study of Japanese women with interval breast cancer found that the tumors were larger (2.6 cm vs. 2.1 cm) and more likely to have greater than four nodal metastases (28.6% vs. 5.8 %) compared with tumors found by screening mammography.[43] Analysis of interval cancers from the randomized Stockholm screening study confirmed the comparison between the interval cancers and screen-detected cancers described previously.[37] In this trial, 45% of the true interval cancers occurred in patients younger than 50 years of age, compared with 21% of the cancers found by screening.[37] The mean size of the true interval cancers was significantly larger than the screen-detected cancers (2.1 cm vs. 1.4 cm). Axillary nodal metastases were present in 59% of the true interval cancers compared with 25% of the screen-detected cancers. Both this study and the West Sussex study found that interval breast cancers had greater than three axillary nodal metastases more frequently than screen-detected breast cancers (17% to 20% vs. 6% to 9%).[23,37] In the Stockholm study, 69% of the true interval cancers presented with advanced stage disease (stage II to IV) compared with 34% of the screen-detected cancers. Low or negative ER content was found in 66% of the true interval cancers compared with 38% of the screen-detected tumors.[37]

The clinical features of the true interval breast cancers compared with the screen-detected cancers described previously suggest that interval cancers are an aggressive subset of breast cancers. Indeed, comparisons of survival of patients with interval breast cancer to those with screen-detected breast cancer have generally confirmed this. In the randomized HIP screening study, the case survival rates for women with interval breast cancer were 62.4% and 46.2% at 5 and 10 years, respectively (Fig. 37-1).[7,8] In contrast, the case survival rates for women with screen-detected breast cancer were 87.1% and 64.4% at 5 and 10 years, respectively.[7] In the BCDDP study, only 29% of patients with interval breast cancer were alive at 6 years compared with greater than 80% of the patients with screen-detected cancer.[39] In the Utrecht DOM study, patients with true interval breast cancer had a 73% 5-year survival and 58% 10-year survival.[51] By contrast, patients with screen-detected cancers had 94% 5-year survival and a 90% 10-year survival.[51] Similarly, a recent analysis of patients with interval breast cancers in the large randomized HIP and CNBSS screening trials found that they had a 53% greater hazard of death than those with screen-detected cancers after adjusting for tumor size, lymph node status, and disease stage.[8] Also, data from the breast cancer screening trial and program in Malmö, Sweden, show that patients with interval breast cancer have increased mortality compared with patients with screen-detected breast cancer.[12] The Malmö study included interval breast cancers detected during the screening trial (conducted from 1976 to 1986) and interval cancers detected in the population-based screening

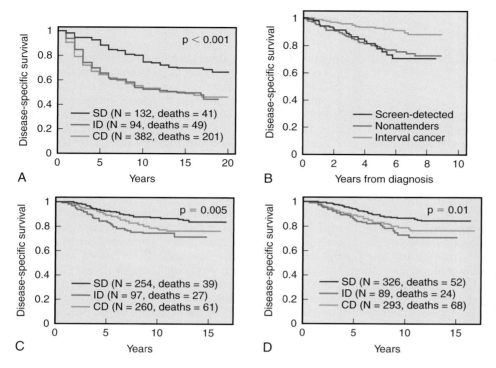

Figure 37-1 Breast cancer survival curves based on mode of detection from representative studies. **A,** Kaplan-Meier curves for breast cancer specific survival from the Health Insurance Plan of New York (HIP) study. **B,** Survival after invasive breast cancer from the Malmö Mammographic Service Screening Programme (MMSSP) study. **C,** Kaplan-Meier curves for breast cancer specific survival from the Canadian National Breast Cancer Screening Studies (CNBSS)-1 study. **D,** Kaplan-Meier curves for breast cancer–specific survival from the CNBSS-2 study. CD, unscreened control population; ID, interval detected; SD, screen detected. (From Shen Y, Yang Y, Inoue LY, et al: Role of detection method in predicting breast cancer survival: Analysis of randomized screening trials. J Natl Cancer Inst 97:1195–1203, 2005; and Zackrisson S, Janzon L, Manjer J, Andersson I: Improved survival rate for women with interval breast cancer—results from the breast cancer screening programme in Malmö, Sweden 1976–1999. J Med Screen 14:138–143, 2007.)

program (with data from 1991 to 1999). Both cohorts of patients with interval breast cancers had worse survival rates than comparable cohorts with screen-detected breast cancer. However, the patients diagnosed with interval breast cancer in the early cohort had a significantly worse prognosis than those in the later cohort (relative risk, 1.99 for death from breast cancer in the early vs. later interval breast cancer cohort).[12] Although the reason for this improved prognosis has not been studied further, it is likely the result of advances in treatment for early-stage breast cancer and the more aggressive use of systemic therapies.[2] Overall, the data support the finding that true interval breast cancers have a worse prognosis than screen-detected breast cancers and that they account for a significant fraction of the breast cancer mortality in a screened population.

Clinical Features and Outcomes of Interval Breast Cancer Compared with Breast Cancer Detected in Control Populations

The data discussed earlier compare interval breast cancers with screen-detected breast cancers. The randomized studies also allow comparison of interval breast cancers with those found in the control, unscreened population. In the Stockholm trial cited previously, the cancers in the control population were also compared with interval and screen-detected cancers.[37] In this trial, 45% of the true interval cancers occurred in patients younger than 50 years of age, compared with 25% of the cancers in the control group and 21% found by screening.[37] The mean sizes of true interval cancers, control cancers, and screen-detected cancers were 2.1 cm, 1.9 cm, and

respectively. Axillary nodal metastases were present in 59% of the true interval cancers, in 40% of the controls, and in 25% of the screen-detected cancers. In the HIP study, 49% of the interval cancers presented as stage II to IV, 51% of the control cancers were advanced stage, but only 24% of the screen-detected cancers were advanced stage.[8] In the CNBSS-1 study, 60% of the interval breast cancers were advanced stage, 53% of the control cancers were advanced stage, and 45% of the screen-detected cancers were advanced stage.[8] In the CNBSS-2 study, 56% of the interval breast cancers were advanced stage, 53% of the control cancers were advanced stage, and 38% of the screen-detected cancers were advanced stage.[8] In the HIP study, 45% of the interval cancers were node positive, 41% of the control cohort cancers were node positive, but only 23% of the screen-detected cancers were node positive.[8] In CNBSS-1, 37% of the interval cancers were node positive, 28% of the control cancers were node positive, and 25% of the screen-detected cancers were node positive.[8] In CNBSS-2, 37% of the interval cancers were node positive, 33% of the control cancers were node positive, and 21% of the screen-detected cancers were node positive.[8] In sum, the cancers found in an unscreened population appear to have features that are intermediate between the screen-detected cancers and the interval cancers. These results are consistent with the idea that the tumors in the control population should include both tumors that would have been detected by mammographic screening as well as those that are detected between screens (i.e., interval cancers).

The most striking results are the comparison of mortality in patients with interval breast cancers compared with mortality in the unscreened populations. Because the tumors in the control populations in the screening trials should contain patients with the tumors that would be detected by screening as well as some interval breast cancers, a logical expectation would be that the control population would have breast cancer mortality curves intermediate between these two. However, studies have consistently found that the mortality curve for the breast cancers found in the control population and the patients with interval breast cancer are not different and both are significantly worse than the patients with screen-detected cancers. In the HIP study, the case survival rate was 59.5% and 46.3% in the control population at 5 and 10 years, respectively.[7] This survival was not significantly different from the interval cancer case survival rate (62.4% and 46.2% at 5 and 10 years, respectively) and was significantly lower than that of the screen-detected cancers (87.1% and 64.4% for the screen detected cancers at 5 and 10 years, respectively; see Fig. 37-1).[7,8] Similarly, in the randomized Swedish two-county screening trial, there was no statistically significant difference between the breast cancer survival or the disease-free survival of the control population compared with the patients with interval breast cancer.[11] An analysis of the CNBSS randomized screening trials also showed no statistical difference between the survival of patients with interval cancers compared with those in the unscreened control group with breast cancer, whereas both groups had a worse survival than the patients with screen-detected cancer.[8] A number of nonrandomized studies have yielded similar results. In the Utrecht DOM study, the survival of the patients with screen-detected and interval cancers was compared with the survival of an unscreened historical control group.[51] There was no significant difference between the survival curves for interval breast cancers and the historical controls. Survival for both of these groups was significantly worse than for the patients with screen-detected breast cancer.[51] Similar results were found when the breast cancer mortality for patients with screen-detected breast cancer, interval breast cancers, and patients who did not attend screening in the Malmö Mammographic Screening program were compared.[12]

Together, these data demonstrating lower mortality in screen-detected breast cancer but similar mortality of the patients with interval breast cancers compared with the mortality of patients with breast cancer in an unscreened control population are consistent with the findings that screening reduces breast cancer mortality cancer by detecting and treating a significant portion of the cancers before they progress to an incurable stage.[4-9] However, an alternative interpretation of the data is that the screen-detected cancers are slow-growing tumors with a relatively good prognosis. Thus, the difference between the breast cancer mortality of the screen-detected cancers and those detected in the unscreened population is the result of a bias due to lead time (defined as the interval between the time of detection by screening and the time when cancer becomes clinically apparent) and not true decreased mortality. According to this interpretation, the interval cancers account for a disproportionate fraction of the mortality due to breast cancer in the unscreened population as well as in the screened population. It should be noted that studies attempting to correct for lead time bias by adjusting for tumor size, stage, and nodal status have found that there is still a decrease in breast cancer mortality in the screened population compared with the unscreened population.[8]

Biologic Features of the Interval Breast Cancers

The clinical features described previously suggest that interval breast cancers are an aggressive subset of breast cancer, and this has motivated a number of studies to investigate the biologic differences between interval breast cancers and screen-detected breast cancer. One of the earliest biologic features to be studied was the proliferation rates of these tumors. As described previously, based on mammographic studies, the doubling time for interval breast tumors has been inferred to be short compared with screen-detected tumors based on their appearance in the interval between screening mammograms.[20,22,35,37-41] Numerous studies using a variety of methods to measure tumor proliferation rates (e.g., thymidine labeling index and flow cytometry to determine the percentage of cells in S-phase) have found correlations between high proliferation rates and high-grade tumors, aneuploidy, and poor prognosis.[52-59] A study comparing the mitotic frequency in interval tumors compared with screen-detected tumors found that the interval tumors were statistically more likely to have a high mitotic frequency.[43] In another study, using flow cytometry to determine S-phase fraction in true interval tumors compared with screen-detected tumors, 38% of interval tumors had a high S-phase fraction whereas only 18% of the screen-detected tumors had a high S-phase fraction.[32] A similar study, measuring tumor proliferation rates by Ki67 staining, found that 33% of interval tumors have high Ki67 staining compared with 20% of the screen-detected cases.[60] Thus, it appears that a greater percentage of true interval breast cancers have a high proliferation rate, consistent with their rapid appearance and poor prognosis. The underlying molecular basis for the increased proliferative rates seen in interval breast cancers is not known. A number of studies of breast cancer samples have found overexpression and/or amplification of several proteins that regulate the cell cycle and proliferation such as cyclin D1, cyclin E, and c-myc.[61-69] Also, loss of expression of negative regulators of the cell cycle such as RB and p16 have been reported in up to 30% of breast cancers.[70-72] However, no studies have directly assessed the expression of these genes in interval breast cancers.

More of the patients with interval breast cancer have increased breast mammographic density.[19,27,28] Increased mammographic density makes the mammographic diagnosis of breast cancer difficult. However, in addition to obscuring the diagnosis, epidemiologic studies and meta-analyses have found that high mammographic density is a strong risk factor for breast cancer, with the magnitude of risk associated with this factor exceeding that of most other identified risk factors.[30,73,74] The basis for the increased breast cancer risk in patients with high mammographic breast density has not been fully elucidated. Studies examining breast density in monozygotic and dizygotic twins have suggested a significant genetic contribution in patients with high mammographic breast density.[75] Histologic examination of breast tissue has correlated greater amounts of epithelium and/or stroma with high mammographic density (reviewed in Boyd and colleagues[76]). A number

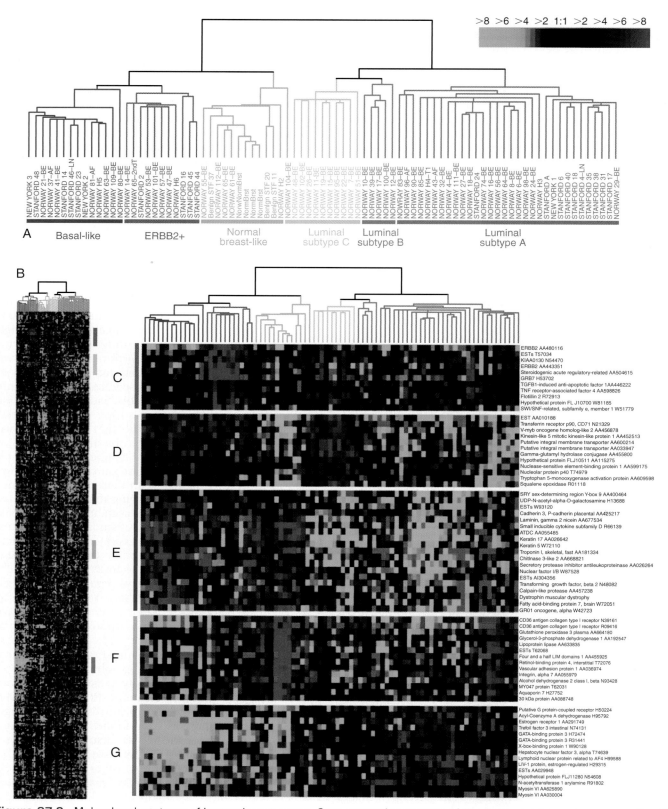

Figure 37-2 Molecular phenotypes of human breast cancer. Gene expression patterns of 85 experimental samples representing 78 carcinoma, three benign tumors, and four normal tissues, analyzed by hierarchical clustering using 476 cDNA intrinsic clone set. **A,** The tumor specimens were divided into subtypes based on gene expression patterns. The tumor subtypes are colored as luminal A (*dark blue*); luminal B (*orange*); luminal C (*light blue*); normal breast-like (*green*); basal-like (*red*); and ERBB2+ (*pink*). **B,** The full cluster diagram scaled down. The colored bars to the right represent the inserts presented in **C–G. C,** ERBB2 amplicon cluster. **D,** Novel unknown cluster. **E,** Basal epithelial cluster. **F,** Normal breast-like cluster. **G,** Luminal epithelial gene cluster containing estrogen receptor. (Adapted from Sorlie T, Perou CM, Tibshirani R, et al: Gene expression patterns of breast carcinomas distinguish tumor subclasses with clinical implications. Proc Natl Acad Sci USA 98:10869–10874, 2001. Copyright 2001. National Academy of Sciences, USA.)

of studies have shown associations between sex hormone–binding globulin, circulating prolactin, and insulin-like growth factor (IGF)-I levels with high mammographic breast density (reviewed in Martin and Boyd[77]). Similarly, studies have found associations between mammographic density and urinary secretion of the carcinogen malondialdehyde (reviewed in Martin and Boyd[77]). This has led one group to hypothesize that mitogenic factors such as IGF-I and prolactin (with levels determined at least in some part genetically) might combine with mutagens to increase the risk of breast cancer in patients with high mammographic density.[77] Further mechanistic studies are needed to understand how high mammographic density contributes to breast cancer development.

Clinically, patients with breast cancer routinely have the expression of ER, progesterone receptor (PR), and amplification of HER2 evaluated because these directly affect the prognosis and treatment of breast cancer.[78] In general, patients whose breast cancers express ER and/or PR have the best prognosis.[78] Interval breast cancers are more likely to be ER negative compared with those found on screening mammography (31% to 35% vs. 14% to 26%).[37,51,60,79] Similarly, one study has reported that interval breast cancers are more likely to be PR negative compared with screen-detected cancers (42% vs. 24%).[60] Only one study has looked at HER2 expression using immunohistochemistry and found that 20% of interval breast cancers had high expression compared with 13% of screen-detected cancers. This difference was not statistically significant. The low expression of hormone receptors seen in studies of interval breast cancers is consistent with their poor prognosis compared with screen-detected breast cancers.

Recent expression profiling of human breast cancers has allowed classification of the tumors based on similarity of expression patterns between normal breast cells and tumors (Fig. 37-2).[78,80,81] The hormone receptor–expressing breast cancers most closely resembled the luminal cells of the breast ducts, whereas cells lacking hormone receptors (and also lacking HER2 amplification) most closely resembled basal cells, cells found on the outside of the breast ducts.[80,81] The basal types of breast cancer (and the less specific category of triple-negative breast cancer subtypes, namely those that are ER−, PR− and HER2−) have a poor prognosis and little is known about the associated underlying oncogenic pathways in this breast cancer subset.[78] Analysis of these basal cancers has found that they share features with tumors that arise in BRCA1 mutation carriers, more frequently expressing cytokeratin 5/6, P-cadherin, and having p53 mutations.[60,82–85] A recent analysis reported an immunohistochemical evaluation of these markers in interval breast cancers compared to screen detected breast cancers (Table 37-1).[60] The interval can-

cers were more likely to be ER negative (31% vs. 14%), express cytokeratin 5/6 (22% vs. 10%), express P-cadherin (24% vs. 10%), and have high p53 expression (27% vs. 7%). Thus, significantly greater fractions of interval cancers have basal phenotypes compared with screen-detected breast cancers. Again, this is consistent with the worse prognosis observed for patients with interval breast cancer.

All of these analyses indicate that the interval breast cancers, like other breast cancers, are a heterogeneous group of breast cancers but consistently the analyses show skewing toward breast cancers with worse features.

Conclusions and Future Directions

Overall, interval breast cancers represent an aggressive subgroup of breast cancers and certainly contribute to a disproportionate fraction of the mortality of the patients who undergo screening for breast cancer. The data from multiple screening trials suggest that shorter screening intervals (e.g., yearly) will decrease the occurrence of interval breast cancer, because the majority appear to be detectable by mammographic screening and the incidence increases with screening interval. In addition, studies indicate that both observer and technical errors contribute to the incidence of false-positive interval breast cancers (i.e., those cancers that should have been detected on the screening mammogram), suggesting that mammographic screening programs require significant attention to quality assurance. Future directions include improved screening procedures (e.g., digital mammography and magnetic resonance imaging [MRI]) that may have a higher sensitivity to detect these cancers earlier in their course. Although no direct analysis of these methods for the detection for interval breast cancer has been reported, digital mammography has been shown to have a higher sensitivity than film mammography for the detection of lesions in younger women and in women with high mammographic density.[86] Similarly, the sensitivity of MRI is higher than film mammography and is not affected by high mammographic breast density.[87,88] As discussed previously, the patients with interval breast cancer are more likely to be younger and have high mammographic density. Thus, both digital mammography and MRI are likely to increase the early detection of interval breast cancer at the time of screening. However, the aggressive features of the interval breast cancers suggest that even if detected early, these tumors still may have a relatively poor prognosis and require improvements in therapy to decrease their associated mortality.

TABLE 37-1

Markers for Interval (*i*) versus Screen-Detected Breast Cancer

Variable	Screen Cases (%; *n* = 95)	Interval Cases (%; *n* = 95)	*i*/*s**	Odds Ratio (95% confidence interval)	*P*[†]	Multivariate Odds Ratio (95% confidence interval)[‡]
Tumor size (mean)[§]	25.1	23.1				
Age (mean)[§]	62	59				
Age (y)						
<60	36 (38)	61 (65)	33/7	1	<0.0001	1
≥60	58 (62)	33 (35)		4.7 (2.1–12.6)		4.4 (1.8–12.7)
Breast density						
Low / moderate (≤70%)	87 (92)	70 (74)	24/7	1	0.004	1
High (>70%)	8 (8)	25 (26)		3.4 (1.4–9.4)		2.9 (1.1–9)
Histologic type						
Ductal	84 (88)	75 (79)	13/6	1	0.17	
Lobular	8 (8)	15 (16)		2.2 (0.8–7)		
Histologic grade						
1 and 2	79 (83)	73 (77)	17/11	1	0.18	
3	16 (17)	22 (23)		1.6 (0.7–3.7)		
Nodal status						
Negative	62 (65)	53 (56)	21/11	1	0.11	
Positive	29 (33)	34 (36)		1.9 (0.9–4.4)		
Locally advanced disease						
No	85 (90)	83 (87)	8/6	1	0.79	
Yes	10 (10)	12 (13)		1.3 (0.4–4.7)		
Metastasis at time of diagnosis						
No	94 (98)	90 (95)	5/1	1	0.22	
Yes	1 (1)	5 (5)		5 (0.6–236.5)		
ER						
Positive	82 (86)	66 (69)	26/10	1	0.01	
Negative	13 (14)	29 (31)		2.6 (1.2–6)		
PR						
Positive	72 (76)	55 (58)	30/13	1	0.01	
Negative	23 (24)	40 (42)		2.3 (1.2–4.8)		
Ki-67						
Low[‖]	76 (80)	64 (67)	24/11	1	0.04	
High	19 (20)	31 (33)		2.2 (1–4.9)		
p53						
Low, score ≤3	88 (93)	69 (73)	24/6	1	0.001	1
High, score >3	7 (7)	26 (27)		4 (1.6–12)		3.2 (1.2–10.4)
C-erbB-2						
Negative, score 0/1	83 (87)	76 (80)	16/9	1	0.23	
Positive, score 2/3	12 (13)	19 (20)		1.8 (0.7–4.6)		
P-cadherin						
Negative, score ≤3	85 (90)	72 (76)	20/8	1	0.04	
Positive, score >3	10 (10)	23 (24)		2.5 (1.1–6.6)		
Cytokeratin 5/6						
Negative, score = 0	86 (91)	74 (78)	21/9	1	0.04	
Positive, score >0	9 (10)	21 (22)		2.3 (1.0–5.8)		

*i, number of matched pairs with high expression in the interval case, low in the screen-detected case; *s*, number of matched pairs with low expression in the interval case, high in the screen-detected case. For age, ER and PR: *s* / *i*.
[†]Exact two-tailed McNemar's test.
[‡]Multivariate conditional logistic regression analysis including p53 status, age, and breast density.
[§]*t*, test for equality of means, *P* = 0.376 and *P* = 0.01 for tumor size and age, respectively.
[‖]Low ≤22.5% (75th percentile).
Modified from Collett K, Stefansson IM, Eide J, et al: A basal epithelial phenotype is more frequent in interval breast cancers compared with screen detected tumors. Cancer Epidemiol Biomarkers Prev 14:1108–1112, 2005.

REFERENCES

1. Jemal A, Siegel R, Ward E, et al: Cancer statistics, 2007. CA Cancer J Clin 57:43–66, 2007.
2. Berry DA, Cronin KA, Plevritis SK, et al: Effect of screening and adjuvant therapy on mortality from breast cancer. N Engl J Med 353:1784–1792, 2005.
3. Ravdin PM, Cronin KA, Howlader N, et al: The decrease in breast-cancer incidence in 2003 in the United States. N Engl J Med 356:1670–1674, 2007.
4. Hendrick RE, Smith RA, Rutledge JH 3rd, Smart CR: Benefit of screening mammography in women aged 40–49: A new meta-analysis of randomized controlled trials. J Natl Cancer Inst Monogr 87–92, 1997.
5. Kerlikowske K, Grady D, Rubin SM, et al: Efficacy of screening mammography. A meta-analysis. JAMA 273:149–154, 1995.
6. Shapiro S, Strax P, Venet L: Periodic breast cancer screening in reducing mortality from breast cancer. JAMA 215:1777–1785, 1971.
7. Shapiro S, Venet W, Strax P, et al: Ten- to fourteen-year effect of screening on breast cancer mortality. J Natl Cancer Inst 69:349–355, 1982.
8. Shen Y, Yang Y, Inoue LY, et al: Role of detection method in predicting breast cancer survival: Analysis of randomized screening trials. J Natl Cancer Inst 97:1195–1203, 2005.
9. Verbeek AL, Hendriks JH, Holland R, et al: Reduction of breast cancer mortality through mass screening with modern mammography. First results of the Nijmegen project, 1975–1981. Lancet 1:1222–1224, 1984.
10. Cronin KA, Yu B, Krapcho M, et al: Modeling the dissemination of mammography in the United States. Cancer Causes Control 16:701–712, 2005.
11. Holmberg LH, Tabar L, Adami HO, Bergstrom R: Survival in breast cancer diagnosed between mammographic screening examinations. Lancet 2:27–30, 1986.
12. Zackrisson S, Janzon L, Manjer J, Andersson I: Improved survival rate for women with interval breast cancer—results from the breast cancer screening programme in Malmö, Sweden 1976–1999. J Med Screen 14:138–143, 2007.
13. Taylor R, Supramaniam R, Rickard M, et al: Interval breast cancers in New South Wales, Australia, and comparisons with trials and other mammographic screening programmes. J Med Screen 9:20–25, 2002.
14. Holland R, Mravunac M, Hendriks JH, Bekker BV: So-called interval cancers of the breast. Pathologic and radiologic analysis of sixty-four cases. Cancer 49:2527–2533, 1982.
15. Martin JE, Moskowitz M, Milbrath JR: Breast cancer missed by mammography. AJR Am J Roentgenol 132:737–739, 1979.
16. de Rijke JM, Schouten LJ, Schreutelkamp JL, et al: A blind review and an informed review of interval breast cancer cases in the Limburg screening programme, the Netherlands. J Med Screen 7:19–23, 2000.
17. Duncan AA, Wallis MG: Classifying interval cancers. Clin Radiol 50:774–777, 1995.
18. Moberg K, Grundstrom H, Tornberg S, et al: Two models for radiological reviewing of interval cancers. J Med Screen 6:35–39, 1999.
19. Taplin SH, Rutter CM, Finder C, et al: Screening mammography: Clinical image quality and the risk of interval breast cancer. AJR Am J Roentgenol 178:797–803, 2002.
20. Andersson I: What can we learn from interval carcinomas? Recent Results Cancer Res 90:161–163, 1984.
21. Buchanan JB, Spratt JS, Heuser LS: Tumor growth, doubling times, and the inability of the radiologist to diagnose certain cancers. Radiol Clin North Am 21:115–126, 1983.
22. Heuser L, Spratt JS Jr, Polk HC Jr, Buchanan J: Relation between mammary cancer growth kinetics and the intervals between screenings. Cancer 43:857–862, 1979.
23. Raja MA, Hubbard A, Salman AR: Interval breast cancer: Is it a different type of breast cancer? Breast 10:100–108, 2001.
24. Porter GJ, Evans AJ, Burrell HC, et al: Interval breast cancers: Prognostic features and survival by subtype and time since screening. J Med Screen 13:115–122, 2006.
25. Bevers TB, Anderson BO, Bonaccio E, et al: NCCN Breast Cancer Screening and Diagnosis Guidelines 2008.
26. Smith RA, Cokkinides V, Brawley OW: Cancer screening in the United States, 2008: A review of current American Cancer Society guidelines and cancer screening issues. CA Cancer J Clin 58:161–179, 2008.
27. Ikeda DM, Andersson I, Wattsgard C, et al: Interval carcinomas in the Malmö Mammographic Screening Trial: Radiographic appearance and prognostic considerations. AJR Am J Roentgenol 159:287–294, 1992.
28. Koivunen D, Zhang X, Blackwell C, et al: Interval breast cancers are not biologically distinct—just more difficult to diagnose. Am J Surg 168:538–542, 1994.
29. Buist DS, Porter PL, Lehman C, et al: Factors contributing to mammography failure in women aged 40–49 years. J Natl Cancer Inst 96:1432–1440, 2004.
30. Vachon CM, van Gils CH, Sellers TA, et al: Mammographic density, breast cancer risk and risk prediction. Breast Cancer Res 9:217, 2007.
31. Cowan WK, Angus B, Gray JC, et al: A study of interval breast cancer within the NHS breast screening programme. J Clin Pathol 53:140–146, 2000.
32. Vitak B, Olsen KE, Manson JC, et al: Tumour characteristics and survival in patients with invasive interval breast cancer classified according to mammographic findings at the latest screening: A comparison of true interval and missed interval cancers. Eur Radiol 9:460–469, 1999.
33. Gershon-Cohen J, Berger SM, Klickstein HS: Roentgenography of breast cancer moderating concept of "biologic predeterminism." Cancer 16:961–964, 1963.
34. Spratt JS, Spratt JA: Growth Rates. In Donegan NL, Spratt JS (eds): Cancer of the breast, 2nd ed. Philadelphia, WB Saunders, 1979, pp 197–220.
35. Heuser L, Spratt JS, Polk HC Jr: Growth rates of primary breast cancers. Cancer 43:1888–1894, 1979.
36. von Fournier D, Weber E, Hoeffken W, et al: Growth rate of 147 mammary carcinomas. Cancer 45:2198–2207, 1980.
37. Frisell J, Eklund G, Hellstrom L, Somell A: Analysis of interval breast carcinomas in a randomized screening trial in Stockholm. Breast Cancer Res Treat 9:219–225, 1987.
38. Andersson I, Aspegren K, Janzon L, et al: Mammographic screening and mortality from breast cancer: the Malmo mammographic screening trial. BMJ 297:943–948, 1988.
39. DeGroote R, Rush BF Jr, Milazzo J, et al: Interval breast cancer: A more aggressive subset of breast neoplasias. Surgery 94:543–547, 1983.
40. Heuser LS, Spratt JS, Kuhns JG, et al: The association of pathologic and mammographic characteristics of primary human breast cancers with "slow" and "fast" growth rates and with axillary lymph node metastases. Cancer 53:96–98, 1984.
41. von Rosen A, Wiege M, Tornberg B, et al: Relationship between certain radiographic and biologic characteristics in breast cancer. Acta Oncol 26:89–93, 1987.
42. Brekelmans CT, Peeters PH, Faber JA, et al: The epidemiological profile of women with an interval cancer in the DOM screening programme. Breast Cancer Res Treat 30:223–232, 1994.
43. Morimoto T, Komaki K, Oshimo K, et al: The characteristics of interval breast cancer in mass screening. Tokushima J Exp Med 39:109–16, 1992.
44. Whitehead J, Cooper J: Risk factors for breast cancer by mode of diagnosis: Some results from a breast cancer screening study. J Epidemiol Community Health 43:115–120, 1989.
45. Chiarelli AM, Kirsh VA, Klar NS, et al: Influence of patterns of hormone replacement therapy use and mammographic density on breast cancer detection. Cancer Epidemiol Biomarkers Prev 15:1856–1862, 2006.
46. Kavanagh AM, Cawson J, Byrnes GB, et al: Hormone replacement therapy, percent mammographic density, and sensitivity of mammography. Cancer Epidemiol Biomarkers Prev 14:1060–1064, 2005.
47. Mandelson MT, Oestreicher N, Porter PL, et al: Breast density as a predictor of mammographic detection: comparison of interval- and screen-detected cancers. J Natl Cancer Inst 92:1081–1087, 2000.
48. Banks E: Hormone replacement therapy and the sensitivity and specificity of breast cancer screening: A review. J Med Screen 8:29–34, 2001.

49. Hofvind S, Moller B, Thoresen S, Ursin G: Use of hormone therapy and risk of breast cancer detected at screening and between mammographic screens. Int J Cancer 118:3112–3117, 2006.
50. Bland KI, Buchanan JB, Mills DL, et al: Analysis of breast cancer screening in women younger than 50 years. JAMA 245:1037–1042, 1981.
51. Brekelmans CT, Peeters PH, Deurenberg JJ, Collette HJ: Survival in interval breast cancer in the DOM screening programme. Eur J Cancer 31A:1830–1835, 1995.
52. Coulson PB, Thornthwaite JT, Woolley TW, et al: Prognostic indicators including DNA histogram type, receptor content, and staging related to human breast cancer patient survival. Cancer Res 44:4187–4196, 1984.
53. Dieterich B, Albe X, Vassilakos P, et al: The prognostic value of DNA ploidy and S-phase estimate in primary breast cancer: A prospective study. Int J Cancer 63:49–54, 1995.
54. McGurrin JF, Doria MI Jr, Dawson PJ, et al: Assessment of tumor cell kinetics by immunohistochemistry in carcinoma of breast. Cancer 59:1744–1750, 1987.
55. Meyer JS, Hixon B: Advanced stage and early relapse of breast carcinomas associated with high thymidine labeling indices. Cancer Res 39:4042–4047, 1979.
56. Meyer JS, Prey MU, Babcock DS, McDivitt RW: Breast carcinoma cell kinetics, morphology, stage, and host characteristics. A thymidine labeling study. Lab Invest 54:41–51, 1986.
57. Silvestrini R, Daidone MG, Del Bino G, et al: Prognostic significance of proliferative activity and ploidy in node-negative breast cancers. Ann Oncol 4:213–219, 1993.
58. Tubiana M, Koscielny S: Cell kinetics, growth rate and the natural history of breast cancer. The Heuson Memorial Lecture. Eur J Cancer Clin Oncol 24:9–14, 1988.
59. Tubiana M, Pejovic MH, Koscielny S, et al: Growth rate, kinetics of tumor cell proliferation and long-term outcome in human breast cancer. Int J Cancer 44:17–22, 1989.
60. Collett K, Stefansson IM, Eide J, et al: A basal epithelial phenotype is more frequent in interval breast cancers compared with screen detected tumors. Cancer Epidemiol Biomarkers Prev 14:1108–1112, 2005.
61. Aulmann S, Adler N, Rom J, et al: c-myc amplifications in primary breast carcinomas and their local recurrences. J Clin Pathol 59:424–428, 2006.
62. Bostner J, Ahnstrom Waltersson M, Fornander T, et al: Amplification of CCND1 and PAK1 as predictors of recurrence and tamoxifen resistance in postmenopausal breast cancer. Oncogene 26:6997–7005, 2007.
63. Deming SL, Nass SJ, Dickson RB, Trock BJ: C-myc amplification in breast cancer: A meta-analysis of its occurrence and prognostic relevance. Br J Cancer 83:1688–1695, 2000.
64. Karlseder J, Zeillinger R, Schneeberger C, et al: Patterns of DNA amplification at band q13 of chromosome 11 in human breast cancer. Genes Chromosomes Cancer 9:42–48, 1994.
65. Keyomarsi K, O'Leary N, Molnar G, et al: Cyclin E, a potential prognostic marker for breast cancer. Cancer Res 54:380–385, 1994.
66. Keyomarsi K, Pardee AB: Redundant cyclin overexpression and gene amplification in breast cancer cells. Proc Natl Acad Sci USA 90:1112–1116, 1993.
67. Nielsen NH, Arnerlov C, Emdin SO, Landberg G: Cyclin E overexpression, a negative prognostic factor in breast cancer with strong correlation to oestrogen receptor status. Br J Cancer 74:874–880, 1996.
68. Ormandy CJ, Musgrove EA, Hui R, et al: Cyclin D1, EMS1 and 11q13 amplification in breast cancer. Breast Cancer Res Treat 78:323–335, 2003.
69. Weinstat-Saslow D, Merino MF, Manrow RE, et al: Overexpression of cyclin D mRNA distinguishes invasive and in situ breast carcinomas from non-malignant lesions. Nat Med 1:1257–1260, 1995.
70. Borg A, Zhang QX, Alm P, et al: The retinoblastoma gene in breast cancer: Allele loss is not correlated with loss of gene protein expression. Cancer Res 52:2991–2994, 1992.
71. Bosco EE, Knudsen ES: RB in breast cancer: At the crossroads of tumorigenesis and treatment. Cell Cycle 6:667–671, 2007.
72. Herman JG, Merlo A, Mao L, et al: Inactivation of the CDKN2/p16/MTS1 gene is frequently associated with aberrant DNA methylation in all common human cancers. Cancer Res 55:4525–4230, 1995.
73. Boyd NF, Guo H, Martin LJ, et al: Mammographic density and the risk and detection of breast cancer. N Engl J Med 356:227–236, 2007.
74. McCormack VA, dos Santos Silva I: Breast density and parenchymal patterns as markers of breast cancer risk: A meta-analysis. Cancer Epidemiol Biomarkers Prev 15:1159–1169, 2006.
75. Boyd NF, Dite GS, Stone J, et al: Heritability of mammographic density, a risk factor for breast cancer. N Engl J Med 347:886–894, 2002.
76. Boyd NF, Lockwood GA, Byng JW et al: Mammographic densities and breast cancer risk. Cancer Epidemiol Biomarkers Prev 7:1133–1144, 1998.
77. Martin LJ, Boyd NF: Mammographic density. Potential mechanisms of breast cancer risk associated with mammographic density: Hypotheses based on epidemiological evidence. Breast Cancer Res 10:201, 2008.
78. Brenton JD, Carey LA, Ahmed AA, Caldas C: Molecular classification and molecular forecasting of breast cancer: Ready for clinical application? J Clin Oncol 23:7350–7360, 2005.
79. Vitak, B, Stal O, Manson JC, et al: Interval cancers and cancers in non-attenders in the Ostergotland Mammographic Screening Programme. Duration between screening and diagnosis, S-phase fraction and distant recurrence. Eur J Cancer 33:1453–1460, 1997.
80. Perou CM, Sorlie T, Eisen MB, et al: Molecular portraits of human breast tumours. Nature 406:747–752, 2000.
81. Sorlie T, Perou CM, Tibshirani R, et al: Gene expression patterns of breast carcinomas distinguish tumor subclasses with clinical implications. Proc Natl Acad Sci USA 98:10869–10874, 2001.
82. Foulkes WD, Stefansson IM, Chappuis PO, et al: Germline BRCA1 mutations and a basal epithelial phenotype in breast cancer. J Natl Cancer Inst 95:1482–1485, 2003.
83. Nielsen TO, Hsu FD, Jensen K, et al: Immunohistochemical and clinical characterization of the basal-like subtype of invasive breast carcinoma. Clin Cancer Res 10:5367–5374, 2004.
84. Palacios J, Honrado E, Osorio A, et al: Immunohistochemical characteristics defined by tissue microarray of hereditary breast cancer not attributable to BRCA1 or BRCA2 mutations: Differences from breast carcinomas arising in BRCA1 and BRCA2 mutation carriers. Clin Cancer Res 9(10 Pt 1):3606–3614, 2003.
85. Sorlie T, Tibshirani R, Parker J, et al: Repeated observation of breast tumor subtypes in independent gene expression data sets. Proc Natl Acad Sci USA 100:8418–8423, 2003.
86. Pisano ED, Gatsonis C, Hendrick E, et al: Diagnostic performance of digital versus film mammography for breast-cancer screening. N Engl J Med 353:1773–1783, 2005.
87. Lehman CD, Gatsonis C, Kuhl CK, et al: MRI evaluation of the contralateral breast in women with recently diagnosed breast cancer. N Engl J Med 356:1295–1303, 2007.
88. Lehman CD, Isaacs C, Schnall MD, et al: Cancer yield of mammography, MR, and US in high-risk women: Prospective multi-institution breast cancer screening study. Radiology 244:381–381, 2007.

chapter 38

Stereotactic Breast Biopsy

MARY MAHONEY | LAWRENCE W. BASSETT

The development of minimally invasive image-guided breast biopsies has changed the management of breast disease.[1] Over the past decade, the percutaneous image-guided biopsy has proved to be an acceptable alternative to surgical excisional biopsy for nonpalpable findings requiring a tissue diagnosis.[2,3]

The stereotactic technique was initially developed for use with fine needle aspiration in Sweden in 1977.[4] Although it was the first of the image-guided techniques to be used in the United States, it did not gain widespread acceptance in this country until 1990, when Parker and colleagues described the use of stereotactic biopsy with an automated large-core needle gun.[1] The technique has evolved over the years, with technologic advances made both in imaging and biopsy instrumentation.

Of the estimated 1.9 million diagnostic breast biopsies to be performed in 2008, 1.4 million are expected to be image-guided biopsies. More than half of these will use stereotactic guidance.[5]

Indications for Stereotactic Biopsy

The indications for stereotactic biopsy are the same as those for needle localization with mammographic guidance. These include nonpalpable suspicious masses, densities, distortions, or microcalcifications identified mammographically. If a lesion is also visualized sonographically, ultrasound-guided biopsy is usually performed, to give the advantage of real-time imaging.[6]

Stereotactic biopsy for sampling of mammographically detected lesions offers a number of advantages over surgical biopsy, including less scarring, fewer complications, lower cost, and faster recovery.[7] But, perhaps even more important, is how the image-guided biopsies have changed the management of patients with breast disease. A large, progressively growing volume of screening mammograms in North America and Europe have generated an increasing number of nonpalpable, image-detected lesions requiring tissue diagnosis.[8] These lesions, referred to as Breast Imaging Reporting and Data System (BI-RADS) category 4 lesions, are suspicious enough to warrant biopsy, but many prove to be benign.[9] Obtaining benign pathology results through image-guided biopsy obviates the need for a surgical procedure.[10]

For patients with highly suspicious mammographic lesions (BI-RADS category 5 lesions), obtaining a preoperative diagnosis via an image-guided biopsy is also advantageous. The number of surgical procedures required for treatment is decreased.[11,12] Once a cancer diagnosis is made percutaneously, the patient undergoes a single operative procedure for resection of the breast malignancy and evaluation of the axilla. Furthermore, the probability of obtaining clear margins at the time of surgery is higher in women with a preoperative diagnosis.[11,12]

Contraindications to Stereotactic Biopsy

Patients who weigh more than 250 pounds are not candidates for the dedicated stereotactic table because of the weight restrictions for these tables.

It is necessary to discontinue certain drugs before a stereotactic biopsy. Anticoagulants are usually discontinued 3 days before and aspirin and nonsteroidal anti-inflammatory agents 1 week before the procedure. Most patients do not require medications for anxiety. An experienced team can usually provide adequate emotional support for patients to successfully complete the procedure.

Equipment

Stereotactically guided biopsy uses x-ray imaging for localizing and targeting a lesion. The stereotactic technique requires targeting equipment, a sampling device, and in most cases, a tissue marker.

TARGETING EQUIPMENT

The stereotactic biopsy procedure may be performed with an upright or prone targeting system. Most systems in the United States are dedicated prone stereotactic tables.[6,8]

Upright Systems

The upright systems are add-on units, which are added onto standard mammographic equipment[13] (Fig. 38-1).

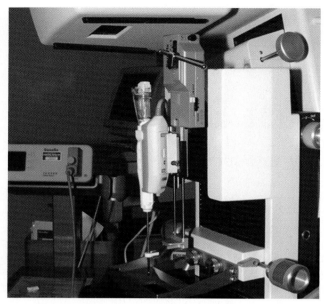

Figure 38-1   Stereotactic biopsy upright device.

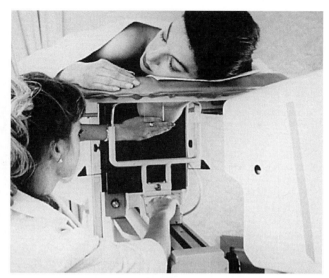

Figure 38-2   Patient is positioned for stereotactic biopsy with prone table.

This is a distinct advantage for centers with a low volume of biopsy procedures, in that the equipment can be revenue generating by performing mammograms when biopsies are not scheduled. The add-on units also have the advantages of requiring less space and are less expensive than the dedicated prone tables. The disadvantage of the upright systems, compared with the prone tables, is the greater incidence of vasovagal reactions because the patient is in the upright position. Adaptations in patient positioning allow decubitus or semireclining positions for the biopsy.[14]

Prone Tables

The dedicated stereotactic systems are designed so that the patient lies prone on the table, with the breast extending through an aperture in the table (Fig. 38-2). The breast is compressed and imaged with mammography equipment beneath the table. There is less patient motion and fewer vasovagal reactions than in an upright unit. The disadvantages of the prone tables, compared with the upright systems, are higher cost and greater space requirements.

SAMPLING DEVICES

The stereotactic technique, initially developed for use with fine needle aspiration, then became widely used with the development of the automated spring-loaded devices. Today, most stereotactic biopsies are performed with vacuum-assisted devices. More recently, a total removal system has been developed.

Automated Spring-Loaded Biopsy Device

The automated, spring-loaded or large core needle devices have a two-step firing mechanism (Fig. 38-3). First, the inner stylet is fired into the lesion. Then, the outer cutting cannula is fired over the stylet to cut the tissue specimen. Although the needles range in size from 20- to 14-gauge, usually a 14-gauge needle is used. This device requires a multipass technique with multiple insertions to obtain sufficient tissue samples. Depending on the gauge of the needle used and the number of tissue cores obtained, underestimation of cancer can occur.[15-17]

Today, the automated large core needle devices are primarily used for ultrasound-guided biopsies. The vacuum-assisted device has largely replaced the automated device for stereotactic biopsy.

Vacuum-Assisted Biopsy Device

The vacuum-assisted device, developed in the mid-1990s, offers a number of advantages. It allows single insertion of the needle and directional sampling. The primary advantage of the vacuum-assisted device is the larger amount of tissue acquired with larger needles and greater sampling efficiency provided by vacuum assistance. This results in more accurate pathology results and fewer upgrades at the time of surgical excision.[17,18]

Vacuum-assisted needles range from 14- to 7-gauge. The needle is positioned in the breast at the site of the

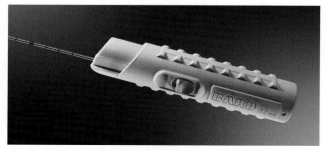

Figure 38-3   Maxcore automated spring-loaded device. (Courtesy of CR Bard, Inc., Murray Hill, NJ.)

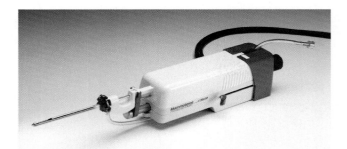

Figure 38-4 Mammotome vacuum-assisted biopsy device. (Courtesy of Ethicon Endo-Surgery, Cincinnati, OH.)

lesion. The vacuum is activated, pulling the tissue into the biopsy aperture. A rotating cutter then is advanced through the needle, shearing off the tissue specimen. The cutter is withdrawn to retrieve the tissue specimen, and the needle is rotated to acquire the next specimen in another area of the lesion. Sampling with this technology allows rapid acquisition of multiple large tissue specimens (Figs. 38-4 to 38-6).

Total Removal System

A breast biopsy system that removes a single, intact, large tissue specimen has been developed recently (Fig. 38-7). This one-pass system collects a specimen in approximately 10 seconds. The probe is inserted into the breast through an 8-mm skin incision. Radiofrequency energy is used to advance the device through the breast to the lesion. Five struts then open to form a basket that circumscribes the lesion. The specimen is withdrawn through the entry channel, which collapses after the specimen is withdrawn. Specimens range in weight from 1 to 3 g and are 10 to 20 mm in diameter, depending on the size of the probe used.

The advantage of this system is that it retrieves an intact specimen, preserving the architecture of the lesion.

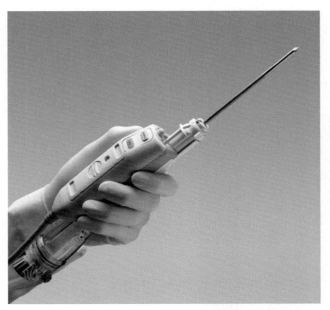

Figure 38-5 EnCor vacuum-assisted biopsy device. (Courtesy of SenoRx, Inc., Aliso Viejo, CA.)

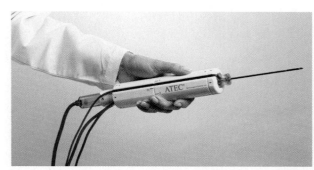

Figure 38-6 Automated Tissue Excision and Collection (ATEC) vacuum-assisted biopsy device. (Courtesy of Hologic: The Women's Company.)

In theory, histologic analysis of this sample should be simpler than evaluating multiple core specimens taken throughout the lesion. Furthermore, retrieving an intact specimen could improve the ability to assess the margins of a lesion. Clinical studies currently are evaluating these potential advantages.

TISSUE MARKERS

Tissue markers, also known as marking clips, are used in two scenarios. One, tissue markers are placed when all mammographic evidence of the lesion is removed at the time of stereotactic biopsy. This facilitates localization of the biopsy site if pathology results require subsequent surgery. Two, markers are used in cases in which neoadjuvant chemotherapy is planned, again to facilitate localization of the malignancy for surgery in the event of a complete imaging response to chemotherapy.

The tissue markers can be placed directly through most biopsy needles into the biopsy cavity. Clip displacement away from the biopsy site with release of compression is not uncommon.[19] A postprocedure mammogram allows identification of the gas-filled biopsy cavity and the relationship of the clip to the cavity. This should be documented in the biopsy procedure report.

Initially, the markers were stainless steel. Most are now composed of titanium embedded in collagen pledgets or biodegradable material similar to Vicryl sutures. The titanium markers are magnetic resonance–compatible, and the pledgets are visible on ultrasound.

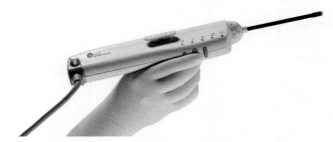

Figure 38-7 EnBloc biopsy device. (Courtesy of Intact, Natick, MA.)

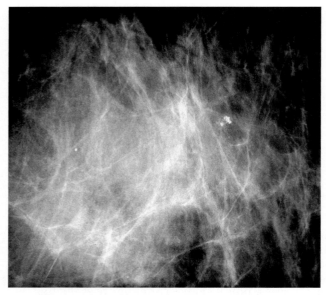

Figure 38-8   Scout view of microcalcifications.

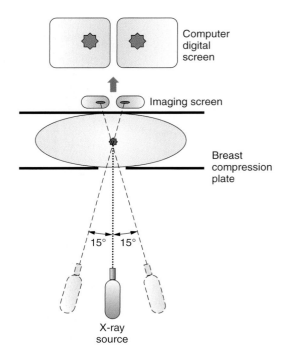

Figure 38-10   Stereotactic views allow triangulation to calculate lesion depth.

Stereotactic Biopsy Procedure

The biopsy needle approach is determined by (1) reviewing the mammograms leading to the biopsy and (2) determining which projection provides the best visualization of the lesion and the shortest distance from the skin to the lesion. The patient is positioned and the breast is compressed between the anterior compression paddle and the image receptor. A scout view is obtained with the lesion located within the 5 × 5 cm open window of the compression paddle. This view provides information on lesion position in the x- and y-axes (Fig. 38-8). Stereo images are then obtained 15 degrees from midline in both positive and negative directions (Fig. 38-9). The depth of the lesion, or the z-axis coordinate, is determined by the targeting computer using the principles of triangulation (Fig. 38-10). It is important to determine whether there is adequate breast tissue to position the needle at the lesion without the needle penetrating the posterior aspect of the breast and striking the image receptor. A distance of 4 mm from the needle tip to back of the breast is considered adequate, and this distance is called the stroke margin.

Once the three-dimensional computer coordinates have been determined, the information is transferred from the computer to the stereotactic table. The needle is then mechanically moved into position for the x- and y-axis coordinates. The z-axis coordinate is manually set by the operator.

The skin overlying the target site is cleansed and anesthetized. A skin incision is made, and the biopsy instrument is introduced into the breast to the prefire position, just proximal to the target. Stereotactic images are obtained to confirm proper needle positioning (Fig. 38-11). The biopsy needle is then fired, and postfire stereotactic images are obtained to confirm that the needle is positioned properly (Fig. 38-12).

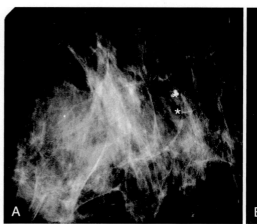
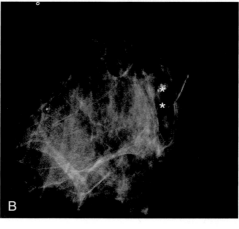

Figure 38-9   **A** and **B**, Stereotactic views.

Figure 38-11 A and **B**, Prefire stereotactic images.

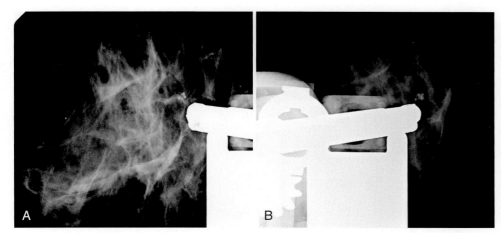

Figure 38-12 A and **B**, Postfire stereotactic images.

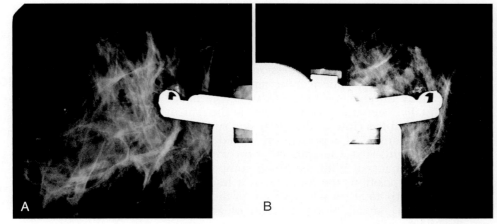

Although tissue specimens are usually obtained in a circumferential manner around the lesion, the vacuum-assisted devices offer the option of selected directional sampling. When the targeted lesion contains calcifications, a specimen radiograph is performed to document the presence of calcifications within the tissue cores (Fig. 38-13). At the completion of the procedure, a tissue marker (marking clip) can be inserted (Fig. 38-14). The needle is then removed, and pressure is held over the biopsy site. The incision is closed with Steri-Strips. Post-procedure mammographic images are taken to confirm that the biopsy site and tissue marker correspond to the targeted lesion initially identified mammographically. Complications are rare and include hematoma or, very rarely, infection. Parker and colleagues reported a 0.2% incidence of hematoma or infection requiring treatment.[2]

Potential Problems and Pitfalls

A number of potential problems can occur with stereotactic biopsy. These include negative or inadequate stroke margins, difficult-to-reach lesions, and targeted calcifications not seen at pathologic evaluation.

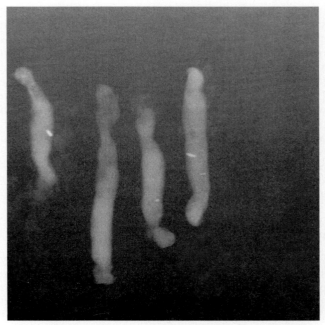

Figure 38-13 Specimen radiograph demonstrates calcifications to be present within the tissue cores.

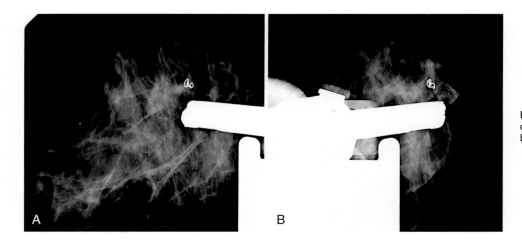

Figure 38-14 **A** and **B**, Postbiopsy stereotactic views demonstrate biopsy cavity and tissue marker.

NEGATIVE STROKE MARGIN

A patient with thin or small breasts may not have an adequate tissue depth after compression to permit the biopsy needle to be positioned for targeting without passing entirely through the breast to strike the image receptor distally. The same problem arises in the patient with a lesion that lies close to the distal skin surface.

There are a number of approaches to remedy a negative stroke margin. First, the planned approach for the needle can be changed. With the breast compressed in the orthogonal position, the location of a lesion may change sufficiently to allow safe insertion of the needle. Second, injecting an additional amount of anesthetic into the tissues may add sufficient depth for a stroke margin that is only slightly negative. Third, the needle may be positioned slightly proximal to the targeted location. Although this places the lesion in the distal aspect of the sampling notch, rather than centered within the sampling notch, adequate tissue samples of the lesion can still be obtained. Fourth, manufacturing adaptations include use of a lateral area to perform the biopsy from an orthogonal approach to the compressed breast (Siemens), or 180-degree rotation of the biopsy site (Hologic). Lastly, the air gap technique may be used in which a second compression plate is placed between the undersurface of the breast and the image receptor, with the open biopsy window of both compression plates in line with the lesion. Once inserted, if the needle passes through the breast and exits the skin on the opposite side, it enters an air space, rather than striking the image receptor.

POSTERIOR AND AXILLARY TAIL LESIONS

Lesions close to the chest wall or high in the axillary tail of the breast may be difficult to sample using the prone stereotactic technique. By rolling the patient toward the table aperture and passing the arm and shoulder through the opening, more of the posterior and axillary tissues can be brought into the biopsy window.

LOST CALCIFICATIONS

When a biopsy is performed for microcalcifications, a specimen radiograph should be performed to confirm the presence of calcifications within the tissue cores. It is helpful to separate and mark the tissue cores containing calcifications prior to sending the tissue to pathology. If microcalcifications cannot be found histologically, the paraffin blocks should be radiographed to direct additional sections for the pathologist, and a polarized lens may be used to identify unstained calcium oxalate crystals. If calcifications are still not identified, the patient should undergo follow-up mammographic images to confirm that the proper site was sampled.

Imaging-Pathology Correlation

One of the most important aspects of any image-guided biopsy is the correlation of the pathology findings with the initial image-detected lesion that prompted the biopsy, to determine concordance. The major limitation of a needle biopsy is sampling error. Therefore, if the pathology results do not explain the imaging findings adequately, the case is discordant, and excisional biopsy should be performed. In addition, there are several pathologic entities that are benign but associated with underestimation of disease. For these pathologic diagnoses, surgical excision is usually recommended.

ATYPICAL DUCTAL HYPERPLASIA

Atypical ductal hyperplasia (ADH) is a proven high risk lesion with potential for underestimation of disease by needle biopsy. Mammographically, ADH presents as microcalcifications that can be indistinguishable from those of ductal carcinoma in situ. Underestimation rates range from 15% to 50%, depending on the needle used; the underestimation rate is lower for vacuum-assisted devices but still too high to preclude excisional biopsy.[16,17]

LOBULAR NEOPLASIA

Lobular neoplasia is a spectrum of lesions including lobular carcinoma in situ and atypical lobular hyperplasia. Several recent studies have shown upgrade rates of 17% to 19% at surgical excision, not significantly different from ADH.[20,21] In addition, no mammographic features have allowed distinction between the patients whose lesions were upgraded at the time of surgery and those whose lesions were not upgraded.[21] Excisional biopsy is recommended for patients with lobular neoplasia diagnosed by stereotactic biopsy.

RADIAL SCAR

A radial scar is identified on mammography as an area of architectural distortion that cannot be differentiated from invasive carcinoma.[22] Radial scars may coexist with carcinoma as well as a number of proliferative breast changes. Therefore, they are considered to be high-risk lesions, and many experts recommend excisional biopsy for radial scars diagnosed by needle biopsy.[23]

PAPILLARY LESIONS

Papillomas (papillary lesions) include large, solitary central duct papillomas and multiple peripheral papillomas. A papilloma is composed of a fibrovascular stalk covered by an epithelial lining. These epithelial cells may undergo hyperplasia and evolve to ADH, ductal carcinoma in situ, or invasive papillary carcinoma.

Mammographically, papillomas may present as small, circumscribed masses or small clusters of calcifications. There are numerous conflicting studies in the literature regarding the rate of underestimation of these lesions when diagnosed at needle biopsy. There is consensus that any atypical papillary lesions should undergo excision, but management of bland-appearing papillary lesions diagnosed by needle biopsy remains controversial.[24]

Summary

Stereotactic core biopsy is a safe, reliable approach for obtaining breast tissue for diagnosis. The indications include any mammographically detected suspicious or indeterminate lesions. Because of the numerous advantages of image-guided biopsy over surgery, this biopsy procedure is now the preferred method of tissue diagnosis for nonpalpable lesions. There are few limitations and complications. Assessment for concordance of radiology and pathology findings and the potential underestimation of disease must be carefully performed to allow proper patient management.

REFERENCES

1. Parker SH, Lovin JD, Jobe WE, et al: Stereotactic breast biopsy with a biopsy gun. Radiology 176:741–747, 1990.
2. Parker SH, Burbank F, Jackman RJ: Percutaneous large-core breast biopsy: A multi-institutional study. Radiology 193:359–364, 1994.
3. Brenner RJ, Bassett LW, Fajardo LL, et al: Stereotactic core-needle breast biopsy: A multi-institutional prospective trial. Radiology 218:866–872, 2001.
4. Bolmgren J, Jacobson B, Nordenstom B: Stereotactic instrument for needle biopsy of the mamma. AJR Am J Roentgenol 129:121–125, 1977.
5. Life Science Intelligence, Inc. #LSI-USOFIWH. 4–31, 2007.
6. Parker SH, Burbank F: A practical approach to minimally invasive breast biopsy. Radiology 1996; 200:11–20, 1996.
7. March DE, Raslavicus A, Coughlin BF, et al: Use of core biopsy in the United States. AJR Am J Roentgenol 169:697–701, 1997.
8. Cady B, Stone MD, Schuler JG, et al: The new era in breast cancer. Invasion, size, and nodal involvement dramatically decreasing as a result of mammographic screening. Arch Surg 131:301–308, 1996.
9. American College of Radiology: Breast imaging reporting and data system (BI-RADS), 3rd ed. Reston, VA, American College of Radiology, 1998.
10. Gisvold JJ, Goellner JR, Grant CS, et al: Breast biopsy: A comparative study of stereotaxically guided core and excisional techniques. AJR Am J Roentgenol 162:815–820, 1994.
11. Kaufman CS, Delbecq R, Jacobson L: Excising the re-excision: Stereotactic core-needle biopsy decreases need for re-excision of breast cancer. World J Surg 22:1023–1028, 1998.
12. Liberman L, Goodstine SL, Dershaw DD, et al: One operation after percutaneous diagnosis of nonpalpable breast cancer: Frequency and associated factors. AJR Am J Roentgenol 178:673–679, 2002.
13. Caines JS, McPhee MD, Konok GP, Wright BA: Stereotactic needle core biopsy of breast lesions using a regular mammographic table with an adaptable stereotactic device. AJR Am J Roentgenol 163:317–321, 1994.
14. Welle GJ, Clark M, Loo SS, et al: Stereotactic breast biopsy: Recumbent breast biopsy using add-on upright equipment. AJR Am J Roentgenol 175:59–63, 2000.
15. Bassett L, Winchester DP, Caplan RB, et al: Stereotactic core-needle biopsy of the breast: A report of the Joint Task Force of the American College of Radiology, American College of Surgeons, and College of American Pathologists. CA Cancer J Clin 47:171–190, 1997.
16. Jackman RJ, Nowels KW, Rodriguez-Soto J, et al: Stereotactic, automated, large-core needle biopsy of nonpalpable breast lesions: False-negative and histologic underestimation rates after long-term follow-up. Radiology 210:799–805, 1999.
17. Burbank F: Stereotactic breast biopsy of atypical ductal hyperplasia and ductal carcinoma in situ lesions: Improved accuracy with directional, vacuum-assisted biopsy. Radiology 202:843–847, 1997.
18. Pfarl G, Helbich TH, Riedl CC, et al: Stereotactic 11-gauge vacuum-assisted breast biopsy: A validation study. AJR Am J Roentgenol 179:1503–1507, 2002.
19. Esserman LE, Cura MA, DaCosta D: Recognizing pitfalls in early and late migration of clip markers after imaging-guided directional vacuum-assisted biopsy. Radiographics 24:147–156, 2004.
20. Foster MC, Helvie MA, Gregory NE, et al: Lobular carcinoma in situ or atypical lobular hyperplasia: Is excisional biopsy necessary? Radiology 231:813–819, 2004.
21. Mahoney MC, Robinson TM, Shaughnessy EA: Lobular neoplasia at 11-gauge vacuum-assisted stereotactic biopsy: Correlation with surgical excision and mammographic follow-up. AJR Am J Roentgenol 187:949–954, 2006.
22. Frouge C, Tristant H, Guinebretiere JM, et al: Mammographic lesions suggestive of radial scars: Microscopic findings in 40 cases. Radiology 195:623–625, 1995.
23. Patterson JA, Scott M, Anderson N, Kirk SJ: Radial scar, complex sclerosing lesion and risk of breast cancer. Analysis of 175 cases in Northern Ireland. Eur J Surg Oncol 30:1065–1068, 2004.
24. Liberman L, Bracero N, Vuolo MA, et al: Percutaneous large-core biopsy of papillary breast lesions. AJR Am J Roentgenol 172:331–337, 1999.

chapter 39

Cytopathology of the Breast

SHAHLA MASOOD

The remarkable changes in the approach to the diagnosis and management of breast cancer in recent years have provided significant opportunities for pathologists to play an active role in patient care. Advances in breast imaging and emphasis on screening programs have led to the increased detection of atypical proliferative lesions and smaller breast cancers.

Minimally invasive procedures such as fine needle aspiration biopsy (FNAB) and core needle biopsy (CNB) have almost replaced open surgical biopsies. Breast conservation therapy and sentinel lymph node biopsy (SLNB) have provided balanced alternatives to mastectomy and total axillary dissection. The advances in molecular testing and recognition of prognostic and predictive factors have contributed to the introduction of molecular targeted therapy and practice of personalized medicine. Above all, enhanced public awareness and recognition of the importance of integrated care via a multidisciplinary approach have resulted in promoting the breast center concept, leading to a better patient care.

Similar to the traditional practice of surgical pathology, the discipline of cytopathology has effectively responded to these changing trends in breast health care. The contribution of cytopathology includes performance of FNAB and interpretation of the results, optimization of new technologies for the small size samples for providing predictive and prognostic information, and the use of imprint cytology in detection of tumor cells at lumpectomy margins and in SLNBs. In addition, imprint cytology has provided an effective tool in the assessment of adequacy of samples obtained from the CNB procedure and the immediate interpretation of test results.

Furthermore, several studies have already confirmed the value of cytomorphology as a breast cancer risk predictor. Recognition of the cytomorphology of high-risk proliferative breast disease and premalignant lesions is an intriguing concept for identifying patients who may benefit from various risk-reduction modalities. FNAB, nipple aspiration fluid (NAF), and ductal lavage, in combination with molecular testing, molecular imaging, and ductoscopy, have provided exciting opportunities for breast cytopathology to become an integral part of breast cancer research and prevention.

This chapter provides a summary of the use of cytopathology in the current practice of breast health care and for the future trend of breast cancer research and prevention.

Diagnosis

FINE NEEDLE ASPIRATION BIOPSY

Introduced in 1930 by Martin and Ellis in New York, FNAB has gone through several ups and downs in United States during the last century.[1] However, in Europe, this procedure has been welcomed as a rapid and cost-effective initial procedure in the evaluation of breast lesions.[2,3] Several years ago, changes in the U.S. medical economy and growing interest in cost containment stimulated a renewed interest in breast FNAB in this country. Breast cytopathology became an integral part of pathology residency training and cytopathology fellowship programs. This change also resulted in numerous series of reports in the literature emphasizing the merits of FNAB.[4-6] Several studies showed superiority of FNAB over CNB in palpable breast lesions by being more accurate, less painful, more rapid, and more cost-effective. This superiority have been attributed to the small diameter of the needle in FNAB, which allows an easy back-and-forth motion in different directions and better sampling of the lesions. In contrast, CNB in a single pass may displace a mobile lesion and miss the target.[7-10]

FNAB is a procedure that is easily accepted by a woman. This acceptance may lead to an earlier detection of breast cancer. In the author's experience, the fear of surgery and the scar on the breast is one of the major causes of delay in seeking medical attention in women who have a breast mass. FNAB relieves the anxiety of a woman who has benign breast disease by providing a rapid diagnosis. In malignant circumstances, FNAB allows a woman to actively participate in her treatment planning prior to any surgical intervention. More importantly, FNAB may be an alternative to surgical biopsy in the evaluation of local occurrences and metastatic lesions, as well as in inoperable conditions. It may also easily provide samples for cases selected for neoadjuvant chemotherapy for diagnostic and predictive/prognostic information.[11-13]

Up to now, despite the previously mentioned advantages of FNAB, the role of this procedure as the sole diagnostic tool in management of patients with breast lesions has remained controversial. It is clear that practice of breast FNAB requires support of the clinicians involved in the care of their patients and their understanding of both merits and limitations of this procedure. Breast FNAB is a simple, yet complex procedure that is influenced by many variables. Accurate interpretation of breast FNAB requires clear guidelines for specimen collection, staining, and preparation. It is also essential to adhere to well-established cytomorphologic criteria for an accurate interpretation. The terminology used for reporting FNAB should be similar to that of surgical biopsy and should include pertinent diagnostic, prognostic, and predictive information. Among various reasons that have contributed to this controversy, casual use of the term *atypia* in benign breast lesions resulting in unnecessary follow-up open biopsies has played a major role.[13,14]

It should be recognized that epithelial atypia is not always a reflection of a prognostically relevant entity. Interpretation of breast cytopathology must be based on recognition of both cellular and architectural features, similar to the well-established "pattern recognition" in surgical pathology. This concept is in contrast to gynecologic cytology where cellular and nuclear features are the most important parameter for diagnostic interpretation.[15]

Recognition of the pattern of presentation of specific benign entities in breast cytology reduces the unnecessary use of the term *atypia* and maximizes the efficiency of cytology. Nuclear atypia is not an uncommon feature in fibroadenoma and proliferative breast disease and is frequently seen in metaplasias, inflammatory/reactive conditions, hormone therapy, or other treatment-induced changes. In contrast, there are several primary breast carcinomas that are associated with insignificant nuclear atypia. These include infiltrating lobular carcinoma, tubular carcinoma, and low-grade lesions.[15,16]

Guidelines have been developed to suggest educational requirements for pathologists interested in performing and interpreting breast FNAB. During the National Cancer Institute (NCI)–sponsored workshop, with participation of an international multidisciplinary panel of experts in breast cancer, the parameters for the practice of breast FNAB were defined and widely published. The NCI published uniform guidelines for breast FNAB, including recommendation for indication, training, credentialing technique, diagnostic terminology, ancillary studies, prognostic and predictive markers, and post-FNAB recommendations. In areas of diagnostic terminology, efforts were made to introduce the category of atypical/indeterminate to underscore the difficulty in interpretation of certain entities. These included the distinction between atypical hyperplasia versus low-grade carcinoma, papilloma versus papillary carcinoma, fibroadenoma versus phyllodes tumor, and mucinous carcinoma versus mucocele. Recommendation was made for a follow-up excisional biopsy when the diagnosis of any of the previously mentioned entities were entertained by breast FNAB.[17,18]

DIFFICULT-TO-DIAGNOSE CASES IN BREAST CYTOPATHOLOGY

Atypical Hyperplasia versus Low-Grade Ductal Carcinoma in Situ

It has been known for many years that women who have undergone a breast biopsy for so-called *fibrocystic disease* have an increased risk of breast cancer.[19] So, attempts have been made to classify the spectrum of fibrocystic disease into reproducible and prognostically relevant categories. These studies have focused on the relative risk of subsequent development of breast disease in patients with fibrocystic disease based on the histologic features in their biopsies. These efforts have resulted in introducing, first, a new terminology of nonproliferative breast disease, proliferative breast disease without atypia and proliferative breast disease with atypia (atypical hyperplasia), and second, defining the specific histologic changes associated with each category. It is generally agreed that nonproliferative breast disease carries no increased risk. Proliferative breast disease without atypia has a slightly increased risk (1.5 to 2 times) and proliferative breast disease with atypia has a moderately increased risk (4 to 5 times) for subsequent development of breast cancer. Patients with carcinoma in situ have 8 to 10 times the risk of eventual development of invasive breast cancer.[20,21]

This information has given a new significance to the recognition of the spectrum of morphologic changes seen in breast disease. It is now possible to separate breast lesions into benign, premalignant, and malignant categories. The precise histologic features of these breast lesions have been well characterized. However, despite the reliability of breast FNAB in separating benign from malignant lesions, the cytologic diagnosis of borderline lesions has remained a challenge.

In a prospective study using mammographically guided fine needle aspirates in 100 nonpalpable breast lesions, we assessed the reliability of a cytologic grading system to define the cytologic features of proliferative and nonproliferative breast disease and to differentiate between benign, premalignant and malignant breast lesions.[22,23] We developed a cytologic grading system evaluating the aspirates for the cellular arrangement, degrees of cellular pleomorphism and anisonucleosis, presence of myoepithelial cells and nucleoli, and status of the chromatin pattern. Values ranging from 1 to 4 were assigned to each criterion, and a score based on the sum of the individual values was calculated for each case. With scores ranging from minimum of 6 to maximum of 24, the cases were divided into nonproliferative breast disease (score, 6–10), proliferative breast disease without atypia (score, 11–14), proliferative breast disease with atypia (score, 15–18), and cancer (score, 19–24). Comparing the cytologic interpretation to the reported histologic diagnosis obtained from needle localization biopsies, we found a high degree of concordance between the results (Tables 39-1 and 39-2).

We believe that by using strict cytologic criteria, it may be possible to define the continuous spectrum of changes in breast lesions and separate hyperplasia from

TABLE 39-1

Masood Cytology Index

Cellular Arrangement	Cellular Pleomorphism	Myoepithelial Cells	Anisonucleosis	Nucleoli	Chromatin Clumping	Score*
Monolayer	Absent	Many	Absent	Absent	Absent	1
Nuclear overlapping	Mild	Moderate	Mild	Micronucleoli	Rare	2
Clustering	Moderate	Few	Moderate	Micro- and/or rare macronucleoli	Occasional	3
Loss of cohesion	Conspicuous	Absent	Conspicuous	Predominately macronucleoli	Frequent	4

*Total scores: 6–10, normal; 11–14, proliferative; 15–18, atypia; ≥19, suspicious for cancer.
Modified from Masood S, Frykberg ER, McLellan GL, et al: Prospective evaluation of radiologically directed fine-needle aspiration biopsy of non-palpable breast lesions. Cancer 66:1480–1487, 1990.

TABLE 39-2

Concordance between Cytologic Evaluation and Histologic Diagnosis in 100 Mammographically Guided Fine Needle Aspirations

Diagnosis	No. of Cases	Concordance (%)
Nonproliferative breast disease	29/34	85
Proliferative breast disease without atypia	15/17	88
Proliferative breast disease with atypia	21/23	91
Cancer	17/20	85

Modified from Masood S, Frykberg ER, McLellan GL, et al: Cytologic differentiation between proliferative and nonproliferative breast disease in mammographically guided fine-needle aspirates. Diagn Cytopathol 7:581–590, 1991.

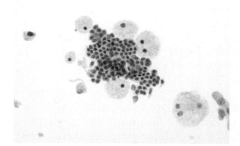

Figure 39-1 Nonproliferative breast disease characterized by a cluster of bland-appearing epithelial and myoepithelial cells and a few macrophages. (Papanicolaou stain, ×40.)

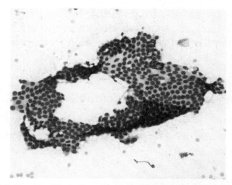

Figure 39-2 Proliferative disease without atypia characterized by a cluster of epithelial and myoepithelial cells with overriding of nuclei. (Diff-Quik stain, ×20.)

neoplasia. This grading system, now recognized as the *Masood Cytology Index*, is commonly used as a surrogate end point biomarker in chemoprevention trials. It has also been used to study the relationship between our defined morphology and the corresponding alterations associated with the pattern of expression of biomarkers and genetic profile in borderline breast lesions.[24–27]

Nonproliferative Breast Disease: Masood Cytology Index, 6–10. The cell yield in these aspirates is variable and depends on the nature of the lesion. In noncystic lesions, the aspirate is scanty or moderate. Frequently, the aspirate consists of clusters of small uniform-appearing epithelial cells arranged in mono-layered sheets with a honeycomb pattern. Foam cells, apocrine cells, single naked cells and fragments of stromal cells are frequently observed. The cells have regular nuclei with fine chromatin pattern. Nucleoli are not commonly seen. Myoepithelial cells are easily identified (Fig. 39-1).

Proliferative Breast Disease without Atypia: Masood Cytology Index, 11–14. Proliferative breast disease differs from nonproliferative breast disease by its higher cell yield and most unique cellular arrangement. The cellularity is moderate to high, depending on the

degree of proliferative epithelial changes. There are increased numbers of tightly cohesive groups of ductal epithelial and myoepithelial cells with some overriding of the nuclei, occasional loss of polarity, and some variability in the nuclear size. Micronucleoli may be seen. Cytologic atypia is inconspicuous. Apocrine cells, histiocytes, and occasional naked nuclei are the accompanying cells in these aspirates (Fig. 39-2).

Proliferative Breast Disease with Atypia (Atypical Hyperplasia): Masood Cytology Index, 15–18. The cellular aspirates are frequently rich and are composed of multiple clustering of epithelial cells. The crowded clusters of cells show conspicuous loss of polarity and overriding of the nuclei. Nucleoli are present and display irregular and coarse chromatin pattern. Variation in nuclear size and cellular pleomorphism are also present. Within the crowded atypical epithelial cells, there is morphologic evidence of myoepithelial cell differentiation (Fig. 39-3).

Ductal Carcinoma in Situ (Masood Cytology Index, 19–24. Ductal carcinoma in situ (DCIS) presents with variable cytologic features, which reflects its morphologic diversity. Divided into low and high nuclear grade DCIS, there are distinct cytologic differences between the two entities.

1. High nuclear grade DCIS. FNAB of high nuclear grade DCIS is usually cellular and displays loosely cohesive clusters of malignant cells with individual cell necrosis and mitosis. Nuclear membrane abnormality, clumping of chromatin, and conspicuous nucleoli are often present. Nuclear pleomorphism and irregularly shaped nucleoli are characteristic features of high nuclear grade DCIS. Microcalcified particles may or may not be present (Fig. 39-4).

2. Low nuclear grade DCIS. Aspirates from low nuclear grade DCIS vary in cellularity and are characterized by a monomorphic cell population of small- to medium-sized epithelial cells arranged singly or as loosely cohesive clusters. The cell clusters may have a solid, cribriform, or papillary pattern with no accompanying myoepithelial cells present. This is in contrast with atypical hyperplasia, where the myoepithelial cells are seen intermingled within the groups of atypical cells and appear as part of the cellular aggregate. Microcalcified particles, foamy histiocytes, and a few isolated myoepithelial cells may be seen in the background (Fig. 39-5).

In Situ versus Invasive Carcinoma

The cytologic features of DCIS are not exclusive and are often seen in invasive lesions. Nevertheless, associated

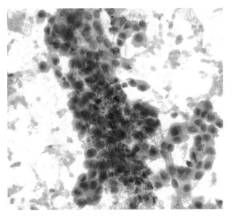

Figure 39-4 High nuclear grade ductal carcinoma in situ characterized by pleomorphic population of neoplastic cells in a necrotic background. (Papanicolaou stain, ×40.)

with specific mammographic features and defined clinical presentations, it may be possible to maximize the utility of FNAB and suggest the correct diagnosis. This includes the recognition of cytologic features of special subtypes of ductal carcinoma such as mucinous, medullary, and small cell carcinoma, which are most often present as an invasive lesion, although rarely in situ mucinous carcinoma and small cell carcinoma can occur. The presence of skin retraction, fixed nipple, ulceration, and inflammatory carcinoma and/or evidence of metastasis are also indicative of invasive breast carcinoma. In our experience, stromal infiltration defined by the presence of neoplastic cells within the stromal elements may predict the status of tumor invasion in breast fine needle aspirates[28] (Fig. 39-6).

Because the recommended management of DCIS may be similar to that of invasive ductal carcinoma, the distinction between these two entities may not be critical. However, this separation becomes essential for those patients selected for preoperative chemotherapy. In these circumstances, assessment of tumor invasion in difficult to diagnose cases should be followed by core needle biopsy.

Lobular Neoplasia

Studies suggest that there are overriding morphologic features between atypical lobular hyperplasia and lobular

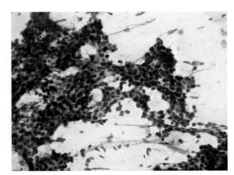

Figure 39-3 Proliferative breast disease with atypia characterized by a cluster of epithelial and myoepithelial cells, with conspicuous overriding of nuclei, loss of polarity, and formation of cribriform-like spaces. (Papanicolaou stain, ×40.)

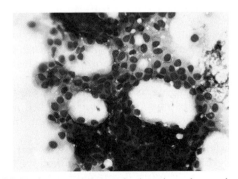

Figure 39-5 Low nuclear grade ductal carcinoma in situ characterized by monotonous population of cells forming cribriform pattern. (Diff-Quik stain, ×40.)

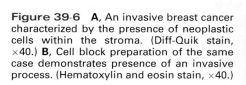

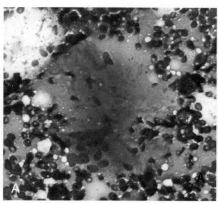

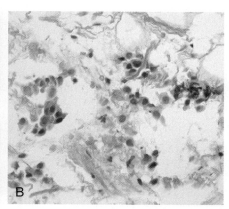

Figure 39-6 A, An invasive breast cancer characterized by the presence of neoplastic cells within the stroma. (Diff-Quik stain, ×40.) **B,** Cell block preparation of the same case demonstrates presence of an invasive process. (Hematoxylin and eosin stain, ×40.)

carcinoma in situ. Therefore the term lobular neoplasia is currently used for these lesions. Lobular neoplasia is now considered as a marker for the subsequent development of breast cancer. The distinction between lobular neoplasia and infiltrating lobular carcinoma is important since the management of these two entities is quite different.[11,29]

Aspirates of lobular neoplasia show loosely cohesive groups of small uniform cells with eccentric regular nuclei and occasional intracytoplasmic lumina. The nuclei are hyperchromatic with fine chromatin clumping and occasional inconspicuous nucleoli. Occasionally, small cell groups forming "cell balls," conforming to acini of lobular neoplasia, may be seen (Fig. 39-7). Aspirates of infiltrating lobular carcinoma show overlapping features but are more cellular and contain more atypical single cells. We believe that the cellular aspirates that contain significant numbers of small uniform cells characteristic of infiltrating lobular carcinoma should be diagnosed accordingly and should be treated definitively. However, patients whose aspirates are scanty in cellularity should undergo an excisional biopsy to confirm the diagnosis.

Infiltrating Lobular Carcinoma. Lobular carcinoma is considered to be a significant contributor to the high false-negative results occurring in breast fine needle aspirates. This is the reflection of the lack of significant nuclear

atypia in the aspirates obtained from this pathologic entity. The smears show a relatively uniform population of small-to medium-sized cells. The cells have scanty, ill-defined cytoplasm with an increased nuclear cytoplasmic ratio and tend to occur singly, in "Indian file," or cords. The cytoplasm may contain sharply punched-out vacuoles and occasionally signet ring forms may be seen. The nuclei have a fine chromatin pattern, which is often eccentric. They contain small nucleoli. Anisonucleosis is minimal[29,30] (Fig. 39-8).

Intraductal Papilloma versus Papillary Carcinoma

Papillary neoplasms are characterized by the formation of three-dimensional epithelial fronds, which are supported by a fibrovascular stroma. The fine needle aspirates are often bloody. The cellularity of the aspirate, varying from highly cellular to sparsely cellular, depends on whether the lesion is solid or cystic, benign or malignant. Benign papillomas tend to be less cellular. On the other hand, their malignant and atypical counterparts have more cohesive clusters of cells. Distinction between benign and malignant lesions can be challenging on cytology. An excision of the lesion is necessary to make this determination, unless features of malignancy, such as a majority population of singly dispersed atypical epithelial cells with eccentrically located nuclei, intact cytoplasm, and high nuclear-to-cytoplasmic ratios are present.[11,13]

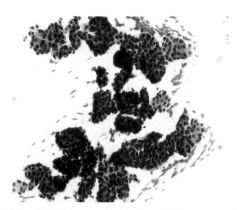

Figure 39-7 Lobular neoplasia characterized by acinar proliferation of small cells with a uniform appearance. (Papanicolaou stain, ×100.) (Reproduced with permission from Masood S: Cytopathology of the breast. Chicago, ASCP Press, 1996. © 1996 American Society for Clinical Pathology.)

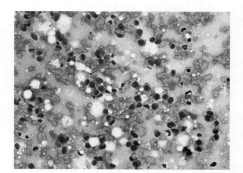

Figure 39-8 Infiltrating lobular carcinoma characterized by dispersed clusters of small cells with eccentric nuclei and cytoplasmic lumen. (Diff-Quik stain, ×60.)

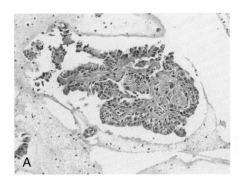

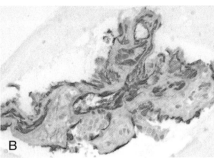

Figure 39-9 A, Cell block preparation obtained from fine needle aspiration biopsy of an intraductal papilloma. (Hematoxylin and eosin stain, ×20.) **B,** Immunostain for calponin demonstrates the presence of myoepithelial cell markers. (Immunostain, ×40.)

One criterion that is useful in distinguishing between a benign and a malignant lesion by histology is to evaluate for the presence or absence of myoepithelial cells. By cytology, benign lesions normally have at least a few myoepithelial cells within the papillary fragments. The presence of myoepithelial cells can be confirmed by immunohistochemical staining with smooth muscle actin or new markers, including calponin and p63. In addition, the presence of apocrine metaplasia, foam cells, and heterogeneous appearance of the cells are also features commonly seen in benign papillary lesions. The epithelial cells arranged around the fibrovascular stroma tend to have a tall columnar morphology with eccentric nuclei[11,31] (Fig. 39-9).

Papillary carcinomas of the breast, whether invasive or noninvasive, probably arise de novo rather than as malignant degeneration of benign papillomas, and they normally have a better prognosis than other malignant neoplasms of the breast. Because of this better prognosis, it is important to recognize potential papillary malignancies by cytology. Noninvasive papillary carcinomas are often completely or partially intracystic, whereas the invasive papillary carcinomas can present either as an infiltrating ductal carcinoma with papillary features or as a pure invasive papillary carcinoma.

Fine needle aspirates of papillary carcinomas are characteristically highly cellular with a monotonous rather than a heterogeneous population of single clusters of short to tall columnar cells (Fig. 39-10). They lack myoepithelial cells, which may be confirmed by the application of immunohistochemical stains. Rarely, tumor cells may show a significant degree of atypia, with an increase in the number of mitotic figures. A necrotic background is also frequently seen. Occasionally, infarction of a papillary lesion can lead to a hemorrhagic and necrotic background. This may cause a false-positive diagnosis of malignancy. There are also issues related to sampling errors, which add to the challenges associated with the diagnosis of papillary lesions by minimally invasive procedures. In these circumstances, total excision of the lesion with inclusion of a rim of normal tissue is advised.

Fibroepithelial Tumors

Fibroadenoma. Fibroadenomas can be accurately diagnosed by FNAB. The aspirates are typically cellular and demonstrate a biphasic pattern consisting of epithelial and stromal elements. A two-cell population exists. There are large sheets of monolayered epithelial cells, which form finger-like projections and fronding with an "antler-horn" pattern. The other cell type is the myoepithelial cells with naked nuclei. These cells may be bipolar or spindle in shape and lie freely in the background. Scattered histiocytes, apocrine cells, and occasional multinucleated giant cells may be intermingled within the cellular aspirate of fibroadenomas[11,13] (Fig. 39-11).

Fibroadenomas have many faces and can display a variety of architectural patterns and cellular features. The cytologic differential diagnosis includes the spectrum of fibrocystic change, including atypical hyperplasia and papillary lesions. Fibroadenomas can also mimic phyllodes tumors and low-grade carcinomas, including tubular carcinoma. The combination of a honeycomb pattern, antler horn-like projections, and numerous bipolar naked nuclei is the most important factor in making the accurate diagnosis of fibroadenoma.[11,13,32]

Fibroadenomas may be associated with significant cytologic atypia, resulting in a false-positive diagnosis. The potential pathogenetic mechanisms for atypia in fibroadenoma include response to hormonal stimulation, focal secretory activity, response to inflammation, squamous and apocrine metaplasia, and atypical epithelial proliferation. We have seen many cases in which the cytologic features of atypical hyperplasia coexisted with histologically proven fibroadenomas. Fibroadenomas may also be characterized by the presence of cell balls and distended cords, simulating lobular neoplasia. Pregnancy and lactational changes increase the cellularity of fibroadenoma and produce moderate nuclear atypia and conspicuous nucleoli. In these circumstances, the cellularity of the aspirate, loose cohesion, occasional papillary structures, anisonucleosis, and macronuclei can simulate carcinoma. The presence of naked nuclei, stromal fragments, and finger-like projections should suggest the benign nature of the lesion. The absence of a necrotic background and isolated, single, pleomorphic epithelial cells are also helpful in distinguishing fibroadenoma from carcinoma.[11,13,32–34]

The cytologic distinction between fibroadenoma and phyllodes tumors may also present a diagnostic challenge. Stromal fragments in phyllodes tumor are conspicuously cellular. Also, the spindle cells in phyllodes

Figure 39-10 **A**, Papillary carcinoma characterized by a cellular aspirate with papillae of various sizes, fibrovascular core and tall columnar cells. (Papanicolaou stain, Immunostain ×100.) **B**, Immunostain for calponin is negative. (Reproduced with permission from Masood S: Cytopathology of the breast. Chicago, ASCP Press, 1996. © 1996 American Society for Clinical Pathology.)

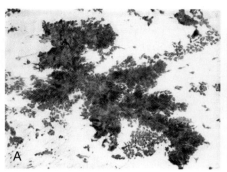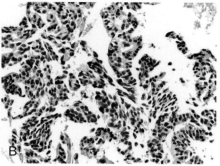

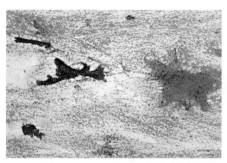

Figure 39-11 Fibroadenoma characterized by biphasic pattern of epithelial/myoepithelial cells and stromal component. (Papanicolaou stain, ×10.)

tumor are embedded in pink-staining, acid mucopolysaccharide of the stroma, which is best demonstrated by metachromatic stains.[11,13,35,36]

Phyllodes Tumor. The cytologic features of phyllodes tumors have been well recognized. Generally, the aspirates from phyllodes tumors are rich in cellularity and demonstrate a distinct biphasic pattern. The smears contain uniform sheets of epithelial cells and associated oval naked nuclei in the background. The second component of the aspirate includes stromal fragments in which there are conspicuous numbers of spindle cells. These cells are enmeshed in material that stains metachromatically with the modified Wright-Giemsa stains. Isolated mesenchymal cells are also present. Foam cells, macrophages, and multinucleated giant cells are frequent companions of phyllodes tumors[13,35] (Fig. 39-12).

The separation between low-grade (benign) from high-grade (malignant) phyllodes tumors is based on the presence of stromal overgrowth, atypical stromal cells, and mitosis. Pleomorphic polygonal or vacuolated stromal cells are the features of malignancy in phyllodes tumors. Blood vessels crossing the stromal fragments previously suggested as characteristic features of malignancy in phyllodes tumors have also been reported in so-called benign phyllodes tumors. Presence or absence of foamy macrophages, multinucleated histiocytes, and apocrine metaplasia are not helpful features to distinguish between low- and high-grade phyllodes tumors. Proliferative changes seen in both low- and high-grade phyllodes tumors can lead to false-positive diagnosis of an invasive breast carcinoma.[13,35]

Mucinous Lesion. Mucinous carcinomas and mucoceles share similar features. Mucinous carcinomas almost always occur in older women. During aspiration, a gelatinous material is obtained, and the smears show abundant mucin, many single cells, and cohesive clusters of small uniform cells with round nuclei, inconspicuous nucleoli, and branching blood vessels (Fig. 39-13). Mucinous carcinomas can also present with a dispersed cell pattern with uniform cell population with eccentric nuclei and mucinous background. In these circumstances, the possibility of a signet ring carcinoma should be considered.

Signet ring carcinoma, although unusual, can present as primary breast carcinoma; however, the possibility of a metastasis to the breast should also be kept in mind. Clues to an accurate diagnosis include the review of the clinical history and of the previous pathology findings as well as the use of ancillary studies such as special stains, electron microscopy, and a panel of immunostains.

Figure 39-12 **A** and **B**, Phyllodes tumor characterized by biphasic pattern of epithelial/myoepithelial cells and cellular stromal component. (Diff-Quik stain, ×40.)

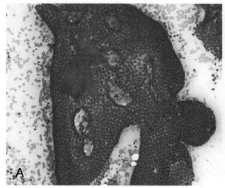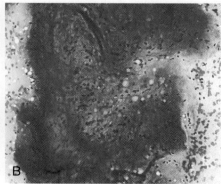

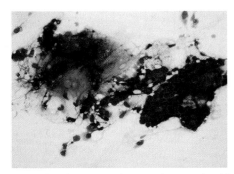

Figure 39-13 Mucinous carcinoma characterized by isolated clusters of neoplastic epithelial cells surrounded by mucinous material. (Diff-Quik stain, ×40.)

Mucinous carcinomas must be distinguished from mucocele-like tumors and myxoid fibroadenomas. Mucocele-like tumor, a rare benign condition of the breast, occurs in premenopausal women.[36] Mucinous carcinoma, in contrast, occurs in postmenopausal women. Therefore, extreme caution should be exercised when considering a diagnosis of mucinous carcinoma in a premenopausal woman. Mucocele-like tumors can also be distinguished from hypocellular variants of mucinous carcinoma by the types of cells embedded in the mucus. In mucocele-like tumors, both epithelial and myoepithelial cells are present, whereas in mucinous carcinomas, only epithelial cells are seen. Immunostaining for myoepithelial markers easily demonstrates the presence of myoepithelial cells in mucocele-like tumors.[13,37]

Another differential diagnosis is fibroadenoma with myxoid stroma, which may mimic the appearance of mucus (Fig. 39-14). Clues to the correct diagnosis are young age of the patient and the presence of two cell populations, bare nuclei, and antler horns in fibroadenoma. Nuclei are reportedly significantly larger in mucinous carcinoma than in benign lesions of the breast.[13,37]

FINE NEEDLE ASPIRATION BIOPSY VERSUS CORE NEEDLE BIOPSY: SIMILARITY IN SAMPLING AND DIAGNOSTIC ISSUES

As more reports appear in the literature, we are beginning to recognize that the limitations with CNB are similar to those previously reported for FNAB. The selection of the patients, the performance of the procedure, the processing of the specimen, and the morphologic interpretation of needle biopsies are issues that require

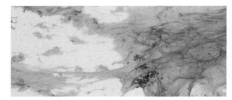

Figure 39-14 Mucocele characterized by ductal/epithelial cells scattered and clustered with collections of mucoid material. (Papanicolaou stain, ×4).

special attention by several specialists interested in breast disease. Further work is necessary to optimize the criteria for selection of the appropriate procedure on an individual basis and refine protocols for follow-up management and assess the long-term outcome of each procedure.

Cost should influence the decision to use FNAB or CNB. This is of critical importance, particularly in countries of limited resources. This procedure may be the only affordable procedure in developing countries that have inadequate health care facilities, a heavy patient load, financial constraints, and an unreliable supply of basic necessities.[38–40]

It is now generally agreed that patients who are diagnosed by CNB as having atypical ductal hyperplasia, lobular lesions, sclerosing lesions such as radial scar, and papillary lesions should undergo a follow-up needle localization excisional biopsy. We are also familiar with discovering invasive lesions in lumpectomy or mastectomy specimens diagnosed as in situ lesions by CNB. Reports in the literature have clearly demonstrated significant frequency of more severe lesions in the follow-up surgical excision of the previously mentioned entities diagnosed by CNB. Similar to FNAB, histologic findings in CNB should be correlated with the mammographic results with consideration of an excisional biopsy if there is any discrepancy[41–44] (Table 39-3).

In addition, small sample size and sampling errors are often common issues. Furthermore, there are reports in the literature about the diagnostic complexity of epithelial displacement simulating pseudoinvasion in core biopsies. In CNB, fragmentation and small size of the specimen may create diagnostic difficulty. Artifactual distortion of the tissue and misplaced epithelial cells occasionally make the distinction between a reactive process and a malignant lesion a serious diagnostic challenge.[45]

Regardless of the limitations of these procedures, both FNAB and CNB provide excellent opportunity to avoid unnecessary open biopsies. Occasionally, more than one technique is needed to make an accurate decision.

NIPPLE CYTOLOGY

Nipple discharge is commonly associated with benign breast lesions; however, it is often associated with a great source of anxiety and frustration for women. Approximately 11% of cases with nipple discharge are caused by malignancy. This incidence increases if the discharge is associated with an underlying mass or abnormality seen in breast imaging.[46] It is critically important to determine whether the discharge is benign or pathologic. Physiologic discharge is often presented as white or green, bilateral nonspontaneous secretions from multiple ducts and may be the result of drugs such as oral contraceptives and antihypertensives, hypothyroidism, or a pituitary adenoma. In addition, puberty, breast nipple stimulation, and elevated levels of prolactin are causes of abnormal physiologic nipple discharge.[46–48]

Pathologic nipple discharge is characterized by serous bloody, unilateral, spontaneous exudate from a single duct, and it occurs in the absence of pregnancy and lactation. It is frequently associated with papilloma. The incidence of carcinoma in patients with nipple discharge

TABLE 39-3
Diagnostic Challenges in Core Needle Biopsy

Pathology Features	Increased Incidence of Malignancy at Excision
Ductal carcinoma in situ	Up to 20%
Atypical ductal hyperplasia	13%–66%
Lobular carcinoma in situ	24.3%
Atypical lobular hyperplasia	22.6%
Atypical papilloma	33%–83%
Papilloma	18%–50%

Reproduced with permission from Masood S: Contemporary issues in breast cytopathology. Clin Lab Med 25:678–688, 2005.

is higher in males.[49] Aside from clinical examination, breast imaging, ductography, and nipple cytology are commonly used in assessment of patients with nipple discharge. However, the presence of a normal ductogram cannot totally exclude the possibility of a significant intraductal lesion.[50]

The value of nipple discharge cytology has remained controversial. Several studies have demonstrated the low sensitivity of this procedure and its limitations as an effective diagnostic tool. However, a few studies have demonstrated up to 85% sensitivity for this technique.[50–52]

The cytologic presentation of nipple discharge varies depending on the underlying cause. The most frequent cause of nipple discharge is fibrocystic change. Smears contain numerous foam cells, a proteinaceous background, and a small numbers of ductal epithelial cells. Similar findings are reported in mammary duct ectasia. However, the secretion may be thick and present with a "paving stone" effect. Nipple discharge associated with mastitis has a significant number of neutrophils.[53]

Papillomas present as tight papillary clusters of slightly atypical ductal cells, columnar epithelial cells, foamy macrophages, and myoepithelial and apocrine cells (Fig. 39-15). Overall, nipple discharge caused by benign

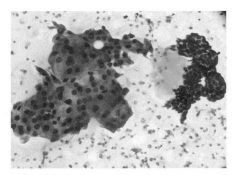

Figure 39-15 Nipple cytology of an intraductal papilloma demonstrating cluster of apocrine metaplasia and ductal epithelial cells forming three-dimensional growth patterns. (Papanicolaou stain, ×40.)

conditions such as fibrocystic change, papillomas, or a physiologic mechanism cannot always be distinguished cytologically. Differentiation between papillary carcinoma versus papilloma in nipple discharge may also be difficult. Similar to FNAB, the term *papillary lesion* may be suggested if the distinction between these two entities is not possible.

IMPRINT CYTOLOGY

Intraoperative Analysis of Sentinel Lymph Nodes

Intraoperative analysis of SLNB is becoming an effective tool in assessment of the presence or absence of metastatic tumor, and therefore influences the treatment offered to the patient.[54,55] This approach will expedite staging and potentially obviate the need for additional surgical procedures. The decision to perform imprint cytology versus frozen section should be based on the level of experience of the pathologist. Small lymph nodes are difficult to assess by frozen section because a significant proportion of tissue may be lost during the frozen section procedure. It is desirable to achieve up to 90% accuracy between intraoperative pathologic analyses of SLNB compared with permanent sections. The Association of Directors of Surgical Pathology recommends that an intraoperative analysis should be performed only if an immediate therapeutic discussion will be made and acted on based on the results. The College of American Pathologists consensus suggests a thorough gross examination and states that imprint cytology is preferable because of its tissue conservation relative to cryostat sectioning[56] (Fig 39-16).

The advantages of imprint cytology over frozen section include preservation of the integrity of the lymph node sample, prevention of loss of micrometastasis, and faster turnaround time. In addition, this procedure costs less and can sample multiple cut surfaces. Imprint cytology is accurate in 100% of grossly abnormal sentinel lymph nodes and allows a single-stage surgery in 50% of patients in several reported series. The disadvantage of imprint cytology include low sensitivity in grossly negative sentinel lymph nodes and high rate of false-negative results in cases with the diagnosis of infiltrating lobular carcinomas. This limitation is secondary to the lack of significant cytologic atypia in infiltrating locular carcinomas. In these circumstances, it may be possible to use intraoperative immunostaining for cytokeratin to improve the accuracy of the test results.[57–60]

Immediate Assessment of Core Needle Biopsy Samples

Imprint cytology has been effectively used as a diagnostic adjunct in intraoperative consultation. It has also been used as a means of assessment of adequacy of samples during image detected CNB procedures.[61,62] In our experience, imprint cytology of breast CNB provides an opportunity for rendering an immediate diagnosis with sensitivity of 97.5% and the specificity of 100%

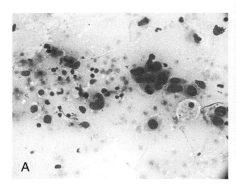

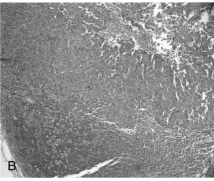

Figure 39-16 **A,** Imprint cytology of a metastatic breast cancer obtained from a sentinel lymph node biopsy during an intraoperative consultation. (Diff-Quik stain, ×20.) **B,** Corresponding tissue section of the same case demonstrating presence of metastatic deposit. (Hematoxylin and eosin stain, ×40.)

(Figs. 39-17 and 39-18; unpublished data). On-site interpretation of CNB is a critical step toward better patient care. Regardless of the diagnosis of benign versus malignant, assessment of the adequacy of the specimen and immediate interpretation of the results leads to better treatment planning and reduction of patient anxiety.

Intraoperative Assessment of Lumpectomy Surgical Margins

Increased local recurrence rates in patients with positive surgical margins highlight the importance of obtaining negative margins in breast conservation surgery.[63,64] The exact width of the resection margin that minimizes the risk of a breast tumor recurrence is unknown. However, a microscopic margin of at least 2 mm seems to ensure the likelihood that local recurrence rates will be less than 7% at 10 years after conservative surgery and radiation therapy.[65] In 1989, Leopold and colleagues studied 10 cases of breast carcinoma with a median follow-up of 64 months.[66] The tumor was completely excised grossly in all 10 patients; however, the microscopic status of the lumpectomy margins was unclear. The local recurrence rate in this group was 40% (4 of 10 patients). In 2003, Kaplan and associates reported a local recurrence rate of 2.8% in microscopically negative lumpectomy specimens.[67] The median follow-up in his study was 98 months, and only 1 of 36 patients with breast carcinoma showed evidence of recurrent carcinoma. In our study, intraoperative imprint cytology showed a sensitivity of 97% and a specificity of 99%, with a positive predictive value of 84% and a negative predictive value of 99%.[68]

The review of the previous studies emphasizes the importance of assessment of the status of lumpectomy margins. Aggressive attempts to optimize margin evaluation at the time of surgery can provide more accurate assessment of margin status. Use of frozen sections to examine the entire breast lumpectomy margins is labor intensive, time consuming, and leads to inevitable tissue loss. Imprint cytology is an alternative to frozen sectioning in assessment of breast lumpectomy margins. It is a simple and quick method to assess relatively entire breast lumpectomy specimen margins. The lumpectomy margins are touched by glass slides, fixed, and stained (Figs. 39-19 and 39-20).

Prognosis and Prediction of Response to Therapy

There is increasing evidence that certain morphologic features and biologic markers found in breast tumors may provide prognostic information by predicting the risk of recurrence and metastasis in early breast cancer. This information may also be important in choosing therapeutic options in patients with advanced disease.[69] FNAB and imprint preparation provide an attractive sample for prognostic and predictive testing. Aside from the assessment of actual tumor size and lymph node status, cytology preparations mainly obtained from breast fine needle aspirates can provide information about nuclear grade, the status of proliferation, hormone receptors, the HER-2/*neu* oncogene, and other emerging biomarkers. This is of particular importance in those patients selected for preoperative chemotherapy.[70]

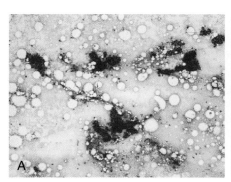

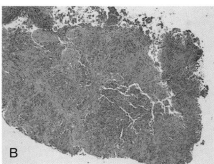

Figure 39-17 **A,** Imprint cytology of core needle biopsy with cytological features of malignancy. (Diff-Quik stain ×20.) **B,** Corresponding core needle biopsy of the same case diagnosed as an invasive breast cancer. (Hematoxylin and eosin stain.)

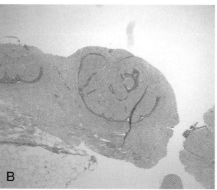
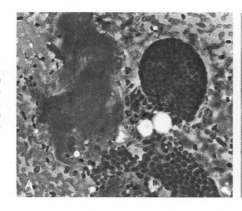

Figure 39-18 **A**, Imprint cytology of core needle biopsy with cytologic features of a fibroadenoma. (Diff-Quik stain, ×40.) **B**, Corresponding tissue section of the core needle biopsy of the same case demonstrates the presence of fibroadenoma.

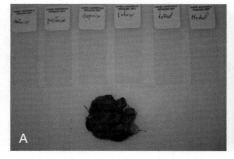
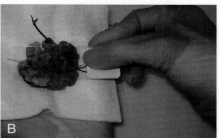

Figure 39-19 **A**, Intraoperative processing of imprint cytology for assessment of the presence of tumor at lumpectomy margins, requiring orientation of the specimen and preparation of slides. **B**, Imprint preparation to recruit cells for immediate interpretation of the test result.

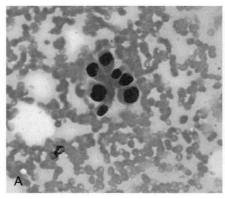
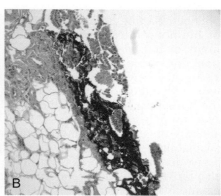

Figure 39-20 **A**, Imprint cytology of a surgical margin during an intraoperative consultation, demonstrating the presence of tumor cells at a margin. (Diff-Quik stain, ×20.) **B**, Corresponding tissue section of the same case showing the presence of tumor cells at the inked surgical margin. (Hematoxylin and eosin stain, ×40.)

NUCLEAR GRADE

The status of nuclear grade can potentially be assessed from breast fine needle aspirates.[71–75] There has been an interest in developing a variety of cytologic scoring systems for breast fine needle aspirates, incorporating variables such as cellular dissociation, cell size, cell uniformity, nucleoli, nuclear margin, chromatin pattern, and pattern of necrosis and inflammatory cells. Similarly, the Scarff-Richardson tumor grading system has been applied to fine needle aspirates of the breast, assessing the reproducibility of nuclear grade, tubule formation, and mitosis.[74] In the majority of these studies, characteristics of nucleus or nuclear grade have shown to be superior to the others. When compared with the corresponding tissue histology, nuclear grading has been the parameter with the highest degree of reproductivity (up to 95%).[75] The relative lack of mitosis may be because these cells are more fragile and less likely to survive smear preparation, or because fewer cells are examined by FNAB than is the case with biopsy material, so that mitoses are less likely to be detected. Similarly, tubular structures are difficult to identify in cytologic preparations. In a retrospective study, we reviewed 110 node-negative breast cancer patients with histologic and clinical follow-up. We found a difference in 5-year survival between patients with nuclear grades 1 and 2 (94%) and those with grade 3 lesions (83%). Because grades 1 and 2 lesions are prognostically similar, it may also be advisable to lump these two grades together and stratify breast fine needle aspirates into low nuclear grade and high nuclear grade[73] (Fig. 39-21).

We believe that information on nuclear grading should be incorporated in breast fine needle aspirates. This is of particular importance for those patients who are treated with neoadjuvant therapy. It has already been suggested that high-grade, fast-growing tumors are more likely to respond to chemotherapy than low-grade, slow-growing tumors, which may be better suited to

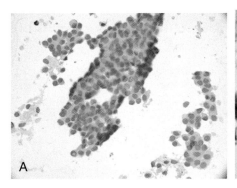
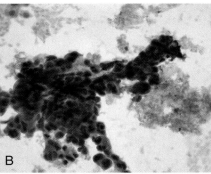

Figure 39-21 Infiltrating duct cell carcinoma; **A**, Low nuclear grade. **B**, High nuclear grade. (Papanicolaou stain, ×60.)

pretreatment with tamoxifen. Thus, potentially, the assessment of biologic aggressiveness of the tumor and the prediction of response to therapy could be ascertained with information about cytologic nuclear grading.

ESTROGEN AND PROGESTERONE RECEPTOR ANALYSIS

Assessment of steroid hormone receptor status in breast cancer patients is a standard practice. The recent availability of monoclonal antibodies for estrogen receptors (ERs) and progesterone receptors (PRs) has provided an attractive alternative for measurement of steroid receptor proteins in small tumors and the samples obtained via fine needle aspirates.[76,77] The visualization of hormone receptors, whether occupied by the hormone or not, at the single-cell level provides information not obtainable by biochemical assays. There are also studies suggesting that hormone receptor determination by immunocytochemistry may be a better predictor of response to hormone therapy.[78] Direct smears and cytospin preparations are suitable for hormone receptor analysis by the immunoperoxidase technique. The adaptability of immunochemical hormone receptor assays to formalin-fixed, paraffin-embedded tissue has also provided an effective means of using cell block preparations for such analysis[76,77] (Fig. 39-22).

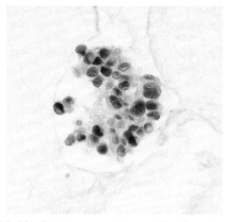

Figure 39-22 Estrogen receptor–positive breast cancer evidenced by nuclear staining. (Immunostain, ×60.)

TUMOR TYPE

According to the 1990 National Institutes of Health Consensus conference, tubular, colloid, and papillary carcinomas are associated with a favorable prognosis and should be recognized in cytologic preparations.[79] The cytologic features of these tumors are well characterized.[13] Tubular carcinomas are relatively rare tumors with a well-differentiated pattern that can potentially be mistaken for a benign proliferative breast lesion. The recognition of tubular carcinomas also has therapeutic implications, because these tumors may not require mastectomy or axillary dissection. It is also important to differentiate between lobular and ductal carcinomas; invasive lobular carcinomas have a different pattern of metastatic spread.

PROLIFERATION RATE

Among the various modalities for assessing the proliferation rate in breast cytology, the techniques most applicable to cytologic preparations are flow cytometry for assessment of the percentage of cells in S phase and immunocytochemical detection of proliferation-associated antigens. Flow cytometry can be applied to cytologic and/or cell block preparations and produces a histogram with information regarding the S-phase fraction of tumor cells. This technique is rapid, and the results are based on the study of large numbers of nuclei. Limitations, however, include the inability of flow cytometry to distinguish between nontumor and tumor cells. In addition, the presence of aneuploid peaks may complicate the established mathematical analysis and result in an inaccurate assessment.

To overcome this shortcoming, S-phase fraction determinations are now complemented by flow cytometric determinations of tumor cell Ki-67 positivity.[80–82] Originally prepared by immunizing mice with a Hodgkin's disease cell line, Ki-67 recognizes a nuclear antigen expressed in cycling cells. Immunostaining with Ki-67 has been applied to routinely prepared, air-dried breast fine needle aspirate smears. Immunostains for Ki-67 can be applied to cell block preparation of breast fine needle aspirate. The expression of Ki-67 is evidenced by the presence of nuclear staining.

HER-2/*neu* ONCOGENE

In the past few years there has been significant interest in assessing HER-2/*neu* oncogene amplification and

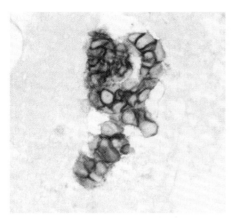

Figure 39-23 Her-2/*neu* oncogene expression demonstrated by membrane staining in a primary breast carcinoma. (Immunostain, ×60.)

overexpression in patients with breast cancer. The Her-2/*neu* oncogene, also known as *c-erb* B2, encodes a 185-kDa transmembrane protein, which is related to the epidermal growth factor receptor. The amplification and overexpression of HER-2/*neu* have been observed in 25% to 30% of human breast cancers.[83,84] HER-2/*neu* overexpression is mainly achieved by gene amplification (increased copies of the normal HER-2 gene), resulting in increased transcription of the gene, increased Her-2 receptors on the cell membrane, and increased cell proliferation. HER-2/*neu* positivity has been correlated with both a shorter disease-free interval and a shorter overall survival time in both node-positive and node-negative breast cancers. Patients with HER-2/*neu* amplification and overexpression are less responsive to cyclophosphamide, methotrexate, and 5-fluorouracil–containing adjuvant therapy and resistant to tamoxifen treatment; however, they are more responsive to dose-intensified, doxorubicin-based therapy.[83–87]

The main reasons for determination of the status of HER-2/*neu* in patients with breast cancer are to assess patient prognosis, to predict the therapeutic outcome to adjuvant chemotherapy and endocrine therapy, and to select patients for trastuzumab (Herceptin) immunotherapy. Among various technologies available to assess the presence or absence of HER-2/*neu* oncogene, immunohistochemistry (IHC) and fluorescent in situ hybridization (FISH) procedures are the most commonly used. The HercepTest (Dako Corporation; Carpinteria, California) is a semiquantitative IHC assay that scores the membrane staining using a scale of 0 to 3. Because IHC is less expensive than FISH technology, it is suggested that cases interpreted by IHC should be followed by FISH to assess the presence or absence of HER-2/*neu* oncogene gene amplification. The concordance between IHC assessment of HER-2/*neu* oncogene and the FISH technology is significant; however, FISH is currently regarded by the U.S. Food and Drug Administration (FDA) as the gold standard method for detection of HER-2/*neu* oncogene amplification. The American Society of Clinical Oncology and the College of American Pathologists have recently published some guidelines to improve the accuracy of HER-2/*neu* oncogene testing in breast cancer.[88,89]

The preliminary studies using cytology cell block preparations for detection of HER-2/*neu* oncogene in breast lesions have shown a good correlation between the expression of this oncogene in cytology and the corresponding tissue sections[12] (Figs. 39-23 and 39-24). Assessment of HER-2/*neu* oncogene in FNAB specimens is particularly important in patients with metastatic breast disease.[90]

Risk Prediction

CYTOMORPHOLOGY AS A PREDICTOR OF BREAST CANCER RISK

Primary prevention of breast cancer requires identification and elimination of cancer-causing agents, which is an incredibly difficult task to follow. It was not until 1998, when the first report of the National Surgical Adjunct Breast and Bowel Project (Breast Cancer Prevention Trial BCPT; P-1) randomized clinical trial appeared in the literature supporting the hypothesis that breast cancer can be prevented. This study showed that administration of tamoxifen reduced the risk of invasive and noninvasive breast cancer by almost 50% in all age groups. In addition, it was found that the breast cancer risk was reduced in women with a history of lobular carcinoma in situ (56%) or atypical hyperplasia (86%). The conclusion of this study was that tamoxifen as a chemopreventive agent is appropriate for many women with increased risk of breast cancer.[91]

This report has been a victory for those interested in chemoprevention. It has also generated a great deal of enthusiasm in those women who are at increased risk for breast cancer. This study, however, also highlighted the side effects of tamoxifen, which includes a threefold increased relative risk of pulmonary emboli and a 2.5-fold increased relative risk of endometrial cancer. In subjects of 50 years of age or older, there was a 1.8-fold increased relative risk of stroke.[91] Other preventive measures such as bilateral prophylactic mastectomy and/or oophorectomy are associated with major financial, psychosocial, and medical implications.[92,93]

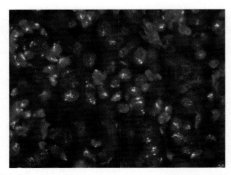

Figure 39-24 Her-2/*neu* oncogene amplification in a primary breast carcinoma. (Fluorescent in situ hybridization, ×100.)

These facts underscore the importance of an accurate risk assessment to better stratify patients who may benefit from chemopreventive intervention. Risk assessment provides the high-risk individuals with an opportunity to take proper and well-balanced measures against breast cancer. If it is not done properly, the process can rapidly destroy the sense of well-being of that individual and can result in premature and hasty decisions.

Risk factors for breast cancer have already been identified.[93,94] These include inherited germline abnormalities or history of previous in situ or invasive breast cancer and proliferative breast disease with and without atypia. It is generally agreed that there is an increasing risk of breast cancer associated with the progression from normal breast epithelium through hyperplasia, atypical hyperplasia, and carcinoma in situ to breast carcinoma. Studies have identified atypical hyperplasia as the specific high-risk precursor lesion for breast cancer. These conclusions have predominately stemmed from retrospective studies using tissue samples. Prospective studies require noninvasive or minimally invasive procedures that could ensure the continuity of monitoring of the biologic and morphologic changes associated with tumorigenesis. Asymptomatic high-risk individuals should also easily accept these procedures.

Despite the significance of breast epithelial proliferation in identifying women at increased risk for breast cancer, only minorities of women who develop breast cancer have undergone previous breast biopsies. Thus, it is likely that occult proliferative breast disease remains undiagnosed. This deprives many women who may be carrying these lesions in their breasts from an accurate assessment and compromises their ability to participate in an appropriate trial or a surveillance program.

With the current availability of tamoxifen as a chemopreventive agent and with the increasing emphasis on early breast cancer detection and prevention, more women seek consultation to determine their risk of breast cancer. However, in the absence of any detectable breast lesion, clinically and mammographically, only a few women may volunteer to have their breasts sampled by surgical biopsy for risk assessment. Other nonsurgical procedures include FNAB, NAF, and the recently introduced ductal lavage. These techniques may provide better alternatives.

In 1999, we reported our experience based on an outcome study of 869 patients, with median follow-up of 5.5 years. We studied cytomorphology of breast FNAB based on the Masood Cytology Index and assessed the predictive value of the results for subsequent development of breast cancer. Follow-up study was available for 61% (n = 530) of cases. The average age ranged from 28 to 75 years. The clinical follow-up ranged from 1.5 to 8 years. In this study overall, 28 of 530 (5%) of women developed breast cancer. The frequency of development of breast cancer was 3.6%, with cases diagnosed as nonproliferative breast disease, 6.7% with proliferative breast disease, and 11.1% with proliferative breast disease with atypia. When adjusted for relative risk by Cox regression analysis and using our previously described cytologic grading system, we demonstrated that a diagnosis of atypical ductal hyperplasia by FNAB imparted a 5.1-fold increased relative risk of developing a subsequent breast carcinoma[95] (Table 39-4).

Similarly, in a recent study of cytology obtained from random FNABs of the breast, and using the Masood Cytology Index, Fabian and colleagues reported a fivefold increase in the relative risk of developing breast cancer in a cohort of high-risk women with atypical hyperplasia. In this study, 15% of high-risk women with a 10-year Gail risk of greater than 4% and atypical hyperplasia by FNAB developed breast cancer within 3 years. It was also reported that an elevated Gail risk and the finding of atypical hyperplasia by FNAB were independent predictors of breast cancer risk[25] (Fig. 39-25).

Interestingly, similar results were reported in 1993 by Wrensch and associates,[96] who analyzed the nipple aspirate fluid collected from 2701 normal women between 1973 and 1980. The median follow-up was 12.7 years. In this study, women with atypical hyperplasia on NAF cytology had a 4.9-fold increased relative risk of developing carcinoma compared with women who did not yield fluid. The greatest increase in relative risk (18-fold) was in women who had both atypical hyperplasia and a

---

TABLE 39-4

Breast Cancer Incidence and Adjusted Relative Risks of Breast Cancer by Fine Needle Aspiration Cytology Diagnosis

Cytologic Diagnosis	No. with Breast Cancer/ Total No.	Percent with Breast Cancer*	Cox Regression	
			Adjusted Relative Risk[†]	95% Confidence Interval
Nonproliferative breast disease	11/307	3.6%	1.2	1.5–5.7
Proliferative breast disease	12/178	6.7%	2.9	3–10.4
Proliferative breast disease with atypia	5/45	11.1%	5.1	1.9–20.3
TOTAL	28/530	5.2%		

*P value = 0.061.
[†]Relative risks adjusted by Cox regression for age.
From Masood S, Rasty G: Potential value of cytology in the detection of breast cancer precursors by fine needle aspiration biopsy: The future Pap smear for breast cancer. Acta Cytol 43:890, 1999.

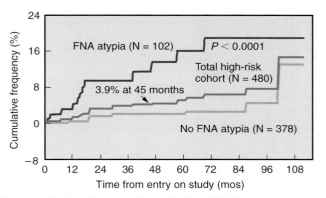

Figure 39-25 Fine needle aspiration (FNA) atypia increases relative risk of breast cancer fivefold. Risk of subsequent development of breast cancer is predicted by cytologic findings from FNA biopsy obtained from women at high risk for development of breast cancer. (From Fabian CJ, Kimler BF, Zalles CM, et al: Short term breast cancer prediction by random periareolar fine needle aspiration cytology and the Gail risk model. J Natl Cancer Inst 92:1217–227, 2000. Used with permission.)

family history of breast cancer in a first-degree relative (Fig. 39-26).

Based on the previous studies, the estimated relative risk of breast cancer development in women with atypical hyperplasia identified by cytology is similar to those reported in histology. In three studies by Page and Dupont,[21,97,98] the relative risk of developing breast cancer conferred by a diagnosis of atypical ductal hyperplasia on tissue biopsy is 4.9- to 5.3-fold higher than in the absence of atypical hyperplasia. These studies also reported a significantly higher increase in relative risk when the patient had atypical hyperplasia and a positive family history of breast cancer (Table 39-5).

Despite these promising reports in the literature, limitations to reliably diagnose atypical hyperplasia by cytology continue to pose a dilemma.[99,100] To a lesser extent, similar issues are also present in surgical pathology.[101,102] In clinical practice, recommendations are made to follow a patient with surgical biopsy if the diagnosis of atypical ductal hyperplasia is obtained

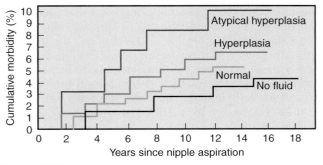

Figure 39-26 Cumulative incidence of breast cancer by cytologic diagnosis in relation to years since nipple aspiration in white volunteer women from the San Francisco Bay area, 1973–1991. Risk of subsequent development of breast cancer is predicted by nipple aspiration fluid. (Wrensch MR, Petrakis NL, King EB, et al: Breast cancer incidence in women with abnormal cytology in nipple aspirates of breast fluid. Am J Epidemiol 135;130–141, 1992. Used with permission.)

by FNAB or CNB. However, the absolute distinction between atypical ductal hyperplasia and low-grade DCIS required in clinical practice might not be a limiting factor in chemoprevention trials that study molecular or morphologic changes over a lifetime in high-risk individuals.

ROLE OF DUCTAL LAVAGE IN RISK ASSESSMENT

Ductal lavage is a minimally invasive procedure that has been developed to identify cellular atypia in breast ducts. A 1.5-cm flexible microcatheter is inserted into the milk ducts through the nipple surface orifices under local anesthesia, and the duct is infused with saline to retrieve cellular material for cytologic analysis. Appearance of turbid fluid in return is often an indication of a successful ductal lavage procedure (Fig. 39-27). Cytologic preparation and interpretation of ductal lavage are somewhat similar to those used for FNAB, nipple discharge, and NAF samples.

Potential uses of ductal lavage include selection of women for risk reduction therapy, monitoring response to a risk reduction intervention, diagnostic workup of a nipple discharge, and early diagnosis of an occult cancer. Currently, data regarding the sensitivity and specify of ductal lavage in detecting breast cancer, its usefulness in risk stratification, and the prognostic significance of mild atypia are not available. Because of these limitations, ductal lavage is best used in the context of clinical trials focused on breast cancer detection and prevention. Other questions include whether cytologic atypia in cells obtained from ductal lavage is truly predictive of cancer development, what proportion of high-risk women will undergo successful ductal lavage, and how the information obtained from ductal lavage cytology might be used to manage high-risk individuals.

Another limitation is the fact that ductal lavage is only able to retrieve cells from intraductal process. However, the finding from the NSABP on 1000 mastectomies have indicated that only 70% of invasive cancers have an intraductal component.[103] Similarly, in their study of 801 mastectomy specimens, Badve and coworkers[104] showed that 14% of invasive cancers lack an intraductal carcinoma. Therefore, ductal lavage is not able to detect at least 14% to 30% of breast cancer cases. Other concerns include the inability of ductal lavage to detect peripherally located lesions and the ambiguity about missing an abnormality in an unyielding duct.

In our own experience, we have found that ductal lavage is a safe, well-tolerated procedure. The cellular yield is limited by old age, prior surgery, radiation, tamoxifen therapy, chemotherapy, and anatomical abnormality of the nipple. Ductal lavage specimens often contain large numbers of foamy histiocytes and occasional multinucleated cells. In a few cases that ductography and tissue biopsy were available following atypical ductal lavage, we have seen a spectrum of changes ranging from proliferative breast disease to atypical ductal hyperplasia, papilloma, and DCIS. It appears

TABLE 39-5

Relative Risk of Breast Cancer in Women Diagnosed with Proliferative Breast Disease with Atypia

Risk	Study	Sample
Cytopathology		
4.9-fold	Wrensch et al.[a]	>2300 women with 12.5 years' follow-up: breast duct fluid cytology
5.1-fold	Masood and Rasty[b]	530 women with 5.5 years follow-up: fine needle aspiration biopsy
4-fold	Fabian et al.[c]	580 women with 45 months' follow-up: fine needle aspiration biopsy
Histopathology		
4.3-fold	Page et al.[d]	Retrospective review of 10,542 biopsies with 17.5 years' follow-up
5.3-fold	Dupont and Page[e]	>3300 women with 17 years' follow-up
4.3-fold	Dupont et al.[f]	>15,000 women with 5–10 years' follow-up

[a]Wrensch M, Petrakis NL, King EB, et al.[96]
[b]Masood S, Rasty G.[95]
[c]Fabian CJ, Kimler BF, Zalles CM, et al.[25]
[d]Page DL, Dupont WD, Rogers W, et al.[97]
[e]Dupont WD, Page DL: Risk factors for breast cancer in women with proliferative breast disease. N Engl J Med 312:146–151, 1985.
[f]Dupont WD, Parl FF, Hartman WH, et al.[98]

that atypia seen in ductal lavage can be associated with recognizable anatomic abnormalities[105,106] (Fig. 39-28).

The most exciting application of ductal lavage is the opportunity to study the genetic alterations associated with breast cancer. In conjunction with the newly identified genetic markers, ductal lavage has the potential to identify early breast cancers before any mammographic changes occur. Currently, there is almost no information as to the earliest genetic changes, which kick-start a cell on the journey toward malignancy. Methylation-specific polymerase chain reaction performed on ductal lavage samples have shown promising results in the early detection of cancer.[107] Other developing gene technologies can be applied to ductal lavage fluid. These include the study of individual genes such as cyclin D2, RAR-B, and Twist. FISH analysis may be performed for the detection of chromosomal aneusomy. Proteonomic analysis, such as surface-enhanced laser desorption/ionization time-of-flight (SELDI-TOF) mass spectrometry potentially provides effective means to study protein expression in biologic fluid such as ductal lavage.[108,109]

Future Perspectives

Breast cytopathology will remain as an integral component of breast cancer diagnosis and management. More importantly, the growing interest in the use of minimally invasive procedures as diagnostic and therapeutic modalities requires integration of morphology with current and emerging molecular testing. This approach is critical in the area of personalized medicine in breast cancer care.

Advances in science will provide unique opportunities to examine the potential of new biomarkers as diagnostic adjuncts in difficult to diagnose cases in cytopathology in order to maximize the efficiency of practice breast cytopathology. This is best evidenced by the report on the diagnostic value of telomerase expression in breast fine needle aspirates[110] (Fig. 39-29).

Enhanced public awareness and the recognition of integrated care via a multidisciplinary approach will result in promoting the establishment of breast health centers across the globe. Within the center concept, the multidisciplinary team will provide the possibility of the use of the FNAB and imprint cytology effectively. Breast cancer screening programs will be enriched by real-time radiologic and pathologic correlation, and patients will benefit from integrated care by qualified physicians.[111,112]

The discipline of cytopathology is uniquely positioned to provide not only diagnostic and predictive information but also to actively participate in risk prediction and breast cancer research. Access to the breast epithelial cells and their surrounding environment via minimally invasive procedures, coupled with contemporary breast imaging and the new surgical interaction,

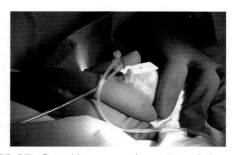

Figure 39-27 Ductal lavage; a microcatheter is inserted into a duct. Lavage fluid in return catheter shows turbid fluid, indicating a successful access to the mammary ductal system.

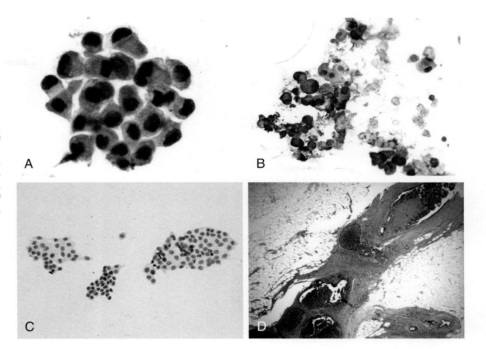

Figure 39-28 Papillary carcinoma diagnosed by ductal lavage: **A,** A cluster of malignant cells. **B,** Positive immunostain for epithelial markers (cytokeratin immunostaining). **C,** Negative immunostain for myoepithelial markers (P63 immunostaining). **D,** Corresponding tissue section of ductectomy specimen demonstrating the presence of ductal carcinoma in situ.

offers an incredible opportunity for an improved understanding of the biology of breast cancer precursors.

There is no doubt that minimally invasive procedures are capable of recruiting cellular material for cytomorphologic interpretation as well as biomarker studies. Reports in the literature also have demonstrated the value of cytomorphology as a risk predictor.[25,95,96] In a prospective study with cytologic-histologic correlation using mammographically directed FNAB and the follow-up needle localization excisional biopsy, the cytomorphology of high-risk proliferative breast disease was defined. We developed a semiquantitative cytologic grading system, which allowed

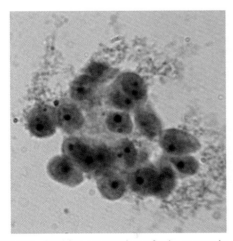

Figure 39-29 Positive expression of telomerase in malignant breast fine needle aspirate evidenced by intranuclear dotlike staining. (Immunostain, ×60.)

us to stratify the spectrum of high-risk proliferative breast disease and to distinguish between hyperplasia and neoplasia.[22,23] As the only prospective study with appropriate cytologic histologic correlation, this system has gained acceptance among oncologists and researchers. This grading system, recognized as the Masood Cytology Index, has been used in several NCI-funded projects and has demonstrated its value as a breast cancer predictor. As a potential surrogate end point biomarker, this index has also been used in the monitoring of the effect of therapy.[24-26]

Recently in a report by Bean and colleagues,[27] the authors studied the pattern of distribution of retinoic acid receptor-beta (RAR beta2P2) promoter methylation in random periareolar fine needle aspiration using the Masood Cytology Index. Results from the study indicated that RAR beta2p2 promoter shows a positive association with increasing cytologic abnormality. The highest level of methylation at M3 and M4 (50%) has observed with cytology score as high as 14 to 15 (atypical ductal hyperplasia). This study is the reflection of the validity of the Masood Cytology Index, which can stratify low-grade proliferation from high-grade proliferation. This promising concept may trigger more interest among other investigators to further assess the potential use of the Masood Cytology Index as a breast cancer predictor (Fig. 39-30).

As has been previously stated, descriptive terms of atypia in breast cytopathology do not always signify malignancy and may not be the reflection of an increased risk of development of breast cancer. The Masood Cytology Index as a panel of several criteria might be a better method for assessment of prognostically relevant atypia in cytologic preparation.

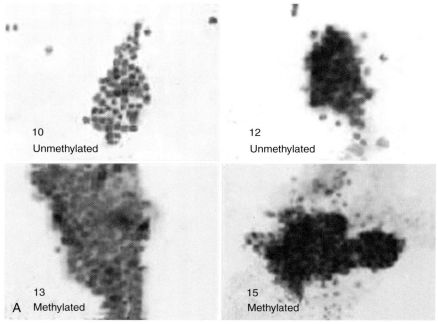

M3 RARBETA P2 METHYLATION

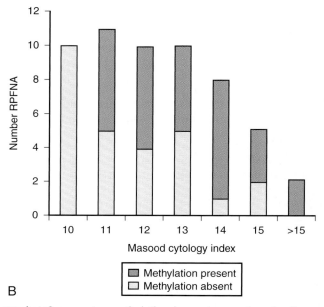

Figure 39-30 Retinoic acid receptor-beta2 promoter methylation in random periareolar fine needle aspiration. (Bean GR, Scott V, Yee L, et al: Retinoic acid reciptor-beta2 promoter methylation in random periareolar fine needle aspiration. Cancer Epidemiol Biomarkers Prev 14: 790–798, 2005.)

REFERENCES

1. Martin HE, Ellis EB: Biopsy of needle puncture and aspiration. Ann Surg 92:169–181, 1930.
2. Saphir O: Early diagnosis of breast lesions. JAMA 150:859–861, 1952.
3. Zajicek J, Franzen S, Jackson P, et al: Aspiration of mammary tumors in diagnosis and research: A critical review of 2,200 cases. Acta Cytol 11:169–175, 1967.
4. Frable WJ: Needle aspiration biopsy: Past, present, and future. Hum Pathol 20:504–517, 1989.
5. Feldman PS, Covell JL: Fine needle aspiration biopsy and its clinical application: Breast and lung. Chicago, ASCP Press, 1985.
6. Linsk JA, Franzen S: Breast aspiration in clinical application cytology. Philadelphia, Lippincott, 1983, pp 105–135.
7. Cheung PS, Yan KW, Alagaratham JT: The complementary role of fine needle aspiration cytology and true-cut needle biopsy in the management of breast masses. Aust NZJ Surg 57:615–620, 1987.
8. Shabot MM, Goldberg IM, Schick P, et al: Aspiration cytology is superior to tru-cut needle biopsy in stabilizing the diagnosis of clinically suspicious breast masses. Ann Surg 196:122–126, 1982.
9. Innes DJ Jr, Feldman PS: Comparison of diagnostic results obtained by fine needle aspiration cytology and tru-cut or open biopsies. Acta Cytol 27:350–354, 1983.
10. Ballo MS, Sneige N: Can core needle biopsy replace fine-needle aspiration cytology in the diagnosis of palpable breast carcinoma? Cancer 78:773–777, 1996.
11. Masood S: Cytopathology of the breast. Chicago, American Society of Clinical Pathology Press, 1996.
12. Masood S: Prognostic factors in breast cancer: Use of cytologic preparations. Diagn Cytopathol 13:388–395, 1995.
13. Masood S: Recent updates in breast fine needle aspiration biopsy. Breast J 2:1–12, 1996.
14. Patel JJ, Gartell PC, Smallwood JA, et al: Fine needle aspiration cytology of breast masses: An evaluation of its accuracy and reasons for diagnostic failure. Ann R Coll Surg Engl 69:156–159, 1987.
15. Masood S: Diagnostic terminology in breast fine needle aspiration biopsy: Redefining the term atypia. Cancer 87:1–4, 1999.
16. Sneige N: Fine-needle aspiration of the breast: A review of 1,995 cases with emphasis on diagnostic pitfalls. Diagn Cytopathol 9:106–112, 1993.
17. The uniform approach to breast fine-needle aspiration biopsy. NCI Fine-Needle Aspiration of Breast Workshop. Diagn Cytopathol 16:295–311, 1997.
18. The uniform approach to breast fine needle aspiration biopsy. NIH Consensus Development Conference. Am J Surg 174:371–385, 1997.
19. Emsler VL: The epidemiology of benign breast disease. Epidemiol Rev 3:184–202, 1981.
20. Page DL: Cancer risk assessment in benign breast biopsies. Hum Pathol 17:871–878, 1986.
21. Dupont WD, Parl FF, Hartman WH, et al: Breast cancer risk associated with proliferative breast disease with atypical hyperplasia. Cancer 71:1258–1265, 1993.
22. Masood S, Frykberg ER, McLellan GL, et al: Prospective evaluation of radiologically detected breast fine needle aspiration biopsy of nonpalpable breast lesions. Cancer 66:1480–1487, 1990.
23. Masood S, Frykberg ER, McLellan GL, et al: Cytologic differentiation between proliferative and nonproliferative breast disease in mammographically guided fine-needle aspirates. Diagn Cytopathol 7:581–590, 1991.
24. Khan SA, Masood S, Miller L, et al: Random fine needle aspiration of the breast of women at increased risk and standard risk controls. Breast J 4:420–425, 1998.
25. Fabian CJ, Kimler BF, Zalles CM, et al: Short term breast cancer prediction by random periareolar fine needle aspiration cytology and the gail risk model. J Natl Cancer Inst 92:1217–1227, 2000.
26. Fabian C, Kilmer BF, Brady D, et al: Phase II chemoprevention trial of DFMO using the random FNA model. Breast Cancer Res Treat 64:48, 2000.
27. Bean GR, Scott V, Yee L, et al: Retinoic acid receptor-beta2 promoter methylation in random periareolar fine needle aspiration. Cancer Epidemiol Biomarkers Prev 14:790–798, 2005.
28. Klijanienko J, Katsahian S, Vielh P, et al: Stromal infiltration as a predictor of tumor invasion in breast fine needle aspiration biopsy. Diagn Cytopathol 30:182–186, 2004.
29. Salhany K, Page DL: Fine needle aspiration of mammary lobular carcinoma in situ and atypical lobular hyperplasia. Am J Clin Pathol 92:22–26, 1989.
30. Hwang S, Ioffe O, et al: Cytology diagnosis of invasive lobular carcinoma: Factors associated with negative and equivocal diagnosis. Diagn Cytopath 31:87–93, 2004.
31. Masood S, Loya A, Khalbuss W: Is core needle biopsy superior to fine needle aspiration biopsy in diagnosis of papillary breast lesions? Diagn Cytopathol 28:329–334, 2003.
32. Bottles K, Chan JS, Holly EA, et al: Cytologic criteria for fibroadenoma. A stepwise logistic regression analysis. Am J Clin Pathol 89:707–713, 1988.
33. Chen KT: Aspiration cytology of breast fibroadenoma with atypia. Diagn Cytopathol 8:309–310, 1992.
34. Stanley MW, Tani EM, Skoog L: Fine needle aspiration of fibroadenomas of the breast with atypia: A spectrum including cases that cytologically mimic carcinoma. Diagn Cytopathol 6:375–382, 1990.
35. Dusenberry D, Frable WJ: Fine needle aspiration cytology of phyllodes tumor: Potential diagnostic pitfalls. Acta Cytol 36:215–221, 1992.
36. Rosen PP: Mucocele-like tumors of the breast. Am J Surg Pathol 10:646, 1986.
37. Bharagava V, Miller TR, Cohen MB: Mucocele-like tumors of the breast. Cytologic findings in two cases. Am J Clin Pathol 95:875–877, 1991.
38. Vargas H, Masood S: Implemenation of a minimal invasive breast biopsy program in countries with limited resources. Breast J 9:81–85, 2003.
39. Masood S: Breast cancer in resource limited countries. Future Med 2:1–4, 2006.
40. Masood S, Vass L, Ibarra JA Jr, et al: Breast pathology guideline implementation in low- and-middle income countries. Cancer 113:2297–2304, 2008.
41. Fornage BD: Percutaneous biopsies of the breast: State of the art. Cardiovasc Intervent Radiol 14:29–39, 1991.
42. Liberman L, Dershaw DD, Rosen PP, et al: Stereotaxic core needle biopsy of breast carcinoma: accuracy at predicting invasion. Radiology 194:379–381, 1995.
43. Dershaw DD, Morris EA, Liberman L, et al: Nondiagnostic sterotactic core needle biopsy: Results of rebiopsy. Radiology 198:323–325, 1996.
44. Liberman L, Sama M, Susnik B, et al: Lobular carcinoma in situ at percutaneous breast biopsy: surgical biopsy finding. AJR Am J Roentgenol 173:300–302, 1999.
45. Youngson BJ, Liberman L, Rosen PP: Displacement of carcinomatos epithelium in surgical breast specimens following stereotaxic core biopsy. Am J Clin Pathol 103:598–602, 1995.
46. Carpenter R, Adamson A, Royle GT: A prospective study of nipple discharge. Br J Clin Pract Suppl. 68:54–57, 1989.
47. Johnson TL, Kini SR: Cytologic and clinical features of abnormal nipple secretions. 225 cases. Diag Cytopatholog 7:17–22, 1991.
48. Carty NJ, Royle GT, Mudan SS, et al: Prospective study of outcome in women presenting with nipple discharge. Ann R Coll Surg Engl 76:387–389, 1994.
49. Goss PE, Reid C, Pintilie M, et al: Male breast carcinoma. Cancer 85:629–639, 1999.
50. Dawes LG, Bowen C, Ventra L, et al: Ductography for nipple discharge: No replacement for ductal excision. Surgery 124:685–691, 1998.
51. Lee WY: Cytology of abnormal nipple discharge: A cytohistological correlation. Cytopathology 14:19–26, 2003.
52. Takeda T, Matsui A, Sato Y, et al: Nipple discharge cytology in mass screening for breast cancer. Acta Cytol 34:161–164, 1990.
53. Masood S, Khalbuss W: Nipple fluid cytology. Clin Lab Med 25:787–794, 2005.
54. Krag D, Weaver DR, Ashikaga T, et al: The sentinel node in breast cancer—a multicenter validation study. N Eng J Med 339:941–946, 1998.
55. Cady B: Consensus on sentinel node biopsy. Breast J 8:123–125, 2002.
56. Association of Directors of Anatomic Surgical Pathology. ADASP recommendations for processing and reporting lymph node specimens submitted for evaluation of metastatic disease. Am J Surg Pathol 25:961–963, 2001.

57. Cox CE, Centeno B, Dickson D, et al: Accuracy of intraoperative cytology for sentinel lymph node evaluation in treatment of breast carcinoma. Cancer 105:13–20, 2005.

58. Litz CE, Bertsch PD, Roberts CA, et al: Intraoperative cytologic diagnosis of breast sentinel lymph nodes in the routine, nonacademic setting: A highly specific test with limited sensitivity. Breast J 10:383–391, 2004.

59. Hakam A, Khin N: Intraoperative imprint cytology in assessment of sentinel lymph nodes and lumpectomy margins. Clin Lab Med 25:795–807, 2005.

60. Weinberg ES, Dickson D, White L, et al: Cytokeratin staining for intraoperative evaluation of sentinel lymph node in patients with invasive lobular carcinoma. Am J Surg 188:419–422, 2004.

61. Green RS, Matthew S: The contribution of cytologic imprints of sterotactically guided core needle biopsy of the breast in the management of patients with mammographic abnormalities. Breast J 7:214–218, 2001.

62. Jacobs TW, Silverman JF, Schroeder B, et al: Accuracy of touch imprint cytology of image-directed breast core needle biopsies. Acta Cytol 43:169–174, 1999.

63. Beriwal S, Schwartz GF, Komarnicky L, et al: Breast-conserving therapy after neoadjuvant chemotherapy: Long-term results. Breast J 12:159–164, 2006.

64. Shimauchi A, Nemoto K, et al: Long-term outcome of breast-conserving therapy for breast cancer. Radiat Med 23:485–490, 2005.

65. Freedman G, Fowble B, Hanlon A, et al: Patients with early stage invasive cancer with close or positive margins treated with conservative surgery and radiation have an increased risk of breast recurrence that is delayed by adjuvant systemic therapy. Int J Radiat Oncol Biol Phys 44:1005–1015, 1999.

66. Leopold KA, Recht A, Schnitt SJ, et al: Results of conservative surgery and radiation therapy for multiple synchronous cancers of one breast. Int J Radiat Oncol Biol Phys 16:11–16, 1989.

67. Kaplan J, Giron G, Tartter PI, et al: Breast conservation in patients with multiple ipsilateral synchronous cancers. J Am Coll Surg 197:726–729, 2003.

68. Bakhshandeh M, Tutuncuoglu O, Fischer G, et al: Use of imprint cytology for assessment of surgical margins is lumpectomy specimens of breast cancer patients. Diagn Cytopathol 35:656–659, 2007.

69. Fisher B, Slack N, Katrych D, et al: Ten year follow-up results of patients with carcinoma in the breast in a cooperative clinical trial evaluating surgical adjuvant chemotherapy. Surg Gynecol Obstet 140:528–534, 1975.

70. Masood S: Prognostic factors in breast cancer: Use of cytologic preparations. Diagn Cytopathol 13:388–395, 1995.

71. Dabbs DJ, Silverman JF: Prognostic factors from the fine needle aspirate: Breast carcinoma nuclear grade. Diagn Cytopathol 10:203–208, 1994.

72. Robinson JA, McKee G, Nichols A, et al: Prognostic value of cytological grading of fine needle aspirates from breast carcinomas. Lancet 343:947–949, 1994.

73. Masood S: Prognostic value of nuclear grading in breast cytology. Mod Pathol 8:1, 21A, 1994.

74. Howell LP, Gandour-Edwards R, O'Sullivan D: Application of the Scarff-Bloom-Richardson tumor grading system to fine needle aspirates of the breast. Am J Clin Pathol 101:262–265, 1994.

75. Cajulis RS, Sneige N, El-Naggar A:Cytologic nuclear grading of fine needle aspirates of the breast carcinomas. Concordance with histopathologic and flow data. Mod Pathol 3:14A, 1990.

76. Masood S: Use of monoclonal antibody for assessment of estrogen receptor content in fine needle aspiration biopsy specimen from patients with breast cancer. Arch Pathol Lab Med 113:26–30, 1989.

77. Masood S: Assessment of progesterone receptor immunocytochemical assay in breast fine needle aspirates. Acta Cytol 34:735, 1990.

78. Pertschuk LP, Eisenberg KB, Carter AC, et al: Immunohistologic localization of estrogen receptors in breast cancer with monoclonal antibodies; correlation with biochemistry and clinical endocrine response. Cancer 55: 1513–1518, 1985.

79. NIH consensus conference: Treatment of early stage breast cancer. JAMA 265:391–395, 1991.

80. Lopez F, Bello F, Lacombe F, et al: Modalities of synthesis of Ki-67 antigen during the stimulation of lymphocytes. Cytometry 10:731–738, 1989.

81. Rishi M, Schwarting R, Kovalich AJ, et al: Detection of growth fraction in tumors by Ki-67 monoclonal antibody in cytologic smears: A prospective study of 40 cases. Diagn Cytopathol 9:52–56, 1993.

82. Henry MJ, Stanley MW, Swenson B, et al: Cytologic assessment of tumor cell kinetics. Applications of monoclonal antibody Ki-67 to fine needle aspiration smears. Diagn Cytopathol 7:591–596, 1991.

83. Slamon DJ, Clark GM, Wong SG, et al: Human breast cancer: Correlation of relapse and survival with amplification of the HER-2/neu oncogene. Science 235:177–182, 1987.

84. Akiyama T, Sudo C, Ogawara SG, et al: The product of the human c-erbB gene: A 185 kilodalton alycoprotein with tyrosine kinase activity. Science 232:1644–1646, 1986.

85. Paik S, Hazan R, Fisher ER, et al: Pathologic findings from the National Surgical Adjuvant Breast Project: Prognostic significance of erbB-2 protein overexpression in primary breast cancer. J Clin Oncol 8:103–112, 1990.

86. Allred D, Clark GM, Tandon AK, et al: HER-2/neu in node negative breast cancer. Prognostic significance of overexpression influenced by presence of in situ carcinoma. J Clin Oncol 10:599–605, 1992.

87. Gancberg D, Lespagnard L, Ronas G, et al: Sensitivity of HER-2/neu antibodies in archival tissue samples of invasive breast carcinomas. Correlation with oncogene amplification in 160 cases. Am J Clin Pathol 113:675–682, 2000.

88. McManus DT, Patterson AH, et al: Fluorescence in situ hybridization detection of erbB2 amplification in breast cancer fine needle aspirates. Mol Pathol 52:75–77, 1999.

89. Wolf AC, Hammond EH, Schwartz JN, et al: American Society of Clinical Oncology/College of American Pathologists guideline recommendations for human epidermal growth factor receptor 2 testing in breast cancer. J Clin Oncol 25:118–145, 2007.

90. Masood S, Bui M: Assessment of Her-2/neu overexpression in primary breast cancers and their metastatic lesions: An immunohistochemical study. Ann Clin Lab Sci 30:259–265, 2000.

91. Fisher B, Constantine JP, Wickerham DL, et al: Tamozifen for prevention of breast cancer: Report of the national surgical adjuvant breast and bowel project P-1 study. J Natl Cancer Inst 90:1371–1388, 1998.

92. Hartman LC, Schaid DJ, Woods JE, et al: Efficacy of bilateral prophylactic mastectomy in women with a family history of breast cancer. N Engl J Med 14:71–84, 1999.

93. Eby N, Chang-Claudej J, Bishop DJ: The familial and genetic susceptibility for breast cancer. Cancer Causes Control 5:458–470, 1994.

94. Narod SA, Ford DA, Devilee P, et al: An evaluation of genetic heterogeneity in 145 breast-ovarian cancer families. Breast cancer linkage consortium. Am J Hum Genet 36:254–264, 1995.

95. Masood S, Rasty G: Potential value of cytology in the detection of breast cancer precursors by fine needle aspiration biopsy: The future Pap smear for breast cancer. Acta Cytol 43:890, 1999.

96. Wrensch M, Petrakis NL, King EB, et al: Breast cancer risk associated with abnormal cytology in nipple aspirates of breast fluids and prior history of breast biopsy. Am J Epidemiol 137:829–833, 1993.

97. Page DL, Dupont WD, Rogers LW, Rados MS: Atypical hyperplastic lesions of the female breast. A long-term follow up study. Cancer 55:2698–2708, 1985.

98. Dupont WD, Parl FF, Hartman WH, et al: Breast cancer risk associated with proliferative breast disease with atypical hyperplasia. Cancer 71:1258–1265, 1993.

99. Silverman J, Masood S, Ducatman BS, et al: Can FNA biopsy separate atypical hyperplasia, carcinoma in situ and invasive carcinoma of the breast? Cytomorphic criteria and limitations in diagnosis. Diagn Cytopathol 9:713–728, 1993.

100. Sidawy M, Stoler M, Frable W, et al: Interobserver variability in the classification of proliferative breast lesions by fine needle aspiration: Results of the Papanicolaou society of cytopathology study. Diagn Cytopathol 18:150–165, 1998.

101. Rosai: Borderline epithelial lesions of the breast. Am J Surg Path 15:209–221, 1991.

102. Schnitt SJ, Connoly JL, Tavassoli FA, et al: Interobserver reproducibility in the diagnosis of ductal proliferative breast lesions using standard criteria. Am J Surg Path 16:1133–1143, 1992.

103. Fisher ER, Gregoria RM, Fisher B, et al: The pathology of invasive breast cancer: A syllabus derived from findings of the national surgical adjuvant breast and bowel project (protocol no. 4). Cancer 36:1–85, 1975.

104. Badve S, Wiley E, Rodriguez N: Assessment of utility of ductal lavage and ductoscopy in breast cancer—a retrospective analysis of mastectomy specimens. Mod Pathol 16:206–209, 2003.

105. Nayar R, Ramakrishnan R, Baird C, et al: Breast ductal lavage (DL): Cytologic findings in 114 samples. Lab Invest 83:76A, 2003.

106. Masood S, Siddiqi AM, Payandeh F, et al: Exfoliative breast cytopathology: An experience with ductal lavage. Mod Pathol 15:79A, 2002.

107. Evron E, Dooley W, Umbricht C, et al: Detection of breast cancer cells in ductal lavage fluid by methylation-specific PCR. Lancet 357:1335–1336, 2001.

108. Yamamoto D, Senzaki H, Nakagawa H, et al: Detection of chromosomal aneusomy by fluorescence in situ hybridization for patients with nipple discharge. Cancer 97:690–694, 2003.

109. Mendrinos SE, Styblo TM, Nolen JDL, et al: Cytologic findings and protein expression profiles associated with ductal carcinoma of the breast in ductal lavage specimen using SELDI-TOF mass spectrometry. Lab Invest 83:76A, 2003.

110. Fischer G, Tutuncuoglu O, Bakhshandeh M, et al: Diagnostic value of telomerase: Expression in breast fine needle aspiration biopsies. Diagn Cytopathol 35:656–659, 2007.

111. Manfrin E, Mariotto R, Romo A, et al: Is there still a role for fine needle aspiration biopsy in breast cancer screening? Experience with real time integrated radiopathologic activity (1999–2004). Cancer Cytopathol 114:74–82, 2008.

112. Sanchez MA, Stahl RE: Fine needle aspiration biopsy of the breast: Obsolete or state of the art? Cancer 114:65–66, 2008.

chapter 40

Breast Ductoscopy

WILLIAM C. DOOLEY

Current screening methods for breast cancer involve clinical breast examination and mammography. Using these methods has resulted in a recent decrease in the age-adjusted death rate from breast cancer as the percentage of patients diagnosed with in situ and small early-stage breast cancers has increased.[1] Our current methods allow breast cancers to be detected late in the clinical evolution of the neoplastic process and still too often when cancers have already begun to metastasize.[2] Estimates from the American Cancer Society suggest that if all women older than 50 years of age were to adhere to screening recommendations for annual mammography and clinical breast examination, the deaths from breast cancer in the United States would fall by only about 25%.[3] New strategies are needed to make a bigger dent in this death rate.[4]

In Japan, fewer women present with mammographic abnormalities and greater numbers present with breast cancers causing a clinical mass or bloody nipple discharge. In fact, the incidence of nipple discharge as the presenting symptom of breast cancer is much higher in all Asian populations. Okazaki and colleagues[5] used a single optical fiber microendoscope to demonstrate the ability to examine the central breast and often isolate the cause of symptomatic nipple discharge. The Japanese experience was limited, however, because of scope size, limitations of air insufflation to distend the ducts, and fragility of the single-fiber scopes. Despite these limitations, breast ductoscopy increased in popularity in Japan, Korea, and China over the following decade.[6-10] Few western investigators were successful at navigating beyond the first 2 to 3 cm, and image quality was so poor that the technique failed to gain acceptance.[11] However, American manufacturers began to develop multifiber submillimeter endoscopes during the 1990s; the images from these endoscopes optically surpassed those from the single-fiber microscopes used in the earliest mammary ductoscopies.[12,13]

By the late 1990s, chemoprevention studies showed the first real success with the National Surgical Adjuvant Breast and Bowel Project (NSABP) P-01 study.[14] These studies defined high risk through the Gail model— depending greatly on close family history, menstrual history, and breast biopsy history. Still, many patients in whom breast cancer ultimately develops have a low Gail model risk. Even with this limitation in selecting patients who are at risk for breast cancer for enrollment in the chemoprevention trial, tamoxifen was shown to decrease the incidence of new cancers substantially. When subsets were analyzed, the group of women with atypical hyperplasia as their primary risk factor had the greatest reduction in new cancer incidence. Although the caveats of subset analysis apply, this does strongly suggest that the best target for chemoprevention might be the stages of hyperplasia and/or atypical hyperplasia. Unfortunately, none of the standard methods of breast cancer screening are optimized to detect hyperplastic noncancerous lesions. These women have been identified as being high risk based on previous unrelated biopsies in which the hyperplasia presence in the specimen was unexpected.

Finally, chemoprevention studies have been hampered by having to wait for the development of a mammographic or clinical breast cancer to prove usefulness. There have been no standard agreed-on biologic intermediates that predict chemoprevention success.[15-17] If health care providers could screen for hyperplastic changes likely to progress, this same technology could be used to monitor women in prevention studies and could potentially be used as that biologic intermediary. To get out of the current stalemate with diagnosis of 66% of breast cancer as invasive, we need to look to the promise of prevention of breast cancer—the 85% reduction with tamoxifen in new events in women with atypical hyperplasia as their increased risk factor for breast cancer.[14] To achieve this, we need to screen for the lesions most sensitive to prevention and prove that we can reverse them or at least stop them from further progression toward breast cancer.

In an effort to develop and define a new method for detection of atypical hyperplasia in the breast, a multicenter clinical trial of a new procedure—ductal lavage— for collecting ductal epithelial cells was designed.[18] In this study, ductal lavage was compared with nipple aspiration with regard to safety, tolerability, and ability to detect abnormal breast epithelial cells in women at high risk for breast cancer who have nonsuspicious mammogram and clinical breast examination results. Women enrolled were at high risk for breast cancer as defined by Gail model risk or a history of contralateral breast cancer and underwent nipple aspiration followed by lavage of fluid-yielding ducts. All statistical tests were two-sided. We enrolled 507 women, including 291 (57%) with a history of breast cancer and 199 (39%) with a 5-year Gail model risk for breast cancer of 1.7% or greater. Nipple aspirate fluid (NAF) samples were evaluated cytologically for 417 women, and ductal lavage samples were evaluated for 383 women. Only 27% of subjects had NAF samples adequate for diagnosis, whereas 78% of subjects had adequate ductal lavage samples. A median of 13,500 epithelial cells per duct (range, 43 to 492,200 cells) was collected with ductal lavage, compared with a median of 120 epithelial cells per breast (range, 10 to 74,300) collected with nipple aspiration. Of women in whom a ductal lavage specimen was obtained, 24% (92 of 383) had abnormal cells that were mildly (17%) or markedly (7%) atypical. Two subjects had ductal lavage samples with malignant cells. Ductal lavage detected abnormal intraductal breast cells 3.2 times more often than nipple aspiration (79 vs. 25 breasts; McNemar's test, $P < 0.001$). No serious procedure-related adverse events were reported. Using a visual pain scale, subjects reported tolerating NAF well. In conclusion, large numbers of ductal cells can be collected with ductal lavage and can then be used to detect atypical cellular changes within the breast. Ductal lavage is a safe and well-tolerated procedure and is a much more sensitive method of detecting cellular atypia than nipple aspiration.[18,19]

This study raised then an important new clinical problem. Repeated lavage of the same duct can be performed and show persistent severe/malignant atypia in 7% of cases of women with normal mammogram and physical examination results. Even when adding ultrasound, Miraluma, and magnetic resonance imaging, other abnormalities were rarely found. Remembering an earlier Japanese experience with ductoscopy[5-10] and combining those techniques with newer American submillimeter scopes and the techniques of ductal distention developed during the lavage trial, researchers undertook a systematic investigation of the potential of ductoscopy to find these lesions.[12] In each of the initial 12 patients with severe atypia, an intraluminal lesion was found; when biopsy was performed, the lesion had the same cytologic cell appearance as the lavaged atypical cells. The cancers found were all in situ, and the noncancerous lesions usually showed severe atypical hyperplasia.

In the course of the lavage research, it was recognized that fluid could often be produced from ducts in the same quadrant of the breast as a newly diagnosed breast cancer. Cytologic analysis could occasionally confirm the presence of tumor cells. Current surgical methods are limited in intraoperative imaging (ultrasound and palpation) during breast conservation procedures. Unsuspected extensive intraductal component (EIC) and more extensive disease are often found in the final pathology of the intended wide excision. It was hypothesized that such fluid-producing ducts would likely connect to the site of the known cancerous/precancerous lesion and that endoscopic evaluation of such ducts might reveal unsuspected additional disease. To test this, women from a single surgeon's practice undergoing lumpectomy for breast conservation from January 2000 to August 2001 were evaluated for fluid production from the nipple at the time

of lumpectomy. If a fluid-producing duct was identified in the same quadrant as the lesion, it was cannulated and dilated using local anesthetic; endoscopy was then performed using a 0.9-mm microendoscope. Of the 201 patients (16 with atypical ductal hyperplasia, 52 with ductal carcinoma in situ [DCIS], and 133 with stage I or II breast cancers) from which fluid could be obtained, 150 (74.6%) could be successfully dilated and their breast ducts navigated beyond multiple divisions. Additional lesions outside the anticipated lumpectomy were identified in 41% (83) of cases. If endoscopy was successful, the chances for a positive margin in DCIS or invasive cancer fell from 23.5% to only 5%. Margins were positive in the nipple direction in only 1 of the 150 cases of successful endoscopy. Endoscopy proved to be a useful adjunct in this series of patients because it identified all cases of EIC in early-stage breast cancer and identified additional noncontiguous DCIS in more than half of the patients with stage 0 lumpectomy who underwent endoscopy (Figs. 40-1 to 40-4). Routine operative breast endoscopy has a great potential to reduce the need for re-excision lumpectomy for initial positive margins. It also finds substantially more cancerous and precancerous disease than anticipated by routine preoperative mammography and ultrasound.[20]

The intraductal approaches to screening with lavage and endoscopy allow collection of both fluid and cells from proliferative epithelial surfaces in the breast. Prior studies suggest that early, relatively large karyotypic events occur in the evolution of a breast cancer.[21] These are often associated with hypermethylation of numerous genes. Cells collected from lavage and endoscopy specimens of the breast ducts were tested with methylation-specific polymerase chain reaction (PCR). Methylated alleles of cyclin D2, *RAR-β*, and *Twist* genes were often detected in fluid from mammary ducts containing endoscopically visualized carcinomas (17 of 20 cases) and DCIS (2 of 7 cases) but rarely in ductal lavage fluid from healthy ducts (5 of 45 cases). Two of the

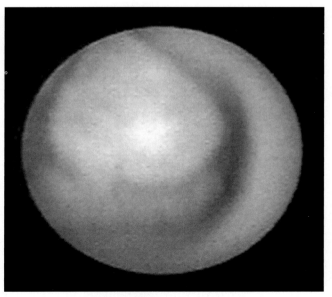

Figure 40-1 Papilloma.

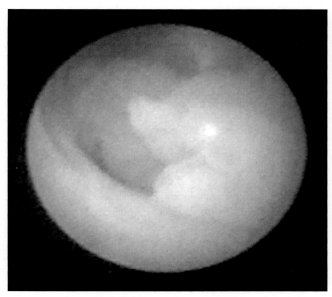

Figure 40-2   Papillomas.

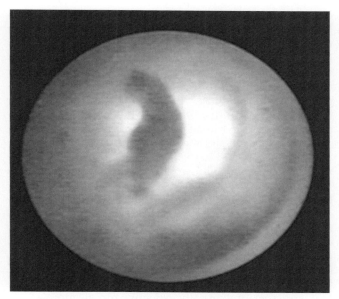

Figure 40-4   High-grade ductal carcinoma in situ.

women with healthy mammograms whose ductal lavage fluid contained methylated markers and cytologically abnormal cells were subsequently diagnosed as having breast cancer. Furthermore, this study demonstrated that carrying out methylation-specific PCR in these fluid samples from lavage or endoscopy may provide a sensitive and powerful addition to mammographic or cytologic screening for early detection of breast cancer.[22]

The two new resources of ductal lavage and endoscopy now need to be refined and developed into the tools that will allow clinicians to screen for, diagnose, and monitor premalignant disease in the breast. Both lavage and endoscopy are time consuming and dependent on a relatively high skill level of the operator, much like gastrointestinal endoscopy. Both may currently be appropriate for patients at highest risk for breast cancer,

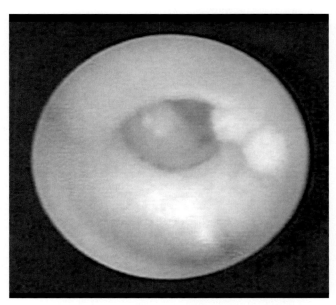

Figure 40-3   Low-grade ductal carcinoma in situ.

but they are not the answer for mass screening. Through examination of the cells and protein obtained from ducts with premalignant and malignant disease, molecular markers of increased risk for atypia may be identified, which are more feasible to test on the few microliters of NAF. By identifying women with suspicious or increased risk by nipple aspirate, the workup can continue with lavage to identify the ductal system producing these changes and then with endoscopy to find the lesions and perform a biopsy.

The burning clinical questions of both lavage and endoscopy are how to best incorporate them into clinical practice. Ductoscopy has a direct and obvious application to investigations of symptomatic nipple discharge. It provides immediate visual intraductal information and direct localization, through transillumination, of the suspect lesion. Beyond this situation, the future of these technologies is less clear. Research that examines the strengths and weaknesses of each technique by collecting data from multiple surgeons performing these techniques at multiple centers is required. The initial lavage study enrolled only patients with breasts considered high risk and that were normal as determined with mammography and clinical examination. It detected significant amounts of atypia cytologically and a few breast cancers. However, this study does not have any long-term comparative data that uses our traditional screening methods to determine direct comparison to standard screening of physical examination and mammography. Ductoscopy has potential to allow surgeons to visually direct lumpectomy procedures or even nonsurgical ablation by determining margin. It is limited because most of our currently identified breast cancers already obstruct the ducts and limit the ability to navigate the scope toward the nipple side only as well as the paucity of submillimeter endoscope manufacturers worldwide.

Optics have improved, allowing more manufacturers the ability to devote a smaller cross-sectional diameter to light and image capture. This leaves available larger working channels for visually directed biopsy in submillimeter endoscopes. These new smaller scopes and new vacuum-assisted biopsy techniques have begun to allow investigators to serially sample up and down the ductal tree and truly begin to map the pathologic changes.[23,24] The value of this is confirmed by Hunerbein and colleagues in Berlin, who have now been able to find extensive intraductal carcinomas beyond what could be seen by traditional external imaging techniques.[25]

The further development of autofluorescence techniques by Jacobs and associates from Munich opens the potential of being able to visually distinguish benign from more suspicious lesions on the basis of simple biologic differences in the ductal lining tissue.[26] The confusion over the overlap in appearance of benign and malignant intraductal lesions has led some authors to question the value of ductoscopy as a current clinical tool.[27-29] The application of autofluorescence as in bronchoscopy will further enhance clinicians' abilities to use this technique and separate confusing intraluminal growths into visually recognizable as more suspicious and less suspicious. Combining ductoscopic findings with results of other imaging techniques seems already to offer substantial benefits in determining the presence and extent of small cancers.[28-30] As the techniques of ductoscopy continue to evolve, some practitioners are using the scopes not just through the nipple but also through direct cyst puncture.[31] Such further refinements of both instrumentation and techniques will further expand both the clinical and research utility of ductoscopy in the near future.[32,33]

The increased incidence of intraluminal disease seen endoscopically than expected with traditional pathologic analysis may account for lower rates of local recurrences following breast conservation. These same endoscopically abnormal lesions may be subclinical and may never progress rapidly enough to limit the patient's life. The hope of the intraductal approach to increase both understandings of breast cancer initiation and progression and design better treatments is great but will be reached only through careful multi-institutional research.

REFERENCES

1. Jemal A, Clegg LX, Ward E, et al (eds): SEER cancer statistics review, Bethesda, MD, 1973-1999, National Cancer Institute. Available at http://seer.cancer.gov/csr/1973_1999/. Accessed November 2002.
2. Tabar L, Duffy SW, Vitak B, et al: The natural history of breast carcinoma: What have we learned from screening? Cancer 86:449-462, 1999.
3. Thomas AG, Jemal A, Thun MJ: Breast cancer facts and figures. Atlanta, GA, American Cancer Society, 2001.
4. Charting the course: Priorities for breast cancer research—the report of the Breast Cancer Progress Review Group, National Cancer Institute. Available at http://prg.nci.nih.gov/breast/default.html. Accessed November 2002.
5. Okazaki A, Okazaki M, Asaishi K, et al: Fiberoptic ductoscopy of the breast: A new diagnostic procedure for nipple discharge. Jpn J Clin Oncol 21:188-193, 1991.
6. Yamamoto D, Ueda S, Senzaki H, et al: New diagnostic approach to intracystic lesions of the breast by fiberoptic ductoscopy. Anticancer Res 21:4113-4116, 2001.
7. Yamamoto D, Shoji T, Kawanishi H, et al: A utility of ductography and fiberoptic ductoscopy for patients with nipple discharge. Breast Cancer Res Treat 70:103-108, 2001.
8. Shen KW, Wu J, Lu JS, et al: Fiberoptic ductoscopy for breast cancer patients with nipple discharge. Surg Endosc 15:1340-1345, 2001.
9. Matsunaga T, Ohta D, Misaka T, et al: Mammary ductoscopy for diagnosis and treatment of intraductal lesions of the breast. Breast Cancer 8:213-221, 2001.
10. Okazaki A, Hirata K, Okazaki M, et al: Nipple discharge disorders: Current diagnostic management and the role of fiber-ductoscopy. Eur Radiol 9:583-590, 1999.
11. Love SM, Barsky SH: Breast-duct endoscopy to study stages of cancerous breast disease. Lancet 348:997, 1996.
12. Dooley WC: Endoscopic visualization of breast tumors, JAMA 284:1518, 2000.
13. Dietz JR, Kim JA, Malyeky JL, et al: Feasibility and technical considerations of mammary ductoscopy in human mastectomy specimens. Breast J 6:161-165, 2000.
14. Fisher B, Costantino JP, Wickerham DL, et al: Tamoxifen for the prevention of breast cancer: Current status of the National Surgical Adjuvant Breast and Bowel Project P-1 Study. J Natl Cancer Inst 97:1652-1662, 2005.
15. Wrensch MR, Petrakis NL, King EB, et al: Breast cancer incidence in women with abnormal cytology nipple aspirates of breast fluid. Am J Epidemiol 135:130-141, 1992.
16. Fabian C, Kimler BF, Zalles CM, et al: Short-term breast cancer prediction by random periareolar fine-needle aspiration cytology and the Gail risk model. J Natl Cancer Inst 92:1217-1227, 2000.
17. Dupont WD, Page DL: Risk factors for breast cancer in women with proliferative breast disease. N Engl J Med 312:146, 1985.
18. Dooley WC, Ljung BM, Veronesi U, et al: Ductal lavage for detection of cellular atypia in women at high risk for breast cancer. J Natl Cancer Inst 93:1624-1632, 2001.
19. O'Shaughnessy JA, Ljung BM, Dooley WC, et al: Ductal lavage and the clinical management of women at high risk for breast carcinoma: A commentary. Cancer 94:292-298, 2002.
20. Dooley WC: Routine operative breast endoscopy during lumpectomy. Ann Surg Oncol 10:38, 2003.
21. Gusev Y, Kagansky V, Dooley WC: Long-term dynamics of chromosomal instability in cancer: a transitional probability model. J Math Comput Model 33:1253, 2001.
22. Evron E, Dooley WC, Umbricht CB, et al: Detection of breast cancer cells in ductal lavage fluid by methylation-specific PCR. Lancet 357:1335-1336, 2001.
23. Jacobs VR, Paepke S, Ohlinger R, et al: Breast ductoscopy: Technical development from a diagnostic to an interventional procedure and its future perspective. Onkologie 11:545-549, 2007.
24. Hunerbein M, Raubach M, Gebauer B, et al: Ductoscopy and intraductal vacuum assisted biopsy in women with pathologic nipple discharge. Breast Cancer Res Treat 3:301-307, 2006.
25. Hunerbein M, Dubowy A, Raubach M, et al: Gradient index ductoscopy and intraductal biopsy of intraductal breast lesions. Am J Surg 4:511-514, 2007.
26. Jacobs VR, Paepke S, Schaaf H, et al: Autofluorescence ductoscopy: A new imaging technique for intraductal breast endoscopy. Clin Breast Cancer 8:619-623, 2007.
27. Louie LD, Crowe JP, Dawson AE, et al: Identification of breast cancer in patients with pathologic nipple discharge. Does ductoscopy predict malignancy? Am J Surg 4:530-533, 2006.
28. Grunwald S, Heyer H, Paepke S, et al: Diagnostic value of ductoscopy in the diagnosis of nipple discharge and intraductal proliferatons in comparison to standard methods. Onkologie 5:243-248, 2007.
29. Grunwald S, Bojahr B, Schwesinger G, et al: Mammary ductoscopy for the evaluation of nipple discharge and comparison with standard diagnostic techniques. Minim Invasive Gynecol 5:418-423, 2006.
30. Makita M, Akiyama F, Gomi N, et al: Endoscopic and histologic findings of intraductal lesions presenting with nipple discharge. Breast J 5:S210-S2177.
31. Uchida K, Toriumi Y, Kawase K, et al: Percutaneous endoscopy-guided biopsy of an intracystic tumor with a mammary ductoscopy. Breast Cancer 2:215-218, 2007.
32. Hunerbein M, Raubach M, Gebauer B, et al: Intraoperative ductoscopy in women undergoing surgery for breast cancer. Surgery 6:833-838, 2006.
33. Valdes EK, Boolbol SK, Cohen JM, et al: Clinical experience with mammary ductoscopy. Ann Surg Oncol 2006 (e-pub).

SECTION X

Clinical Trials: Biostatistical Applications

chapter 41

Design and Conduct of Clinical Trials for Breast Cancer

YU SHYR

What Are Clinical Trials?

A clinical trial can be defined as a prospective study evaluating the clinical effect or benefit of treatment in human beings to answer specific clinical questions. The word *clinical* is derived from the Greek *kline*, which means bed. In modern usage, *clinical* refers not only to the bedside but also more generally to the care of human patients. The Code of Federal Regulations defines a clinical investigation as "any experiment in which a drug is administered or dispensed to, or used involving, one or more human subjects."[1] Meinert defines a clinical trial as

> ....a planned experiment designed to assess the efficacy of a treatment in man by comparing the outcomes in a group of patients treated with the test treatment with those observed in a comparable group of patients receiving a control treatment, where patients in both groups are enrolled, treated, and followed over the same time period.[2]

Chow and Liu use three key terms in their definition of clinical trial: *experimental unit*, *treatment*, and *evaluation* of the treatment.[3] In this definition, an *experimental unit* usually refers to a subject from the target population under study; a *treatment* can be a placebo or any combination of a new pharmaceutical identity, diagnostic test, or medical device; and *evaluation* focuses on the efficacy of a test treatment.

In recent years, clinical trials have demonstrated the value of treatment for many diseases, including breast cancer. With the development of more detailed statistical theories and applications, experimental design and biostatistical analysis have become more important in evaluating the effectiveness of diagnostic techniques, as well as treatments. Several key components of well-performed clinical trials, such as trial design, randomization, sample size determination, interim monitoring, and evaluation of clinical effects, are highly dependent on successful application of biostatistics and an understanding of probabilities.

The application of biostatistics is relevant throughout phase I, II, III, and IV clinical trials. Phase I trials introduce investigational drugs to humans. The primary objectives of a phase I trial are to generate preliminary information on the biochemical properties of a drug, such as metabolism, pharmacokinetics, and bioavailability, and to determine a safe drug dose, dosing ranges, or schedule of administration. Phase I studies also may provide preliminary evidence of a drug's activity by means of a pharmacodynamic or biomarker response. The focus of the phase I trial is assessment of safety; a phase I trial is usually a nonrandomized dose-escalation study with no more than 20 to 80 normal volunteers or patients with disease.

In oncology trials, the goal of phase I is usually to determine a safe and/or potentially effective dose to be used in phase II. For cytotoxic agents, the primary objective of the phase I trial is to determine the maximum tolerated dose (MTD) for a new drug and to evaluate qualitative and quantitative toxicities. For noncytotoxic agents, the primary objective of the phase I trial is to identify the optimum biologically effective dose (OBED). For target or novel agents, the phase I trial is designed to determine the minimum effective blood concentration level of the agent or minimum expression level of a molecular target.

Phase II trials provide preliminary information on the efficacy of a drug and additional information on safety and dosing ranges. These trials may be designed to include a control or may use a single-arm design, enrolling 20 to 200 or more patients with disease. It is important that phase II studies provide data on the doses to be used in phase III, although this may not be as easy as it appears. For phase II oncology trials, tumor response rate is usually the primary end point. Time to progression also may serve as the primary end point, when the estimated median time to progression is relatively short

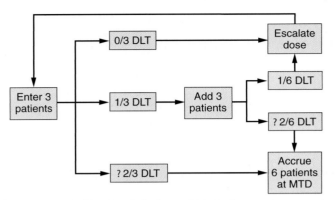

Figure 41-1 The 3 + 3 design, which is the most commonly used phase I oncology trial design. DLT, dose-limiting toxicity; MTD, maximum tolerated dose.

for the study agent. In addition, an early stopping rule is very common in phase II oncology trials, to prevent the testing of ineffective drugs or agents in more patients.

The phase III trial is a full-scale treatment evaluation, with the primary goal of comparing efficacy of a new treatment with that of the standard regimen. Phase III trials are usually randomized controlled studies enrolling several hundred to several thousand patients with disease. For oncology phase III trials, overall survival is usually the primary end point; however, time to progression also may serve as the primary end point if the estimated median overall survival time is relatively long for the study agent.

To look for uncommon long-term side effects, phase IV or postregistration trials may be conducted after regulatory approval of a new treatment or drug. Thus, phase IV trials evaluate agents or drugs already available for physicians to prescribe, rather than new drugs still being developed. These trials can be designed as randomized studies, but they are usually observational studies with thousands of patients.

Trial Design for Phase I Oncology Studies

As mentioned in the previous section, the primary objective of the phase I oncology trial is usually to determine the MTD of a new drug or agent. The most common phase I oncology trial design is the 3 + 3 design (Fig. 41-1). In this design, at least three patients are studied at each dose level and evaluated for toxicity. At any given dose level, three patients are accrued. If none of these patients experiences a dose-limiting toxicity (DLT), the dose is escalated. If one of these patients experiences a DLT, three additional patients are treated. If none of the additional patients develops a DLT, the dose is escalated; otherwise, escalation ceases. If at any

time at least two patients (≥ 2 of 3 or ≥ 2 of 6) experience a DLT, the MTD has been exceeded. For a dose level at which a patient has a high probability of developing a DLT, the probability of escalation to a higher dose level should be low. As shown in Table 41-1, the probability of escalating a certain dose is only 3%, if the dose level has a true DLT rate of 70%.

Another commonly used phase I oncology trial design is the continual reassessment method, introduced by O'Quigley, Pepe, and Fisher.[4] Like the 3 + 3 design, the continual reassessment method is designed to determine MTD. This method can be described as a one-parameter Bayesian-based logit model (Fig. 41-2), which describes the association between dose level (x-axis) and toxicity level (y-axis). The investigator picks a target toxicity level for the study agent, for example, 30%. Given this target toxicity, the investigator then selects a first or starting dose associated with this toxicity, using a prior dose-toxicity curve, which may be based on an animal model, results from a similar study, or the investigator's experience. After testing the first dose, the investigator recalculates the dose associated with the target probability of toxicity. This estimated dose is used to treat the next patient(s). The process of treating, evaluating toxicity, statistical model fitting, and dose estimation is repeated until the model converges (i.e., data from additional patients do not improve the model). The advantages of the continual reassessment method are that it is somewhat more efficient than the 3 + 3 design and has an unbiased estimation method.

Trial Design for Phase II Oncology Studies

One of the primary objectives of a phase II oncology trial of a new drug or agent is to determine whether the agent has sufficient antitumor activity to warrant more extensive development. Two-stage phase II designs are widely used in oncology studies. Several two-stage designs will be discussed in this section: Gehan's, Fleming's, Simon's optimal, Simon's minimax, and Fei and Shyr's balanced two-stage designs.

GEHAN'S DESIGN

Gehan's design[5] is a two-stage design that estimates response rate while providing for early termination if the drug shows insufficient antitumor activity. The design is most commonly used with a first stage of 14 patients. If no responses (completed or partial) are observed, the trial is terminated. The rationale for stopping is that if the true response probability were at least 20%, at least one response would very likely be observed in the first

TABLE 41-1								
Probability of Escalating a Dose with a Particular Dose-Limiting Toxicity Rate in the 3 + 3 Trial Design								
True dose-limiting toxicity rate	10%	20%	30%	40%	50%	70%	80%	90%
Probability of escalating	0.91	0.71	0.49	0.31	0.17	0.03	0.01	0.001

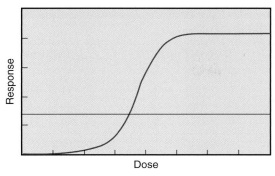

Figure 41-2 Dose-response curve. With the continual reassessment method, the response of interest is toxicity.

14 patients; if no responses are seen, it is unlikely that the true response rate is at least 20%. If at least one response is observed in the first 14 patients, then a second stage of accrual is carried out to obtain an estimate of the response rate. The number of patients to accrue in the second stage depends on the number of responses observed in the first stage and the precision desired for the final estimate of response rate. If the first stage consists of 14 patients, the second stage consists of between 1 and 11 patients if a standard error of 10% is desired and between 45 and 86 patients if a standard error of 5% is desired. A common use of Gehan's design is to accrue 14 patients in the first stage and an additional 11 patients in the second stage, for a total of 25 patients. This provides an estimate of response rate with a standard error of about 10%, which corresponds to very broad confidence limits. For example, if three responses are observed among 25 patients, a 95% confidence limit for the true response rate is from about 3% to about 30%.

A limitation of Gehan's design is that a very poor drug may be allowed to move to the second stage. For example, if a drug has a response rate of only 5%, there exists a 51% chance of at least one response among the first 14 patients. Thus, the first stage of 14 patients will not effectively screen out all inactive drugs.

FLEMING'S DESIGN

Fleming presented a multistage design for testing the hypothesis that the probability of a true response is less than some uninteresting level (e.g., 5% response rate) against the hypothesis that the probability of a true response is at least as large as a target level (e.g., 20% response rate).[6] Table 41-2 shows two examples of Fleming's design.

As a third example, consider a design with an uninteresting level of a 5% response rate and a clinically interesting (i.e., clinically significant) level of a 20% response rate, for which both error limits (type I and type II) are to be less than 10%. These constraints can be met with a two-stage Fleming's design with 15 patients in the first stage and 20 in the second stage, as follows:

1. If no responses are observed in the first 15 patients, then the trial is terminated and the drug is rejected.
2. If at least three responses are observed in the first 15 patients, then the trial is terminated and the drug is accepted.
3. If one to two responses are observed in the first 15 patients, then 20 more patients are accrued.
4. After all 35 patients are evaluated, the drug is accepted if the response rate is 11.4% or greater ($\geq$4 responses in 35 patients), and the drug is rejected if the response rate is 8.6% or less ($\leq$3 in 35 patients).

Fleming's design is the only two-stage design covered here that may terminate early with an "accept the drug" conclusion.

SIMON'S OPTIMAL DESIGN

Simon's optimal two-stage designs[7] are optimal in the sense that the expected sample size is minimized if the regimen has low activity subject to type I and type II error probability constraints. The following values provide an example of Simon's optimal design:

Clinically uninteresting level = 5% response rate
Clinically interesting level = 20% response rate
Type I error (α) = 0.05
Type II error (β) = 0.20
Power = 1 − type II error = 0.80
Stage I: Reject the drug if the response rate $\leq$0/10
Stage II: Reject the drug if the response rate $\leq$3/29

In this example, the first stage consists of 10 patients. If no responses are seen in the first 10 patients, the trial is terminated. Otherwise, accrual continues to a total of 29 patients. If there are at least four responses in the total of 29 patients, the trial may move to a phase III study. The average sample size is 17.6, and the probability of early termination is 60% for a drug with a response rate of 5% (low activity). Simon's optimal design is the most commonly used two-stage design.

TABLE 41-2									
Examples of Fleming's Two-Stage Design									
				Reject Drug If Response Rate		**Accept Drug If Response Rate**			
P_0	P_1	n_1	n	$\leq r_1/n_1$	$\leq r/n$	$\geq r_1/n_1$	$\geq r/n$	α	β
0.05	0.20	15	35	0/15	3/35	3/15	4/35	0.10	0.08
0.05	0.25	15	25	1/15	2/25	3/15	3/25	0.09	0.09

P_0, uninteresting response rate; P_1, clinically interesting response rate; n_1, stage I sample size; n, total sample size; r_1, number of responses observed in stage I; r, total number of responses observed at end of stage II; α, type I error rate; β, type II error rate.

TABLE 41-3										

Examples of Balanced Two-Stage Design, with Comparison to Optimal Design

				Optimal Design			Balanced Design		
P_0	P_1	α	β	n_1	n_2	$n_1{:}n_2$	n_1	n_2	$n_1{:}n_2$
0.75	0.95	0.05	0.20	3	19	0.16	11	11	1
0.35	0.50	0.10	0.20	19	68	0.28	43	44	0.98
0.70	0.90	0.05	0.20	6	21	0.29	14	14	1

P_0, uninteresting response rate; P_1, clinically interesting response rate; α, type I error rate; β, type II error rate; n_1, stage I sample size; n_2, stage II sample size.

SIMON'S MINIMAX DESIGN

Simon's minimax two-stage design[7] minimizes maximum sample size subject to type I and type II error probability constraints. The following values provide an example of Simon's minimax design:

Clinically uninteresting level = 5% response rate
Clinically interesting level = 20% response rate
Type I error (α) = 0.05
Type II error (β) = 0.20
Power = 1 − type II error = 0.80
Stage I: Reject the drug if the response rate $\leq 0/13$
Stage II: Reject the drug if the response rate $\leq 3/27$

In this example, the first stage consists of 13 patients. If no responses are seen in the first 13 patients, the trial is terminated. Otherwise, accrual continues to a total of 27 patients. If there are at least four responses in the total of 27 patients, the trial may move to a phase III study. The average sample size is 19.8, and the probability of early termination is 51% for a drug with a response rate of 5% (low activity).

COMPARISONS OF THE OPTIMAL AND MINIMAX DESIGNS

Simon's optimal two-stage design minimizes *expected* sample size, but it does not necessarily minimize *maximum* sample size, subject to error probability constraints. As a result, the minimax design may be more attractive when the difference in expected sample sizes is small and the accrual rate is low. Consider, for example, the case of distinguishing the uninteresting response rate of 10% from the clinically interesting response rate of 30% with $\alpha = \beta = 10\%$. The optimal design has an expected sample size of 19.8 and a maximum sample size of 35. The minimax design has an expected sample size of 20.4 and a maximum sample size of 25. If the accrual rate is only 10 patients per year, it could take one year longer to complete the optimal design than the minimax design. This may be more important than the slight reduction in expected sample size.

FEI AND SHYR'S BALANCED DESIGN

As discussed in the previous subsections, Simon's optimal and minimax two-stage designs are commonly used for phase II oncology trials. The optimal design minimizes expected sample size, and the minimax design minimizes maximum sample size. Neither method, however, considers balance between sample sizes in stages I and II (n_1 and n_2, respectively). For example, with the minimax design, if the investigator is testing a 15% improvement (0.50 vs. 0.65) in response rate, 66 patients are required in stage I but only two patients in stage 2 ($n_1/n_2 = 33$). Thus, there is little value in early termination; this saves enrolling only two patients. As another example, with the optimal design, if the investigator is testing a 15% improvement (0.35 vs. 0.50) in response rate, 19 patients are required in stage I and 68 additional patients in stage II ($n_1/n_2 = 0.28$). In a case such as this, clinical investigators may resist early termination, given that stage I includes only 22% of the total target accrual. To address issues such as these, Fei and Shyr proposed a balanced two-stage design focused on balancing the sample size ratio (n_1/n_2), subject to type 1 and type 2 error probability constraints.[8] With Fei and Shyr's balanced two-stage design, expected sample size is less than that of the minimax design and/or maximum sample size is less than that of the optimal design. Tables 41-3 and 41-4 provide examples of balanced design, with comparison to optimal design

TABLE 41-4										

Examples of Balanced Two-Stage Design, with Comparison to Minimax Design

				Minimax Design			Balanced Design		
P_0	P_1	α	β	n_1	n_2	$n_1{:}n_2$	n_1	n_2	$n_1{:}n_2$
0.45	0.60	0.05	0.10	93	2	46.5	58	58	1
0.50	0.65	0.05	0.20	66	2	33	39	39	1
0.70	0.90	0.05	0.20	6	21	0.29	14	14	1

P_0, uninteresting response rate; P_1, clinically interesting response rate; α, type I error rate; β, type II error rate; n_1, stage I sample size; n_2, stage II sample size.

(see Table 41-3) or minimax design (see Table 41-4); Tables 41-5 and 41-6 provide a more detailed comparison of stage I sample sizes, total sample sizes, expected sample sizes, probability of early termination, and sample size ratios for optimal, minimax, and balanced designs.

Balanced design provides an additional two-stage design choice. This choice allows investigators to stop a trial near the half-way point.

Trial Design for Phase III Randomized Controlled Studies

The most common types of randomized controlled study design are the parallel design, crossover design, and factorial design. Figure 41-3 illustrates parallel design. After patients are recruited, they are randomly assigned to either the intervention group or the control group (i.e., placebo group); after the course of therapy is completed, outcomes are measured in each group. Advantages of this study design are that (1) randomization tends to produce comparable groups and removes bias in the allocation of participants to intervention group versus control group, and that (2) the validity of statistical tests of significance is likely guaranteed. One major problem with parallel design is that patients vary both in their initial disease state and in their response to therapy. Because of this interpatient variability, the investigator needs substantial groups of patients in each treatment to estimate reliably the magnitude of any treatment difference (see Sample Size Determination and Power Analysis for a discussion of sample size determination).

The crossover design is also a randomized controlled study design, in which patients cross from one therapy (e.g., intervention) to another (e.g., placebo). The difference between crossover and parallel designs is that patients in crossover trials are studied twice. For example, as illustrated in Figure 41-4, patients assigned to order I receive treatment A (e.g., intervention) followed by treatment B (e.g., placebo). Patients assigned to order II receive treatment B followed by treatment A. Between the two treatment periods, all patients enter what is called a *washout*, to ensure they return to their pretreatment baseline before starting the second assigned treatment. The advantages of this design are that (1) interpatient variability is reduced due to the fact that each patient serves as his or her own control, and that (2) study sample size tends to be reduced. Disadvantages are that (1) a fairly strict assumption about treatment carryover must be made (i.e., the effects of the intervention during the first period must not carry over into the second period), and that (2) it is very difficult to design a crossover study for oncology trials.

The other commonly used randomized controlled study is the factorial design. Figure 41-5 shows the details of the factorial design. The patients in this design are randomized to one of four study groups: patients assigned to group I receive treatment A (e.g., chemotherapy) and treatment B (e.g., radiation therapy) together;

patients assigned to group II or group III receive treatment B or treatment A only, respectively; and group IV is the true placebo or control group. Advantages of this study design are that (1) the investigator is able to evaluate two interventions compared with a control in a single experiment, and that (2) study sample size tends to be reduced. A concern with factorial design is the possibility of interaction between the two interventions and the impact of potential interaction on the sample size.

Randomization Process

One of the strengths of randomized clinical trials is reduction in bias. Bias may be defined as systematic error or the difference between the true value and that obtained due to all causes other than sampling variability. The randomization process is one of the best tools to reduce bias in clinical trials. Through randomization, each subject has the same chance of being assigned to either intervention or control; to remove investigator bias, neither the subject nor the investigator should know the treatment assignment before the subject's decision to enter the study. Randomization tends to produce groups that are comparable with respect to known or unknown risk factors, prognostic variables, and covariates; it also tends to guarantee the validity of statistical tests.

There are several methods for making random treatment assignments. Many attempt to balance treatment groups over time, over stratification factors, or both. In the following, we assume equal allocation of patients to each treatment (i.e., 1:1 randomization). Complete randomization is the most elementary form of randomization. One simple method of complete randomization is to toss an unbiased coin. Another common method is to generate a random digit table using a computer program and assign patients with even digits to treatment A and odd digits to treatment B. The advantage of complete randomization is that it is easy to implement; the disadvantage is that, at any point in time, there may be an imbalance in the number of subjects on each treatment. For instance, with n = 20, the chance of a 12:8 split or worse is approximately 50%; with n = 100, the chance of a 60:40 split or worse is still greater than 5%. Thus, it is desirable to restrict randomization to ensure similar treatment numbers throughout the trial. We will look at three approaches to restricting randomization: replacement randomization, random permuted block randomization, and biased coin randomization.

In replacement randomization, the investigator prespecifies an amount of imbalance that would be unacceptable during the trial. For example, with n = 100 patients on each treatment, the treatment imbalance (number on treatment A minus number on treatment B) should be less than six at any point in time. A simple randomization method is then used to generate a randomization list. If the imbalance is unacceptable based on the prespecified criterion, a new list is generated. This process is repeated as necessary until an acceptable list is obtained.

Random permuted block randomization was described by Hill.[9] This technique is used to avoid serious imbalance

TABLE 41-5
Optimal, Minimax, and Balanced Designs for Independent Data, $p_1 - p_0 = 0.15$

		Optimal Design					Minimax Design					Balanced Design				
		Reject Drug If Response Rate					Reject Drug If Response Rate					Reject Drug If Response Rate				
p_0	p_1	$\leq r_1/n_1$	$\leq r/n$	EN (p_0)	PET (p_0)	$n_1{:}n_2$	$\leq r_1/n_1$	$\leq r/n$	EN (p_0)	PET (p_0)	$n_1{:}n_2$	$\leq r_1/n_1$	$\leq r/n$	EN (p_0)	PET (p_0)	$n_1{:}n_2$
0.05	0.20	0/12	3/37	23.5	0.54	0.48	0/18	3/32	26.4	0.4	1.29	1/19	3/38	23.7	0.75	1
		0/10	3/29	17.6	0.6	0.53	0/13	3/27	19.8	0.51	0.93	0/14	3/28	21.2	0.49	1
		1/21	4/41	26.7	0.72	1.05	1/29	4/38	32.9	0.57	3.22	1/21	4/42	26.9	0.72	1
0.10	0.25	2/21	7/50	31.2	0.65	0.72	2/27	6/40	33.7	0.48	2.08	2/24	7/48	34.5	0.56	1
		2/18	7/43	24.7	0.73	0.72	2/22	7/40	28.8	0.62	1.22	2/21	7/42	28.4	0.65	1*
		2/21	10/66	36.8	0.65	0.47	3/31	9/55	40	0.62	1.29	4/32	10/64	38.8	0.79	1*
0.20	0.35	5/27	16/63	43.6	0.54	0.75	6/33	15/58	45.5	0.5	1.32	6/32	16/62	45.9	0.54	1.07
		5/22	19/72	35.4	0.73	0.44	6/31	15/53	40.4	0.57	1.41	7/31	17/62	39.4	0.73	1*
		8/37	22/83	51.4	0.69	0.8	8/42	21/77	58.4	0.53	1.2	8/39	21/78	53.7	0.62	1*
0.3	0.45	9/30	29/82	51.4	0.59	0.58	16/50	25/69	56	0.68	2.63	12/39	28/78	53.9	0.62	1*
		9/27	30/81	41.7	0.73	0.5	16/46	25/65	49.6	0.81	2.42	11/34	26/68	44.4	0.69	1*
		13/40	40/110	60.8	0.7	0.57	27/77	33/88	78.5	0.86	7	18/53	39/106	64.4	0.78	1*
0.4	0.55	16/38	40/88	54.5	0.67	0.76	18/45	34/73	57.2	0.56	1.61	19/44	40/80	56.2	0.72	1*
		11/26	42/88	46.2	0.67	0.42	28/59	34/70	60.1	0.9	5.36	17/39	38/78	49.3	0.73	1*
		19/45	49/104	64	0.68	0.76	24/62	45/94	78.9	0.47	1.94	23/53	50/105	66.7	0.74	1
0.5	0.65	18/35	47/84	53	0.63	0.71	19/40	41/72	58	0.44	1.25	20/39	44/78	53.6	0.63	1*
		15/28	48/83	43.7	0.71	0.51	39/66	40/68	66.1	0.95	33	21/39	46/78	49.2	0.74	1*
		22/42	60/105	62.3	0.68	0.67	28/57	54/93	75	0.5	1.58	25/50	58/100	72.2	0.56	1*
0.6	0.75	21/34	47/71	47.1	0.65	0.92	25/43	43/64	54.4	0.46	2.05	24/38	50/76	49	0.71	1
		17/27	46/67	39.3	0.69	0.68	18/30	43/62	43.8	0.57	0.94	22/34	46/67	41.7	0.77	1.03
		21/34	64/95	55.6	0.65	0.56	48/72	57/84	73.2	0.9	6	28/45	61/90	59.7	0.67	1*
0.7	0.85	14/20	45/59	36.2	0.58	0.51	15/22	40/52	36.8	0.51	0.73	18/26	40/52	38	0.54	1
		14/19	46/59	30.3	0.72	0.47	16/23	39/49	34.4	0.56	0.88	21/28	44/56	34.2	0.78	1*
		18/25	61/79	43.4	0.66	0.46	33/44	53/68	48.5	0.81	1.83	28/38	59/76	47.7	0.74	1*
0.80	0.95	5/7	27/31	20.8	0.42	0.29	5/7	27/31	20.8	0.42	0.29	5/7	27/31	20.8	0.42	0.29
		7/9	26/29	17.7	0.56	0.45	7/9	26/29	17.7	0.56	0.45	7/9	26/29	17.7	0.56	0.45
		16/19	37/42	24.4	0.76	0.83	31/35	35/40	35.3	0.94	7	18/22	39/44	29.3	0.67	1

p_0, uninteresting response rate; p_1, clinically interesting response rate; r_1, lower bound for number of responses observed in stage I; n_1, stage I sample size; r, lower bound for total number of responses observed at end of stage II; n, total sample size; EN, expected sample size; PET, probability of early termination.

*Balanced design has both expected and maximum sample sizes between those of optimal and minimax designs.

Reproduced from Fei Y, Shyr Y: Balanced two-stage designs for phase II clinical trials. Clin Trials 4: 514–524, 2007.

TABLE 41-6

Optimal, Minimax, and Balanced Designs for Independent Data, $p_1 - p_0 = 0.20$

p_0	p_1	Optimal Design					Minimax Design					Balanced Design				
		Reject Drug If Response Rate					Reject Drug If Response Rate					Reject Drug If Response Rate				
		$\leq r_1/n_1$	$\leq r/n$	EN(p_0)	PET(p_0)	$n_1{:}n_2$	$\leq r_1/n_1$	$\leq r/n$	EN(p_0)	PET(p_0)	$n_1{:}n_2$	$\leq r_1/n_1$	$\leq r/n$	EN(p_0)	PET(p_0)	$n_1{:}n_2$
0.05	0.25	0/9	2/24	14.5	0.63	0.6	0/13	2/20	16.4	0.51	1.86	0/11	2/22	15.7	0.57	1*
		0/9	2/17	12	0.63	1.13	0/12	2/16	13.8	0.54	3	1/12	3/25	13.5	0.88	0.92
		0/9	3/30	16.8	0.63	0.43	0/15	3/25	20.4	0.46	1.5	1/15	3/30	17.6	0.83	1
0.10	0.3	1/12	5/35	19.8	0.66	0.52	1/16	4/25	20.4	0.51	1.78	2/17	5/34	21	0.76	1
		1/10	5/29	15	0.74	0.53	1/15	5/25	19.5	0.55	1.5	1/13	5/26	17.9	0.62	1*
		2/18	6/35	22.5	0.73	1.06	2/22	6/33	26.2	0.62	2	3/22	8/44	25.8	0.83	1
0.20	0.4	3/17	10/37	26	0.55	0.85	3/19	10/36	28.3	0.46	1.12	4/20	11/40	27.4	0.63	1
		3/13	12/43	20.6	0.75	0.43	4/18	10/33	22.3	0.72	1.2	4/18	11/36	23.1	0.72	1
		4/19	15/54	30.4	0.67	0.54	5/24	13/45	31.2	0.66	1.14	5/24	14/48	32.3	0.66	1
0.3	0.5	7/22	17/46	29.9	0.67	0.92	7/28	15/39	35	0.36	2.55	6/21	16/42	30.4	0.55	1*
		5/15	18/46	23.6	0.72	0.48	6/19	16/39	25.7	0.67	0.95	7/21	17/42	26.8	0.72	1
		8/24	24/63	34.7	0.73	0.62	7/24	21/53	36.6	0.56	0.83	9/28	22/56	36.9	0.68	1
0.4	0.6	7/18	22/46	30.2	0.56	0.64	11/28	20/41	33.8	0.55	2.15	10/24	23/48	32.4	0.65	1
		7/16	23/46	24.5	0.72	0.53	17/34	20/39	34.4	0.91	6.8	12/25	25/50	28.8	0.85	1
		11/25	32/66	36	0.73	0.61	12/29	27/54	38.1	0.64	1.16	13/30	30/60	38.6	0.71	1
0.5	0.7	11/21	26/45	29	0.67	0.88	11/23	23/39	31	0.5	1.44	12/23	27/46	30.8	0.66	1
		8/15	26/43	23.5	0.7	0.54	12/23	23/37	27.7	0.66	1.64	12/21	26/43	25.2	0.81	0.95
		13/24	36/61	34	0.73	0.65	14/27	32/53	36.1	0.65	1.04	16/29	35/59	35.9	0.77	0.97*
0.6	0.8	6/11	26/38	25.4	0.47	0.41	18/27	24/35	28.5	0.82	3.38	10/18	25/36	28.1	0.44	1*
		7/11	30/43	20.5	0.7	0.34	8/13	25/35	20.8	0.65	0.59	11/18	26/36	24.7	0.63	1
		12/19	37/53	29.5	0.69	0.56	15/26	32/45	35.9	0.48	1.37	16/25	35/50	31.8	0.73	1*
0.7	0.9	6/9	22/28	17.8	0.54	0.47	11/16	20/25	20	0.55	1.78	11/15	24/30	19.5	0.7	1
		4/6	22/27	14.8	0.58	0.29	19/23	21/26	23.2	0.95	7.67	10/14	23/28	19	0.64	1
		11/15	29/36	21.2	0.7	0.71	13/18	26/32	22.7	0.67	1.29	13/17	31/39	21.4	0.8	0.77

p_0, uninteresting response rate; p_1, clinically interesting response rate; r_1, lower bound for number of responses observed in stage I; n_1, stage I sample size; r, lower bound for total number of responses observed at end of stage II; n, total sample size; EN, expected sample size; PET, probability of early termination.

*Balanced design has both expected and maximum sample sizes between those of optimal and minimax designs.

Reproduced from Fei Y, Shyr Y: Balanced two-stage designs for phase II clinical trials. Clin Trials 4:514–524, 2007.

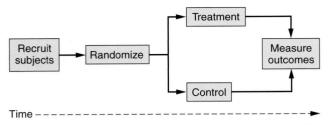

Figure 41-3 Parallel design. Patients are randomized to either treatment or control.

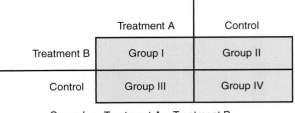

Group I = Treatment A + Treatment B
Group II = Treatment B + Control
Group III = Treatment A + Control
Group IV = Control

Figure 41-5 Factorial design. Patients are randomized to treatment A plus treatment B, treatment A only, treatment B only, or control.

in the number of participants assigned to each group and to equalize the number of subjects on each treatment. A block of size b is specified. For each block of b subjects enrolled in the study, $b/2$ are assigned to each treatment. In the case of block size four, there are six possible combinations of group assignments: AABB, ABAB, BAAB, BABA, BBAA, and ABBA. One of these arrangements is selected at random, and the four participants are assigned accordingly. This process is repeated as many times as needed. The advantage of blocking is that balance between the numbers of participants in each group is guaranteed throughout the course of randomization; thus, if the trial is terminated before enrollment is completed, balance exists in terms of number of participants randomized to each group.

Biased coin randomization is a baseline adaptive randomization procedure, originally discussed by Efron.[10] This technique attempts to balance the number of participants in each treatment group based on previous assignments, but it does not take participant responses into consideration. The purpose of the algorithm is basically to randomize the allocation of participants to groups A and B with equal probability, as long as the number of participants in each group is equal or nearly equal. If an imbalance occurs and the difference in the number of participants is greater than some prespecified value c, the allocation probability p needs to be adjusted to increase the probability of allocation to the group with fewer participants. In other words, if the number of subjects already on each treatment (n_A and n_B) is equal ($n_A \approx n_B$), then we randomize to either treatment with $p = \frac{1}{2}$. If $n_A > n_B + c$, then we increase the probability of allocation to treatment B to be greater than 50%. If $n_B > n_A + c$, then we increase the probability of allocation to treatment A to be greater than 50%. Advantages of this method include that (1) the next treatment assignment cannot be predicted, and that the (2) statistical power is greater with equal allocation.

Sample Size Determination and Power Analysis

Clinical trials should have sufficient statistical power to detect differences in treatment outcomes considered to be of clinical interest. Therefore, calculation of sample size to ensure statistical significance and adequate power is an essential part of planning. Power can be defined as the probability of rejecting the null hypothesis if a specific alternative (e.g., clinically significant improvement) is true. The biggest danger of low study power (i.e., insufficient sample size) is that no conclusion can be made if a statistically significant difference is not found. Instead of discussing the statistical techniques involved in calculating power, this section focuses on the principles that may affect power analysis. The following questions should be considered before the power analysis:

- What is the main purpose of the trial? Is it a superiority trial, clinical equivalence trial, or noninferiority trial? Superiority trials are designed to detect a difference between treatments. Clinical equivalence trials are designed to confirm the absence of a difference between treatments. Noninferiority trials are designed to show that a new treatment is not much worse than an existing treatment (i.e., active control).
- What study design will be used to achieve the study goal? How many arms are needed? Will the study use a two-arm parallel design, crossover design, or four-arm factorial design?
- What is the study's principal measure of interest (i.e., primary end point)? What is the study's primary outcome variable? Is it an interval variable, categorical variable, or time-to-event variable?

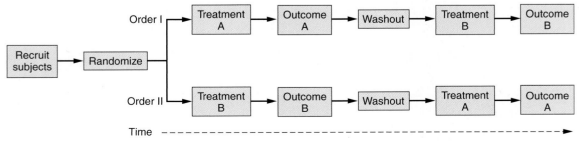

Figure 41-4 Crossover design. Patients are randomized to either treatment A followed by treatment B or treatment B followed by treatment A.

- What result is anticipated with standard treatment, possibly based on other similar studies?
- How small a treatment difference is it important to detect (i.e., what is the smallest clinically significant level of difference between treatments)? With what degree of certainty must this difference be detected?
- Which statistical method will be used to estimate sample size? Is the method to be used a statistical test, confidence interval method, or computer simulation?
- What is the ratio of treatment assignments? Will patients be randomized to intervention and control in a 1:1 ratio, or will more participants be assigned to the intervention group than to the control group?
- Will the intent-to-treat principle be used in the final data analysis? Is there any drop-in or drop-out adjustment?
- What technique for interim monitoring will be used? Is the technique to be used a group sequential method, a stochastic curtailment method, a repeated confidence interval method, or a Bayesian approach? All methods except the Bayesian approach will affect sample size adjustment; the group sequential method and stochastic curtailment is discussed further in the next section.

Sample size calculations are approximate. They are often based on roughly estimated parameter values from mathematical models, which only approximate truth. Because of the approximate nature of sample size calculations, it is best to be liberal when estimating sample size (i.e., overestimate rather than underestimate).

Monitoring Response Variables

The investigator's ethical responsibility to the subjects of a study demands that results be monitored during a trial. Interim monitoring is used to check protocol compliance, make sure that data management and forms submission are up to date, and report adverse effects (e.g., treatment toxicity) and summary statistics (e.g., numbers of patients and distribution by prognostic factors). In addition, if treatment groups are combined, overall outcome results may be reported. More importantly, interim analyses should monitor the response variables of interest to identify early dramatic benefits of the new treatment, potential harmful effects, or an outcome difference between treatments so unimpressive that showing a statistically significant difference at the end of the trial is very unlikely; any of these results should be reported to the study's data safety and monitoring committee only, not to study investigators or to the public.

This section focuses on techniques for interim monitoring of treatment differences. One of the problems of interim analysis is the repeated testing for significance. Under the null hypothesis H_0 (no difference between treatment groups), repeated testing at a type I error level of α yields a probability of finding a significant result greater than α, as shown in Table 41-7 (the figures in Table 41-7 hold for either a test for equality of binomial proportions or a t-test for the difference in means

TABLE 41-7

Type I Error Rates with Repeated Testing

No. of Tests	P(rejection) under H_0 with $\alpha = 0.05$
1	0.05
2	0.08
5	0.14
10	0.19
20	0.25
50	0.32
1000	0.53
∞	1

between two normal populations, assuming that roughly equal numbers of patients are added between each interim test). In this section, we look at three techniques for addressing the problem of repeated testing for significance: the group sequential method, the alpha-spending function, and the curtailed sampling procedure.

The Haybittle-Peto procedure[11] is one of the group sequential methods that favors using a large critical value, such as $Z_i = \pm 3$, for all interim tests (where $i < k$, with k = total number of patient groups that will be monitored over the course of the trial, and i = number of groups with completed data at a given point in time). With this method, any adjustment for repeated testing at the final test ($i = k$) is negligible, and the conventional critical value can be used. This method is ad hoc in the sense that no precise type I error level is guaranteed. It might, however, be viewed as a precursor to the more formal procedures described in the following section.

Pocock[12] modified the repeated testing methods of McPherson and Armitage[13,14] and developed a group sequential method for clinical trials that avoids many of the limitations of the Haybittle-Peto procedure. Pocock's method divides the participants into a series of k equal-sized groups with $2n$ participants in each, n assigned to intervention and n to control. The number of groups, k, is the number of times that data will be monitored during the course of the trial, and the total expected sample size is $2nk$. The test statistic used to compare control and intervention is computed as soon as data for the first group of $2n$ participants are available, and recomputed when data from each successive group become known. Under the null hypothesis, the distribution of the test statistic, Z_i, is assumed to be approximately normal with zero mean and unit variance, where i indicates the number of groups ($i \leq k$) with completed data. This statistic Z_i is compared with the stopping boundaries, $\pm Z'_k$, where Z'_k has been determined such that for up to k repeated tests, the overall significance level for the trial will be α. Table 41-8 shows the normal significance levels required for repeated two-sided significance testing. For example, for $k = 5$ and $\alpha = 0.05$ (two-sided), we use a normal significance value of 0.0160 for each test, yielding $Z'_k = 2.413$ (instead of $Z_1 = 1.96$ for a single test at $\alpha = 0.05$).

O'Brien and Fleming also discussed a group sequential procedure.[15] Using the preceding notation, their

TABLE 41-8

Normal Significance Level Required to Achieve Overall α = 0.05 or 0.01 with Repeated Two-Sided Significance Testing

No. of Tests	Significance Level for Each Test to Achieve Overall α = 0.05	Significance Level for Each Test to Achieve Overall α = 0.01
2	0.0290	0.0056
3	0.0220	0.0041
4	0.0180	0.0033
5	0.0160	0.0028
10	0.0106	0.0018
15	0.0086	0.0015
20	0.0075	0.0013

stopping rule compares the statistic Z_i with $Z^*(k/i)^{1/2}$ where Z^* is determined so as to achieve the desired significance level. Table 41-9 shows the values of Z^* for overall α = 0.05. For example, if $k = 5$ and α = 0.05 (two-sided), $Z^* = 2.04$. One attractive feature of the O'Brien-Fleming procedure is that the critical value used at the last test ($i = k$) is approximately the same as that used if a single test were done.

The O'Brien-Fleming model is unlikely to lead to stopping in the early stages of a trial. Later on, however, this procedure leads to a greater chance of stopping prior to the end of a study than does the Pocock or Haybittle-Peto procedure. Both the Haybittle-Peto and the O'Brien-Fleming boundaries avoid the awkward situation of accepting the null hypothesis when the observed statistic at the end of the trial is much larger than the conventional critical value (i.e., 1.96 for a two-sided 5% significance level). There is a slight loss of power with multiple testing. For example, if the investigator is testing a binomial hypothesis (H_0: $P_1 = P_2$ versus H_a: $P_1 \neq P_2$) and wants 90% power to detect a difference of $P_1 = 0.50$ versus $P_2 = 0.70$ with α = 0.05, the required sample size for a single test is 262. With increasing numbers of tests, the sample sizes required to maintain the same power are shown in Table 41-10.

Lan and DeMets introduced the alpha-spending function.[16] This function allows the investigator to determine how he or she wants to "spend" the type I error (i.e., alpha) during the course of a trial. The alpha-spending function guarantees that at the end of the trial, the overall type I error will be the prespecified value of α; thus, this approach is a generalization of the group sequential method, such that the Pocock and O'Brien-Fleming monitoring procedures become special cases. To understand the alpha-spending function, we must first distinguish between calendar time and information fraction.

At any particular calendar time t in the study, a certain fraction t^* of the total information is observed. The value for t^* must be between 0 and 1. The information fraction is more generally defined in terms of the ratio of the inverse of the variance of the test statistic at the particular interim analysis to that at the final analysis. The alpha-spending function, $\alpha(t^*)$, determines how the prespecified α is allocated at each interim analysis as a function of the information fraction. At the beginning of the trial, $t^* = 0$ and $\alpha(t^*) = 0$, whereas at the end of the trial, $t^* = 1$ and $\alpha(t^*) = \alpha$. The relationships between the alpha-spending function and the O'Brien-Fleming method and the Pocock method are described as follows:

$$\text{O'Brien-Fleming method}: \alpha_{O-F}(t^*) = 2 - 2\Phi(Z_{\alpha/2}/t^*)$$

$$\text{Pocock method}: \alpha_P(t^*) = \alpha \bullet ln[1 + (e - 1)t^*]$$

The advantage of the alpha-spending function is that neither the number nor the time of interim analyses needs to be specified in advance, thereby giving group sequential monitoring the flexibility that is often required in the actual clinical trial setting.

Whereas group sequential methods focus on existing data, curtailed sampling methods consider future data. With curtailed methods, multiple checks for the possibility of early curtailment do not cause problems of repeated testing. Two curtailed sampling procedures are discussed in this section: the simple curtailment method and the stochastic curtailment method.

The principle of simple curtailment is that a study should be stopped as soon as the result is inevitable (i.e., the trend toward a final outcome cannot be reversed). For example, in a two-sample t-test, suppose all values must be between A and B ($A < B$), and that after sampling n^* out of n total observations, we have observed no significant result. We may assign values to the remaining $n - n^*$ observations as follows:

1. Assign all As to group 1, all Bs to group 2, and recompute the test statistic.
2. Assign all Bs to group 1, all As to group 2, and recompute the test statistic.

If both recomputations yield no significance, we can be sure that the final result of all sampling will not reach statistical significance, and the trial may be stopped.

Similarly, if a significant difference is observed after sampling n^* out of n total observations, we also may perform the preceding recomputations. If both lead to significance, then the trial may be stopped. With this method, the requirement of absolute certainty is very conservative and does not give much opportunity for early stopping.

By contrast, stochastic curtailment is less conservative, allowing the trial to be stopped as soon as the result is highly probable based on calculation of conditional

TABLE 41-9

Values of Z* Required to Achieve Overall α = 0.05 with Repeated Testing

No. of tests	1	2	3	4	5	6	7	8	9	10
Z	1.96	1.98	2	2.02	2.04	2.05	2.06	2.07	2.08	2.09

TABLE 41-10

Sample Sizes Required to Maintain 90% Power to Detect a Difference of $P_1 = 0.50$ vs. $P_2 = 0.70$ with $\alpha = 0.05$ after Repeated Testing

No. of tests	1	2	3	4	5	10
Sample size	262	264	266	267	268	271

power; if the conditional power is very low, the trial may be stopped. For example, let $S(t)$ be the test statistic at time t. If T = the end of the trial, then $S(T)$ is the final test statistic. There are two conditions to consider:

1. Suppose the result in the intervention group is significantly better than that in the control group at $t < T$. Then compute

   $\pi_0 = P$ (rejecting $H_0 \mid H_0$ true and observed data from the study).

   π_0 is equal to the probability of still rejecting H_0 if the rest of the data come in reflecting no treatment effect. If π_0 is large (≈ 1), then the trend is unlikely to disappear.

2. Suppose the result in the intervention group is not significantly different from that in the control group at $t < T$. Then compute, for a set of reasonable values of difference (δ) between the intervention group and control group

   $\pi_1 = P$ (rejecting $H_0 \mid H_1$ true and observed data from the study).

How large must the true effect (δ) be to reverse the current decision? If δ must be unrealistically large and the probability of reversal is small, then terminating the trial may be considered.

Because there is a small probability that the results will change, a slightly greater risk of type I or type II error will exist if a trial is curtailed than would exist if the trial continued to the scheduled end; however, the type I error is bounded by α/π_0, and the type II error by β/π_1.

Conclusions

Bull indicated that the clinical trial is "the most definitive tool for evaluation of the applicability of clinical research," representing "a key research activity with the potential to improve the quality of health care and control costs through careful comparison of alternative treatment."[17] Study design, randomization, sample size determination, and interim monitoring analysis are key factors for a successful trial. Without solid biostatistical support, these trial features cannot be addressed in full. In other words, without careful and adequate biostatistical input, clinical trials are unable to answer the research questions for which they are designed.

Acknowledgments

The author wishes to thank Lynne Berry for her editorial suggestions.

REFERENCES

1. 21 Code of Federal Regulations 312.3(b). Revised as of April 1, 2003.
2. Meinert CL: Clinical trials: Design, conduct, and analysis. Oxford, England, Oxford University Press, 1986, p 3.
3. Chow SC, Liu JP: Design and analysis of clinical trials: Concepts and methodologies. New York, Wiley, 1998.
4. O'Quigley J, Pepe M, Fisher L: Continual reassessment method: A practical design for phase I clinical trials in cancer. Biometrics 46:33–48, 1990.
5. Gehan EA: The determination of the number of participants required in a follow-up trial of a new chemotherapeutic agent. J Chronic Dis 13:346–353, 1961.
6. Fleming TR: One-sample multiple testing procedure for phase II clinical trials. Biometrics 38:143–151, 1982.
7. Simon R: Optimal two-stage designs for phase II clinical trials. Control Clin Trials 10:1–10, 1989.
8. Fei Y, Shyr Y: Balanced two-stage designs for phase II clinical trials. Clin Trials 4:514–524, 2007.
9. Hill AB: The clinical trial. Br Med Bull 71:278–282, 1951.
10. Efron B: Forcing a sequential experiment to be balanced. Biometrika 58:403–417, 1971.
11. Haybittle JL: Repeated assessment of results in clinical trials of cancer treatment. Br J Radiol 44:793–797, 1971.
12. Pocock SJ: Clinical trials: A practical approach. New York, Wiley, 1984.
13. Armitage P: Sequential tests in prophylactic and therapeutic trials. Q J Med 23:255–274, 1954.
14. Armitage P: Interim analysis in clinical trials. Stat Med 10:925–937, 1991.
15. O'Brien PC, Fleming TR: A multiple testing procedure for clinical trials. Biometrics 35:549–556, 1979.
16. Lan KKG, DeMets DL: Discrete sequential boundaries for clinical trials. Biometrika 70:659–663, 1983.
17. Bull JP: The historical development of clinical therapeutic trials. J Chronic Dis 10:218–248, 1959.

Index

Page numbers followed by *b*, *f*, or *t* indicate boxes, figures, or tables, respectively.